Brief Contents

UNIT 1 QUALITY AND SAFETY IN NURSING PRACTICE

UNIT 2 PATIENT ASSESSMENT SKILLS

UNIT 3 BASIC HUMAN NEEDS

UNIT 4 ACTIVITY AND MOBILITY

UNIT 5 PROMOTING ELIMINATION

UNIT 6 MEDICATION ADMINISTRATION

UNIT 7 DRESSINGS AND WOUND CARE

UNIT 8 COMPLEX NURSING INTERVENTIONS

UNIT 9 SUPPORTIVE NURSING INTERVENTIONS

APPENDIXES

SEVENTH EDITION 7

NURSING INTERVENTIONS & CLINICAL SKILLS

ANNE GRIFFIN PERRY, RN, MSN, EdD, FAAN
Professor Emerita
School of Nursing
Southern Illinois University—Edwardsville
Edwardsville, Illinois

PATRICIA A. POTTER, RN, MSN, PhD, FAAN
Formerly, Director of Research
Patient Care Services
Barnes-Jewish Hospital
St. Louis, Missouri

WENDY R. OSTENDORF, RN, MS, EdD, CNE
Contributing Faculty
Master's of Science in Nursing
Walden University
Minneapolis, Minnesota

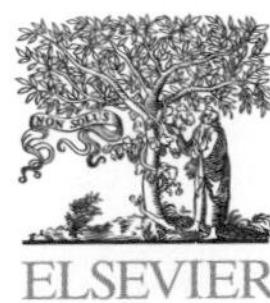
ELSEVIER

NURSING INTERVENTIONS AND CLINICAL SKILLS, SEVENTH EDITION ISBN: 978-0-323-54701-7

Notice

Practitioners and researchers must always rely on their own experience and knowledge in evaluating and using any information, methods, compounds or experiments described herein. Because of rapid advances in the medical sciences, in particular, independent verification of diagnoses and drug dosages should be made. To the fullest extent of the law, no responsibility is assumed by Elsevier, authors, editors or contributors for any injury and/or damage to persons or property as a matter of products liability, negligence or otherwise, or from any use or operation of any methods, products, instructions, or ideas contained in the material herein.

Previous editions copyrighted 2016, 2012, 2007, 2004, 2000, 1996.

International Standard Book Number: 978-0-323-54701-7

Director: Tamara Myers
Content Development Manager: Lisa P. Newton
Senior Content Development Specialist: Tina Kaemmerer, Melissa Rawe
Publishing Services Manager: Julie Eddy
Senior Project Manager: Jodi M. Willard
Design Direction: Renee Duenow

Printed in China.

Last digit is the print number: 9 8 7 6 5 4 3 2 1

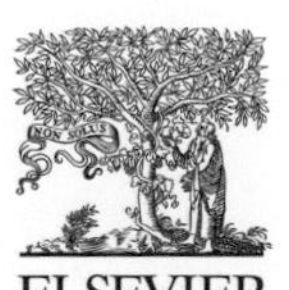

3251 Riverport Lane
St. Louis, Missouri 63043

About the Authors

ANNE GRIFFIN PERRY, RN, MSN, EdD, FAAN

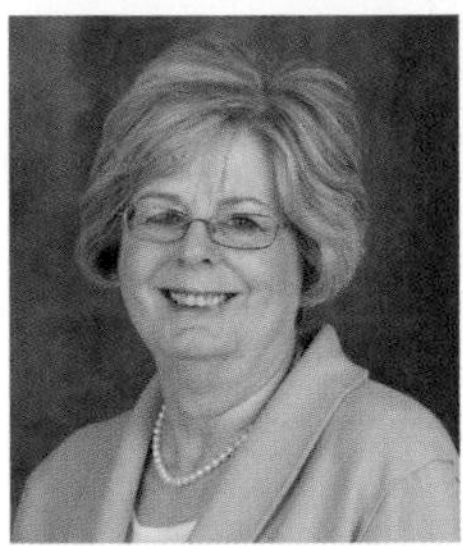

Dr. Anne G. Perry is Professor Emerita and Former Interim Dean and Associate Dean of Nursing at Southern Illinois University—Edwardsville. Dr. Perry was also a Professor and taught at Saint Louis University School of Nursing for over 30 years and is a Fellow in the American Academy of Nursing. She received her BSN from the University of Michigan, her MSN from Saint Louis University, and her EdD from Southern Illinois University at Edwardsville. Dr. Perry is a prolific and influential author and speaker. Her work includes four major textbooks (*Essentials for Nursing Practice*, *Fundamentals of Nursing*, *Nursing Interventions and Clinical Skills*, and *Clinical Nursing Skills and Techniques*), multiple journal articles abstracts, and nursing research and education grants. She has presented multiple papers at conferences across the United States. She has acted as an editorial board member of numerous journals (*Journal of Nursing Measurement*, *Intensive Care Medicine*, *AACN Clinical Issues*, and *Perspectives in Respiratory Nursing*), and she was one of a few key consultants on *Mosby's Nursing Skills Videos* and *Mosby's Nursing Skills Online*.

PATRICIA A. POTTER, RN, MSN, PhD, FAAN

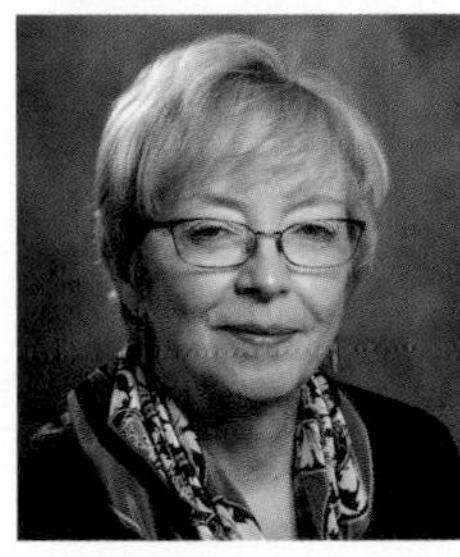

Dr. Patricia Potter received her diploma in nursing from Barnes School of Nursing; her BSN at the University of Washington in Seattle, Washington; and her MSN and PhD at Saint Louis University in St. Louis, Missouri. A ground-breaking author for more than 30 years, her work includes four major textbooks (*Essentials for Nursing Practice*, *Fundamentals of Nursing*, *Nursing Interventions and Clinical Skills*, and *Clinical Nursing Skills and Techniques)* and multiple journal articles. She has been an unceasing advocate of evidence-based practice and quality improvement in her roles as administrator, educator, and researcher.

Dr. Potter has devoted a lifetime to nursing education, practice, and research. She spent a decade teaching at Barnes Hospital School of Nursing and Saint Louis University. She entered into a variety of managerial and administrative roles, ultimately becoming the director of nursing practice for Barnes-Jewish Hospital. In that capacity she sharpened her interest in the development of nursing practice standards and measurement of patient outcomes in defining nursing practice. Her most recent passion has been in the area of nursing research, specifically cancer family caregiving, the effects of compassion fatigue on nurses, and fall prevention. Dr. Potter was most recently the Director of Research for Patient Care Services at Barnes-Jewish Hospital in St. Louis, Missouri, before her retirement in 2017.

WENDY R. OSTENDORF, RN, MS, EdD, CNE

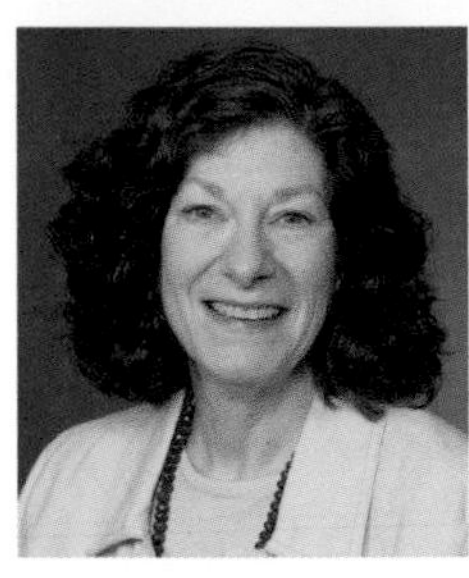

Dr. Wendy R. Ostendorf received her BSN from Villanova University, her MS from the University of Delaware, and her EdD from the University of Sarasota. She currently serves as a contributing faculty in the Master's of Science in Nursing at Walden University. She has contributed over 26 chapters to multiple nursing textbooks and has served as co-author for *Clinical Nursing Skills and Techniques* and *Nursing Interventions & Clinical Skills*. She has presented over 25 papers at conferences at the local, national, and international levels.

Professionally, Dr. Ostendorf has a diverse background in pediatric and adult critical care. She has taught at the undergraduate, master's, and doctoral level for over 30 years. With decades of practice as a clinician, her educational experiences have influenced her teaching philosophy and perceptions of the nursing profession. Dr. Ostendorf's current interests include the history and image of nursing as it has been represented in film, as well as the use of dedicated units and preceptors on students' transition to practice.

Contributors

SECTION EDITOR

Nancy Laplante, PhD, RN, AHN-BC
Associate Professor
School of Nursing
Widener University
Chester, Pennsylvania

CONTRIBUTORS TO THE SEVENTH EDITION

Carolyn Wright Boon, MSN, BSN
Assistant Professor, Nursing
Saint Francis Medical Center College of Nursing
Peoria, Illinois

Janice Colwell, MS, CWOCN, FAAN
Advanced Practice Nurse
General Surgery
University of Chicago Medicine
Chicago, Illinois

M. Elayne DeSimone, PhD, RN, NP-C, FAANP
Clinical Professor, Director Master's Program
Nursing
Widener University
Chester, Pennsylvania

Jane Fellows, MSN, CWOCN-AP
Wound/Ostomy CNS
Advanced Clinical Practice
Duke University Health System
Durham, North Carolina

Susan Fetzer, BA, BSN, MSN, MBA, PhD
Professor
College of Health and Human Services
University of New Hampshire
Durham, New Hampshire;
Director of Research
Patient Care Services
Southern New Hampshire Medical Center
Nashua, New Hampshire

Paula A. Gray, DNP, CRNP, NP-C
Director, Family (Individual Across the Lifespan) CRNP Program
Nursing
Widener University
Chester, Pennsylvania;
Clinical Associate Professor of Nursing
School of Nursing
Widener University
Chester, Pennsylvania;
Nurse Practitioner
Family Physicians at Middletown
Crozer-Keystone Health Systems
Media, Pennsylvania

Christina Gresh, MSN, RN
Nurse Care Coordinator, Nursing
Abington Jefferson Health
Abington, Pennsylvania

Carol Ann Liebold, RN, BSN, CRNI
President/Owner
Operations
CarolAnn Liebold, Inc.
Earlton, New York

Amy Luckowski, PhD RN CCRN CNE
Assistant Professor, Nursing
Neumann University
Aston, Pennsylvania;
RN, Postanesthesia Care Unit
Chester County Hospital
West Chester, Pennsylvania

Nelda Martin, MSN
Clinical Nurse Specialist
Heart and Vascular
Barnes-Jewish Hospital
St. Louis, Missouri

Carrie Monson, ADN, BSN, MSN
Registered Nurse
5D Medical
Christiana Care Health System
Newark, Delaware

Pamela Ostby, PhD, RN, OCN, CLT
Research Specialist, Nursing
University of Missouri—Columbia
Columbia, Missouri

Theresa Pietsch, PhD, RN, CRRN, CNE
Associate Professor & Associate Dean of the Undergraduate Nursing Program
Division of Nursing & Health Sciences
Neumann University
Aston, Pennsylvania

Cherie R. Rebar, PhD, MBA, RN, COI
Professor of Nursing
Wittenberg University
Springfield, Ohio;
Adjunct Faculty, Nursing
Mercy College
Toledo, Ohio;
Affiliate Faculty, Nursing
Indiana Wesleyan University
Marion, Indiana

Jackie Saleeby, PhD, RN
Associate Professor
Catherine McAuley School of Nursing
Maryville University
St. Louis, Missouri

Beth Taylor, DCN, RD-AP, CNSC, FCCM
Research Scientist
Department of Research for Patient Care Services
Barnes-Jewish Hospital
St. Louis, Missouri

CONTRIBUTORS TO PREVIOUS EDITIONS

Elizabeth A. Ayello, RN, BSN, MS, PhD, CS, CETN
Margaret R. Benz, RN, MSN(R), BC, APN
Barbara J. Berger, MSN, RN
V. Christine Champagne, APRN, BC
Aurelie Chinn, RN, MSN
Kelly Jo Cone, PhD, RN, CNE
Patricia Conley, RN, MSN, PCCN
Karen S. Conners, RNC, MSN
Eileen Costantinou, MSN, RN
Deborah Crump, RN, MS, CHPN
Sheila A. Cunningham, BSN, MSN
Ruth Curchoe, RN, MSN, CIC
Wanda Cleveland Dubuisson, PhD, RN
Julie Eddins, RN, BSN, MSN, CRNI
Deborah Oldenburg Erickson, RN, BSN, MSN
Joan O. Ervin, RN, BSN, MN, CCRN
Melba J. Figgins, MSN, BSN
Janet B. Fox-Moatz, RN, BSN, MSN
Lynn C. Hadaway, MEd, RNC, CRNI
Amy Hall, RN, PhD
Roberta L. Harrison, PhD, RN, CRRN
Susan A. Hauser, RN, BSN, BA, MS
Diane M. Heizer, MSN, RN
Anne Marie Herlihey, DNP, RN, CNOR
Mimi Hirshberg, RN, MSN
Carolyn Chaney Hoskins, RN, BSN, MSN
Maureen B. Huhmann, MS, RD
Meredith Hunt, MSN, RNC, NP
Nancy Jackson, RN, BSN, MSN(R), CCRN
Linda L. Kerby, RN-C-R, BSN, MA, BA
Marilee Kuhrik, BSN, MSN, PhD
Nancy Kuhrik, BSN, MSN, PhD
Amy Lawn, BSN, MS, CIC
Kristine M. L'Ecuyer, RN, MSN, CCNS
Antoinette Kanne Ledbetter, RN, BSN, MS, TNS
Catherine Limbaugh, RN, BSN, MSN, ACNS-BC, OCN
Mary MacDonald, RN, MSN
Mary Kay Knight Macheca, MSN(R), RN, CS, ANP, CDE
Cynthia L. Maskey, RN, MS
Constance C. Maxey, RN-BC, MSN
Barbara Maxwell, MS, RN, LNC
Angela McConachie, DNP, FNP-C
Barbara McGeever, RN, RSM, BSN, MSN, DNSc
Mary "Dee" Miller, RN, BSN, MS, CIC
Peter R. Miller, RN, MSN, ONC
Rose M. Miller, RN, BSN, MSN, MPA, ACLS
Karen Montalto, RN, DNSc
Kathleen Mulryan, RN, BSN, MSN
Elaine K. Neel, RN, BSN, MSN
Kim Campbell Oliveri, RN, MS, CS
Marsha Evans Orr, RN, MS
Shirley E. Otto, MSN, RN, AOCN
Deborah Paul-Cheadle, RN
Elizabeth S. Pratt, DNP, RN, ACNS-BC
Roberta J. Richmond, MSN, RN, CCRN
Paulette D. Rollant, RN, BSN, MSN, PhD, CCRN
Linette M. Sarti, RN, BSN, CNOR
Lynn Schallom, RN, MSN, CCRN, CCNS
Kelly Schwartz, RN, BSN
Julie Snyder, RN, MSN, BC
Amy Spencer, MSN, RN-BC
Phyllis G. Stallard, BSN, MSN, ACCE
Victoria Steelman, PhD, RN, CNOR
Patricia A. Stockert, RN, PhD
E. Bradley Strecker, PhD, RN, CRRN
Virginia Strootman, RN, MSN, CRNI
Sue G. Thacker, RNC, BSN, MS, PhD
Donna L. Thompson, MSN, CRNP, FNP-BC, CCCN
Nancy Tomaselli, RN, MSN, CS, CRNP, CWOCN, CLNC
Stephanie Trinkl, BSN, MSN
Kathryn Tripp, BSN
Paula Vehlow, RN, MS
Pamela Becker Weilitz, MSN(R), RN, CN, ANP
Jana L. Weindel-Dees, RN, BSN, MSN
Joan Domigan Wentz, MSN, RN
Trudie Wierda, RN, MSN
Laurel A. Wiersema-Bryant, MSN, RN, CS
Terry L. Wood, PhD, RN, CNE
Rita Wunderlich, MSN, PhD
Rhonda Yancey, BSN, RN
Valerie J. Yancey, PhD, RN, HNC, CHPN

Reviewers

Michelle Aebersold, PhD, RN, CHSE, FAAN
Clinical Associate Professor
Director-Simulation and Education Innovation
School of Nursing
University of Michigan
Howell, Michigan

Jennifer Brunworth, BA, MSN, RN
Assistant Professor of Nursing
Coordinator, Nursing Learning Labs
Maryville University
St. Louis, Missouri

Kimberly Clevenger, EdD, MSN, RN, BC
Associate Professor of Nursing
Morehead State University
Morehead, Kentucky

Eileen Costantinou, MSN, RN-BC
Practice Specialist, Program Coordinator
Barnes-Jewish Hospital Center for Practice Excellence
St. Louis, Missouri

Holly Johanna Diesel, PhD, RN
Associate Professor and Academic Chair of the Accelerated and RN to BSN Program
Goldfarb School of Nursing at Barnes-Jewish College
St. Louis, Missouri

Amber Essman, DNP, MSN, FNP-BC
Visiting Professor
Chamberlain College of Nursing
Moses Lake, Washington

Margaret M. Gingrich, MSN, CRNP
Professor of Nursing
Harrisburg Area Community College
Harrisburg, Pennsylvania

Jacqueline A. Guhde, MSN, RN
Senior Instructor
School of Nursing
The University of Akron
Akron, Ohio

Vickey Keathly, MSN, RN
ABSN Clinical Nurse Educator
School of Nursing
Duke University
Durham, North Carolina

Christina D. Keller, MSN, RN, CHSE
Instructor of Nursing
Radford University Clinical Simulation Center
Radford, Virginia

Patricia T. Ketcham, RN, MSN
Director of Nursing Laboratories
School of Nursing
Oakland University
Rochester, Michigan

Vicky J. King, RN, MS, CNE
Nursing Faculty
Cochise College
Sierra Vista, Arizona

Janis Longfield McMillan, RN, MSN, CNE
Associate Clinical Professor
Northern Arizona University
Flagstaff, Arizona

Sarah E. Newton, PhD, RN
Associate Professor
School of Nursing
Oakland University
Rochester, Michigan

Rebecca Otten, EdD, RN
Professor Emeritus
California State University
Fullerton, California

Jill R. Reed, PhD, APRN-NP
Assistant Professor
College of Nursing
University of Nebraska Medical Center
Kearney Division
Omaha, Nebraska

Diane M. Rudolphi, MSN, RN
Medical-Surgical Clinical Faculty
School of Nursing
University of Delaware
Newark, Delaware

Susan Parnell Scholtz, RN, PhD
Associate Professor of Nursing
Moravian College
Bethlehem, Pennsylvania

Benjamin A. Smallheer, PhD, RN, ACNP-BC, FNP-BC, CCRN, CNE
Assistant Professor of Nursing
Lead Faculty, Adult-Gerontology Acute Care Nurse Practitioner Program
School of Nursing
Duke University
Durham, North Carolina

Peter D. Smith, BA, MSN, RN
Clinical Education Specialist
Barnes-Jewish Hospital
St. Louis, Missouri

Lynne L. Tier, MSN, RN, LNC
Assistant Director of Simulation
Adventist University of Health Sciences
Orlando, Florida

Heidi Tymkew, PT, DPT, MHS, CCS
Research Scientist
Barnes-Jewish Hospital
St. Louis, Missouri

Susan A. Wheaton, RN, BSN, MSN
Lecturer in Nursing
Learning Resource Director
School of Nursing
University of Maine
Orono, Maine

Paige D. Wimberly, PhD, CNS-BS, CNS
Associate Professor of Nursing
Arkansas State University
Jonesboro, Arkansas

Jean Yockey, PhD, FNP, CNE
Assistant Professor
University of South Dakota
Vermillion, South Dakota

Acknowledgments

Thanks to the talented and dedicated professionals at Elsevier: Tamara Myers, Director, who has provided support, leadership, enthusiasm, and a healthy sense of humor during the revision process; Tina Kaemmerer, Senior Content Development Specialist, and Melissa Rawe, Content Development Specialist, who spent countless hours keeping the author team informed and organized. Their commitment to accuracy and dedication to quality kept the project on target; Jodi Willard, Senior Project Manager, whose organization, careful editing, kindness, and continuous support for this project throughout the production process helped to ensure an accurate, high quality, consistent book; Julie Eddy, Publishing Services Manager, who contributed support throughout the process; and Renee Duenow, whose creativity provides an attractive and unique visual appeal to the text. These contributions significantly enhance the learning process.

NOTES FROM THE AUTHORS

I wish to acknowledge the nurse educators at Saint Louis University and Southern Illinois University—Edwardsville School of Nursing. Their knowledge of the discipline and commitment to nursing education help to shape the practice of nursing in the region. These educators skillfully integrate the science and the art of nursing into their classes and clinical experiences. These faculty, together with the expert nursing staff in the clinical settings, provide the initial foundation for caring clinical practice.

Anne Griffin Perry

The past thirty years of writing foundational textbooks have been enriching and enlightening. I hope that our author team can continue to produce the high-quality textbook that faculty and students expect. My personal thanks to Anne, Wendy, and Nancy for making this particular edition a joy. Thanks as always to all of my dear friends for their ongoing support.

Patricia A. Potter

It is my pleasure to contribute to a book that continues to support the nursing education of so many nurses. I always want to acknowledge the contribution of my husband, who has endless patience as I take so much of our time to work on my career. I also want to thank Toba and Harris, who would be so proud of this book.

Wendy R. Ostendorf

Preface to the Instructor

The evolution of knowledge and technology influences the way we teach clinical skills to nursing students. The foundation for success in performing nursing skills remains a competent and well-informed nurse who thinks critically and asks the right questions at the right time to provide appropriate, high-quality nursing care. This edition of *Nursing Interventions & Clinical Skills* retains the successful elements of previous editions but incorporates material key to this shift in how nurses practice.

Emphasis on QSEN Competencies may be easily found throughout the text. You will find sections on *Safety* and *Evidence-Based Practice* at the beginning of each chapter. Information on *Delegation and Collaboration*, *Safe Patient Care*, and *Recording/Hand-off Reporting* appear in each skill and procedure as needed. We have retained the concise format, clear language, and streamlined approach that were hallmarks of previous editions. New photos and line drawings update the generous illustration program. All skills and procedures are presented within the framework of the nursing process.

KEY FEATURES

- **Comprehensive coverage** of nursing skills ranges from basic skills such as measuring temperature to complex, advanced skills such as intravenous therapy and management of endotracheal tubes.
- **Extensive full-color art program** includes dozens of new photographs.
- **Safe Patient Care boxes** incorporated into skills inform students when to take special precautions and the specific risks to consider when performing a skill.
- **Delegation and Collaboration guidelines** are included in the planning section for each skill and procedure.
- **Step-by-step presentation of steps** are given each skill and include supporting rationales that are often evidence-based.
- **Recording guidelines** include what should be reported and documented after performing skills.
- **Hand-off Reporting** sections list important and relevant information to include for better overall patient care during the hand-off report.
- **Special Considerations** sections provide information on how to adapt skills in specific circumstances, such as in the home care setting or when caring for a child or older adult.
- **Teach-Back** step shows how to evaluate the success of patient teaching so you can be sure that the patient understands a task or topic or whether to consider additional teaching.

NEW TO THIS EDITION

- **Chapter 6, Disaster Preparedness,** focuses on caring for patients after biological, chemical, or radiation exposure.
- **Practice Reflections** sections give students an opportunity to reflect on their clinical and simulation experiences with a clinical scenario and questions.
- A new Appendix on **Integrative Practice Reflections** helps student synthesize skill performance with overall patient care to develop a better understanding of the "big picture." Scenarios with a pediatric patient and a gerontological patient are included.

ANCILLARIES

- The **Evolve Instructor Resources** (available online at http://evolve.elsevier.com/Perry/nursinginterventions/) are a collection of the most important tools instructors need, including the following:
  - **TEACH for Nurses** ties together every chapter resource you need for the most effective class presentations, with sections dedicated to objectives, teaching strategies, nursing curriculum standards (including QSEN/NLN Competencies, BSN Essentials, and Nursing Concepts), instructor chapter resources, student chapter resources, and an in-class case study discussion. Teaching Strategies include relationships between the textbook content and discussion items. Examples of student activities, online activities, and large group activities are provided for more "hands-on" learning.
  - The **Test Bank** contains a revised set of more than 850 questions, with answers coded for NCLEX Client Needs category, nursing process, and cognitive level. The ExamView software allows instructors to create new tests; edit, add, and delete test questions; sort questions by NCLEX category, cognitive level, nursing process step, and question type; and administer/grade online tests.
  - **PowerPoint Presentations** are provided for each chapter.

The Evolve Student Resources are available online at http://evolve.elsevier.com/Perry/nursinginterventions/ and include the following valuable learning aids organized by chapter:

- Audio Glossary
- Animations
- Answers to Text Review Questions
- Tutorial for Fluids and Electrolytes and Drug Calculations
- Case Studies with Questions
- Interactive Skills Performance Checklists for each skill in an interactive PDF format
- Review Questions
- Video Clips

Also available:

- **Nursing Skills Online 4.0** contains 19 modules rich with animations, videos, interactive activities, and exercises to help students prepare for their clinical lab experience. The instructionally designed lessons focus on topics that are difficult to master and pose a high risk to the patient if done incorrectly. Lesson quizzes allow students to check their learning curve and review as needed, and the module exams feed out to an instructor grade book. Modules cover Airway Management, Blood Therapy, Bowel

Elimination/Ostomy, Cardiac Care, Closed Chest Drainage Systems, Enteral Nutrition, Infection Control, Maintenance of IV Fluid Therapy, IV Fluid Therapy, Administration of Parenteral Medications: Injections and IV Medications, Nonparenteral Medication Administration, Safe Medication Preparation, Safety, Specimen Collection, Urinary Catheterization, Caring for Central Vascular Access Devices (CVAD), Vital Signs, and Wound Care.

- **Mosby's Nursing Video Skills: Basic, Intermediate, Advanced, 4th edition,** provides 126 skills with overview information covering skill purpose, safety, and delegation guides; equipment lists; preparation procedures; procedure videos with printable step-by-step guidelines; appropriate follow-up care; documentation guidelines; and interactive review questions. Available online, as a student DVD set, or as a networkable DVD set for the institution.

Contents

UNIT 9 SUPPORTIVE NURSING INTERVENTIONS

APPENDIXES

1 Using Evidence in Nursing Practice

OUTLINE

EVOLVE WEBSITE/RESOURCES LIST

http://evolve.elsevier.com/Perry/nursinginterventions

Audio Glossary • Case Studies • Clinical Review Questions • Answers and Rationales for Clinical Review Questions

INTRODUCTION

What is evidence? Basically, it is a body of facts or information that proves a concept, belief, or physical event is true and valid. Evidence allows us to form conclusions and make decisions about some phenomenon. For example, evidence shows that the earth rotates as it revolves around the sun; thus scientists apply the evidence in other interplanetary science studies, including sending people into space. Evidence shows a link between smoking and the occurrence of head, neck, and lung cancer; thus scientists and public health professionals apply the evidence in developing smoking prevention strategies. In nursing, evidence has demonstrated that safe patient-handling techniques coupled with good body mechanics reduce patient and nurse injuries during patient transfers. Evidence regarding safe patient handling led to the development of numerous transfer devices to reduce the physical burden of patient transfers. The use of evidence improves our world by applying what is known to be true and factual to create better public health policies, improve health care delivery, and improve clinical practices.

All health care providers desire the same thing: being able to deliver safe, patient-centered, evidence-based care. Evidence-based practice (EBP) is a framework to ensure that the best available scientific evidence from research studies, the expertise of clinicians, and patient values and preferences influence decisions about health care practices (Phillips, 2015). So basically, there are three forms of evidence (Puddy and Wilkins, 2011):

Scientific evidence: This comprises the data obtained after testing questions about phenomena through well-designed, systematically conducted research studies. What we learn from research is the strongest form of evidence because it has been shown to be relevant, accurate, and current (at the time of the study). Scientific evidence is represented in research articles as well as clinical guidelines that incorporate research findings.

Experiential evidence: This type of evidence is based on professional insight, understanding, skill, and expertise that is gathered over time. It is often referred to as intuitive knowledge. A clinical nurse specialist (CNS) who has spent a career studying and caring for older-adult patients has experiential evidence in gerontology.

Contextual evidence: This type of evidence is based on factors that address whether a strategy (evidence-based intervention) is useful, feasible to implement, and accepted by a particular community (e.g., the ethnic population served by a community clinic; the type of staffing used on a nursing unit).

As a nurse, you cannot simply take a single scientific finding and apply it in practice without considering what you have learned as a nurse with respect to the finding and the values and preferences of patients that will affect how you apply the scientific finding. Here is a case example of this concept:

Nurses on a colo-rectal surgical unit are considering a strategy to reduce the incidence of wound infections on their unit. One option is the use of chlorhexidine gluconate (CHG) for daily patient bathing. Patients on the unit have surgical incisions, and some have abdominal stomas (see Chapter 21). There is scientific evidence that CHG is highly effective in reducing health care–associated infections because of its antimicrobial activity against gram-positive organisms, rapid onset, and prolonged residual effect on the skin (Choi et al., 2015; Wang and Layon, 2017). One might think you would recommend using CHG to bathe all patients. However, the CNS who has worked on the surgery unit for several years knows from experience and after checking the drug information pamphlet on CHG that the antiinfective should not be applied directly to a stoma because of potential irritation of tissues. The nurse has also observed mild inflammation develop over the stoma of one patient when CHG was used for cleansing. However, research also has shown that CHG causes minimal skin irritation (Popp et al., 2014). Patients occasionally report that CHG causes the skin to feel sticky and prefer soap and water for bathing. Because the nurse knows the evidence to support the use of CHG in bathing is strong and that its use can potentially reduce infection rates (Wang and Layon, 2017), the following changes in practice are recommended to the unit EBP committee: implementing CHG bathing every other day, alternating with soap-and-water baths; avoiding use of CHG on stomas and other mucous membranes; and giving nurses on the unit information to explain to those patients who prefer soap and water the important advantages of using CHG while in the hospital.

Evidence from scientific studies is not to be used in isolation. Nurses are most successful in establishing EBPs when they respect the experience of colleagues and make informed decisions based on the unique needs of their patients. Remember, too, that you should never automatically accept the findings of any study simply because it was published; critically appraise all studies yourself using the criteria outlined in this chapter.

STEPS IN THE EBP FRAMEWORK

EBP is a systematic approach to rational decision making that aligns nursing practices with the best available scientific knowledge. If you are just learning about EBP, understanding this framework is critical for making EBP a knowledge-based approach involving critical thinking. Graduate nurses who read this text will find the framework a useful summary to prepare for the application of EBP in daily practice.

Following the seven basic steps of the EBP framework ensures that you obtain the strongest available scientific evidence and apply it appropriately in nursing practice. Melnyk and Fineout-Overholt (2015) recommend a seven-step process (Steps 0 through 6) for EBP:

0. Cultivate a spirit of inquiry.
1. Ask a clinical question in PICO(T) format.
2. Search for the most relevant and best evidence.
3. Critically appraise the evidence you gather.
4. Integrate the best evidence with your clinical expertise and patient preferences and values in making a practice decision or change.
5. Evaluate the outcomes of the practice decision or change based on the evidence.
6. Communicate the outcomes of the EBP decision or change.

Fleiszer and colleagues (2016) offer a critical additional step for sustaining knowledge use and practice changes. This means continuing practices or procedures within an agency that successfully lead to the routine use of evidence in practice. *In the previous case example, the CNS will monitor the use of CHG for bathing to determine if staff are adherent to the new bathing practice. In addition, the CNS will track the infection control report for the surgical unit to evaluate whether health care–associated infection rates decline over the next several months.*

Cultivate a Spirit of Inquiry

Always ask questions. If you are a beginning student, seek new knowledge and challenge ideas that are unclear. Nurses in practice must routinely ask, "Why do we practice this way?" when there does not seem to be a clear reason for decisions that affect patient care. Nurses naturally practice a certain way because it is what they learn in school or observe from others. However, there is new nursing knowledge being reported each day; what was once a best practice just a few years ago may now be outdated. Students can learn to develop a spirit of inquiry by forming study groups or posing thoughtful questions during clinical experiences. In the practice setting, nurses use time during staff meetings and clinical practice sessions to discuss their questions.

Ask a Clinical Question

Questions tend to arise from two sources: recurrent problems (e.g., repeated infections on a nursing unit, incidence of patient falls, patients being readmitted to the health care agency in less than 30 days) and new knowledge from the literature or from clinical experts. There is a suggested format for phrasing a question, using the PICO(T) acronym. Using as many of the PICO(T) elements as you can to phrase your question ensures that when you next go to the literature to search for articles (evidence), you will likely find what you want. The PICO(T) elements are as follows:

P = Patient population or area of interest
Identify the patients (family, clinical staff) by age, gender, ethnicity, disease, and experience, or identify a health problem or knowledge area of interest.

I = Intervention of interest
Which intervention do you think you want to use in practice (e.g., a new treatment, educational approach)?

C = Comparison of interest
What is the usual standard of care or current intervention that you now use in practice?

O = Outcome
What result do you wish to achieve or observe as a result of an intervention (e.g., change in patient/family caregiver behavior, a physical finding, patient perception)?

T = Time
This element is optional, but it allows you to identify the time you believe is needed to demonstrate an outcome (e.g., the time it takes for an intervention to achieve an outcome).

Here are some examples of PICO(T) questions:

1. Does the use of early mobility protocols (**I**) for postoperative patients undergoing general surgery (**P**) compared with standard activity guidelines (**C**) improve time to ambulation (**O**) during patient length of stay (**T**)?
2. What educational approach for presenting information about human papillomavirus (HPV) (**I**) is preferred by young adult males (**P**) to improve their adherence to HPV vaccinations (**O**)?
3. Does the rate of falls with injury (**O**) among inpatient adult oncology patients (**P**) change as a result of using a family coach (**I**) compared with a standard fall prevention protocol (**C**)?

Note that not every question you raise will include all of the PICO(T) elements. If you want to learn about patients' or health care providers' perceptions about a concept, it is less likely you will have a comparison group or time element. Use as many of the elements as you can so that your literature search will be focused.

Search for the Most Relevant and Best Evidence

After framing a PICO(T) question concisely, you will use each element to build a search approach for finding evidence in the literature. Thousands of resources are available to aid in your search, including government and professional websites, agency procedure manuals, performance improvement data, existing clinical practice guidelines, and computerized bibliographical databases. Using bibliographical databases is not a simple task. The way each element is worded or phrased can make a difference in the number of articles you can obtain.

Here is an example: Take the following key words to gather articles about early mobility: **early mobility, surgical patients, time to ambulation, standard activity**. When these key words were entered into the MEDLINE database for the period of 2013 through June 2017, a total of 2970 articles was returned from the full search. No clinician has time to read 2970 articles. However, when you enter the key words by combining them—early mobility **and** surgical patients **and** time to ambulation **and** standard activity—you obtain the number of

TABLE 1.1

Searchable Scientific Literature Databases and Sources

Database/Source	Description
CINAHL	Cumulative Index of Nursing and Allied Health Literature; includes studies in nursing, allied health, and biomedicine http://www.cinahl.com/
MEDLINE	Studies in medicine, nursing, dentistry, psychiatry, veterinary medicine, and allied health http://www.ncbi.nim.nih.gov
PsycINFO	Psychology and related health care disciplines http://www.apa.org/psycinfo/
Cochrane Database of Systematic Reviews	Full text of regularly updated systematic reviews prepared by the Cochrane Collaboration; includes completed reviews and protocols http://www.cochrane.org/reviews
National Guidelines Clearinghouse	Repository for structured abstracts (summaries) about clinical guidelines and their development; also includes condensed version of guidelines for viewing http://www.guideline.gov/
PubMed	Health science library at the National Library of Medicine offers free access to journal articles http://www.nlm.nih.gov
Worldviews on Evidence-Based Nursing	Electronic journal containing articles that provide a synthesis of research and an annotated bibliography for selected references

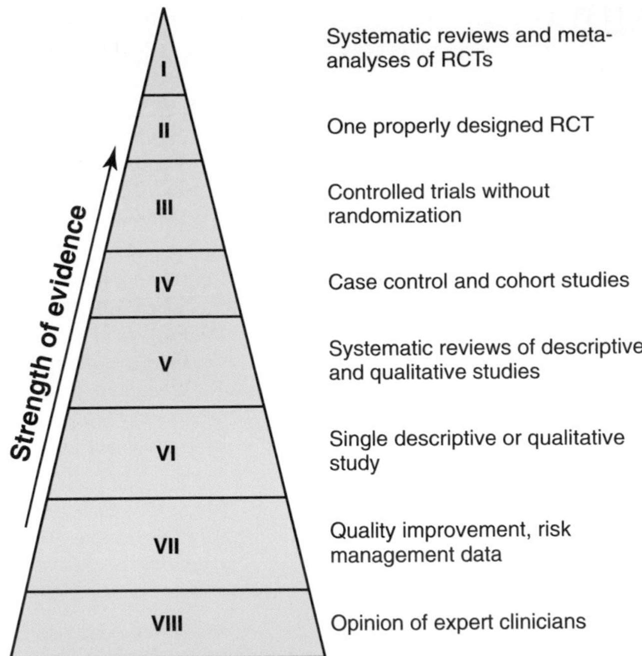

FIG 1.1 The evidence hierarchy pyramid. *RCT*, Randomized controlled trial. *(Modified from Guyatt G, Rennie D: User's guide to the medical literature, Chicago, 2002, AMA Press; Harris RP et al.: Current methods of the U.S. Preventive Services Task Force: a review of the process,* Am J Prev Med *20[3 Suppl]:21, 2001.)*

articles that contain all three terms. In this example, zero articles were retrieved. That is not helpful either. If you manipulate the wording, such as changing *surgical patients* to *surgery*, and focus just on the two most important key words, *surgery* ***and*** *early mobility*, you obtain eight articles. That is a great place to start! You will have obtained a practical number of articles to review on your topic.

When you conduct a literature search, an important resource in clinical settings is a medical librarian who knows the databases that are available to you (Table 1.1). In the academic setting, seek assistance from the reference librarian. The databases store published scientific studies, including peer-reviewed research. A **peer-reviewed** article is one submitted for publication and reviewed by a panel of experts familiar with the topic or subject matter of the article. The librarian is able to translate your PICO(T) question into the language or key words that will yield the best evidence and the articles that most likely address your topic of interest. For the purpose of EBP, you are trying to find a limited number of the best articles available so that you can move to the next step in determining if you can use the available evidence in your practice.

Critically Appraise the Evidence

The next step in EBP is to critically review and analyze the available articles from your search and other sources to evaluate the strength and relevance of evidence. This requires a systematic approach. You will appraise each source of evidence (research article, clinical guideline, expert summary) to determine its value, feasibility, and utility of evidence for making a practice change. Often the review of multiple articles is most effective within a group such as a study group in school or a hospital practice committee, where each member reviews one or two articles. The pyramid in Fig. 1.1 represents an example of the hierarchy of available evidence. The level of rigor or the amount of confidence you have in the findings of a study decreases as you move down the pyramid (Ingham-Broomfield, 2016).

It is impossible to be an expert on all aspects of the types of research studies conducted. But you can learn enough about the types of studies to help you know which ones have the best scientific evidence (Table 1.2). Understanding the hierarchy of evidence helps you decide if evidence from a source is relevant, valid, and appropriate for use in practice. Your aim is to determine the worth of any evidence you obtain by considering the following:

- What is the level of evidence?
- How well was a study (if research article) conducted?
- How useful are the findings to practice?

When rating the evidence from a research study, you determine the strength of evidence based on the evidence hierarchy and by using a numbering system (Box 1.1) for rating. For example, evidence from a systematic review would be rated a 1, evidence from a randomized trial is rated a 2, whereas published clinical articles are rated at the lower level of 6 (LoBiondo-Wood and Haber, 2017). Combining all articles gives you a sense of the highest level of evidence you have to address your clinical question. You do not average the numbers for rating. Instead, you appraise what evidence is consistent in all articles and the strength and relevance of that evidence to apply in your practice.

For example, you may review three different randomized controlled trials (RCTs) and find that the evidence for early mobility protocols that use specific screening criteria for eligible patients and have levels of mobility to use to progress patients is consistent and strong in all studies. Thus you would create such a program on your unit. If instead, the review showed no consistency in the evidence for

TABLE 1.2

Types of Studies in the Evidence Hierarchy

Study Type	Description
Systematic review	Synthesis of primary scientific evidence on a particular topic or question Summarizes the best evidence on a specific clinical, educational or administrative question Critically appraises primary studies, extracts data, reviews methodology and validity of results, and reports conclusions on whether evidence is generalizable and can be applied in practice (Oh, 2016)
Randomized controlled trial (RCT)	Highest level of experimental research Involves the testing of an intervention (e.g., early mobility protocol or patient education method) against the usual standard of care Participants in an RCT are randomly assigned to either a control or a treatment group. In other words, all of the subjects have an equal chance of being in either group. The treatment group receives the experimental intervention. The control group receives the usual standard of care. Both groups are measured for the same outcomes (using analytic statistics) preintervention and postintervention to see if the experimental intervention made a significant difference.
Quasiexperimental study	Study aims to determine whether a program or intervention has the intended effect on its participants. An RCT includes (1) a *pretest–posttest design*, (2) a *treatment group* and a *control group*, and (3) *random assignment* of study participants; however, quasiexperimental studies lack one or more of these design elements.
Descriptive study	Study that describes phenomena affecting patients or health care professionals Study does not try to quantify the relationship between groups but tries to give a picture of what is happening in a population. Uses simple descriptive statistics such as frequency, prevalence, or incidence
Case control study	Study compares patients who have a disease or outcome of interest with patients who do not have the disease or outcome. The researcher looks back (retrospectively) to compare how frequently the exposure to a risk factor is present in each group to determine the relationship between the risk factor and disease.
Qualitative	Analysis of interviews, observations, and/or surveys to measure people's perceptions, feelings, or views of phenomena Results describe common themes.

BOX 1.1

Rating Evidence

Evidence-based practice is ranked by the way the evidence was collected by the researcher or clinician. The following is an example of a rating system from strongest to weakest evidence (LoBiondo-Wood and Haber, 2017):

Level 1: Systematic reviews or meta-analyses of randomized and nonrandomized clinical trials; evidence-based clinical practice guidelines based on systematic reviews

Level 2: Well-designed single randomized and nonrandomized clinical trials

Level 3: Controlled trials without randomization (quasiexperimental studies)

Level 4: Single nonexperimental studies such as correlational, cohort, or case control studies

Level 5: Systematic review of descriptive and qualitative studies

Level 6: Single descriptive or qualitative studies

Level 7: Opinions from authorities and/or reports from expert committees

how early mobility protocols are developed and used, then you would be more reluctant to adopt such a protocol.

Read each article carefully to decide how well a study was conducted. When reading through a scientific study, summarize key elements. You may choose to use critical appraisal guides or useful checklists for evaluating studies (Spruce et al., 2016). A guide lists questions about the essential elements of research (e.g., purpose, sample size, setting, method of study, approach to data analysis). It is important to know the elements of scientific articles to decide the value and relevance to your PICO(T) question.

Integrate the Best Evidence

Once you complete an evidence appraisal, you decide if the evidence is strong enough to be used in practice immediately. The easiest approach is to apply the evidence in a plan of care for a patient. For instance, you are assigned to work in a long-term care nursing center, and you care for a patient with dementia who wanders. Your review of the literature reveals clinical guidelines and results of research that offer strong evidence on techniques that can successfully reduce wandering (e.g., providing a secure place for patients to wander, enhancing the patient's environment visually and tactilely, and making exits less accessible [Futrell et al., 2010]). You decide to use several techniques from the articles you reviewed during your next clinical assignment to see if it reduces wandering in your assigned patient. You use the approaches that work best for the particular setting. If you need to submit a written plan of care, use the source of evidence as the scientific rationale for the intervention you plan to try.

Nurses in practice often become part of a hospital committee or task force, adopting EBP on a larger scale than just a patient-focused care plan. One strategy for nurses to become involved in the EBP process is the formation of a nursing clinical effectiveness committee (McKeever et al., 2016). Once the committee has identified evidence to make a practice change, an organized collaborative effort is needed to bring appropriate administrators and staff on board. The nursing clinical effectiveness committee can overcome barriers to implementation of EBP (McKeever et al., 2016). This requires bringing all stakeholders (individuals who have an interest or concern in the practice change) together to explain why the evidence-based interventions are important. For example, administrators want to know if the practice change improves patient outcomes and lowers costs. Staff nurses want to know if the practice change improves patient outcomes and how it will affect the way they provide care. Health care providers also want to know how the practice change affects the way they provide care. To integrate evidence into practice, education of all those involved in the practice change must occur. This requires approaches such as teaching seminars, informational newsletters, and ongoing discussions during staff and clinical effectiveness meetings.

The actual way in which nurses integrate evidence into practice can involve the development of teaching tools, clinical practice guidelines or protocols, and new assessment or documentation tools. Depending on the amount of change needed to apply evidence in practice, it becomes necessary to involve a number of staff members from a given nursing unit. It is important to consider the setting in which to apply the evidence. Is there support from all staff? Does/do the practice change(s) fit within the scope of practice in the clinical setting? Are there resources (time, equipment, staff) available to make a change? To integrate evidence, it is important to apply the best evidence to improve the care that nurses directly provide their patients.

A common approach used for integrating evidence into practice is to incorporate new evidence into policies and procedures (P&Ps). Many health care agencies have adopted an EBP approach when reviewing all P&Ps. A key feature of a practice environment that supports the use of best evidence is requiring clinical practice P&Ps to be evidence-based (Hanrahan et al., 2015; Jun et al., 2016). P&Ps are important tools for supporting nurses in using evidence in their everyday practice and promoting positive patient outcomes. **This is the approach used throughout the chapters of this textbook. Each skill incorporates the best evidence available.**

Evaluate the Outcomes of the Practice Change

When you plan to integrate the evidence you discover into practice, it is essential to decide how you will evaluate the outcomes (Table 1.3). Remember the "O" in your PICO(T) question. It represents the outcomes you choose to measure after you integrate the evidence. These outcomes tell you how well the evidence-based intervention works. Consider the example of adopting guidelines to reduce wandering in a patient with dementia. The nursing agency tracks incidents of wandering for each patient. Thus, you would evaluate your level of success by comparing the number of wandering incidents before you adopted strategies for wandering prevention to the number of incidents following your intervention. You might choose to gather measures for several days following your intervention to also determine if any change was sustained.

When an EBP change occurs on a larger scale, for example, changing a protocol on a nursing unit, an evaluation of outcomes is more formal. Nurses who adopt EBP on a unit must have an evaluation plan that includes outcome measurement at least 3 months before implementing the practice change, followed by another 3 months after the practice change. This provides a prepractice and postpractice change comparison that determines the effects of the practice change and whether modifications are necessary. If outcomes do not improve, the staff may decide to not continue the practice change. Outcomes chosen for measurement should reflect whether or not the practice change had an effect. Examples of outcome measures include the following:

- Symptoms (e.g., pain, fatigue, nausea)
- Functional status (e.g., activity tolerance, ability to perform activities of daily living)
- Learning (e.g., ability to demonstrate a skill, complete a written quiz, and describe precautions to take after surgery)
- Safety (e.g., incidence of falls, infections, pressure injuries, staff injuries)
- Psychological distress (e.g., anxiety, depression)
- Physiological measures (e.g., vital signs, weight, blood glucose)

When identifying an outcome to evaluate a practice change, consider the type of measurement to use. Will you observe a patient behavior (e.g., taking a medication or performing an exercise or skill) or collect a physiological measure (e.g., weight or blood pressure)? Will measurement require you to conduct an interview, audit an existing medical record, or check results in a laboratory report? If you choose to use some form of survey or assessment tool, try to use one that has already been developed and shown to be valid.

Outcome measurement plans are more successful when the approach is acceptable and important to the clinicians involved. Before any formal implementation and evaluation of EBP, it is important to include all staff members who will be affected by an EBP project from the beginning. It is also important to be consistent and accurate when collecting outcome measures. Any clinicians who are involved in outcome measurement should receive proper training in data measurement and collection. For example, if outcome measurement involves a new device such as a pulse oximeter, each data collector must show competence in the use of the oximeter. Those who collect outcome data must collect it in the same way each time.

TABLE 1.3

Outcome Measurement

Outcome	Measurement Approach
Patient able to ambulate after surgery within 12 hours postoperatively.	Time when ambulation begins postoperatively
Patient loses 4.5 kg (10 lb) in 2 months.	Weight measured each clinic visit
Patient describes side effects of antihypertensive medication.	Patient interview
Patient is satisfied with nursing care.	Patient satisfaction survey
Patient expresses less fatigue after a 4-week exercise program.	Self-report fatigue scale
Incidence of methicillin-resistant *Staphylococcus aureus* drops among surgical patients.	Medical record laboratory reports

Communicate the Outcomes

Once you have implemented and evaluated the outcomes of an EBP change, communicate the results. There are several options for communicating practice changes successfully:

- After adopting an evidence-based approach to care, report the results to the nurse in charge and the oncoming nurse assuming care for your patient. Record the result of the approach in the appropriate section of the electronic health record (EHR).
- Share the results of an evidence-based approach with fellow students during a postclinical discussion.
- As a staff nurse, share information about the change and the results in unit staff meetings, clinical effectiveness team meetings, and leadership meetings.

- Present results at a staff inservice.
- Present results at an EBP workshop or conference (poster or podium presentation).
- Write an article about the practice change and results.

SAFE AND EFFECTIVE NURSING SKILLS AND PROCEDURES

Scientific evidence is central to making nursing skills and procedures safe and effective. As new research adds to the body of nursing knowledge, it becomes important to update any skills and procedures. New evidence appears almost daily, more so on certain topics than others. For example, the research directed toward pain management and infection control is extensive. In contrast, less evidence is available on eye and ear care. As a nurse, you want to be familiar with agency procedures but also know the newest evidence to determine if changes in practice need to be made in your agency.

Evidence Integrated Into Skills

The aim of this textbook is to introduce and incorporate the newest evidence available into the skills presented. This is achieved in two ways.

First, the **Practice Standards** section at the beginning of each chapter includes clinical standards relevant to skills on the chapter topic. A bulleted list provides the actual source of the standard (e.g., professional organization, government agency, author), followed by the year it was published and the name of the standard. A brief statement describes the content included in the skills that relates to the standard. This feature ensures that the skills within the text contain updated and relevant clinical standards from professional organizations. Here is an example:

PRACTICE STANDARDS

- Institute for Safe Medication Practices (ISMP), 2017: List of error-prone abbreviations, symbols, and dose designations—Medication safety
- Institute for Safe Medication Practices (ISMP), 2016: 2016–2017 targeted medication safety best practices for hospitals—Medication safety
- Institute for Safe Medication Practices (ISMP), 2016: Oral dosage forms that should not be crushed—Medication safety
- The Joint Commission (TJC), 2019: National Patient Safety Goals—Patient identification

Second, you will then find the standards incorporated appropriately within the chapter. Here is an example from a portion of the skill *Administering Oral Medications;* italics and bold show the incorporation of the ISMP 2016–2017 targeted medication safety best practices for hospitals:

i. Prepare liquids.

(1) Unit-dose container with correct amount of medication; gently shake container. Administer medication packaged in a single-dose cup directly from the single-dose cup. Do not pour medicine into another cup.	Using unit-dose container with correct dosage of medication provides most accurate dose of medication (ISMP, 2016). Shaking container ensures that medication is mixed before administration.

Safe Patient Care *On the basis of current best practice (ISMP, 2016), liquid medications that are not available or are not in correct dose in a unit-dose container should be dispensed by the pharmacy in special oral syringes marked "Oral Use Only." These syringes do not connect to any type of parenteral (e.g., intravenous [IV]) tubing. In addition, current evidence shows that liquid measuring devices on patient care units result in inaccurate dosing. Having oral medications prepared in the pharmacy ensures that you give the most accurate dose of a medication possible and prevents parenteral administration of oral medications.*

When you read a skill in the text, look for references cited with the rationales. The authors update these skills and ensure the newest evidence-based practices. Another example comes from the Infusion Nurses Society (2016). This is a professional organization that routinely updates its standards of practice to ensure high-quality infusion practices. This can be found in the chapter on intravenous and vascular access therapy:

PRACTICE STANDARDS

- Infusion Nurses Society (INS), 2016: Infusion therapy standards of practice—Insertion of peripheral catheters

Safe Patient Care *Short extension sets may be used on short-peripheral catheters. Reduces catheter manipulation. For patient safety, all connections should be of Luer-Lok type (INS, 2016). Many agencies use short extension tubing for continuous infusions and standalone saline locks (capped catheters).*

8. Prepare IV tubing and solution for continuous infusion.

a. Check IV solution using seven rights of medication administration (see Chapter 22) and review label for name and concentration of solution, type and concentration of any additives, volume, beyond-use and expiration dates, sterility state. If using bar code, scan code on patient's wristband and then on IV fluid container. Be sure that prescribed additives such as potassium and vitamins have been added. Check solution for color and clarity. Check bag for leaks.	Reviewing label for accuracy reduces risk for medication errors (INS, 2016). Bar-code system reduces human error (INS, 2016). Risk for medication errors can be reduced with safe medication practices, including (INS, 2016): • Do not add medications to infusing containers of IV solutions (INS, 2016). • Do not use IV solutions that are discolored, contain precipitates, or are expired. • Risk for transmission of infection can be reduced by: • Not using leaking bags because integrity has been compromised.

Developing and Reviewing Nursing Policies and Procedures

The daily work that nurses do in performing skills and procedures is too important to not be supported by the current and most relevant evidence. Health care agencies are required by regulating groups such as the Centers for Medicare and Medicaid Services and The Joint Commission (TJC) to review all P&Ps routinely. Each health care agency has committees (e.g., pharmacy, physical therapy, nursing) that are given the responsibility for reviewing their department P&Ps. In the case of nursing P&Ps, the committee is usually composed of clinical nurse experts, experienced staff nurses, and consultants from education and practice departments.

Each agency conducts policy and procedure review differently. However, Table 1.4 offers a step-by-step review of what most agencies

TABLE 1.4

Policy and Procedure Algorithm Steps

Review Steps	Actions
1. Policy and procedure committee selects the policy/procedure for revision or creates new policy if none available on topic.	Perform a routine review (every 2 or 3 years) of practice changes. The following process is also applicable for new policies.
2. Using the procedure and population to which it is delivered as key terms, search for available evidence.	Suggested sites for searching: • CINAHL and MEDLINE databases • Cochrane Library • American College of Physicians • National Guideline Clearinghouse • Professional association guidelines/standards of care (e.g., American Association of Colleges of Nursing, Association of periOperative Registered Nurses, Oncology Nursing Society) • University Health Consortium for other academic hospital policies/procedures • Local standards or policies • Expert opinion/clinical expertise • Clinical articles and Web search
3. Critique and evaluate the evidence.	Appraise the research evidence and assign a level of evidence for each source. Consider a mechanism for organizing the evidence (e.g., an evidence table).
4. Compare the evidence to current policy and procedure and make a decision.	Decision point: • Make no changes (update references). • Make language more precise. • Revise policy/procedure to include new evidence. • Develop new policy or procedure based on evidence, if indicated. • Retire or delete policy if outdated or no longer effective for quality patient care.
5. Have new/revised policy reviewed by stakeholders and experts.	Send revised policy to stakeholders (those who have reviewed prior versions of the policy or those who should review) with revisions deadline and timeline goal for presentation of policy to the policy and procedure committee.
6. Make any revisions recommended by stakeholders or experts.	If stakeholders make major revisions, resend new revision (with stakeholder suggestions) back to original distribution list for approval, again including approval deadline date.
7. Obtain approval signatures.	Changes are usually signed by the nursing executive(s) responsible for nursing practice.
8. Submit policy/procedure to full committee.	Final recommendations and approval made by committee.
9. Provide staff education as needed.	

Adapted from Houser J, Oman KS: *Evidence-based practice: an implementation guide for healthcare organizations*, Sudbury, MA, 2011, Jones & Bartlett.

follow. Note that the steps follow the basic seven steps of EBP. The search for the best evidence, careful evidence review, and thoughtful determination of whether to revise or discontinue an existing procedure or create a new one are the key roles of any policy and procedure committee. The legal implications are significant. If nurses do not follow the current practices outlined in P&Ps, any errors or deletions can create liability.

BENEFITS OF EBP

Working within an organization that makes EBP a priority is rewarding and professionally stimulating. The American Nurses Credentialing Center (ANCC) established the Magnet Recognition® Program to recognize health care agencies that achieve excellence in nursing practice (ANCC, 2016). Health care agencies that apply for Magnet® status must demonstrate quality patient care, nursing excellence, and innovations in professional practice. One of the criteria that must be met for institutions to achieve Magnet® status is the presentation of extensive evidence showing that nurses are involved in evidence-based practice and research activities.

There are five ways evidence-based health care adds value to health care systems (Haughom, 2016):

- Helps clinicians remain current on standardized, evidence-based protocols
- Uses nearly real-time scientific data to make care decisions
- Improves transparency, accountability, and value (e.g., safe care)
- Improves quality of care
- Improves outcomes

Advocate for EBP in your practice to benefit staff, professional colleagues, and your patients. Always be mindful of the importance of EBP, remain inquisitive, and pursue the new knowledge that exists.

✦ PRACTICE REFLECTIONS

Consider a patient you are assigned to care for in a clinical area. What is significant about the patient's medical history, nursing history, and recent assessment? What are the patient's primary problems identified by the health care team? What does the patient want to learn about his or her main health concerns, and what is expected of the health care team?

1. What are the patient's primary problems or clinical concerns that you would focus on? Why?
2. What area of scientific knowledge applies to the patient situation?
3. Write a PICO(T) question for this situation, and discuss the key terms you would use to search for literature.
4. Based on the PICO(T) question you chose, how would you plan to evaluate the outcome of an evidence-based approach?

✦ CLINICAL REVIEW QUESTIONS

1. A monthly report for a neurosurgical unit shows that there have been three, five, and six falls, respectively, for the past 3 months. A staff nurse on the unit discusses with a colleague a summary of an article about hourly nursing rounds. Could this be a way to improve patient care? The two nurses decide to bring the issue up in their next clinical effectiveness meeting. What would be the most appropriate PICO(T) question for this situation?
   1. Do staff nurses who work with neurosurgical patients conduct hourly rounding compared with nurses on nonneurosurgical areas?
   2. Does hourly rounding compared with standard rounding improve patient satisfaction?
   3. Do staff nurses on neurosurgical units perceive hourly rounding to be effective?
   4. In neurosurgical patients, does hourly rounding compared with standard rounding affect fall incidence?
2. Which of the following are examples of contextual evidence? (Select all that apply.)
   1. An orthopedic nurse's knowledge of postoperative pain after working in orthopedics for 10 years
   2. The literacy level of patients visiting a medicine clinic
   3. The results of a quasiexperimental study
   4. A clinical practice guideline from a professional nursing association
   5. The percentage of patient care technicians working on a nursing unit
3. Match the category of outcome with the appropriate measurement.

Category	Measurement
1. Symptom	A. A patient describes schedule for taking medications at home
2. Safety	B. Pulse oximeter reading
3. Learning	C. Shortness of breath
4. Physiological	D. Number of medication errors

Answers and Rationales for Clinical Review Questions can be found on the Evolve website.

REFERENCES

American Nurses Credentialing Center (ANCC): Magnet Model, 2016. http://www.nursecredentialing.org/Magnet/ProgramOverview/New-Magnet-Model.

Choi EY, et al: Efficacy of chlorhexidine bathing for reducing healthcare associated bloodstream infections: a meta-analysis, *Ann Intensive Care* 5:31, 2015.

Fleiszer AR, et al: Nursing unit leaders' influence on the long-term sustainability of evidence-based practice improvements, *J Nurs Manag* 24:309, 2016.

Futrell M, et al: Evidence-based guideline: wandering, *J Gerontol Nurs* 36(2):6–14, 2010.

Hanrahan K, et al: Sacred cow gone to pasture: a systematic evaluation and integration of evidence-based practice, *Worldviews Evid Based Nurs* 12(1):3, 2015.

Haughom J: 5 Reasons the practice of evidence-based medicine is a hot topic, HealthCatalyst, 2016. https://www.healthcatalyst.com/5-reasons-practice-evidence-based-medicine-is-hot-topic.

Infusion Nurses Society (INS): Infusion therapy standards of practice, *J Intraven Nurs* 39(1S):2016.

Ingham-Broomfield R: A nurses' guide to the hierarchy of research designs and evidence, *Aust J Adv Nurs* 33(3):38, 2016.

Jun J, et al: Barriers and facilitators of nurses' use of clinical practice guidelines: an integrative review, *Int J Nurs Stud* 60:54, 2016.

LoBiondo-Wood G, Haber J: *Nursing research: methods and critical appraisal for evidence-based practice*, ed 9, St. Louis, 2017, Elsevier.

McKeever S, et al: Engaging a nursing workforce in evidence-based practice: introduction of a nursing clinical effectiveness committee, *Worldviews Evid Based Nurs* 13(1):85, 2016.

Melnyk BM, Fineout-Overholt E: *Evidence-based practice in nursing and healthcare: a guide to best practice*, ed 3, Philadelphia, 2015, Lippincott Williams & Wilkins.

Oh EG: Synthesizing quantitative evidence for evidence-based nursing: systematic review, *Asian Nursing Res* 10(2):89–93, 2016.

Phillips C: Relationships between duration of practice, educational level, and perception of barriers to implement evidence-based practice among critical care nurses, *Int J Evid Based Healthc* 13(4):224–232, 2015.

Popp JA, et al: Hospital-acquired infections and thermally injured patients: chlorhexidine gluconate baths work, *Am J Infect Control* 42:129–132, 2014.

Puddy RW, Wilkins N: *Understanding evidence part 1: best available research evidence. A guide to the continuum of evidence of effectiveness*, Atlanta, GA, 2011, Centers for Disease Control and Prevention. https://www.cdc.gov/violenceprevention/pdf/understanding_evidence-a.pdf.

Spruce L, et al: AORN's revised model for evidence appraisal and rating, *AORN J* 103:60, 2016.

Wang EW, Layon AJ: Chlorhexidine gluconate use to prevent hospital acquired infections—a useful tool, not a panacea, *Ann Transl Med* 5(1):14, 2017.

2 Communication and Collaboration

SKILLS AND PROCEDURES

EVOLVE WEBSITE/RESOURCES LIST

http://evolve.elsevier.com/Perry/nursinginterventions

Audio Glossary • Case Studies • Checklists • Clinical Review Questions • Answers and Rationales for Clinical Review Questions

INTRODUCTION

Communication is a basic human need and the foundation for establishing a caring relationship between a nurse and patient (Fig. 2.1). It involves the expression of emotions, ideas, and thoughts through verbal (words or written language) and nonverbal (e.g., behaviors) exchanges. Verbal communication includes both the spoken and the written word. Nonverbal communication includes body movement, physical appearance, personal space, touch, and facial expression. As a nurse, be aware of techniques that facilitate or inhibit communication (Table 2.1). Essential interpersonal skills include having empathy and a nonjudgmental attitude, being aware of both verbal and nonverbal communication, using appropriate body language, being patient and sensitive to patients' cues, and giving feedback appropriately. Many factors influence the complex process of communication (Box 2.1).

PRACTICE STANDARDS

- Agency for Healthcare Research and Quality (AHRQ), 2013: Strategy 4: Care transitions from hospital to home: IDEAL discharge planning—Discharge planning guidelines
- Occupational Safety and Health Administration (OSHA), 2015: Guidelines for preventing workplace violence for healthcare and social service workers—Guidelines for reporting violent incidents
- The Joint Commission (TJC), 2013: The need for collaboration across entire care continuum—Risk factors for readmission after discharge
- The Joint Commission (TJC), 2015a: Transitions of care: engaging patients and families—Recommendations for patient and family engagement
- The Joint Commission (TJC), 2015b: Sentinel event data—Root causes by event type, 2004–2015—Sentinel event root causes
- The Joint Commission (TJC), 2019: National Patient Safety Goals—Patient identification

EVIDENCE-BASED PRACTICE

Workplace Violence

Workplace violence against nurses is at epidemic levels, with up to 50% of nurses being victims at some point in their career (Moore et al., 2018). According to a recent study, three in four nurses experienced verbal or physical abuse such as yelling, cursing, grabbing, scratching, or kicking from patients as well as visitors (Speroni et al., 2014). Nurses are at higher risk of exposure when caring for patients with dementia or Alzheimer disease, patients with drug-seeking behavior, or drug- or alcohol-influenced patients. Hospitals are implementing workplace violence prevention programs to maintain a safe work environment because it is a legal and ethical responsibility of health care administrators and nursing leaders (Copeland et al., 2017). These prevention programs have multiple goals: to help raise the overall safety and health knowledge across the workforce, to provide employees with the tools needed to identify workplace safety and security hazards, and to address potential problems before they arise and ultimately reduce the likelihood of workers being assaulted (Moore et al., 2018). General prevention measures that can be instituted to prevent or manage violence include:

- Learning effective de-escalation techniques involving personal space, body language, and listening skills
- Having a well-trained security workforce
- Using a tiered alarm system to contact trained personnel
- Limiting access to areas such as the emergency department that are at higher risk for potential violence
- Regularly educating staff on techniques to prevent and manage violence

SAFETY GUIDELINES

Miscommunication, between health care providers and between provider and patient, can adversely affect patient safety. Listen to what and how a patient communicates, including content and verbal

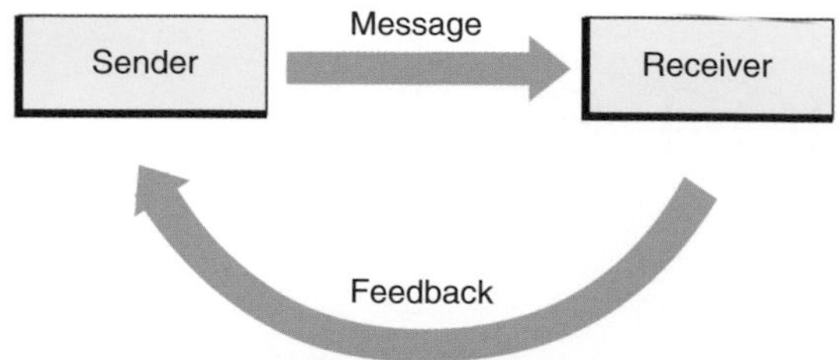

FIG 2.1 Communication is a two-way process.

BOX 2.1

Factors That Influence Communication

- *Perceptions:* Personal views based on past experiences.
- *Values:* Beliefs that a person considers important in life.
- *Emotions:* Subjective feelings about a situation (e.g., anger, fear, frustration, pain, anxiety, personal appearance).
- *Sociocultural background:* Language, gestures, and attitudes common for a specific group of people relating to family origin, occupation, or lifestyle.
- *Knowledge level:* Level of education and experience influences a person's knowledge base.
- *Roles and relationships:* Conversation between two nurses differs from conversation between the nurse and a patient.
- *Environment:* Noise, lack of privacy, and distractions influence effectiveness.
- *Space and territoriality:* A distance of 18 inches to 4 feet is ideal for sitting with a patient for an interaction. Patients from different cultures often have different needs for personal space.

and nonverbal messages. Barriers to effective communication techniques exist in the form of ineffective responses and behaviors (Box 2.2). Consider your personal safety when interacting with patients who are potentially violent. Patients who are angry and frustrated and believe that no one is listening may be more likely to behave in a violent manner. The illness experience is a stressor, and some patients have trouble coping. Safety principles relevant to the skills in this chapter are as follows:

- Control external factors in both the environmental setting (temperature of room, privacy issues) and psychological setting (emotional state of the nurse and patient) that facilitate or hinder communication.
- Establish and understand the purpose of an interaction.
- Involve family caregivers during patient teaching because family caregivers may be providing support to patients at home.
- Do not be offended by challenging and difficult patients; approach them by being calm, patient, and respectful, and acknowledge their distress.
- When facing a violent patient, try to move the person away from other people to an environment where he or she can feel safe and that is also safe for you. Also, position yourself correctly by standing in a position of safety—usually between the person and the doorway, but not directly in front of the door so that the individual also has an escape route.
- Always express genuine concern and acknowledge a patient's beliefs and fears (Delbanco et al., 2013).

BOX 2.2

Ineffective Responses and Behaviors

- Not listening
- Talking too much
- Using clichés
- Seeming uncomfortable with silence
- Laughing nervously
- Not paying attention
- Showing disapproval
- Avoiding sensitive topics
- Belittling feelings
- Arguing
- Minimizing problems
- Being superficial
- Being defensive
- Changing the subject
- Focusing on personal problems of the nurse
- Having a closed posture
- Making false promises

From Keltner N, et al: *Psychiatric nursing: a psychotherapeutic management approach*, ed 7, St. Louis, 2015, Mosby.

✦ SKILL 2.1 Discharge Planning and Transitional Care

Purpose

Discharge planning is an important part of patient care during hospitalization. The discharge process is complex and can be hazardous to a patient, most likely because of inadequate communication, which can lead to patient errors and other negative outcomes. Developing an agreed-on discharge plan based on the needs and preferences of a patient and family is essential to the discharge process (Graham et al., 2013). During this era of value-based and accountable care, hospitals are focusing on discharge planning to place patients in the most appropriate care setting on the health-care continuum as well as to avoid hospital readmissions. The Joint Commission (TJC) and AHRQ (2013) have developed standards for discharge planning. The standards include patient education; patients and family caregivers must be told how to obtain the services they need. There are also requirements for communicating with the receiving provider (TJC, 2016). Transitional care refers to the actions of the health care team to ensure the coordination and continuity of care as patients move between various health locations and settings, depending on their health status. Elderly patients and patients with a chronic illness are examples of the types of patients who require transitional care. Examples of health care settings include hospitals, nursing homes, long-term care facilities, and patients' homes.

Delegation and Collaboration

The skill of discharge planning cannot be delegated to nursing assistive personnel (NAP). The nurse directs the NAP to:

- Assist in gathering patient belongings when being discharged from the agency.
- Assist patient with any final hygiene needs before actual discharge.

ASSESSMENT

1. Identify patient using at least two identifiers (e.g., name and birthday or name and medical record number) according to agency policy. *Rationale: Complies with The Joint Commission standards and improves patient safety (TJC, 2019).*

TABLE 2.1

Facilitating and Inhibiting Communication

Technique	Examples	Rationale
Initiating and Encouraging Interaction		
Giving information	"It is time for me to ...." "I will be here until ...."	Informs patient of facts needed to understand situation Provides a means to build trust and develop a knowledge base for patients to make decisions
Stating observations	"You're smiling." "I see you're up already."	By calling patient's attention to what is observed, encourages patient to be aware of behavior
Listening	Remain quiet and listen.	Allows you to be attentive to what a patient is saying verbally and nonverbally
Open questions/ comments	"What is your biggest concern?" "Tell me about your health."	Allows patient to choose the topic of discussion according to circumstances and needs
General leads	"And then?" "Go on ...." "Tell me more ...."	Encourages patient to continue talking
Focused questions/ comments	"Tell me about your pain or comfort." "What did your doctor say?" "How has your family reacted?" "What is your biggest fear?"	Encourages patient to give more information about specific topic of concern
Helping Patient Identify and Express Feelings		
Sharing observations	"You look tense." "You seem uncomfortable when ...."	Promotes patient's awareness of nonverbal behavior and feelings underlying behavior; helps clarify meaning of behavior
Paraphrasing	Patient: "I couldn't sleep last night." Nurse: "You've had trouble sleeping?"	Encourages patient to describe the situation more fully; demonstrates that nurse is listening and concerned
Reflecting feelings	"You were angry when that happened?" "You seem upset ...."	Focuses patient on identified feelings based on verbal or nonverbal cues
Focused comments	"That seems worth talking about more." "Tell me more about ...."	Encourages patient to think about and describe a particular concern in more detail
Ensuring Mutual Understanding		
Seeking clarification	"I don't quite follow you ...." "Do you mean ...?" "Are you saying that ...?"	Encourages patient to expand on a topic that is not yet clear or that seems contradictory
Summarizing	"So there are three things that you're upset about: your family being too busy, your diet, and being in the hospital so long."	Reduces the interaction to three or four points identified by nurse as significant; allows patient to agree or add other concerns
Validation	"Did I understand you correctly that ...?" "What made you decide to eat that when you know it gives you stomach pain?"	Allows clarification of ideas that nurse may have interpreted differently than intended by patient
Inhibiting Communication		
"Why" questions	"Why did you go back to bed?"	Asks patient to justify reasons; implies criticism and makes patient feel defensive; better to state what happened and encourage telling the whole story (e.g., "I noticed you went back to bed.")
Sidestepping or changing subject	Patient: "I'm having a hard time with my family." Nurse: "Do you have any grandchildren?"	Eases nurse's own discomfort and avoids exploring topic identified by patient
False reassurance	"Everything will be okay." "Surgery is no big deal."	Vague and simplistic and tends to belittle patient's concerns; does not invite a response
Giving advice	"You really should exercise more." "You shouldn't eat fast food every day."	Keeps patient from actively engaging in finding a solution; often patient knows what should or should not be done and needs to explore alternative ways of dealing with issue
Stereotyped responses	"You have the best doctor in town." "All patients with cancer worry about that."	Does not invite patient to respond
Defensiveness	"The nurses here work very hard." "Your doctor is extremely busy."	Moves focus away from patient's feelings without acknowledging concerns

2. From time of admission, assess patient's discharge needs using nursing history data, including assessments of patient's physical health, functional status, psychosocial support system, financial resources, health values, cultural and ethnic background, level of education, and barriers to care that are needed. *Rationale: Planning for discharge begins at admission and continues throughout patient's stay in an agency. The discharge planning assessment determines patient's continuing care needs after leaving an acute care hospital/post–acute care agency setting.*
3. Review ongoing assessment data during your shift of care, including physical examinations and discussions with patient and health care provider. Be sure that the discharge plan is culturally appropriate (e.g., learn the patient's preferences and values about continuing health care after discharge). *Rationale: A patient-centered discharge plan is likely to be more successful.*
4. Identify risk factors for readmission post discharge: diagnoses associated with high readmissions (e.g., heart failure, chronic lung disease); co-morbidities; the need for numerous medications; a history of readmissions, psychosocial and emotional factors (e.g., problems with mental illness, interpersonal relationships, or family matters); the lack of a family caregiver; older age; financial distress or deficient living environment (e.g., water supply, heating). *Rationale: Knowing risk factors for readmission after discharge (TJC, 2013) allows you to better prioritize interventions that manage these risk factors during patient's hospital stay.*
5. If patient's destination at discharge will be the home, assess patient's and family caregiver's learning needs as soon as possible (e.g., psychomotor skills, ability to manage medications for patient or recognize symptoms). Engage patient and family as partners in the discharge teaching plan by having them identify their concerns about discharge. *Rationale: Improves understanding of patient's health care needs and ability to achieve self-care at home. Inclusion of family caregiver in teaching sessions provides patient with more reliable resource. Engaging patient and family in the assessment supports patient- and family-centered nursing (TJC, 2015a).*
6. Assess for current barriers to learning (e.g., age, fatigue, pain, lack of motivation). Assess patient's health literacy. *Rationale: Determines timing and approach to instruction. Different types of educational materials are effective with different individual learning styles. If printed material is to be used, be sure that material is written at proper reading level.*
7. Ask patient and/or family caregiver to describe the home environment and assess for environmental factors that may interfere with self-care (e.g., size of rooms, doorway clearances for wheelchair, steps, lighting, bathroom facilities). (A home care nurse is usually available on referral to help with assessment; see Chapter 32.) *Rationale: Environmental factors within patient's home pose safety risks or problems for self-care.*
8. Collaborate with interprofessional team to determine patient's anticipated needs after discharge and his or her eligibility for home care reimbursement. Ask these questions: Does patient have an injury or illness that makes it difficult to leave home (e.g., requires the aid of supportive devices such as a wheelchair or walker; require the use of special transportation; need the assistance of a family caregiver)? Does the patient have a "skilled need" that requires skills from a specific health care provider? *Rationale: These conditions are needed for Medicare reimbursement of home health services. Patient must have a "skilled need" that requires the skills of a licensed nurse, speech therapist, or physical therapist to perform. A health care provider's order is also needed.*
9. Assess patient's and family's perceptions of continued health care needs outside the hospital and family caregivers' perceived ability to provide care to patient, including their level of social and community support and their ability to manage multiple medications with which the patient is discharged. *Rationale: Family caregiving is a highly stressful experience. Family members who are not properly prepared for caregiving are frequently overwhelmed by the patient's needs, which can lead to unnecessary hospital readmissions.*

Safe Patient Care *It is often necessary to talk with patient and family separately to learn about true concerns or doubts.*

10. Assess patient's acceptance of health problems and related restrictions. *Rationale: Affects motivation to learn and adhere to health care recommendations.*
11. Assess patient's or family caregiver's knowledge, experience, and health literacy. *Rationale: Ensures patient or family caregiver has the capacity to obtain, communicate, process, and understand basic health information (CDC, 2016).*

STEP	RATIONALE
PLANNING	
1. Expected outcomes following completion of procedure:	
• Patient can demonstrate self-care activities (or family caregiver is able to administer care measures).	Feedback ensures learning.
• Obstacles to patient's mobility and hazards to ambulation in home setting are removed.	Patient is often physically weakened or has physical changes resulting from illness that predispose to injury.
• Patient or family caregiver explains how health care is to continue in home (or other agency), for which problems to observe and what to do, which treatments or medications patient needs, and when to go to next medical appointment.	Increases likelihood of care not being interrupted in home (or other agency) and reduces chances of unplanned readmission to the hospital.

STEP	RATIONALE
IMPLEMENTATION	
1. Preparation before day of discharge:	
a. Partner with patient and family caregiver in identifying ways to prepare physical arrangement of home that will be required to meet patient's needs (see Chapter 32).	Maintains patient's level of independence and ability to retain function within safe environment.
b. Provide patient and family caregiver with information about community health care resources (e.g., medical equipment companies, Meals on Wheels, adult day care). Referrals are usually made while patient is in hospital.	Community resources offer services that patient or family cannot provide.
c. Conduct teaching sessions with patient and family caregiver as soon as possible during hospitalization. Cover these topics: description of what life at home will be like; review of medications and dosing schedules; warning signs of possible health problems; explanation of test results; explanation of how to provide therapies or use home medical equipment; review of restrictions resulting from health alterations; and when to make follow-up appointment (Agency for Healthcare Research and Quality [AHRQ], 2013). Use appropriate materials such as pamphlets, books, or multimedia resources. Refer patient to reliable and current resources on the Internet.	Gives patient opportunities to practice new skills, ask questions, and obtain necessary feedback to ensure learning. A combination of written and verbal information is effective in improving patient satisfaction and knowledge (TJC, 2015a). In some settings, electronic programs are available that allow you to tailor patient-specific media instructions.
d. Communicate patient's and family caregiver's response to teaching and proposed discharge plan to other health care team members.	Facilitates continuity and achievement of an individualized discharge plan.
2. Procedure on day of discharge:	
a. Encourage patient and family caregiver to ask questions or discuss issues related to home care. A final opportunity to demonstrate learned skills is helpful.	Allows for final clarification of information previously discussed. Helps relieve anxiety.
b. Check health care provider's discharge orders for prescriptions, change in treatments, or need for special medical equipment. (Make sure that orders are written as early as possible.) Arrange for delivery and setup of equipment (e.g., hospital bed, oxygen) before patient arrives home.	Only a health care provider can authorize a discharge. Early check of orders permits you to attend to any last-minute treatments or procedures well before discharge.
c. Determine whether patient or family caregiver has arranged for transportation.	Patient's condition at discharge determines method of transport.
d. Provide privacy and assistance as patient dresses and packs all personal belongings. Check closets and drawers for belongings. Obtain copy of list of valuables signed by patient and have security or appropriate administrator deliver valuables to patient.	Prevents loss of personal items. Patient's signature verifies receipt of items and relieves nursing department of liability for losses.
e. Complete medication reconciliation per agency policy. Check discharge medication orders against the medication administration record and home medication list. Provide patient with prescriptions or pharmacy-dispensed medications ordered by health care provider. Offer a final review of information needed to facilitate safe medication self-administration.	Medication reconciliation is the process of creating the most accurate list possible of all medications a patient is taking and comparing that list against the physician's admission, transfer, and/or discharge orders, with the goal of providing correct medications to the patient at all transition points of care (Institute for Healthcare Improvement [IHI], 2017). Decreases risk of medication errors (TJC, 2019). Review provides feedback to determine patient's success in learning about medications
f. Provide information on follow-up appointments to health care provider's office.	Provides patient with contact for questions that arise after discharge. Ensures continuity of care to prevent hospital readmission.
g. Contact agency business office to determine whether patient needs to finalize arrangements for payment of bill. Arrange for patient or family to visit business office. *Option:* Refer patient to case manager.	Source of concern for many patients is whether agency has accepted insurance or other payment forms.

STEP	RATIONALE
h. Have NAP acquire utility cart to move patient's belongings. Obtain wheelchair for patient. Transport patients leaving by ambulance on ambulance stretchers.	Provides for safe transport.
i. Help patient to wheelchair or stretcher using safe patient handling and transfer techniques (see Chapter 17). Escort patient to entrance of agency where source of transportation is waiting (see agency policy). Lock wheelchair wheels. Help patient transfer into transport vehicle (see illustration). Help place personal belongings in vehicle.	Prevents injury to nurse and patient. Agency policy requires escort to ensure patient's safe exit. Agency's liability ends once patient is safely in vehicle.

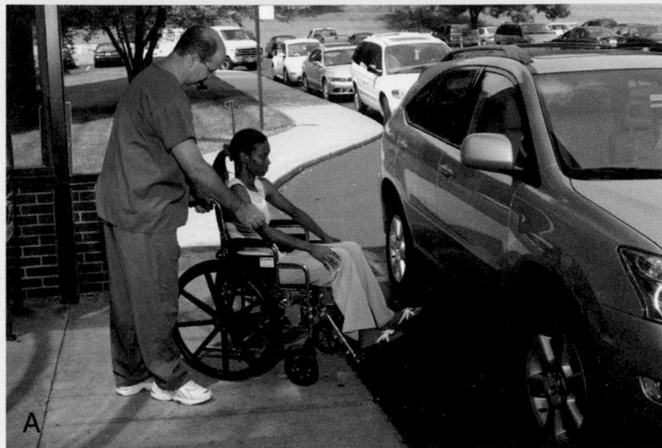

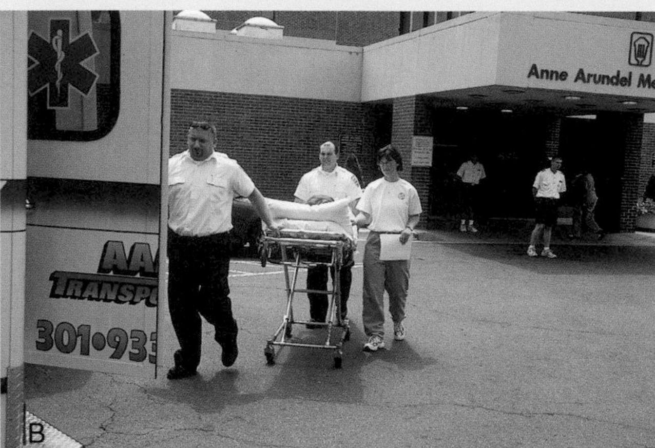

STEP 2i (A) Nurse escorts patient to transport vehicle at time of discharge via a wheelchair. (B) Many patients are discharged via stretcher.

STEP	RATIONALE
j. Return to division. Notify admitting or appropriate department of time of discharge. Notify housekeeping of need to clean patient's room.	Allows agency to prepare for admission of next patient.

EVALUATION

1. Ask patient or family caregiver to describe nature of illness, treatment and medication regimens, and physical signs or symptoms to be reported to a health care provider.	Measures patient's or family caregiver's learning.
2. Have patient or family caregiver perform any treatments that will continue in the home.	Return demonstrations allow you to evaluate level of learning.
3. Home care nurse inspects home, identifies obstacles that pose risks for patient, and recommends revisions.	Provides continuity of care.
4. **Use Teach-Back:** "I want to be sure you understand when your follow-up appointment is. Can you tell me when you are coming back to the clinic?" Revise your instruction now or develop a plan for revised patient/family caregiver teaching if patient/family caregiver is not able to teach back correctly.	Determines patient's/family caregiver's level of understanding of instructional topic.

Unexpected Outcomes	Related Interventions
1. Patient or family caregiver is unable to explain or demonstrate self-care measures.	• Provide immediate clarification or additional instruction. • Plan additional time to demonstrate treatment measures. • Ask patient to explain which aspect of procedure is difficult to perform and why. • If patient or family caregiver continues to be unable to correctly demonstrate treatment measures, request referral for home care services.
2. Environmental risks are still present in home.	• Reassess reason for changes not being implemented. • Home care nurse will problem solve and seek appropriate solution.
3. Patient or family caregiver resists discharge plans and refuses assimilation of new roles needed for home care.	• Contact additional resources (e.g., social worker, home care, pastoral care).

Recording

- Record strategies used and topics covered during discharge teaching with the patient.
- Report verbal and nonverbal responses by the patient and family caregiver.
- Document your evaluation of patient learning.

Hand-Off Reporting

- Use a standardized process/structured format to relay information to ensure coordinated, safe, quality patient care as the patient moves between locations or experiences a change in level of care (written, verbal hand-off).
- Provide clear, effective communication between the health care team members; minimize noise, other distractions, and interruptions.
- Include relevant patient information related to discharge or transitional care (medications, procedures, devices required).
- Provide time for the receiver to clarify information and read back relevant points to ensure patient safety.
- Discuss the use of patient summaries in clinical decision making to ensure patient ownership; patient summaries, both in written and spoken formats, should include a summary statement, events leading to admission, hospital course, and ongoing assessment plan (Lane-Fall et al., 2014).

✦ SKILL 2.2 Workplace Violence and Safety

Purpose

Workplace violence targeting health care workers is a widely recognized problem. Examples of workplace violence include direct physical assaults (with or without weapons), written or verbal threats, physical or verbal harassment, and homicide (Occupational Safety and Health Administration [OSHA], 2015). The American Organization of Nurse Executives and the Emergency Nurses Association support a zero-tolerance workplace violence policy that sends a clear message to everyone working in a hospital that all threats or incidents of violence will be taken seriously (AONE and ENA, n.d.). Exposure to violence negatively impacts the emotional and physical health of all members of the health care team. Consequently, it is imperative that workplace violence prevention programs be implemented to ensure a safe working environment. A workplace violence hazard assessment must be conducted to assess risk factors prior to implementing de-escalation techniques. De-escalation is the ability to organize one's thinking and calmly respond to a threatening situation that helps one avoid a potential crisis (Crisis Prevention Institute [CPI], 2017; Moore et al, 2018). Services should be implemented to investigate any violent incident as well as to provide debriefing for health care staff involved in an incident.

Delegation and Collaboration

The skill of workplace safety can be delegated to nursing assistive personnel (NAP). The nurse assists the NAP by:

- Directing the NAP to assess for potential hazards and risk factors for patient violence
- Confirming understanding of de-escalation techniques

ASSESSMENT

1. Assess baseline knowledge of hospital staff regarding workplace violence. *Rationale: It is imperative that staff are aware of the agency's emergency management plan to maintain a safe environment for patients, family caregivers, and health care staff.*
2. Identify organizational risk factors for workplace violence. *Rationale: Identifies factors in a work setting that if not addressed makes health care staff unequipped to manage violent situation.*
   - Lack of agency policies and staff training for recognizing and managing escalating hostile and assaultive behaviors from patients, clients, visitors, or staff
   - Working when understaffed—especially during mealtimes and visiting hours
   - High worker turnover
   - Inadequate security and mental health personnel (OSHA, 2015)
3. Identify patient- and setting-related risk factors for workplace violence: patients who are experiencing pain, showing mood-altering behaviors, or impaired due to ethyl alcohol (ETOH)/drugs. High-risk settings include the emergency department, psychiatric units, and geriatric long-term care facilities (OSHA, 2015). *Rationale: Identifies factors within a work setting that increase risk of health care workers being exposed to violent behavior.*
4. Assess patient for signs and symptoms of potentially violent behavior: recent stressors or losses (e.g., job loss, divorce); history of confirmed psychiatric disorder; history of drug or ETOH abuse or aggression; content of speech and tone of voice indicating agitated state (loud voice, angry tone); escalating verbal and nonverbal behaviors, including cursing or name-calling, pacing, and clenched fists. *Rationale: All are risk factors for violence.*

STEP	RATIONALE
PLANNING	
1. Expected outcomes following completion of procedure:	
• Staff are educated on violence prevention and de-escalation strategies.	De-escalation training raises the overall safety and health knowledge across the workforce and provides employees with the tools needed to identify workplace safety and security hazards.

STEP	RATIONALE
• Potentially violent patient situations are avoided and/or minimized.	Participation in workplace violence prevention programs helps nurses to address potential problems before they arise and ultimately reduces the likelihood of workers being assaulted (Sinnott et al., 2014).
• Incident reporting and debriefing occurs when indicated.	Established policies ensure the reporting, recording, and monitoring of incidents and near misses to help identify the root cause and help prevent future incidents of violence (OSHA, 2015).

IMPLEMENTATION

STEP	RATIONALE
1. Use notification system for identifying high-risk patients: label or color-code medical records; supply potentially violent patients with different colored socks.	Indicates to health care team patients most likely to commit a violent act. Acknowledges the value of a safe, healthful, violence-free workplace.
2. Remove opportunity for any type of weapon to be used by patients or visitors (fists, teeth, bodily fluids, medical supplies, meal tray, furniture). Be aware of personal space with patient who may try to bite, hit with fists, or throw bodily fluids. Observe body stance (clenched fists, feces in hands).	Managing threats of violence involves recognizing potential weapons and taking a proactive approach to minimizing use of those items (HCPRO, 2015). Removing the potential risk and stimulus can eliminate and block the opportunity to act.
3. Do not work alone if feeling uncomfortable with a patient. Use measures to prevent or control workplace hazards.	Use of physical barriers (guards, door locks), metal detectors, panic buttons, better lighting, and accessible exits can reduce employee exposure.
4. Make sure all staff are trained to cope with physical and verbal abuse using the following de-escalation techniques (CPI, 2016; Moore et al., 2018):	Victims of hospital violence are most often untrained or newly hired nurses, so prepare by training them with proven strategies for safely defusing anxious, hostile, or violent behavior at the earliest possible stage. This includes teaching them to look for warning signs, ask for help if they feel unsafe, and report any violent or suspicious behavior to a supervisor.
a. Be empathetic and nonjudgmental.	When someone says or does something you perceive as weird or irrational, try not to judge or discount his or her feelings. Whether you think those feelings are justified, they are real to the other person. Pay attention to them (CPI, 2016).
b. Respect personal space.	If possible, stand 1.5 to 3 feet away from a person who is escalating. Allowing personal space tends to decrease a person's anxiety and can help you prevent acting-out behavior (CPI, 2016; Moore et al., 2018).
c. Use nonthreatening nonverbal behaviors.	The more a person loses control, the less he or she hears your words—and the more the person reacts to your nonverbal communication. Be mindful of your gestures, facial expressions, movements, and tone of voice (CPI, 2016).
d. Avoid overreacting. Remain calm, rational, and professional.	While you cannot control the person's behavior, how you respond to that behavior will have a direct effect on whether the situation escalates or defuses (CPI, 2016; Moore et al., 2018).
e. Focus on feelings.	Facts are important, but how a person feels is the heart of the matter. Yet some people have trouble identifying how they feel about what is happening to them (CPI, 2016).
f. Ignore challenging questions.	Answering challenging questions often results in a power struggle. When a person challenges your authority, redirect his or her attention to the issue at hand (CPI, 2016).
g. Set limits.	If a person's behavior is belligerent, defensive, or disruptive, give him or her clear, simple, and enforceable limits. Offer concise and respectful choices and consequences (CPI, 2016).

STEP	RATIONALE
h. Choose wisely what you insist upon.	It is important to be thoughtful in deciding which rules are negotiable and which are not. For example, if a person doesn't want to shower in the morning, try to allow him or her to choose the time of day that feels best (CPI, 2016).
i. Allow silence for reflection.	Although it may seem counterintuitive to let moments of silence occur, sometimes it is the best choice. It can give a person a chance to reflect on what is happening and how he or she needs to proceed (CPI, 2016).
j. Allow time for decisions.	When a person is upset, he or she may not be able to think clearly. Give him or her a few moments to think through what you have said (CPI, 2016).
k. Use concise, simple language	Elaborate and technical terms are difficult for an impaired person to understand (Moore et al., 2018).
5. Notify security staff to intervene if patient begins unruly behavior or if additional information is needed to determine potential for violence.	If a patient begins to exhibit unruly behavior, you may request a security consultation to determine whether the patient poses a threat. If officers identify danger, a patient will undergo a safety assessment including a detailed search of personal effects for any weapons or dangerous items.
6. If an incident occurs, initial steps are first aid and emergency care for the injured workers and prevention of further injury.	Following a violent incident, first determine the extent of injuries and establish priorities of treatment.
7. Debrief using standard post-incident procedures and services. The purpose of an investigation should be to identify the "root cause" of the incident.	Root causes refer to all possible causes associated with the incident of violence. If the root cause is not addressed and/or corrected, it will inevitably re-create the conditions for another incident to occur (OSHA, 2015).
8. Implement comprehensive program of medical and psychological counseling and debriefing for staff who have experienced and witnessed assaults/violent incidents.	A strong follow-up program for these workers will not only help them address these problems but also help prepare them to confront or prevent future incidents of violence (OSHA, 2015).

EVALUATION

1. Evaluate staff comprehension of workplace violence program and de-escalation strategies.	Ensures staff preparation for any violent events. Require annual certification for all staff in safety training.
2. Monitor prevention impact. Evaluate prevalence of such incidents on a regular basis.	Data determine need to revise training or to assist select individuals with prevention techniques.
3. If there is a violent incident, evaluate safety of all persons involved. Provide prompt medical treatment for victims of workplace violence.	Worker well-being is critical to maintain safety and stability of work environment.
4. If there is an incident, immediately evaluate the effectiveness of the de-escalation techniques implemented. Victims of an assault, as well as their co-workers, need the opportunity to discuss their concerns and feelings about the event.	A critical incident debriefing suggests ways to prevent similar incidents in the future. Critical incidents can cause emotional reactions that affect health care workers' ability to function.
5. **Use Teach-Back:** "Tell me about the use of de-escalation techniques (from a patient/family caregiver and staff perspective) used to prevent an incident of workplace violence. How effective were they?" Revise your instruction now or develop a plan for revised patient/family caregiver and staff teaching if patient/family caregiver and staff are not able to teach back correctly.	Determines health care staff's as well as patient's/family caregiver's level of understanding of instructional topic.

Unexpected Outcomes	Related Interventions
1. There is a violent incident between patient and nursing staff.	• Notify the agency's multidisciplinary response team. • Provide immediate treatment to persons injured. • Report the presence of a weapon immediately to a manager, a supervisor, or security (ANOE and ENA, n.d.). • Implement post-incident procedures (root cause analysis and follow-up debriefing for staff).
2. De-escalation techniques are ineffective.	• Further workplace violence prevention training is necessary for staff.

Recording

- Record staff attendance at workplace violence prevention programs.
- Record hazard assessment and strategies used to promote a safe environment.
- Record escalating behaviors exhibited by patient.
- Record any injuries and treatments offered.
- Record root cause analysis of violent incident.
- Record follow-up program services offered.

Hand-Off Reporting

- Provide detailed assessment of potentially hazardous situation.
- Report patients who are flagged as high risk for potentially violent behaviors.
- Report strategies implemented to prevent escalating behaviors.
- Report any violent incidents and outcomes associated with the incidents.

PROCEDURAL GUIDELINE 2.1 *Hand-Off Communication*

Purpose

In addition to written documentation, a nurse provides a change-of-shift report to the next nurse who assumes responsibility for patient care. The purpose of the report is to provide continuity of care for a specific patient. A hand-off report is more than a list of tasks the next nurse must assume. Instead it is the story of what occurred to a patient during a shift that is essential to convey so that the receiving nurse has a full picture of a patient's situation and can anticipate care needs (Birmingham et al., 2015). Inaccurate or incomplete shift reports contribute to sentinel events. Potential for patient harm from minor to severe exists when a receiver gets information that is inaccurate, incomplete, not timely, misinterpreted, or otherwise not what is needed (TJC, 2017). Whether a nurse conveys or receives incomplete or inaccurate information is affected by time constraints, distractions, noise, and interpersonal tensions (Carroll et al., 2012; Birmingham et al., 2015). Nurses give hand-off reports face-to-face, through a written report or the electronic health record (EHR), or during walking rounds at each patient's bedside. It is important to have some type of guidelines for reporting to avoid repetitive, irrelevant, and speculative communication (Eberhardt, 2014; Foster-Hunt et al., 2015). Regardless of the form of the hand-off report, always maintain a patient's confidentiality.

Delegation and Collaboration

The skill of giving a hand-off report cannot be delegated to nursing assistive personnel (NAP). Licensed practical nurses (LPNs) may report on patients for whom they care directly. The nurse directs the NAP to:

- Report to the nurse clinical or behavioral changes (e.g., increased pain, changes in vital signs, restlessness) so that there can be assessment, validation, and reporting of any changes later in the hand-off report.

Equipment

Electronic or printed worksheets; patient care summary or nursing Kardex; plan of care, critical pathway, or interprofessional treatment plan

Procedural Steps

1. Identify patient using at least two identifiers (e.g., name and birthday or name and medical record number) according to agency policy (TJC, 2019).
2. Gather information from your most recent patient assessments and interactions, documentation sources, NAP report, or other relevant documents. Cue into critical details of the patient's story during the shift of care to ensure a relevant and timely report.

Safe Patient Care *Report only relevant information to next shift to ensure staff's timely responsiveness.*

3. Prioritize information to report based on the patient's needs and problems.
4. Reduce distractions: Close room doors when entering patient room, notify other staff you are conducting a hand-off report, and reduce any extraneous noise in or around room if possible.
5. Use an organized format such as a mnemonic, checklist, or template for delivering the report that provides a comprehensive description of patient needs and problems. Options include SBAR (Situation, Background, Assessment, Recommendation [see Procedural Guideline 2.2]; Cornell et al., 2014) and the I-PASS mnemonic (AHRQ, 2017). I-PASS stands for the following:
   - **I**llness severity: one-word summary of patient acuity ("stable," "watcher," or "unstable")
   - **P**atient summary: brief summary of the patient's diagnoses and treatment plan
   - **A**ction list: to-do items to be completed by the clinician receiving patient
   - **S**ituation awareness and contingency plans: directions to follow in case of changes in the patient's status, often in an "if, then" format
   - **S**ynthesis by receiver: an opportunity for the receiver to ask questions and confirm the plan of care
6. Critical information to include in any format or mnemonic includes the following: patient's history, current status, and relevant demographic and diagnostic information; critical details regarding most recent shift of care; interventions, follow-up, and plan of care (Blaz and Staggers, 2012; Birmingham et al., 2015).
7. Ask the staff member who is assuming patient's care from oncoming shift if he or she has any questions regarding information provided.
8. Oncoming nurse then sees patient to conduct an assessment and make a connection with information reported. Cues into critical details to identify any signs of clinical worsening (Birmingham et al., 2015).

PROCEDURAL GUIDELINE 2.2 *SBAR Communication*

Purpose

In health care settings, communicating is a key part of everyday practice. The quality of these interactions is a key component of error prevention; clarity, comprehension, and adherence to treatment plans; and positive patient outcomes. TJC publishes National Patient Safety Goals, one of which is to "improve the effectiveness of communication among caregivers" (TJC, 2019).

Standardized communication using the SBAR (Situation-Background-Assessment-Recommendation) format is structured to optimize effective communication among all members of the health care team in any situation, such as patient injury or complaint, change of shift, change in patient clinical status, or patient transfer to different care unit. SBAR can be used nurse to nurse, physician to nurse, nurse to technician, administrator to physician, social worker to nurse, and so forth. Using SBAR, nurses are better prepared to outline the most important points in a situation and thus better collaborate successfully with professional colleagues. Improved communication using structured communication techniques with the SBAR framework streamlines information exchanges and promotes patient safety (Boykins, 2014; Panesar et al., 2016; Titzer et al., 2015).

Delegation and Collaboration

The skill of communicating using the SBAR format can be delegated to nursing assistive personnel (NAP) who become involved in clinical incidents. The nurse instructs the NAP about:

- The proper communication skills needed to effectively interact verbally and nonverbally with colleagues

Equipment

Electronic or printed worksheets; patient care summary or nursing Kardex; plan of care, critical pathway, or interprofessional treatment plan

Procedural Steps

1. Identify purpose of interaction with colleague (e.g., reporting lab test results, status of intravenous [IV] treatments, fall incident, change in patient's clinical condition).
2. Assess factors influencing communication with others (e.g., environment, timing, presence of others' cultural beliefs and values, prior experiences).
3. Be aware of your nonverbal cues that affect communication with others. Remain nonjudgmental.
4. Prepare environment physically; go to a quiet, calm area. Reduce distractions such as external noises.
5. Be aware of hierarchical differences among members of the health care team as a common barrier to effective communication and collaboration.
6. Provide brief, simple introduction; introduce yourself and explain purpose of interaction.
7. Be aware of your own body language and tone. Assume an open stance; do not fold arms across your chest. Maintain eye contact.
8. Use oral communication skills such as the following: ask open-ended questions; do not assume; do not interrupt; do not blame others. Provide feedback. Use active listening and recognize nonverbal triggers. Ask for clarification when necessary.
9. Use a range of workplace written communication methods, such as the SBAR method, to provide relevant patient information to colleagues.
10. For each patient, include the following (example reviews details in a hand-off report):
    S—Situation: Patient's name, gender, age, chief complaint on admission, and current situation
    B—Background information: Allergies, emergency code status (i.e., do not resuscitate [DNR]), medical and surgical histories, special needs as related to any physical challenges (e.g., blind, hearing deficit, amputee), and vaccinations
    A—Assessment data: Objective observations and measurements that pertain to the current situation; emphasis on any recent changes. Include any relevant information reported by patient, family caregiver, or health care team members, such as laboratory data and diagnostic test results. Include therapies or treatments administered during shift and expected outcomes (e.g., medication changes, use of oxygen, referral visits). Describe education given in the teaching plan and patient's/family caregiver's ability to demonstrate learning. Report on evaluation by explaining patient's response and whether outcomes are met.
    R—Recommend: Explanation of the priorities to which receiving nurse must attend, including referrals, nursing orders, and core measures.
11. Review patient's progress toward discharge during each change-of-shift report.

SPECIAL CONSIDERATIONS

Patient-Centered Care

High-quality communication between the nurse, patient, and family facilitates patient-centered care. It is important to recognize cultural diversity and demonstrate respect for people as unique individuals. Culture is just one factor that influences communication between two people. Awareness of cultural norms or values enhances understanding of nonverbal cues. Be aware of your own cultural values and expectations and how they may "filter" or direct your care. Consider any potential communication barriers with people from other cultures, including cultural perspective, heritage, and health traditions of both you and the patient. Know yourself—one's personality, values, beliefs, and ethics—when caring for patients who are different from oneself (Purnell, 2013). Guidelines include the following:

- *Use of language, gestures, and vocal emphasis of words:* Taking care to determine if understanding was achieved is important. Avoid overly technical jargon or terms unique to a culture (Box 2.3). If the patient is not English speaking, have a professional interpreter present or available (Giger, 2016).
- *Eye contact:* Direct eye contact is valued in some cultures, whereas other cultures find it improper and intrusive (e.g., it may be improper to make eye contact with an authority figure).

BOX 2.3

Special Approaches for a Patient Who Speaks a Different Language

- Use a caring tone of voice and facial expression to help alleviate the patient's fears.
- Speak slowly and distinctly but not loudly.
- Use gestures, pictures, and role playing to help the patient understand.
- Repeat the message in different ways if necessary.
- Be alert to words the patient seems to understand, and use them frequently.
- Keep messages simple and repeat them frequently.
- Avoid using medical terms that the patient may not understand.
- Use an appropriate language dictionary, or have a medical interpreter make flash cards to communicate key phrases.

Modified from Giger J: *Transcultural nursing: assessment and intervention*, ed 7, St. Louis, 2016, Mosby.

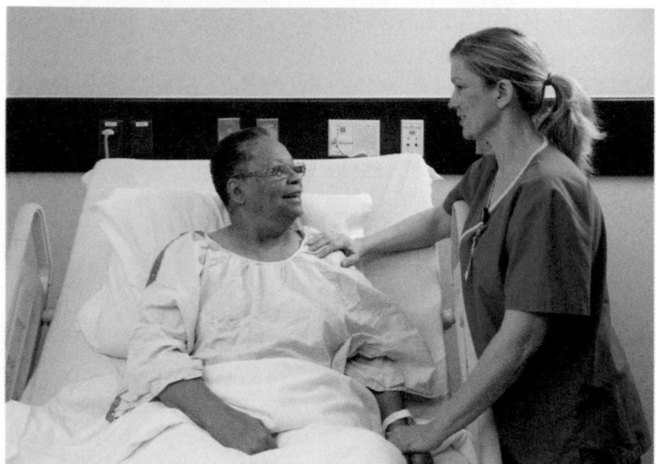

FIG 2.2 Therapeutic use of touch needs to take cultural factors into consideration.

- *Use of touch and personal space:* Some cultures are "noncontact" cultures and have needs for clear boundaries; other cultures value close contact, handshakes, and embracing (Fig. 2.2).
- *Time orientation:* Many cultures are oriented to the present; some cultures value planning for the future.
- *Nonverbal behaviors:* Use gestures with shared meaning.

Patient Education

- Consider health literacy, the degree to which persons have the capacity to understand basic health information and services needed to make appropriate decisions about their health, when planning and implementing patient education.
- Consider patients' access to the Internet; recommend sites that are reliable for patients and family members to access health information and health self-management tools (Boykins, 2014).

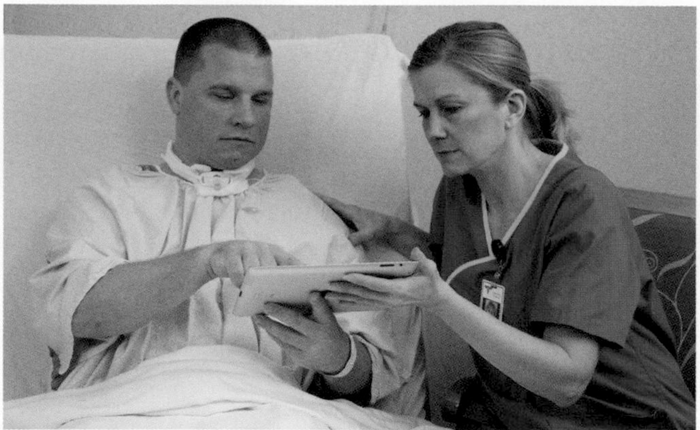

FIG 2.3 Communication tools are available for patients who cannot speak because of a tracheostomy.

Age-Specific

Pediatric

- Use vocabulary that is familiar to the child based on child's level of understanding and usual patterns of communication.
- Consider the child's developmental level when interacting with the child.
- Include parents or guardians in the discharge or transfer-of-care process.

Gerontological

- Be aware of any cognitive or sensory impairment that may affect patient's understanding and ability to convey clear messages.
- Speak face-to-face with the patient with hearing impairment, articulate clearly in a moderate tone of voice, and assess whether the patient hears and understands the words.
- Ensure that patients with visual impairments have any necessary assistive devices, such as eyeglasses and large-print reading material.
- Encourage patients with auditory, physical, or visual impairments to use assistive devices to aid in communication, for example: pad and felt-tipped pen or magic slate; communication board with words, letters, or pictures denoting basic needs (e.g., water, bedpan, pain medication); sign language; use of eye blinks or movement of fingers for simple responses (e.g., "yes" or "no"); flash cards that contain pictures rather than words; computer or electronic devices.

Home Care

- Identify a primary caregiver for the patient. This individual may be a family member, friend, or neighbor.
- Assess the level of understanding of patient and primary caregiver regarding the patient's condition and impact on self-care.
- Incorporate the patient's usual daily habits and routines into the communication event (e.g., bathing and dressing patient).
- Assess for the presence of any cognitive or physical impairments that may hinder communication (Fig. 2.3).

✦ PRACTICE REFLECTIONS

You are assigned to care for a patient who was transferred from a nursing home. The patient arrived at your agency alone via ambulance without any collateral information about the patient's baseline behavior. This patient has both auditory and visual impairments, which makes communication difficult. In addition, the change in environment has caused the patient to experience increased agitation.

1. What are some of the communication challenges you face with this patient?
2. What strategies can you use to communicate effectively with this patient?
3. What communication techniques can you use to reduce the patient's agitation?

✦ CLINICAL REVIEW QUESTIONS

1. A nurse working in a long-term care facility is reviewing the status of patients on her assigned unit. Patients most likely to be at risk for displaying violence toward nursing staff include which of the following? (Select all that apply.)
   1. 72-year-old patient admitted to facility in the past 48 hours
   2. 81-year-old patient who is transferred back to long-term care after being hospitalized for 4 days
   3. 75-year-old patient who has cancer pain and is receiving minimal relief from ordered analgesics
   4. 90-year-old patient with progressive dementia
   5. 69-year-old patient admitted with advanced Parkinson's disease
2. The nurse in the mental health unit reviews therapeutic and nontherapeutic communication techniques with a nursing student. Which of the following are therapeutic communication techniques? (Select all that apply.)
   1. Paraphrasing
   2. Listening
   3. Asking the patient "Why?"
   4. Summarizing a discussion
   5. Giving advice
   6. Reflecting patient's feelings
3. The nurse in the intensive care unit (ICU) is planning to discharge a patient who is going to be transferred to a skilled nursing facility for further care after suffering a stroke. What are the steps during the assessment phase of the discharge planning process? (Select all that apply.)
   1. Identify risk factors that may increase the chances of being readmitted after discharge.
   2. Assess current barriers to learning.
   3. Ask patient and family caregiver to describe the home environment.
   4. Assess the need for supportive devices related to mobility.
   5. Assess family's willingness to participate in home care regimen.

Answers and Rationales for Clinical Review Questions can be found on the Evolve website.

REFERENCES

Agency for Healthcare Research and Quality (AHRQ): Strategy 4: Care transitions from hospital to home: IDEAL discharge planning, 2013. http://www.ahrq.gov/professionals/systems/hospital/engagingfamilies/strategy4/index.html.

Agency for Healthcare Research and Quality (AHRQ): Patient Safety Network: handoffs and signouts, 2017. https://psnet.ahrq.gov/primers/primer/9/handoffs-and-signouts.

American Organization of Nurse Executives (AONE), Emergency Nurses Association (ENA): Toolkit for mitigating violence in the workplace, n.d. http://www.aone.org/resources/final_toolkit.pdf.

Birmingham P, et al: Handoffs and patient safety: grasping the story and painting a full picture, *West J Nurs Res* 37(11):1458–1478, 2015.

Blaz JW, Staggers N: The format of standard tools for nursing handoff: an integrative review, *Nurs Inform* 2012:023, 2012.

Boykins A: Core communication competencies in patient-centered care, *ABNF J* 25(2):40, 2014.

Carroll JS, et al: The ins and outs of change of shift handoffs between nurses: a communication challenge, *BMJ Qual Saf* 21:586–593, 2012.

Centers for Disease Control and Prevention (CDC): What is health literacy, 2016. https://www.cdc.gov/healthliteracy/learn/index.html.

Copeland D, et al: Workplace violence and perceptions of safety among emergency department staff members: experiences, expectations, tolerance, reporting, and recommendations, *J Traum Nurs* 24(2):65–77, 2017.

Cornell P, et al: Impact of SBAR on nurse shift reports and staff rounding, *Medsug Nurs* 23(5):335–341, 2014.

Crisis Prevention Institute (CPI): CPI's top 10 de-escalation tips, 2016. https://www.crisisprevention.com/CPI/media/Media/download/PDF_DT.pdf.

Crisis Prevention Institute (CPI): De-escalation techniques, 2017. https://www.crisisprevention.com/Blog/June-2011/De-escalation-Techniques.

Delbanco T, et al: A patient-centered view of the clinician-patient relationship, UpToDate, 2013. http://www.uptodate.com/contents/a-patient-centered-view-of-the-clinician-patient-relationship.

Eberhardt S: Improve handoff communication with SBAR, *Nursing* 2014:17–19, 2014.

Foster-Hunt T, et al: Information structure and organisation in change of shift reports: an observational study of nursing hand-offs in a paediatric intensive care unit, *Intensive Crit Care Nurs* 31(3):156, 2015.

Giger J: *Transcultural Nursing: Assessment & Intervention*, ed 7, St. Louis, 2016, Mosby.

Graham J, et al: Nurses' discharge planning and risk assessment: behaviours, understanding and barriers, *J Clin Nurs* 22(15–16):2338, 2013.

HCPRO: Preventing workplace violence: handbook for health care workers, March 2015. http://hcmarketplace,com/preventing-workplace-violence-handbook-for-health-care-workers.

Institute for Healthcare Improvement: Medication reconciliation to prevent adverse drug events, 2017. http://www.ihi.org/Topics/ADEsMedicationReconciliation/Pages/default.aspx.

Lane-Fall M, et al: Addressing the mandate for hand-off education: a focused review and recommendations for anesthesia resident curriculum development and education, *Anesthes* 120(1):218–229, 2014.

Moore G, et al: Assessment and emergency management of the acutely agitated and violent adult, UpToDate, 2018. https://www.uptodate.com/contents/assessment-and-emergency-management-of-the-acutely-agitated-or-violent-adult.

Occupational Safety and Health Administration (OSHA): Guidelines for preventing workplace violence for healthcare and social service workers. U.S. Department of Labor Occupational Safety and Health Administration, 2015. https://www.osha.gov/Publications/osha3148.pdf.

Panesar R: The effect of an electronic SBAR communication tool on documentation of acute events in the pediatric intensive care unit, *Am J Med Qual* 31(1):64–68, 2016.

Purnell L: *Transcultural health care: a culturally competent approach*, ed 4, Philadelphia, 2013, FA Davis.

Sinnott M, et al: Introducing the safety score audit for staff member and patient safety, *J AORN* 100:91–95, 2014.

Speroni K, et al: Incidence and cost of nurse workplace violence perpetrated by hospital patients or patient visitors, *J Emerg Nurs* 4(40):218–228, 2014.

The Joint Commission (TJC): The need for collaboration across entire care continuum. In Hot Topics in Healthcare: Issue number 2, Transitions of care: the need for collaboration, 2013. http://www.jointcommission.org/assets/1/6/toc_hot_topics.pdf.

The Joint Commission (TJC): Transitions of care: engaging patients and families, 2015a. http://www.jointcommission.org/assets/1/23/Quick_Safety_Issue_18_November_20151.PDF.

The Joint Commission (TJC): Sentinel event data—root causes by event type 2004-2014, 2015b. http://www.tsigconsulting.com/tolcam/wp-content/uploads/2015/04/TJC-Sentinel-Event-Root_Causes_by_Event_Type_2004-2014.pdf.

The Joint Commission (TJC): Transitions of care portal, 2016. https://www.jointcommission.org/toc.aspx.

The Joint Commission (TJC): Sentinel event: inadequate hand-off communication, 2017. https://www.jointcommission.org/assets/1/18/SEA_58_Hand_off_Comms_9_6_17_FINAL_(1).pdf.

The Joint Commission (TJC): *2019 National Patient Safety Goals*, Oakbrook Terrace, IL, 2019, The Commission. http://www.jointcommission.org/standards_information/npsgs.aspx.

Titzer J, et al: Interprofessional education: lessons learned from conducting an electronic health record assignment, *J Interprof Car* 29(6):536–540, 2015.

3 Documentation and Informatics

SKILLS AND PROCEDURES

EVOLVE WEBSITE/RESOURCES LIST

http://evolve.elsevier.com/Perry/nursinginterventions
Audio Glossary • Case Studies • Checklists • Clinical Review Questions • Answers and Rationales for Clinical Review Questions

INTRODUCTION

Health care documentation is anything entered in written or electronic format into a patient's medical record. Documentation is an essential component of health care delivery because when it is done correctly and appropriately, it is a form of communication that ensures better continuity of care to patients, increases interaction among care providers, and improves patient safety (Charalambous and Goldberg, 2016). Electronic documentation is the desired standard because it integrates all relevant patient information in real time (HealthIT.gov, 2014; Hoover, 2016). Informatics refers to the property and structure of information or data. It is important that nurses know how to record and report data and apply the information for patient care. Nursing informatics is a specialty that integrates nursing science, computer science, and information science to manage and communicate data, information, and knowledge in nursing practice (American Nurses Association [ANA], 2014; Healthcare Information and Management Systems Society, 2017).

PRACTICE STANDARDS

- American Nurses Association (ANA), 2014: Nursing informatics scope and standards of practice—Standards of practice for nursing informatics
- The Joint Commission (TJC), 2017: 2017 comprehensive accreditation manual for hospitals: the offical handbook—Patient identification

ELECTRONIC HEALTH RECORD

The traditional paper medical record is episode oriented, with a separate record for each patient visit to a health care agency. Key information, such as patient allergies, current medications, and complications from treatment, may be lost from one episode of care to the next. The electronic health record (EHR) is a longitudinal electronic record of patient health information generated by one or more encounters in any care delivery setting (Chung and Cho, 2017). It automates and streamlines the care provider's workflow in real time. The EHR can generate a complete record of a clinical patient encounter and use that information to support other care-related activities, including evidence-based decision support, quality management, and outcomes reporting. For example, if a patient develops hypoglycemia, the blood sugar level entered into the EHR may trigger an automatic alert that informs nurses of the need to follow a treatment protocol. Electronic forms and flow sheets are designed by nursing and other health care providers. Professional nursing standards, regulatory requirements, and evidence-based practice are incorporated into the content of many forms. Designing forms that collect pertinent information aims to improve communication among health care providers and ultimately safer patient care.

You must obtain patient consent before information in the EHR is transferred or shared with another agency. Use precautions to protect the patient's information. Facilities have developed guidelines and policies to ensure the privacy and confidentiality of the information consistent with federal and state regulations such as the Health Insurance Portability and Accountability Act of 1996 (HIPAA, 1999). Patients can access their EHRs through patient portals that permit access, printing, and sending of one's own health record (Hoover, 2016).

EVIDENCE-BASED PRACTICE

Rapid Response Team

A rapid response team (RRT) is a group of clinical experts that quickly responds to a deterioration in a patient's status on a patient care unit. The purpose of an RRT is to provide early intervention to prevent a patient transfer to a higher level of care, such as an intensive care unit or a cardiac arrest. The nurse at the bedside must recognize early warning signs of clinical deterioration, such as a change in vital signs, to activate an RRT. EHRs can assist the nurse with identifying warning signs; considerations include the following:

- Clinical changes are sometimes subtle, and they often go unrecognized. EHRs can alert nurses about early warning signs of patient deterioration (Heal et al., 2017; Kang et al., 2016).
- By predetermining early warning values, the EHR notifies the nurse of a clinical change that may meet the criteria to

activate an RRT. Computer screen pop-ups and dashboards are examples of EHR alerts.

- Data such as the patient's vital signs can be used to populate an early warning sign system in an EHR (Heal et al., 2017).
- Data must be entered into EHRs at the time of data collection to capture early warning data in real time (Heal et al., 2017).
- Continuity of nurse assignments also provide support toward a nurse's recognition of clinical deterioration (Hart et al., 2016).
- Patient outcomes can be improved when an electronic early warning system is part of an EHR (Heal et al., 2017; Kang et al., 2016).

SAFETY GUIDELINES

A patient's medical record is a legal document that reflects all aspects of the patient's care while in a health care setting. As a result, there are standards that all health care agencies integrate into a documentation system to ensure that the care delivered represents safe practices. Considerations include the following:

- Standard documentation categories include allergy entries, fall risk information, intravenous (IV) fluid rates, and identifying information.
- Information entered into the medical record must be accurate, thorough, and current because all care providers rely on the information to deliver and coordinate patient care.
- Inaccurate or incomplete documentation or falsification of information can result in medical or nursing therapies that are unnecessary, inappropriate, and delayed, all potentially resulting in negative patient outcomes.

CONFIDENTIALITY

Nurses are legally and ethically obligated to keep information about patients confidential. Do not disclose information about a patient's status to other patients, family members (unless the patient grants permission), or health care staff not involved in the patient's care. In 1996, HIPAA legislation to protect the privacy of patient health information was proposed; HIPAA was finalized in 2003 with specific guidelines for communication of patients' personal health information (U.S. Department of Health and Human Services [USDHHS], 2003). Under HIPAA, patients have access to their medical records, and providers must obtain patient consent before information is released for health-related purposes. HIPAA requires the USDHHS to establish national standards for electronic health care transactions and national identifiers for providers, health plans, and employers. These standards are designed to improve the efficiency and effectiveness of the U.S. health care system by encouraging the widespread use of electronic data interchange in health care. HIPAA also addresses the security and privacy of health data.

Only health care providers directly involved in a specific patient's care have legitimate access to the medical record. Other professionals may use records for data gathering, research, or education only with permission and according to established agency, state, and federal guidelines. Many states require reporting of certain infectious or communicable diseases through the public health department, which must be done through proper channels.

Computerized documentation poses risks to patient confidentiality (Rezaeibagha et al., 2015). Most security mechanisms for information systems use a combination of passwords and physical restrictions such as firewalls and antivirus spyware to protect information. However, there are also guidelines for care providers to use to protect patient information, such as proper use of passwords and ensuring a computer terminal is never left unattended when patient information is still displayed. It is important to follow an agency's policy if backup files are accidentally deleted. Confidentiality procedures also should be followed for documenting sensitive patient information.

LEGAL GUIDELINES IN DOCUMENTATION

Accurate documentation is one of the best defenses for legal claims associated with nursing care. To limit nursing liability, documentation must clearly indicate that individualized, goal-directed nursing care was provided to a patient based on a nursing assessment. The record needs to describe exactly what happens to a patient. This is best achieved by charting immediately after providing care to a patient. Although nursing care may have been excellent, in a court of law, "care not documented is care not provided." Know your agency's policies for documenting, either in paper format or electronically.

Common charting mistakes that may result in malpractice include failure to record pertinent health information, drug information, nursing interventions, and acuity changes (DeMilliano, 2017). The documentation problem of unreadable handwriting has been reduced with EHRs (Hoover, 2016). Although EHRs can minimize documentation problems, the nurse is still responsible for adhering to documentation standards for care delivered.

STANDARDS

Current TJC (2017) standards require that all patients who are admitted to a health care agency have an assessment of physical, psychosocial, environmental, self-care, patient education, and discharge planning needs. Documentation within the context of the nursing process provides structure. The nursing process shapes your approach, the direction of care, and how you document care:

- Record assessments that offer a database from which health care team members can draw conclusions about the patient's health problems.
- Record information about the patient's concerns or condition to assist caregivers in problem identification, planning, and setting priorities.
- Describe care activities in detail to reflect the implementation of the plan of care.
- Evaluate patient responses to nursing care to show the patient's progress in achieving expected outcomes of care.

GUIDELINES FOR QUALITY DOCUMENTATION

Nurses practice in a variety of settings and use various forms and formats to communicate specific information about a patient's health care. The use of standard documentation guidelines ensures more efficient, safe, individualized patient care. Ideally, forms are designed to make data easy to enter, find, and interpret and to avoid unnecessary duplication. For example, most nursing forms have a place for patient identification, date and times, and a key to indicate the meaning of abbreviations or entries used and the type of information required. Because of legal requirements, you must follow agency documentation standards. Regardless of the documentation method, all nurses must follow certain basic guidelines.

Factual

A factual record or report contains descriptive and objective information about what a health care provider sees, hears, feels, or smells. An example of an objective description is "pulse 108 beats/

minute, strong, and irregular." Avoid using words such as *good, adequate, fair,* or *poor* that are subject to interpretation. Inferences are conclusions based on factual data. An example of an inference is "The patient has a poor appetite," which would be based on factual data, including the amount of food the patient ate during a meal and his or her fluid intake. For example, "The patient ate only two bites of toast for breakfast, with 180 mL of apple juice." The recording of factual data leads to appropriate inferences from which clinical decisions are made.

The only subjective data included in a record or report are what a patient actually verbalizes. Document subjective information using the patient's words in quotes; for example, "Patient states, 'I feel sick to my stomach'" or "Patient states, 'I do not like the food choices here.'" In both cases, document the actual food intake and the patient's subjective report.

Accurate

The use of exact, precise measurements is a means to make comparisons and determine when a patient's condition has changed. Charting that an "abdominal wound is 6 cm (2.4 inches) in length, without redness, edema, or discharge" is more accurate than the statement "abdominal wound is healing." Accurate charting requires you to use only those abbreviations approved by your health care agency and write out all terms that may be confusing. Correct spelling is essential because terms are easy to misinterpret (e.g., *accept* or *except, dysphagia* or *dysphasia*). The Institute for Safe Medicine Practice (2017) publishes a list of abbreviations, symbols, and words that are prone to misinterpretation during medication preparation and administration (see Chapter 22).

Records need to reflect your accountability during the time frame that you care for a patient. You must chart your own observations and actions. Your signature holds you accountable for any information recorded. When you report observations to another caregiver and interventions are performed by someone else, that fact must be clearly indicated (e.g., "Surgical drain removed by Dr. Smith. Pulse 100, BP 132/64 reported to J. Kemp, RN"). Each written entry must end with your first name or first initial, last name, and title. Electronic entries document your name and title. Nursing students sign off using the approved abbreviation for the school and the program level on any signature.

Complete

The information within a recorded entry must be complete, containing appropriate and essential information. There are criteria for thorough communication for certain health situations. For example, when recording discharge planning, measurable patient goals or expected outcomes, progress toward goals, and need for referrals are always included. When documenting patient behavior, onset, behaviors exhibited, and precipitating factors are included. The following is an example of what may occur when a note has not been recorded completely:

> A nurse explains and demonstrates a teaching session about giving insulin injections. The patient eagerly expresses a desire to give the next injection when it is due. Documentation is as follows: "Discussed learning about injection technique." During the next shift, another nurse spends time demonstrating the injection technique and assessing the patient's readiness to give the injection because the previous teaching was not completely communicated. As a result, time is wasted repeating information that the patient learned previously instead of coaching the patient through a self-injection.

Another example of following criteria for complete documentation involves hourly rounding. Recently many hospitals have adopted intentional hourly rounding to decrease patient falls and improve patient satisfaction (Brosey and March, 2015). Documentation of a patient visit during rounding includes the 4 *P*s of care: pain, position, possession, and potty (Brosey and March, 2015; Emerson et al., 2014; Hicks, 2015; Box 3.1).

BOX 3.1

Documenting the Four Ps of Care

Focus of Care	Documentation
Pain	Level of pain using a pain scale of 0 to 10. Include interventions to reduce pain.
Position	Change in the patient's position and interventions to improve comfort.
Possessions	Possessions are within reach. Include nurse call system, bedside table, and adaptive devices (e.g., eyeglasses).
Potty	Assistance to use the toilet or bedpan. Record output.

Concise

Concise documentation facilitates efficient retrieval of pertinent information. EHRs reduce narrative writing and improve accuracy (Hoover, 2016). When you learn to write concisely, less time is needed for documentation. A comparison of a concise and a lengthy note follows:

Concise, Factual Entry	Lengthy Entry Using Vague Terms
1500 Left toes cool and pale, without inflammation, capillary return >5 sec; left pedal pulse 1+; right pedal pulse 4+. Patient responds to tactile stimulation and is able to wiggle toes on left foot. Describes pain in left foot as dull, aching 3 (scale 0–10).	1500 The patient's left toes are cool, with pale color. There is no inflammation. There is slow capillary return present greater than 5 seconds. Dorsalis pedis pulse in left foot is weak, and the patient complains of some discomfort. The pain in left foot is described as throbbing without any relief.

Current

Making timely entries in a patient's record avoids omissions and delays in patient care. Many health care agencies keep records and computers near patients' bedsides to facilitate immediate documentation of care activities. Document the following activities or findings at the time of occurrence:

- Acute change in medical condition
- Pain assessment
- Administration of medications and treatments
- Preparation for diagnostic tests or surgery
- Change in patient status and who was notified
- Patient response to an intervention
- Admission, transfer, discharge, or death of a patient

Writing notes on a work pad at the time of an event helps ensure accuracy when you later complete your formal documentation. Often, nurses on a care unit design worksheets that incorporate their standards of care.

Many facilities use military time, a 24-hour time system, to avoid misinterpretation of AM and PM times. The military clock ends with midnight at 2400 and begins at 1 minute after midnight at 0001. The following examples compare standard with military time: 10:22 AM is 1022 military time; 3:15 PM is 1515 military time (Fig. 3.1).

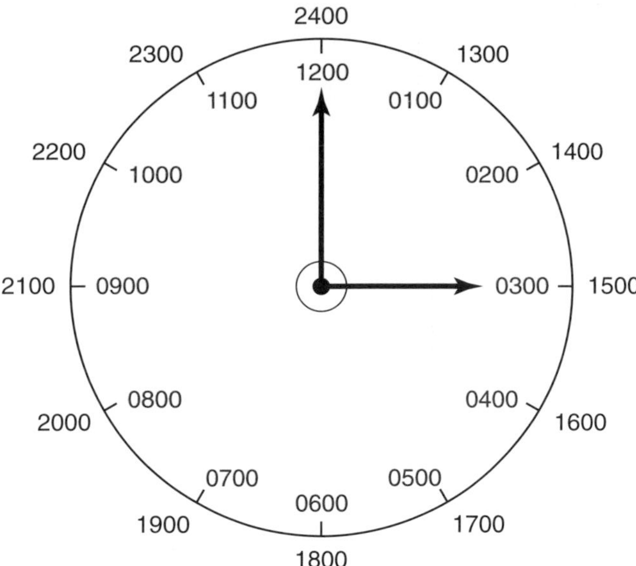

FIG 3.1 Comparison of military time and standard time.

Organized

Organized notes are written in a logical order. For example, an organized note follows the nursing process to describe the assessment, interventions, and patient response for each patient problem or nursing diagnosis in a sequence. Communication is also more effective when it is organized. When making a record entry, make a list of what to include before beginning to write in the permanent legal record. Identifying relevant content is helpful in deleting unnecessary words. The following compares a well-organized note with a disorganized note:

Organized Note	Disorganized Note
7/17 0630 Patient reports sharp pain 7 (scale 0–10) in left lower quadrant of abdomen, worsened by turning onto right side. Positioning on left side decreases pain to 4 (scale 0–10). Abdomen is tender to touch and rigid. Bowel sounds absent in all 4 quadrants. Dr. Phillips notified. To x-ray for CT scan of abdomen. T. Reis, RN	7/17 0630 Patient experiencing sharp pain in lower quadrant of abdomen. MD notified. Abdomen tender to touch, rigid, with bowel sounds absent. Positioning on left side offers minimal relief of pain. CT scan ordered of the abdomen. J. Adams, RN

Methods of Recording

The method of recording selected by a nursing administration often reflects the philosophy of the department. Staffs use the same method of recording throughout an agency. There are several acceptable methods for recording health care data.

The problem-oriented medical record (POMR) is a structured method of documentation that emphasizes and organizes data by a patient's problems or diagnoses. Any notes about a patient's care are organized using the nursing process. Ideally, each member of the health care team contributes to a single list of identified patient problems. Each recording includes a database, problem list, care plan, and progress notes.

A source record is a way to organize chart information by each discipline instead of by patient problems. The advantage of a source record is that caregivers can easily locate the section of the chart to make entries. Members of each discipline can go to sections such as nurse's notes, physician or health care provider's notes, or laboratory results. A disadvantage of the source record is fragmented data. Source records are less common.

Charting by exception (CBE) is a method of recording that eliminates redundancy and makes documentation of routine care more concise. The emphasis is on recording abnormal findings and trends in clinical care. It is a shorthand method for documenting based on defined standards for normal nursing assessments and interventions. CBE simply involves completing a flow sheet that incorporates these standards, minimizing the need for lengthy narrative notes. However, the CBE system can be used inappropriately when nurses fail to enter notes that describe abnormal findings or unexpected changes in a patient's condition.

Communication

Structured communication using the ISBAR approach is a popular technique that provides a framework for communication among members of the health care team. The ISBAR approach offers an easy-to-remember mechanism that you can use to frame conversations, especially critical ones that require a clinician's immediate attention and action. Some health care institutions provide tools for staff to easily use the ISBAR approach (IHI, 2018). ISBAR is a mnemonic for the following:

I: Identify (identify yourself and the patient to be discussed)
 Example: Dr. Sullivan, this is Ed Cashmere, RN on 7200 unit. I am contacting you about Mrs. Denise Thomas, date of birth 12/15/1965.

S: Situation (state what is happening at the present time)
 Example: The patient is having a drop in her blood pressure.

B: Background (explain the circumstances leading up to the situation)
 Example: Mrs. Thomas is 1 day postop, and her BP before surgery was 132–144/80. She had a colectomy performed. She is receiving IV fluids of D5½NS at 80 mL/hr.

A: Assessment (what you think the problem is)
 Example: Her BP was 120/78 at 5 AM, now at 6 AM it is 100/60. She has become increasingly restless over the past hour. Her heart rate is 90 and regular, and BP is now 100/48; respiratory rate is 22. I am concerned she might be bleeding. There is no increase in drainage from her wound.

R: Recommendation (what you would do to correct the problem)
 Example: I would like to increase her IV rate and ask that you come take a look at her.

ISBAR promotes the provision of safe, efficient, timely, and patient-centered communication (Kitney et al., 2016).

Incident Occurrence

An incident occurrence is an adverse event not consistent with the routine operation of a health care unit or routine care of a patient. Adverse event reports are important sources of data for enhancing the understanding of underlying causes of events that, when analyzed, can improve patient safety (Westbrook et al., 2015). Nurses are active participants in examining the cause of errors and redesigning systems to minimize the same type of errors in the future. By focusing on systems rather than individual failures, there is greater opportunity to improve patient safety (Henneman, 2017; Pronovost et al., 2017). For example, when a patient is administered the wrong medication by a nurse, a review of the event focuses primarily on the medication process as opposed to blaming the nurse for the error.

The National Quality Forum (2017) identified a standardized list of preventable, serious adverse events that facilitate reporting of such events (Box 3.2). Completion of an occurrence report happens when there is actual or potential patient injury (near miss) that is not part of the patient record. Document in the patient's record an objective description of what you observed and follow-up actions taken without reference to the incident report/occurrence report.

BOX 3.2

Examples of Serious Reportable Events Occurring Within a Health Care Agency

- Surgery or other invasive procedure performed on the wrong patient or wrong site
- Patient death or serious injury associated with use of restraints or bedrails
- Patient death or serious injury associated with use or function of a device in patient care in which device is used for or functions other than intended
- Patient death or serious injury associated with a fall
- Patient death or serious injury associated with electrical shock
- Unintended retention of foreign object in a patient after surgery or invasive procedure
- Patient death or serious injury associated with elopement
- Patient death or serious injury associated with medication error
- Patient death or serious injury associated with unsafe administration of blood products
- Stage 3, 4, or unstageable pressure injury acquired after admission to a health care agency

Data from the National Quality Forum, 2017: List of SREs, http://www.qualityforum.org/Topics/SREs/List_of_SREs.aspx.

PROCEDURAL GUIDELINE 3.1 *Documenting an Incident Occurrence*

Purpose

An occurrence report is used by health care providers to document an adverse event. You complete the report even if an injury does not occur or is not apparent. The information from the reports helps nursing staff find solutions to prevent repeated incidents. The reports are an important part of the quality improvement program of a unit and the health care institution.

Delegation and Collaboration

The skill of adverse event reporting cannot be delegated to nursing assistive personnel (NAP). The nurse instructs the NAP to:

- Report to the nurse any event such as a fall, incorrect treatment, or adverse reaction.
- Report to the nurse any pertinent information about the event so that a report can be completed.

Equipment

Adverse event report form or computer screen; black pen or digital technology

Procedural Steps

1. Identify patient using at least two identifiers (e.g., name and birthday or name and medical record number) according to agency policy (TJC, 2019).
2. Use clinical reasoning skills to systematically and carefully determine what was involved in the event. Either report the event as witnessed or determine from NAP specifically what occurred. Record the exact sequence of events involved, including time and type of event; injury to patient, nurse, or other staff; and observation of factors that possibly contributed to the event (e.g., wet floor discovered in area of patient fall). Notify risk management per agency protocol.

Safe Patient Care *Prepare the report on any questionable event. Do not avoid reporting because of concerns that punitive actions will occur if reports are filed.*

3. Assess extent of any injury to patient or others, including patient's subjective report and objective physical examination findings.
4. If the adverse event involves an injury, take steps to restore individual's safety, such as stabilizing patient's position after a fall and assessing for further injuries.
5. When patient sustains an injury, call the health care provider immediately.
6. When visitor or staff member sustains an injury, refer to emergency department or appropriate treatment setting.
7. Complete the adverse event report form.

Safe Patient Care *Document on the report form as quickly as possible. The closer to the event, the more accurate the recording.*

   a. Record time of event and describe exactly what occurred or was observed, using objective findings and observations. Use language that does not allow for subjective interpretation. Do not include personal opinions or feelings. Document victim's interpretation of event by using quotes.
   b. Objectively describe patient's or staff member's condition when event was discovered or observed.
   c. Describe measures taken by any caregivers at time of event.
   d. Send completed report to designated department.
8. When a patient is involved, document events of incident in patient's chart.
   a. Only enter objective description of what happened.
   b. Record any assessment and intervention activities initiated as a result of event.
   c. Do not duplicate all information from report.
   d. Do not record that report was completed.
9. Submit the report properly with the risk-management department or designated people.
10. Communicate the occurrence and recommendation for priorities of care during hand-off reporting.

SPECIAL CONSIDERATIONS

Patient-Centered Care

- If a patient speaks a language different from your own, have a professional interpreter present or available during care. Document the name and contact information of the interpreter in the EHR.
- Document on the occurrence report the name(s) of any family caregiver(s) present during an adverse event.
- Patient-centered care involves nurses individualizing care delivered to patients and being responsive in meeting patient needs (Clark, 2017).
- Thorough documentation is central to patient-centered care. A nurse is responsible for documenting detailed information about the care that is provided to patients, including aspects of care that are individualized.

- When you provide a level of detail, the medical record becomes a valuable resource for all health care providers.
- Communication among members of the health care team through documentation is essential for accurate and timely delivery of therapies.
- When you record an entry in a patient record, it must convey information about the patient's status, the specific type of interventions delivered, patient responses to care, and other critical information that allows all care providers to deliver an organized and comprehensive plan of care.

✦ PRACTICE REFLECTIONS

Consider a time in your practice when you may care for a patient who is injured during a fall in the hospital. Because of the fall, the patient needs surgery. Instead of returning home as planned, your patient will be transferred from the hospital to a rehabilitation unit.

1. What are some of the challenges you will face in hand-off reporting to the rehabilitation nurse?
2. What is the most difficult aspect of the adverse event to discuss with the rehabilitation nurse?
3. Will the adverse event affect what you document about your hand-off report?
4. What do you think might have contributed to this fall, and how might it be prevented in the future?

✦ CLINICAL REVIEW QUESTIONS

1. The patient has an adverse reaction to a medication. Which actions will the nurse perform? (Select all that apply.)
   1. Identify the patient using at least two patient identifiers.
   2. Document your clinical assessment and interventions in the EHR.
   3. Complete an occurrence report as close to the actual event as possible.
   4. Document the occurrence report in the EHR.
   5. Assess extent of injury to the patient.
2. The patient is being transferred from an acute patient care unit to a skilled nursing unit. Place the following in correct order for an ISBAR report.
   1. State your name and the patient's full name and date of birth.
   2. Recommend the priorities of care to the next health care provider.
   3. Communicate medical history, allergies, code status, and isolation status.
   4. Describe what is occurring with the patient at this time.
   5. Communicate the current clinical assessment.
3. The nurse is caring for a patient over a 10-hour shift. She conducts her routine assessment at the beginning of the shift and assists the patient with toileting. At 1000, the nurse assesses the patient's surgical wound and notes increased erythema and drainage. At 1500, the patient reports shoulder pain at a level of 8 on a pain scale of 0 to 10, and the nurse administers pain medication. A reassessment of pain occurs at 1530. At 1600, the dietitian visits the patient to review food allergies. The dietitian informs the nurse of a new food allergy, which the nurse confirms. Which of the activities performed by the nurse should be recorded immediately? (Select all that apply.)
   1. Food allergy
   2. Medication administration
   3. Assistance in toileting
   4. Pain assessment
   5. Wound assessment

Answers and Rationales for Clinical Review Questions can be found on the Evolve website.

REFERENCES

American Nurses Association (ANA): *Nursing informatics scope and standards of practice*, ed 2, Silvers Spring, MD, 2014.

Brosey L, March K: Effectiveness of structured hourly nurse rounding on patient satisfaction and clinical outcomes, *J Nurs Care Qual* 30(2):153–159, 2015.

Charalambous L, Goldberg S: 'Gaps, mishaps and overlaps'. Nursing documentation: how does it affect care? *J Res Nurs* 21(8):638–648, 2016.

Chung J, Cho I: The need for academic electronic health record systems in nurse education, *Nurse Educ Today* 54:83–88, 2017.

Clark A: A paradigm shift for patient/family-centered care in intensive care units: bring in the family, *Crit Care Nurse* 37(2):96–99, 2017.

DeMilliano D: *8 Common charting mistakes to avoid*, 2017. http://www.nso.com/risk-education/individuals/articles/8-Common-Charting-Mistakes-To-Avoid.

Emerson B, et al: Administration of emergency medicine: hourly rounding in the pediatric emergency department: patient and family safety and satisfaction rounds, *J Emerg Med* 47:99–104, 2014.

Hart P, et al: Medical-surgical nurses' experiences as first responders during deterioration events: a qualitative study, *J Clin Nurs* 25(21–22):3241–3251, 2016.

Heal M, et al: Design and development of a proactive rapid response system, *Comput Inform Nurs* 35(2):77–83, 2017.

Healthcare Information and Management Systems Society: *What is nursing informatics*, 2017. http://www.himss.org/what-nursing-informatics.

HealthIT.gov: *Learn EHR basics*, 2014. https://www.healthit.gov/providers-professionals/learn-ehr-basics.

Henneman E: Recognizing the ordinary as extraordinary: insight into the "way we work" to improve patient safety outcomes, *Am J Crit Care* 6(4):272–277, 2017.

Hicks D: Can rounding reduce patient falls in acute care? An integrative literature review, *Medsurg Nurs* 24(1):51, 2015.

Hoover R: Benefits of using an electronic health record, *Nursing* 46(7):21–22, *2016*.

Institute for Healthcare Improvement (IHI): *ISBAR trip tick*, 2018. http://www.ihi.org/resources/Pages/Tools/ISBARTripTick.aspx.

Institute for Safe Medicine Practice: *List of error-prone abbreviations*, 2017. https://www.ismp.org/recommendations/error-prone-abbreviations-list.

Kang M, et al: Real-time risk prediction on the wards: a feasibility study, *Crit Care Med* 44(8):1468–1473, 2016.

Kitney P, et al: Handover between anaesthetists and post-anaesthetic care unit nursing staff using ISBAR principles: a quality improvement study, *J Periop Nurs Aust* 29(1):30–35, 2016.

National Quality Forum: *List of SREs*, 2017. http://www.qualityforum.org/Topics/SREs/List_of_SREs.aspx.

Pronovost P, et al: Changing the narratives for patient safety, *Bull World Health Organ* 95(6):478–480, 2017.

Rezaeibagha F, et al: A systematic literature review on security and privacy of electronic health record systems: technical perspectives, *Health Inf Manag* 44(3):23–38, 2015.

The Joint Commission: *2017 Comprehensive accreditation manual for hospitals: the official handbook*, Oakbrook Terrace, IL, 2017. The Commission.

The Joint Commission (TJC): *2019 National Patient Safety Goals*, Oakbrook Terrace, IL, 2019. The Commission. http://www.jointcommission.org/standards_information/npsgs.aspx.

U.S. Department of Health and Human Services: *Standards for privacy of individually identifiable health information, Health Insurance Portability and Accountability Act of 1996*, Fed Reg 64:60053, revised 2003, http://www.hhs.gov/ocr/privacy/hipaa/administrative/privacyrule/index.html.

Westbrook J, et al: What are incident reports telling us? A comparative study of two Australian hospitals of medication errors identified at audit, detected by staff and reported to an incident system, *Int J Qual Health Care* 27(10):1–9, 2015.

4 Patient Safety and Quality Improvement

SKILLS AND PROCEDURES

EVOLVE WEBSITE/RESOURCES LIST

http://evolve.elsevier.com/Perry/nursinginterventions
Audio Glossary • Checklists • Clinical Review Questions • Answers and Rationales for Clinical Review Questions • Case Studies • Video Clips

INTRODUCTION

Ensuring patient safety is an important nursing responsibility. Patient safety is the prevention of physical and psychological harm to patients. The Institute for Healthcare Improvement (Frankel et al., 2017) defines safety as freedom from accidental injury. Patient safety requires effective communication, teamwork, critical thinking, and timely clinical decisions. As part of the health care team, professional nurses engage in all activities that support a patient-centered safety culture. This means recognizing each patient as the source of control and full partner in providing compassionate and coordinated care based on respect for each patient's preferences, values, and needs (Quality and Safety Education for Nurses [QSEN], 2018). The QSEN safety competency is stated as "Minimizes risk of harm to patients and providers through both system effectiveness and individual performance." The QSEN skills for safety competency include the following:

- Demonstrate effective use of technology and standardized practices that support quality and safety.
- Demonstrate effective use of strategies to reduce the risk of harm to self or others.
- Use appropriate strategies to reduce reliance on memory.
- Communicate observations or concerns related to hazards and errors to patients, families, and the health care team.

In this chapter, the focus is on how to protect patients from injuries related to falls; use of physical restraints; seizures; and exposure to electrical, chemical, and fire hazards.

PRACTICE STANDARDS

- Agency for Healthcare Research and Quality (AHRQ), 2013: Preventing falls in hospitals—Evidence-based interventions for fall prevention
- American Epilepsy Society (Glauser et al.), 2016: Evidence-based guideline: treatment of convulsive status epilepticus in children and adults—Treatment of status epilepticus
- National Institute for Health and Care Excellence (NICE), 2014: NICE guidelines on antiepileptic drugs—Antiepileptic drugs for seizures
- The Joint Commission (TJC), 2015: Preventing falls and fall-related injuries in health care agencies—Fall prevention
- The Joint Commission (TJC), 2019: National Patient Safety Goals—Patient identification

EVIDENCE-BASED PRACTICE

Self-Perception of Fall Risk

Self-perception of fall risk can be a factor in whether patients fall while hospitalized. One patient population at high risk for falls with injuries is oncology patients. Researchers are examining whether involving patients by informing them of their fall risks and then offering targeted education based on those risks reduces the incidence of falls. Huang and colleagues (2015) explored the effect of patient knowledge and self-efficacy of fall prevention on fall incidence on an oncology hospital unit. Patients who received a 20-minute program on fall prevention had greater knowledge and self-efficacy about fall prevention after the intervention, and the fall rate on the hospital unit declined (comparing pre- with postintervention). Research shows that education of patients about fall prevention and activities associated with falling increases their awareness of the potential of falling and promotes patient safety. Considerations include the following:

- Education of patients about fall risk factors and discussion regarding fall prevention strategies strengthens patients' knowledge of fall risks and participation in their own risk management (Huang et al., 2015).
- Inform patients that the bedside is the most frequent location for falling in hospitals (Huang et al., 2015).

- Clarify for patients the proper use of hospital equipment (e.g., crutches, wheelchairs) that can prevent falls (Huang et al., 2015).
- The Joint Commission (2016) recommends all patients receive targeted education about their specific fall risks.
- Tailor education to the patients' perceived risk of falls (Kuhlenschmidt et al., 2016).

SAFETY GUIDELINES

Hospitalized patients are at risk for injury partly as a result of unfamiliar environments. Normal life cues, such as a bed without side rails and the direction one usually takes to walk to the bathroom, are absent. Thought processes and coping mechanisms can be affected by illness and associated treatments and emotional responses. Patients are often more vulnerable to injury due to changes related to illness, such as fatigue, visual alterations, or lower extremity weakness. Considerations include the following:

- Always check and confirm patient identification before any procedure. Use at least two patient identifiers (TJC, 2019).
- In a health care setting, always keep a patient bed in the low position when unattended, and use the standard fall prevention strategies of the agency. If a patient is at high risk of falling, a bed alarm needs to be activated at all times. Options also include the use of a chair alarm in a recliner or wheelchair.
- In the home setting, partner with the patient and family caregiver to conduct a home safety checklist (see Chapter 32).
- Be alert for conditions within a patient's environment that pose risks for injury (e.g., personal care items out of the patient's reach, hazards along walking paths, pets at home, electrical equipment not functioning correctly, liquid spilled on floors).
- Use safe patient-handling techniques (see Chapter 17) when transferring and assisting patients with ambulation to reduce the risk of a patient fall.
- When seizure precautions are necessary, explain and demonstrate precautions to the patient and family caregiver.

✦ SKILL 4.1 Fall Prevention in a Health Care Setting

Purpose

Patient falls continue to be a challenging issue for health care agencies. Every year approximately 700,000 to 1,000,000 people in the United States fall in hospitals (AHRQ, 2018). Patient falls are multifactorial; many different conditions can contribute to a single patient fall (Berry and Kiel, 2018; TJC, 2016). The risk factors for falls include two categories: patient related (intrinsic) and health care agency environment and working process related (extrinsic). In an international systematic review of studies examining risk factors for falls, common risks were found for all patients (Berry and Kiel, 2018; Severo et al., 2014; Table 4.1). In an effort to anticipate a patient's fall risk, health care agencies use fall risk assessment tools that include risk factors that have been identified from the scientific literature. The number of risks identified for a specific patient is computed into a fall risk score, for example, high, medium, and low. The most common risk assessment tools used in health care agencies are the Morse Fall Scale, the STRATIFY scale, and the Hendrich II Fall Risk Model (Berry and Kiel, 2018; Severo et al., 2014). Once a patient's fall risks are identified, a nurse's responsibility is to partner with the patient to affirm those risks and to select evidence-based interventions (usually multiple strategies) that appropriately target the patient's risks (Berry and Kiel, 2018; Box 4.1).

Delegation and Collaboration

The skill of assessing and communicating a patient's risks for falling cannot be delegated to nursing assistive personnel (NAP). Skills used to prevent falls can be delegated. The nurse directs the NAP by:

- Explaining a patient's specific fall risks and associated prevention measures needed to minimize risks
- Explaining environmental safety precautions to use
- Explaining specific patient behaviors (e.g., disorientation, wandering) that are precursors to falls and that should be reported to the registered nurse (RN) immediately

Equipment

- Standardized and valid fall risk assessment tool (Berry and Kiel, 2018; TJC, 2016)
- Hospital bed with side rails; *Option*: low bed
- Wedge cushion
- Nurse call system
- Gait belt for assisting with ambulation
- Wheelchair and seat belt (as needed)
- Optional safety devices: bed alarm pad, no-slip floor mat, protective headgear, hip protector

ASSESSMENT

1. Identify patient using at least two identifiers (e.g., name and birthday or name and medical record number) according to agency policy. *Rationale: Ensures correct patient. Complies with The Joint Commission standards and improves patient safety (TJC, 2019).*
2. Review medical record and determine if patient has a recent history of a fall and risks for injury (ABCS) (IHI, 2017):
   - Age over 85
   - Bone disorders (e.g., metastasis, osteoporosis)
   - Coagulation disorders (e.g., leukemia, thrombocytopenia, anticoagulant use)
   - Surgery (specifically thoracic or abdominal surgery or lower limb amputation)

   Rationale: Conditions increase likelihood of serious injury from a fall such as fracture or internal hemorrhage.
3. Perform hand hygiene. Assess for fall risks using a validated fall risk assessment tool. Compute fall risk score. Conduct a comprehensive individualized patient assessment and consider patient's unique fall risks (Berry and Kiel, 2018; Kiel et al., 2018; TJC, 2017b; see Table 4.1) Perform a fall risk assessment in general acute care settings on admission, on transfer from one unit to another, or with a significant

TABLE 4.1

Risk Factors for Hospitalized Patient Falls

Intrinsic Factors	Extrinsic Factors
History of previous fall	Frequency of rounding
Altered cognition	Physical hazards: liquids on floor, electrical cords, compression stocking cords
Altered mobility Lower extremity weakness Abnormal gait Shuffling and stumbling Requires assistance with mobility and/or assistive device	Increased use of restraints (Berry and Kiel, 2018)
Sensory deficit	Footwear with greater heel height (Kiel et al., 2018)
Medications: Benzodiazepines Antipsychotics Antidepressants Opiates Barbiturates Antihistamines Anticonvulsants Sedatives Antihypertensives Diuretics	

change in a patient's condition, or after a fall (AHRQ, 2013; Kiel et al., 2018). *Rationale: Reduces transmission of microorganisms. A variety of intrinsic physiological factors predispose patients to falls. Tools based on the risk factors of a population (e.g., elderly, oncology, or neurological patient) are more likely sensitive to predicting falls.*

4. Perform the Banner Mobility Assessment Tool (BMAT; Boynton et al., 2014) or the timed "get up and go" (TUG) test (CDC, 2017; Kiel et al., 2018) if patient is able to ambulate. At a minimum, observe an ambulatory patient walk in room (with or without help). *Rationale: The BMAT assesses four functional tasks to identify the level of mobility a patient can achieve, revealing if assistance is needed (Boynton et al., 2014). The TUG test measures the progress of balance, sit to stand, and walking.*

Safe Patient Care *Do not ask patient to provide a self-report of balance, gait, or ability to ambulate. Ask patient to walk a short distance using timed "get up and go," or complete the BMAT assessment and observe each factor.*

5. Assess patient's pain severity (use rating scale ranging 0 to 10). *Rationale: Pain, especially when it is associated with lower extremities (e.g., arthritis, injury) is a fall risk factor.*
6. Ask patient or family caregiver if patient has a history of recent falls or other injuries within the home. Assess previous falls using the acronym SPLATT (Touhy and Jett, 2018):
   - Symptoms at time of fall
   - Previous fall
   - Location of fall
   - Activity at time of fall
   - Time of fall
   - Trauma after fall

BOX 4.1

Evidence-Based Fall Prevention Interventions in Health Care Settings

- Universal fall precautions, including scheduled rounding protocols (AHRQ, 2013)
  - Familiarize the patient with the environment.
  - Have the patient demonstrate call system use.
  - Be sure nurse call system is accessible to patient.
  - Keep the patient's personal possessions within patient's safe reach.
  - Have patient use sturdy handrails in patient bathrooms, room, and hallway.
  - Place the hospital bed in low position when a patient is resting in bed; raise bed to a comfortable height when the patient is transferring out of bed.
  - Keep hospital bed brakes locked.
  - Keep wheelchair wheel locks in locked position when stationary.
  - Keep nonslip, comfortable, well-fitting footwear on the patient (Berry and Kiel, 2018).
  - Use night-lights or supplemental lighting.
  - Keep floor surfaces clean and dry. Clean up all spills promptly.
  - Keep patient care areas uncluttered.
  - Follow safe patient-handling practices.
- Care planning and interventions that address the identified risk factors within the overall care plan for the patient (AHRQ, 2013)
  - Encourage patients with sensory deficits to use eyeglasses, hearing aids, footwear, and mobility devices.
  - Institute toileting and comfort rounds based on patient need (Berry and Kiel, 2018).
  - Review patient's individual medications, and provide interventions that minimize risks created by medication side effects.
  - Encourage early mobility with appropriate assistance.
  - Consider use of rooms designated for cognitively impaired patients requiring (1) closer supervision and (2) specialty equipment and activities.
  - Assess patient risk for orthostatic hypotension, and assist patient to get out of bed safely.
  - Provide patient and family education regarding patient's unique fall risks (Berry and Kiel, 2018).

Rationale: Symptoms are helpful in identifying cause of fall. Onset, location, and activity offer details on how to prevent future falls.

7. Review patient's medications (including over-the-counter [OTC] medications and herbal products) for drugs that create risk for falls (see Table 4.1) Also assess for polypharmacy (unnecessary use of multiple and/or redundant medications in management of the same condition and drugs inappropriate for condition; De Jong et al., 2013). *Rationale: Effects of certain medications increase risk for falls (Berry and Kiel, 2018; Kiel et al., 2018; Severo et al., 2014).*
8. Assess patient's fear of falling: consider those over 70 years of age, female, lower income, or single and have poor perceived general health (Kiel et al., 2018). *Rationale: Fear of falling is interrelated with incidence of falls, inability to rise from a chair of knee height, lower household income, using a walking aid, difficulty in using public transport, self-reported balance problems, lower educational level, and a higher body mass index (BMI; Kumar et al., 2014).*

9. Assess condition of equipment (e.g., legs on bedside commode, end tips on a walker). *Rationale: Equipment in poor repair increases risk for fall.*
10. Use patient-centered approach to determine what patient already knows about risks for falling. Show patient and family caregiver results of fall risk assessment, and explain significance of risk factors. Explain how a plan for fall prevention will be developed. Assess patient's or family caregiver's experience and health literacy level. *Rationale: Knowledge of fall risks influences one's ability to take necessary precautions in reducing falling. Matching interventions with factors that patient perceives as relevant may increase success in preventing falls. Ensures patient has the capacity to obtain, communicate, process, and understand basic health information (Berry and Kiel, 2018; CDC, 2016).*
11. If patient is a fall risk, apply color-coded wristband (see illustration). Some agencies institute fall risk signs on doors, whereas others may use color-coded socks or gowns. *Rationale: Color-coded yellow bands, socks, and gowns are easily recognizable.*

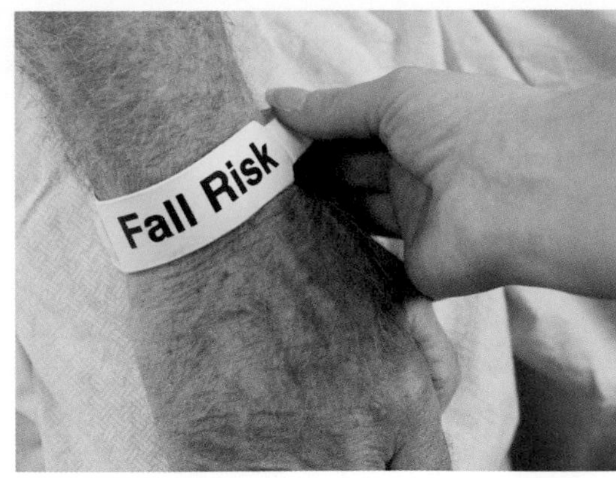

STEP 11 Fall risk armband alerts health care staff to patient's risk of falling.

12. If patient is in a wheelchair, assess his or her level of comfort, fatigue, boredom, mental status, or level of engagement with others. *Rationale: These factors can cause patient to make an attempt to exit wheelchair without help.*

STEP	RATIONALE

PLANNING

STEP	RATIONALE
1. Expected outcomes following completion of procedure:	
• Patient's environment is free of hazards.	Hazards predispose to tripping and falls.
• Patient and/or family caregiver is able to identify fall risks.	Awareness of risks promotes cooperation and understanding of fall prevention plan.
• Patient and/or family caregiver verbalizes understanding of fall prevention interventions to be planned.	Includes patient and family caregiver in decisions about preventive strategies.
• Patient does not experience a fall or injury.	Fall precautions successfully prevent falls.
2. Provide privacy, be sure patient is comfortable, and prepare environment.	Reduces patient anxiety and facilitates an organized procedure.
3. Perform hand hygiene and gather equipment.	Reduces transmission of microorganisms and organizes care.
4. Explain what fall prevention measures you plan to provide in relation to patient's risks. Also plan for time to discuss fall prevention in the home (see Chapter 32).	Results in fall prevention measures that are patient centered and not just routine. Younger patients are very independent and often believe that they are not likely to fall.
5. Educate patients and family caregivers on medication side effects that increase risk for falls (TJC, 2016).	Certain medications have side effects that alter a patient's balance, level of consciousness, and other factors and thus increase a patient's fall risk. Family caregivers need this information to reduce falls.

IMPLEMENTATION

STEP	RATIONALE
1. Conduct hourly rounds on all patients to determine status of pain, need to toilet, and need to relocate personal items for easy reach; provide pain-relief intervention.	Provides nurses with surveillance mechanism to purposefully keep patients safe and comfortable by proactively meeting their needs.
2. Implement early mobility protocols within health care agency (see Chapter 18). Follow protocols to ensure patient increases level of mobility progressively. Consider use of accelerometers, small devices that can be worn by a patient and quantify biomechanical body movement and number of steps per shift (Growdon et al., 2017).	A patient's functional decline (loss of the ability to perform self-care activities or activities of daily living) may result from deconditioning, which is associated with inactivity (Gorman et al., 2014; Grass et al., 2018). Deconditioning is a risk for hospitalized patients who spend most of their time in bed, even when they are able to walk.

STEP	RATIONALE
3. Adjust bed to low position with wheels locked (see illustration; Berry and Kiel, 2018). Place nonslip padded floor mats at exit side of bed.	Height of bed allows ambulatory patient to get in and out of bed easily and safely. Mats provide nonslippery surface for preventing falls and injuries.

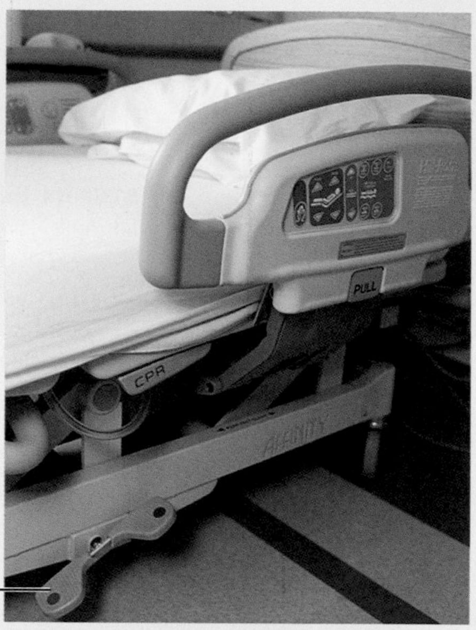

STEP 3 Hospital bed should be kept in lowest position, with wheels locked and side rails up (as appropriate).

STEP	RATIONALE
4. Encourage use of properly fitted skid-proof footwear (Berry and Kiel, 2018; Kiel et al., 2018). *Option:* Place nonslip padded floor mat on exit side of bed.	Prevents falls from slipping on floor.
5. Orient patient to surroundings, nurse call system, and routines to expect in plan of care (AHRQ, 2013).	Orientation to room and plan of care provides familiarity with environment and activities to anticipate.
a. Provide patient's hearing aid and glasses. Be sure that each is functioning/clean (AHRQ, 2013). If patient complains of visual or hearing problems, refer to appropriate health care provider.	Enables patient to remain alert to conditions in environment.
b. Place nurse call system in an accessible location within patient's reach. Explain and demonstrate how to use system at bedside and in bathroom. Have patient perform return demonstration.	Knowledge of location and use of call system is essential for patient to be able to call for help quickly. Reaching for an object when in bed can lead to an accidental fall.
c. Explain to patient/family caregiver when and why to use nurse call system (e.g., report pain, assistance needed to get out of bed or go to bathroom). Provide clear instructions regarding mobility restrictions.	Increases likelihood that patient/family caregiver will call for help and of nurse being able to respond to patient's needs in a timely way.
6. Safe use of side rails:	
a. Explain to patient and family caregiver reason for patient to use side rails: moving and turning self in bed.	Promotes a feeling of comfort and security. Aids in turning and repositioning and provides easy access to bed controls (U.S. Food and Drug Administration [FDA], 2014).
b. Check agency policy regarding side-rail use.	
(1) Dependent, less mobile patients: In two-side-rail bed, keep both rails up. (**Note:** Rails on newer hospital beds allow for room at foot of bed for patient to safely exit bed.) In four-side-rail bed, leave two upper rails up.	Side rails are restraint devices if they restrict a patient's freedom of movement and therefore do not promote the individual's independent functioning (TJC, 2017c).
(2) Patient able to get out of bed independently: In four-side-rail bed, leave two upper side rails up. In two-side-rail bed, keep only one rail up.	Allows for safe exit from bed.

STEP	RATIONALE
7. Make patient's environment safe:	
a. Remove excess equipment, supplies, and furniture from rooms and halls.	Reduces likelihood of falling or tripping over objects.
b. Keep floors free of clutter and obstacles (e.g., intravenous [IV] pole, electrical cords), particularly path to bathroom (AHRQ, 2013).	Reduces likelihood of falling or tripping over objects.
c. Coil and secure excess electrical, telephone, and any other cords or tubing.	Reduces risk of entanglement.
d. Clean all spills on floors promptly (Berry and Kiel, 2018). Post sign indicating wet floor. Remove sign when floor is dry (usually done by housekeeping).	Reduces risk of falling on slippery, wet surfaces.
e. Ensure adequate glare-free lighting; use a night-light at night.	Glare may be problem for older adults because of vision changes.
f. Have assistive devices (e.g., cane, walker, bedside commode) on exit side of bed. Have chair back of a bedside commode placed against wall of room if possible.	Provides added support when transferring out of bed. Stabilizes commode.
g. Arrange personal items (e.g., water pitcher, telephone, reading materials, dentures) within patient's easy reach and in logical way (AHRQ, 2013).	Facilitates independence and self-care; prevents falls related to reaching for hard-to-reach items.
h. Secure locks on beds, stretchers, and wheelchairs (Berry and Kiel, 2018).	Prevents accidental movement of devices during patient transfer.
8. Provide comfort measures, offer ordered analgesics for patients experiencing pain.	Pain can cause patients to exit bed; thus pain relief is essential. Be cautious because opioids increase fall risk.
9. Interventions for patients at moderate to high risk for falling (based on fall risk assessment):	
a. Prioritize nurse call system responses to patients at high risk; use a team approach, with all staff knowing responsibility to respond.	Ensures rapid response by care provider when patient calls for help; decreases chance of patient trying to get out of bed on own.
b. Establish elimination schedule, using bedside commode when appropriate.	Proactive toileting keeps patients from being unattended with sudden urge to use toilet.

Safe Patient Care *Toileting is a common event leading to a patient's fall (Berry and Kiel, 2018).*

STEP	RATIONALE
c. Stay with patient during toileting (standing outside bathroom door).	Patients often try to get up to stand and walk back to their beds from the bathroom without help.
d. Place patient in a geri chair or wheelchair with wedge cushion. Use wheelchair only for transport, not for sitting for an extended time.	Maintains alignment and comfort and makes it difficult to exit chair.
e. Consider use of a low bed that has lower height than standard hospital bed. Apply nonskid floor mats.	Low beds may reduce fall-related injuries. Low beds can make it difficult for patients with lower extremity weakness or pain in lower joints to exert effort needed to stand.
f. Activate a bed alarm for patient.	Alarm activates when patient rises off sensor. Alarm sounds alert to staff.

Safe Patient Care *Use judgment in choosing the use of a bed alarm. Bed alarms alert nursing staff so that if a patient exits a bed, a quick response may prevent a fall. If a patient exits a bed quickly and falls, the alarm alerts staff to respond so that further injury does not occur while the patient lies on floor. However, bed and chair alarms can restrict patient activity. Reports have shown that patients perceive that an alarm makes them feel restrained (Growdon et al., 2017). Determine if use of bed or chair alarm is limiting frequency of patient getting up and remaining active.*

STEP	RATIONALE
g. Confer with physical therapy about gait training, strength and balance training, and regular weight-bearing activities.	Exercise can reduce falls, fall-related fractures, and several risk factors for falls in individuals with low bone density and older adults (Berry and Kiel, 2018). Strength and balance training reduces the rate of injurious falls in older adults (Uusi-Rasi et al., 2015).
h. Use sitters or restraints only when alternatives are exhausted.	A sitter is a nonprofessional staff member or volunteer who stays in a patient room to closely observe patients who are at risk of falling. Restraints should be used only as a final option (see Skill 14.2).

STEP	RATIONALE
i. Consider having patient wear protective headgear (e.g., oncology patient or patients at risk for bleeding) or hip protectors.	Contains impact-resistant material within the hat that surrounds the head and protects against head injury. Hip protectors have padding to reduce fall impact.
10. When ambulating patient, have patient wear a gait belt or walking sling, and walk along his or her side (see Chapter 17).	Safe patient-handling techniques allow for safe patient ambulation and prevention of injury to you and patient.
11. Safe use of wheelchair:	
a. Be sure that wheelchair is correct fit for patient: Patient thighs are level while sitting, feet flat on floor; back of chair comes up to mid-shoulder, elbows rest on armrests without leaning over or tucking arms in, and two finger widths of space between patient and side of chair.	Correctly fitted chair promotes comfort, making it less likely for patient to try to exit it.
b. Transfer patient to wheelchair using safe handling techniques (see Chapter 17). Use a wedge cushion in chair (see illustration).	Cushion prevents patient from slipping out of chair.
c. Back wheelchair into and out of elevator or door, leading with large rear wheels first (see illustration).	Prevents smaller front wheels from catching in crack between elevator and floor, causing chair to tip.
d. Manage patient's pain, and do not allow him or her to sit in wheelchair for an extended amount of time; provide alternative sitting option.	Reduces restlessness and discomfort that can lead to wheelchair exit.
12. Schedule oral medication administration for at least 2 hours before "bedtime" (TJC, 2016).	Reduces risk created by medications that can cause patients to have to use bathroom during night.
13. Remove unnecessary supplies at bedside from patient room. Perform hand hygiene.	Reduces clutter. Reduces transmission of microorganisms.

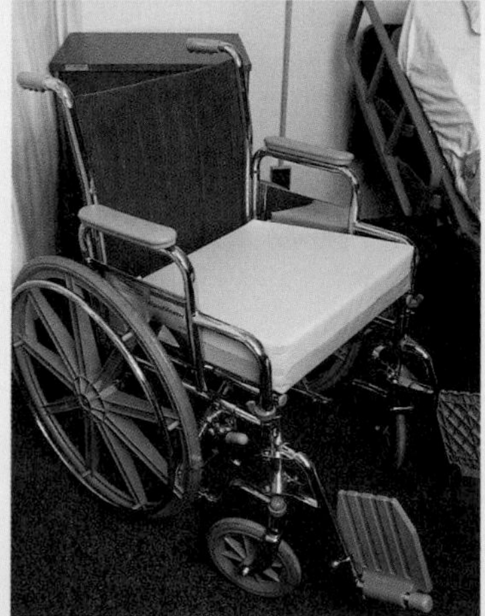
STEP 11b Wheelchair with footplates raised and wedge cushion in place.

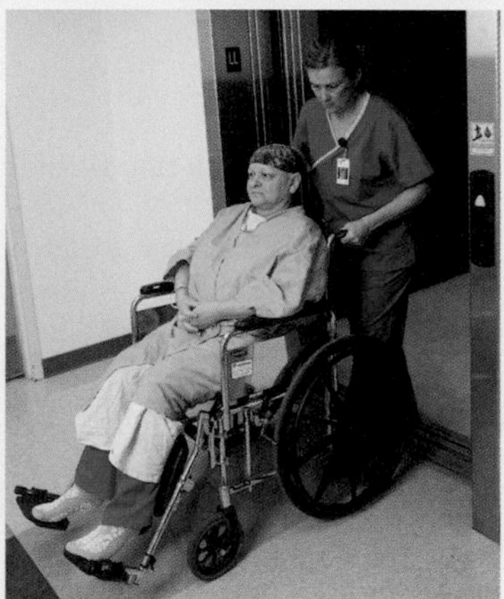
STEP 11c Nurse backing wheelchair into elevator.

EVALUATION

1. Ask patient/family caregiver to identify patient's fall risks.	Demonstrates learning.
2. Ask patient/family caregiver to describe fall prevention interventions to implement.	Demonstrates learning.
3. Evaluate patient's ability to use assistive devices such as walker or bedside commode at different times during the day.	Adjustments in devices may become necessary. Evaluating at different times can help identify strengths and weaknesses.
4. Evaluate for changes in motor, sensory, and cognitive status, and review if any falls or injuries have occurred.	May require different interventions to be added. Fall outcomes determine success of plan.

STEP	RATIONALE
5. **Use Teach-Back:** "I want to be sure I explained clearly to you (example) why you are at risk for falls. Tell me some of those reasons." Revise your instruction now or develop plan for revised patient/family caregiver teaching if patient/family caregiver is not able to teach back correctly.	Determines patient's/family caregiver's level of understanding of instructional topic.

Unexpected Outcomes	Related Interventions
1. Patient/family caregiver unable to identify fall risks or fall prevention strategies.	• Reinforce identified risks with patient, and review safety measures with family caregiver. • Consider using other instructional options.
2. Patient starts to fall while ambulating with nurse or other caregiver.	• Put both arms around patient's waist or grasp gait belt. • Stand with feet apart to provide broad base of support. • Extend one leg and let patient slide against it to floor (Fig. 4.1A). Use caution because patient weight can cause hyperextension of your knee. • Bend knees and lower body as patient slides to floor (see Fig. 4.1B).
3. Patient found after falling.	• Call for assistance. • Assess patient for injury, and stay with him or her until help arrives. • Notify primary health care provider and family caregiver. • Complete an agency occurrence or sentinel event report (see agency policy). • Conduct a **postfall huddle/debrief** as soon as possible after the fall. Involve staff at all levels and the patient if possible. Discuss whether appropriate interventions were in place, considerations as to why fall occurred, staffing at time of fall, which environment-of-care factors were in place, and how care plan will change (TJC, 2016).

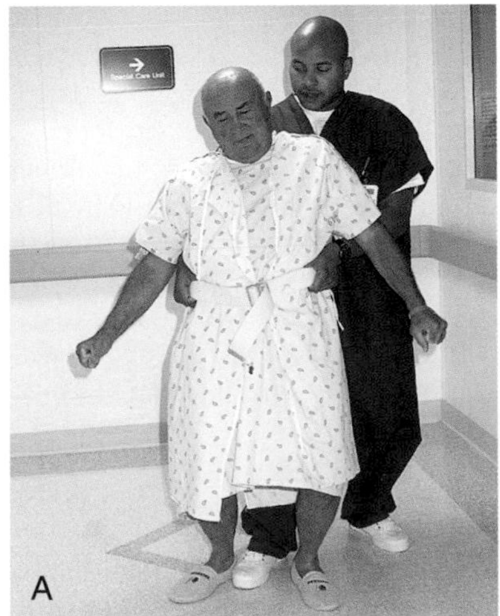

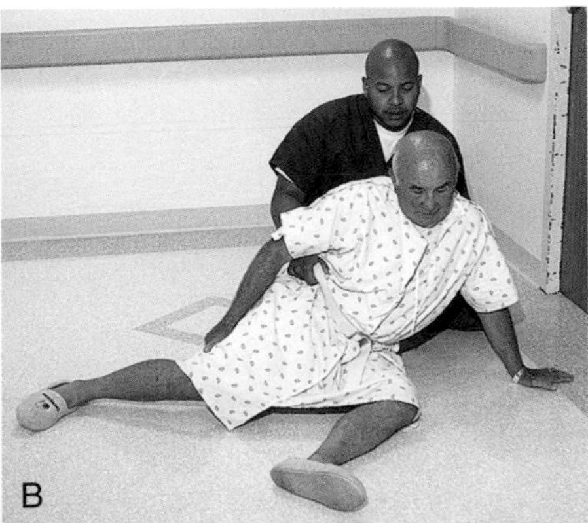

FIG 4.1 (A) Stand with feet apart to provide broad base of support; extend one leg against which patient can slide to floor. (B) Bend knees and lower body as patient slides to floor.

Recording

- Record in the plan of care specific fall prevention interventions. Use whiteboards in patient rooms to communicate fall risks to staff on all shifts.
- Document what patient is able to explain or not explain about fall risks and interventions taken.
- Utilize whiteboards to communicate patient fall risks to all staff (TJC, 2016).
- Complete an agency safety event or incident report noting objective details of fall (time, location, patient's condition, treatment, treatment response). Do not place the report in patient's medical record.

Hand-Off Reporting

- Use a standardized hand-off communication regarding specific patient risks for falls and falls with injury between caregivers. Discuss patient-specific interventions taken (TJC, 2016).
- Report immediately to the physician or health care provider if patient sustains a fall or an injury.

✦ SKILL 4.2 Designing a Restraint-Free Environment

Purpose

A restraint is any method (chemical or physical) of restricting an individual's freedom of movement, including physical activity or normal access to his or her body that (1) is not a usual part of a medical diagnostic or treatment procedure, (2) is not indicated to treat the individual's medical condition, or (3) does not promote the individual's independent functioning (TJC, 2017b). Serious and often fatal complications can result from the use of restraints. Because of the risks associated with the use of restraints, current legislation emphasizes reducing this use. The Centers for Medicare and Medicaid Services (CMS) set the original standard that restraint or seclusion may be imposed only to ensure the immediate physical safety of a patient and must be discontinued at the earliest possible time (CMS, 2008). When trying to create a restraint-free environment, patients at risk for falling or wandering present special safety challenges. Wandering is aimless pacing, attempts at elopement, or getting lost on one's own that exposes a patient to harm and is frequently in conflict with boundaries, limits, or obstacles (Butcher et al., 2018). Wandering is common among patients who are confused or disoriented (e.g., delirium) or have dementia. Interrupting a wandering patient can increase his or her distress. *A restraint-free environment is the first goal of care for all patients.*

Delegation and Collaboration

The skills of assessing patient behaviors and orientation to the environment and determining the type of restraint-free interventions to use cannot be delegated to nursing assistive personnel (NAP). Actions that provide a safe environment can be delegated to NAP. The nurse directs the NAP about:

- Using specific diversional or activity measures for making the environment safe
- Applying appropriate monitoring or alarm devices
- Reporting patient behaviors and actions (e.g., confusion, getting out of bed unassisted) to the nurse

Equipment

- Visual or auditory stimuli meaningful to patient (e.g., photos, music [MP3 player, radio], calendar, piece of art, television)
- Diversional activities (e.g., puzzle, game, audiobook, DVD)
- Wedge cushion
- Wraparound belt
- *Options:* Electronic bracelet or pressure pad alarm sensor; bed enclosure system

ASSESSMENT

1. Identify patient using at least two identifiers (e.g., name and birthday or name and medical record number) according to agency policy. *Rationale: Ensures correct patient. Complies with The Joint Commission standards and improves patient safety (TJC, 2019).*
2. Assess patient's medical history for memory impairment and underlying causes of agitation and cognitive impairment (e.g., delirium, dementia, depression). Also assess for the following: considered dangerous to self or others; gravely disabled as result of mental disorder; lacks cognitive ability (permanently or temporarily) to make relevant decisions; alcohol or substance withdrawal; fluid and electrolyte imbalance; or has physical limitations that increase risk. *Rationale: Causes of agitation and wandering are commonly associated with these conditions (Berry and Kiel, 2018; Cipriani et al., 2014; Rainier 2014; Stewart et al., 2014).*
3. Review patient's medications for over-the-counter (OTC) and prescribed medications (see Table 4.1) that pose risk for falling. Assess for interactions and untoward effects. *Rationale: Medication interactions or side effects often contribute to falling or altered mental status.*
4. Perform hand hygiene. Perform patient assessment, including patient's behavior (e.g., orientation, level of consciousness, ability to understand and follow directions), balance and gait, vision and hearing, bowel/bladder routine, level of pain, electrolyte and blood count values, and presence of orthostatic hypotension. *Rationale: Reduces transfer of microorganisms. Accurate assessment identifies patients' safety risks and the physiological causes for patient behaviors. Proper selection of nonrestraint interventions can be targeted toward conditions.*
5. For patients who wander or have known dementia, assess for cognitive decline using a validated patient assessment tool, such as the General Practitioner Assessment of Cognition (GPCOG), the Memory Impairment Screen (MIS), the Mini-Mental State Exam (MMSE), or the Mini-Cog™ Mini-Mental State Examination (MMSE) (Alzheimer's Association, n.d.). Assess patient during time of day when cognition normally decreases (e.g., at the end of the day) or at night. *Rationale: Assessments aid in determining patient's mental status, predisposition to wandering, and potential interventions.*

   Option: Assess degree of wandering behavior. Use the Algase Wandering Scale Version 2 (AWS-V2; Martin et al., 2015; Nelson and Algase, 2007). *Rationale: The AWS-V2 is a valid and reliable measure overall and for persistent walking, spatial disorientation, and eloping behavior subscales.*
6. For patient with dementia, ask family about his or her usual communication style and cues to indicate pain,

fatigue, hunger, and need to urinate or defecate. *Rationale: Enables you to use best method to determine patient needs, which often prompt wandering or agitation when need is unmet.*

7. Assess daily to determine if a medical device is necessary or can be discontinued. Consider alternative therapy (e.g., oral medications instead of intravenous) when possible. *Rationale: Patients who are agitated often attempt to remove medical devices.*
8. Inspect condition of any therapeutic medical devices. *Rationale: Patients who become restless, agitated, or confused will try to remove medical devices and then become candidates for physical restraint.*
9. Assess patient's or family caregiver's knowledge, experience, and health literacy in relation to patient's condition and need for precautions. *Rationale: Ensures patient has the capacity to obtain, communicate, process, and understand basic health information (CDC, 2016).*

STEP	RATIONALE
PLANNING	
1. Expected outcomes following completion of procedure: • Patient is injury-free and/or does not inflict injury on others while in restraint-free environment. • Patient does not remove a therapeutic medical device.	Alternatives are successful in reducing agitation and preventing injury.
2. Provide privacy, be sure patient is comfortable, and prepare environment	Reduces patient anxiety and facilitates an organized procedure.
3. Perform hand hygiene and gather any necessary supplies.	Reduces transmission of microorganisms and organizes care.
IMPLEMENTATION	
1. Orient patient and family caregiver to surroundings, introduce to staff, and explain all treatments and procedures. Be sure that patient is able to read your name badge.	Promotes patient understanding and cooperation.
2. Assign same staff to care for patient as often as possible. Encourage family and friends to stay with patient. In some agencies, volunteers are effective companions.	Increases familiarity with individuals in patient's environment, decreasing anxiety and restlessness. Companions are helpful and prevent patient from being alone.
3. Place patient in room that is easily accessible to caregivers, close to nurses' station.	Allows for frequent observation to reduce falls in high-risk patients.
4. Follow all universal fall precautions (see Box 4.1) to create a safe environment (AHRQ, 2013).	Reduces environmental risks for falls/injuries.
5. Provide visual and auditory stimuli meaningful to patient (e.g., clock, calendar, radio/MP3 player [with patient's choice of music], television, and family pictures).	Orients patient to day, time, and physical surroundings. Individualizes stimuli for this to be effective.
6. Anticipate patient's basic needs (e.g., toileting, relief of pain, relief of hunger) as quickly as possible; conduct hourly rounds (Nuckols et al., 2017).	Providing basic needs in timely fashion decreases patient discomfort, anxiety, restlessness, and incidence of falls.
7. Provide scheduled ambulation, chair activity, and toileting (e.g., ask patient every hour during rounds about toileting needs). Organize treatments so that patient has uninterrupted rest periods throughout the day. Consider using a bedside commode for toileting (but insist that patient be assisted).	Early mobility is essential for all patients (see Chapter 18). Regular opportunity to void lowers risk of patient trying to reach bathroom alone. Constant activity overstimulates and can tire patients. Commode makes toileting more accessible.

Safe Patient Care *Caution: A bedside commode can sometimes encourage patients to get up unassisted. Reinforce to patient and family caregiver that assistance is necessary.*

STEP	RATIONALE
8. Position intravenous (IV) catheters, urinary catheters, and tubes/drains out of patient view. Use commercial tube holders, camouflage with bandage or stockinette (e.g., wrapping IV site with stockinette), long-sleeved robes, and commercial sleeves over arms (Bradas et al., 2016). Place undergarments on patient with urinary catheter, or cover abdominal feeding tubes/drains with loose abdominal binder.	Reduces patient access to tubes/lines so that treatment delivery can be maintained and restraints are unnecessary.

STEP	RATIONALE
9. Decrease wandering: Eliminate stressors from environment such as cold at night, changes in daily routines, and extra visitors.	Reduced stress allows patient's energy to be channeled more appropriately.
10. Use stress-reduction techniques such as back rub, massage, and guided imagery (see Chapter 15).	Reduces level of anxiety and restlessness.
11. Use diversional activities: puzzles, games, music therapy, pet therapy, performing purposeful activity (e.g., folding towels, drawing/coloring). Be sure that it is an activity in which patient has interest. Involve family caregiver (if appropriate).	Meaningful diversional activities provide distraction, help to reduce boredom, and provide tactile stimulation. Minimize occurrences of wandering.
12. Position patient on wedge cushion and apply wraparound belt (see illustration).	Cushion prevents slipping in chair and makes it difficult for patient to get out of chair without help. Wraparound belt allows patient to lift flap for self-release.

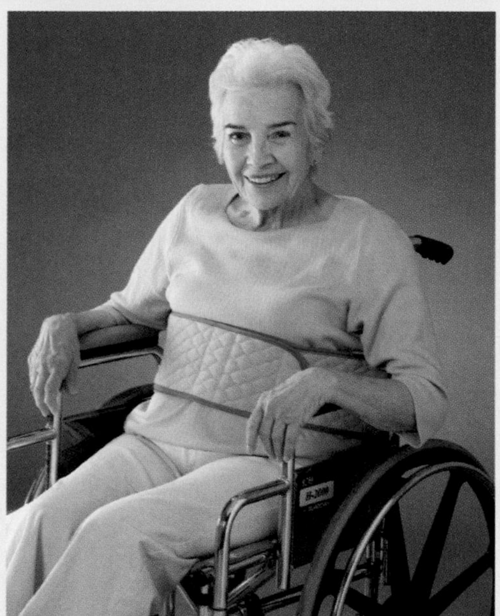

STEP 12 Wraparound belt. *(Courtesy Posey Company, Arcadia, CA.)*

STEP	RATIONALE
13. Use pressure-sensitive bed or chair pad with alarms:	Alarms alert staff to patient who is standing or rising from bed or chair without help.
a. Explain use of device to patient and family caregiver.	Reduces any misunderstanding; promotes cooperation.
b. When in bed, position device so that it is correctly positioned under patient's mid-to-low back or buttocks.	Alarm activates sooner if placed under patient's back. By the time buttocks are off sensor, patient may be almost out of bed.
c. Test alarm by applying and releasing pressure.	Ensures that alarm is audible through nurse call system.
Option: Place electronic monitoring bracelet on wrist of patient with dementia.	Tag in bracelet contains radio-frequency circuit that communicates with detection sensor installed at an exit door or elevator. Distance between tag and monitor is constantly measured, with an alarm sounding when predetermined distance is exceeded.
14. Consult with physical, speech, and occupational therapy for activities that provide stimulation and exercise.	Involvement in meaningful and purposeful activities reduces tendency to wander. Exercise improves balance and coordination.
15. Minimize invasive treatments (e.g., tube feedings, blood sampling) as much as possible.	Stimuli increase patients' restlessness.

STEP	RATIONALE

EVALUATION

1. Monitor patient's behavior routinely.	Will determine if agitation, wandering, or attempt to remove medical devices has been prevented.
2. Observe patient for any injuries.	Patient should be injury-free.
3. Observe patient's behavior toward staff, visitors, and other patients.	Ensures that patient's behavior does not cause injury to others.
4. **Use Teach-Back:** "We have talked about what we are doing to reduce your husband's wandering. Tell me ways you can help. I want to be sure you understand." Revise your instruction now or develop plan for revised family caregiver teaching if family caregiver is not able to teach back correctly.	Determines family caregiver's level of understanding of instructional topic.

Unexpected Outcomes	Related Interventions
1. Patient displays behaviors that increase risk for injury to self or others.	• Review episodes for pattern (e.g., activity, time of day) that indicates alternatives that would eliminate behavior. • Discuss alternative interventions with all caregivers and family.
2. Patient sustains injury or is agitated and places others at risk for injury.	• Notify health care provider, and complete occurrence report. • Treat injury as ordered. • Identify alternative measures for safety or behavioral control. • Apply physical restraint (see Skill 4.3) only after all other interventions are unsuccessful.
3. Patient wanders away from health care agency.	• Be prepared to follow agency policy, which should include: whom to notify; who will search for patient; which areas will be searched and their priority; who will notify authorities, if necessary; who will notify family members; who will coordinate search efforts.

Recording

- Record all behaviors that relate to cognitive status and ability to maintain safety: orientation to time, place, and person; ability to follow directions; mood and emotional status; understanding of condition and treatment plan; medication effects related to behaviors; restraint alternatives used; and patient response.
- Document evaluation of patient learning.

Hand-Off Reporting

- Report to other health care providers all interventions being used to prevent agitation or wandering and any occurrences of wandering or other behavior that places the patient at risk for injury.

✦ SKILL 4.3 Applying Physical Restraints

Purpose

Physical restraints are most commonly used in health care agencies to prevent a patient from injuring self and/or others, to prevent falls, and to protect medically necessary devices (e.g., drainage tubes, catheters, IV catheters; Rainier, 2014). The use of restraints is most common in the critical care setting, where patients who are acutely ill often unknowingly try to remove their medical devices (Rainier, 2014; Suliman et al., 2017). The process of using restraints requires continuous assessment to determine the appropriateness of use and the type of restraint/safety device to use. The CMS (2015, 2016) and TJC (2017b) have standards for reducing the use of restraints in health care settings. Properly and cautiously applied physical restraints enhance patient safety and reduce the risk of patient injury or even death (Chang et al., 2016).

The CMS standards (CMS, 2016) for the safe use of restraints in hospitals require that restraints can only be used (1) to ensure the immediate physical safety of a patient, staff member, or others; (2) when less restrictive interventions have been ineffective; (3) in accordance with a written modification to a patient's plan of care; (4) when a restraint is the least restrictive intervention that will be effective to protect a patient, staff member, or others from harm; and (5) in accordance with safe and appropriate restraint techniques determined by agency policy and procedure;

additionally, (6) restraints must be discontinued at the earliest possible time.

Restraints are a temporary way to keep patients safe. Research has shown that patients suffer fewer injuries if left unrestrained (Berry and Kiel, 2018). Know your agency's policies for the use of restraints. A licensed health care provider's order based on a face-to-face assessment is needed to implement the use of restraints. A patient's or family caregiver's informed consent is necessary in the long-term care setting.

ASSESSMENT

1. Identify patient using at least two identifiers (e.g., name and birthday or name and medical record number) according to agency policy. *Rationale: Ensures correct patient. Complies with The Joint Commission standards and improves patient safety (TJC, 2019).*
2. Review medical record to assess for underlying cause(s) of agitation and cognitive impairment leading to patient-initiated medical device removal (Bradas et al., 2016). If there is abrupt change in perception, attention, or level of consciousness:
   a. Assess for life-threatening physiological impairments. Physiological alterations might lead to accidental patient-initiated medical device removal (Bradas et al., 2016). *Rationale: Identification of conditions might lead to more appropriate medical or pharmacological treatment, eliminating need for restraints* (see Skill 4.2).
   b. Perform hand hygiene. Assess for respiratory and neurological alterations, fever and sepsis, hypo- and hyperglycemia, alcohol or substance withdrawal, and fluid and electrolyte imbalance. *Rationale: Reduces transmission of microorganisms. Factors affect patient cognition.*
   c. Notify health care provider of change in mental status and compromised physiological status.
3. Obtain baseline or premorbid cognitive function from family caregivers. *Rationale: Excellent sources of information for patient's behavior patterns and past history.*
4. Establish whether patient has history of dementia or depression. *Rationale: Cognitively impaired are at risk for exiting bed without asking for assistance.*
5. Review medications that cause risk for falling (see Table 4.1). *Rationale: Medications can alter cognition, cause postural hypotension, and create other risks.*
6. Review current laboratory values (e.g., electrolytes, blood glucose, blood culture, urinalysis). *Rationale: May reveal a fluid and electrolyte imbalance or other problems such as a blood glucose imbalance or an infection, all of which can cause sudden confusion in the elderly (National Health Service [NHS], 2015).*
7. Assess patient's current behavior (e.g., confusion, disorientation, agitation, restlessness, combativeness, inability to follow directions, or repeated removal of therapeutic devices). Does patient create a risk to other patients? *Rationale: If patient's behavior continues despite treatment or restraint alternatives, use of least restrictive restraint might be indicated.*

Safe Patient Care *In the case of alcohol withdrawal, the use of restraints can increase agitation and worsen neuropsychiatric disturbances (Hoffman and Weinhouse, 2018; Rainier, 2014).*

8. If restraint alternatives failed earlier, confer with health care provider. Review agency policies and state laws regarding restraints. **Obtain current health care provider's order for restraint,** including purpose, type, location, and time or duration of restraint. Determine if signed consent for use of restraint is necessary (long-term care). For nonviolent/non–self-destructive patients, orders are renewed per agency policy. A restraint order that is being used for violent or self-destructive behavior has a definite time limit (e.g., every 4 hours for adults, every 2 hours for children); these orders may be renewed according to the prescribed time limits for a maximum of 24 consecutive hours (TJC, 2017a). *Rationale: A health care provider's order for least restrictive type of restraint is required (TJC, 2017b).*

Safe Patient Care *A licensed independent health care provider responsible for the care of the patient evaluates the patient in person within 1 hour of the initiation of restraint used for the management of* ***violent or self-destructive behavior*** *that jeopardizes the physical safety of the patient, staff, or others. A registered nurse or a physician assistant may conduct the in-person evaluation if he or she is trained in accordance with the requirements and consults with the above health care provider after the evaluation as determined by agency policy (TJC, 2017b).*

9. Review manufacturer instructions for restraint application. Determine most appropriate size restraint. Be familiar with all devices. *Rationale: Incorrect application of restraint device results in patient injury or death.*
10. Assess patient's or family caregiver's knowledge about use of restraints, experience, and health literacy level. *Rationale: Ensures patient has the capacity to obtain, communicate, process, and understand basic health information (CDC, 2016).*

STEP	RATIONALE
PLANNING	
1. Expected outcomes following completion of procedure:	
• Patient maintains intact skin integrity, pulses, temperature, color, and sensation of restrained body part.	Restraints applied and monitored correctly.
• Patient is free from injury.	Restraints removed in a timely manner.

STEP	RATIONALE
• Patient's therapy (e.g., intravenous [IV] tube, catheters) is uninterrupted.	Disruption of therapy causes patient injury, pain, or discomfort and increases risk of infection.
• Patient maintains self-esteem and sense of dignity.	Physical restraints have detrimental effect on psychosocial well-being of patient. A sense of coerciveness and powerlessness has been experienced by psychiatric patients who were restrained (Fugger et al., 2016).
• Restraint is discontinued as soon as possible.	Limits period of time patient is at risk for injury.
2. Provide privacy, be sure patient is comfortable, and prepare environment.	Reduces patient anxiety and facilitates an organized procedure.
3. Perform hand hygiene. Gather equipment.	Reduces transmission of microorganisms and organizes care.
4. Explain to patient and family caregiver the choice of restraint, how it is to be applied, and the monitoring that will be conducted.	Reduces patient and family caregiver anxiety and promotes cooperation.

IMPLEMENTATION

STEP	RATIONALE
1. Adjust bed to proper height and lower side rail on side of patient contact. Be sure that patient is comfortable and in proper body alignment.	Allows you to reposition patient during restraint application without injuring self or patient. Proper alignment prevents contracture formation when restraints are in place.
2. Perform hand hygiene. Inspect area where restraint is to be placed. Note if there is any nearby tubing or device. Assess condition of skin, sensation, adequacy of circulation, and range of joint motion.	Restraints sometimes compress and interfere with functioning of devices or tubes. Assessment provides baseline to monitor patient's response to restraint.
3. Pad skin and bony prominences (as necessary) that will be under restraint.	Reduces friction and pressure from restraint to skin and underlying tissue.
4. Apply proper-size restraint. **NOTE:** Refer to manufacturer directions.	
a. *Mitten restraint:* Thumbless mitten device restrains patient's hands. Place hand in mitten, being sure that Velcro strap is around wrist and not forearm (see illustration).	Prevents patient from dislodging or removing medical device, removing dressings, or scratching but allows greater movement than wrist restraint. It is considered a restraint alternative if untethered and patient is physically and cognitively able to remove it.
b. *Elbow restraint (freedom splint):* Restraint consists of rigidly padded fabric that wraps around arm and is closed with Velcro. The upper end has a clamp that hooks to sleeve of patient's gown or shirt (see illustration). Insert arm so that elbow joint rests against padded area, keeping joint extended.	The restraint makes it difficult to remove or disrupt a medical device near the face or neck. It does not impede removing abdominal or urinary medical devices.

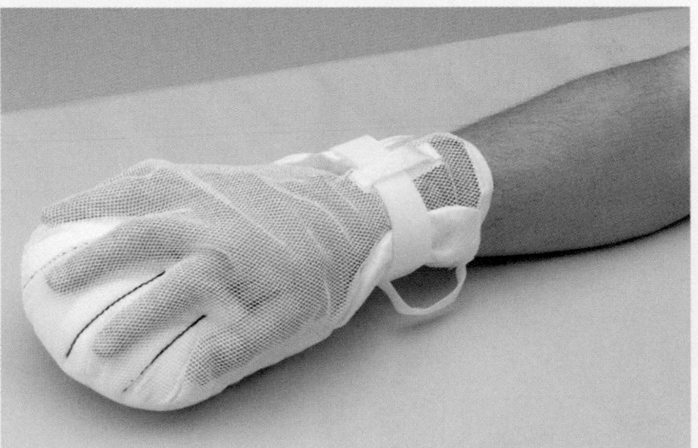

STEP 4a Mitten restraint. *(Courtesy Posey Company, Arcadia, CA.)*

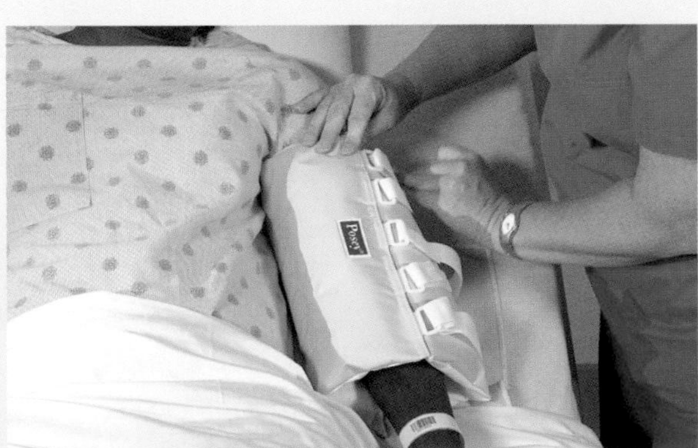

STEP 4b Freedom elbow restraint.

STEP	RATIONALE
c. *Belt or body restraint:* Have patient in sitting position in bed. Apply belt over clothes, gown, or pajamas. Be sure to place restraint at waist, not chest or abdomen. Slot in belt may be positioned in front for limited movement or rear for increased movement. Remove wrinkles or creases in clothing. Bring ties through slots in belt. Help patient lie down in bed. Have patient roll to side, and avoid applying belt too tightly. Ensure that straps secured to bedframe are snug so that belt does not slide to sides of bed (see illustrations). *Option:* Apply restraint net if intent is to limit patient turning.	Restrains center of gravity and prevents patient from rolling off stretcher, sitting up while on stretcher, or falling out of bed. Tight application interferes with ventilation if belt moves up over abdomen or chest.
d. *Soft extremity (ankle or wrist) restraint:* Restraint made of soft quilted material or sheepskin with foam padding. Wrap limb restraint around wrist or ankle with soft part toward skin and secure snugly (not tightly) in place by Velcro strap (see illustration). Insert two fingers under secured restraint (see illustration).	Restraint designed to immobilize one or all extremities. Maintain immobilization of extremity to protect patient from fall or accidental removal of therapeutic device (e.g., IV tube, Foley catheter). Tight application interferes with circulation and potentially causes neurovascular injury.

Safe Patient Care *Patient with wrist and ankle restraints is at risk for aspiration if positioned supine. Place patient in lateral position or with head of bed elevated rather than supine.*

STEP	RATIONALE
5. Attach restraint straps to part of bedframe that moves when raising or lowering head of bed. Be sure that straps are secure. *Do not attach to side rails.* Attach restraint to chair frame for patient in chair or wheelchair, ensuring that buckle is out of patient's reach.	Properly positioned strap does not tighten and restrict circulation when bed is raised or lowered.

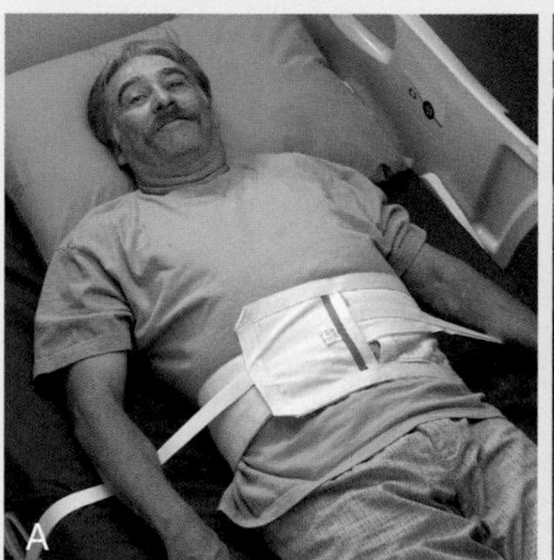

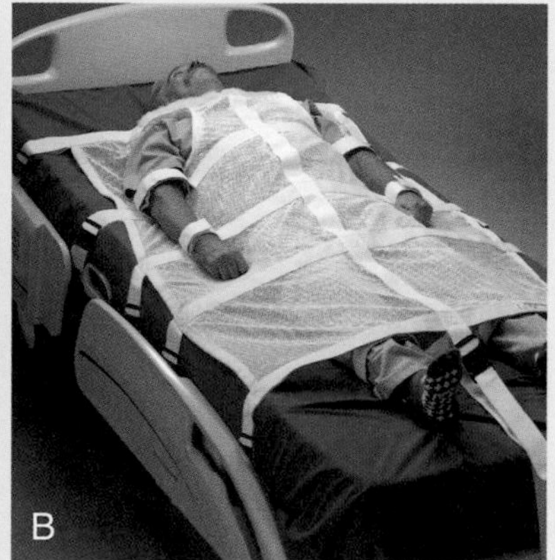

STEP 4c (A) Properly applied belt restraint allows patient to turn in bed. (B) *Option:* Restraint with net limits patient's ability to turn.

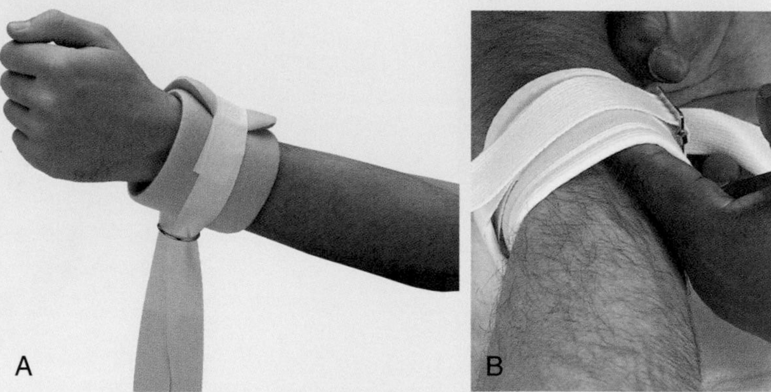

STEP 4d (A) Soft extremity restraint. (B) Check restraint for constriction by inserting two fingers under restraint. *(Courtesy Posey Company, Acadia, CA.)*

STEP	RATIONALE
6. Secure restraints on bedframe with quick-release buckle (see illustration). *Do not tie strap in a knot.* Be sure that buckle is out of patient reach.	Allows for quick release in emergency.

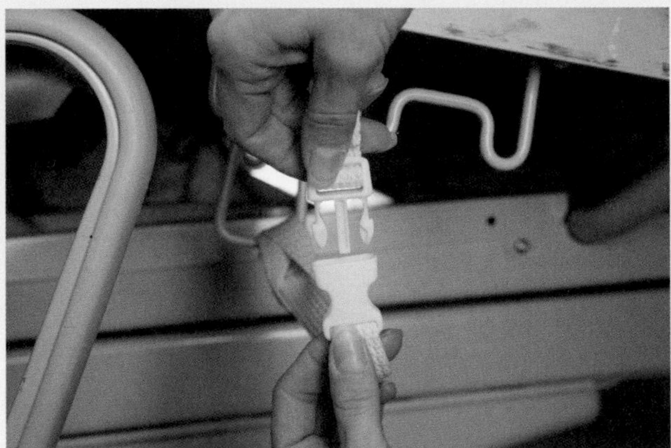

STEP 6 Quick-release buckle makes it easier to disconnect and evacuate patients in an emergency.

STEP	RATIONALE
7. Double-check and insert two fingers under secured restraint one more time. Assess proper placement of restraint, including skin integrity, pulses, skin temperature and color, and sensation of restrained body part. Place bed in lowest position after restraint(s) applied.	Provides baseline to later evaluate if injury develops from restraint. Provides safest environment in which to leave a patient who is restrained.
8. Perform hand hygiene. Remove restraint at least every 2 hours (TJC, 2017b) or more frequently as determined by agency policy. Reposition patient, provide comfort and toileting measures, and evaluate patient condition each time. If patient is violent or noncompliant, remove one restraint at a time and/or have staff assistance while removing restraints.	Provides opportunity to attend to patient's basic needs and determine need for continuation of restraints.

Safe Patient Care *Do not leave a patient who is violent or aggressive unattended while restraints are off. Monitoring of violent/self-destructive patients placed in restraints is continuous (by way of video or audio) versus every 2 hours for nonviolent patients.*

STEP	RATIONALE
9. Be sure nurse call system is within patient's reach.	Allows patient, family, or caregiver to get help quickly.
10. Leave bed or chair with wheels locked. Keep bed in lowest position.	Prevents bed or chair from moving if patient tries to get out. If patient falls with bed in lowest position, this reduces chance of injury.
11. Remove and dispose of any supplies. Perform hand hygiene.	Reduces transmission of microorganisms.

EVALUATION

STEP	RATIONALE
1. After restraint application, evaluate patient's response to restraints: **a.** Nonviolent patients—conduct evaluation for signs of injury (e.g., circulation, range of motion [ROM], vital signs, skin condition), behavior and psychologic status, and readiness for discontinuation (frequency based on agency policy) (TJC, 2017b). **b.** For violent/self-destructive patients, conduct same evaluation every 15 minutes. Perform visual checks if patient is too agitated to approach (TJC, 2017b).	Frequent evaluation prevents injury to patient and ensures removal of restraint at earliest possible time. Frequency of monitoring guides staff in determining appropriate intervals for evaluation based on patient's needs and condition, type of restraint used, risk associated with use of chosen intervention, and other relevant factors.
2. Evaluate patient's need for toileting, nutrition and fluids, hygiene, and elimination and release restraint at least every 2 hours.	Prevents injury to patient and attends to basic needs.

STEP	RATIONALE
3. Evaluate patient for any complications of immobility.	Early detection of skin irritation, restricted breathing, or reduction in mobility prevents serious adverse events.
4. Renewal of restraints: **a.** Nonviolent patients may have renewal of restraints based on agency policy. However, the restraint must be discontinued at the earliest possible time, regardless of the scheduled expiration of the order **b.** Violent/self-destructive patients may have restraints renewed within the following limits: • 4 hours for adults 18 years of age or older • 2 hours for children and adolescents 9 to 17 years of age • 1 hour for children under 9 years of age These orders may be renewed according to the time limits for a maximum of 24 consecutive hours	Ensures that restraint application continues to be medically appropriate.
5. Observe IV catheters, urinary catheters, and drainage tubes to determine that they are positioned correctly and that therapy remains uninterrupted.	Reinsertion is uncomfortable and increases risk for infection or interrupts therapy.
6. Use Teach-Back: "We have talked about the reason we are using restraints on your father. Tell me that reason. I want to be sure you understand." Revise your instruction now or develop a plan for revised family caregiver teaching if family caregiver is not able to teach back correctly.	Determines family caregiver's level of understanding of instructional topic.

Unexpected Outcomes	Related Interventions
1. Patient experiences impaired skin integrity.	• Evaluate need for continued use of restraint and if alternatives can be used. • If restraint is still needed, be sure that it is applied correctly, and provide adequate padding. • Check skin under restraint for abrasions, and remove restraints more often. Provide appropriate skin care, and change wet or soiled restraints.
2. Patient becomes more confused or agitated.	• Determine cause of behavior and eliminate if possible; consult with health care provider. • Determine need for more or less sensory stimulation, and make any stimulation meaningful. • Reorient as needed, and try restraint-free options.
3. Patient has neurovascular injury (e.g., cyanosis, pallor, and coldness of skin or complains of tingling, pain, or numbness).	• Remove restraint immediately, stay with patient, and have health care provider notified. • Protect extremity from further injury.

Recording

- Record restraint alternatives tried, patient's behavior, level of orientation, and patient or family member's statement of understanding of the purpose of restraint and consent for application (if required by agency).
- Record placement and purpose for restraint, type and location of restraint, time applied, time restraint ended, and all routine assessments made in nurses' notes and flow sheet.
- Record patient's behavior after restraint application. Record times patient was assessed, attempts to use alternatives to restraint and patient's response, times restraint was released (temporarily and permanently), and patient's response when restraint was removed.
- Document evaluation of patient learning.

Hand-Off Reporting

- Immediately report any injury resulting from a restraint to RN in charge and health care provider.
- During hand-off, report location of restraint, last time assessment was conducted, and findings.

✦ SKILL 4.4 Seizure Precautions

Purpose

Seizure precautions are guidelines that health care providers follow to minimize injury to a patient during any type of seizure. Observation during a seizure is critical. A seizure is a sudden, abnormal electrical discharge in the brain causing alterations in behavior, sensation, or consciousness. Anything that interrupts the normal connections between neurons in the brain can cause a seizure, including a high fever, low blood sugar, high blood sugar, alcohol or drug withdrawal, or a brain concussion (Johns Hopkins Medicine, n.d.). Anyone can have one or more seizures; however, a person who has two or more seizures is considered to have epilepsy. The two broad categories of epileptic seizures are generalized seizures (involving both sides of the brain) and partial seizures (involving one or more areas of one side of the brain; Box 4.2).

Status epilepticus is an emergent situation and involves more than 30 minutes of continuous seizure activity or two or more sequential seizures without full recovery of consciousness between each seizure (Glauser et al., 2016; Hill et al., 2017). Status epilepticus can be convulsive (shown by rhythmic jerking of the extremities) or nonconvulsive (seizure activity shown on an EEG). The American Epilepsy Society released practice guidelines for patients with status epilepticus (Glauser et al., 2016; NICE, 2014). Within the first 2 minutes, establishing and protecting the airway when a patient loses consciousness is a priority. Noninvasive airway protection and gas exchange with head positioning should be done immediately, keeping the airway patent and administering oxygen. When the seizure begins to subside, intubation (insertion of an artificial airway) should be attempted only if gas exchange is compromised or if the patient is believed to have increased intracranial pressure.

Delegation and Collaboration

The skill of assessing a patient's risk for seizures cannot be delegated to nursing assistive personnel (NAP). However, the interventions for making a patient's environment safe and the ongoing care of patients on seizure precautions can be delegated. The nurse directs the NAP about:

- The patient's prior seizure history and factors that may trigger a seizure
- Taking immediate action in the event of a seizure by protecting the patient from falling or injury, not trying to restrain the patient, and not placing anything into patient's mouth
- Informing the nurse immediately when a seizure activity develops
- Observing the patient's behaviors during a seizure

BOX 4.2

Phases of a Seizure

- Aura—the start of a partial seizure. If an aura is the only phase a patient experiences, the patient has had a simple partial seizure. If the seizure spreads and affects consciousness, it is a complete partial seizure. If the seizure spreads to the rest of the brain, it is a generalized seizure.
- Ictus—meaning "attack." Ictus is another word for the physical seizure involving a series of muscle contractions, called tonic and clonic contractions.
- Postictal—meaning "after the attack." Postictal refers to the aftereffects of a seizure (e.g., arm numbness, altered consciousness, partial paralysis, loss of memory).

Equipment

- Seizure pads for side rails and headboard
- Suction machine, oral Yankauer suction catheter, oral airway (see Chapter 16)
- Oxygen via nasal cannula or face mask
- Equipment for vital signs, pulse oximetry, and blood glucose testing (see Chapters 7 and 9)
- Equipment for IV insertion (see Chapter 28); bag of 0.9% normal saline solution
- Emergency antiepileptic medications:
  - First-line treatment (tried first and usually used on its own):
    - Focal seizure: carbamazepine, lamotrigine
    - Generalized seizures: sodium valproate, lamotrigine
  - Alternative first-line treatment (added to a first-line treatment [so are used in combination])
    - Focal seizure: levetiracetam, oxcarbazepine, sodium valproate
    - Generalized seizures: carbamazepine, oxcarbazepine
- Clean gloves
- *Option:* protective headgear

ASSESSMENT

1. Identify patient using at least two identifiers (e.g., name and birthday or name and medical record number) according to agency policy. *Rationale: Ensures correct patient. Complies with The Joint Commission standards and improves patient safety (TJC, 2019).*
2. Review medical record for medical and surgical conditions that may contribute to or be a cause of a seizure (Box 4.3) and for any bleeding tendencies. *Rationale: Common conditions that lead to seizures or worsen existing seizure condition. Bleeding conditions predispose patient to injury during a seizure.*
3. Assess record for patient's seizure history (e.g., new diagnosis, seizure within past year), knowledge of precipitating factors (e.g., emotional stress, sleep deprivation), frequency of seizures, presence of an aura (e.g., metallic taste, sense of breeze blowing on face, or noxious odor), symptoms during a seizure (Box 4.4), and sequence of seizure events known. Use a family caregiver as resource if needed. *Rationale: Allows you to eliminate triggers that can cause seizure, anticipate onset of seizure activity and take appropriate safety precautions.*
4. Assess medication history (e.g., antidepressants and antipsychotics). Ask patient about adherence to anticonvulsants, and review therapeutic drug levels if laboratory test results are available. *Rationale: Certain medications lower seizure threshold. Seizure medications must be taken as prescribed and not stopped suddenly; otherwise, may precipitate seizure activity.*
5. Inspect patient's environment for potential safety hazards (e.g., extra furniture or equipment). Keep bed in low position, with side rails up at head of bed. *Rationale: Protects patient from injury sustained by striking head or body on furniture or equipment.*

BOX 4.3

Possible Precipitating Factors for or Causes of Seizures

Acute Processes

- Metabolic disturbances: electrolyte abnormalities, hypoglycemia, renal failure
- Central nervous system (CNS) infection: meningitis, encephalitis, abscess
- Stroke: ischemic, intracerebral or subarachnoid hemorrhage, cerebral sinus thrombosis
- Head trauma with or without epidural or subdural hematoma
- Drug issues/toxicity: Withdrawal from opioid, benzodiazepine, barbiturate, or alcohol; noncompliance with antiepileptic drugs (AEDs)
- Hypoxia, cardiac arrest
- Encephalopathy

Chronic Processes

- Preexisting epilepsy: breakthrough seizures or discontinuation of AEDs
- Chronic alcohol abuse; ethanol intoxication or withdrawal
- CNS tumors

Factors in Children

- Prolonged febrile seizures are the most frequent cause of status epilepticus in children.
- CNS infections, especially bacterial meningitis; inborn errors of metabolism; and ingestion are frequent causes of status epilepticus

Data from Glauser T et al: Evidence-based guideline: Treatment of convulsive status epilepticus in children and adults: Report of the Guideline Committee of the American Epilepsy Society. *Epilepsy Curr* 16(1):48, 2016; and Schachter, S: Evaluation and management of the first seizure in adults, *UpToDate*, 2018. https://www.uptodate.com/contents/evaluation-and-management-of-the-first-seizure-in-adults.

BOX 4.4

Symptoms or Warning Signs of Seizures

- Loss of bowel or bladder function
- Breathing problems
- Staring
- Eyes rolling backward
- Changes in smell or taste
- Jerking movements of the arms and legs
- Stiffening of the arms and legs
- Loss of consciousness
- Falling suddenly for no apparent reason, especially when associated with loss of consciousness
- Periods of rapid eye blinking and staring

6. Assess patient's individual and cultural perspective about the meaning of seizures and their treatment. *Rationale: Some cultures follow different caring practices for a person with seizures.*
7. Assess patient's or family caregiver's knowledge about seizures and seizure precautions, experience, and health literacy level. *Rationale: Ensures patient has the capacity to obtain, communicate, process, and understand basic health information (CDC, 2016).*

STEP	RATIONALE
PLANNING	
1. Expected outcomes following completion of procedure:	
• Patient remains free of traumatic injury while experiencing seizure.	Seizure precautions prevent patient from incurring injury from a fall or seizure.
• Patient's airway remains patent during seizure activity.	Airway occlusion and aspiration are potential complications of seizure activity.
• Patient does not experience lowered sense of self-esteem following seizure episode.	Loss of bowel or bladder control is common in generalized seizures, causing patient to feel embarrassed.
• Patient or family caregiver can identify triggers that lead to patient having a seizure.	Knowledge can help in preventing seizure activity.
2. Provide privacy, be sure patient is comfortable, and prepare environment.	Reduces patient anxiety and facilitates an organized procedure.
3. Perform hand hygiene and prepare equipment.	Reduces transmission of microorganisms and organizes care.
4. Inform patient and appropriate family caregiver that patient is on seizure precautions. Discuss the possible triggers that result in patient's seizure activity. Include discussion of approaches to adopt seizure precautions in the patient's home environment.	May help to relieve patient and family caregiver anxiety and aid in their participation in patient care.

STEP	RATIONALE

IMPLEMENTATION

1. For patients with history of seizures, keep bed in lowest position, with side rails up (see agency policy). Pad rails if patient is at risk for head injury, and offer protective headgear as an option. Have oral suction and oxygen equipment ready for use (see illustration).

Modifications to environment minimize risk of injury from seizure activity or related fall. Use padded side rails and headgear only when patient is at risk for head injury.

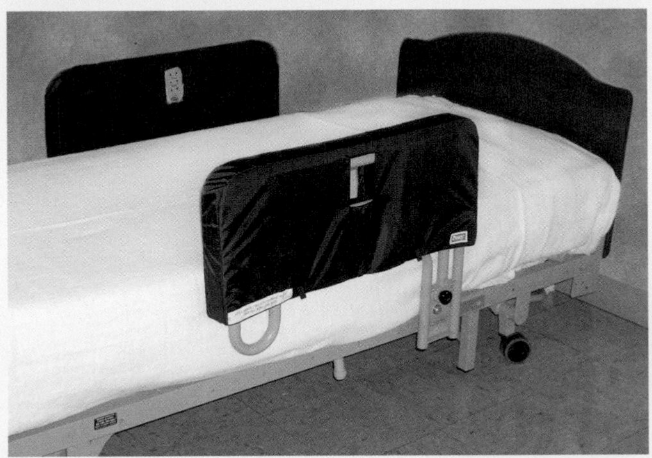

STEP 1 Padded side rails for patients at risk for head injury.

2. Place patient with history of seizures in room close to nurses' station or room with video monitor (if available).

Improves likelihood of quick identification of seizure and response with emergency equipment.

3. **Partial or general seizure response:**
   a. Position patient safely.
      (1) Guide a patient who is standing or sitting to the floor and protect head by cradling in your lap or placing pillow under head. Position patient so as to keep head tilted to maximize breathing (if able). Try to position patient on side *but do not force*. Do not lift patient from floor to bed during seizure.

      Position protects patient from aspiration and traumatic injury, especially head injury.

      (2) If patient is in bed, turn him or her onto side *(do not force)* and raise side rails.
   b. Note time the seizure began, and call for help immediately to have staff member bring emergency cart to bedside and clear surrounding area of furniture. Provide airway protection and gas exchange by positioning head. Have health care provider and rapid response team notified immediately.

   Timing and description of seizure may help in ultimate identification of type of seizure. Establishing and protecting airway when patient loses consciousness must occur in first 2 minutes (Glauser et al., 2016).

Safe Patient Care *Activate your agency's rapid response team. When a patient demonstrates signs of imminent clinical deterioration, a team of providers is summoned to the bedside to immediately assess and treat the patient, with the goal of preventing intensive care unit transfer, cardiac arrest, or death* (AHRQ, 2017).

   c. Keep patient in side-lying position (if possible), supporting head and keeping it flexed slightly forward.

   Position prevents tongue from blocking airway and promotes drainage of secretions, reducing risk of aspiration.

   d. Do not restrain patient; if patient is flailing limbs, hold them loosely. Loosen restrictive clothing/gown to aid breathing.

   Prevents musculoskeletal injury. Promotes free ventilatory movement of chest and abdomen.

   e. *Never force any object into patient's mouth*, such as fingers, medicine, tongue depressor, or airway, when teeth are clenched.

   Prevents injury to mouth and possible aspiration.

Safe Patient Care *Injury can result from forcible insertion of a hard object into the mouth. Soft objects can break and become aspirated. Insert a bite block or oral airway in advance if you recognize the possibility of a generalized seizure.*

STEP	RATIONALE
f. If possible, provide privacy. Have staff control flow of visitors in area.	Embarrassment is common after a seizure, especially if others witnessed it.
g. Observe sequence and timing of seizure activity. Note type of seizure activity (tonic, clonic, staring, blinking); whether more than one type of seizure occurs; sequence of seizure progression; level of consciousness; character of breathing; presence of incontinence; presence of autonomic signs of lip smacking, mastication, or grimacing; rolling of eyes.	Continued observation helps document, diagnose, and treat seizure disorder.
h. As patient regains consciousness, assess vital signs and reorient and reassure him or her. Explain what happened and answer patient's questions. Stay with patient until fully awake.	Informing patients of type of seizure activity experienced helps them to participate knowledgeably in their care. Some patients remain confused for a period of time after a seizure or become violent.
4. Status epilepticus is a medical emergency.	
a. Follow Steps 3a to 3e to protect patient and call rapid response team.	Ensures rapid management of airway and breathing.
b. Assist health care provider with intubation (introduction of endotracheal tube or oral airway; see Chapter 30) if oxygen saturation is compromised or elevated intracranial pressure is suspected. (**NOTE:** Apply clean gloves if timing allows.) Physician on team will intubate patient when jaw is relaxed (between seizure activity).	Airway establishes oxygenation (Glauser et al., 2016; Smith et al., 2015).
c. Access and administer oxygen; turn on suction equipment; keep airway patent with oral suctioning (if possible).	Maintains oxygenation.

Safe Patient Care *Never place hands in patient's mouth during a seizure. The patient may accidentally bite your fingers. Do not force any type of airway into mouth.*

STEP	RATIONALE
d. Have another nurse on team measuring blood pressure, heart rate, respirations, and oxygen saturation immediately and then every 2 minutes, and have team member perform fingerstick to check blood glucose (Schachter, 2018; Smith et al., 2015).	Necessary to monitor and support baseline vital signs and determine if patient is hypoglycemic (common cause of seizure).
e. Member of team will prepare for and insert IV catheter (if one is not in place) with 0.9% sodium chloride infusing and administer IV antiseizure medications (see Chapter 28).	Provides route for IV medication to stop seizure and for fluid resuscitation (Schachter, 2018; Smith et al., 2015).
f. As seizure subsides, suction patient's airway if secretions have accumulated. If oral airway was inserted, be sure that it remains in correct position. Continue oxygen administration.	Maintains open airway, decreases chance of aspiration, and promotes oxygenation.
g. Keep patient in side-lying position of comfort in bed with side rails up and bed in lowest position.	Provides for continued safety to reduce risk of aspiration of secretions as patient regains consciousness and lessens risk of fall with injury if patient tries to exit bed.
h. As patient regains consciousness, reorient and reassure. Explain what happened and provide quiet, nonstimulating environment (e.g., lights low, minimal care interruptions). Place nurse call system within reach. Instruct patient not to get out of bed without help.	Provides for continued safety. Patients are often confused and lethargic following seizure (postictal). At risk for falls if they attempt to get out of bed.
5. Clean up patient care area; dispose of used supplies. Perform hand hygiene.	Reduces transmission of microorganisms.

EVALUATION

STEP	RATIONALE
1. Check vital signs and oxygen saturation every 15 minutes during postictal phase, and maintain patent airway.	Determines patient's cardiopulmonary status and response to seizure episode.
2. Recheck blood glucose per health care provider order or agency protocol.	Determines if normal blood glucose level has been reached.

STEP	RATIONALE
3. Examine patient for injury, including oral cavity (broken teeth, laceration of tongue or mucosa) and extremities.	Determines presence of any traumatic injuries resulting from seizure activity.

Safe Patient Care *If onset of seizure was not witnessed and you suspect that patient fell and struck head, treat as a closed head injury or spinal injury. Place a cervical collar on patient before attempting to turn or reposition.*

STEP	RATIONALE
4. Evaluate patient's mental status after seizure (level of consciousness, confusion, hallucinations). Encourage him or her to verbalize feelings.	Temporary mental status changes are common following seizure. Therapeutic interaction enables patient to recognize feelings associated with having a seizure disorder.
5. Help health care provider conduct neurological examination of patient and collect any ordered blood tests (see Chapter 7).	Evaluates for any intracranial lesions, bleeding, and life-threatening metabolic condition (Schachter, 2018; Smith et al., 2015).
6. **Use Teach-Back:** "We talked about what to do if your father has a seizure at home. Tell me what steps you would take." Revise your instruction now or develop a plan for revised teaching if family caregiver is not able to teach back correctly.	Determines family caregiver's level of understanding of instructional topic.

Unexpected Outcomes	Related Interventions
1. Patient suffers traumatic injury.	• Continue to protect patient from further injury. • Notify health care provider immediately. • Administer prescribed treatments. • Reassess patient's environment and eliminate any safety hazards. • Complete agency occurrence report.
2. Patient aspirates oral secretions.	• Turn onto side, insert oral airway, and apply suction to remove material in oral pharynx and maintain patent airway (see Chapter 16). • Administer oxygen as needed per order.

Recording

- Record timing of seizure activity, sequence of events, presence of aura (if any), level of consciousness, vital signs, posture, color, movements of extremities, incontinence, and patient's status (physical and emotional) immediately after seizure.
- Record evaluation of family caregiver learning.

Hand-Off Reporting

- Report seizure to health care provider immediately, including timing of seizure, number of seizures, and sequence of relevant events. Note a status epilepticus, which is an emergency.

PROCEDURAL GUIDELINE 4.1 *Fire, Electrical, and Chemical Safety*

Purpose

Structural fires in health care agencies have been on the decline, but from 2009 to 2013, U.S. fire departments responded to over 5500 fires in health care properties (National Fire Protection Association [NFPA], 2016). Fortunately, most of the fires were very small. The leading causes of fires in health care agencies involve cooking equipment in cafeterias, electrical distribution and wiring, intentional causes, and smoking materials (NFPA, 2016). Smoking-related fires pose a significant risk because of unauthorized smoking in beds or bathrooms by patients and visitors. Health care agencies routinely check and maintain all electrical devices. Every biomedical device (e.g., suction machine, infusion pump) must have a safety inspection sticker with an expiration date applied to it. Electrical equipment in good working order requires a three-prong electrical plug for proper grounding. If a patient brings an electrical device to a health care agency an engineer must inspect the device for safe wiring and function before use. Prevention is the key to fire safety. Always comply with agency smoking policies, use equipment correctly, and keep combustible materials away from heat sources.

Chemicals in medications (e.g., chemotherapy drugs), anesthetic gases, cleaning solutions, and disinfectants are potentially toxic. They injure the body after skin or mucous membrane (e.g., eyes) contact, ingestion, or vapor inhalation. Health care agencies provide

Continued

PROCEDURAL GUIDELINE 4.1 *Fire, Electrical, and Chemical Safety—cont'd*

employees access to a safety data sheet (SDS) (previously called material safety data sheet) for each hazardous chemical in the workplace (U.S. Department of Labor, 2015). An SDS form contains information about the properties of the particular chemical and how to handle the substance safely (Box 4.5).

Delegation and Collaboration

The skill of fire, electrical, and chemical safety can be delegated to nursing assistive personnel (NAP). A nurse leads the health care team in an emergency response. In the event of fire, a nurse collaborates with the fire department. In the event of an electrical or chemical event, the team collaborates with the safety officer of the agency. Knowing where all staff and patients are is essential during these types of emergencies in case of need for evacuation. The nurse directs the NAP to:

- Identify patients requiring the most help to evacuate or protect.
- Be aware of any risks for chemical exposure.

Equipment

Fire: Appropriate fire extinguisher for fire: type A, B, C, or ABC

Chemical: Appropriate personal protective equipment (PPE): clean gloves, mask, gown; SDS form

Procedural Steps

1. Review agency policies for rapid response to fire, electrical, and chemical emergency. Know your responsibilities, such as initiating fire alarm and patient evacuation.
2. Know the location of fire alarms, emergency equipment (e.g., fire extinguishers), SDS forms, emergency eyewash stations, and emergency exit routes on your work unit.
3. Be alert to situations that increase the risk of fire (e.g., a patient on oxygen charging a cell phone while in bed). Regularly check a patient room for electrical or fire hazards.
4. Know which patients are on oxygen. Oxygen delivery may be shut off in the event of a severe fire; be aware of location and who has access to the shut-off valve.
5. Inspect equipment for current maintenance sticker. Check electrical equipment for basic safety features (i.e., intact cords and plugs, intact casing). Know agency process for tagging and reporting broken or unsafe equipment.
6. Know your patient's mental status and ability to ambulate, transfer, or move so that if a fire occurs, you can anticipate the procedures needed for evacuation.
7. Fire safety:
   a. In the event of a fire, follow the acronym **RACE**.
      (1) Rescue patient from immediate injury by removing from area or shielding from fire to avoid burns.
      (2) Activate fire alarm immediately. Follow agency policy for alerting staff to respond. (In many situations perform Steps 1 and 2 simultaneously by using call system to alert staff while you help patients at risk.)
      (3) Contain the fire by doing the following:
         (a) Closing all doors and windows
         (b) Turning off oxygen and electrical equipment
         (c) Placing wet towels along base of doors
      (4) Evacuate patients:
         (a) Direct ambulatory patients to walk by themselves to a safe area. Know the fire exits and emergency evacuation route.
         (b) If patient is on life support, maintain respiratory status manually (Ambu bag) until you remove him or her from fire area.
         (c) Move bedridden patients by stretcher, bed, or wheelchair.
         (d) For patients who cannot walk or ambulate use these options:
            (i) Place on blanket and drag patient out of area of danger.
            (ii) *Use two-person swing*: Place patient in sitting position and have two staff members form a seat by clasping forearms together. Lift patient into "seat" and carry out of area of danger (see illustrations A and B).

Safe Patient Care *Consider the patient's weight and size when choosing an evacuation carry. Use safe patient-handling techniques. Have a staff member help to avoid injury.*

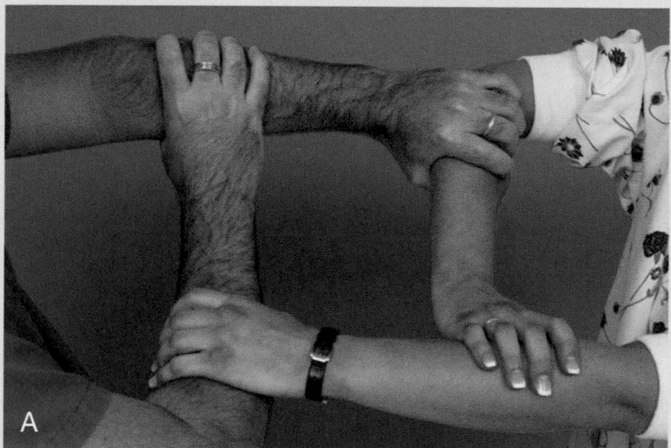

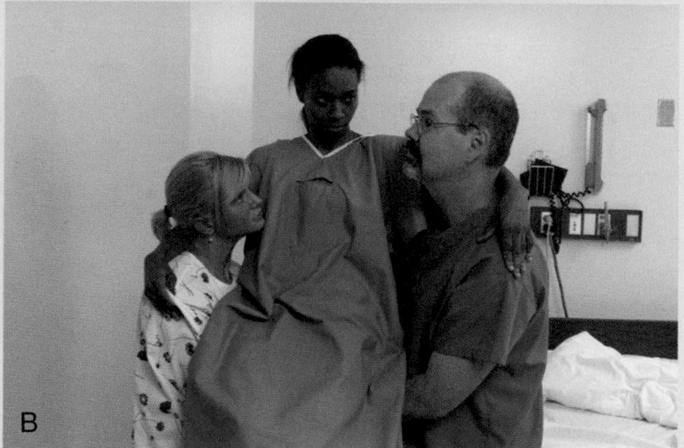

STEP 7a(4)(d)(ii) (A) Hands positioned to form two-person evacuation swing. (B) Patient seated firmly on swing and holding shoulders of nurses for evacuation.

PROCEDURAL GUIDELINE 4.1 *Fire, Electrical, and Chemical Safety—cont'd*

(e) If fire department personnel are on scene, they will help with patient evacuation.

b. Extinguish fire using appropriate fire extinguisher: **type A** for ordinary combustibles (e.g., wood, cloth, paper, most plastics); **type B** for flammable liquids (e.g., gasoline, grease, paint, anesthetic gas); **type C** for electrical equipment; **type ABC** for any type of fire (most common extinguisher in use). To use an extinguisher, follow the acronym **PASS.**

(1) **P**ull the pin (see illustration A).

(2) **A**im nozzle at base of fire (see illustration B).

(3) **S**queeze extinguisher handles (see illustration C).

(4) **S**weep from side to side to coat area evenly.

c. Most agencies have fire doors that are held open by magnets and close automatically when a fire alarm sounds. Fire doors should never be blocked.

8. Once patient has been evacuated, make the patient comfortable. Keep locks on wheelchairs or beds locked. Perform hand hygiene.

9. Electrical safety:

a. If patient receives an electrical shock, immediately turn off power to electrical source and assess for presence of a pulse. *Caution:* When disengaging electrical source, check for presence of water on floor.

Safe Patient Care *Do not touch a person who is being shocked while he or she is still engaged with the electrical source. If unable to turn off power, call emergency number for help.*

b. Once the source of electricity is disconnected, provide appropriate assistance. If patient is pulseless, institute emergency resuscitation (see Chapter 30).

c. Notify emergency personnel and patient's health care provider.

d. If patient has a pulse and remains alert and oriented, obtain vital signs and assess the skin for signs of thermal injury.

10. Chemical safety (the following steps apply to the nurse):

a. If you or a work colleague are exposed to a chemical, treat chemical splashes to the eyes immediately. Flush eyes with water using clean, lukewarm tap water for 15 to 20 minutes. Stand under a shower or place head under running faucet. Remove contact lenses if flushing does not remove them (see Chapter 12). Treat exposure of the skin by flushing with clean, lukewarm tap water for 15 minutes.

b. Notify people in the immediate area of the spill, and evacuate all nonessential personnel from area.

c. Refer to SDS form for chemical; if the spilled material is flammable, turn off electrical and heat sources.

d. Avoid breathing vapors of spilled material; apply appropriate respirator.

e. Use appropriate personal protective equipment (refer to SDS form) to clean up a spill.

f. Dispose of any materials used in cleanup as hazardous waste.

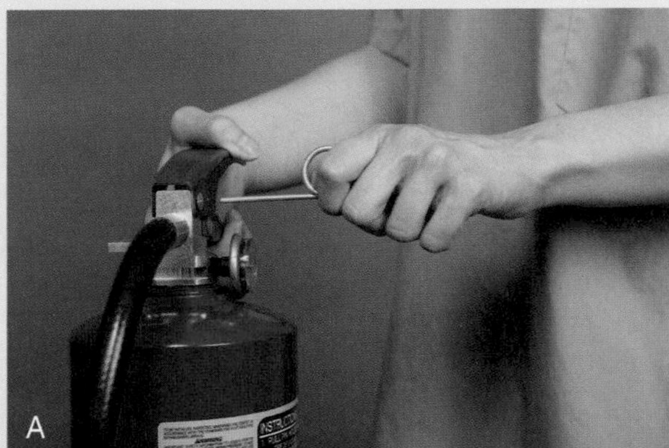

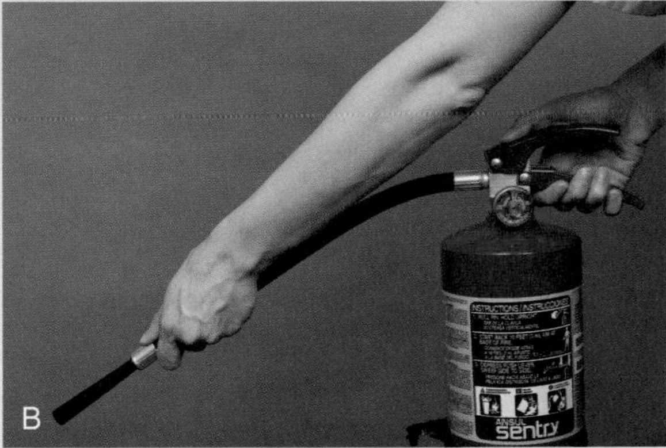

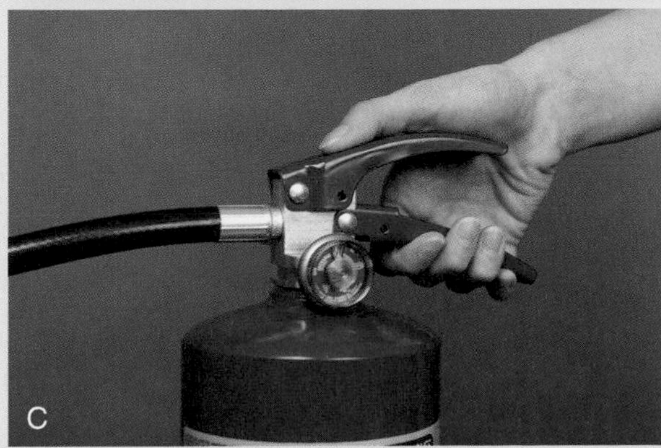

STEP 7b (A) Pull safety pin from fire extinguisher. (B) Aim nozzle of hose at base of fire. (C) Squeeze handle while sweeping side to side with nozzle.

BOX 4.5

Information Required on OSHA Safety Data Sheets

- **Identification:** Product identifier; manufacturer or distributor name, address, phone number; emergency phone number; recommended use; restrictions on use
- **Hazard(s):** All hazards regarding the chemical; required label element
- **Composition/information on ingredients:** Chemical ingredients; trade secret claims
- **First-aid measures:** Symptoms/effects, acute, delayed; required treatment
- **Fire-fighting measures:** Suitable extinguishing techniques, equipment; chemical hazards from fire
- **Accidental release measures:** Emergency procedures; protective equipment; proper methods of containment and cleanup
- **Handling and storage:** Precautions for safe handling and storage, including incompatibilities
- **Exposure controls/personal protection:** OSHA's Permissible Exposure Limits (PELs) and any other exposure limit used or recommended by the chemical manufacturer, importer, or employer and appropriate engineering controls; personal protective equipment (PPE)
- **Physical and chemical properties:** Lists characteristics of chemical
- **Stability and reactivity:** Lists chemical stability and possibility of hazardous reactions
- **Toxicological information:** Routes of exposure; related symptoms, acute and chronic effects; numerical measures of toxicity

OSHA, Occupational Safety and Health Administration.

Adapted from U.S. Department of Labor: OSHA quickcard: hazard communication safety data sheets, 2015. https://www.osha.gov/Publications/HazComm_QuickCard_SafetyData.html.

SPECIAL CONSIDERATIONS

Patient-Centered Care

- Respect patient values, preferences, and expressed needs when selecting interventions for patient safety. Partner closely with patients and their family caregivers in making decisions about fall prevention and restraint reduction interventions.
- A recent Australian study of patients' and family members' perceptions of poor practices in the use of restraints revealed six themes: human rights, trauma, control, isolation, dehumanization, and antirecovery. Examples of poor practices included the use of excessive force, lack of empathy/paternalistic attitudes, lack of communication and interaction, and lack of alternative strategies to the use of restraints (Brophy et al., 2016).
- Adverse events are closely tied to failures of communication. Be attentive in communicating with patients from diverse cultural backgrounds. Be sure you have assessed their injury risks accurately and that the patients and family caregivers understand the risks for injury. Be sure they understand the plan of care. Use of a professional interpreter can improve the clarity of communication.
- When restraints are needed, clarify their meaning to the patient and family caregiver. Some patients will see restraining of older adults as disrespectful. Survivors of war or persecution may view restraints as a form of imprisonment or punishment.
- Remove restraints (if possible) when family members are present to show respect and caring for the patient.
- Be familiar with agency restraint protocol. Identify potential areas for negotiation with a patient's and family's preferences, such as using mittens instead of arm restraints.

Patient Education

- Teach family caregivers (as appropriate) what to observe for with respect to symptoms of wandering and the behaviors that often occur before and during seizures.
- Educate patients and family caregivers on steps to take to make their homes safe to reduce falls, to reduce unsupervised wandering outside of the home, and to have a fire response plan in the home (see Chapter 32).
- Educate parents about a child's risk of falling when the child is hospitalized.

Age-Specific

Pediatric

- When caring for an infant, keep a hand on the infant when you turn away from the bedside.
- Encourage children with severe atonic seizures (seizures that produce an abrupt loss of muscle tone, also called a drop attack) to wear head helmets.
- Have patients (any age) with a history of seizures wear a medical alert bracelet.
- Distraction techniques such as having a child hold a stuffed animal while inserting an IV catheter or blowing bubbles when removing a surgical drain can decrease the need for even temporary restraints.
- Developmentally and age-appropriate safety interventions for infants, toddlers, and preschoolers, such as net enclosures on beds, crib domes and side rails, and highchair lap safety belts, are generally not considered restraints (Hockenberry and Wilson, 2017).
- The use of restraints can often be avoided with adequate preparation of the child or parent.
- Limit the use of restraints to clinically appropriate and adequately justified situations (e.g., examination or treatment involving head and neck).
- When a child needs to be restrained for a procedure, it is best that the person applying the restraint not be the child's parent or guardian. Allow the parents to be in the supportive parental role.

Gerontological

- Patients with short-term memory loss or cognitive dysfunction may be unable to follow directions and may attempt to climb out of bed or get up from a chair unassisted.
- Physical therapy for improving balance, lower body strength, and gait can be beneficial to older patients (Touhy and Jett, 2018).
- The use of physical restraints was found in an international study to be predictive of longer hospital stay; thus physical restraints should be used with more caution and be reduced for older patients in the health care setting (Bai et al., 2014).
- Confusion can often lead to wandering and restlessness, leading patients to perform activities without assistance and increasing

the risk for falls. A sudden onset of confusion, weakness, and functional decline in a previously oriented older adult patient may indicate the presence of an underlying illness (e.g., an infection). Assess for physical causes of behavior changes, such as urinary or respiratory infection, hypoxia, fever, fluid and electrolyte imbalance, side effects of multiple drug administration, depression, anemia, hypothyroidism, or fecal impaction.

- Reminiscence helps older adults remain oriented (Touhy and Jett, 2018).
- Restrained older adults often respond with anger, fear, depression, humiliation, demoralization, discomfort, and resignation.
- Consider the risks associated with use of restraints (e.g., pressure ulcers, impaired strength) for older adults (Touhy and Jett, 2018). Complications of immobility are amplified, leading to a greater chance for functional decline.
- Older adults who have had a seizure may have symptoms such as confusion lasting several days, receptive and expressive speech problems, and unusual behaviors that may make it difficult to recognize a seizure.
- Older adults metabolize anticonvulsants more slowly; drugs accumulate and cause toxicity. Monitor therapeutic blood levels of drugs closely.
- Do not try to remove dentures during a seizure. If dentures loosen, tilt patient's head slightly forward and remove after seizure.

Home Care

- Assess patient's home environment for hazards, and institute safety measures as appropriate for fall reduction and reduction in wandering (see Chapter 32). Have the family caregiver set up an area in the home where it is safe for an older adult to wander. Be aware that pets can be a fall risk for patients.
- Personal items should be kept in their familiar positions and within easy reach in rooms frequently used.
- If a patient has a history of falls and lives alone, recommend that he or she wear an electronic Safe Patient Care device. The device is turned on by the wearer to alert a monitoring site to call emergency services for help.
- Patients at risk for self-injury or violence toward others need intensive supervision. The family caregiver must recognize this need and be able to provide necessary supervision.

PRACTICE REFLECTIONS

Select a patient that you are assigned to care for in an inpatient setting: hospital, rehabilitation facility, or extended care. Complete the Morse Fall Scale on your patient. Connect to http://networkofcare.org/library/Morse%20Fall%20Scale.pdf. Once you have computed a fall risk score, also assess the patient's medication history and the use of sensory assist devices. Consider the following questions:

1. What evidence-based fall prevention strategies would be appropriate to use for your patient?
2. Using the patient you assessed, conduct the Banner Assessment Mobility Tool available at https://www.americannursetoday.com/wp-content/uploads/2014/09/ant9-Patient-Handling-Supplement-821a_Implementing.pdf. Does this information suggest any additional strategies you should use?
3. When a patient does have a history of confusion or cognitive changes, name three behaviors that can indicate risk for wandering.

CLINICAL REVIEW QUESTIONS

1. A nurse working on an oncology unit is preparing a dose of chemotherapy that is to be given intravenously. The nurse accidentally spills a small amount (less than 1 mL) of the medication but also touches it with her bare hand. Arrange the following steps in the order the nurse should perform them.
   _____ a. Applies gloves to clean up spill
   _____ b. Notifies other staff nurses of the spill
   _____ c. Washes exposed hand in clean lukewarm water for 15 minutes
   _____ d. Disposes of cleanup materials into hazardous waste container
   _____ e. Refers to safety data sheet form about the chemotherapy medication
2. A nurse enters a patient's room and observes the patient lying on the floor having tonic and clonic contractions. After calling for help immediately, what first steps should the nurse take to protect the patient's airway and prevent aspiration? (Select all that apply.)
   1. Places patient supine with neck extended
   2. Cradles the patient's head in his or her lap
   3. Gently removes the patient's dentures
   4. Suctions the patient's airway secretions
   5. Keeps patient in the side-lying position
3. A nurse is caring for a 78-year-old man, Mr. Bernardo, who has been hospitalized for liver disease. The nurse learns that Mr. Bernardo fell in his bedroom at home 6 months ago after getting up at night to go to the bathroom. He had not fallen previously. At the time of the fall, approximately 1 AM, the patient felt a bit lightheaded when he stood to walk to the bathroom. He also admits he could not see clearly because he did not put his glasses on. Mr. Bernardo, fortunately, did not injure himself, but he felt "a bit scared" when he did fall. He takes an antihistamine to help him sleep at night, and he said that when he awakens, he is always a bit groggy. Use the SPLATT format to complete this patient's fall assessment.
   S -
   P -
   L -
   A -
   T -
   T -

Answers and Rationales for Clinical Review Questions can be found on the Evolve website.

REFERENCES

Agency for Healthcare Research and Quality (AHRQ): Preventing falls in hospitals: A toolkit for improving quality of care, AHRQ Publication No. 13-0015-EF, 2013. https://www.ahrq.gov/sites/default/files/publications/files/fallpxtoolkit.pdf.

Agency for Healthcare Research and Quality (AHRQ): Rapid response systems, 2017. https://psnet.ahrq.gov/primers/primer/4/rapid-response-systems.

Agency for Healthcare Research and Quality (AHRQ): Preventing falls in hospitals a toolkit for improving quality of care, 2018. https://www.ahrq.gov/professionals/systems/hospital/fallpxtoolkit/index.html.

Alzheimer's Association: Cognitive assessment toolkit, n.d. https://www.alz.org/documents_custom/141209-CognitiveAssessmentToo-kit-final.pdf.

Bai X, et al: Physical restraint use, and older patient's length of hospital stay, *Health Psychol Behav Med* 2(1):160, 2014.

Berry S, Kiel D: Falls: prevention in nursing care facilities and the hospital setting, UpToDate, 2018. http://www.uptodate.com/contents/falls-prevention-in-nursing-care-facilities-and-the-hospital-setting.

Boynton K, et al: Banner mobility assessment tool for nurses: instrument validation, *Am J Safe Patient Handl Mov* 4(3):86, 2014.

Bradas CM, et al: Physical restraints and side rails in acute and critical care settings. In Boltz M, et al, editors: *Evidence-based geriatric nursing protocols for best practice*, ed 5, New York, 2016, Springer Publishing Company, pp 229–245.

Brophy LM, et al: Consumers and their supporters' perspectives on poor practice and the use of seclusion and restraint in mental health settings: results from Australian focus groups, *Int J Ment Health Syst* 10(7):2016. https://www.ncbi.nlm.nih.gov/pmc/articles/PMC4744440/.

Butcher H: *Nursing Interventions Classification (NIC)*, ed 7, St. Louis, 2018, Elsevier.

Centers for Disease Control and Prevention (CDC): What is health literacy, 2016. https://www.cdc.gov/healthliteracy/learn/index.html.

Centers for Disease Control and Prevention (CDC): The timed get up and go test (TUG), 2017. https://www.cdc.gov/steadi/pdf/TUG_Test-print.pdf.

Centers for Medicare and Medicaid Services (CMS): Department of Health and Human Services: Revisions to Medicare conditions of participation, 37, Bethesda, MD, 2008, U.S. Department of Health and Human Services.

Centers for Medicare and Medicaid Services (CMS): Guidance to surveyor's appendix M, Bethesda, MD, 2015, U.S. Department of Health and Human Services. https://www.cms.gov/Regulations-and-Guidance/Guidance/Manuals/downloads/som107ap_m_hospice.pdf.

Centers for Medicare and Medicaid Services (CMS): *Survey protocol, regulations and interpretive guidelines for critical access hospitals*, Bethesda, MD, 2016, US Department of Health and Human Services. https://www.cms.gov/Regulations-and-Guidance/Guidance/Manuals/downloads/som107ap_w_cah.pdf.

Chang YY, et al: The efficacy of an in-service education program designed to enhance the effectiveness of physical restraints, *J Nurs Res* 24(1):79, 2016.

Cipriani G, et al: Wandering and dementia, *Psychogeriatrics* 14(2):135, 2014.

de Jong MR, et al: Drug-related falls in older patients: implicated drugs, consequences, and possible preventions strategies, *Ther Adv Drug Saf* 4(4):147, 2013.

Frankel A, et al: *A framework for safe, reliable, and effective care: White Paper*, Cambridge, MA, 2017, Institute for Healthcare Improvement and Safe & Reliable Healthcare.

Fugger G, et al: Psychiatric patients' perception of physical restraint, *Acta Psychiatr Scand* 133(3):221–231, 2016.

Glauser T, et al: Evidence-based guideline: Treatment of convulsive status epilepticus in children and adults: Report of the Guideline Committee of the American Epilepsy Society, *Epilepsy Curr* 16(1):48, 2016.

Gorman G, et al: Physical activity, exercise and aging, *Wellbeing* 4(7):1–19, 2014.

Grass G, et al: Feasibility of early postoperative mobilisation after colorectal surgery: A retrospective cohort study, *Int J Surg* 56:161, 2018.

Growdon ME, et al: Viewpoint: the tension between promoting mobility and preventing falls in the hospital, *JAMA Intern Med* 177(6):759–760, 2017.

Hill CE, et al: Timing is everything: where status epilepticus treatment fails, *Ann Neurol* 82:155, 2017.

Hockenberry MJ, Wilson D: *Wong's essentials of pediatric nursing*, ed 10, St. Louis, 2017, Mosby.

Hoffman R, Weinhouse G: Management of moderate and severe alcohol withdrawal syndromes. UpToDate, 2018. https://www.uptodate.com/contents/management-of-moderate-and-severe-alcohol-withdrawal-syndromes#!

Huang LC, et al: The effectiveness of a participatory program on fall prevention in oncology patients, *Health Educ Res* 30(2):298–308, 2015.

Institute for Healthcare Improvement (IHI): Patient safety, 2014. http://www.ihi.org/explore/patientsafety/Pages/default.aspx.

Institute for Healthcare Improvement (IHI): The ABCs of reducing harm from falls, 2017. http://www.ihi.org/resources/Pages/ImprovementStories/ABCsofReducingHarmfromFalls.aspx.

Johns Hopkins Medicine: Health Library–Epilepsy and seizures, n.d. http://www.hopkinsmedicine.org/healthlibrary/conditions/nervous_system_disorders/epilepsy_and_seizures_85,P00779/.

Kiel D, et al: Falls in older persons: Risk factors and patient evaluation. UpToDate, 2018. https://www.uptodate.com/contents/falls-in-older-persons-risk-factors-and-patient-evaluation.

Kuhlenschmidt ML, et al: Tailoring education to perceived fall risk in hospitalized patients with cancer: a randomized, controlled trial, *Clin J Oncol Nurs* 20(1):84–89, 2016.

Kumar A, et al: Which factors are associated with fear of falling in community-dwelling older people?, *Age Ageing* 43(1):76–84, 2014.

Martin E, et al: French validation of the revised algase wandering scale for long-term care, *Am J Alzheimers Dis Other Demen* 30(8):762, 2015.

National Fire Protection Association: Fires in healthcare facilities, 2016. http://www.nfpa.org/news-and-research/fire-statistics-and-reports/fire-statistics/fires-by-property-type/health-care-facilities/fires-in-health-care-facilities.

National Health Service (NHS): Sudden confusion: delirium, 2015. https://www.nhs.uk/conditions/confusion/.

National Institute for Health and Care Excellence (NICE): NICE guidelines on antiepileptic drugs, 2014. https://www.epilepsysociety.org.uk/nice-guidelines-anti-epileptic-drugs#.WWpIIM-Wypo.

Nelson AL, Algase DL: *Evidence-based protocols for managing wandering behavior*, New York, 2007, Springer Publishing.

Nuckols T, et al: Clinical effectiveness and cost of a hospital-based fall prevention intervention: The importance of time nurses spend on the front line of implementation, *J Nurs Adm* 47(11):571, 2017.

Quality and Safety Education for Nurses (QSEN): QSEN competencies, 2018. http://qsen.org/competencies/.

Rainier NC: Reducing physical restraint use in alcohol withdrawal patients: a literature review, *Dimens Crit Care Nurs* 33(4):201–206, 2014.

Schachter S: Evaluation and management of the first seizure in adults. *UpToDate*, 2018. https://www.uptodate.com/contents/evaluation-and-management-of-the-first-seizure-in-adults.

Severo IM, et al: Risk factors for falls in hospitalized adult patients: an integrative review, *Rev Esc Enferm USP* 48(3):537, 2014.

Smith G, et al: Epilepsy update: part 2: nursing care and evidence-based treatment, *Am J Nurs* 115(6):34, 2015.

Stewart TV, et al: Practice patterns, beliefs, and perceived barriers to care regarding dementia: a report from the American Academy of Family Physicians (AAFP) national research network, *J Appl Biomater Funct Mater* 27(2):275, 2014.

Suliman M, et al: Knowledge, attitude and practice of intensive care unit nurses about physical restraint, *Nurs Crit Care* 22(5):264, 2017.

The Joint Commission (TJC): 2015: Preventing falls and fall-related injuries in health care facilities—Issue 55, September 28, 2015. https://www.jointcommission.org/assets/1/6/SEA_55_Falls_4_26_16.pdf.

The Joint Commission (TJC): Preventing patient falls: a systematic approach from the Joint Commission Center for Transforming Healthcare Project, October 2016. http://www.hpoe.org/Reports-HPOE/2016/preventing-patient-falls.pdf.

The Joint Commission (TJC): Joint Commission Resources Quality & Safety Network (JCRQSN) Resource Guide: be prepared: maximizing behavioral healthcare-related tracer activities, April 27, 2017a.

The Joint Commission (TJC): *2017 Comprehensive accreditation manual for hospitals: the official handbook*, Oakbrook Terrace, IL, 2017b, The Commission.

The Joint Commission (TJC): Standards FAQ details: restraint and seclusion-side rails, 2017c. https://www.jointcommission.org/standards_information/jcfaqdetails.aspx?StandardsFaqId=1362&ProgramId=46.

The Joint Commission (TJC): *2019 National Patient Safety Goals*, Oakbrook Terrace, IL, 2019, The Commission. https://www.jointcommission.org/assets/1/6/2018_HAP_NPSG_goals_final.pdf.

Touhy T, Jett K: *Ebersole and Hess' gerontological nursing and health care*, ed 5, St. Louis, 2018, Mosby.

U.S. Department of Labor: OSHA quickcard: hazard communication safety data sheets, 2015. https://www.osha.gov/Publications/HazComm_QuickCard_SafetyData.html.

U.S. Food and Drug Administration (FDA): A guide to bed safety bed rails in hospitals, nursing homes and home health care: the facts, 2014. https://www.fda.gov/MedicalDevices/ProductsandMedicalProcedures/GeneralHospitalDevicesandSupplies/HospitalBeds/ucm123676.htm.

Uusi-Rasi K, et al: Exercise and vitamin D in fall prevention among older women: a randomized clinical trial, *JAMA Intern Med* 175(5):703, 2015.

5 | Infection Control

SKILLS AND PROCEDURES

EVOLVE WEBSITE/RESOURCES LIST

http://evolve.elsevier.com/Perry/nursinginterventions

Audio Glossary • Checklists • Clinical Review Questions • Answers and Rationales for Clinical Review Questions • Video Clips

INTRODUCTION

Infection control and prevention pertain to efforts made by nurses and other health care providers to control and prevent the spread of disease by breaking links in the chain of infection (Fig. 5.1). This is accomplished when nurses and other health care providers utilize medical asepsis, or clean technique, which consists of procedures to reduce the number of infectious organisms (Box 5.1); and surgical asepsis, which consists of procedures to eliminate all microorganisms from an area (Box 5.2). Nurses are responsible for teaching patients and their family caregivers about the signs and symptoms of infection, modes of transmission, and methods of prevention. Infection control and prevention are vitally important to nursing because it is estimated that 1 in 25 patients will contract a health care–associated infection (HAI), which is defined as an infection that a patient acquires in a health care agency (Centers for Disease Control and Prevention [CDC], 2016c). HAIs result in approximately 75,000 deaths at a direct medical cost to health care facilities of almost $10 billion annually (Hsu, 2014; Zimlichman et al., 2013).

PRACTICE STANDARDS

- Association of Perioperative Registered Nurses (AORN), 2017: Guidelines for perioperative practice—Evidence-based guidelines for perioperative and invasive procedures
- Centers for Disease Control and Prevention (CDC), 2015: Isolation precautions—Summary of recommendations, including hand hygiene, personal protective equipment, and droplet and airborne precautions
- Centers for Disease Control and Prevention (CDC), 2016c: Management of multidrug-resistant organisms in healthcare settings—Identification and control of MDROs in health care facilities
- Centers for Disease Control and Prevention (CDC), 2017a: Clean hands count for healthcare providers—Hand-hygiene guidelines, including gloving, surgical hand antisepsis, and hand-skin health
- Centers for Disease Control and Prevention (CDC), 2017b: HAI data and statistics—Sequence for donning and doffing personal protective equipment (PPE)
- The Joint Commission (TJC), 2019: National Patient Safety Goals—Patient safety guidelines
- World Health Organization (WHO), 2017: Clean care is safer care—Five moments for hand hygiene

EVIDENCE-BASED PRACTICE

Multidrug-Resistant Organisms

Multidrug-resistant organisms (MDROs) are microorganisms that are resistant to at least one class of antibiotics. MDROs common to health care facilities include methicillin-resistant *Staphylococcus aureus* (MRSA), vancomycin-resistant enterococci (VRE), *Clostridium difficile* (*C. difficile*), and other gram-negative bacilli (GNB) (CDC, 2015). An emerging threat is the carbapenem-resistant Enterobacteriaceae (CRE) (CDC, 2015; Hayden, 2015). Common vehicles of infection transmission are the hands and stethoscopes of health care providers (Holleck et al., 2017). Health care providers' uniforms frequently become contaminated during routine patient care and may also serve as a vehicle for the transmission of infectious microorganisms (Anderson et al., 2017). Contact with infected patients and contaminated surfaces can result in transmission of the infectious organism up to 45% of the time (AORN, 2017). Nurses play an important role in preventing the spread of MDROs. Methods nurses use include the following:

- Judicious use of hand hygiene—alcohol-based hand rubs are ineffective in eliminating *C. difficile* spores; soap and water must be used (CDC, 2017a).
- Swift and accurate identification of colonized patient
- Isolation of patient in a private room or cohorting with a patient infected by the same MDRO
- Utilizing standard precautions and appropriate contact precautions

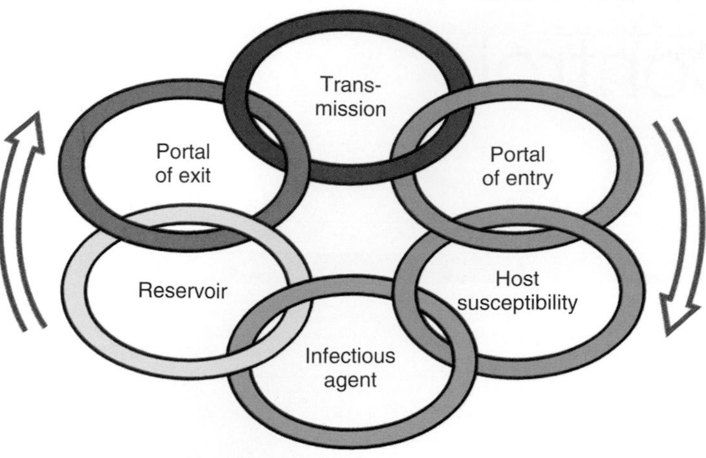

FIG 5.1 Chain of infection.

BOX 5.1

Medical Asepsis Principles

- Before and after patient contact, perform hand hygiene with an alcohol-based hand rub or soap and water as an essential part of patient care and infection prevention.
- Always assess a patient's susceptibility to infection, specifically, age, nutritional status, response to stress, disease processes, and so forth, as these may place patients at higher risk.
- Recognize the elements of the chain of infection, and implement interventions to prevent the onset and/or spread of infection.
- Consistently incorporate the basic principles of asepsis into all patient care.
- Protect nurses and other health care providers from exposure to infectious agents through proper use, cleaning, and disposal of equipment.
- Understand the chain of infection that can lead to health care–associated infections because this enables the implementation of interventions to prevent their occurrence.

BOX 5.2

Surgical Asepsis Principles

- All items used within a sterile field must be sterile.
- A sterile barrier that has been permeated by punctures, tears, or moisture is considered contaminated.
- When a sterile package is opened, a 2.5-cm (1-inch) border around the edges is considered unsterile.
- Tables draped with a sterile field are considered sterile only at table level.
- If there is any question or doubt about the sterility of an item, the item is considered unsterile.
- Sterile persons and/or items may contact only sterile items; unsterile persons or items may contact only unsterile items.
- Movement around or in the sterile field must not compromise or contaminate the sterile field.
- A sterile object or field out of the range of vision or an object held below a person's waist is considered to be contaminated.
- A sterile object or field becomes contaminated by prolonged exposure to air. Be organized and complete patient procedures as soon as possible.

- Use of room-dedicated medical devices such as thermometers, blood pressure cuffs, and stethoscopes
- Monitoring use of antibiotics (CDC, 2017b)
- Sterile insertion, maintenance, and removal of indwelling medical devices according to hospital policy (Booth, 2016)
- Application of appropriate personal protective equipment (PPE) on patient during transport within the hospital or to another agency (AORN, 2017)
- Proper cleaning and disinfection of environment and medical equipment, using appropriate cleaning agent (CDC, 2016e; Livshiz-Riven et al., 2015)
- Disinfecting stethoscopes before and after use on patient and not using fabric stethoscope covers
- Not wearing scrubs, shoes, and other attire worn during patient care in public places such as restaurants and grocery stores (AORN, 2017)
- Providing patient and family caregiver with infection prevention education

SAFETY GUIDELINES

It is imperative that nurses adhere to precautions and guidelines established by health protection agencies, such as the CDC, the World Health Organization (WHO), and professional nursing organizations, as well as agency policies, in order to contain and control the spread of infection. Nurses must help ensure that all health care providers (e.g., respiratory, physical, occupational, and speech therapists; physicians; other nurses) working with patients, support staff (e.g., housekeepers), and family caregivers maintain infection-prevention practices at all times.

- Hand hygiene is known to be the most effective method to prevent the transmission of infectious microorganisms (AORN, 2017).
- Alcohol-based hand rubs reduce the number of microorganisms on hands that are not visibly dirty.
- Health care providers should keep their natural nails less than ¼ inch long and should not wear artificial fingernails or extensions because microorganisms can live under them after handwashing and using alcohol-based hand rubs (CDC, 2017a).
- Use tier one, standard-based precautions, and place patients on tier two, transmission-based precautions (airborne, droplet, and contact) as determined by the nature of the patient's illness to contain and prevent the spread of illness (CDC, 2015; Table 5.1).
- Proper donning and doffing of PPE is important to prevent contamination of skin or clothing (CDC, 2016a).
- Use of a bundle, or group, of evidence-based interventions, has been demonstrated to reduce the spread of infection more effectively than the use of individual interventions (Hsu, 2014).
- Health care providers, patients, and family caregivers must practice respiratory and cough hygiene by covering nose and mouth with a tissue or sleeve when coughing or sneezing, properly disposing used tissues, and performing hand hygiene.
- Masks and eye protection must be worn when contact with spray, splashes, blood droplets, or other infectious materials is anticipated.
- Gloves must be worn when contact with infectious materials, blood, mucous membranes, or nonintact skin may occur (AORN, 2017).

TABLE 5.1

Centers for Disease Control and Prevention Isolation Guidelines

Standard Precautions (Tier One) for Use With All Patients

- Standard precautions apply to blood, blood products, all body fluids, secretions, excretions (except sweat), nonintact skin, and mucous membranes.
- Perform hand hygiene before direct contact with patients; between patient contacts; after contact with blood, body fluids, secretions, and excretions and with equipment or articles contaminated by them; and immediately after gloves are removed.
- When hands are visibly soiled or contaminated with blood or body fluids, wash them with either a nonantimicrobial soap or antimicrobial soap and water.
- When hands are not visibly soiled or contaminated with blood or body fluids, use an alcohol-based hand rub to perform hand hygiene.
- Wash hands with nonantimicrobial or antimicrobial soap and water if contact with spores (e.g., *C. difficile*) is likely to have occurred.
- Do not wear artificial fingernails or extenders if duties include direct contact with patients at high risk for infection and associated adverse outcomes.
- Wear gloves when touching blood, body fluids, secretions, excretions, nonintact skin, mucous membranes, or contaminated items or surfaces. Remove gloves and perform hand hygiene between patient care encounters and when going from a contaminated to a clean body site.
- Wear PPE when your anticipated patient interaction will likely involve contact with blood or body fluids.
- A private room is unnecessary. Check with the infection prevention and control professional of your agency.
- Discard all contaminated sharp instruments and needles in a puncture-resistant container. Health care facilities must make needleless devices available. Activate the mechanical safety device, if present. If needle recapping is necessary, use the one-handed scoop method and dispose of the capped needle as soon as possible.
- Respiratory hygiene and cough etiquette: Have patients cover the nose or mouth when sneezing or coughing; use tissues to contain respiratory secretions, and dispose in nearest waste container; perform hand hygiene after contacting respiratory secretions and contaminated objects or materials; contain respiratory secretions with procedure or surgical mask; sit at least 3 feet away from others if coughing.

Transmission-Based Precautions (Tier Two) for Use With Specific Types of Patients

Category	Disease	Barrier Protection
Airborne Precautions	Droplet nuclei < 5 μm, measles, chickenpox (varicella), disseminated herpes zoster, *Mycobacterium tuberculosis,* rubeola	Private room, negative-pressure airflow of at least 6–12 exchanges per hour via HEPA filtration, mask or respiratory protection device, N95 respirator
Droplet Precautions	Droplets > 5 μm; being within 3 feet of the patient; influenza, adenovirus, group A streptococcus, *Neisseria meningitides,* pertussis, rhinovirus, *Mycoplasma pneumoniae*, pertussis, diphtheria, pneumonic plague, rubella, mumps, respiratory syncytial virus	Private room or cohort patients, mask or respirator (refer to agency policy)
Contact Precautions	Direct patient or environmental contact, colonization or infection with multidrug-resistant organisms, such as VRE and MRSA, *Clostridium difficile,* shigella and other enteric pathogens, major wound infections, herpes simplex, scabies, varicella zoster (disseminated), respiratory syncytial virus	Private room or cohort patients (see agency policy), gloves, gowns
Protective Environment	Allogeneic hematopoietic stem cell transplants	Private room; positive airflow with ≥ 12 air exchanges per hour; HEPA filtration for incoming air; mask, gloves, gowns

HEPA, high-efficiency particulate air; *MRSA,* methicillin-resistant *Staphylococcus aureus;* VRE, vancomycin-resistant enterococcus.

Modified from Centers for Disease Control and Prevention (CDC): Hospital Infection Control Practice Advisory Committee: Guidelines for isolation precautions in hospitals, 2017, https://www.cdc.gov/infectioncontrol/guidelines/isolation/index.html; Association of Operating Room Nurses (AORN): AORN guidelines for perioperative practice, Denver, 2017, AORN; U.S. Food and Drug Administration (FDA), What to do if you can't find a sharps disposal container, 2018, https://www.fda.gov/MedicalDevices/ProductsandMedicalProcedures/HomeHealthandConsumer/ConsumerProducts/Sharps/default.htm.

✦ SKILL 5.1 Hand Hygiene

Purpose

Hand hygiene pertains to cleaning hands by handwashing with soap and water, with an antiseptic hand wash, with an alcohol-based hand rub, or surgical hand antisepsis to prevent the spread of infection (CDC, 2017a). According to the WHO's (2017) *My 5 Moments for Hand Hygiene* protocol, health care providers should wash their hands before and after patient contact, before clean or aseptic procedures, after actual or presumed contact with body fluids, and after touching patient surroundings. The CDC also recommends that hands be washed if hands move from a contaminated body site to a clean site and after glove removal. Hands that are not visibly dirty should be cleaned with an alcohol-based hand rub because it takes less time, is more effective, and is less irritating to the hands than washing with soap and water. Soap and water should be used when hands are visibly dirty, before eating, after using the restroom, and after known or suspected exposure to C. *difficile*, *Bacillus anthracis*, and infectious diarrhea during norovirus outbreaks (CDC, 2017b).

Delegation and Collaboration

The skill of hand hygiene is performed by all caregivers. Hand hygiene is not optional.

Equipment

- Antiseptic hand rub
  - Alcohol-based waterless antiseptic
- Handwashing
  - Easy-to-reach sink with warm running water
  - Antimicrobial or regular soap
  - Paper towels
  - Disposable nail cleaner *(optional)*

ASSESSMENT

1. Inspect surface of hands for breaks or cuts in skin or cuticles. Cover any skin lesions with a dressing before providing care. If lesions are too large to cover, you may be restricted from direct patient care. *Rationale: Open cuts or wounds can harbor high concentrations of microorganisms. Agency policy may prevent nurses from caring for high-risk patients if open lesions are present on hands (WHO, 2017).*
2. Inspect hands for visible soiling. *Rationale: Visible soiling requires handwashing with soap and water (CDC, 2017a).*
3. Inspect condition of nails. Natural tips should be no longer than 0.625 cm (¼ inch) long. Be sure that fingernails are short, filed, and smooth. *Rationale: Microorganisms can live under artificial nails after handwashing and using an alcohol-based sanitizer and should not be worn by health care providers having direct contact with patients (CDC, 2017b).*

STEP	RATIONALE
PLANNING	
1. Expected outcomes after completion of procedure:	
• Hands and areas under fingernails are clean and free of debris.	Infectious microorganisms have been removed.
• Patient and/or family caregiver have been instructed about the importance of hand hygiene for themselves and making sure that all health care providers clean their hands before touching the patient (CDC, 2014).	Education improves patient outcomes.
IMPLEMENTATION	
1. Push wristwatch and long uniform sleeves above wrists. Avoid wearing rings. If worn, remove during hand hygiene.	Provides complete access to fingers, hands, and wrists. The skin underneath jewelry may carry a higher bacterial count (AORN, 2017).
2. Antiseptic hand rub	
a. According to manufacturer directions, dispense ample amount of product into palm of one hand (see illustration).	Use enough product to cover hands thoroughly.
b. Rub hands together for 15–20 seconds, covering all surfaces of hands and fingers with antiseptic (see illustration).	Provides enough time for product to work (CDC, 2017a).
c. Rub hands together until alcohol is dry. Allow hands to dry completely before applying gloves.	Ensures complete antimicrobial action.
3. Handwashing using regular or antimicrobial soap:	
a. Stand in front of sink, keeping hands and uniform away from sink surface. (If hands touch sink during handwashing, repeat sequence.)	Inside of sink is a contaminated area. Reaching over sink increases risk of touching edge, which is contaminated.
b. Turn on water. Turn on faucet (see illustration). It is best if sinks have knee, foot, or electronic sensor controls.	Knee pads within operating room and treatment areas are preferred to prevent hand contact with faucet. Faucet handles are likely to be contaminated with organic debris and microorganisms (AORN, 2017).
c. Avoid splashing water against uniform.	Microorganisms travel and grow in moisture.
d. Regulate flow of water so that temperature is warm.	Warm water removes less of protective oils on hands than hot water.
e. Wet hands and wrists thoroughly under running water. Keep hands and forearms lower than elbows during washing.	Hands are most contaminated parts to wash. Water flows from least to most contaminated area, rinsing microorganisms into sink.

STEP	RATIONALE
f. Apply the amount of antiseptic soap recommended by the manufacturer and rub hands together (see illustration).	Ensure that all surfaces of hands and fingers are cleaned.

Safe Patient Care *The decision whether to use an antiseptic soap or an alcohol-based hand rub depends on whether the hands are visibly soiled, the type of infectious microorganism, the procedure you will perform, and the patient's immune status.*

STEP	RATIONALE
g. Perform hand hygiene using plenty of lather and friction for at least 15 seconds. Interlace fingers and rub palms and back of hands with circular motion at least 5 times each. Keep fingertips down to facilitate removal of microorganisms.	Soap cleans by emulsifying fat and oil and lowering surface tension. Friction and rubbing mechanically loosen and remove dirt and transient bacteria. Interlacing fingers and thumbs ensures that all surfaces are cleaned. Adequate time is needed to expose skin surfaces to antimicrobial agent.
h. Areas underlying fingernails are often soiled. Clean them with fingernails of other hand and additional soap or with disposable nail cleaner.	Area under nails can be highly contaminated, which increases risk for transmission of infection from nurse to patient.
i. Rinse hands and wrists thoroughly, keeping hands down and elbows up (see illustration).	Rinsing mechanically washes away dirt and microorganisms.
j. Dry hands thoroughly from fingers to wrists with paper towel or single-use cloth.	Drying from cleanest (fingertips) to least clean (wrist) avoids contamination. Drying hands prevents chapping and roughened skin. Do not tear or cut skin under or around nail.
k. If used, discard paper towel in proper receptacle.	Prevents transfer of microorganisms.

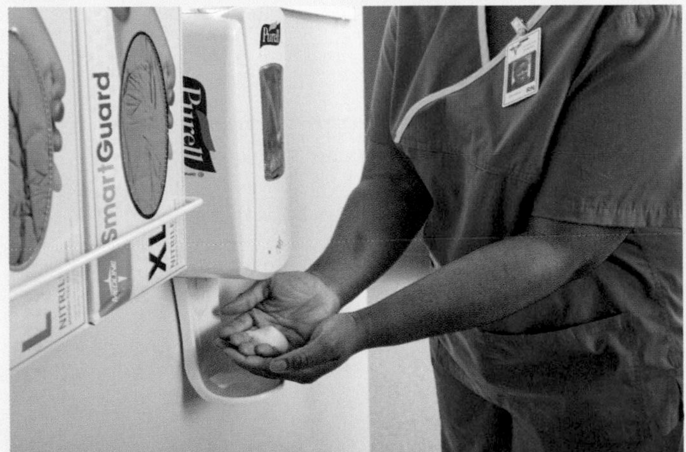

STEP 2a Apply waterless antiseptic to hands.

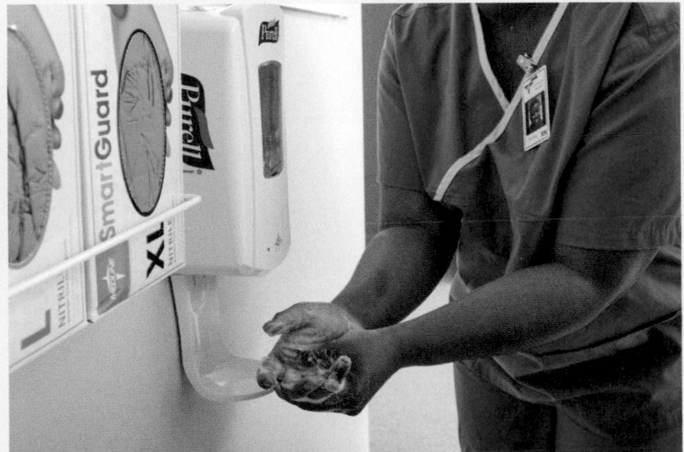

STEP 2b Rub hands thoroughly.

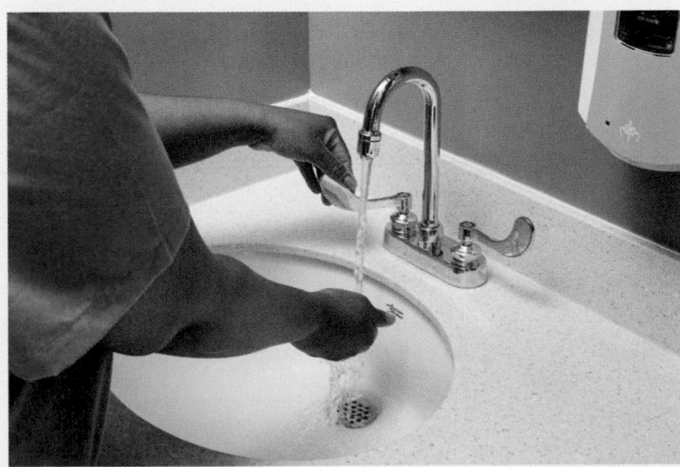

STEP 3b Turn on water.

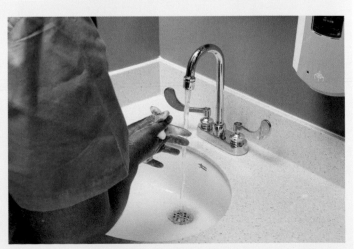

STEP 3f Lather hands thoroughly.

STEP	RATIONALE
l. To turn off hand faucet, use clean, dry paper towel; avoid touching handles with hands (see illustration). Turn off water with foot or knee pedals (if applicable).	Wet towel and hands allow transfer of pathogens from faucet by capillary action.
m. If hands are dry or chapped, use small amount of lotion or barrier cream.	Helps minimize skin dryness. Only use lotions or creams approved by your health care agency because they have been selected to not interact with hand-sanitizing products (CDC, 2017a).

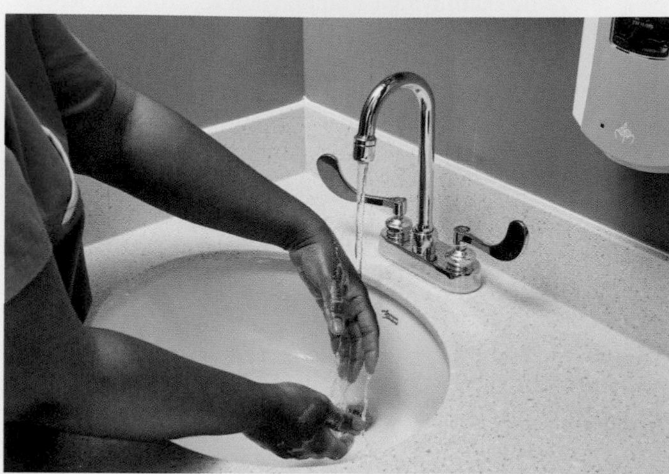

STEP 3i Rinse hands.

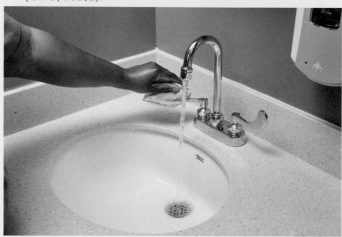

STEP 3l Turn off faucet.

EVALUATION

1. Inspect surface of hands for obvious signs of dirt or other contaminants.	Determines whether hand hygiene is adequate.
2. Inspect hands for dermatitis or cracked skin.	Breaks in skin integrity increase risk for transmission of microorganisms.
3. Use Teach-Back: "I want to be sure I adequately explained why hand hygiene is important. Please describe to me when you and your family caregiver should perform hand hygiene and the different kinds of ways you can wash your hands." Revise your instruction now or develop a plan for revised patient/family caregiver teaching if patient/family caregiver is not able to teach back correctly.	Determines patient's/family caregiver's level of understanding of instructional topic.

Unexpected Outcomes	Related Interventions
1. Hands or areas under fingernails remain soiled.	• Repeat handwashing with soap and water.
2. Repeated use of soaps or antiseptics causes dermatitis or cracked skin.	• Rinse and dry hands thoroughly after using soap and water; avoid excessive amounts of soap or antiseptic; try various products. • Use approved hand lotions or barrier creams that will not interfere with hand-sanitizing products (CDC, 2017a).

Recording

- It is unnecessary to document handwashing.

Hand-Off Reporting

- Report dermatitis, psoriasis, and/or cuts to agency employee health or infection control department.

✦ SKILL 5.2 Applying Personal Protective Equipment

Purpose

Certain procedures performed at the bedside require the application of personal protective equipment (PPE), such as gloves, gowns, caps, masks, and/or eyewear. Standard precautions require nurses to wear clean gloves before coming in contact with blood, body fluids, secretions and excretions (except sweat), nonintact skin, mucous membranes, and other potentially infectious material. Transmission-based precautions are used in addition to standard precautions when special patient placement is required and additional supplies are needed to prevent the spread of infection. Which PPE to use varies depending on the level of precautions required (standard, contact, droplet, or airborne), type and mode of transmission of the infectious microorganism, and the kind of procedure to be performed (Booth, 2016; CDC, 2015). PPE is applied and removed in a specific sequence to prevent unnecessary adjusting of items during the process, which increases the risk of contamination (Beam et al., 2015; CDC, 2016d).

Delegation and Collaboration

The skill of properly applying and removing PPE can be delegated to nursing assistive personnel (NAP). The nurse instructs the NAP to:

- Perform hand hygiene before putting on gloves and after removal.
- Be available to hand off equipment or assist with patient positioning during a sterile procedure.

Equipment

- Clean gloves
- Gown (may be either disposable or reusable depending on agency protocol)
- Mask or respirator (N95, N99, N100, PAPR)
- Protective eyewear (e.g., goggles or face shield)

ASSESSMENT

1. Review type of procedure to be performed and consult agency policy regarding use of PPE. *Rationale: Not all procedures require PPE. PPE ensures that you and patient are properly protected.*
2. If you have symptoms of a respiratory infection, either avoid performing the procedure or apply a mask. *Rationale: A greater number of pathogenic microorganisms reside within the respiratory tract when infection is present.*
3. Assess patient's risk for infection (e.g., older adult, neonate, or immunocompromised patient). *Rationale: Some patients are at a greater risk for acquiring an infection; thus use additional protective barriers.*
4. Assess patient's or family caregiver's knowledge, experience, and health literacy level. *Rationale: Ensures patient has the capacity to obtain, communicate, process, and understand basic health information (CDC, 2016b).*

STEP	RATIONALE
PLANNING	
1. Expected outcome is the prevention of localized or systemic infection: • Patient remains afebrile 24–48 hours after a procedure or during repeated procedures. • Patient does not develop signs of localized infection (e.g., redness, tenderness, edema, drainage) or systemic infection (e.g., fever, change in white blood cell [WBC] count) 24 hours after procedure.	Indicates minimal microorganism transfer to patient.
2. Provide patient and family caregiver education as to why PPE is utilized and if it will be required when the patient returns home.	Education improves patient outcomes.
IMPLEMENTATION	
1. Perform hand hygiene	Reduces transmission of microorganisms on skin.
2. Apply gown. a. Opening to the back and covering torso from neck to knees, arms to end of wrists, and wrapping around to the back. b. Tie securely behind neck and waist (see illustration).	Protects skin and clothing and prevents contamination during procedures when contact with bodily fluids is likely.
3. Apply a cap. (**NOTE:** Only required for some sterile procedures; refer to agency policy.)	
a. If hair is long, comb back behind ears and secure.	Hair can be a source of microorganism transmission (AORN, 2017).
b. Cap should cover all of the hair, scalp, and ears (see illustration).	Minimizes skin and hair shedding and protects patients from shedding (Spruce, 2014).

STEP	RATIONALE
4. Apply surgical mask or fitted respirator around mouth and nose (type and fit-testing depend on type of isolation and agency policy). You must have a medical evaluation and be fit-tested before using a respirator.	Protects the mucous membranes of the eyes, nose, and mouth of the nurse during procedures when splashes or sprays of bodily fluids are likely. Prevents exposure to airborne microorganisms.
a. Find top edge of mask, which usually has a thin metal strip along the edge.	Pliable metal fits securely against bridge of nose.
b. Hold mask by top two strings or loops, keeping top edge above bridge of nose.	Position prevents contact of hands with clean facial part of mask. Mask covers all of nose.
c. Tie two top strings in a bow at top of back of head with strings above the ears (see illustration).	Position of ties at top of head provides tight fit. Strings over ears may cause irritation.
d. Tie two lower ties in a bow securely around neck, with mask well under chin (see illustration).	Tying prevents escape of microorganisms through sides of mask as you talk and breathe.
e. Gently pinch upper metal band around bridge of nose.	Pinching prevents microorganisms from escaping around nose and eyeglasses from steaming up.

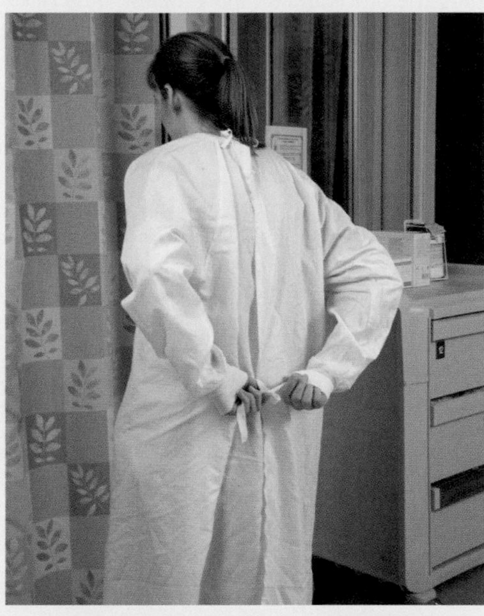

STEP 2b Tie isolation gown at waist.

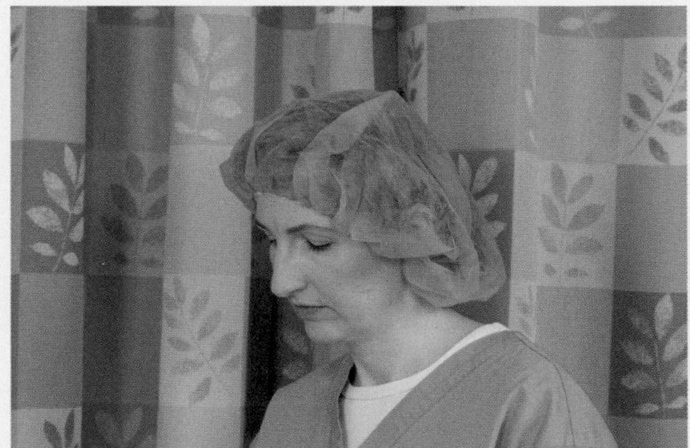

STEP 3b Apply cap over head, covering all hair.

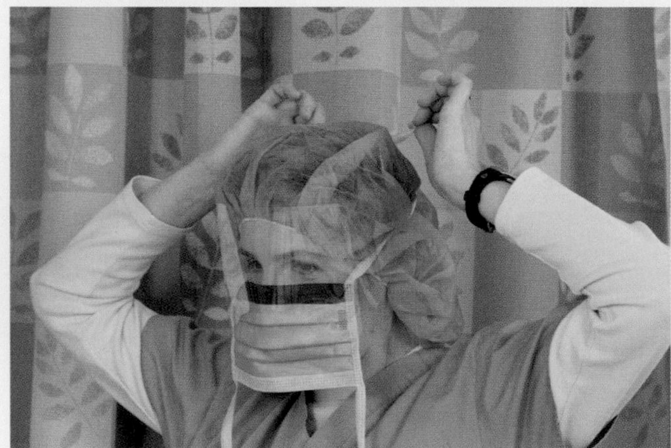

STEP 4c Tie top strings of mask.

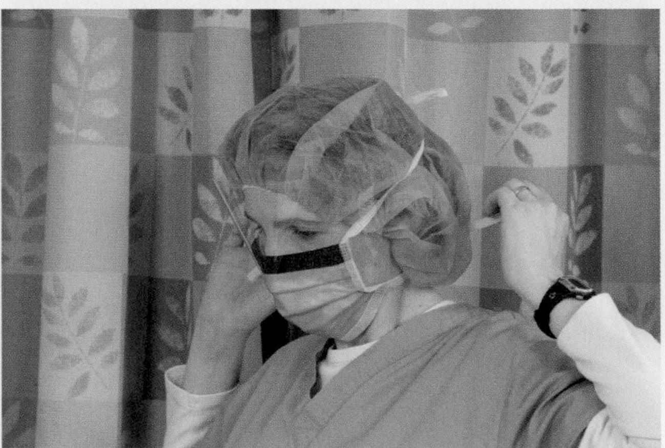

STEP 4d Tie bottom strings of mask.

STEP	RATIONALE
5. Apply protective eyewear.	
a. Apply protective glasses, goggles, or face shield comfortably over eyes and check that vision is clear (see illustration). If you wear prescription glasses, side shields may be used.	Positioning affects clarity of vision.
b. Be sure that face shield fits securely around forehead and face.	Secure fitting ensures that eyes are fully protected.
6. Apply clean gloves.	Prevents the transmission of microorganisms.
a. Extend gloves up to cover the wrist of the gown. (**NOTE:** Wear unpowdered, latex-free gloves if you, the patient, or another health care worker has latex allergy.) Bring glove cuffs over edge of gown sleeves (see illustration).	
7. Removal of PPE	
a. Nondisposable Gown:	
(1) Remove gloves. Remove one glove by grasping cuff and pulling glove inside out over hand. Hold removed glove in gloved hand. Slide fingers of ungloved hand under remaining glove at wrist (see illustration). Peel glove off over first glove. Discard gloves in proper container.	Proper removal of gloves prevents contamination of hair, neck, and facial area from contaminated gloves.

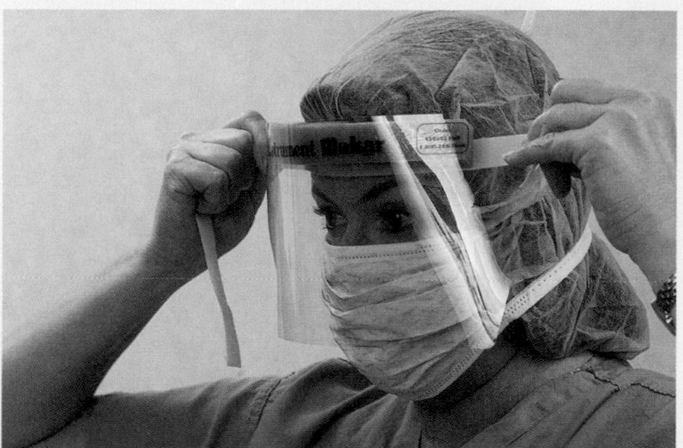

STEP 5a Apply face shield over cap.

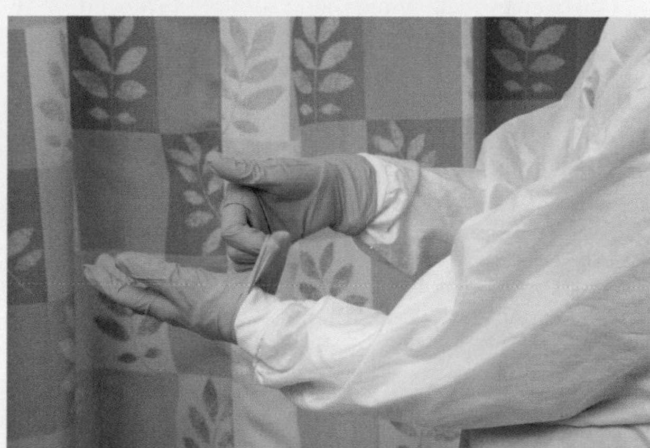

STEP 6a Apply gloves over edge of gown sleeves.

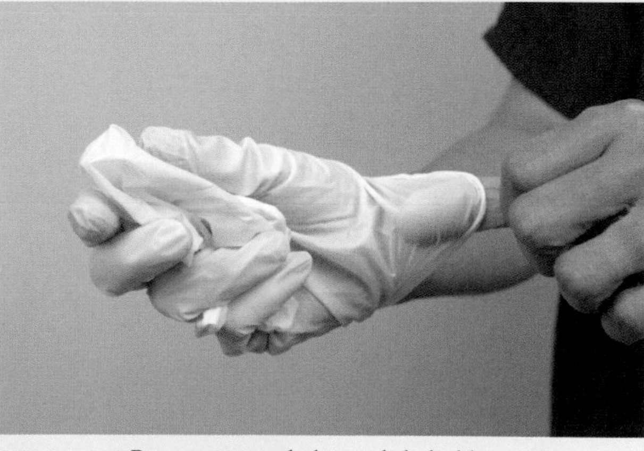

STEP 7a(1) Remove second glove while holding soiled glove.

STEP	RATIONALE
(2) Remove eyewear, face shield, or goggles. Avoid placing hands over soiled lens. Remove googles or face shield from the back by lifting up the earpieces or head band. Discard in proper container.	Proper removal of eyewear, face shield, or goggles prevents transmission of microorganisms.
(3) Remove gown. Unfasten neck ties and then untie back strings of gown. Allow gown to fall from shoulders touching only inside of gown. Remove hands from sleeves without touching outside of gown. Hold gown inside shoulder seams and fold inside out into a bundle; discard in laundry bag (see illustration). **NOTE:** If gown is soiled with body fluids, discard in red soiled-linen bag.	Front and sleeves of gown are contaminated. This method of disposal prevents transmission of infection.
(4) Remove mask or respirator. If mask secures over ears, remove elastic from ears and pull mask away from face. For tie-on mask, untie *bottom* mask string and then top strings, pull mask away from face (see illustration A), and drop into plastic-lined trash receptacle (see illustration B). (Do not touch outer surface of mask.) If respirator is worn, remove once outside patient room and door is closed.	Proper removal prevents top part of mask from falling down over uniform. If mask falls and touches uniform, uniform will be contaminated. The respirator is removed outside of the patient's room to prevent the inhalation of infectious microorganisms.
(5) Remove cap. Grasp outer surface of cap and lift from hair. Discard in proper receptacle.	Minimizes contact of hands with hair. Reduces transmission of microorganisms.
b. Disposable Gown:	
(1) Remove gown and gloves. Grasp gown in the front with gloved hand and pull forward until the ties break, being careful to only touch the outside of gown. Allow gown to fall from shoulders touching only inside of gown (see illustration). While removing the gown, fold and roll inside-out into a bundle while simultaneously removing gloves, taking care to only touch the inside of gloves and gown with bare hands. Dispose in proper container.	The gown is torn off so that gown and gloves can be removed simultaneously (CDC, 2016a).

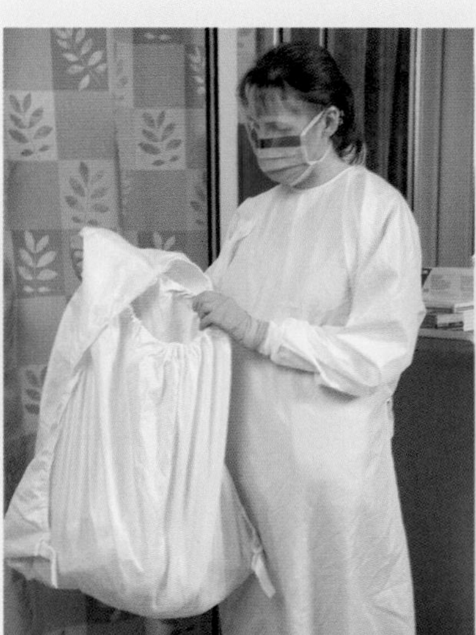

STEP 7a(3) Tie bag securely.

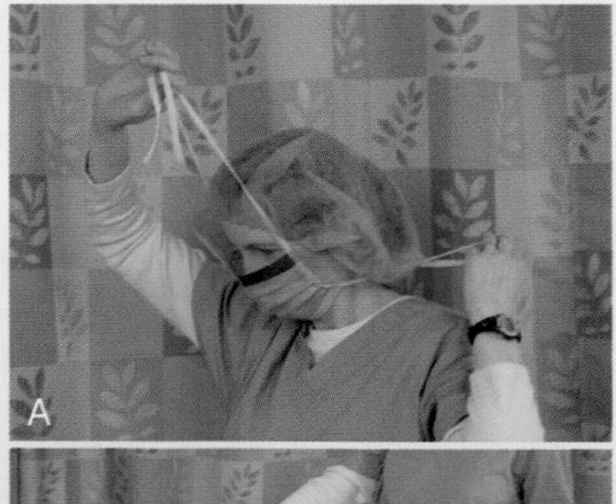

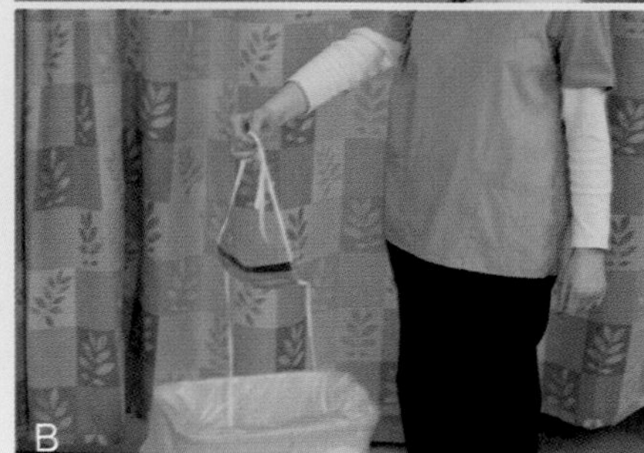

STEP 7a(4) (A) Pull mask away from face. (B) Drop into trash receptacle.

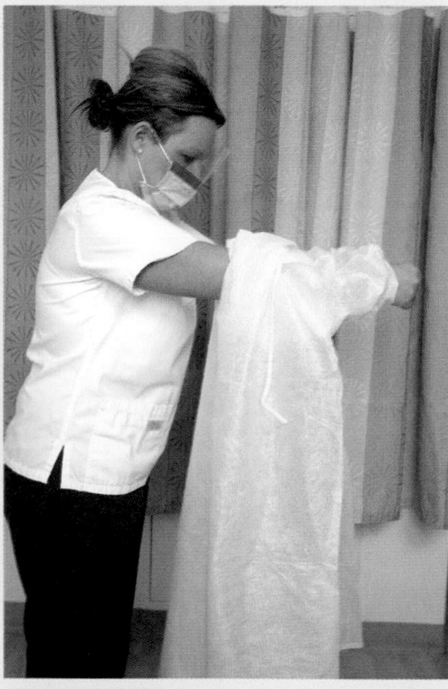

STEP 7b(1) Remove gown by allowing it to fall from shoulders.

STEP	RATIONALE
(2) Remove eyewear, face shield, or goggles. Handle by headband or earpieces. Discard in proper waste container.	Outside of goggles is contaminated. Hands will not be soiled if properly removed.
(3) Remove mask or respirator. See Step 7a(4).	Proper removal prevents top part of mask from falling down over uniform. If mask falls and touches uniform, uniform will be contaminated. The respirator is removed outside of the patient's room to prevent the inhalation of infectious microorganisms.
(4) Remove cap. Grasp outer surface of cap and lift from hair. Discard in proper receptacle.	Minimizes contact of hands with hair. Reduces transmission of microorganisms.
8. Perform hand hygiene.	Reduces transmission of microorganisms.

EVALUATION

1. After the procedure is completed, assess the patient during your course of care for any signs and symptoms of infection. Depending on what the PPE equipment was used for, the evaluation will vary.	Assessment rules out presence of localized infection.
2. **Use Teach-Back:** "I want to be sure I explained why personal protective equipment is used. Please explain to me why you and your family caregiver need to wear personal protective equipment and show me how you will put it on." Revise your instruction now or develop a plan for revised patient/family caregiver teaching if patient/family caregiver is not able to teach back correctly.	Determines patient's/family caregiver's level of understanding of instructional topic.

Unexpected Outcomes	Related Interventions
1. Hands become contaminated at any point during PPE removal.	Immediately wash hands with soap and water or with an alcohol-based hand rub, as appropriate.
2. Redness, heat, edema, pain, or purulent drainage develops at wound or treatment site, indicating possible infection.	Notify health care provider of change in patient's condition and initiate appropriate interventions as prescribed.

Recording

- It is unnecessary to document use of PPE.

✦ SKILL 5.3 Caring for Patients Under Isolation Precautions

Purpose

When a patient has an infection, nurses and other health care providers follow specific infection prevention and control practices to reduce the risk of cross-contamination to other patients. Body substances, such as feces, urine, mucus, and wound drainage, contain potentially infectious organisms. Tier two isolation precautions, or transmission-based precautions, are used in addition to standard precautions for patients with suspected or known colonization or infection with particularly virulent microorganisms that are transmitted by the contact, droplet, or airborne route (see Table 5.1). Isolation precautions include the use of PPE (see Skill 5.2). When caring for a patient with tuberculosis (TB), a special set of guidelines must be followed (Box 5.3).

Delegation and Collaboration

Basic care for patients on isolation precautions can be delegated to nursing assistive personnel (NAP). However, the nurse is responsible for knowing the patient's status and isolation indications. The nurse instructs the NAP about:

- Reason patient is on isolation precautions
- Use of the correct PPE for the specific isolation
- Precautions for bringing equipment into the patient's room, if appropriate
- Reporting abnormal findings and any high-risk behaviors (e.g., patient does not adhere to secretion control when coughing) for infection transmission that pertain to the patient
- Special precautions regarding individual patient needs, such as transportation to diagnostic tests

Equipment

- PPE determined by type of isolation required: clean gloves; cap, mask, eyewear or goggles; face shield; and gown (gowns may be disposable or reusable depending on agency policy)
- Other patient care equipment as appropriate (e.g., hygiene items, medications, dressing supplies, sharps container, disposable blood pressure cuff, thermometer, and stethoscope)
- Soiled-linen bag and trash receptacle

BOX 5.3

Special Tuberculosis Precautions

Tuberculosis (TB) is a deadly disease infecting one-third of the world's population. In 2015 there were 9557 TB cases reported in the United States. Individuals with weakened immune systems (e.g., transplant recipients, patients with HIV infection) are especially susceptible to developing TB. The current Centers for Disease Control and Prevention (CDC) guidelines for preventing and controlling TB focus on early detection of TB infection, protecting close contacts of patients with active TB disease, and applying effective infection control measures in health care settings.

- A patient who has respiratory symptoms lasting longer than 3 weeks, unexplained weight loss, pain in the chest, night sweats, fever, or a productive cough (might be streaked with blood) should be suspected of having TB.
- Isolation for patients with suspected or confirmed TB includes placing the patient on airborne infection precautions in a single-patient airborne infection isolation room with negative pressure.
- Occupational Safety and Health Administration (OSHA) and CDC guidelines require health care providers who care for patients with suspected or confirmed TB to wear special respirators (e.g., N95 or P100). These respirators are high-efficiency particulate masks that filter particles at a 95% or better efficiency. Health care workers who use these respirators must be fit-tested, a procedure to determine adequate fit to minimize leakage into the face piece and to provide better protection.
- OSHA requires employers to provide training concerning the transmission of TB, especially in areas where the risk of exposure is high (OSHA, 2015).
- There are two methods of TB testing: the skin and blood. The Mantoux tuberculin skin test requires two visits to a health care provider: one to have the skin test placed, and a second visit 48 to 72 hours later to have it read. There are two blood tests available: the QuantiFERON®-TB Gold and the T-SPOT®. An individual's health care provider will decide which is best to use. Testing an individual with both tests is not recommended (CDC, 2016e).
- When caring for patients on isolation precautions for TB, they will be in a negative-pressure isolation room that needs to have the door closed at all times.
- Provide instruction to the patient and family related to TB and how it is transmitted and how to prevent the spread of infection to others.

- Sign for door indicating type of isolation and/or for visitors to come to the nurses' station before entering room
- TB isolation
- Room with negative airflow
- N95, N99, or P100 respirator to be worn by nurses/NAP

ASSESSMENT

1. Identify patient using at least two identifiers (e.g., name and birthday or name and medical record number) according to agency policy. *Rationale: Ensures patient safety. Complies with The Joint Commission (TJC) standards and improves patient safety (TJC, 2019).*
2. Assess patient's health history for possible indications for isolation (e.g., TB, diarrhea, major draining wound, or purulent productive cough). Review precautions for specific isolation system, including appropriate barriers to apply (see Table 5.1). *Rationale: Mode of transmission for infectious microorganism determines type and degree of precautions followed. Ensures adequate protection.*
3. Review laboratory test results (e.g., wound culture, acid-fast bacillus [AFB] smears, changes in WBC count). *Rationale: Reveals type of microorganism for which patient is being isolated, body fluid in which it was identified, and whether patient is immunosuppressed.*
4. Review agency policies and isolation precautions necessary for type of isolation ordered and consider types of care measures that you will perform while in patient's room (e.g., medication administration or dressing change). *Rationale: Allows you to organize care items for procedures and time spent in patient's room.*
5. Assess patient's or family caregiver's knowledge, experience, and health literacy level. *Rationale: Ensures patient has the capacity to obtain, communicate, process, and understand basic health information (CDC, 2016b).*
6. Review nursing care plan/nursing documentation notes regarding patient's emotional state and reaction/adjustment to isolation. Assess patient's understanding of purpose of isolation. *Rationale: Provides opportunity to implement interventions for patient's need for emotional support and teaching about infection transmission/rationale for isolation.*
7. Assess whether patient has known latex allergy. If allergy is present, refer to agency policy and resources available to provide full latex-free care. *Rationale: Protects patient from serious allergic response.*

STEP	RATIONALE
PLANNING	
1. Expected outcomes focus on preventing transmission of infection to nurse and other patients.	The spread of infection is controlled and contained.
2. Provide patient and family caregiver with information about infection transmission and purpose of isolation.	Instruction about precautions improves patient and family caregiver's ability to cooperate in care.
3. Teach patient and family caregiver how to use appropriate barrier techniques in the home, as necessary.	Instruction about precautions improves patient and family caregivers' abilities to cooperate with care.
4. Prepare all equipment to be taken into patient's room. In many cases dedicated equipment, such as stethoscopes, blood pressure (BP) equipment, and thermometers should remain in room until patient is discharged. If patient is infected or colonized with a resistant organism (e.g., VRE, MRSA), equipment remains in room and is thoroughly disinfected before removal (see agency policy).	Prevents providers from making multiple trips into room. The CDC recommends use of dedicated noncritical patient care equipment (CDC, 2016b).

STEP	RATIONALE
IMPLEMENTATION	
1. Perform hand hygiene (see Skill 5.1).	Reduces transmission of microorganisms.
2. Prepare for entrance into isolation room. Ideally, before applying PPE, step into patient's room and stay by door. Introduce yourself and explain care that you are providing. If this is not possible, apply PPE outside of the room.	Allows patient to see you without PPE and personalizes care without exposing yourself to risk of infection transmission.
a. Apply gown, being sure that it covers all outer garments. Pull sleeves down to wrist. Tie securely at neck and waist.	Prevents transmission of infection; protects you when patient has excessive drainage or discharge.
b. Apply either surgical mask or fitted respirator around mouth and nose (type and fit-testing depend on type of isolation and agency policy). You must have a medical evaluation and be fit-tested before using a respirator.	Prevents exposure to airborne microorganisms or microorganisms from splashing of fluids.
c. If needed, apply eyewear, goggles, or face shield securely around face and eyes. If you wear prescription glasses, side shields may be used.	Protects you from exposure to microorganisms that may occur during splashing of fluids.
d. Apply clean gloves. (**NOTE:** Wear unpowdered, latex-free gloves if you, patient, or another health care worker has latex allergy.) Secure glove cuffs over edge of gown sleeves.	Reduces transmission of microorganisms.
3. Enter patient's room. Arrange supplies and equipment. (**NOTE:** If equipment will be reused, set aside on clean surface.)	Prevents extra trips entering and leaving room. Minimizes contamination of care items.
4. Explain purpose of isolation and precautions patient and family caregiver are to take. Offer opportunity for patient and family caregiver to ask questions. If TB precautions are in use, instruct patient to cover mouth with tissue when coughing and to wear disposable surgical mask when leaving room.	Improves patient's and family caregiver's ability to participate in care and minimizes anxiety. Identifies opportunity for planning social interaction and diversional activities. Reduces TB microorganism transmission.
5. Assess vital signs (see Chapter 7).	
a. If patient is infected or colonized with resistant organism (e.g., VRE, MRSA), use disposable or dedicated equipment that remains in room, including thermometer, stethoscope, and BP cuff (CDC, 2016a).	Decreases risk of infection being transmitted to another patient and/or health care provider.
b. If stethoscope is to be reused, clean diaphragm, bell, and ear tips with alcohol or alcohol-based hand rub. Set aside on clean surface.	Stethoscopes are a common vehicle for transmission of infection. This action decreases the presence of microorganisms (Holleck et al., 2017).
c. Use an individual electronic or disposable thermometer.	Prevents cross-contamination.
6. Administer medications (see Chapters 22, 23, and 24).	
a. Give oral medication in wrapper or cup.	
b. Dispose of wrapper or cup in plastic-lined receptacle.	Handle and discard supplies to minimize transfer of microorganisms.
c. Wear gloves when administering an injection.	Reduces risk of exposure to patient's blood.
d. Discard needleless syringe or safety sheathed needle into designated sharps container.	Needleless devices should be used to reduce risk of needlesticks and sharps injuries to nurses and other health care providers.
7. Administer hygiene; encourage patient to ask questions or express concerns about isolation. Provide patient teaching.	Hygiene practices further minimize transfer of microorganisms. Develops caring relationship with patient.
a. Avoid allowing isolation gown to become wet; carry washbasin outward away from body; avoid leaning against wet surfaces (e.g., table, sink).	Moisture allows organisms to travel through gown to uniform.
b. Help patient remove own gown; discard in leak-proof linen bag.	Reduces transfer of microorganisms.
c. Remove linen from bed; avoid contact with isolation gown. Place in leak-proof linen bag.	Handle linen soiled by patient's body fluids to prevent contact with clean items.

STEP	RATIONALE
d. Provide clean bed linen.	Decreases presence of microorganisms and moisture. Improves patient's self-image and comfort.
e. Change gloves and perform hand hygiene. If gloves become excessively soiled and further care is necessary, reglove.	Change gloves between exposures to body sites and patient equipment. Inadequate glove changes and hand hygiene can lead to contamination, increasing the risk of health care–associated infections (HAIs) (CDC, 2017a).
8. Collect specimens (see Chapter 9).	
a. Place specimen container on clean paper towel in patient's bathroom and follow procedure for collecting specimen of body fluids.	Container will be taken out of patient's room; prevents contamination of outer surface.
b. Follow agency procedure for collecting specimen of body fluids (see Chapter 9).	
c. Transfer specimen to container without soiling outside of container. Place container in biohazard bag and place label on outside of bag or per agency policy (see illustration). Label specimen in front of patient (TJC, 2019). Perform hand hygiene and reglove if additional procedures are needed.	Specimens of blood and body fluids are placed in well-constructed containers with secure lids to prevent leaks during transport. Proper labeling prevents diagnostic error.
d. Check label on specimen for accuracy. Send to laboratory (warning labels are often used, depending on agency policy). Label containers of blood or body fluids with biohazard sticker.	Ensures that health care providers who transport or handle containers are aware of infectious contents.
9. Assist patient to comfortable position.	Gives patient sense of well-being.
10. Be sure nurse call system is in an accessible location within patient's reach. Instruct patient in its use.	Provides for patient comfort and safety.
11. Raise side rails (as appropriate) and lower bed to lowest position.	Provides for patient comfort and safety.
12. Dispose of linen, trash, and disposable items.	Reduces transmission of microorganisms.
a. Use sturdy moisture-impervious single bags to contain soiled articles. Use double bag if outer bag is torn or contaminated.	
b. Tie bags securely at top in knot.	
13. Retrieve and clean nondedicated equipment in room according to agency policy.	Reduces transmission of microorganisms.
14. Resupply room as needed. Have nursing staff/NAP hand new supplies to you.	Limiting trips of personnel into and out of room reduces patient's and health care providers' exposure to microorganisms.

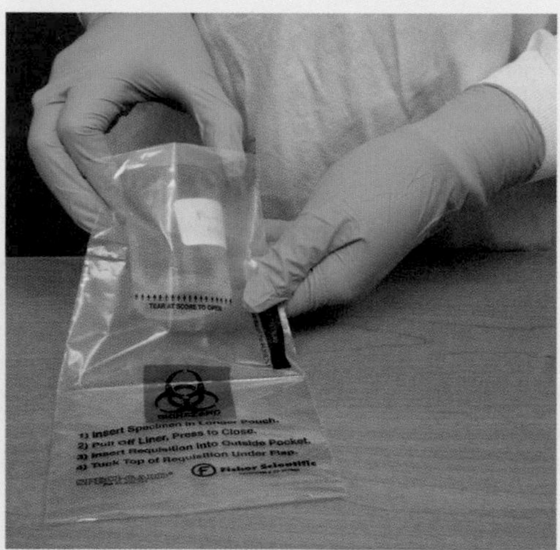

STEP 8c Place specimen container in biohazard bag.

STEP	RATIONALE
15. Leave isolation room. The order of removal of PPE depends on what is worn and if gown is disposable or nondisposable. Skill 5.2, Steps 7a and 7b describe steps to take if all barriers are worn. PPE worn in room must be removed before leaving room.	Order of removal minimizes exposure to microorganisms and/or infectious material on PPE (CDC, 2016d).

Safe Patient Care *All PPE, except respirator, should be removed before leaving patient's room. Remove and properly dispose of respirator after leaving patient's room and the door is closed to prevent inhalation of infectious microorganisms.*

STEP	RATIONALE
16. Perform hand hygiene.	Reduces transmission of microorganisms.

Safe Patient Care *If patient is being treated for* C. difficile *infection, wash hands with soap and water. Alcohol-based hand rubs are not effective against* C. difficile *spores.*

STEP	RATIONALE
17. Explain to patient when you plan to return to room. Ask whether patient requires any personal care items. Offer books, magazines, audiotapes.	Diversions can help to minimize boredom and feeling of social isolation.
18. Be sure nurse call system is in an accessible location within patient's reach.	Ensures patient can call for assistance if needed.
19. Raise side rails (as appropriate) and lower bed to lowest position.	Ensures patient safety.
20. Leave room and close door, if necessary. Always close door if patient is on airborne precautions or in negative-airflow room.	Maintains negative-airflow environment and reduces transmission of microorganisms.

EVALUATION

1. Observe patient's and family caregivers' use of isolation precautions when they are visiting.	Identifies any improper use of PPE/precautions.
2. Use Teach-Back: "I want to be sure I explained why isolation precautions are used. Please explain to me why isolation precautions are used." Revise your instruction now or develop a plan for revised patient/family caregiver teaching if patient/family caregiver is not able to teach back correctly.	Determines patient's/family caregivers' level of understanding of instructional topic.

Unexpected Outcomes	Related Interventions
1. Patient does not engage in social and/or therapeutic discussions.	• Work to develop a caring and therapeutic relationship with patient and family caregivers. Assess if patient is lonely or depressed. Assess patient's need for diversional activities.
2. Patient or health care provider may have an allergy to latex gloves.	• Notify health care provider/employee health and treat sensitivity or allergic reaction appropriately. • Use latex-free gloves for future care activities.
3. Infectious organism spreads to other patients.	• Notify health care provider and others according to agency policy. • Determine appropriate isolation precautions for other affected patients.

Recording

- Record assessment data, procedures performed (including patient education), and patient's response(s) to care.
- Record type of isolation in use and the rationale (e.g., microorganism, if known).
- Record patient's response to social isolation.
- Record evaluation of interventions/care implemented.

Hand-Off Reporting

Discuss the following with nurses and other pertinent health care providers:

- Patient and family caregiver education provided regarding the infection and need for isolation.
- Any ongoing patient and family caregiver needs and concerns.

✦ SKILL 5.4 Preparing a Sterile Field

Purpose

Performing sterile aseptic procedures requires a work area in which objects can be handled with minimal risk of contamination. A sterile field is an area free of microorganisms and provides a sterile surface for placement of sterile equipment. A field may consist of the inside of a sterile commercial kit or tray, the surface of an opened sterile linen-wrapped package, or the surface of a large sterile drape. Sterile drapes establish a sterile field around a treatment site such as a surgical incision, venipuncture site, or site for introduction of an indwelling urinary catheter. Sterile drapes also provide a work surface for placing sterile supplies and manipulating items with sterile gloves. After you create a sterile field, you are responsible for making sure that the field is not contaminated while performing the procedure.

Delegation and Collaboration

Nurses prepare sterile fields for some sterile procedures, such as urinary catheter insertion and performing tracheostomy care and suctioning, whereas other health care providers usually prepare sterile fields in the operating room (see agency policy). The skill of preparing a sterile field cannot be delegated to nursing assistive personnel (NAP). The nurse can direct the NAP to:

- Help with patient positioning and obtaining any necessary supplies.

Equipment

- Sterile pack (commercial or facility wrapped)
- Sterile drape or kit that will be used as a sterile field
- Sterile gloves (if not included in kit)
- Sterile solution and equipment specific to procedure
- Waist-high table/countertop surface
- Appropriate PPE: gown, mask, cap, protective eyewear (see agency policy)

ASSESSMENT

1. Identify patient using at least two identifiers (e.g., name and birthday or name and medical record number) according to agency policy. *Rationale: Ensures correct patient. Complies with The Joint Commission standards and improves patient safety (TJC, 2019).*
2. Assess type of aseptic technique needed for procedure. *Rationale: Some procedures require medical aseptic technique, whereas others require surgical aseptic technique.*
3. Assess patient's comfort, positioning, oxygen requirements, and elimination needs before preparing for procedure. *Rationale: Certain procedures requiring a sterile field may last a long time. Anticipates patient's needs so patient can relax and avoid any unnecessary movement that might disrupt procedure.*
4. Instruct patient (and family caregiver, if present) not to touch work surface or equipment during procedure. *Rationale: Prevents contamination of sterile field.*
5. Assess patient for latex allergies. *Rationale: A review of the patient's health history may reveal a latex allergy. Determine the need to use latex-free supplies.*
6. Check sterile package integrity for punctures, tears, discoloration, moisture, or any other signs of contamination. Check the expiration date. Check sterile package for sterilization indicator (marker that changes color when exposed to heat or steam). *Rationale: Inspection of packaging ensures that sterile field is not contaminated (AORN, 2017).*
7. Anticipate supplies needed for procedure. *Rationale: Not all sterile kits contain sufficient amounts or types of supplies needed for all procedures. Failure to have the proper supplies may cause you to leave the sterile field, increasing the risk for contamination and potential need to set up another sterile field.*
8. Assess patient's or family caregiver's knowledge, experience, and health literacy level. *Rationale: Ensures patient has the capacity to obtain, communicate, process, and understand basic health information (CDC, 2016b).*

STEP	RATIONALE
PLANNING	
1. Expected outcomes after completion of procedure:	
• Sterile field is not contaminated.	Correct aseptic technique is performed.
• Patient is not exposed to microorganisms.	Lack of exposure minimizes infection transmission.
2. Complete all other nursing interventions (e.g., medication administration, repositioning patient) before beginning procedure.	Prepare sterile field as close as possible to time of use to reduce potential for contamination (AORN, 2017).
3. Suggest that visitors step out briefly during procedure. Discourage movement of staff assisting with procedure.	Traffic or movement can increase potential for contamination through spread of microorganisms by air currents.
4. Arrange equipment/supplies at bedside or in a location convenient to the procedure.	Ensures availability before procedure and prevents break in sterile technique during procedure (**NOTE:** Povidone-iodine and chlorhexidine are not considered sterile solutions and require separate work surfaces for preparation.)
5. Position patient comfortably for specific procedure to be performed. If a body part is to be examined or treated, position patient so area is accessible. Have NAP help with positioning as needed.	Patient should be able to lie still in one position comfortably during procedure. Movement can disrupt the sterile field.

STEP	RATIONALE
6. Explain to patient purpose of procedure and importance of sterile technique.	Performing patient teaching before procedure increases patient understanding and may reduce the need to talk during procedure, which can cause air-droplet contamination of sterile area.

IMPLEMENTATION

STEP	RATIONALE
1. Perform hand hygiene (see Skill 5.1).	Hand hygiene reduces number of microorganisms on hands, thus reducing transmission to patient. Do not allow rinse water to run down arms onto clean hands (i.e., arms are considered contaminated).
2. Apply PPE as needed (check agency policy) (see Skill 5.2).	PPE controls microorganism transmission.
3. Select a clean, flat, dry work surface above waist level.	A dry surface is needed for a sterile field. A sterile object placed below a person's waist is considered contaminated.
4. Prepare sterile work surface.	
a. Use sterile commercial kit or package containing sterile items.	
(1) Place sterile kit or package on the prepared work surface.	
(2) Open outside cover (see illustration) and remove package from dust cover. Place on work surface.	Outside of kit is not sterile. Inner kit remains sterile.
(3) Grasp outer surface of tip of outermost flap.	Outer surface of package is considered unsterile. There is a 2.5-cm (1-inch) border around any sterile drape or wrap that is considered contaminated and can be touched with clean fingers.
(4) Open outermost flap away from body, keeping arm outstretched and away from sterile field (see illustration).	Reaching over sterile field contaminates it.
(5) Grasp outside surface of edge of first side flap.	Outer border is considered unsterile.
(6) Open side flap, pulling to side, allowing it to lie flat on table surface. Keep arm to side and not over sterile surface (see illustration).	Drape or wrapper should lie flat so it does not accidentally rise up and contaminate inner surface or sterile contents.
(7) Repeat Step 4a(6) for second side flap (see illustration).	
(8) Grasp outside border of last and innermost flap (see illustration). Stand away from sterile package and pull flap back, allowing it to fall flat on table. Kit is ready to be used.	Outer border is considered unsterile. Never reach over a sterile field.
b. Open sterile linen-wrapped package.	
(1) Place package on clean, dry, flat work surface above waist level.	Sterile items placed below waist level are considered contaminated.

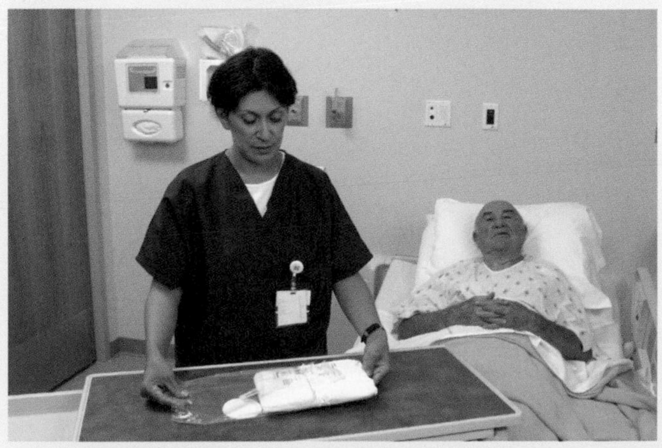

STEP 4a(2) Open outside cover of sterile kit.

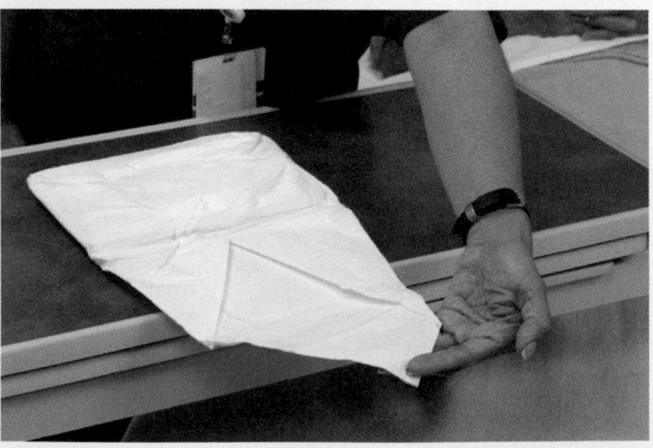

STEP 4a(4) Open outermost flap of sterile kit away from body.

STEP	RATIONALE
(2) Remove sterilization tape seal and unwrap both layers following same steps (see Steps 4a [2] through 4a [8]) as for sterile kit (see illustration).	Linen-wrapped items have two layers. The first is a dust cover. The second layer must be opened to view sterilization indicator.
(3) Use opened package wrapper as sterile field.	Inside of package wrapper is considered sterile.
c. Prepare sterile drape.	
(1) Place pack containing sterile drape on flat, dry surface and open as described (see Steps 4a [2] through 4a[8]) for sterile package.	Packaged drape remains sterile.
(2) Apply sterile gloves (*optional*, see agency policy). The outer 2.5-cm (1-inch) border of drape may be touched without wearing gloves.	Sterile object remains sterile only when touched by another sterile object. Gloves are not necessary as long as fingers grasp the 2.5-cm (1-inch) unsterile border of the drape.
(3) Using fingertips of one hand, pick up folded top edge of drape along 2.5 cm (1-inch) border. Gently lift drape up from its wrapper without touching any object. Discard wrapper with other hand.	If sterile object touches any nonsterile object, it becomes contaminated.
(4) With other hand, grasp an adjacent corner of drape and hold it straight up and away from body. Allow drape to unfold, keeping it above waist and work surface and away from body (see illustration).	An object held below a person's waist or above chest is contaminated. Drape can now be placed properly with two hands.

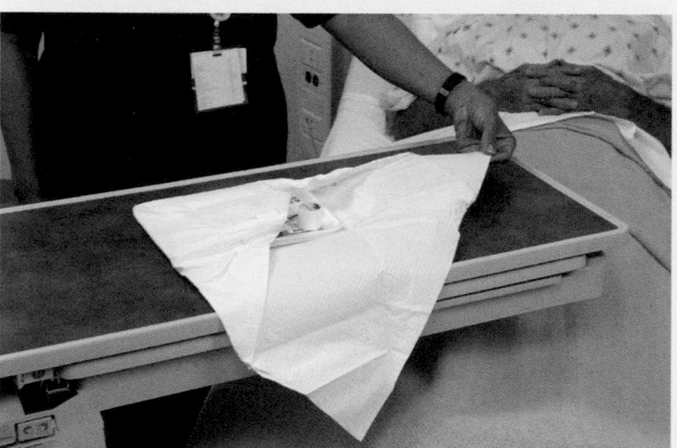

STEP 4a(6) Open first side flap, pulling to side.

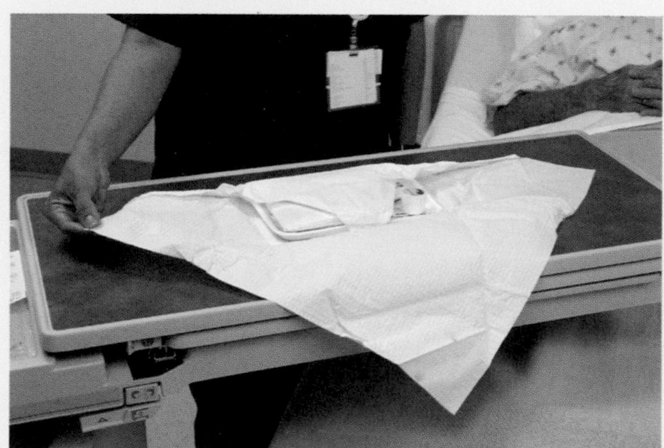

STEP 4a(7) Open second side flap, pulling to side.

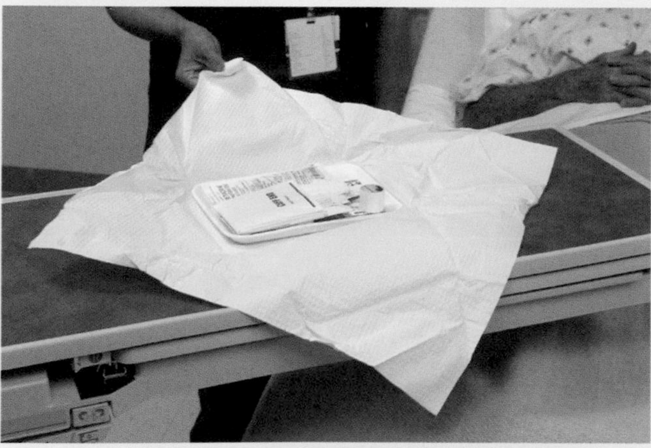

STEP 4a(8) Open last and innermost flap.

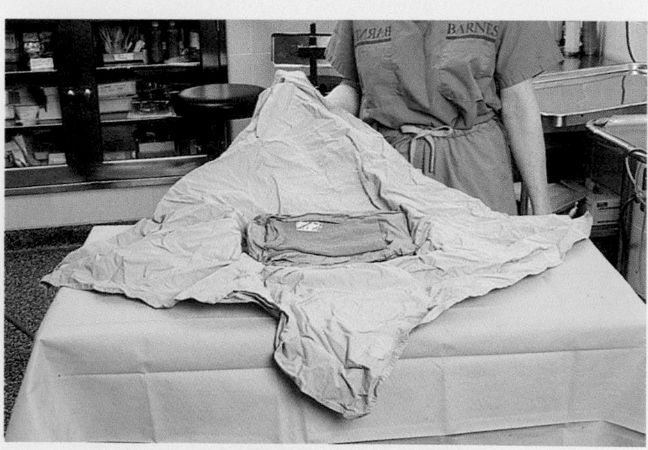

STEP 4b(2) Open sterile linen-wrapped package.

STEP	RATIONALE
(5) Holding drape, position bottom half over top half of intended work surface (see illustration).	Proper positioning prevents nurse from reaching over sterile field.
(6) Allow top half of drape to be placed over bottom half of work surface (see illustration).	Proper positioning creates flat, sterile work surface for placement of sterile supplies.

Safe Patient Care *Use slow movements when setting up sterile drapes. Fast movements can stir up dust, lint, and infectious microorganisms that can contaminate the sterile field.*

STEP	RATIONALE
5. Add sterile items to sterile field.	
a. Open sterile item (following package directions) while holding outside wrapper in nondominant hand.	Use of nondominant hand frees dominant hand for unwrapping outer wrapper.
b. Carefully peel wrapper over nondominant hand.	Item remains sterile. Inner surface of wrapper covers hand, making it sterile.
c. Be sure that the wrapper does not fall onto the sterile field. Place the item onto the field at an angle (see illustration). Do not hold arms over sterile field.	Secured wrapper edges prevent flipping wrapper and contaminating contents of sterile field (AORN, 2017). Arms are contaminated.
d. Dispose of outer wrapper.	Disposal prevents accidental contamination of sterile field.
6. Pour sterile solutions.	
a. Verify contents and expiration date of solution.	Verification ensures proper solution and sterility of contents.
b. Place receptacle for solution near table/work surface edge. Sterile kits have cups or plastic molded sections into which fluids can be poured.	Proper placement prevents reaching over sterile field during pouring of solution.

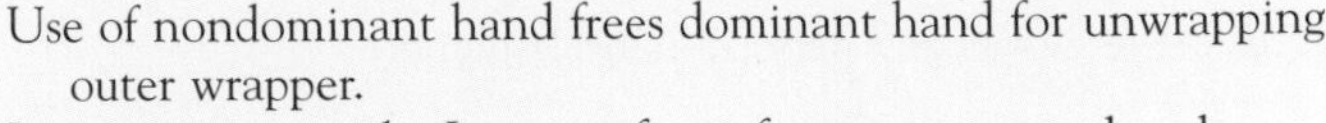

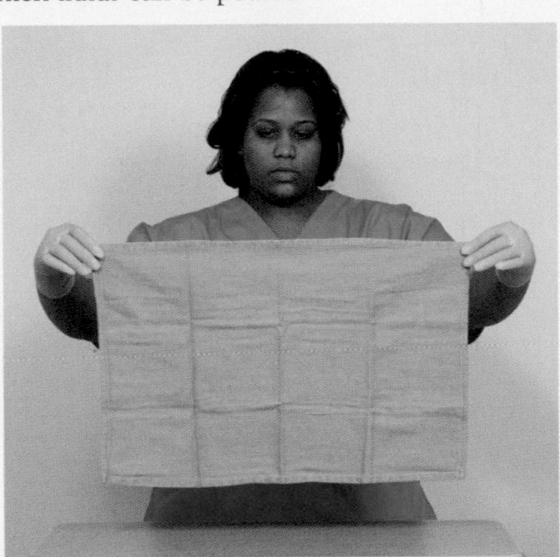

STEP 4c(4) Grasp corners of sterile drape, then hold up and away from body.

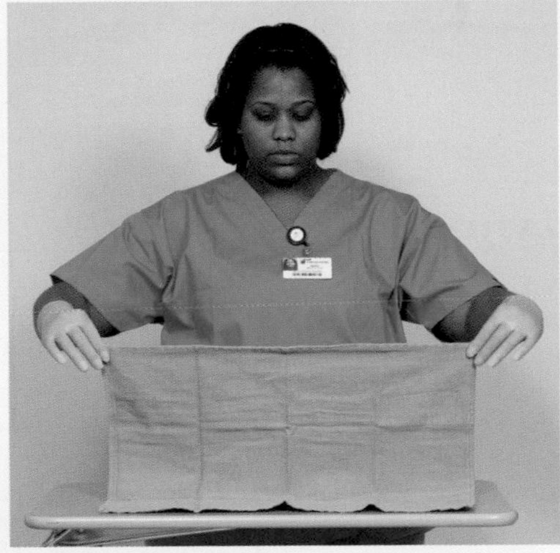

STEP 4c(5) Position bottom half of sterile drape over top half of work space.

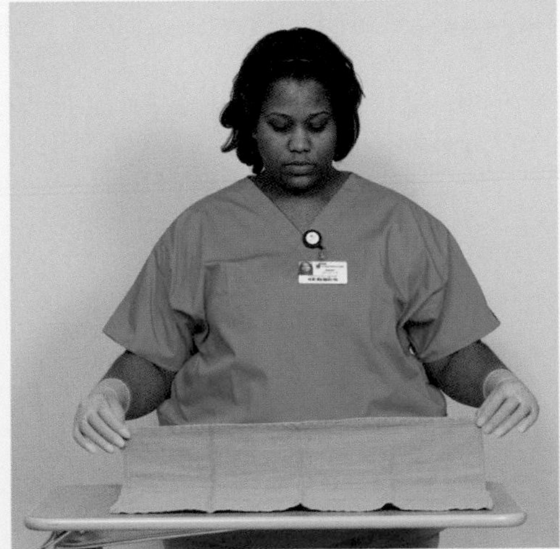

STEP 4c(6) Allow top half of drape to be placed over bottom half of work surface.

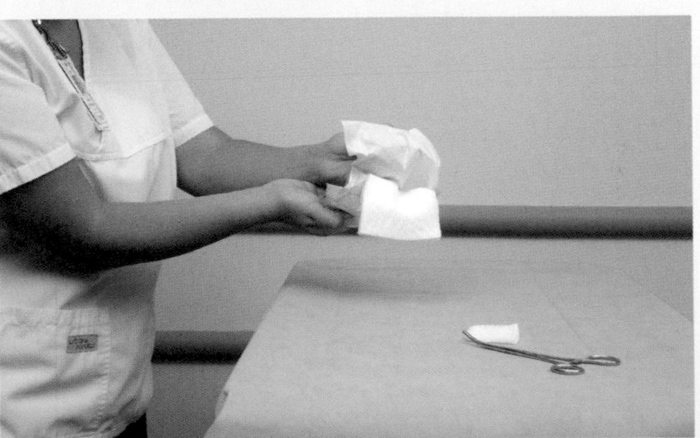

STEP 5c Add items to sterile field.

STEP	RATIONALE
c. Remove sterile seal and cap from bottle in upward motion.	Upward movement prevents contamination of bottle lip.
d. With solution bottle held away from field and bottle lip 2.5–5 cm (1–2 inch) above inside of sterile receiving container, slowly pour needed amount of solution into container. Hold bottle with label facing palm of hand (see illustration).	Edge and outside of bottle are considered contaminated. Slow pouring prevents splashing. Sterility of contents cannot be ensured if cap is replaced. Prevents label from becoming wet and illegible.

Safe Patient Care *When liquids permeate sterile field or barrier, it is called a strikethrough, resulting in contamination of the sterile field.*

STEP	RATIONALE
7. Remove gloves and perform hand hygiene.	Reduces transmission of infection.

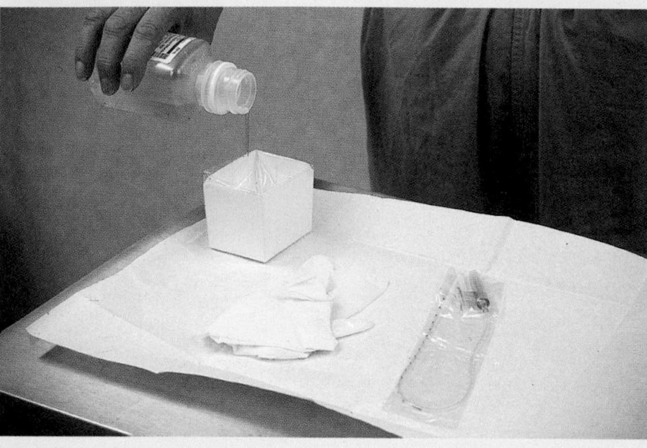

STEP 6d Pour solution into receiving container on sterile field.

EVALUATION

1. Observe for breaks in sterile technique throughout the procedure.	A break in sterile technique requires you to repeat the procedure.
2. **Use Teach-Back:** "I want to be sure I explained the procedure that was performed and the steps used to prevent infection. Please tell me some things that can be done to prevent infection." Revise your instruction now or develop a plan for revised patient/family caregiver teaching if patient/family caregiver is not able to teach back correctly.	Determines patient's/family caregiver's level of understanding of instructional topic.

Unexpected Outcomes	Related Interventions
1. Sterile field comes in contact with contaminated object or liquid splatters onto drape, causing strikethrough.	• Discontinue field preparation and start over with new equipment.
2. Sterile item falls off sterile field.	• Open another package containing new sterile item and add to field. Apply a new pair of sterile gloves. If field becomes contaminated, a new sterile field would need to be established. Apply a new pair of sterile gloves.

Recording

- Record the procedure performed and that sterile technique was used.

Hand-Off Reporting

- Discuss with nurses and other pertinent health care providers the sterile procedure performed, outcome, patient's response, and any necessary follow-up. This ensures quality continuation of care and provides for optimal patient outcomes.

✦ SKILL 5.5 Sterile Gloving

Purpose

Sterile gloves act as a barrier against the transmission of pathogens and are applied before performing sterile procedures, such as a sterile dressing change or urinary catheter insertion. Sterile gloves do not replace hand hygiene. The open-glove application method is used for procedures not requiring a sterile gown. Choose gloves that are the correct size—tight enough for objects to be picked up easily, but not so tight that they can easily tear. Contaminated or torn gloves need to be replaced immediately after performing hand hygiene. If you or the patient has a latex allergy (Box 5.4), choose latex-free or synthetic gloves.

Delegation and Collaboration

Assisting with skills that include the application and removal of sterile gloves may be delegated to nursing assistive personnel (NAP). However, most procedures that require the use of sterile gloves cannot be delegated to NAP. The nurse instructs the NAP about:

- The reason sterile gloves are being used for a specific procedure

Equipment

- Package of proper-size sterile gloves, latex or synthetic nonlatex. If patient has a latex allergy, ensure that gloves are latex-free and powder-free.

ASSESSMENT

1. Consider the type of procedure to be performed and consult agency policy on use of sterile gloves. In some facilities, double gloving is recommended for the operating room (OR) and if exposure to blood, body fluids, or infectious microorganisms is anticipated (AORN, 2017). *Rationale: Ensures proper use of sterile gloves. Evidence supports the use of double gloving and double gloving with an indicator glove system to decrease the risk of percutaneous injury and therefore is an effective barrier to bloodborne pathogen exposure (AORN, 2017).*
2. Consider patient's risk for infection (e.g., preexisting condition, immunosuppressed, type of procedure). *Rationale: Knowledge of risk directs you to follow necessary precautions (e.g., use of additional protective barriers) if necessary.*
3. Select correct size and type of gloves and examine glove package to determine whether it is dry and intact with no visible stains. *Rationale: Torn or wet package is considered contaminated. Visible stains on package indicate previous contamination by water or other liquid.*
4. Use nonpowdered gloves. *Rationale: The U.S. Food and Drug Administration (FDA) passed a ruling that powdered gloves may no longer be used due to increased risks of hypersensitivity and allergic reactions (FDA, 2016).*
5. Inspect condition of hands for cuts, hangnails, open lesions, or abrasions. In some settings, you can cover any open lesion with a sterile, impervious transparent dressing (check agency policy). In some cases, presence of such lesions may prevent you from participating in a procedure. *Rationale: Cuts, abrasions, and hangnails tend to ooze serum, which possibly contains pathogens. Breaks in skin integrity permit microorganisms to enter and increase the risk of infection for both patient and nurse (AORN, 2017).*
6. Assess patient for the following risk factors before applying latex gloves. *Rationale: Risk factors determine level of patient's risk for latex allergy (see Box 5.4).*
   a. Previous reaction to the following items within hours of exposure: adhesive tape, dental or face mask, golf club grip, ostomy bag, rubber band, balloon, bandage, elastic underwear, intravenous (IV) tubing, rubber gloves, condom. *Rationale: Items are known to lead to latex allergy.*
   b. Personal history of asthma, contact dermatitis, eczema, urticaria, rhinitis. *Rationale: Patients with a history of these conditions are at higher risk of having a reaction.*
   c. History of food allergies, especially avocado, banana, peach, chestnut, raw potato, kiwi, tomato, papaya. *Rationale: Patients with a history of food allergies are at higher risk of developing a reaction.*
   d. Previous history of adverse reactions during surgery or dental procedure. *Rationale: Previous history suggests allergic response.*
   e. Previous reaction to latex product. *Rationale: Previous reaction suggests allergic response.*
7. Assess patient's or family caregiver's knowledge, experience, and health literacy level. *Rationale: Ensures patient has the capacity to obtain, communicate, process, and understand basic health information (CDC, 2016b).*

BOX 5.4

Risk Factors for Latex Allergy

- Patients with spina bifida
- Patients with congenital or urogenital defects
- Patients with a history of indwelling catheters or repeated catheterization
- Patients with a long-term history of using condom catheters
- Individuals with high latex exposure (e.g., nurses, housekeepers, food handlers, tire manufacturers, other workers in industries that use gloves routinely)
- Patients with a history of multiple childhood surgeries
- People with a family history of allergies, such as hay fever or hives
- People with a history of food allergies, especially banana, avocado, chestnut, kiwi, apple, carrot, papaya, potato, tomato, and melons

Modified from Kahn SL, et al: Natural rubber latex allergy, *Dis Mon,* 62(1):5-17, 2016; Mayo Clinic Staff: *Latex allergy*, October 2014, http://www.mayoclinic.org/diseases-conditions/latex-allergy/basics/risk-factors/con-20024233.

STEP	RATIONALE
PLANNING	
1. Expected outcomes after completion of procedure:	
• Patient does not develop signs or symptoms of infection after procedure.	Indicates that microorganisms were not introduced into sterile body cavities or sites (such as skin or urinary tract) during procedure.
• Patient does not develop latex sensitivity or latex allergy reaction.	Patient at risk for latex allergy is not exposed to latex proteins.
• Explain to patient or family caregiver that sterile gloves are being used to prevent the transmission of infection.	Patient education is an important aspect of nursing care.
IMPLEMENTATION	
1. Apply sterile gloves.	
a. Perform thorough hand hygiene. Place glove package near work area.	Hand hygiene reduces number of microorganisms on skin surfaces and transmission of infection. Proximity to work area ensures availability before procedure.
b. Remove outer glove package wrapper by carefully separating and peeling apart sides (see illustration).	Proper removal prevents inner glove package from accidentally opening and touching contaminated objects.
c. Grasp inner package and place on clean, dry, flat surface at waist level. Open package, keeping gloves on inside surface of wrapper (see illustration).	Sterile object held below waist is contaminated. Inner surface of glove package is sterile.
d. Identify right and left glove. Each glove has a cuff approximately 5 cm (2 inches) wide. Glove dominant hand first.	Proper identification of gloves prevents contamination by improper fit. Gloving of dominant hand first improves dexterity.
e. With thumb and first two fingers of nondominant hand, grasp glove for dominant hand by touching only inside surface of cuff.	Inner edge of cuff will lie against skin and thus is not sterile.
f. Carefully pull glove over dominant hand, leaving a cuff and being sure that cuff does not roll up wrist. Be sure that thumb and fingers are in proper spaces (see illustration).	If outer surface of glove touches hand or wrist, it is contaminated.
g. With gloved dominant hand, slip fingers underneath cuff of second glove (see illustration).	Cuff protects gloved fingers. Sterile touching sterile prevents glove contamination.
h. Carefully pull second glove over fingers of nondominant hand (see illustration).	Contact of gloved hand with exposed hand results in contamination.

Safe Patient Care *Do not allow fingers and thumb of gloved dominant hand to touch any part of exposed nondominant hand. Keep thumb of dominant hand abducted back.*

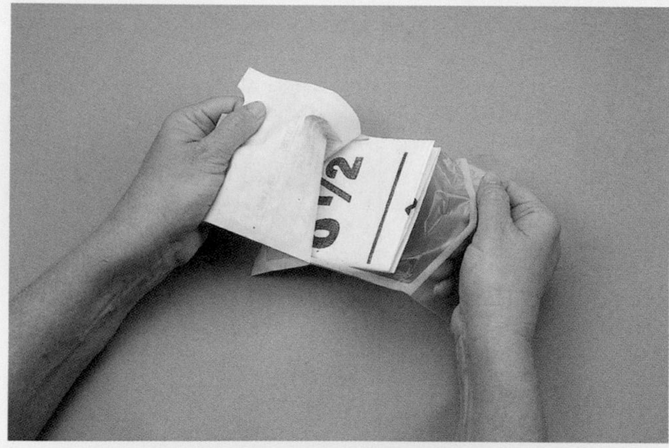

STEP 1b Open outer glove package wrapper.

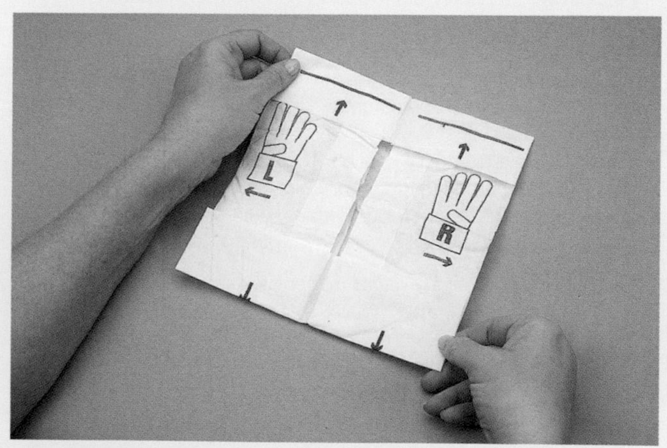

STEP 1c Open inner glove package on work surface.

STEP	RATIONALE
i. After second glove is on, interlock hands together and hold away from body above waist level until beginning procedure (see illustration).	Ensures smooth fit over fingers and prevents contamination.
2. Perform procedure.	
3. Remove gloves.	
a. Grasp outside of one cuff with other gloved hand; avoid touching wrist.	Procedure minimizes contamination of underlying skin.
b. Pull glove off, turning it inside out, and place it in gloved hand.	Outside of glove does not touch skin surface.
c. Take fingers of bare hand and tuck inside remaining glove cuff (see illustration). Peel glove off inside out and over previously removed glove. Discard both gloves in trash receptacle.	Fingers do not touch contaminated glove surface.
d. Perform thorough hand hygiene.	Hand hygiene protects health care provider from contamination resulting from any unseen tears or pinholes in gloves.

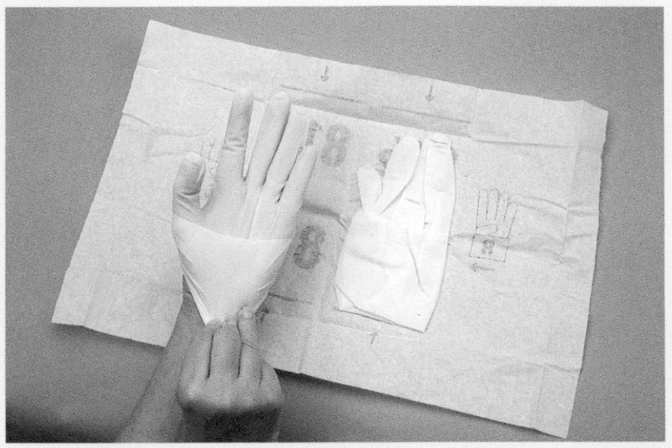

STEP 1f Pick up glove at cuff of dominant hand and insert fingers. Pull glove completely over dominant hand (example is for left-handed person).

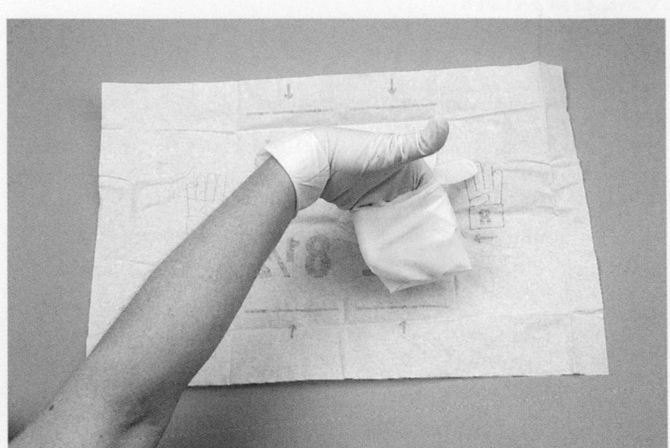

STEP 1g Pick up glove for nondominant hand.

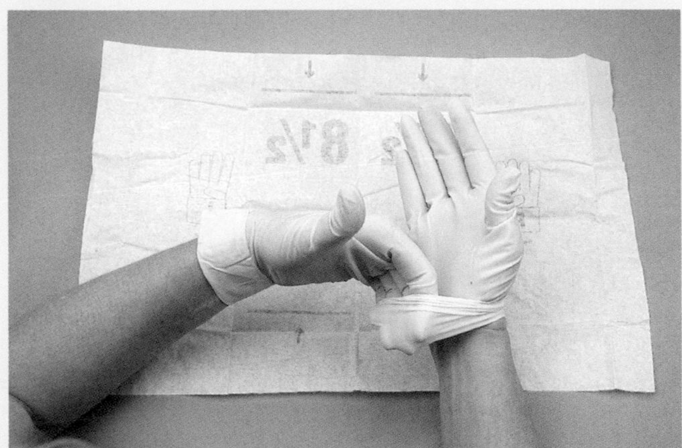

STEP 1h Pull second glove over nondominant hand.

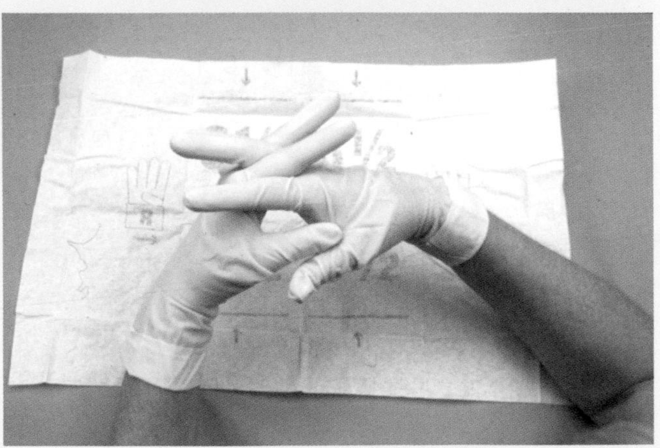

STEP 1i Interlock gloved hands.

STEP	RATIONALE

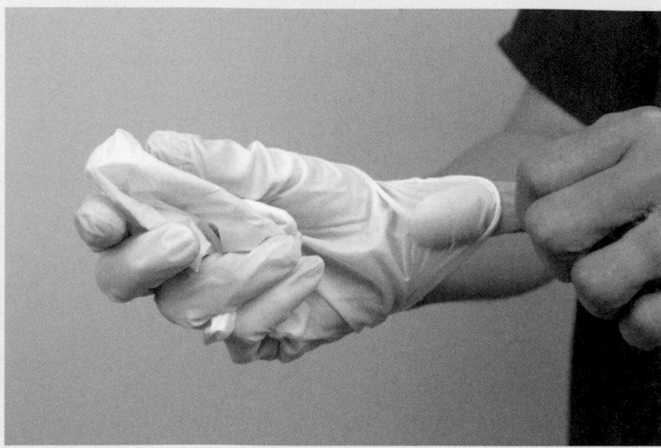

STEP 3c Remove second glove by turning it inside out.

EVALUATION

1. Assess patient for signs/symptoms of infection, focusing on area treated.	Improper sterile technique contributes to development of an infection.
2. Assess patient for signs/symptoms of latex allergy.	Assessment establishes baseline for patient's reaction to latex.
3. **Use Teach-Back:** "I want to be sure I explained why I used sterile gloves for this procedure. Please explain to me why I needed to use sterile gloves." Revise your instruction now or develop a plan for revised patient/family caregiver teaching if patient/family caregiver is not able to teach back correctly.	Determines patient's/family caregiver's level of understanding of instructional topic.

Unexpected Outcomes	Related Interventions
1. Patient develops localized signs of infection (e.g., urine becomes cloudy or odorous; wound becomes painful, edematous, or reddened).	• Contact health care provider and implement appropriate interventions as prescribed.
2. Patient develops systemic signs of infection (e.g., fever, malaise, increased white blood cell count). • Patient develops allergic reaction to latex (Box 5.5).	• Contact health care provider and implement appropriate interventions as prescribed. • Immediately remove source of latex, if known. • Bring emergency equipment to bedside. Have epinephrine injection ready for administration, and be prepared to initiate IV fluids and oxygen. • Alert the health care team after agency protocol.

BOX 5.5

Levels of Latex Reactions

The three levels of symptoms are mild, more-severe, and anaphylactic shock symptoms. Symptoms are listed in order of increasing severity.

1. *Mild symptoms:* Itching, skin redness, hives or rash.
2. *More-severe symptoms:* Sneezing, runny nose, itchy or watery eyes, scratchy throat, difficulty breathing, wheezing and coughing.
3. *Anaphylactic shock symptoms:* Difficulty breathing, wheezing, hives or swelling, decrease in blood pressure, dizziness, loss of consciousness, confusion, rapid or weak pulse. A true latex allergy can be life-threatening, and emergency care is recommended.

Modified from Mayo Clinic Staff: *Latex allergy,* October 2014, http://www.mayoclinic.org/diseases-conditions/latex-allergy/basics/symptoms/con-20024233.

Recording

- No recording or reporting is required for sterile gloving.
- Record the procedure performed and patient's response.

Hand-Off Reporting

- Discuss with nurses and other pertinent health care providers the sterile procedure performed, patient's response, outcome, and any necessary follow-up.

SPECIAL CONSIDERATIONS

Patient-Centered Care

- If patient does not speak English, use a professional interpreter if available, agency-approved video, or telephone translation service to educate patient and family caregiver.

- Isolation in a private room can cause loneliness, and suffering from an infectious disease can also cause self-concept and body-image issues (AORN, 2017). Health care providers enter isolation rooms less frequently than nonisolation rooms (CDC, 2016c). The patient's needs must be assessed and interventions implemented to appropriately care for the patient.

Patient Education

- Explain the need for PPE to patients and family caregivers.
- Demonstrate to family caregivers how to apply and remove PPE.
- Teach patients and family caregivers to observe for signs of infection.
- Explain the purpose of isolation to patients and family caregivers.
- Teach family caregivers about the isolation-related precautions that must be taken before entering an isolation room (AORN, 2017).
- Teach patients and family caregivers about the importance of hand hygiene. Providing patients with hand wipes or alcohol-based hand rub at the bedside has been shown to decrease the occurrence of HAIs (Haverstick et al., 2017).

Age-Specific

- The use of PPE can be confusing and frightening to children and the elderly, especially those who have signs and symptoms of confusion or depression. Provide age- and developmentally appropriate teaching and demonstrations related to the need for, and application of, PPE. Assess for understanding and provide follow-up instructions, as needed, especially because patients often become more confused when cared for by a nurse using PPE or when left in a room with the door closed. Assess the patient's health history and whether the door needs to be closed (negative-airflow room) as well as any safety measures required.
- Memory and sensory deficits may impair an older patient's ability to understand the need for a procedure. Provide patient-specific interventions (e.g., music therapy) while a patient is in isolation.
- The risk for and impact of infection is greater for children and the elderly. Diligent hand hygiene is crucial when caring for patients in these age groups.
- When caring for a child, show the child all the PPE to be used, and explain why it is needed. Involve parents in any explanations. Nurses should let children see their faces before applying masks so that children do not become frightened (Hockenberry and Wilson, 2017) and to personalize the care.
- Isolation creates a sense of separation from family. The strange environment can confuse a child. Preschoolers are often unable to understand the rationale for isolation.
- Depending on their level of developmental maturity, children may be unable to cooperate during a sterile procedure.
- Family members may wish to assist during a sterile procedure so that the child remains calm and does not contaminate the sterile field (Hockenberry and Wilson, 2017).

Home Care

- Patients and family caregivers should be encouraged to make the practice of hand hygiene an important part of everyday life.
- Instruct family caregivers as to how and when to use PPE, if necessary.
- Teach family caregiver about the signs of infection and whom to contact if symptoms develop.
- Patients are generally not isolated in the home, but patients and family caregivers should be taught how to prevent infection in the home environment (e.g., by not sharing personal items and receiving recommended vaccinations).
- Clean technique is used for most procedures performed in the home, such as self-catheterization and tracheostomy care. If sterile technique will be required, teach patients and family caregivers how to perform sterile procedures well before discharge so that the skills can be learned and reinforced with professional assistance. Assess for understanding via return demonstration and teach-back methods.
- Limit the amount of reusable equipment brought into the home if patients are infected or colonized with MDROs. If removing equipment from the home after a visit (e.g., stethoscope), clean the items before removing with a low- to intermediate-strength disinfectant (CDC, 2016c).

✦ PRACTICE REFLECTIONS

You are caring for a 76-year-old woman requiring isolation precautions for *C. difficile.* She is upset that you and the NAP take a long time to respond to the nurse call system because you first must apply PPE. She is concerned about the use of PPE by everyone who enters her room because she believes it suggests that she is offensive to others.

1. What are the priority diagnoses applicable for this patient?
2. What patient education should be provided to meet the needs of this patient?
3. What information should be communicated to nurses and other health care providers caring for this patient?

✦ CLINICAL REVIEW QUESTIONS

1. Which of the following are examples of proper hand hygiene? (Select all that apply.)
   1. Washing hands for at least 15 seconds.
   2. Washing hands with hot water.
   3. Using a paper towel to turn off the faucet.
   4. Keeping hands and forearms higher than elbows during washing and rinsing.
   5. Rubbing hands together until alcohol-based hand rub is completely dry.

2. Place the steps for removing PPE when wearing a disposable gown in order:
   1. Remove goggles, eyewear, or face shield.
   2. Remove mask or respirator.
   3. Remove cap (if worn).
   4. Remove gown and gloves simultaneously.
   5. Perform hand hygiene.

3. Which of the following demonstrate that a nurse knows how to properly care for a patient who has an MDRO? (Select all that apply.)
   1. Judicious use of hand hygiene
   2. Utilizing standard and appropriate contact precautions
   3. Cohorting a patient diagnosed with MRSA and a patient diagnosed with VRE
   4. Applying appropriate PPE on a patient being transported for a procedure or test

Answers and Rationales for Clinical Review Questions can be found on the Evolve website.

REFERENCES

Anderson DJ, et al: The antimicrobial scrub contamination and transmission (ASCOT) trial: a three-arm, blinded, randomized controlled trial with crossover design to determine the efficacy of antimicrobial-impregnated scrubs in preventing healthcare provider contamination, *Infect Control Hosp Epidemiol* 38(10): 1147–1154, 2017.

Association of periOperative Registered Nurses (AORN): *Guidelines for perioperative practice*, Denver, 2017, AORN.

Beam E, et al: Clinical challenges in isolation care, *Am J Nurs* 115(4):44–49, 2015.

Booth K: Preventing healthcare associated infections (HAIs), *J Contin Educ Nurs Topics Issues* 18(1):18–23, 2016.

Centers for Disease Control and Prevention (CDC): Patient safety: what you can do to be a safe patient, 2014. https://www.cdc.gov/hai/patientsafety/patient-safety.html.

Centers for Disease Control and Prevention (CDC): Isolation precautions, 2015. https://www.cdc.gov/infectioncontrol/guidelines/isolation/index.html.

Centers for Disease Control and Prevention (CDC): Carbapenem-resistant Enterobacteriaceae in healthcare settings, 2016a. https://www.cdc.gov/hai/organisms/cre/index.html.

Centers for Disease Control and Prevention (CDC): What is health literacy, 2016b. https://www.cdc.gov/healthliteracy/learn/index.html.

Centers for Disease Control and Prevention (CDC): Management of multidrug-resistant organisms in healthcare settings, 2016c. https://www.cdc.gov/infectioncontrol/guidelines/mdro/recommendations.html.

Centers for Disease Control and Prevention (CDC): Sequence for putting on personal protective equipment (PPE), 2016d. https://www.cdc.gov/hai/pdfs/ppe/PPE-Sequence.pdf.

Centers for Disease Control and Prevention (CDC): Tuberculosis (TB), 2016e. https://www.cdc.gov/tb/default.htm.

Centers for Disease Control and Prevention (CDC): Clean hands count for healthcare providers, 2017a. https://www.cdc.gov/handhygiene/providers/index.html.

Centers for Disease Control and Prevention (CDC): HAI data and statistics, 2017b. https://www.cdc.gov/hai/surveillance/index.html.

Haverstick S, et al: Patients' hand washing and reducing hospital-acquired infection, *Crit Care Nurse* 37(3):e1–e8, 2017.

Hayden M: Measuring carbapenem-resistant Enterobacteriaceae in the United States: a critical step for control, *JAMA* 314(14):1455–1456, 2015.

Hockenberry MJ, Wilson D: *Wong's essentials of pediatric nursing*, ed 10, St. Louis, 2017, Mosby.

Holleck JL, et al: Can education influence stethoscope hygiene? *Am J Infect Control* 45(7):811–812, 2017.

Hsu V: Prevention of healthcare-associated infections, *Am Fam Physician* 90(6): 377–382, 2014.

Livshiz-Riven I, et al: Relationship between shared patient care items and healthcare-associated infections: a systematic review, *Int J Nurs Stud* 52:380–392, 2015.

Occupational Safety and Health Administration (OSHA): Enforcement procedures and scheduling for occupational exposure to tuberculosis, 2015. https://www.osha.gov/OshDoc/Directive_pdf/CPL_02-02-078.pdf.

Spruce L: Back to basics: surgical attire and cleanliness, *AORN J* 99(1):138–146, 2014.

The Joint Commission (TJC): *2019 National Patient Safety Goals*, Oakbrook Terrace, IL, 2019, The Commission. http://www.jointcommission.org/standards_information/npsgs.aspx.

U.S. Food & Drug Administration (FDA): Medical device bans, 2016. https://www.fda.gov/MedicalDevices/Safety/MedicalDeviceBans/default.htm.

World Health Organization (WHO): Clean care is safer care: save lives: clean your hands, 2017. http://www.who.int/gpsc/5may/background/5moments/en/.

Zimlichman E, et al: Healthcare-associated infections: A meta-analysis of costs and financial impact on the US health care system, *JAMA Intern Med* 173(22): 2039–2046, 2013.

6 Disaster Preparedness

SKILLS AND PROCEDURES

EVOLVE WEBSITE/RESOURCES LIST

http://evolve.elsevier.com/Perry/nursinginterventions

Audio Glossary • Checklists • Clinical Review Questions • Answers and Rationales for Clinical Review Questions

INTRODUCTION

A disaster can lead to significant destruction and/or adverse consequences (Box 6.1). The terrorist attacks on the World Trade Center and Pentagon on September 11, 2001, caused severe physical and emotional destruction, impacting the sense of security felt by citizens of the United States. The National Terrorism Advisory System (NTAS) was developed to facilitate public awareness by providing government officials, first responders, and public citizens with information regarding the nature and degree of terrorist threat (Fig. 6.1) (Department of Homeland Security [DHS], 2016).

Natural disasters, including hurricanes Harvey and Irma in 2017 and disease outbreaks, such as the Ebola outbreak of 2014 (Box 6.2), further reinforce the need for public health education on disaster preparedness and response. The incident command system (ICS) is a standardized, on-scene, all-hazards incident management approach, which provides organization so that all members of the health care team and community know their roles and know the chain of command in an emergency situation (Emergency Management System, 2017) (Fig. 6.2).

Nurses play a key role in the coordination and implementation of an interprofessional approach to prepare for and respond to disaster through education and delivery of care to diverse populations at times of crisis. Some states are enacting new laws that require disaster training as part of the continuing education requirement for licensure (American Nurses Association [ANA], 2017), and nurses may deliver care during emergencies in states where they are not licensed. The ANA (2017) is continually working to create laws to protect providers. In addition, nurses and other professionals are at risk for the physical and psychological effects of disasters; therefore they need to have the knowledge and skill to protect themselves from physical and emotional harm.

PRACTICE STANDARDS

- American Nurses Association (ANA), 2017: Disaster preparedness and response
- American Red Cross, 2017: How to prepare for emergencies
- Centers for Disease Control and Prevention (CDC), 2017c: Emergency preparedness and response
- Federal Emergency Management Agency (FEMA), 2018: 2018–2022 strategic plan: a guide for disaster planning and response

TRIAGE, TREAT, AND EVACUATE

Triage is the process of sorting individuals by the IDME categories (immediate, delayed, minimal, expectant) for seriousness of their condition and the likelihood of their survival (Box 6.3). In an epidemic situation, triage is also used to prevent secondary spread of a disease. Be compassionate and respectful, and learn your patients' concerns and fears. Disaster triage can be accomplished with the SALT (Sort–Assess–Lifesaving interventions–Treatment/transport) triage system. All victims are first sorted into groups based on mobility. They are then individually assessed, sorted into categories, and evacuated for treatment as needed (Fig. 6.3). The goal is to sort, assess, and perform lifesaving measures as quickly as possible for large numbers of victims. Using simple language, explain to patients the process of triage:

Step One in the SALT triage model is to "sort" individuals into one of three major categories before they are assessed individually. Category one includes people who are not moving and have obvious life-threatening injuries. Category two includes people who can wave or have purposeful movements. Category three includes people who can walk.

Step Two of the SALT triage system involves individual assessment and further patient sorting into categories that include

(1) those minimally injured, (2) people who will survive even with delayed treatment, (3) those who need immediate intervention, and (4) people expected to die. Lifesaving interventions will be administered according to which category the person is labeled.

Step Three of SALT triage involves treatment and/or transport of victims. As with any emergency, reassessment is always necessary. During reassessment, rescue workers consider patient conditions, resources, and scene safety.

During triage, the focus may shift to psychological support of survivors or transport to specific agencies.

BOX 6.1

Disaster Definitions and Types

- **Disaster:** A catastrophic and/or destructive event (e.g., tsunamis, terrorist attacks) that disrupts normal functioning; may include any anticipated or unexpected event, the effects of which lead to significant destruction and/or adverse consequences
- **Mass-casualty incident or event (MCI):** Any event or situation (e.g., bombing of a public area) that results in multiple casualties and/or deaths; exists when health care needs exceed health care resources
- **All-hazards event:** Multiple manmade or natural events with destructive capacity to cause multiple casualties
- **All-hazards preparedness:** The comprehensive preparedness necessary to manage casualties resulting from a disaster, regardless of etiology
- **Casualty:** Any individual who is ill, injured, missing, or killed as a result of an MCI
- **Medical disasters:** Catastrophic events (e.g., mass shootings) that result in human casualties that overwhelm the available health care resources
- **Natural/environmental disasters:** Catastrophic events that result from an ecological event that exceeds the capacity of the community (e.g., the impact of hurricanes or tornados on a community)
- **Manmade disasters:** Catastrophic events (e.g., wildfires) the principal direct cause of which is attributable to human action
- **Technological disasters:** Catastrophic events in which people, property, community infrastructure, and economic welfare are adversely affected by the disruption of technology (e.g., industrial accidents, unplanned release of nuclear waste)

EVIDENCE-BASED PRACTICE

Disaster Nursing Competence

Although nurses play a key role in disaster preparedness and response, research suggests that nurses may not be functioning to the extent of their abilities in these situations and are not optimally prepared. A recent study examined the self-reported competence of nursing students and registered nurses (RNs), focusing on their readiness

BOX 6.2

Ebola Virus Disease

- Ebola virus disease (EVD), formerly known as Ebola hemorrhagic fever, is a severe, often fatal illness in humans.
- It is transmitted to people from blood, secretions, organs, or other bodily fluids of infected animals such as chimpanzees, gorillas, fruit bats, monkeys, forest antelope, and porcupines found ill or dead or in the rain forest.
- It spreads by human-to-human contact via direct contact with the blood, secretions, organs, or other bodily fluids of infected people and with surfaces and materials.
- Ebola was first discovered in 1976. The 2014–2016 outbreak in West Africa was the largest and most complex Ebola outbreak since the virus was first discovered.
- The incubation period is 2 to 21 days; humans are not infectious until they develop symptoms.
- Early symptoms include sudden onset of fever, fatigue, muscle pain, headache, and sore throat, followed by vomiting, diarrhea, rash, symptoms of impaired kidney and liver function, and in some cases, both internal and external bleeding.
- Early supportive care with rehydration and symptomatic treatment improves survival. There is no licensed treatment proven to neutralize the virus, but blood, immunological, and drug therapies are under development.
- Prevention and control focus on reducing the risk of transmission and outbreak containment measures.
- Health care providers take standard precautions and apply extra infection control measures when caring for a patient with EVD.
- When in close contact (within 1 meter) of patients with EVD, wear face protection (a face shield or a medical mask and goggles); a clean, nonsterile long-sleeved gown; and gloves (sterile gloves for some procedures).

Data from World Health Organization (WHO): *Ebola virus disease,* 2017, http://www.who.int/mediacentre/factsheets/fs103/en/.

Alert Is Issued		
Elevated Threat Alert Warns of a credible terrorist threat against the United States	**Imminent Threat Alert** Warns of a credible, specific, and impending terrorist threat against the United States	
Information Included in Alert		
Summary	Details, including affected areas	Duration of alert
How you can help	Steps to stay prepared	How to stay informed
Sunset Provision An individual threat alert is issued for a specific time period and then automatically expires. It may be extended if new information becomes available or the threat evolves.		

FIG 6.1 National Terrorism Advisory System overview. (*Adapted from Department of Homeland Security: National Terrorism Advisory System bulletin, 2017.* https://www.dhs.gov/sites/default/files/ntas/alerts/16_1115_NTAS_bulletin.pdf.)

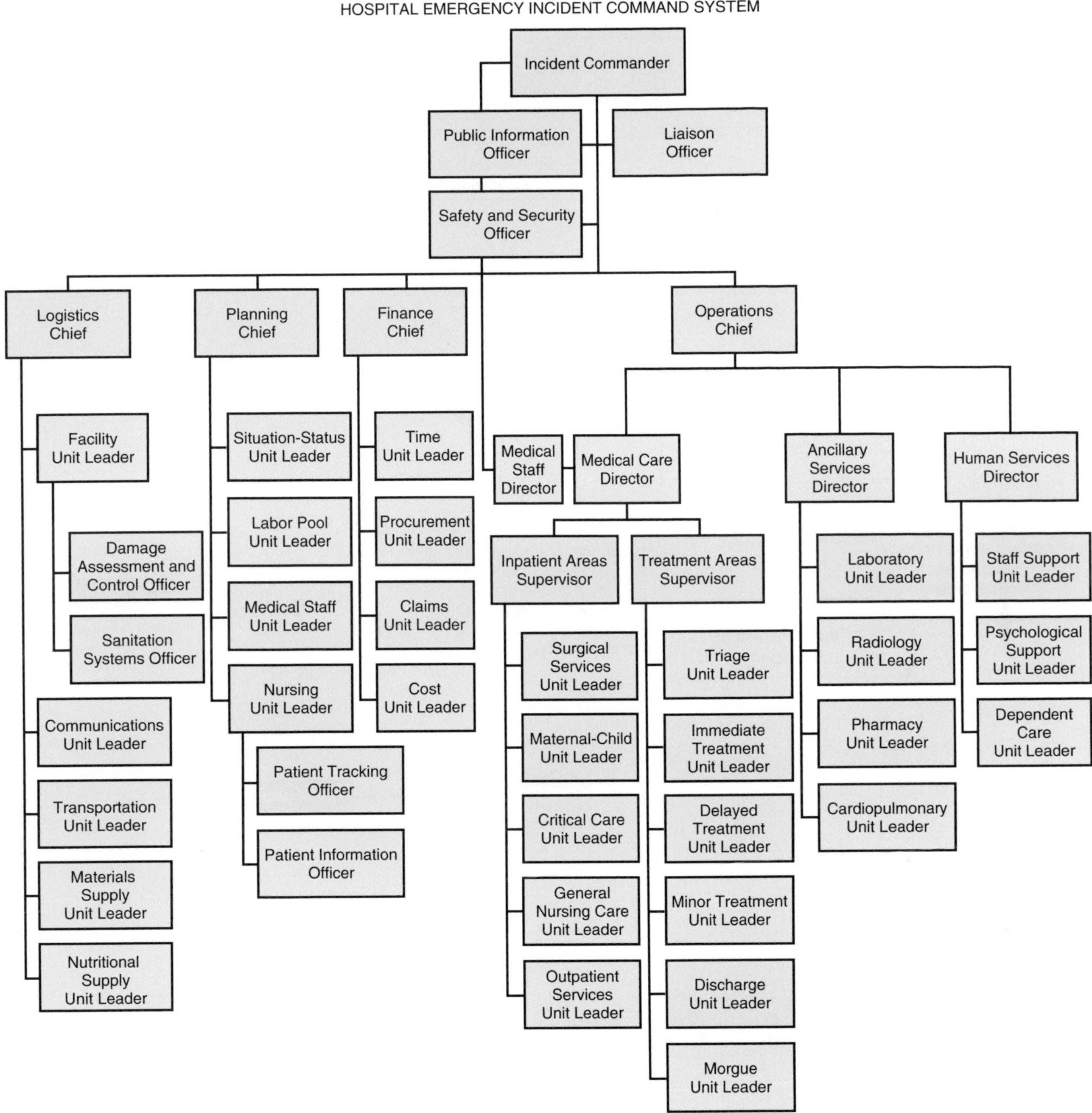

FIG 6.2 The hospital emergency incident command system prepares all response teams to work smoothly in a disaster situation.

BOX 6.3

IDME—Assess, Treat, and Send

Immediate (Red)

- Unconscious or unresponsive
- Altered mental status
- Experiencing hypoxia or near-hypoxia
- Chest pain
- Chest wounds
- Full-thickness burns over 20% to 60% of the body
- Uncontrollable bleeding
- Amputations above elbow or knee
- Rapid or weak pulse
- Open abdominal wounds

Delayed (Yellow)

- Deep lacerations
- Open fractures with controlled bleeding and strong pulses
- Multiple fractures
- Finger amputations
- Abdominal injuries with stable vital signs
- Closed head injuries without altered level of consciousness

Minimal (Green)

- Abrasions
- Contusions
- Sprains
- Minor lacerations
- No apparent injuries
- Other injuries of similar severity

Expectant (Black)

- Victims still alive but so severely injured as to have little chance of survival
- Victims who have died

IDME, Immediate, delayed, minimal, expectant.

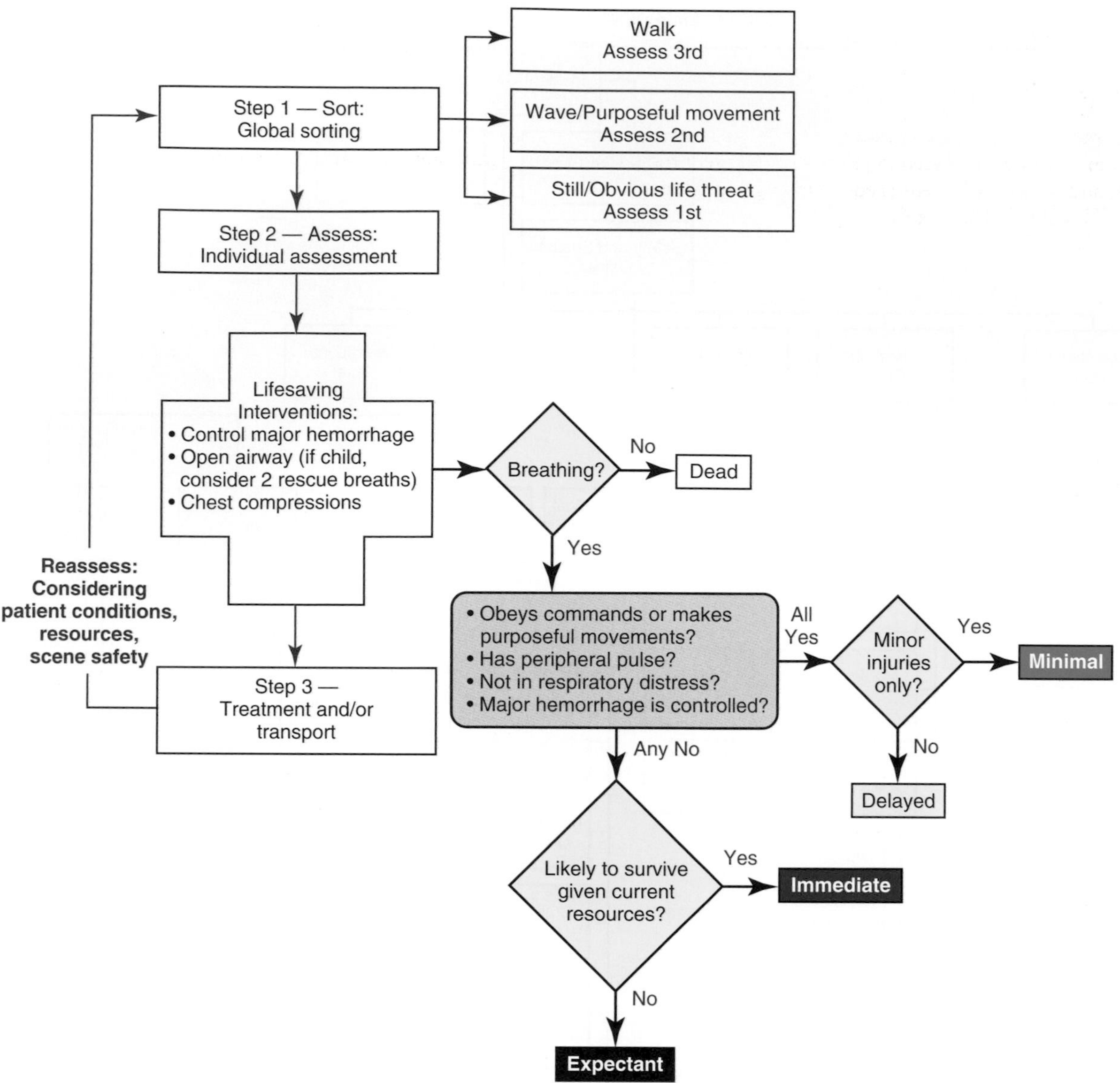

FIG 6.3 SALT (Sort, Assess, Lifesaving interventions, Treatment/transport) mass-casualty triage algorithm. (*Adapted from Lerner EB et al.: Mass casualty triage: an evaluation of the science and refinement of a national guideline*, Disaster Med Public Health Prep *5[2]:129, 2011.*)

to manage violence, serious events, and disasters (Nilsson et al., 2016). Participants were asked about their ability to handle situations involving violence, to act in accordance with regulations specific to fire and disaster situations, and to apply principles of disaster medicine. Findings from Nilsson et al. highlight the need for education and practice to support the development of these competencies and bridge the gaps in knowledge and preparedness in disaster nursing management and include the following:

- RNs scored significantly higher than nursing students in their ability to handle situations involving violence and threats of violence/harm and application of disaster medicine.
- RNs working in emergency care scored higher than nurses working in non-emergency care, supporting the importance of RNs being exposed to disaster nursing.
- Higher competence was also reported by RNs who had completed some graduate education, who worked the night shift, and who were in a relationship at the time of the study.
- Students who lived alone, had extra work experience in health care during their nursing education, and had a preference for working in emergency care scored higher in competence. Male students also scored higher than female students.
- Additional hours of disaster nursing are needed in undergraduate education to better prepare RNs for disaster management.
- Varied teaching methods can help engage students and prepare them to respond to violence and disasters.

Nilsson et al. (2016) also concluded that opportunities for RNs to maintain and improve competence in disaster nursing are needed and that simulation can be one means to accomplish this. A study by Jung et al. (2016) utilized simulation by examining the effect of in situ simulation on health care providers' knowledge and skill in disaster response. During the simulation, there were issues of communication resulting in a disruption of the flow of patients through triage. This was in part due to communication devices failing, a lack of gurneys to transport patients, and participants not utilizing the disaster resources, including the disaster manual. Real patients also continued to be treated in the emergency department (ED), also impacting the flow of triage. Both studies support the need for continued education and evaluation of competence in disaster response.

SAFETY GUIDELINES

When considering all forms of disaster, there are basic safety guidelines for a nurse or other health care providers to follow:

- The first priority at any disaster scene is to protect yourself and other team members. The second priority is to protect the public, patients, and the environment (Federal Emergency Management Agency [FEMA], 2018; Box 6.4).
- It is essential that rescue and health care workers avoid becoming victims. This may go against your initial instinct to help others, but first responders must wait until a disaster scene is secured and all safety precautions are taken (FEMA, 2018).
- Assessing hazards is more important than knowing the exact cause of a disaster; a mass-casualty incident (MCI) can result in secondary hazards that come in many forms (Box 6.5).
- The potential for public alarm and major disruption of everyday life is enormous. Know crisis intervention and stress-management techniques.
- In an MCI, most people, whether contaminated, exposed, or not, will self-triage and go directly to a local hospital, bypassing triage and treatment. Plans are needed to transfer patients to other medical facilities.
- Personal protective equipment (PPE) minimizes the risk for contact with contaminated materials or individuals. Proper use of advanced forms of PPE requires training, fitting, and an understanding that not all PPE protects against all potential hazards.
- When used inappropriately, PPE becomes a hazard (e.g., dehydration, decreased vision, mobility, and ability to communicate). Some of these hazards result from the fact that the user is unable to eat, drink, or go to the bathroom while using advanced forms of PPE.
- PPE is categorized by levels A to D for the level of safety provided:
  - Level A—Selected when the greatest level of skin, respiratory, and eye protection is required. It provides maximum protection because it offers a self-contained breathing apparatus, total encapsulating chemical-protective suit, coveralls, undergarments, chemical-resistant boots and gloves, hard hat, and disposable protective suit worn over the encapsulating suit (Fig. 6.4). Highly trained personnel use level A protection

BOX 6.4

Safety and Security

- Trained emergency personnel (e.g., firefighters and police) are responsible for the safety and security of a disaster scene.
- Nurses stay out of a disaster scene unless well trained and invited. Call 9-1-1 if emergency personnel have not already been notified.
- Do not disturb the scene; key evidence could be lost or contaminated.
- A health care agency becomes a secondary disaster site when contaminated by the agent from the original disaster scene. For example, a patient has been exposed to mustard gas, an oily chemical that is difficult to remove from a patient's body. If not properly decontaminated, the victim contaminated by the mustard gas will inadvertently contaminate health care providers and others (CDC, 2013).

BOX 6.5

Potential Hazards at the Scene of a Disaster

- Downed powerlines
- Smoke/toxic gases
- Debris that can result in trauma
- Fractured/leaking gas lines
- Fire resulting in burns
- Structural collapse
- Blood and other body fluids
- Inclement weather
- Hazardous materials
- Nuclear, biological, or chemical exposure
- Flooding and the threat of drowning
- Radiation exposure
- Explosion, particularly secondary explosions
- Snipers
- Darkness
- Infection
- High-velocity projectiles and the pressure wave after an explosion
- Becoming incapacitated and unable to protect yourself or your patient

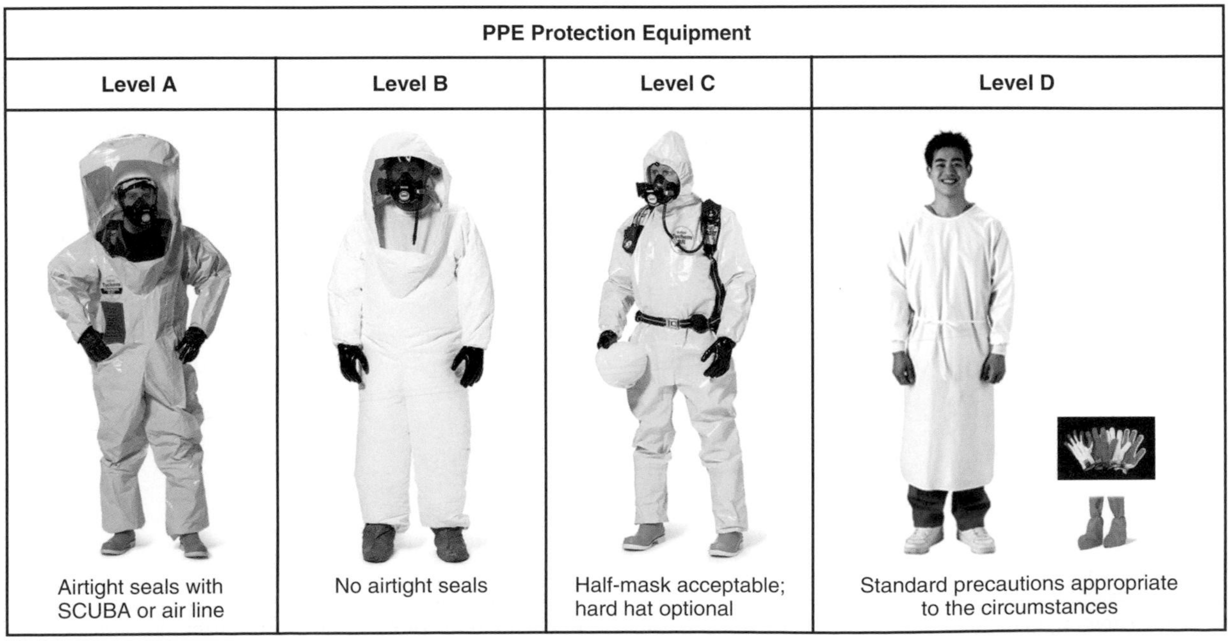

PPE Protection Equipment			
Level A	Level B	Level C	Level D
Airtight seals with SCUBA or air line	No airtight seals	Half-mask acceptable; hard hat optional	Standard precautions appropriate to the circumstances

FIG 6.4 The Occupational Safety and Health Administration (OSHA) defines personal protective equipment for the four levels of hazardous exposure. *PPE*, Personal protective equipment; *SCUBA*, self-contained underwater breathing apparatus.

in heavily contaminated areas. If you are not wearing this type of protection and you are near an area where level A PPE is being used, get out or do not enter.
- Level B—Provides the highest level of respiratory protection but less skin protection. Used by trained responders, this PPE includes a self-contained breathing apparatus; hooded chemical-resistant suit; and face, boot, and glove protection. Level B protection also requires training and fitting.
- Level C—First responders (emergency personnel first on the scene) and hospital personnel are trained and fitted to use level C protection, which involves knowing the concentration and type of airborne substance(s) and the criteria for using air-purifying respirators. Level C constitutes the use of full-face or half-mask air-purifying respirators (approved by the National Institute for Occupational Safety and Health [NIOSH]), hooded chemical-resistant clothing, and protective gloves and boots. Because of the garment protection worn with levels A, B and C, the user is at risk for dehydration and hyperthermia.
- Level D—Standard work uniforms or work clothes are appropriate and used for nuisance contamination only. The users must wear coveralls and chemical-resistant shoes; depending on the contaminant, gloves, goggles, mask, face shield, and hard hats may also be worn. There is no respiratory protection. It is important to take standard precautions when using level D protection. Depending on the circumstances, some health care providers also choose to use a fluid-impermeable gown, cap, eye protection, mask, gloves, and shoe covers (Occupational Safety and Health Administration [OSHA], 2011).
- The most recently labeled level of protection is BioPPE. BioPPE requires the use of standard work clothes along with contact and respiratory protection. Double gloving and an N95 mask (see Chapter 5) or a better respirator are recommended. BioPPE protection is not adequate when caring for patients exposed to toxic chemicals; however, it provides adequate protection against radiological and biological agents.
- Hand hygiene that includes washing with soap and water followed by use of an alcohol gel is important at all levels (see Chapter 5).

✦ SKILL 6.1 Care of a Patient After Biological Exposure

Purpose

In a bioterrorism attack, there is a deliberate release of viruses, bacteria, or other germs with the intent to cause illness or death (National Institutes of Health [NIH], 2017). The use of biological agents is a considerable terrorist threat because they are easy to disperse and affect large numbers of people at a relatively low cost; sometimes several agents are disseminated at the same time (Box 6.6). Some biological attacks are unannounced or covert, and the onset of symptoms is delayed by an incubation period (i.e., the time between exposure and onset of symptoms), during which some of these agents may be transmitted as an infected patient exposes others. Recognition of bioterrorism is a challenge because early signs and symptoms mimic the flu or produce a rash mistaken for a viral illness (Fig. 6.5A–B). To understand how to protect yourself from becoming a victim, you need to understand the mode of transmission and precautions to take for biosafety (Table 6.1).

BOX 6.6

Potential Bioterrorism Agents/Diseases

- Anthrax (*Bacillus anthracis*)
- Botulism (*Clostridium botulinum toxin*)
- Brucellosis (*Brucella* species)
- *Chlamydia psittaci* (psittacosis)
- Ebola virus hemorrhagic fever
- Emerging infectious diseases such as Nipah virus and Hantavirus
- Epsilon toxin of *Clostridium perfringens*
- *Escherichia coli* O157:H7 (*E. coli*)
- Food safety threats (e.g., *Salmonella* species, *E. coli* O157:H7, *Shigella*)
- Plague (*Yersinia pestis*)
- Q fever (*Coxiella burnetii*)
- *Salmonella* species (salmonellosis)
- Staphylococcal enterotoxin B
- Tularemia (*Francisella tularensis*)
- Typhoid fever (*Salmonella typhi*)
- Variola major (smallpox)
- *Vibrio cholerae* (cholera)
- Viral encephalitis (alphaviruses [e.g., Venezuelan equine encephalitis, eastern equine encephalitis, western equine encephalitis])
- Water safety threats (e.g., *V. cholerae*, *Cryptosporidium parvum*)

Data from Centers for Disease Control and Prevention (CDC): *Bioterrorism agents/diseases,* 2017, http://www.emergency.cdc.gov/agent/agentlist.asp.

Delegation and Collaboration

The skill of assessing a patient exposed to a biological agent cannot be delegated to nursing assistive personnel (NAP). The nurse directs the NAP to:
- Use appropriate PPE to prevent exposure during care activities.
- Use proper techniques for handling a body after death to prevent contamination.

Equipment

Choice of equipment depends on the route of transmission of the infectious agent. The following is a general list of supplies that might be used in the event of release of the most contagious biological agents:
- Biohazard bags with label
- Soap and water
- 0.5% diluted bleach or Environmental Protection Agency (EPA)–approved germicidal agent
- Negative-pressure room (high-efficiency particulate air [HEPA] filtration may be required) with anteroom
- Clean gloves
- Gown
- Shoe covers
- Head covers
- Mask
- Standard face mask
- N95 mask
- Face shield
- Equipment for physical examination
- Oxygen therapy
- Airway maintenance supplies
- Intravenous therapy supplies

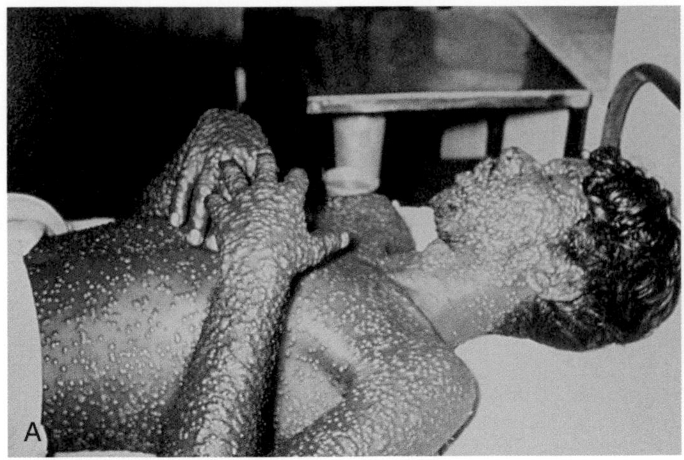

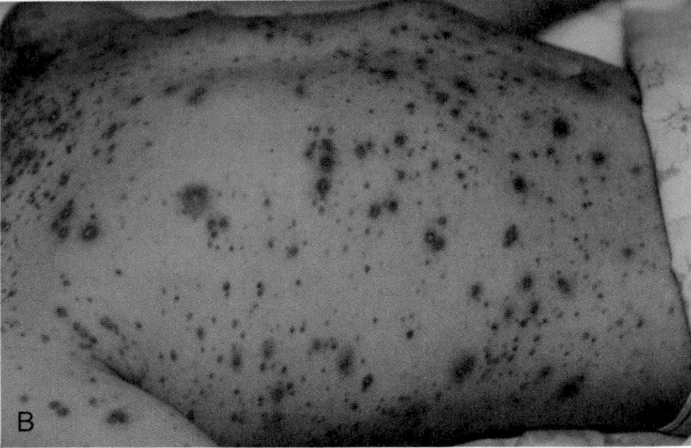

FIG 6.5 Differences in distribution of smallpox versus chickenpox. (A) Man with smallpox. *(Courtesy CDC/NIP/Barbara Rice.)* (B) Chickenpox covering patient torso. *(Courtesy David Effron, MD.)*

TABLE 6.1

Summary of Selected Class A Biological Warfare Agents

Disease/ Infectious Agent	Form and Incubation/Onset of Symptoms	Untreated Course of Disease: Early-Onset Symptoms	Untreated Course of Disease: Late-Onset Symptoms	Probable Route of Contamination for Use as a Biological Warfare Agent	Treatment of Mass Casualties	Prophylaxis/ Vaccine
Bacterial Biological Agents						
Anthrax *Bacillus anthracis*, a gram-positive bacillus that can remain stable in spore form	Inhalation or pulmonary (usually within 48 hours but may incubate for up to 60 days)	Febrile flulike symptoms (malaise, low-grade fever, dry cough, and headache)	Severe respiratory distress, hemodynamic failure, and death	Aerosol; no person-to-person transmission	Ciprofloxacin or doxycycline	Ciprofloxacin or, if susceptible, doxycycline; vaccine available but in short supply
	Cutaneous (1–12 days)	Local urticaria; painless papular lesions usually located on head, forearms, or hands	Papular lesions become vesicular, later developing black eschar and edema	Person-to-person transmission with direct contact with skin lesions		
	Gastrointestinal (1–7 days)	Abdominal pain, nausea, vomiting, and diarrhea	Gastrointestinal bleeding, fever; usually followed by toxic sepsis and death	Contaminated food and/or water		
Plague Acute, severe bacterial infection secondary to a gram-negative bacillus, *Yersinia pestis*	Bubonic Onset of symptoms dependent on route of transmission (1–6 days)	Swollen, tender lymph nodes (most notable femoral and inguinal), high fever, rapid pulse	Hypotension, extreme exhaustion, death	Aerosol and then human-to-human by droplet inhalation	Ciprofloxacin or doxycycline	Ciprofloxacin or doxycycline; no vaccine available at present time
	Pneumonic (1–6 days)	High fever, chills, tachycardia, headache	Fulminate pneumonia (foamy hemoptysis, tachypnea, and dyspnea), sepsis, and death			

Continued

TABLE 6.1
Summary of Selected Class A Biological Warfare Agents—cont'd

Disease/ Infectious Agent	Form and Incubation/Onset of Symptoms	Untreated Course of Disease: Early-Onset Symptoms	Untreated Course of Disease: Late-Onset Symptoms	Probable Route of Contamination for Use as a Biological Warfare Agent	Treatment of Mass Casualties	Prophylaxis/ Vaccine
Botulism Anaerobic gram-positive bacillus that produces a potent muscle-paralyzing neurotoxin	Foodborne (12–36 hours)	Nausea, vomiting, diarrhea	Symmetrical cranial nerve paralysis, descending flaccid paralysis (progressive paralysis of arms, respiratory muscles, and legs), and death	Contaminated food	Passive immunization (antitoxin); supportive care	Passive immunization (antitoxin); antitoxin available in short supply
	Inhalational (2 hours–8 days)	No fever, no changes in mental status	Symmetrical cranial nerve paralysis, descending flaccid paralysis (progressive paralysis of arms, respiratory muscles, and legs), and death	Inhalation of aerosolized toxin		
Typhoidal tularemia *Francisella tularensis*, an extremely infectious bacterium	Contaminated water or food or via aerosol distribution (1–14 days)	Flulike symptoms (headache, cough, fever and chills, malaise)	Pharyngeal ulcers, pleuritic chest pain, pneumonia, pericarditis, respiratory failure, sepsis, and death	Inhalation of aerosolized bacteria	Ciprofloxacin or doxycycline	Ciprofloxacin or doxycycline; vaccine available, only limited supply; vaccine offers incomplete protection
Major Viral Biological Agent of Concern						
Smallpox variola virus	Distribution via airborne droplets, aerosols, and fomites (7–17 days; weaponized smallpox when delivered aerosolized has an incubation period of only 3–5 days)	Acute viral symptoms (high fever, myalgia, headache, and backache)	Continued viral symptoms, high fever, prostration, synchronous onset of rash progressing from macules to papules to vesicles, and eschar formation Vesicles more abundant on extremities and face, and all develop at the same time; pustules appear on palms of hands and soles of feet (unlike chickenpox)	Transmitted person to person by large droplets; therefore spread may be by inhalation of aerosolized virus, oral secretions, infected human vector exposure, or exposure to contaminated objects	Supportive therapy only (ventilator)	None; vaccine available in short supply

ASSESSMENT

1. Perform hand hygiene. Don proper PPE. *Rationale: Proper PPE provides safety to personnel and helps prevent spread of infectious agent to health care provider.*
2. Identify patient using at least two identifiers (e.g., name and birthday or name and medical record number) according to agency policy. *Rationale: Ensures correct patient. Complies with The Joint Commission (TJC) standards and improves patient safety (TJC, 2019).*
3. Conduct focused health history and physical examination (e.g., skin assessment; pulmonary assessment—oxygen saturation, lung sounds, sputum character; cardiac—heart sounds; gastrointestinal [GI]—nausea, vomiting, diarrhea; neurological—movement of extremities, Glasgow Coma Scale, reflexes). Review history of patient's presenting symptoms and determine if pattern exists (see Chapter 8). *Rationale: Symptom identification and clustering of data help to accurately determine exposure to type of biological agent and patient's response.*
4. Measure patient's vital signs and include assessment of pain on a scale of 0 to 10. *Rationale: Provides baseline to later evaluate patient's response to therapy.*
5. Review results of diagnostic tests and consult with health care provider. *Rationale: Initial signs and symptoms of exposure to biological agent suggest common disorders (e.g., flu). Further review of diagnostic findings helps to rule out other common disorders.*
6. Assess patient for health risks (e.g., history of heart disease, pulmonary disease, cancer) that complicate effects of

exposure to biological agent. *Rationale: Patients with preexisting medical conditions often require additional treatment or are at greater risk for death.*

7. Stay calm. Listen and assess patient's immediate psychological response after exposure. Some patients present with dissociative symptoms (e.g., feeling as though "not there" or sensing that everything is outside of the person): disorientation, depression, anxiety, psychosis, and inability to care for self. Even without direct exposure to a biological agent, many individuals, spurred by feelings of fear and doom, present for emergency services. *Rationale: Aids in providing appropriate crisis intervention and stress management. Remaining calm and projecting confidence while assessing individuals for clinical symptoms will reduce the anxiety of the ill and worried as they experience the general sense of panic associated with a biological event.*
8. Identify and gather all patient contacts (names, addresses, and phone numbers) before the patient leaves the ED. *Rationale: All patient contacts need to be identified for proper follow-up by public health department. Often patients will self-triage and transport to ED.*
9. Identify agency resources available (e.g., critical-incident stress-debriefing teams, counselors, psychiatric/mental health nurse practitioners). *Rationale: Expert resources help to assess extent of impact the disaster has on patient's psychological health.*
10. If possible, assess patient's or family caregiver's knowledge, experience, and health literacy level. *Rationale: Ensures patient and family caregiver have the capacity to obtain, communicate, process, and understand basic health information (Centers for Disease Control and Prevention [CDC], 2016c).*

STEP	RATIONALE
PLANNING	
1. Expected outcomes following completion of procedure:	
• Patient is comforted.	In some cases, care is only palliative, with comfort as the focus. Do not underestimate the value of *comfort* as *care*.
• Patient's vital signs return to baseline.	When there are no underlying medical conditions and *if* the patient's disease process is responsive to treatment (when available), vital signs will normalize. However, this may take days or weeks.
• Patient's work of breathing decreases.	Indicates improved gas exchange and cardiac output.
• Patient's skin integrity returns to baseline.	Antibiotic and antitoxin therapy will aid in resolution/healing of lesions over time.
• Patient's level of consciousness (LOC) returns to baseline.	Treatment measures restore neurological function and oxygenation status.
• Patient's mental health status returns to pre-trauma level of functioning.	Crisis intervention successfully reduces patient's anxiety, fear, and dissociative symptoms.
2. Explain care to patient and family, including decontamination and treatment. Explain your role, orient to location and activities to perform, explain what patient has experienced, and ask, "How are you feeling right now?" Assure them that a medical professional will see them shortly.	Information helps to calm anxiety and fear.
IMPLEMENTATION	
1. Continue wearing PPE applied before assessment. Follow transmission-based isolation precautions (see Chapter 5). (See Table 6.1 for route of contamination.) Use strict isolation with smallpox because of its communicability from person to person. Use airborne precautions, contact precautions, and a negative-pressure room for patients suspected of having smallpox.	Reduces transmission of microorganisms and the likelihood of additional secondary sites of contamination.
2. Decontaminate (see emergency policies). If you suspect anthrax, have patient remove clothing and place in labeled plastic biohazard bag. **CAUTION:** *Do not pull over patient's head; instead, cut garments off.* Instruct patient to shower thoroughly with soap and water.	Handle clothing minimally to avoid agitation. Showering with soap and water helps decontaminate and reduce exposure (CDC, 2014a).
3. Establish intravascular access (see Chapter 28). Administer appropriate antibiotics and/or antitoxins.	Various biological agents are commonly treated with ciprofloxacin and/or doxycycline.
4. Administer immunizations (in the event of smallpox). In the event of a smallpox outbreak, public health officials will determine who needs the vaccine.	Anyone who has been directly exposed to the virus (e.g., had prolonged face-to-face contact) should receive the vaccine (CDC, 2017e).
5. Administer intravenous fluids (oral if tolerated) and appropriate nutrition therapy.	Biological agents commonly cause gastrointestinal (GI) disturbances that sometimes result in dehydration.

STEP	RATIONALE
6. Administer oxygen therapy.	Various biological agents (e.g., pulmonary anthrax) commonly cause respiratory symptoms that result in altered gas exchange.
7. Provide supportive care (e.g., comfort measures, including pain and nausea management).	Some victims of a biological attack will not survive; end-of-life care is essential (see Chapter 31).
8. After leaving patient area, remove most heavily contaminated items first. Peel off gown and gloves, roll inside out, and dispose. Perform hand hygiene. Remove face shield from behind and dispose of safely. Remove goggles and mask from behind. Place goggles in container for reprocessing; dispose of mask safely. Perform hand hygiene.	Avoids contamination of self, others, and environment. Reduces transmission of microorganisms.
9. Counsel patient and family about acute and potential long-term psychological effects of exposure. Offer access to trained counselors. Support survivors of a disaster by identifying resources available.	Reaction of patients will include shock, fear, and immobilization. Long-term psychological effects can arise without proper counseling. Social support networks foster coping in the days following a disaster.

Safe Patient Care *Collaborate with the health care provider and other rescue workers for an ongoing plan for managing patients exposed to a biological agent while caring for other patients who are already present in the health care agency seeking care for illness unrelated to the current MCI.*

EVALUATION

1. Observe for improved airway maintenance, breathing, circulation, LOC, and neurological functioning.	Evaluates patient's response to available treatment and/or supportive care.
2. Evaluate vital signs and level of pain.	Evaluates patient's response to treatment.
3. Inspect condition of patient's skin; note character of remaining lesions.	Evaluates patient's response to antibiotic therapy.
4. Query patient, "Tell me how you feel right now." Check level of orientation and ability to conduct conversation.	Evaluates patient for changes that suggest either improvement or deterioration of psychological status.

Unexpected Outcomes	Related Interventions
1. Patient's physical or psychological symptoms progress.	• Notify health care provider. • Notify mental health treatment team. • Remain calm, offer reassurance, and protect self and others from physical harm. • Continue to provide comfort care.
2. Patient death occurs.	• When handling bodies, consider there is continued risk for contamination; make sure that everyone is fully informed regarding proper procedure (see Chapter 31).
3. Secondary contamination of rescue workers.	• Rescue workers immediately report symptoms to a health care provider or nursing supervisor.

Recording

- Use disaster checklists to quickly record specific data regarding patient status, treatment administered, and response to treatment and/or comfort measures.

Hand-Off Reporting

- Report suspected cases of a biological incident to health care provider or ED officer. In the event of an ED exposure to a communicable disease, the department will be locked down immediately. Public health officials (e.g., the emergency officer) will determine if the hospital should be locked down.
- Report any unexpected outcome to health care provider in charge.

✦ SKILL 6.2 Care of a Patient After Chemical Exposure

Purpose

The mechanism of dispersal of a chemical agent is not always known. In fact, the dispersal mechanism, such as an explosion or fire, can be a secondary terrorist attack designed to create greater fatalities. Because symptoms are almost immediate, evacuate victims as quickly as possible from a contaminated zone to a decontamination zone (Table 6.2).

Chemical events are generally confined to small areas, although larger dispersal of these agents may occur (e.g., via a crop duster). The nature and scale of contamination depends on the state of the

TABLE 6.2

Summary of Selected Chemical Warfare Agents

Chemical Agent	Onset of Symptoms	Untreated Course of Chemical Exposure
"Lethal" agents—nerve agents (tabun, sarin, soman, and VX)	Symptoms are generally immediate.	Pinpoint pupils and shortly thereafter, salivation, runny nose, dyspnea, chest tightness, nausea, muscle twitching, coma, seizures, and death
"Blood" agents—hydrogen cyanide	Rapid onset of symptoms; cyanide poisoning is often associated with the smell of bitter almonds.	Death caused by asphyxiation
"Blister" agents—mustard and lewisite	Symptoms may be immediate or delayed.	Skin irritation and blistering
"Choking" agents—phosgene and chlorine	Symptoms can be immediate or delayed up to 24 hours.	Coughing, choking, and disruption in pulmonary function that can lead to death

agent used (e.g., gas versus liquid), characteristics of the chemical used (e.g., heavy or lighter than air), and where the event occurs (e.g., indoors, where ventilation systems affect dispersal; or outdoors, where wind and velocity affect speed and direction of dispersal). For safety reasons, rescue workers should be upwind and uphill from a toxic chemical disaster scene to avoid exposure. The exception is when cyanide gas has been released. Cyanide is lighter than air and thus will travel uphill. It has the unique smell of bitter almonds. If you detect the smell, evacuate the area immediately, although exposure may have already occurred (CDC, 2015).

Delegation and Collaboration

The skill of assessing and caring for a patient exposed to a chemical agent cannot be delegated to nursing assistive personnel (NAP). The nurse directs the NAP to:

- Use appropriate PPE to prevent chemical exposure.
- Use techniques for handling a body after death to prevent contamination.

Equipment

- Decontamination room or area (adult decontamination rooms may not meet the needs of children requiring decontamination; decontamination areas for ambulatory victims will not meet the needs of those who are not ambulatory)
- Scissors or a tool to cut off clothing
- Biohazard bags with labels
- Large volumes of water, decontamination shower (Fig. 6.6)
- Appropriate PPE
- Equipment for physical examination

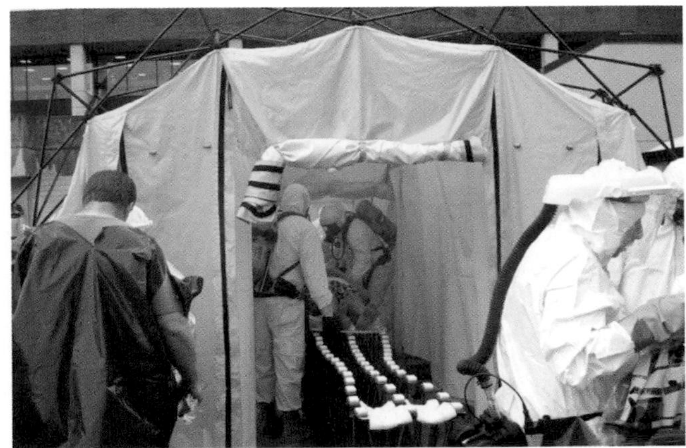

FIG 6.6 Portable decontamination shower for ambulatory victims. *(From Roberts JR, et al:* Roberts and Hedges' clinical procedures in emergency medicine and acute care, *ed 7, Philadelphia, 2019, Elsevier.)*

ASSESSMENT

1. Perform hand hygiene. Don proper PPE. *Rationale: Provides safety to personnel and helps prevent spread of infectious agent to health care provider.*
2. Identify patient using at least two identifiers (e.g., name and birthday or name and medical record number) according to agency policy. *Rationale: Ensures correct patient. Complies with The Joint Commission standards and improves patient safety (TJC, 2019).*
3. Conduct focused physical assessment (see Chapter 8) (e.g., skin assessment; pulmonary assessment—oxygen saturation, lung sounds; cardiac—heart sounds; gastrointestinal—nausea, vomiting) (see Skill 6.1). Observe for presence of liquid on patient's skin, mucous membranes, or clothing and odor (e.g., chlorine). *Rationale: Detects common conditions present when chemical exposure has occurred. Skin assessment reveals severity of exposure. Symptoms vary, depending on type of chemical used.*
4. Assess patient for preexisting medical conditions that will complicate effects of toxic chemical exposure. *Rationale: These patients will likely require additional treatment and sometimes are at greater risk for death.*

Safe Patient Care *Consider a toxic chemical event when large numbers of ill persons present who have unexplained yet similar symptoms. The primary objective for initial care is decontamination (i.e., the removal of harmful contaminants from the skin surface). You achieve this by removing clothing; scrubbing the skin; and hydrolysis, a process of chemical dilution using large volumes of water.*

5. Remain calm. Listen and assess patient's immediate psychological response after exposure. Some patients present with dissociative symptoms: disorientation, depression, anxiety, psychosis, and inability to care for self. Even without direct exposure to a chemical agent, many individuals, spurred by feelings of fear and doom, will present for emergency services and quickly overwhelm available emergency services. *Rationale: Aids in being able to provide*

appropriate crisis intervention and stress management. Remaining calm and projecting confidence reduces anxiety of the ill and worried as they experience the general sense of panic associated with chemical exposure.

6. Identify agency resources available (e.g., critical-incident stress-debriefing teams, counselors, psychiatric/mental health nurse practitioners). *Rationale: Expert resources help to assess extent of impact the disaster has on patient's psychological health.*
7. If possible, assess patient's or family caregiver's knowledge, experience, and health literacy level. *Rationale: Ensures patient and family caregiver have the capacity to obtain, communicate, process, and understand basic health information (CDC, 2016c).*

STEP	RATIONALE
PLANNING	
1. Expected outcomes following completion of procedure:	
a. Patient is comforted.	Because of fatal nature of many chemical agents, the only care available may be palliative.
b. Patient's vital signs return to baseline.	When there are no underlying medical conditions and *if* patient's condition is responsive to treatment (when available), vital signs will return to normal within days or weeks.
c. Patient's work of breathing decreases.	Indicates improved gas exchange and cardiac output.
d. Patient's skin integrity returns to baseline, or no new injury develops.	Minimizing exposure of skin to chemical agent reduces severity and extent of lesions.
e. Patient's LOC returns to baseline.	Neurological stability is achieved by minimizing exposure to chemical and giving antitoxin quickly.
f. Patient's mental health status returns to a pre-trauma level of functioning.	Crisis intervention successfully reduces patient's anxiety, fear, and dissociative symptoms.
2. Explain care to patient and family, including decontamination and treatment. Explain your role, orient to location and activities to perform, explain what patient has experienced, and ask, "How are you feeling right now?" Assure them that a medical professional will see them shortly.	Information helps to calm anxiety and fear.
IMPLEMENTATION	
1. Continue wearing PPE applied during assessment. Prepare for decontamination.	Before decontamination, victims are a potential source of contamination. Use of PPE reduces transmission of and injury from toxic chemicals. Secondary contamination is high with toxic chemical incidents. PPE reduces likelihood of secondary toxic chemical contamination to untrained personnel attempting decontamination.

Safe Patient Care *Only trained personnel using required PPE may decontaminate patients with toxic chemical contamination. Hold victim outside decontamination area until preparations are completed for decontamination. If patient is grossly contaminated, consider decontamination before entry into building. A hospital provides decontamination when a contaminated individual presents for treatment.*

STEP	RATIONALE
2. Provide for patient privacy by closing room curtains or door.	Prevents discomfort and embarrassment when clothing is removed.
3. Decontaminate patient:	
a. Act quickly; avoid touching contaminated parts of clothing as much as possible.	The rapid decontamination of victims is more important than determining the exact toxic chemical. Prevents your own contamination.
b. Remove all of patient's clothing. **CAUTION:** *Do not pull over patient's head; instead, cut garments off.*	Cutting off clothing prevents contamination of head and hair.
c. Use large amounts of soap and water to wash patient thoroughly.	Leads to chemical dilution and in some cases, prevents patient death.
d. If eyes are burning or vision is blurred, rinse eyes with plain water for 10 to 15 minutes. If patient wears contacts, remove and place with contaminated clothing; do not reinsert in eyes. Wash eyeglasses with soap and water; reapply when completed.	Flushes toxins from eye.
4. Dispose of patient's contaminated clothing in appropriate biohazard bag and seal. Place bag in another plastic bag and seal (see agency policy).	Reduces likelihood of secondary chemical contamination.

STEP	RATIONALE
5. Initiate treatment for chemical agent using appropriate chemical agent protocol.	Appropriate chemical agent protocol varies with patient exposure (e.g., linesterase, mustard, nerve agent, chlorine, and lewisite) (Box 6.7).
6. Establish airway if needed; administer oxygen therapy (see Chapter 16).	Various chemical agents commonly cause respiratory problems that will result in altered gas exchange.
7. Control bleeding.	Various chemical agents cause extensive bleeding.
8. Establish intravascular access. Administer fluid and parenteral nutrition therapy (see Chapters 14 and 28).	Various chemical agents commonly cause gastrointestinal disturbances that can result in dehydration.
9. Provide supportive care (e.g., comfort measures, including pain and other symptom management; see Chapters 15 and 31).	Some victims will not survive; it is essential for a nurse to provide palliative symptom control.
10. Remove most heavily contaminated items first. Peel off gown and gloves, roll inside out, and dispose. Perform hand hygiene. Remove face shield from behind and dispose of safely. Remove goggles and mask from behind. Place goggles in container for reprocessing; dispose of mask safely. Perform hand hygiene.	Avoids contamination of self, others, and environment. Reduces transmission of microorganisms.
11. Counsel patient and family on both acute and potential long-term psychological effects of exposure. Offer access to trained counselors.	Reaction of patients to exposure includes shock, immobilization, and fear. Long-term psychological effects can arise without proper counseling.

Safe Patient Care *Collaborate with the health care provider and other rescue workers for an ongoing plan to manage patients exposed to a toxic chemical agent. You will need to do this while also caring for other patients who are already present in the health care agency seeking care for illness unrelated to the current MCI.*

EVALUATION

1. Observe status of airway maintenance, breathing, circulation, LOC, and neurological functioning. Assess vital signs.	Evaluates patient's physical response to available treatment and/or supportive care.
2. Ask patient to rate pain level on a scale of 0 to 10.	Determines if comfort measures are effective.
3. Inspect condition of skin; note extent of blistering.	Determines extent of healing.
4. Evaluate patient's level of orientation, ability to problem solve, and perception of condition.	Evaluates patient's psychological status and ability to make decisions.

Unexpected Outcomes	Related Interventions
1. Secondary contamination of rescue workers occurs.	• Rescue workers immediately remove their clothing, scrub their bodies, and use copious amounts of soap and water. • Contain clothes in appropriate biohazard bags. • Provide clean clothes.
2. Patient's physical symptoms progress despite appropriate treatment.	• Notify health care provider in charge. • Continue to provide comfort care.
3. Patient's psychological symptoms progress despite appropriate treatment. Patient exhibits anxiety, disorientation, and suicidal ideation.	• Notify mental health treatment team. • Remain calm, offer reassurance, and protect self and others from physical harm. • Continue to provide comfort measures.
4. Patient death occurs.	• When handling bodies, there is continued risk for contamination; make sure that everyone is fully informed regarding proper procedures (see Skill 31.3). When delegating preparation of the deceased, always consider the level of training of those managing the body.

BOX 6.7

Examples of Chemical Exposure Protocols

Chlorine Protocol

1. Dyspnea?
   Try bronchodilators
   Admit to hospital
   Oxygen by mask
   Chest x-ray film examination
2. Treat other problems and reevaluate (consider phosgene)
3. Respiratory system OK?
   Yes—Go to 5
4. Is phosgene poisoning possible?
   Yes—Go to Phosgene Protocol on CDC website
5. Give supportive therapy: treat other problems or discharge

Mustard Protocol

1. Airway obstruction?
   Yes—Tracheostomy
2. If there are large burns:
   Establish intravenous line—Do not push fluids as for thermal burns
   Drain vesicles—Unroof large blisters and irrigate area with topical antibiotics
3. Treat other symptoms appropriately:
   Antibiotic eye ointment
   Sterile precautions prn
   Morphine prn (generally not needed in emergency treatment; might be appropriate for in-patient treatment)

Data from the Centers for Disease Control and Prevention (CDC): *Emergency room procedures in chemical hazard emergencies: a job aid*, 2013, http://www.cdc.gov/nceh/demil/articles/initialtreat.htm#CHLORINEPROTOCOL.

Recording

- Record patient's status, decontamination and treatment procedures, and response to treatment and/or comfort measures.

Hand-Off Reporting

- Report suspected cases of a toxic chemical event to health care provider or emergency officer
- Report any unexpected outcome to health care provider in charge.

✦ SKILL 6.3 Care of a Patient After Radiation Exposure

Purpose

Radiological events differ from nuclear events. A radiological event is the dispersal of radioactive material via a "dirty bomb," by deliberate contamination of food or water supplies, or over the terrain. A nuclear event involves a device that releases nuclear energy in an explosive manner as a result of a nuclear chain reaction. Radiation affects the body in many ways, depending on the level of exposure. High levels of radiation exposure cause a person to develop acute radiation syndrome (ARS) with symptoms of nausea, vomiting, and diarrhea (CDC, 2016b).

Radiation comes in a variety of forms. Alpha particles are the least dangerous, traveling only a few centimeters. They do not penetrate materials easily and are harmful only if ingested. An individual's clothing blocks alpha particles from reaching the skin. Beta particles penetrate a short distance into the skin. Protective clothing is necessary for protection. Gamma rays pose the greatest health risk because the waves penetrate deeply, causing severe burns and internal injury. Lead shielding protects against gamma rays. Blasts caused by a nuclear explosion cause not only injury from radiation exposure but also traumatic injuries and burns. Some victims will present with many combined forms of injury requiring treatment. The sooner symptoms begin to appear, the greater a patient's exposure to the radiation. Early symptoms (i.e., within a few hours) suggest that an individual has received a lethal dose of radiation.

Nuclear incidents usually result in wide destruction requiring specialized equipment and resources at the scene to assess structural damage and levels of radioactivity. Radiological events usually cover much smaller areas, but they are often difficult to define. Specialized equipment and training are required to assess the source of radioactivity, determine the scope of contamination, and perform decontamination. The principles to follow to protect individuals from exposure include get inside, stay inside, and stay tuned (CDC, 2014b).

Delegation and Collaboration

The skill of assessment and care of a patient exposed to a radiological agent cannot be delegated to nursing assistive personnel (NAP). The nurse directs the NAP to:

- Use appropriate PPE to prevent exposure.
- Use techniques for handling a body after death to prevent contamination.

Equipment

- Decontamination room or area (adult decontamination rooms do not always meet the needs of children requiring decontamination; decontamination of ambulatory victims will not meet the needs of those who are not ambulatory)
- Scissors or some other tool to cut off clothing
- Clothing containers; type depends on the kind of radiological exposure
- Appropriate PPE for use by personnel in area of radiation release
- Appropriate PPE for health care workers in hospital setting (i.e., surgical masks, N95 masks recommended if available)
- Radiation meter available to survey hands and clothing at frequent intervals
- Equipment for select specimen collection
- Equipment for physical examination
- Plastic wrap or bag

ASSESSMENT

1. Perform hand hygiene. Don proper PPE. *Rationale: Provides safety to personnel and helps prevent spread of infectious agent to health care provider.*
2. Identify patient using at least two identifiers (e.g., name and birthday or name and medical record number) according to

agency policy. *Rationale: Ensures correct patient. Complies with The Joint Commission standards and improves patient safety (TJC, 2019).*

Safe Patient Care *Before assessment a specially trained technician conducts a radiation survey of the patient, initially scanning the face, hands, and feet with a radiation survey instrument. If meter results are positive, a thorough survey (5 to 8 minutes per person) is conducted.*

3. Assess patient's symptoms by performing a focused physical examination (see Skill 6.1). *Rationale: Symptom identification and clustering of data are first steps to determine patient's condition and response to radiation.*
4. Measure patient's vital signs and include assessment of pain on a scale of 0 to 10. *Rationale: Provides baseline to later evaluate patient's response to therapy.*

Safe Patient Care *Do not touch a wound if you suspect that radioactive fragments are present.*

5. Assess patient for preexisting medical conditions that will complicate effects of the radiological exposure. Symptoms of acute radiation syndrome include nausea, vomiting, headache, and diarrhea (CDC, 2016b). *Rationale: Patients with preexisting medical conditions can require additional treatment or are at greater risk for death.*
6. Review results of diagnostic testing (e.g., complete blood count). *Rationale: Data offer a baseline to evaluate injury progression or response to treatment.*
7. Determine patient's allergies, specifically allergy for iodine sensitivity. *Rationale: Patients with iodine sensitivity need to avoid taking potassium iodide, the treatment of choice for radioactive iodine exposure.*
8. Assess individual psychological response to radiological event. Some patients present with dissociative symptoms (e.g., feeling as though "not there," sensing that experiences are outside the person): disorientation, depression, anxiety, psychosis, and an inability to care for self. Ask patient, "How do you feel now?" Determine level of orientation, ability to follow conversation. *Rationale: Allows you to provide appropriate crisis intervention and stress management. Remaining calm and projecting confidence while assessing individuals for clinical symptoms versus feeling of panic goes a long way toward reducing the anxiety of the ill and worried as they experience the general sense of panic associated with a radiological event.*
9. Identify agency resources available (e.g., critical-incident stress-debriefing teams, counselors, psychiatric/mental health nurse practitioners). *Rationale: Expert resources help to assess extent of impact the disaster has on patient's psychological health.*

Safe Patient Care *A radiological event is the disaster event most feared by most individuals. Many are uneducated regarding the dangers of and differences among radiation materials. Health care agencies will likely have many anxious, frightened individuals who can potentially create a danger to the environment. Assess individual for signs of psychological distress. Early identification of symptoms and stress-management interventions can help prevent an individual or mass-panic response (CDC, 2016b).*

10. If possible, assess patient's or family caregiver's knowledge, experience, and health literacy level. *Rationale: Ensures patient and family caregiver have the capacity to obtain, communicate, process, and understand basic health information (CDC, 2016c).*

STEP	RATIONALE
PLANNING	
1. Expected outcomes following completion of procedure:	
a. Patient is comforted.	In some cases, the only care that is available is palliative.
b. Patient is successfully decontaminated.	Decontamination procedures remove radioactive materials from patient's skin.
c. Patient's vital signs return to baseline.	When there are no underlying medical conditions and *if* the patient's disease process is responsive to treatment (when available), vital signs will return to normal within days or weeks.
d. Patient is free of nausea and diarrhea.	Gastrointestinal (GI) alterations following radiation exposure typically respond to antidiarrheal and antiemetic medications.
e. Patient's skin integrity returns to baseline.	Radiological burns are minimized through successful decontamination procedures.
f. Patient's immune system (e.g., complete blood count [CBC]) returns to baseline.	Exposure to radiation is minimized successfully.
g. Patient's work of breathing decreases.	Indicates improved gas exchange and cardiac output.
2. Explain care to patient and family. Explain your role, orient to location and activities to perform, explain what patient has experienced, and ask, "How are you feeling right now?" Assure them that medical personnel will see them shortly.	Crisis intervention reestablishes patient's orientation and sense of reality.

STEP	RATIONALE
IMPLEMENTATION	
1. Continue wearing PPE applied during assessment. Prepare for decontamination. *Only trained personnel use required PPE to decontaminate patients with radiological contamination.*	Reduces likelihood of secondary radiological contamination to untrained personnel attempting decontamination.
2. Provide for patient privacy by closing room curtains or door.	Prevents anxiety or embarrassment when clothes are removed.
3. Decontaminate patient:	
a. Remove patient's clothing.	Normally eliminates up to 90% of contamination.
b. Wash patient's skin thoroughly with water and soap, taking care not to abrade or irritate the skin. Use tepid decontamination water. Cover wounds with waterproof dressings to avoid spread of radioactivity (Radiation Emergency Medical Management [REMM, 2017a).	Use of large amounts of water is critical in decontamination. Water that is too cold will close pores, and water that is too hot enhances absorption of radioactive materials (REMM, 2017a).
c. Have radiation technician resurvey patient after washing. Rewash as necessary.	Determines if radiation residual is present.
d. Isolate and cover any area of skin that is still positive for radiation by using plastic bag or wrap.	Area is washed until no further reduction in contamination is achieved (verified by survey instrumentation) and then covered to reduce exposure of health care workers.
4. Bag and tag patient's contaminated clothing for further evaluation and place in appropriate biohazard container.	Reduces likelihood of secondary contamination when you use containers designed to contain radiological particles.

Safe Patient Care *Collaborate with the health care provider and other rescue workers for an ongoing plan to manage patients exposed to radiological materials. You will need to do this while also caring for other patients who are already present in the health care agency seeking care for illness unrelated to the current nuclear or radiological event.*

STEP	RATIONALE
5. Prepare for possibly obtaining a CBC, urinalysis, fecal specimen, and swabs of body orifices (see Chapter 9).	CBC establishes baseline to determine patient's immunological status over time. A health care provider who suspects internal contamination will order collection of urine, feces, and body orifice swabs to analyze for radionuclides.
6. Treat symptoms according to ordinary treatment practices: provide intravenous fluid support, antidiarrheal therapies, antiemetic medications, and potassium iodide tablets.	Patient exposed to radiation is at risk for GI alterations and fluid imbalance. Treatment is directed at limiting or removing internal contamination, depending on type of radioactive material (CDC, 2016a).
7. Remove most heavily contaminated items first. Peel off gown and gloves, roll inside out, and dispose. Perform hand hygiene. Remove face shield from behind and dispose of safely. Remove goggles and mask from behind. Place goggles in container for reprocessing; dispose of mask safely. Perform hand hygiene.	Avoids contamination of self, others, and environment. Reduces transmission of microorganisms.
8. Counsel patient and family on psychological effects of exposure. Offer access to trained counselors.	Reaction of patients to exposure includes shock, immobilization, and fear. Long-term psychological effects can arise without proper counseling.
EVALUATION	
1. Observe skin integrity, fluid balance, respiratory and GI status, level of consciousness, and neurological functioning. Look for improvement of other radiological agent-specific symptoms. Evaluate vital signs.	Evaluates patient's physical response to available treatment and/or supportive care.
2. Monitor CBC and other laboratory tests.	Determines patient's immune response.
3. Evaluate patient's level of consciousness, orientation, and ability to relate events. Ask if patient remembers what has occurred; observe affect.	Determines if psychological status has improved.

STEP	RATIONALE
Unexpected Outcomes	**Related Interventions**
1. Secondary contamination of rescue workers occurs.	• Institute appropriate decontamination of worker.
2. Patient's symptoms progress despite appropriate treatment.	• Notify health care provider in charge. • Continue to provide comfort care.
3. Patient's psychological state deteriorates, with development of disorientation, suicidal ideation, violence toward others.	• Notify mental health treatment team. • Remain calm, offer reassurance, and protect self and others from physical harm. • Continue to provide comfort care.
4. Patient death occurs.	• When handling bodies, consider there is continued risk for contamination; make sure that everyone is fully informed about proper procedure. • If the deceased is known or suspected to be contaminated, all people handling the body will wear PPE and a personal dosimeter. A Disaster Mortuary Operations Response Teams (DMORTs) may need to be called to assist (REMM, 2017b). • When delegating preparation of the deceased, consider the level of training of those managing the body.

Recording

- Record patient's status and response to treatment and/or comfort measures.

Hand-Off Reporting

- Report presence of open wound and any suspected radioactive fragment to health care provider in charge.
- Report any unexpected outcomes to health care provider.

SPECIAL CONSIDERATIONS

Patient-Centered Care

- The 2018–2022 FEMA Strategic Plan provides the best possible support to the American people before, during, and after disasters (FEMA, 2018).
- Detection and surveillance focus on an awareness of the environment, recognizing what is unusual or different, and knowing what these differences possibly mean for the purpose of mitigation or prevention (DHS, n.d.).
- Detection is the first goal in an MCI and includes (a) determining the presence of an MCI or public health emergency (PHE), (b) recognizing the cause of the incident, and (c) becoming aware of the environment or more specifically changes in the environment (e.g., an unusual pattern of patient presentation or unusual smells).
- Remain calm and assess a patient's immediate psychological response. Some patients present with dissociative symptoms such as disorientation, depression, anxiety, psychosis, and an inability to care for self.
- Physical injuries may be similar across cultures; however, the psychological responses usually differ among cultures (Sterling, 2014).
- A lack of cultural considerations of victims leads to the impression of insensitivity and biases toward patients who are different racially, sexually, or ethnically.
- Regardless of cultural differences and perhaps language difficulties, it is important to convey compassion and respect while working closely with people within the community for disaster recovery. Professional interpreters become an invaluable resource.
- Some disaster events result in a changed culture for individuals, families, and communities. Once a disaster has struck, there can be a sense of vulnerability that causes increased fear and a sense of insecurity.

Patient Education

- Nurses provide public health education to empower resilience in communities by focusing on individual self-accountability and responsibility and knowing how to access community, state, and federal resources. In terms of a disaster, support means, "Give me what I need to get the job done." The earlier you ask for support, the better.
- Preparation for an MCI goes a long way toward preventing casualties and chaos. Public education of the likelihood of a mass-casualty biological event is necessary and includes information about types of biological agents, mode of transmission, symptoms, treatment, and locations of shelters and disaster treatment sites.
- Preparedness includes teaching individuals, families, and communities resilience and the ability to care for themselves when support services are not available or inaccessible.
- Education of the public includes locations of shelters and disaster treatment sites.
- Health care providers need an opportunity to debrief after a disaster to help avoid psychological complications such as post-traumatic stress disorder.

Age-Specific

Pediatric

- Children are one of the most vulnerable populations, and many facets influence the impact of disaster on children. These facets often include age, gender, family dynamics, and the level of and direct exposure to disaster (Hockenberry and Wilson, 2017).
- Children have both physical and emotional needs during disasters. They often show stress-related symptoms and may have temporary changes in behavior after a disaster (Hockenberry and Wilson, 2017).

- Many disasters result in the need to relocate, which creates stress and unique challenges in children. Stress may be increased by changes in children's cultural, psychological, and social environment. Reactions of their parents and other family members contribute to how well children will cope with relocation and whether or not they will be able to stay connected with friends and familiar activities (Hockenberry and Wilson, 2017).
- Outbreaks of communicable diseases have been reported after natural disasters, and children are more likely to develop infections secondary to their immature immune systems (Hockenberry and Wilson, 2017).
- Keep families together after a disaster. Family togetherness offers reassurance to a child and lessens fears of being abandoned and unprotected (Hockenberry and Wilson, 2017).
- Media have an enormous influence on children and may impact development and behavior. Encourage parents to limit their children's exposure to media reports of the disaster and to watch television with them whenever possible to clarify information and answer questions (Hockenberry and Wilson, 2017).
- The death of a child is always traumatic; parents may have a compelling need to be present during pediatric resuscitation and at the time of death; ideally, you should allow it. It is important for a nurse to be present to explain what is happening and facilitate the grieving process (Hockenberry and Wilson, 2017).
- Children are vulnerable to radiation because (1) their organ systems are more sensitive than those of adults, and (2) they have more years of life expectancy over which to develop complications from the radiological exposure.
- To avoid becoming a secondary victim, emergency responders need to consider potential contamination of children before picking them up and holding them. Often, decontamination consists of providing fresh air and a large volume of low-pressure warm water. Observe children for potential hypothermia because they are more susceptible.
- Adult decontamination facilities are not always appropriate to meet the needs of children. The special PPE worn by rescue workers may frighten young children. The cleaning process and possible separation from uncontaminated parents will likely cause considerable stress and anxiety. Additional health care workers are often necessary to ensure that adequate decontamination has taken place. Verbal encouragement and praise are effective in facilitating the process.

Gerontological

- Under disaster conditions, triage older adults according to injuries, not age.
- Older adults may have impaired mobility, diminished sensory awareness, multiple chronic health conditions, and social and economic limitations that may impact their ability to prepare for, respond to, and adapt during MCIs (CDC, 2012).
- Because some older adults have many concurrent illnesses, radiological agents can worsen these conditions and result in the older adult needing more immediate care than an initial triage had indicated (CDC, 2016b).

Home Care

- Community engagement is key to successfully controlling people's responses during disasters; establishing trust is essential.
- Assemble a disaster kit before disaster strikes. FEMA (2018) and the American Red Cross (2017) offer free literature on establishing home care preparedness (Boxes 6.8 and 6.9).

BOX 6.8

Basic Disaster Supply Kit

- Water: 1 gallon of water per person per day (minimum of 3-day supply for evacuation/2-week supply for home)
- Food: nonperishable, easy to prepare (minimum of 3-day supply for evacuation/2-week supply for home)
- Manual can opener
- Plastic resealable bags
- Utility knife
- Disposable cups, plates, and utensils
- Several flashlights
- Battery-powered or hand-cranked radio
- Fresh batteries
- Matches in waterproof container
- First-aid kit
- Medications (7-day supply) and medical items
- Map of the area
- Emergency blanket
- Sanitation and hygiene items (e.g., hand sanitizer, toilet paper)
- Cell phone and chargers
- Copies of personal documents (e.g., birth certificates, deed to home, passport)
- Family and emergency contact

Additional Considerations

- Items for infants, seniors, or disabled people
- Pet supplies (leash, food, ID collar, carrier, bowl)
- Entertainment items/games for small children
- Extra set of keys and identification
- Copies of medical prescriptions in plastic sealable bags

Additional Supplies for Sheltering-in-Place (in the Event of a Chemical or Radiological Hazard)

- Roll of duct tape and scissors
- Plastic sheeting precut to fit shelter-in-place room openings (10 square feet per person will provide sufficient air to prevent carbon dioxide buildup for up to 5 hours.)
- Additional supplies in preparation for a pandemic flu (Have a 2-week supply of basic items so you can survive without outside help or going out in public.)
- Thermometer, nonaspirin pain reliever, prescription medication
- Household-cleaning supplies (e.g., disinfectant sprays, bleach)
- Extra bath and hand soap

Data adapted from American Red Cross (ARC) and Centers for Disease Control and Prevention (CDC): *Plan and prepare,* 2017, http://www.redcross.org/prepare/location/home-family/get-kit.

BOX 6.9

Suggested Foods for a Disaster Supply Kit

- Foods that last about 1 year:
- Canned soups, canned nuts
- Canned fruits, fruit juices, vegetables
- Peanut butter, jelly
- Ready-to-eat cereals and uncooked instant cereals
- If stored in proper conditions/containers, foods kept indefinitely:
  - Dried corn, dried pasta
  - Instant coffee, tea, cocoa
  - Rice; bouillon products, seasoning packets

Data from Centers for Disease Control and Prevention (CDC): *Emergency food supplies,* 2017, http://emergency.cdc.gov/preparedness/kit/food/.

- Individuals with special needs (e.g., hearing impairment, impaired mobility, special diets) and individuals without vehicles require additional planning to be prepared for a disaster.
- Post emergency telephone numbers by the telephone and teach children how and when to call 9-1-1.

- Family members need to establish a meeting place away from the home in case they cannot stay in their home or cannot reach their home during a disaster.
- Remain isolated and advise friends and relatives not to visit if family members are symptomatic. Instruct family to use the appropriate PPE needed to protect the family; this can include sheltering-in-place.
- Maintain strict hand hygiene for both well and symptomatic family members after using the bathroom, before eating and drinking, and after contact with pets.
- When a sick individual's symptoms worsen, transport to the nearest designated hospital.
- Change a sick person's clothing and bed linens frequently; wash them separately from those of other family members, using any commercial detergent. Disinfect surfaces with which the symptomatic person comes in contact. Use an appropriate disinfectant (e.g., Lysol), especially when soiled with blood or other body fluids.
- Family caregivers need to get plenty of rest, drink fluids frequently, and eat a healthy diet. If the caregiver develops symptoms, obtain appropriate medical care immediately.
- When a radiological or nuclear event becomes a reality, listen to the radio or television for special instructions, including appropriate means for maintaining a safe shelter.
- Instruct community members to keep upwind and uphill from the release of the radioactive materials and toxic chemical unless it is cyanide.
- Through the clinician outreach and communication activity (COCA) resource, the CDC helps health care providers respond to emergencies by communicating relevant and timely information (CDC, 2017a).
- The CDC (2017c) and the American Red Cross (2017) advocate preparedness and coordination of prompt, effective emergency efforts. This includes outreach to other agencies or groups through mutual aid agreements (e.g., willingness of an agency to provide shelter [school or church]), clothing (e.g., department store, Salvation Army), or care for the deceased (funeral homes).
- The CDC's (2017b) Crisis and Emergency Risk Communication provides resources to help health communicators, emergency responders, and leaders of organizations communicate effectively during emergencies.
- Disaster planning is an interprofessional and multiagency task. In addition to nurses, average citizens, government agencies, and other health care workers play a vital role in disaster preparedness.
- First responders quickly distinguish between actual victims with exposure to the weapon of mass destruction (chemical, biological, or nuclear) that led to the MCI and the worried well.
- Support resources necessary during a disaster include human resources, agencies, facilities, supplies, and vehicles.
- Support is for the victims of disaster and all health care providers involved. Support is holistic, encompassing the body, mind, and spirit. Health care providers (including nurses, first responders, and physicians) are at risk for posttraumatic stress disorder (PTSD).
- Once local and federal authorities confirm the need for medicine and supplies, the CDC's strategic national stockpile (SNS) is accessed, and items are delivered to the state in need. Each state has a plan to receive and distribute SNS items (CDC, 2017d).
- Health care providers care for the worried well (those injured and able to transport themselves to a hospital and those frightened by the events) and the sick and injured individuals already admitted to the hospital or ED.

✦ PRACTICE REFLECTIONS

What started off as an already busy morning in the ED quickly turned to chaos when a chemical explosion occurred four blocks away from the hospital. The ED staff began to organize for incoming victims of the explosion while also continuing to care for their current patients and mobilize resources.

1. What type of PPE would you expect to need to protect you as you care for these victims?
2. How will you approach triaging the victims of the chemical explosion?
3. Consider what the most urgent needs will be for the victims of the chemical explosion and what resources you should plan to gather.

✦ CLINICAL REVIEW QUESTIONS

1. In the case of a biological exposure, the nurse can direct the NAP to do which of the following? (Select all that apply.)
   1. Conduct a focused health history.
   2. Handle the body after death.
   3. Review diagnostic test results.
   4. Gather and wear PPE.
   5. Administer a decontamination shower.
2. The nurse is caring for a patient who has been diagnosed with botulism from a foodborne source. Signs and symptoms the nurse is likely to observe include which of the following? (Select all that apply.)
   1. Swollen lymph nodes
   2. Nausea and vomiting
   3. Progressive paralysis of arms
   4. Gastrointestinal bleeding
   5. Dry cough and headache
3. Your patient was exposed to a chemical agent and needs to be decontaminated. Place the following steps in the correct order.
   1. Wash patient with soap and water.
   2. Dispose of contaminated clothing.
   3. Remove contaminated clothing.
   4. Administer intravenous (IV) fluids.
   5. Rinse eyes with plain water.
   6. Initiate treatment for chemical agent.

Answers and Rationales for Clinical Review Questions can be found on the Evolve website.

REFERENCES

American Nurses Association (ANA): Disaster preparedness and response, 2017. http://www.nursingworld.org/disasterpreparedness.

American Red Cross: How to prepare for emergencies, 2017. http://www.redcross.org/get-help/how-to-prepare-for-emergencies.

Centers for Disease Control and Prevention (CDC): Identifying vulnerable older adults and legal options for increasing their protection during all-hazards emergencies: a cross-sector guide for states and communities, 2012. http://www.cdc.gov/aging/emergency/pdf/guide.pdf.

Centers for Disease Control and Prevention (CDC): Emergency room procedures in chemical hazard emergencies: a job aid, 2013. http://www.cdc.gov/nceh/demil/articles/initialtreat.htm.

Centers for Disease Control and Prevention (CDC): Anthrax overview, 2014a. http://www.cdc.gov/niosh/topics/anthrax/default.html.

Centers for Disease Control and Prevention (CDC): Radiation emergencies: what should I do? 2014b. http://emergency.cdc.gov/radiation/whattodo.asp.

Centers for Disease Control and Prevention (CDC): Facts about cyanide, 2015. http://emergency.cdc.gov/agent/cyanide/basics/facts.asp.

Centers for Disease Control and Prevention (CDC): Medical countermeasures (treatments) for radiation exposure and contamination, 2016a. https://emergency.cdc.gov/radiation/countermeasures.asp.

Centers for Disease Control and Prevention (CDC): Radiation emergencies and your health, 2016b. http://emergency.cdc.gov/radiation/healthandsafety.asp.

Centers for Disease Control and Prevention: What is health literacy, 2016c. https://www.cdc.gov/healthliteracy/learn/index.html.

Centers for Disease Control and Prevention (CDC): Clinician outreach and communication activity (COCA), 2017a. http://emergency.cdc.gov/coca/index.asp.

Centers for Disease Control and Prevention (CDC): Crisis and emergency risk communication, 2017b. https://emergency.cdc.gov/cerc/index.asp.

Centers for Disease Control and Prevention (CDC): Emergency preparedness and response, 2017c. http://emergency.cdc.gov/.

Centers for Disease Control and Prevention (CDC): Strategic national stockpile (SNS), 2017d. http://www.cdc.gov/phpr/stockpile/stockpile.htm.

Centers for Disease Control and Prevention (CDC): Who should get vaccination, 2017e. https://www.cdc.gov/smallpox/vaccine-basics/who-gets-vaccination.html.

Department of Homeland Security (DHS): If you see something say something campaign, n.d., https://www.dhs.gov/see-something-say-something.

Department of Homeland Security (DHS): National terrorism advisory system, 2016. https://www.dhs.gov/sites/default/files/ntas/alerts/16_1115_NTAS_bulletin.pdf.

Emergency Management System: Incident command system (ICS) and the National Incident Management System (NIMS), 2017. https://mil.wa.gov/emergency-management-division/training-and-exercise/incident-command-system-ics-and-the-national-incident-management-system-nims.

Federal Emergency Management Agency (FEMA): FEMA strategic plan, 2018. https://www.fema.gov/media-library-data/1533052524696-b5137201a4614ade5e0129ef01cbf661/strat_plan.pdf.

Hockenberry M, Wilson D: *Wong's essentials of pediatric nursing*, ed 10, St. Louis, 2017, Mosby.

Jung D, et al: Disaster preparedness in the emergency department using in situ simulation, *Adv Emerg Nurs J* 38(1):56–68, 2016.

National Institutes of Health (NIH): Biodefense and bioterrorism, 2017. http://www.nlm.nih.gov/medlineplus/biodefenseandbioterrorism.html.

Nilsson J, et al: Disaster nursing: self-reported competence of nursing students and registered nurses, with focus on their readiness to manage violence, serious events and disasters, *Nurse Educ Pract* 17:102, 2016.

Occupational Safety and Health Administration (OSHA): OSHA fact sheet: personal protective equipment (PPE) reduces exposure to bloodborne pathogens, 2011. www.osha.gov/OshDoc/data_BloodborneFacts/bbfact03.pdf.

Radiation Emergency Medical Management (REMM): Decontamination procedures, 2017a. http://www.remm.nlm.gov/ext_contamination.htm.

Radiation Emergency Medical Management (REMM): Management of the deceased, 2017b. http://www.remm.nlm.gov/deceased.htm.

Sterling YM: Nursing 'caring' during catastrophic events: theoretical, research, and clinical insights, *Int J Human Caring* 18(1):60, 2014.

The Joint Commission (TJC): *2019 National Patient Safety Goals*, 2019. Oakbrook Terrace, IL, The Commission. http://www.jointcommission.org/standards_information/npsgs.aspx.

7 Vital Signs

SKILLS AND PROCEDURES

EVOLVE WEBSITE/RESOURCES LIST

http://evolve.elsevier.com/Perry/nursinginterventions
Audio Glossary • Animations • Case Studies • Checklists • Clinical Review Questions • Answers and Rationales for Review Questions • Video Clips

INTRODUCTION

Vital signs include temperature, pulse, respirations, and blood pressure (Table 7.1). These are indicators of the ability of the body to regulate body temperature, oxygenate body tissues, and maintain blood flow. Pain assessment is considered a fifth vital sign (see Chapter 15). A change in one vital sign (e.g., pulse) can reflect changes in the other vital signs (temperature, respirations, and blood pressure). Likewise, a change in pain intensity can alter pulse and blood pressure. As a nurse, use clinical judgment to determine which vital signs to measure, when to take measurements (Box 7.1), and when measurements can be delegated safely. Keeping patients informed of their vital signs promotes understanding of their health status.

PRACTICE STANDARDS

- The Joint Commission (TJC), 2019: National Patient Safety Goals—Patient identification
- Whelton et al., 2017: Guideline for the prevention, detection, evaluation, and management of high blood pressure in adults—Blood pressure assessment

EVIDENCE-BASED PRACTICE

Mobile Applications for Electronic Heart Rate

Nurses educate patients to palpate and record their own heart rate before or after exercise or cardiac medications and during tele-assessment. Applications (apps) for mobile electronic devices such as smartphones or tablets offer electronic heart rate determination (Poh and Poh, 2017). A study by Coppetti and colleagues (2017) compared the monitored heart rates of adult emergency room patients with the heart rates measured by apps using finger contact with the device or a noncontact camera. The accuracy of the app-obtained heart rate varied; the noncontact camera measurements resulted in a difference of as much as a 20 beats/min. The fingertip-based app obtained a heart-rate assessment comparable to pulse oximetry. Guidelines for using apps include the following:

- Be aware of the method patients use to self-measure heart rate.
- Observe patients using an app to measure pulse.
- Analyze app accuracy prior to use in clinical practice (Boudreaux et al., 2014).
- Instruct patients to compare app-obtained heart rates with palpated heart rates at high, low, or irregular heart rates (Poh and Poh, 2017).

SAFETY GUIDELINES

Assessing vital signs requires equipment that is clean and in working order. The biomedical department of a hospital routinely inspects electronic blood pressure machines for electrical safety. Know how to use each device; if you are unsure, ask for instructions. It is important to use each device correctly and appropriately to ensure patient safety and to obtain correct, complete patient information. Other guidelines include the following:

- Carefully clean stethoscopes, thermometers, and blood pressure cuffs before and after use with each patient to avoid contamination by microorganisms.
- Control or minimize environmental factors that affect vital signs. For example, assessing the patient's temperature in a warm, humid room may yield a value that is not a true indicator of the patient's condition.
- Ensure that patients with latex allergies are provided with latex-free equipment, including blood pressure cuffs and pulse oximeter probes.
- Continuous blood pressure or pulse oximetry readings can compromise skin integrity and cause device-related pressure injuries (DRPIs). Remove equipment at least every 2 hours and assess underlying skin.

TABLE 7.1

Vital Signs: Acceptable Ranges

Vital Signs	Acceptable Range
Temperature	36–38°C (96.8–100.4°F)
Oral/tympanic	37.0°C (98.6°F)
Rectal	37.5°C (99.5°F)
Axillary	36.5°C (97.7°F)
Pulse	Adult: 60–100 beats/min, strong and regular
Respirations	Adult: 12–20 breaths/min, deep and regular
Blood pressure*	
Systolic	<120 mm Hg
Diastolic	<80 mm Hg
Pulse pressure	30–50 mm Hg
Pulse oximetry	Normal SpO_2: 95%–100%

*In some patients, blood pressure is measured consecutively with the patient lying, sitting, and standing or in both arms. In normal individuals, the change from lying to standing causes a decrease in systolic blood pressure of <15 mm Hg. Record the position and extremity and compare the measurements for significant differences.

BOX 7.1

When to Take Vital Signs

- On admission to a health care facility
- When assessing a patient during home health visits
- In a hospital or care facility on a routine schedule according to the health care provider's order or standards of practice of the agency
- Before, during, and after a surgical procedure or invasive diagnostic procedure
- Before, during, and after a transfusion of any type of blood product
- Before, during, and after administration of medications or application of therapies that affect cardiovascular, respiratory, and temperature-control functions
- When a patient's general physical condition changes (e.g., loss of consciousness, increased severity of pain)
- Before and after nursing interventions influencing a vital sign (e.g., before and after a patient previously on bed rest ambulates, before and after patient performs range-of-motion exercises)
- When a patient reports specific symptoms of physical distress (e.g., feeling "funny" or "different")

✦ SKILL 7.1 Measuring Body Temperature

Purpose

Body temperature measurements provide an average of the core temperature of body tissues. Body tissues and cell processes function best within a relatively narrow temperature range of 36° to 38°C (96.8° to 100.4°F), with average body temperature depending on the measurement site used. Each site and type of thermometer (Box 7.2) has unique techniques, contraindications, or limitations and norms (Table 7.2). You can measure temperature on a Celsius or Fahrenheit scale. Although some electronic thermometers can display both Celsius and Fahrenheit readings, conversion charts are also available to convert from one scale to the other.

Delegation and Collaboration

The skill of temperature measurement can be delegated to nursing assistive personnel (NAP). The nurse instructs the NAP by:

- Communicating the appropriate route, device, and frequency of temperature measurement
- Explaining any precautions needed in positioning the patient (e.g., for rectal temperature measurement)
- Reviewing the usual temperature values and significant changes to report to the nurse

Equipment

- Thermometer (selected on the basis of site used)
- Soft tissue or wipe
- Alcohol swab
- Water-soluble lubricant (for rectal measurements only)
- Pen and vital sign flow sheet, record form, or electronic health record (EHR)
- Clean gloves (optional), plastic thermometer sleeve, disposable probe or sensor cover
- Towel

ASSESSMENT

1. Identify patient using at least two identifiers (e.g., name and birthday or name and medical record number) according to agency policy. *Rationale: Ensures patient safety. Complies with The Joint Commission standards and improves patient safety (TJC, 2019).*
2. Obtain data from patient's EHR to determine need to measure patient's body temperature:
   a. Note patient's risks for temperature alterations. *Rationale: Certain conditions place patients at risk for temperature alterations and require more frequent temperature measurement and nursing assessment.*
      - Expected or diagnosed infection
      - Open wounds or burns
      - White blood cell count below 5000/mm^3 or above 12,000/mm^3
      - Immunosuppressive drug therapy
      - Injury to hypothalamus
      - Exposure to temperature extremes
      - Blood product infusion
      - Hypothermia or hyperthermia therapy
      - Postoperative status
   b. Assess for other signs and symptoms that accompany temperature alteration. *Rationale: Physical signs and symptoms alert you to alterations in body temperature.*
      - *Hyperthermia:* Decreased skin turgor, dry mucous membranes; tachycardia; hypotension; decreased venous filling; concentrated urine
      - *Heatstroke:* Body temperature of 40°C (104°F) or more (Goforth and Kazman, 2015); hot, dry skin; tachycardia; hypotension; excessive thirst; muscle cramps; visual disturbances; confusion or delirium

BOX 7.2

Types of Thermometers

Electronic Thermometers

- Thermometer consists of a rechargeable battery-powered display unit with a thin wire cord and a temperature-processing probe covered by a disposable cover
- Within 1 minute after placement, thermometer displays a digital temperature reading.
- Separate probes are available for oral and axillary temperature measurement (blue tip) and rectal temperature measurement (red tip) (see illustration A).

Tympanic Thermometers

- Probe consists of an otoscope-like speculum with an infrared sensor tip that detects heat radiated from the tympanic membrane of the ear (see illustration B).
- Within seconds after placement in the ear canal and depressing the scan button, a digital reading appears on the display unit; a sound signals when the peak temperature has been measured.

Temporal Artery Thermometers

- Infrared scanner displays a digital reading within seconds after scanning while sweeping across the forehead and just behind the ear (see illustration C).

Chemical Dot Single-Use or Reusable Thermometers

- Thermometer consists of a thin strip of plastic with a temperature sensor at one end that contains chemically impregnated dots formulated to change color to reflect temperature reading, usually within 60 seconds (see illustration D).

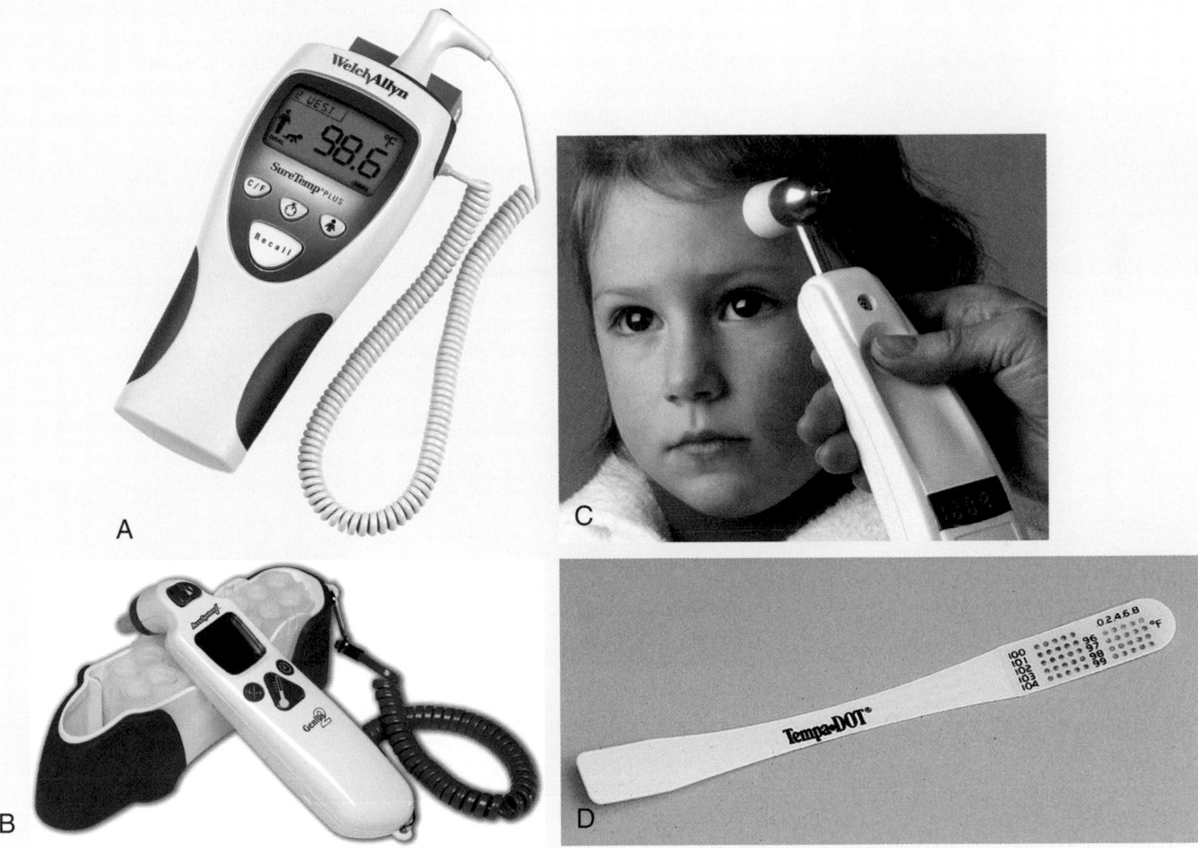

(A) Electronic thermometer (Sure Temp PLUS). (B) Electronic tympanic membrane thermometer (Genius 2 Thermometer). (C) Temporal artery thermometer measures heat from blood flowing through the superficial temporal artery. (D) Chemical dot disposable single-use thermometer. (**B,** *Genius 2 Thermometer used with permission of Covidien. All rights reserved.* **C,** *Photo courtesy Exergen.)*

- *Hypothermia:* Pale skin; skin cool or cold to touch; bradycardia and dysrhythmias; uncontrollable shivering; reduced level of consciousness; shallow respirations

c. Assess for factors that normally influence temperature. *Rationale: Allows you to accurately assess for presence and significance of temperature alteration.*
   - Age. *Rationale: Older adults have narrower range of temperature than younger adults.*

Safe Patient Care *No single temperature is normal for all people. A temperature within an acceptable range in an adult may reflect a fever in an older adult. Undeveloped temperature-control mechanisms in infants and children cause temperature to rise and fall rapidly.*

   - Exercise. *Rationale: Muscle activity increases metabolism, which increases heat production and raises temperature.*

TABLE 7.2

Advantages and Limitations of Selected Temperature Measurement Sites

Site Advantages	Site Limitations
Oral	
Easily accessible—requires no position change Comfortable for patient Provides accurate surface temperature reading Reflects rapid change in core temperature Reliable route to measure temperature for intubated patients	Causes delay in measurement if patient recently ingested hot or cold fluids or foods, smoked, or chewed gum Not used with patients who have had oral surgery; are unable to position thermometer in mouth; or have trauma, shaking or chills, or history of epilepsy Not used with infants; small children; or confused, unconscious, or uncooperative patients Risk of body fluid exposure
Tympanic Membrane	
Easily accessible site Minimal patient repositioning required Obtained without disturbing, waking, or repositioning patient Used for patients with tachypnea without affecting breathing Sensitive to core temperature changes Very rapid measurement (2–5 seconds) Unaffected by oral intake of food or fluids or smoking Used in newborns to reduce infant handling and heat loss	More variability of measurement than with other core temperature devices Requires removal of hearing aids at least 2 minutes before measurement Requires disposable sensor cover with only one size available Readings distorted by otitis media and cerumen impaction Not used with patients who have had surgery of the ear or tympanic membrane; ear drainage; or blood, cerebrospinal fluid, or foreign bodies in the ear canal Does not accurately measure core temperature changes during and after exercise Affected by ambient temperature devices such as incubators, radiant warmers, and facial fans Difficult to position correctly in neonates, infants, and children <3 years old because of anatomy of ear canal Inaccuracies reported caused by incorrect positioning of handheld unit
Rectal	
Argued to be more reliable when oral temperature is difficult or impossible to obtain	Lags behind core temperature during rapid temperature changes Not used for patients with diarrhea or patients who have had rectal surgery, rectal disorders, bleeding tendencies, or neutropenia Requires positioning and is a source of patient embarrassment and anxiety Risk of body fluid exposure Requires lubrication Not used for routine vital signs in newborns Readings sometimes influenced by impacted stool
Axilla	
Safe and inexpensive Used with newborns and unconscious patients	Long measurement time Requires continuous positioning Measurement lags behind core temperature during rapid temperature changes Not recommended for detecting fever in infants and young children (Forrest et al., 2017) Requires exposure of thorax, which results in temperature loss, especially in newborns Affected by exposure to the environment, including time to place thermometer Underestimates core temperature
Skin	
Inexpensive Provides continuous reading Safe and noninvasive Used for neonates	Useful for screening temperatures, especially in infants; during invasive procedures; and in orally intubated patients in the critical care unit; not appropriate for monitoring fever in acutely ill patients or monitoring temperature therapies May underestimate oral temperature by 0.4° C (32.7° F) or more in 50% of adults Disposable, easy to store, and can be used for patients requiring isolation Measurement lags behind other sites during temperature changes, especially during hyperthermia Adhesion impaired by diaphoresis or sweat Affected by environmental temperature Cannot be used on patients with allergy to adhesives
Temporal Artery	
Easy to access without position change Very rapid measurement Eliminates need to disrobe or unbundle Comfortable for patient with no risk of injury Less disruptive for premature infants, newborns, and children (Opersteny et al., 2017) Reflects rapid change in core temperature Sensor cover not required	Inaccurate with head covering or hair on forehead Affected by skin moisture such as diaphoresis or sweating

- Hormones. *Rationale: Women have wider temperature fluctuations than men because of menstrual cycle hormonal changes, because body temperature varies during menopause, and because women have a thicker layer of subcutaneous fat.*
- Stress. *Rationale: Stress elevates temperature.*
- Environmental temperature. *Rationale: Infants and older adults are more sensitive to environmental temperature changes.*
- Medications. *Rationale: Some drugs impair or promote sweating, vasoconstriction, or vasodilation or interfere with ability of hypothalamus to regulate temperature.*
- Daily fluctuations. *Rationale: Body temperature normally changes 0.5° to 1°C (0.9° to 1.8°F) during a 24-hour period. Temperature is lowest during early morning. Most patients have maximum temperature elevation between 5 PM and 7 PM; temperature falls gradually during night.*

3. Determine appropriate measurement site and device for patient (see Box 7.2). Use disposable thermometer for patient on isolation precautions. *Rationale: Determines if patient's status contraindicates selection of a specific method or site.*
4. Determine previous baseline temperature and measurement site (if available) from patient's electronic health record. *Rationale: Allows you to assess for change in condition. Provides comparison with future temperature measurements.*
5. Assess patient's or family caregiver's knowledge, experience, and health literacy level. *Rationale: Ensures patient has the capacity to obtain, communicate, process, and understand basic health information (Centers for Disease Control and Prevention [CDC], 2016).*

STEP	RATIONALE
PLANNING	
Expected outcomes following completion of procedure:	
1. Body temperature is within acceptable range for patient's age-group.	Thermoregulation is maintained.
Body temperature returns to baseline range following therapies for abnormal temperature.	Environmental factors that alter temperature are controlled.
2. Provide privacy and prepare environment.	Maintains confidentiality and minimizes embarrassment. Helps patient relax.
3. Prepare and organize equipment.	Ensures an organized procedure for obtaining body temperature measurement.
4. Verify that patient has not had anything to eat or drink and has not chewed gum or smoked within the past 20 minutes (if having oral temperature measured).	Oral food and fluids, smoking, and gum can alter oral temperature measurement.
5. Explain to patient or family caregiver how you will measure temperature and importance of maintaining proper position until reading is complete.	Promotes patient cooperation and increases compliance. Patients are often curious about their temperatures and should be cautioned against prematurely removing thermometer to read results.
IMPLEMENTATION	
1. Perform hand hygiene.	Reduces transmission of infection.
2. Obtain temperature reading.	
a. **Oral temperature (electronic):**	
(1) Help patient to supine position in bed or chair.	
(2) *Optional:* Apply clean gloves when there is risk for exposure to respiratory secretions or facial or mouth wound drainage.	An oral probe cover is removable without physical contact and thus does not require gloves.
(3) Remove thermometer pack from charging unit. Attach oral thermometer probe stem (blue tip) to thermometer unit. Grasp top of probe stem, being careful not to apply pressure on ejection button.	Charging provides battery power. Ejection button releases plastic cover from probe stem.
(4) Slide disposable plastic probe cover over thermometer probe stem until cover locks in place (see illustration).	Soft plastic cover will not break in patient's mouth and prevents transmission of infection between patients.
(5) Ask patient to open mouth; gently place thermometer probe under tongue in posterior sublingual pocket lateral to center of lower jaw (see illustration).	Heat from superficial blood vessels in sublingual pocket produces temperature reading. With electronic thermometer, temperatures in right and left posterior sublingual pocket are significantly higher than in area under front of tongue.

STEP	RATIONALE
(6) Ask patient to hold thermometer probe with lips closed.	Maintains proper position of thermometer during recording.
(7) Leave thermometer probe in place until audible signal indicates completion and patient's temperature appears on digital display; remove thermometer probe from under patient's tongue.	Probe must stay in place until signal occurs to ensure accurate reading.
(8) Push ejection button on thermometer probe stem to discard plastic probe cover into appropriate receptacle.	Reduces transmission of infection.
(9) If wearing gloves, remove, dispose in appropriate receptacle, and perform hand hygiene.	Reduces transmission of infection.
(10) Return thermometer probe stem to storage position of thermometer unit.	Protects probe stem from damage. Returning thermometer probe stem automatically causes digital reading to disappear.
b. **Rectal temperature (electronic):**	
(1) Draw curtain around bed and/or close room door. Help patient to side-lying or Sims' position with upper leg flexed. Move aside bed linen to expose only anal area. Keep patient's upper body and lower extremities covered with sheet or blanket.	Maintains patient's privacy, minimizes embarrassment, and promotes comfort.
(2) Apply clean gloves. Cleanse anal region when feces and/or secretions are present. Remove soiled gloves and reapply clean gloves.	Maintains standard precautions when exposed to items soiled with body fluids (e.g., feces).
(3) Remove thermometer pack from charging unit. Attach rectal thermometer probe stem (red tip) to thermometer unit. Grasp top of probe stem, being careful not to apply pressure on ejection button.	Ejection button releases plastic cover from probe stem.
(4) Slide disposable plastic probe cover over thermometer probe stem until cover locks in place.	Soft plastic probe cover prevents transmission of infection between patients.
(5) Using a single-use package, squeeze a liberal amount of lubricant on tissue. Dip probe cover of thermometer, blunt end, into lubricant, covering 2.5 to 3.5 cm (1 to 1½ inches) for adult.	Lubrication minimizes trauma to rectal mucosa during insertion. Tissue avoids contamination of remaining lubricant in container.
(6) With nondominant hand, separate patient's buttocks to expose anus. Ask patient to breathe slowly and relax.	Fully exposes anus for thermometer insertion. Relaxes anal sphincter for easier thermometer insertion.

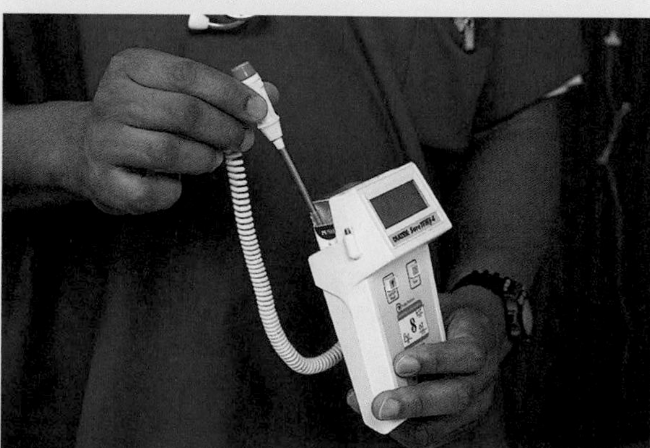

STEP 2a(4) Nurse inserts electronic thermometer probe stem into probe cover. Cover snaps in place.

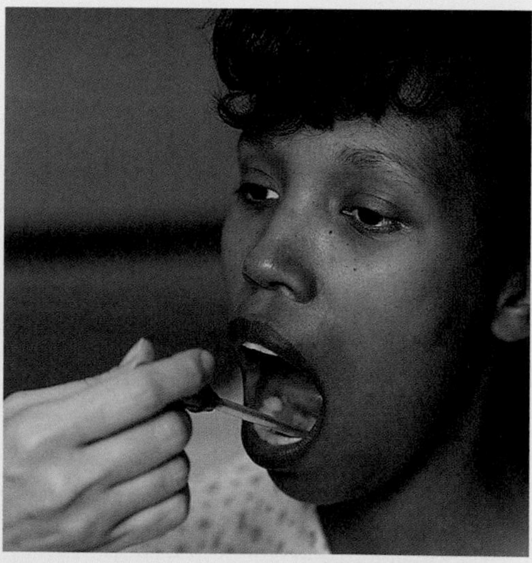

STEP 2a(5) Probe placed under tongue in posterior sublingual pocket.

STEP	RATIONALE
(7) Gently insert thermometer into anus in direction of umbilicus 3.5 cm (1½ inches) for adult. Do not force thermometer.	Ensures adequate exposure against blood vessels in rectal wall.
(8) If you feel resistance during insertion, withdraw immediately. Never force thermometer.	Prevents trauma to mucosa.

Safe Patient Care *If you cannot adequately insert thermometer into rectum or resistance is felt during insertion, remove thermometer and consider alternative method for obtaining temperature.*

STEP	RATIONALE
(9) Once positioned, hold thermometer probe in place until audible signal indicates completion and patient's temperature appears on digital display; remove thermometer probe from anus (see illustration).	Probe must stay in place until signal occurs to ensure accurate reading.

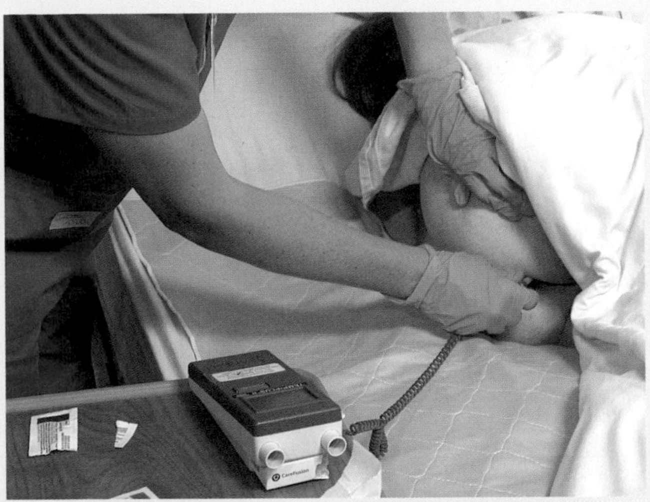

STEP 2b(9) Probe inserted into anus. *(Copyright © Mosby's Clinical Skills: Essentials Collection.)*

STEP	RATIONALE
(10) Push ejection button on thermometer stem to discard plastic probe cover into appropriate receptacle. Wipe probe stem with alcohol swab, paying particular attention to ridges where probe stem connects to probe.	Reduces transmission of infection.
(11) Return thermometer stem to storage position of recording unit.	Protects probe stem from damage. Returning thermometer stem automatically causes digital reading to disappear.
(12) Wipe patient's anal area with soft tissue to remove lubricant or feces and discard tissue. Perform perineal hygiene as needed.	Provides for comfort and hygiene.
(13) Remove and dispose of gloves in appropriate receptacle. Perform hand hygiene.	Reduces transmission of infection.
c. **Axillary temperature (electronic):**	
(1) Draw curtain around bed and/or close room door. Help patient to supine or sitting position. Move clothing or gown away from shoulder and arm.	Maintains patient's privacy, minimizes embarrassment, and promotes comfort. Exposes axilla for correct thermometer probe placement.
(2) Remove thermometer pack from charging unit. Attach oral thermometer probe stem (blue tip) to thermometer unit. Grasp top of thermometer probe stem, being careful not to apply pressure on ejection button.	Charging provides battery power. Ejection button releases plastic cover from probe stem.
(3) Slide disposable plastic probe cover over thermometer stem until cover locks in place.	Soft plastic probe cover prevents transmission of infection between patients.

STEP	RATIONALE
(4) Raise patient's arm away from torso. Inspect for skin lesions and excessive perspiration; if needed, dry axilla or select alternative site. Insert thermometer probe into center of axilla (see illustration), lower arm over probe, and place arm across patient's chest.	Maintains proper position of thermometer against blood vessels in axilla.

Safe Patient Care *Do not use axilla if skin lesions are present because local temperature is sometimes altered, and area may be painful to touch.*

STEP	RATIONALE
(5) Once thermometer probe is positioned, hold it in place until audible signal indicates completion and patient's temperature appears on digital display; remove thermometer probe from axilla.	Thermometer probe must stay in place until signal occurs to ensure accurate reading.
(6) Push ejection button on thermometer stem to discard plastic probe cover into appropriate receptacle.	Thermometer probe must stay in place until signal occurs to ensure accurate reading.
(7) Return thermometer stem to storage position of recording unit.	Returning thermometer stem to storage position automatically causes digital reading to disappear. Protects stem from damage.
(8) Replacing linen or gown.	Restores comfort and sense of well-being.
(9) Perform hand hygiene.	Reduces transmission of infection.
d. **Tympanic membrane temperature:**	
(1) Assist patient to assume comfortable position with head turned toward side, away from you. If patient has been lying on one side, use upper ear. Note if there is an obvious presence of cerumen (earwax) in patient's ear canal.	Ensures comfort and facilitates exposure of auditory canal for accurate temperature measurement. Heat trapped in ear facing down causes false-high temperature reading. Cerumen impedes lens cover of speculum. Switch to other ear or select alternative measurement site.
(2) Obtain temperature from patient's right ear if you are right-handed. Obtain temperature from patient's left ear if you are left-handed.	The less acute the angle of approach, the better the probe seal.
(3) Remove thermometer handheld unit from charging base, being careful not to apply pressure to ejection button.	Charging base provides battery power. Removal of handheld unit from base prepares it to measure temperature. Ejection button releases plastic probe cover from thermometer tip.
(4) Slide disposable speculum cover over otoscope-like lens tip until it locks in place. Be careful not to touch lens cover.	Soft plastic probe cover prevents transmission of infection between patients. Lens cover should not have dust, fingerprints, or cerumen obstructing optical pathway.
(5) Insert speculum into ear canal following manufacturer instructions for tympanic probe positioning (see illustration):	Correct positioning of probe with respect to ear canal allows maximal exposure of tympanic membrane.

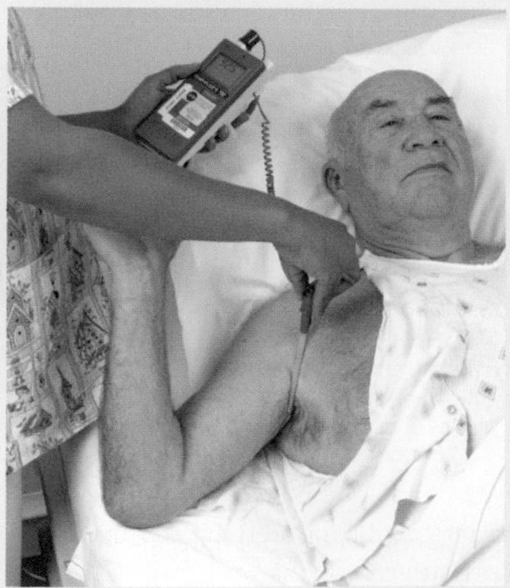

STEP 2c(4) Insert thermometer probe into center of axilla.

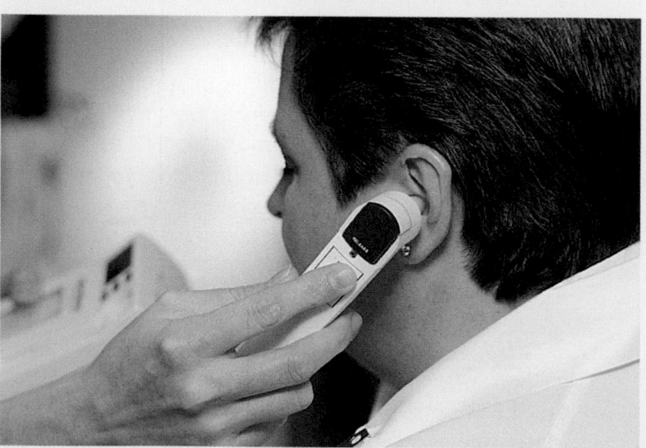

STEP 2d(5) Tympanic membrane thermometer with probe cover placed in patient's ear.

STEP	RATIONALE
(a) Pull ear pinna backward, up, and out for an adult. For children less than 3 years of age, pull pinna down and back; point covered probe toward midpoint between eyebrow and sideburns. For children older than 3 years, pull pinna up and back (Hockenberry et al., 2017).	Ear tug straightens external auditory canal, allowing maximum exposure of tympanic membrane and therefore correctly positioning speculum (Hockenberry et al., 2017).
(b) Fit speculum tip snug in canal, pointing toward nose.	Gentle pressure seals ear canal from ambient air temperature, which alters readings as much as 2.8°C (5°F).
Optional: Move thermometer in figure-eight pattern.	Some manufacturers recommend movement of speculum tip in figure-eight pattern that allows sensor to detect maximum tympanic membrane heat radiation.
(6) Once positioned, press scan button on handheld unit. Leave speculum in place until audible signal indicates completion and patient's temperature appears on digital display.	Pressing scan button causes detection of infrared energy. Speculum probe tip must stay in place until device has detected infrared energy noted by audible signal.
(7) Carefully remove speculum from auditory meatus. Push ejection button on handheld unit to discard speculum cover into appropriate receptacle.	Reduces transmission of infection. Automatically causes digital reading to disappear.
(8) If temperature is abnormal or second reading is necessary, replace probe cover and wait 2 minutes before repeating in same ear or repeat measurement in other ear. Consider an alternative temperature site or instrument.	Lens cover must be free of cerumen to maintain optical path. Time allows ear canal to regain usual temperature.
(9) Return handheld unit to thermometer base.	Protects sensor tip from damage.
(10) Perform hand hygiene and assist patient to a comfortable position.	Reduces transmission of infection.
e. **Temporal artery temperature:**	
(1) Assist patient to assume sitting position. Ensure that forehead is dry; dry with towel if needed.	Moisture interferes with thermometer sensor.
(2) Place sensor firmly on patient's forehead.	Firm contact avoids measurement of ambient temperature.
(3) Press red scan button with your thumb. Slowly slide thermometer straight across forehead while keeping sensor flat and firmly on skin (see illustration). Keeping scan button depressed, lift sensor after sweeping the forehead and touch sensor on neck just behind earlobe. Read temperature when clicking sound during scanning stops. Release scan button.	Thermometer continuously scans for highest temperature when scan button is depressed. Area behind earlobe is less affected by diaphoresis and verifies temperature.

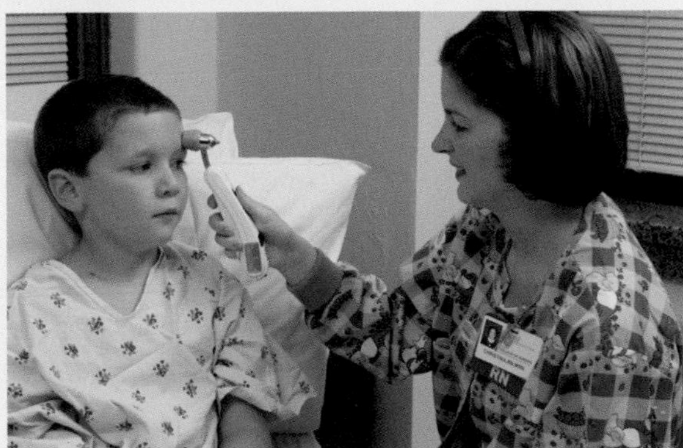

STEP 2e(3) Scanning the forehead with a temporal thermometer.

STEP	RATIONALE
(4) Gently clean sensor with alcohol swab, return to storage unit, and perform hand hygiene.	Reduces transmission of infection.
(5) Return thermometer to charger.	Maintains battery charge of thermometer unit.
3. Assist patient to comfortable position.	Ensure comfort and well-being.
4. Inform patient of temperature reading and record per agency policy.	Promotes participation in care and understanding of health status.

STEP	RATIONALE
5. Place nurse call system within reach; instruct patient in use.	Promotes safety and prevents falls.
6. Raise side rails (as appropriate) and lower bed to lowest position.	Promotes safety and prevents falls.

EVALUATION

STEP	RATIONALE
1. If you are assessing temperature for the first time, establish it as baseline if it is within acceptable range.	Used to compare future temperature measurements.
2. Compare temperature reading with patient's previous baseline and acceptable temperature range for patient's age-group.	Body temperature fluctuates within narrow range; comparison reveals presence of abnormality. Improper placement or movement of thermometer can cause inaccuracies. Second measurement confirms initial findings of abnormal body temperature.
3. If patient has fever, take temperature approximately 30 minutes after administering antipyretics and every 4 hours until temperature stabilizes.	Determines if temperature begins to fall in response to therapy.
4. **Use Teach-Back:** "I want to be sure I explained how to check your child's temperature at home. Show me how to swipe his forehead using the temporal thermometer." Revise your instruction now or develop a plan for revised patient/family caregiver teaching if patient/family caregiver is not able to teach back correctly.	Determines patient's/family caregiver's level of understanding of instructional topic.

Unexpected Outcomes	Related Interventions
1. Patient has temperature 1° C (1.8° F) or more above usual range.	Initiate measures to lower body temperature: • Cool room environment. • Reduce external covering on patient's body to promote heat loss but do not induce shivering. • Keep clothing and bed linen dry. • Limit physical activity and sources of emotional stress. • Administer antipyretics as ordered. • Increase fluid intake to at least 3 L daily (unless contraindicated). • Initiate measures to stimulate appetite and provide nutrients to meet increased energy needs. • Prevent or control spread of infection. • Perform pulmonary hygiene (see Chapter 16). • Promote adequate urinary elimination (see Chapter 19). • Apply hypothermia blanket as ordered.
2. Patient has temperature 1° C (1.8° F) or more below usual range.	Initiate measures to raise body temperature: • Remove wet clothing or linen. • Apply warm blankets and, unless contraindicated, offer warm liquids. • Apply hyperthermia blankets if ordered.
3. Unable to obtain temperature.	• Reassess correct placement of temperature probe or sensor. • Choose alternative temperature measurement site. • Obtain alternative temperature measurement device.

Recording

- Record temperature and route and any signs or symptoms of temperature alterations.
- Record temperature after administration of specific therapies, such as blood or blood product transfusions.
- Document your evaluation of patient learning.

Hand-Off Reporting

- Report abnormal findings, including route of assessment.
- Report measures to reduce or increase temperature and need for reassessment.

✦ SKILL 7.2 Assessing Apical Pulse

Purpose

Assessing the pulse provides indications of heart function and tissue perfusion (circulation). The apical pulse is the most accurate noninvasive measure of heart rate and requires correct use of a stethoscope (Box 7.3). A stethoscope magnifies heart sounds as they are transmitted from the chest wall through the tubing to the listener.

Delegation and Collaboration

The skill of apical pulse measurement cannot be delegated to nursing assistive personnel (NAP). Often you measure the apical pulse

BOX 7.3

Exercises for Learning to Use a Stethoscope

1. Place earpieces in both ears with tips of earpieces turned toward the face. Lightly blow against the diaphragm (flat side of chest piece). Next, place earpieces in both ears with the tips turned toward the back of the head and again blow against the diaphragm. Compare comfort in the ears and amplification of sounds with earpieces in both directions. Earpieces pointing toward the face should fit snugly and comfortably.
2. If the stethoscope has both a diaphragm (flat side) and a bell (bowl-shaped with a rubber ring) (see illustration A), put earpieces in ears and lightly blow against the diaphragm to learn the difference in sound transmission. The chest piece can be turned to allow sound to be carried through either side (bell or diaphragm) of the chest piece. If sound is faint, lightly blow into the bell. Next, turn the chest piece and blow again against both the diaphragm and the bell. The diaphragm is used for higher-pitched heart sounds, bowel sounds, and lung sounds (see illustration B). The bell is used for lower-pitched heart sounds and vascular sounds (see illustration C).
3. With earpieces in place and using the diaphragm, move the diaphragm lightly over the hair on your arm. The bristling sound mimics a sound heard in the lungs. When listening for significant sounds, hold the diaphragm still and firmly make a tight seal against the skin to eliminate extraneous sounds.
4. Place the diaphragm over the front of your chest directly on your skin and listen to your own breathing, comparing the bell and the diaphragm. Repeat the process while listening to your heartbeat. Ask someone to speak in a conversational tone and note how the speech detracts from hearing clearly. When using a stethoscope, both the patient and the examiner should remain quiet.
5. With the earpieces in your ears, gently tap the tubing. Tapping also generates extraneous sounds. When listening to a patient, maintain a position that allows the tubing to extend straight and hang free. Tubing that rubs or bumps objects creates extraneous sounds. Kinked tubing muffles sounds.

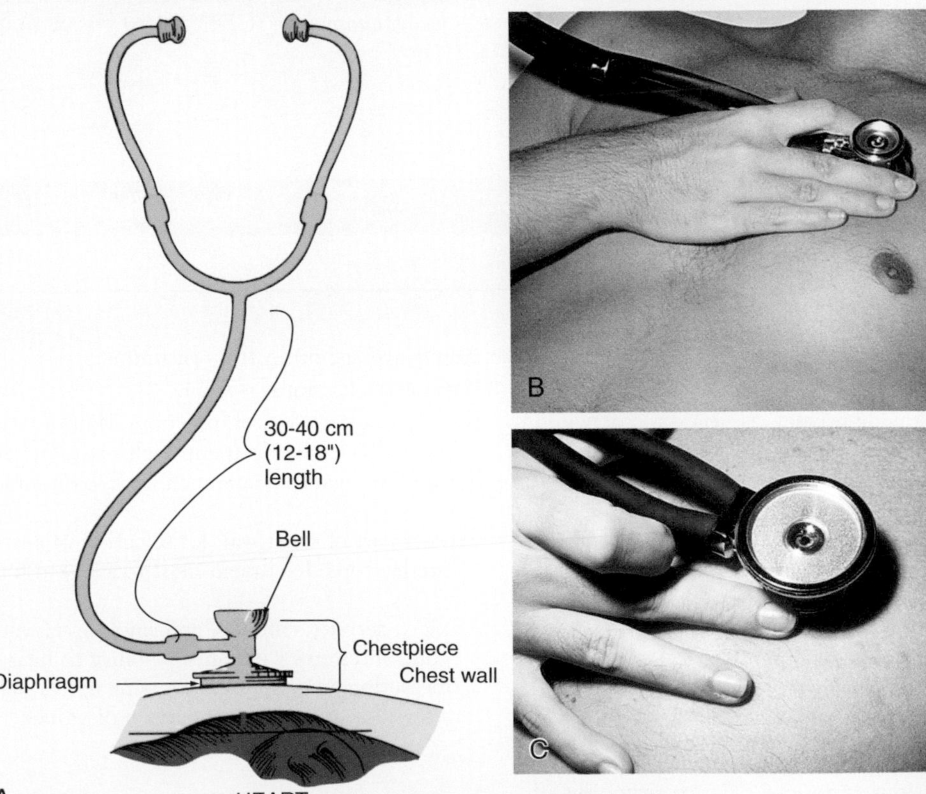

(A) Parts of a stethoscope. (B) The diaphragm is placed firmly and securely when auscultating high-pitched lung and bowel sounds. (C) The bell must be placed lightly on the skin to hear low-pitched vascular and heart sounds.

when you suspect an irregularity in the radial pulse or when a patient's condition requires a more accurate assessment.

Equipment

- Stethoscope
- Wristwatch with second hand or digital seconds display
- Pen and vital sign flow sheet in chart or EHR
- Alcohol swab

ASSESSMENT

1. Identify patient using at least two identifiers (e.g., name and birthday or name and medical record number) according to agency policy. *Rationale: Ensures patient safety. Complies with The Joint Commission standards and improves patient safety (TJC, 2019).*
2. Obtain data from patient's EHR to determine need to assess patient's apical pulse:
   a. Assess for any risk factors for apical pulse alteration: heart disease, onset of sudden chest pain or acute pain from any site, invasive cardiovascular diagnostic tests, surgery, sudden infusion of large volume of intravenous (IV) fluid, internal or external hemorrhage, administration of medications that alter heart function. *Rationale: Certain conditions place patients at risk for pulse alterations.*
   b. Assess for signs and symptoms of altered cardiac function such as dyspnea, fatigue, chest pain, orthopnea, syncope, palpitations, edema of dependent body parts, cyanosis, or pallor of skin (see Chapter 8). *Rationale: Physical signs and symptoms indicate alteration in cardiac output or stroke volume.*
   c. Assess for factors that normally influence apical pulse rate and rhythm. *Rationale: Allows you to anticipate factors that alter apical pulse, ensuring an accurate interpretation:*
      - Age. *Rationale: Infant's heart rate (HR) at birth ranges from 100 to 160 beats/min at rest; by age 2, pulse rate slows to 70 to 120 beats/min; by adolescence, rate varies between 60 and 90 beats/min and remains so throughout adulthood (Hockenberry et al., 2017).*
      - Exercise. *Rationale: Physical activity increases HR; a well-conditioned patient may have a slower-than-usual resting HR that returns more quickly to resting rate after exercise.*
      - Position changes. *Rationale: HR increases temporarily when changing from lying to sitting or standing position.*
      - Medications. *Rationale: Antidysrhythmics, sympathomimetics, and cardiotonics affect rate and rhythm of pulse; large doses of opioid analgesics can slow HR; general anesthetics slow HR; central nervous system stimulants such as caffeine can increase HR.*
      - Temperature. *Rationale: Fever or exposure to warm environments increases HR; HR declines with hypothermia.*
      - Sympathetic stimulation. *Rationale: Emotional stress, anxiety, or fear stimulates sympathetic nervous system, which increases HR.*
   d. Determine previous baseline apical rate (if available). *Rationale: Allows you to assess for change in condition.*
3. Determine any report of latex allergy. If patient has latex allergy, ensure that stethoscope is latex-free. *Rationale: Reduces risk of allergic reaction to stethoscope.*
4. Assess patient's or family caregiver's knowledge, experience, and health literacy level. *Rationale: Ensures patient has the capacity to obtain, communicate, process, and understand basic health information (CDC, 2016).*

STEP	RATIONALE
PLANNING	
1. Expected outcomes following completion of procedure:	
• Apical HR is within acceptable range.	Adults average 60 to 100 beats/min.
• Rhythm is regular.	Cardiovascular status is stable.
2. Perform hand hygiene. Provide privacy, as necessary; draw curtain around bed and/or close door.	Reduces transmission of infection. Maintains confidentiality and minimizes embarrassment. Helps patient relax.
3. Collect and bring appropriate supplies to patient's bedside.	Ensures an organized approach for assessing radial pulse.
4. Help patient to supine or sitting position. Move aside bed linen and gown to expose sternum and left side of chest.	Exposes part of chest wall for selection of auscultatory site. Stethoscope diaphragm must touch skin for best sounds.
5. Explain to patient or family caregiver that you will assess apical pulse rate. Encourage patient to relax and not speak. **NOTE:** If patient has been active, wait 5 to 10 minutes before assessing pulse. If he or she has been smoking or ingesting caffeine, wait 15 minutes before assessing pulse.	Anxiety, activity, caffeine, and smoking elevate HR. Patient's voice interferes with nurse's ability to hear sound when measuring apical pulse. Assessing apical pulse rate at rest allows for objective comparison of values.

STEP	RATIONALE

IMPLEMENTATION

1. Perform hand hygiene.
   Reduces transmission of infection.
2. Locate anatomical landmarks to identify point of maximal impulse (PMI), also called *apical impulse* (see Chapter 8). The heart is located behind and to left of sternum with base at top and apex at bottom. Find angle of Louis just below suprasternal notch between sternal body and manubrium; it feels like a bony prominence (see illustration A). Slip fingers down each side of angle to find second intercostal space (ICS) (see illustration B). Carefully move fingers down left side of sternum to fifth ICS and laterally to left midclavicular line (MCL) (see illustration C). A light tap felt within area 1 to 2.5 cm (½ to 1 inch) of PMI is reflected from apex of heart (see illustration D).
   Use of anatomical landmarks allows correct placement of stethoscope over apex of heart. This position enhances ability to hear heart sounds clearly. If unable to palpate PMI, reposition patient on left side. In presence of serious heart disease, you may locate PMI to left of MCL or at sixth ICS. PMI may not be palpated in obese adults or patients with severe pulmonary disease that has changed shape of thorax.

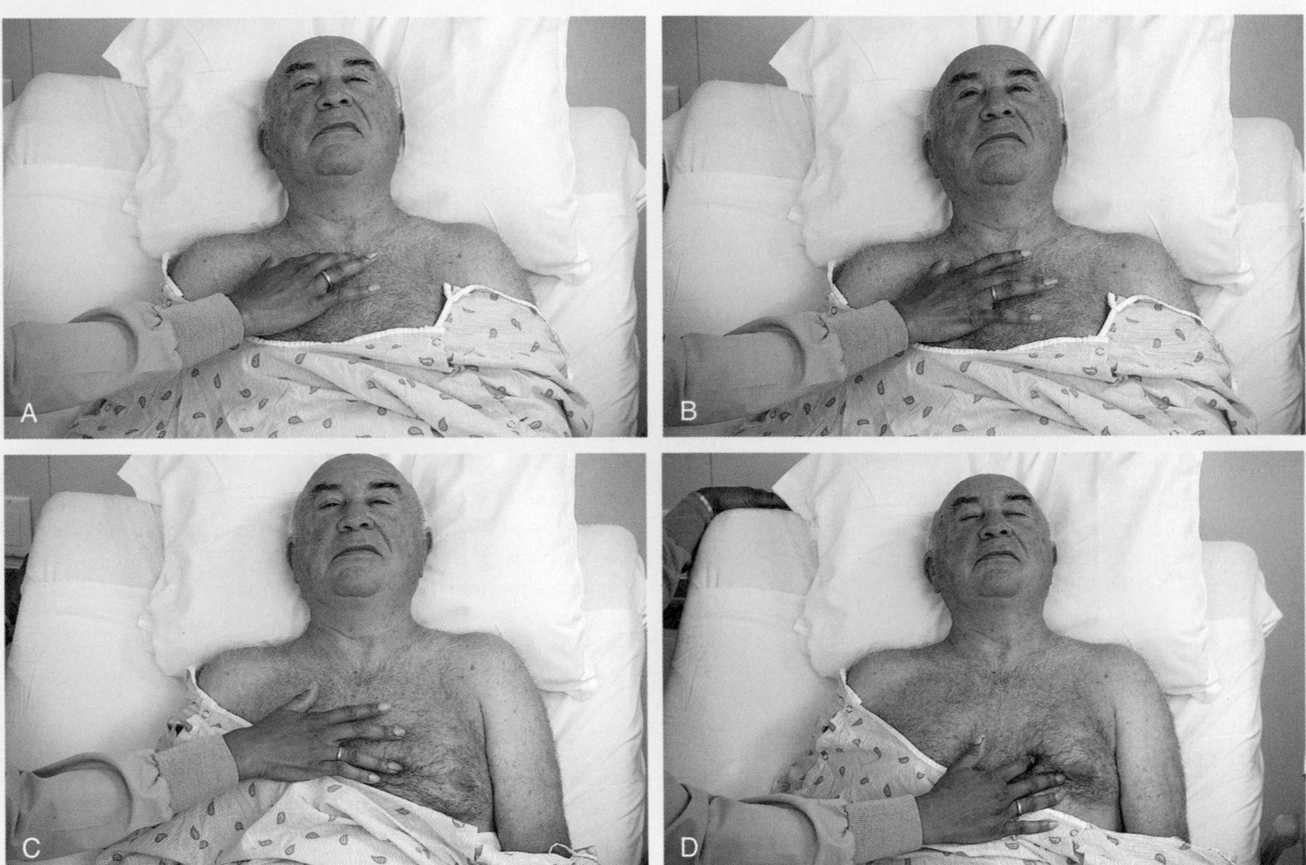

STEP 2 (A) Nurse locates sternal notch. (B) Nurse locates second intercostal space. (C) Nurse locates fifth intercostal space. (D) Nurse locates point of maximal impulse at fifth intercostal space at left midclavicular line.

3. Place diaphragm of stethoscope in palm of hand for 5 to 10 seconds.
   Warming of metal or plastic diaphragm prevents patient from being startled and promotes comfort.
4. Place diaphragm of stethoscope over PMI at fifth ICS, at left MCL, and auscultate for normal S_1 and S_2 heart sounds (heard as "lub-dub") (see illustration).
   Allow stethoscope tubing to extend straight without kinks that would distort sound transmission. Normal sounds S_1 and S_2 are high-pitched and best heard with diaphragm.
5. When you hear S_1 and S_2 with regularity, use second hand of watch and begin to count rate: when sweep hand hits number on dial, start counting with zero, then one, two, and so on.
   Apical rate is determined accurately only after you are able to auscultate sounds clearly. Timing begins with zero. Count of one is first sound auscultated after timing begins.
6. If apical rate is regular, count for 30 seconds and multiply by 2.
   You can assess regular apical rate within 30 seconds.

STEP	RATIONALE

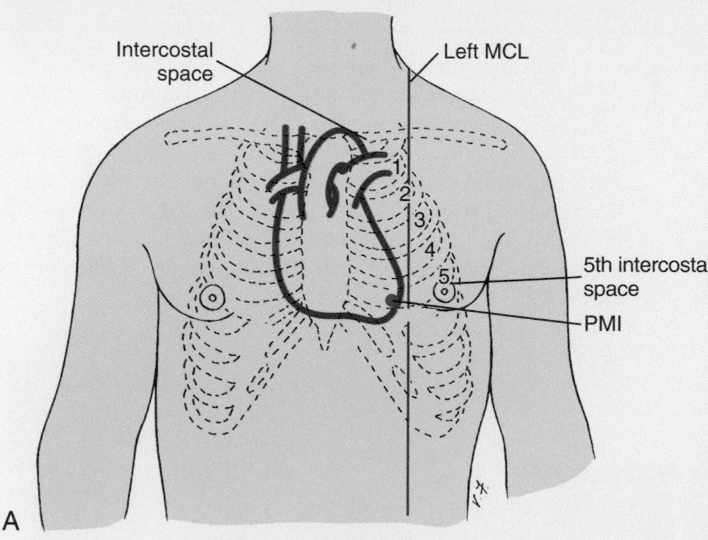

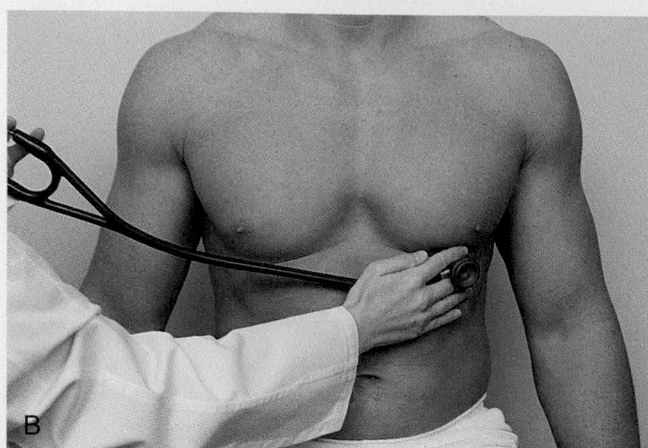

STEP 4 (A) Location of point of maximal impulse (PMI) in adult. (B) Listening to PMI in adult. *MCL*, Misclavicular line.

STEP	RATIONALE
7. If HR is irregular or patient is receiving cardiovascular medication, count for a full 1 minute (60 seconds).	Irregular rate is more accurately assessed when measured over longer interval.
8. Note regularity of any dysrhythmia (S_1 and S_2 occurring early or late after previous sequence of sounds) (e.g., every third or every fourth beat is skipped).	Regular occurrence of dysrhythmia within 1 minute indicates inefficient contraction of heart and potential alteration in cardiac output.

Safe Patient Care *If apical rate is abnormal or irregular, repeat measurement or have another nurse conduct measurement. Original measurement may be incorrect. Second measurement confirms initial findings of an abnormal HR.*

STEP	RATIONALE
9. Replace patient's gown and bed linen.	Restores comfort and promotes sense of well-being.
10. Assist patient to comfortable position.	Ensures comfort and well-being.
11. Place nurse call system within reach; instruct patient in use and perform hand hygiene.	Promotes safety and prevents falls. Reduces transmission of infection.
12. Discuss findings with patient.	Promotes participation in care an understanding of health status
13. Clean earpieces and diaphragm of stethoscope with alcohol swab routinely after each use. Perform hand hygiene.	Stethoscopes are frequently contaminated with microorganisms. Regular disinfection can control nosocomial infections.

EVALUATION

STEP	RATIONALE
1. If assessing pulse for first time, establish apical rate as baseline if it is within an acceptable range.	Used to compare future pulse assessments.
2. Compare apical rate and character with patient's previous baseline and acceptable range of HR for patient's age.	Allows you to assess for change in patient's condition and for presence of cardiac alteration.
3. **Use Teach-Back:** "I want to be sure I explained why it is important to check your heart rate at home. Tell me which medication you are taking that would decrease your heart rate." Revise your instruction now or develop a plan for revised patient/family caregiver teaching if patient/family caregiver is not able to teach back correctly.	Determines patient's and family caregiver's level of understanding of instructional topic.

Unexpected Outcomes	Related Interventions
1. Adult patient's apical pulse is greater than 100 beats/min (tachycardia).	• Identify related data, including fever, pain, fear or anxiety, recent exercise, low blood pressure, blood loss, or inadequate oxygenation. • Observe for signs and symptoms associated with abnormal cardiac function, including dyspnea, fatigue, chest pain, orthopnea, syncope, palpitations, edema of body parts, cyanosis, or dizziness.

Unexpected Outcomes	Related Interventions
2. Patient's apical pulse is less than 60 beats/min (bradycardia).	• Assess for factors that decrease HR such as beta blockers and antiarrhythmic drugs. • Observe for signs and symptoms associated with abnormal cardiac function, including dyspnea, fatigue, chest pain, orthopnea, syncope, palpitations, edema of body parts, cyanosis, or dizziness. • Have another nurse assess apical pulse. • Report findings to nurse in charge and/or health care provider. It may be necessary to withhold prescribed medications that alter HR until health care provider can evaluate need to alter dosage.
3. Patient's apical rhythm is irregular.	• Assess for signs and symptoms of decreased cardiac output (see Chapter 8). • Report findings to nurse in charge and/or health care provider, who may order an electrocardiogram to detect cardiac conduction alteration.

Recording

- Record apical pulse rate after administration of specific therapies.
- Record any signs and symptoms of alteration in cardiac function.
- Document your evaluation of patient learning.

Hand-Off Reporting

- Report bradycardia, tachycardia, or irregular pulse to nurse in charge or health care provider immediately.

✦ SKILL 7.3 Assessing Radial Pulse

Purpose

The pulse is a palpable bounding of blood flow caused by pressure-wave transmission from the left ventricle of the heart to the peripheral arteries. Assessing the pulse provides indications of heart function and tissue perfusion (circulation). The radial pulse in an adult is the easiest to access and provides a quick, accurate assessment of peripheral circulation and heart function. The brachial or apical pulse is the site for routine pulse assessment in infants.

Delegation and Collaboration

The skill of radial pulse measurement can be delegated to nursing assistive personnel (NAP) if a patient's condition is stable. The skill cannot be delegated when a patient's condition is unstable, because the patient is at high risk for acute or serious cardiac problems, or when the nurse is evaluating a patient's response to a treatment or medication. The nurse instructs the NAP by:

- Indicating the appropriate site for measuring pulse rate; frequency of measurement; and factors related to the patient history such as risk for abnormally slow, rapid, or irregular pulse
- Reviewing patient's usual pulse rate and significant changes to report to the nurse
- Reviewing the specific changes or abnormalities to report to the nurse for further assessment

Equipment

- Wristwatch with second hand or digital seconds display
- Pen and vital sign flow sheet in chart or EHR

ASSESSMENT

1. Identify patient using at least two identifiers (e.g., name and birthday or name and medical record number) according to agency policy. *Rationale: Ensures patient safety. Complies with The Joint Commission standards and improves patient safety (TJC, 2019).*
2. Obtain data from patient's EHR to determine need to assess patient's radial pulse:
   a. Assess for any risk factors for pulse alterations. *Rationale: Certain conditions place patients at risk for pulse alterations. A history of peripheral vascular disease often alters pulse rate and quality.*
      - History of heart disease
      - Cardiac dysrhythmia
      - Onset of sudden chest pain or acute pain from any site
      - Invasive cardiovascular diagnostic tests
      - Surgery
      - Sudden infusion of large volume of IV fluid
      - Internal or external hemorrhage
      - Administration of medications that alter cardiac function
   b. Assess for signs and symptoms of altered cardiac function such as presence of dyspnea, fatigue, chest pain, orthopnea, syncope, palpitations, edema of dependent body parts, cyanosis, or pallor of skin (see Chapter 8). *Rationale: Physical signs and symptoms often indicate alteration in cardiac function, which affects radial pulse rate and rhythm.*

c. Assess for signs and symptoms of peripheral vascular disease such as pale, cool extremities; thin, shiny skin with decreased hair growth; thickened nails. *Rationale: Physical signs and symptoms indicate alteration in local arterial blood flow.*
d. Assess for factors that influence radial pulse rate and rhythm: age, exercise, position changes, fluid balance, medications, temperature, sympathetic stimulation (e.g., caffeine or nicotine). *Rationale: Can anticipate factors that alter pulse, ensuring accurate interpretation. Dysrhythmics, cardiotonics, antihypertensives, vasodilators, and vasoconstrictors affect pulse rate and rhythm.*

3. Determine patient's previous baseline pulse rate (if available) or perform hand hygiene and measure pulse. *Rationale: Allows you to assess for change in condition. Provides comparison with future pulse measurements.*
4. Assess patient's or family caregiver's knowledge, experience, and health literacy. *Rationale: Ensures patient has the capacity to obtain, communicate, process, and understand basic health information (CDC, 2016).*

STEP	RATIONALE
PLANNING	
1. Expected outcomes following completion of procedure:	
• Radial pulse is palpable, within usual range for patient's age.	Usual range for adults is 60 to 100 beats/min.
• Rhythm is regular.	Cardiac status is stable.
• Radial pulse is strong, firm, and elastic.	Radial artery is patent.
2. Perform hand hygiene. Provide privacy and prepare environment.	Reduces transmission of infection. Maintains confidentiality and minimizes embarrassment. Ensures a more organized procedure.
3. Collect appropriate equipment and bring to patient's bedside.	Ensures an organized approach for assessing a radial pulse.
4. Explain to patient or family caregiver that you will assess radial pulse rate (heart rate [HR]). Encourage patient to relax as much as possible.	Anxiety, activity, caffeine, and smoking elevate heart rate. Assessing radial pulse rate at rest allows for objective comparison of values.
NOTE: If patient has been active, wait 5 to 10 minutes before assessing pulse. If patient has been smoking or ingesting caffeine, wait 15 minutes before assessing pulse.	
IMPLEMENTATION	
1. Perform hand hygiene.	Reduces transmission of infection.
2. Help patient to assume a supine or sitting position.	Provides easy access to pulse sites.
3. If patient is supine, place his or her forearm straight alongside or across lower chest or upper abdomen (see illustration A). If sitting, bend patient's elbow 90 degrees and support lower arm on chair or on your arm. Place tips of first two or middle three fingers of hand over groove along radial or thumb side of patient's inner wrist (see illustration B). Slightly extend or flex wrist with palm down until you note strongest pulse.	Fingertips are most sensitive parts of hand to palpate arterial pulsation. Your thumb has pulsation that interferes with accuracy.

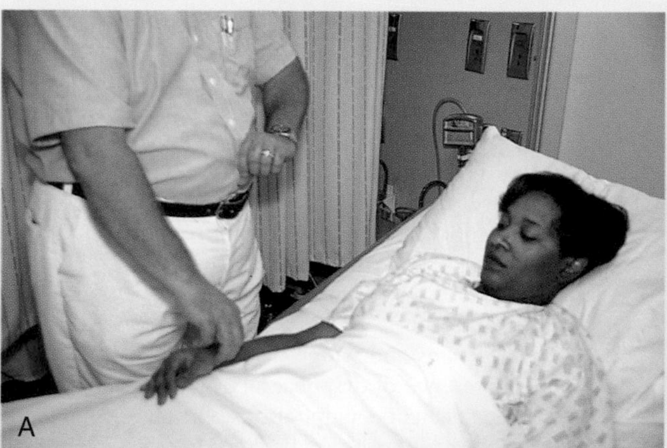

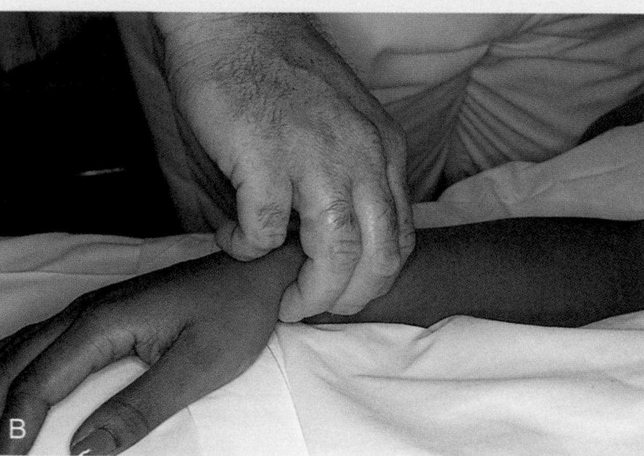

STEP 3 (A) Pulse check with patient's forearm at side with wrist extended. (B) Hand placement for pulse check.

STEP	RATIONALE
4. Lightly compress pulse against radius, losing pulse initially; relax pressure so pulse becomes easily palpable.	Pulse assessment is more accurate when using moderate pressure. Too much pressure occludes pulse and impairs blood flow.
5. Determine strength of pulse. Note whether thrust of vessel against fingertips is bounding (4+); full increased, strong (3+); expected (2+); barely palpable, diminished (1+); or absent, not palpable (0).	Strength reflects volume of blood ejected against arterial wall with each heart contraction. Accurate description of strength improves communication among nurses and other health care providers.
6. After palpating a regular pulse, look at watch second hand and begin to count rate. Count the first beat after the second hand hits the number on the dial; count as one, then two, and so on.	Rate is determined accurately only after pulse has been palpated. Timing begins with zero. Count of one is first beat palpated after timing begins.
a. If pulse is regular, count rate for 30 seconds and multiply total by 2.	A 30-second count is accurate for rapid, slow, or regular pulse rates.
b. If pulse is irregular, count rate for a full 60 seconds. Assess frequency and pattern of irregularity.	Inefficient contraction of heart fails to transmit pulse wave, resulting in irregular pulse. Longer time ensures accurate count.
c. When pulse is irregular, compare radial pulses bilaterally and compare with apical pulse.	A marked difference between pulses indicates that arterial flow is compromised to one extremity and as a nurse you need to take action.
7. Assist patient to comfortable position.	Promotes comfort and sense of well-being.
8. Place nurse call system within reach; instruct patient in use.	Promotes safety and prevents falls.
9. Discuss findings with patient.	Promotes participation in care and understanding of health status.
10. Perform hand hygiene.	Reduces transmission of infection.

EVALUATION

1. If assessing pulse for first time, establish this radial pulse measure as baseline if it is within acceptable range.	Used to compare future pulse assessments.
2. Compare pulse rate and character with patient's previous baseline and acceptable range for patient's age.	Allows for assessment of change in patient's condition and presence of cardiac alteration.
3. **Use Teach-Back:** "You are taking a medication that can affect your pulse rate, and you must check your pulse daily. I want to be sure you know how to do this. Show me how you will check your pulse rate." Revise your instruction now or develop a plan for revised patient/family caregiver teaching if patient/family caregiver is not able to teach back correctly.	Determines patient's/family caregiver's level of understanding of instructional topic.

Unexpected Outcomes	Related Interventions
1. Patient has irregular pulse.	• Auscultate apical pulse (see Skill 7.2). • Assess for **pulse deficit**: (a) one nurse auscultates apical pulse while second provider palpates radial pulse; (b) nurse begins 60-second pulse count by calling out loud when to begin counting pulses; (c) the two pulse rates are compared. If pulse count differs by more than 2, a deficit exists; assess for other signs and symptoms of decreased cardiac output (see Chapter 8).
2. Patient has weak, thready, or difficult-to-palpate radial pulse.	• Assess both radial pulses and compare findings. • Observe for symptoms associated with ineffective tissue perfusion, including pallor and cool skin distal to weak pulse. • Assess for swelling in surrounding tissues or any encumbrance (e.g., dressing or cast) that may impede blood flow. • Obtain Doppler or ultrasound stethoscope to detect low-velocity blood flow (see Chapter 8). • Have another nurse assess pulse.

Unexpected Outcomes	Related Interventions
3. An adult patient's pulse rate is less than 60 beats/min (bradycardia) or more than 100 beats/min (tachycardia).	• Identify related data, including fever, pain, fear or anxiety, recent exercise, low blood pressure, blood loss, or inadequate oxygenation. • Observe for signs and symptoms associated with abnormal cardiac function, including dyspnea, fatigue, chest pain, orthopnea, syncope, palpitations, edema of body parts, cyanosis, or pallor of skin. • Auscultate apical pulse (see Skill 7.2). • Confer with health care provider and be prepared to order/obtain electrocardiogram.

Recording

- Record pulse rate and rhythm with assessment site and any signs and symptoms of altered cardiac function.
- Record pulse rate after administration of specific therapies.
- Document your evaluation of patient learning.

Hand-Off Reporting

- Report bradycardia, tachycardia, or irregular pulse to nurse in charge or health care provider immediately.

✦ SKILL 7.4 Assessing Respirations

Purpose

Respiration involves evaluating the exchange of oxygen and carbon dioxide between the environment, the blood, and the cells. Assessment of respirations includes determining respiratory rate, depth, and rhythm of respiratory movements. Abnormal respirations can be the first indication of patient deterioration. On inspiration the diaphragm contracts, the abdominal organs move downward, and the chest cavity expands. On expiration the diaphragm relaxes upward, and the ribs and sternum return to the relaxed position (Fig. 7.1).

Delegation and Collaboration

The skill of counting respirations can be delegated to nursing assistive personnel (NAP) unless the patient is considered unstable (i.e., complaints of dyspnea). The nurse instructs the NAP by:

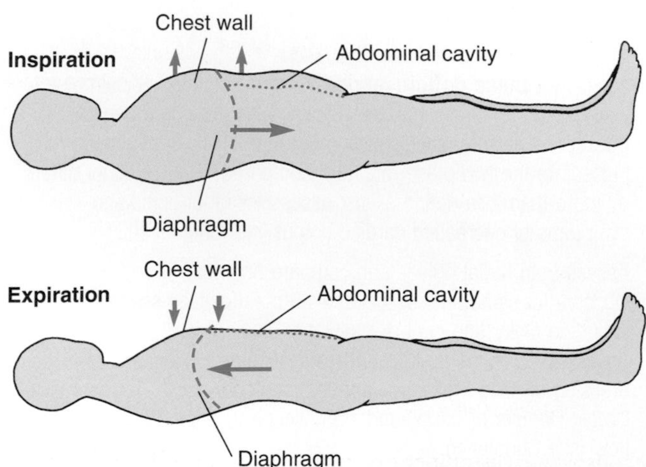

FIG 7.1 Diaphragmatic and chest wall movement during inspiration and expiration.

- Communicating the frequency of measurement and factors related to patient history or risk for increased or decreased respiratory rate or irregular respirations
- Reviewing any unusual respiratory values and significant changes to report to the nurse

Equipment

- Wristwatch with second hand or digital seconds display
- Pen and vital sign flow sheet in chart or EHR

ASSESSMENT

1. Identify patient using at least two identifiers (e.g., name and birthday or name and medical record number) according to agency policy. *Rationale: Ensures patient safety. Complies with The Joint Commission standards and improves patient safety (TJC, 2019).*
2. Obtain data from patient's EHR to determine need to assess patient's respirations:
   a. Assess for factors that influence character of respirations. *Rationale: Allows you to anticipate factors that influence respirations, ensuring a more accurate interpretation.*
      - Fever. *Rationale: Elevated body temperature increases oxygen demand and increases respiration rate and depth.*
      - Exercise. *Rationale: Respirations increase in rate and depth to meet need for additional oxygen and rid body of carbon dioxide.*
      - Anxiety. *Rationale: Anxiety increases oxygen demand and causes increase in respiration rate and depth because of sympathetic nervous system stimulation.*
      - Diseases/trauma of chest wall or muscles. *Rationale: Certain conditions (e.g., fractured ribs, thoracic surgery, asthma, acute or chronic lung disease, pulmonary edema, pulmonary emboli) affect inspiration and/or expiration.*

- Constrictive chest, presence of chest tube, or abdominal incisions or dressings. *Rationale: These can impact the ease with which a patient is able to breathe deeply.*
- Acute pain. *Rationale: Pain increases oxygen demand and alters rate and rhythm of respirations; breathing becomes shallow. Patient inhibits or splints chest wall movement when pain is in area of chest or abdomen.*
- Smoking. *Rationale: Chronic smoking changes pulmonary airways, resulting in increased respiratory rate at rest when not smoking.*
- Medications. *Rationale: Opioid analgesics, general anesthetics, and sedative-hypnotics depress rate and depth; amphetamines and cocaine increase rate and depth; bronchodilators dilate airways, which ultimately slows respiratory rate.*
- Body position. *Rationale: Standing or sitting erect promotes full ventilatory movement and lung expansion; stooped or slumped posture impairs ventilatory movement; lying flat prevents full chest expansion.*
- Neurological injury. *Rationale: Damage to brainstem impairs respiratory center and inhibits rate and rhythm.*
- Anemia, decreased hemoglobin. *Rationale: Decreased hemoglobin levels lower amount of oxygen carried in blood, which results in increased respiratory rate to increase oxygen delivery. An increase in altitude lowers amount of saturated hemoglobin, which increases respiratory rate and depth.*

b. Assess for signs and symptoms of respiratory alterations such as the following. *Rationale: Physical signs and symptoms indicate alterations in respiratory status (see Chapter 8).*
- Bluish or cyanotic appearance of nail beds, lips, mucous membranes, and skin
- Restlessness, irritability, confusion, reduced level of consciousness
- Pain during inspiration
- Labored or difficult breathing
- Orthopnea
- Use of accessory muscles
- Adventitious breath sounds (see Chapter 8)
- Inability to breathe spontaneously
- Thick, frothy, blood-tinged, or copious sputum production

3. Assess pertinent laboratory/clinical values:
   a. Arterial blood gases (ABGs): Normal ranges (values vary slightly among agencies).
   - pH, 7.35–7.45
   - $PaCO_2$, 35–45 mm Hg
   - HCO_3, 22–28 mEq/L
   - PaO_2, 80–100 mm Hg
   - SaO_2, 95%–100%

   Rationale: ABG values measure arterial blood pH, partial pressure of oxygen and carbon dioxide, and arterial oxygen saturation, which reflect patient's ventilation and oxygenation status.

   b. Pulse oximetry (SpO_2): Normal SpO_2 95% to 100%; less than 90% is a clinical emergency (see Procedural Guideline 7.2). *Rationale: SpO_2 less than 90% is often accompanied by changes in respiratory rate, depth, and rhythm.*

   c. Complete blood count (CBC): Normal CBC for adults (values vary within agencies).
   - Hemoglobin: 14 to 18 g/100 mL, males; 12 to 16 g/100 mL, females
   - Hematocrit: 42% to 52%, males; 37% to 47%, females
   - Red blood cell count: 4.7 to 6.1 million/mm^3, males; 4.2 to 5.4 million/mm^3, females

   Rationale: CBC measures red blood cell count; volume of red blood cells; and concentration of hemoglobin, which reflects patient's capacity to carry oxygen.
4. Determine previous baseline respiratory rate (if available). *Rationale: Assesses for change in condition. Provides comparison with future respiratory measurements.*
5. Assess patient's or family caregiver's knowledge, experience, and health literacy level. *Rationale: Ensures patient has the capacity to obtain, communicate, process, and understand basic health information (CDC, 2016).*

STEP	RATIONALE
PLANNING	
1. Expected outcomes following completion of procedure:	
• Respiratory rate is within acceptable range.	Adults average 12 to 20 breaths/min.
• Respirations are regular and of normal depth.	Respiratory status is stable.
2. Perform hand hygiene. Provide privacy and prepare environment.	Reduces transmission of microorganisms. Maintains confidentiality and minimizes embarrassment. Ensures a more organized procedure.
3. Collect and bring appropriate supplies to patient's bedside.	Ensures an organized approach for assessing radial pulse.
4. If patient has been active, wait 5 to 10 minutes before assessing respirations.	Exercise increases respiratory rate and depth. Assessing respirations while patient is at rest allows for objective comparison of values.
5. Be sure that patient is in comfortable position, preferably sitting or lying with head of bed elevated 45 to 60 degrees.	Sitting erect promotes full ventilatory movement. Position of discomfort causes patient to breathe more rapidly.

Safe Patient Care *Assess patients with difficulty breathing (dyspnea), such as those with heart failure or abdominal ascites or in late stages of pregnancy, in the position of greatest comfort. Repositioning may increase the work of breathing, which increases respiratory rate.*

STEP	RATIONALE
6. Assess respirations after pulse measurement in an adult.	Inconspicuous assessment of respirations immediately after pulse assessment prevents patient from consciously or unintentionally altering rate and depth of breathing.

STEP	RATIONALE
IMPLEMENTATION	
1. Perform hand hygiene.	Reduces transmission of infection.
2. Be sure that patient's chest is visible. If necessary, move bed linen or gown.	Ensures clear view of chest wall and abdominal movements.
3. Place patient's arm in relaxed position across abdomen or lower chest or place your hand directly over patient's upper abdomen.	A similar position used during pulse assessment allows respiratory rate assessment to be inconspicuous. Patient's or your hand rises and falls during respiratory cycle.
4. Observe complete respiratory cycle (one inspiration and one expiration).	Rate is accurately determined only after viewing a complete respiratory cycle.
5. After observing a cycle, look at second hand of watch and begin to count rate: when sweep hand hits number on dial, begin time frame, counting one with first full respiratory cycle.	Timing begins with count of one. Respirations occur more slowly than pulse; thus, timing does not begin with zero.
6. If rhythm is regular, count number of respirations in 30 seconds and multiply by 2. If rhythm is irregular, less than 12, or greater than 20, count for 1 full minute.	Respiratory rate is equivalent to number of respirations per minute. Suspected irregularities require assessment for at least 1 minute (Table 7.3).
7. Note depth of respirations by observing degree of chest wall movement while counting rate. In addition, assess depth by palpating chest wall excursion or auscultating posterior thorax after you have counted rate (see Chapter 8). Describe depth as shallow, normal, or deep.	Character of ventilatory movement reveals specific disease states restricting volume of air from moving into and out of lungs.
8. Note rhythm of ventilatory cycle. Normal breathing is regular and uninterrupted. Do not confuse sighing with abnormal rhythm.	Character of ventilations reveals specific types of alterations. Periodically people unconsciously take single deep breaths or sighs to expand small airways prone to collapse.

Safe Patient Care *Any irregular respiratory pattern or periods of apnea (cessation of respiration for several seconds) are symptoms of underlying disease in the adult, and you need to report this to the health care provider or nurse in charge. Further assessment and immediate intervention are often necessary.*

STEP	RATIONALE
9. Replace bed linen and patient's gown.	Restores comfort and promotes sense of well-being.
10. Assist patient to comfortable position.	Promotes comfort and sense of well-being.
11. Place nurse call system within reach and instruct patient in use.	Promotes safety and prevents falls.
12. Raise side rails (as appropriate) and lower bed to lowest position.	Promotes safety and prevent falls.
13. Perform hand hygiene.	Reduces transmission of infection.
14. Discuss results with patient.	Promotes participation in care and understanding of health.

TABLE 7.3

Alterations in Breathing Pattern

Alteration	Description
Apnea	Respirations cease for several seconds. Persistent cessation results in respiratory arrest.
Biot's respiration	Respirations are abnormally shallow for two to three breaths, followed by irregular period of apnea.
Bradypnea	Rate of breathing is regular but abnormally slow (<12 breaths/min).
Cheyne-Stokes respiration	Respiratory rate and depth are irregular, characterized by alternating periods of apnea and hyperventilation. Respiratory cycle begins with slow, shallow breaths that gradually increase to abnormal rate and depth. The pattern reverses; breathing slows and becomes shallow, concluding in apnea before respiration resumes.
Hyperpnea	Respirations are increased in depth. Hyperpnea occurs normally during exercise.
Hyperventilation	Rate and depth of respirations increase. Hypocarbia may occur.
Hypoventilation	Respiratory rate is abnormally low, and depth of ventilation may be depressed. Hypercarbia may occur.
Kussmaul's respiration	Respirations are abnormally deep but regular.
Tachypnea	Rate of breathing is regular but abnormally rapid (>20 breaths/min).

STEP	RATIONALE

EVALUATION

STEP	RATIONALE
1. If assessing respirations for first time, establish rate, rhythm, and depth as baseline if within acceptable range.	Used to compare future respiratory assessment.
2. Compare respirations with patient's previous baseline and usual rate, rhythm, and depth.	Allows you to assess for changes in patient's condition and presence of respiratory alterations.
3. Correlate respiratory rate, depth, and rhythm with data obtained from pulse oximetry and ABG measurements if available.	Evaluations of ventilation, perfusion, and diffusion are interrelated.
4. **Use Teach Back:** "I want to be sure I explained why you will be reminded to take deep breaths after surgery. Tell me why deep breathing is important." Revise your instruction now or develop a plan for revised patient/family caregiver teaching if patient/family caregiver is not able to teach back correctly.	Determines patient's/family caregiver's level of understanding of instructional topic.

Unexpected Outcomes	Related Interventions
1. Adult patient's respiratory rate is below 12 breaths/min (bradypnea) or above 20 breaths/min (tachypnea). Breathing pattern is sometimes irregular (see Table 7.3). Depth of respirations is increased or decreased. Patient complains of dyspnea.	• Assess for related factors, including obstructed airway, abnormal breath sounds, productive cough, restlessness, anxiety, and confusion (see Chapter 8). • Help patient to supported sitting position (semi- or high-Fowler's) unless contraindicated. • Provide oxygen as ordered (see Chapter 16). • Assess for environmental factors that influence patient's respiratory rate such as secondhand smoke, poor ventilation, or gas fumes. • Notify health care provider or nurse in charge if alteration continues.
2. Patient demonstrates Kussmaul's, Cheyne-Stokes, or Biot's respirations (see Table 7.3).	• Notify health care provider for additional evaluation and possible medical intervention.

Recording

- Record respiratory rate and character, noting any abnormalities.
- Record respiratory rate after administration of specific therapies.
- Record type and amount of oxygen therapy if used by patient during assessment.
- Document your evaluation of patient learning

Hand-Off Reporting

- Report bradypnea, tachypnea, or abnormal depth or rhythm to nurse in charge or health care provider immediately.

✦ SKILL 7.5 Assessing Blood Pressure

Purpose

Accurate blood pressure measurement is critical for making decisions about fluid volume replacement and need for medications and for assessing rapidly changing clinical conditions. Blood pressure trends, not individual measurements, guide nursing interventions. There are four categories of blood pressure in adults: normal, elevated, hypertension stage 1, and hypertension stage 2 (Whelton et al., 2017). Measuring blood pressure using the auscultatory method requires detecting the sounds of the rush of blood (Korotkoff phases) as blood resumes its flow through an artery (Fig. 7.2). The auscultatory method is performed manually with the use of a sphygmomanometer and a stethoscope or electronically with an electronic blood pressure machine using a microphone to detect the Korotkoff phases.

Delegation and Collaboration

The skill of blood pressure (BP) measurement can be delegated to nursing assistive personnel (NAP) unless the patient is considered unstable (i.e., hypotensive). The nurse instructs the NAP by:

- Explaining the appropriate limb to use for measurement, BP cuff size, and equipment (manual or electronic) to be used
- Communicating the frequency of measurement and factors related to the patient's history, such as risk for orthostatic hypotension
- Reviewing the patient's usual BP values and significant changes or abnormalities to report to the nurse

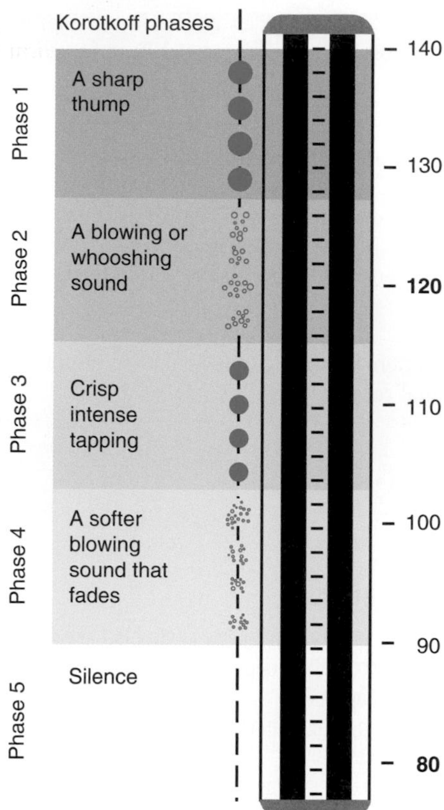

FIG 7.2 Sounds auscultated during blood pressure measurement can be differentiated into five Korotkoff phases. In this example, the blood pressure is 140/90 mm Hg.

Equipment

- Aneroid sphygmomanometer or electronic blood pressure machine
- Cloth or disposable vinyl pressure cuff of appropriate size for patient's extremity (see Step 3a)
- Stethoscope
- Alcohol swab
- Pen and vital sign flow sheet in chart or EHR

ASSESSMENT

1. Identify patient using at least two identifiers (e.g., name and birthday or name and medical record number) according to agency policy. *Rationale: Ensures patient safety. Complies with The Joint Commission standards and improves patient safety (TJC, 2019).*
2. Obtain data from patient's EHR to determine need to assess patient's BP.
   a. Assess risk factors for BP alterations. *Rationale: Certain conditions place patients at risk for BP alteration.*
      - History of cardiovascular disease
      - Renal disease
      - Diabetes mellitus
      - Circulatory shock (hypovolemic, septic, cardiogenic, or neurogenic)
      - Acute or chronic pain
      - Rapid IV infusion of fluids or blood products
      - Increased intracranial pressure
      - Postoperative status
      - Toxemia of pregnancy
   b. Assess for signs and symptoms of BP alterations. In patients at risk for high BP (HBP), assess for headache (usually occipital), flushing of face, nosebleed, and fatigue in older adults. Hypotension is associated with dizziness; mental confusion; restlessness; pale, dusky, or cyanotic skin and mucous membranes; and cool, mottled skin over extremities. *Rationale: Physical signs and symptoms indicate alterations in BP. Hypertension is often asymptomatic until pressure is very high.*
   c. Assess for factors that influence BP. *Rationale: Allows you to anticipate factors that influence blood pressure, ensuring a more accurate interpretation.*
      - Age. *Rationale: Acceptable values for BP vary throughout life (see Age-Specific section). Older patients experience greater "white coat" effect as BP increases when in the presence of a provider (Kallioinen et al., 2017).*
      - Gender. *Rationale: During and after menopause, women often have higher BPs than men of same age.*
      - Daily (diurnal) variation. *Rationale: BP varies throughout day; pressure is highest during the day between 10:00 AM and 6:00 PM and lowest in early morning.*
      - Position. *Rationale: BP falls as person moves from lying to sitting or standing position; normally postural variations are minimal (Hale et al., 2017).*
      - Exercise. *Rationale: Increases in oxygen demand by body during activity increases BP. BP increases if patients do not rest at least 5 minutes prior to measurement (Kallioinen et al., 2017).*
      - Weight. *Rationale: Obesity is an independent predictor of hypertension.*
      - Sympathetic stimulation. *Rationale: Pain, anxiety, or fear stimulates sympathetic nervous system, causing BP to rise. A full bladder increases systolic and diastolic BP (Kallioinen et al., 2017).*
      - Medications. *Rationale: Antihypertensives, diuretics, beta-adrenergic blockers, vasodilators, calcium channel blockers, angiotensin-converting enzyme (ACE) inhibitors, angiotensin receptor blockers (ARBs), and antidysrhythmics lower BP; opioids and general anesthetics also cause a drop in BP (Soyal et al., 2016).*
      - Smoking. *Rationale: Smoking results in vasoconstriction, a narrowing of blood vessels. Systolic BP (SBP) and diastolic BP (DBP) rise acutely and return to baseline approximately 20 to 30 minutes after stopping smoking, 30 minutes after snuff chewing, and 40 to 60 minutes after a nicotine tablet (Kallioinen et al., 2017).*
      - Ethnicity. *Rationale: Incidence of hypertension is higher in African Americans than in European Americans. African Americans tend to develop more severe hypertension at an earlier age and have twice the risk for the complications of hypertension (i.e., stroke and heart attack). Hypertension-related deaths are also higher among African Americans (Moughrabi, 2017).*
      - Temperature. *Rationale: Cold exposure increases SBP (Kallioinen et al., 2017).*
   d. Determine best site for BP assessment. Avoid applying cuff to extremity when IV fluids are infusing, an arteriovenous shunt or fistula is present, or breast or axillary surgery has been performed on that side. In addition, avoid applying cuff to traumatized or diseased extremity or one that has a cast or bulky bandage. Use lower extremities when brachial arteries are inaccessible. *Rationale: Inappropriate site selection may result in poor amplification of sounds,*

causing inaccurate readings. Application of pressure from inflated cuff bladder temporarily impairs blood flow and can further compromise circulation in extremity that already has impaired blood flow.

e. Determine previous baseline BP and site (if available). Determine any report of latex allergy. *Rationale: Assesses for change in condition. Provides comparison with future BP measurements. If patient has latex allergy, verify that stethoscope and BP cuff are latex-free.*

3. Assess patient's or family caregiver's knowledge, experience, and health literacy level. *Rationale: Ensures patient has the capacity to obtain, communicate, process, and understand basic health information (CDC, 2016).*

STEP	RATIONALE

PLANNING

STEP	RATIONALE
1. Expected outcome following completion of procedure: • BP is within acceptable range for patient's age.	Cardiovascular status is stable.
2. Perform hand hygiene. Provide privacy and prepare environment.	Reduces transmission of infection. Promotes confidentiality and relaxes patient. Ensures a more organized procedure.
3. Prepare and organize equipment. a. Select appropriate cuff size (Table 7.5; see illustration) and ensure that other equipment is in patient's room.	Use of improper-size cuff causes false-low or false-high reading (American Association of Critical-Care Nurses [AACN], 2016) (Table 7.4).
4. Assist patient to a sitting or lying position. Be sure that room is warm, quiet, and relaxing.	Maintains patient's comfort during measurement. Patient's perceptions that physical or interpersonal environment is stressful affect BP.
5. Be sure that patient has not exercised, ingested caffeine, or smoked for 30 minutes before assessment of BP.	Smoking increases BP immediately and lasts up to 30 minutes. The effects of coffee or caffeine increase BP up to 3 hours (Kallioinen et al., 2017).

TABLE 7.4
Common Mistakes in Blood Pressure Assessment

Error	Effect
Bladder or cuff too wide	False-low reading
Bladder or cuff too narrow or too short	False-high reading
Cuff wrapped too loosely or unevenly	False-high reading
Deflating cuff too slowly	False-high diastolic reading
Deflating cuff too quickly	False-low systolic and false-high diastolic reading
Arm below heart level	False-high reading
Arm above heart level	False-low reading
Arm not supported	False-high reading
Stethoscope that fits poorly or impairment of examiner's hearing, causing sounds to be muffled	False-low systolic and false-high diastolic reading
Stethoscope applied too firmly against antecubital fossa	False-low diastolic reading
Inflating too slowly	False-high diastolic reading
Repeating assessments too quickly	False-high systolic reading
Inadequate inflation level	False-low systolic reading
Multiple examiners using different Korotkoff sounds for diastolic readings	False-high systolic and false-low diastolic reading

TABLE 7.5
Proper Cuff Size for Electronic Monitor

Cuff Type	Limb Circumference (cm)
Small adult	17–25
Adult	23–33
Large adult	31–40
Thigh	38–50

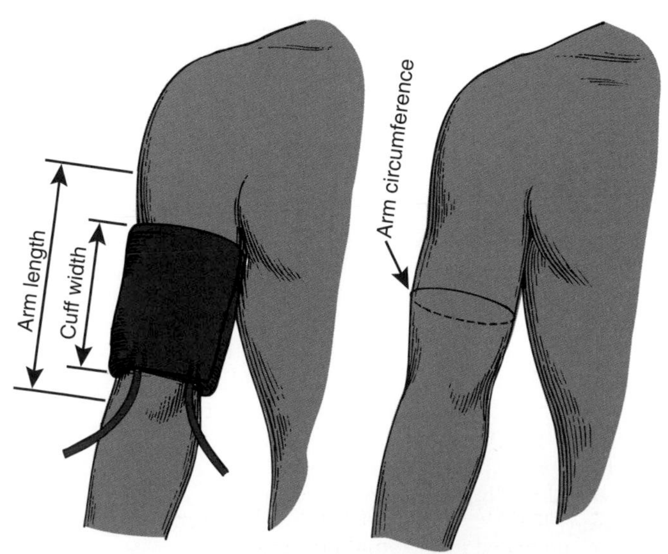

STEP 3a Proper cuff size. Length of bladder is 80% of arm circumference; cuff width is at least 40% larger than arm diameter.

STEP	RATIONALE
6. Explain to patient or family caregiver that you will assess BP. Have patient rest at least 5 minutes before measuring lying or sitting BP and 1 minute before measuring standing (Drawz, 2017). Ask patient not to speak while you are measuring BP.	Reduces anxiety that falsely elevates readings. Exercise causes false elevations in BP. Deep breathing lowers BP. Talking during assessment increases BP (Kallioinen et al., 2017).

IMPLEMENTATION

STEP	RATIONALE
1. Perform hand hygiene.	Reduces transmission of infection.
2. Assess BP by auscultation:	
a. *Upper extremity:* With patient sitting or lying, position his or her forearm at heart level with palm turned up (see illustration). Support arm on a table or under your arm. If sitting, support back and instruct patient to keep feet flat on floor without legs crossed. If supine, patient should not have legs crossed.	If arm is extended and not supported, patient will perform isometric exercise that can increase diastolic pressure. Placement of arm above level of heart causes false-low reading; arm below the level of the heart creates a false-high reading (Kallioinen et al., 2017). Not providing a support for the arm can falsely elevated SBP (Gunes and Efteli, 2016). BP measured with the back unsupported are higher than those with the back supported (Ringrose et al., 2017). Legs crossed at the knees can significantly increase BP (Kallioinen et al., 2017).

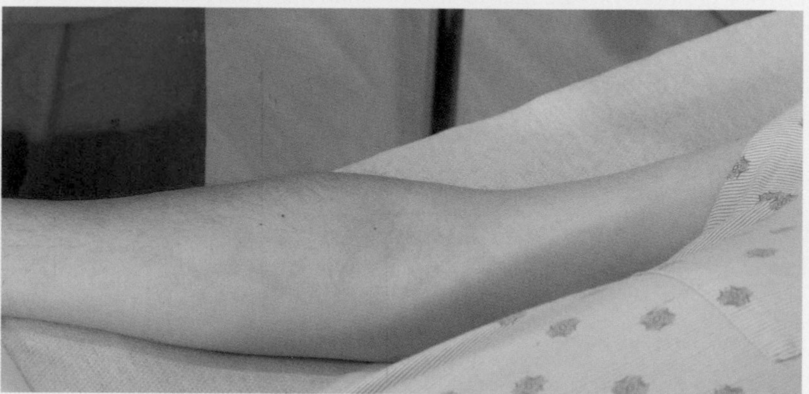

STEP 2a Patient's forearm supported on bed. *(Copyright © Mosby's Clinical Skills: Essentials Collection.)*

STEP	RATIONALE
b. *Lower extremity:* With patient prone, position patient so knee is slightly flexed. If the patient cannot be placed in prone position, position him or her supine with knee slightly bent.	
3. Expose extremity (arm or leg) fully by removing constricting clothing. Cuff may be placed over a sleeve as long as stethoscope rests on skin (Kallioinen et al., 2017).	Ensures proper cuff application.
4. Palpate brachial artery (arm, see illustration A) or popliteal artery (leg). With cuff fully deflated, apply bladder of cuff above artery by centering arrows marked on cuff over artery (see illustration B). If cuff does not have any center arrows, estimate center of bladder and place this center over artery. Position cuff 2.5 cm (1 inch) above site of pulsation (antecubital or popliteal space). With cuff fully deflated, wrap it evenly and snugly around upper arm (see illustration C) or leg (see illustration D).	Brachial artery is along groove between biceps and triceps muscles above elbow at antecubital fossa. Popliteal artery is just below patient's thigh, behind knee. Placing bladder directly over artery ensures that you apply proper pressure during inflation. Loose-fitting cuff causes false-high readings.
5. Position manometer gauge vertically at eye level. You should be no farther than 1 meter (approximately 1 yard) away.	Looking up or down at scale can result in distorted readings.

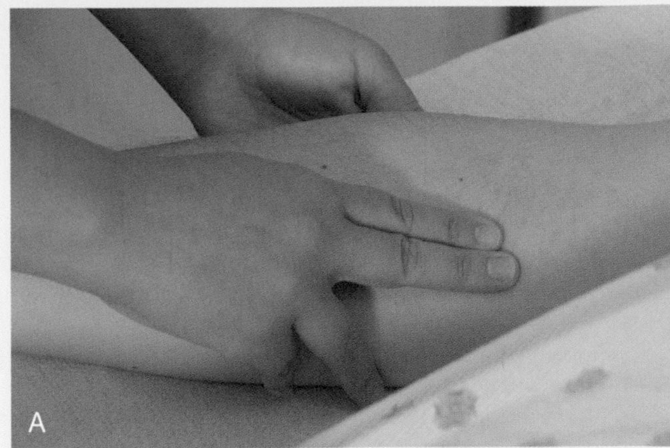

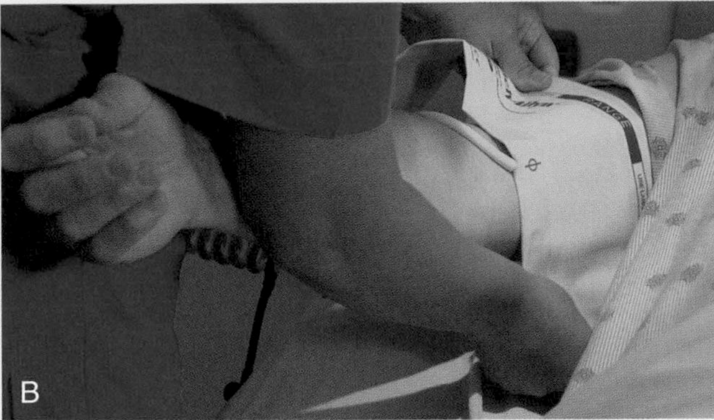

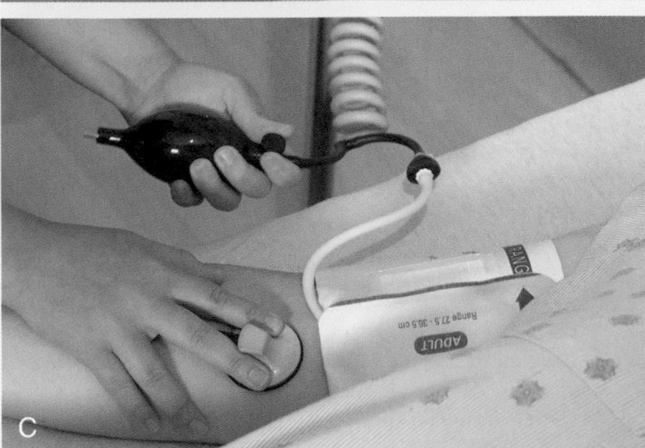

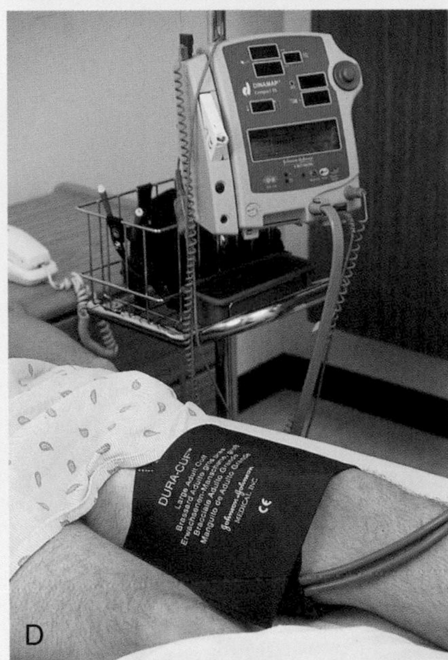

STEP 4 (A) Palpating brachial artery. (B) Aligning blood pressure cuff arrow with brachial artery. (C) Blood pressure cuff wrapped around upper arm. (D) Blood pressure cuff applied around thigh. *(A-C, Copyright © Mosby's Clinical Skills: Essentials Collection.)*

STEP	RATIONALE
a. **Measure BP using two-step method:**	
(1) Relocate brachial or popliteal pulse. Palpate artery distal to cuff with fingertips of nondominant hand while inflating cuff rapidly to pressure 30 mm Hg above point at which pulse disappears. Slowly deflate cuff and note point when pulse reappears. Deflate cuff fully and wait 30 seconds.	Palpation helps determine maximal inflation point. Ultrasonic stethoscopes are used when artery cannot be palpated due to weak pulse. Completely deflating cuff and waiting 30 seconds prevents venous congestion and false-high readings.
(2) Place stethoscope earpieces in ears and be sure that sounds are clear, not muffled.	Ensures that each earpiece follows angle of ear canal to facilitate hearing.
(3) Relocate artery and place bell or diaphragm chest piece of stethoscope over it. Do not allow chest piece to touch cuff or clothing.	Proper stethoscope placement ensures best sound reception. Stethoscope improperly positioned causes muffled sounds that often result in false-low systolic and false-high diastolic readings. The bell provides better sound reproduction, whereas the diaphragm is easier to secure with fingers and covers a larger area. Placing the stethoscope under the cuff increases the systolic and decreases the diastolic BP measurement (Kallioinen et al., 2017).
(4) Close valve of pressure bulb clockwise until tight. Quickly inflate cuff to 30 mm Hg above patient's estimated systolic pressure.	Tightening valve prevents air leak during inflation. Rapid inflation ensures accurate measurement of systolic pressure.

STEP	RATIONALE
(5) Slowly release pressure bulb valve and allow manometer needle to fall at rate of 2 to 3 mm Hg/second.	A too-rapid decline decreases systolic BP and increases diastolic BP measurement (Kallioinen et al., 2017).
(6) Note point on manometer when you hear first clear sound. Sound will slowly increase in intensity.	First sound reflects systolic BP.
(7) Continue to deflate cuff gradually, noting point at which sound disappears in adults. Note pressure to nearest 2 mm Hg. Listen for 20 to 30 mm Hg after last sound and allow remaining air to escape quickly.	Beginning of last or fifth sound is indication of diastolic pressure in adults (Thomas et al., 2017). In children distinct muffling of sounds indicates diastolic pressure (Thomas et al., 2017).
b. **Measure BP using one-step method:**	
(1) Place stethoscope earpieces in ears and be sure that sounds are clear, not muffled.	Earpieces should follow angle of ear canal to facilitate hearing.
(2) Relocate brachial or popliteal artery and place bell or diaphragm chest piece of stethoscope over it. Do not allow chest piece to touch cuff or clothing.	Proper stethoscope placement ensures optimal sound reception. Stethoscope improperly positioned causes muffled sounds that often result in false readings. Bell provides better sound reproduction, whereas diaphragm is easier to secure with fingers and covers larger area. Placing the stethoscope under the cuff increases the systolic and decreases the diastolic BP measurement (Kallioinen et al., 2017).
(3) Close valve of pressure bulb clockwise until tight. Quickly inflate cuff to 30 mm Hg above patient's usual systolic pressure.	Tightening valve prevents air leak during inflation. Inflation above systolic level ensures accurate measurement of systolic pressure.
(4) Slowly release pressure bulb valve and allow manometer needle to fall at rate of 2 to 3 mm Hg/second. Note point on manometer when you hear first clear sound. Sound will slowly increase in intensity.	Too-rapid a decline decreases systolic BP and increases diastolic BP measurement (Kallioinen et al., 2017). First sound reflects systolic pressure.
(5) Continue to deflate cuff gradually, noting point at which sound disappears in adults. Note pressure to nearest 2 mm Hg. Listen for 10 to 20 mm Hg after last sound and allow remaining air to escape quickly.	Beginning of fifth sound is indication of diastolic pressure in adults (Thomas et al., 2017). In children, distinct muffling of sounds indicates diastolic pressure (Thomas et al., 2017).
6. The American Heart Association recommends average of two sets of BP measurement, 2 minutes apart. Use second set of BP measurements as baseline. If readings are different by more than 5 mm Hg, additional readings are necessary.	Two sets of BP measurements help to prevent false-positive readings based on patient's sympathetic response (alert reaction). Averaging minimizes effect of anxiety, which often causes first reading to be higher than subsequent measures (Kallioinen et al., 2017).
7. Remove cuff from patient's arm or leg unless you need to repeat measurement.	Continuous cuff inflation causes arterial occlusion, resulting in numbness and tingling of patient's arm/leg.
8. If this is first assessment of patient, repeat procedure on other arm or leg.	Comparison of BP in both arms or legs detects circulatory problems. (Normal difference of 5 to 10 mm Hg exists between arms.) Use arm with higher pressure for repeated measurements (AACN, 2016).
9. Assess systolic BP by palpation:	
a. Follow Steps 2a through 2b of auscultation method.	
b. Locate and then continually palpate brachial, radial, or popliteal artery with fingertips of one hand. Inflate cuff to pressure 30 mm Hg above point at which you can no longer palpate pulse.	Ensures accurate detection of true systolic pressure once pressure valve is released.

Safe Patient Care *If unable to palpate artery because of weakened pulse, use a Doppler ultrasonic stethoscope (see Chapter 8).*

STEP	RATIONALE
c. Slowly release valve and deflate cuff, allowing manometer needle to fall at rate of 2 mm Hg/second. Note point on manometer when pulse is again palpable.	A too-rapid decline decreases systolic BP and increases diastolic BP measurement (Kallioinen et al., 2017). Palpation helps identify systolic pressure only.
d. Deflate cuff rapidly and completely. Remove cuff from patient's extremity unless you need to repeat measurement.	Continuous cuff inflation causes arterial occlusion, resulting in numbness and tingling of extremity.
10. Assist patient return to comfortable position and cover upper arm or leg if previously clothed.	Restores comfort and provides sense of well-being.
11. Discuss results with patient.	Promotes participation in care and understanding of health.
12. Place nurse call system with reach and instruct patient in use.	Promotes safety and prevents falls.

STEP	RATIONALE
13. Raise side rails (as appropriate) and lower bed to lowest position.	Promotes safety and prevents falls.
14. Wipe cuff with agency-approved disinfectant if used between patients. Clean and store electronic blood pressure machine according to agency protocol.	Reduces transmission of infection.
15. Clean earpieces and diaphragm of stethoscope with alcohol swab as needed.	Reduces transmission of infection when nurses share stethoscope.
16. Perform hand hygiene.	Reduces transmission of infection.

EVALUATION

1. If assessing BP for first time, establish whether baseline BP is within acceptable range.	Used to compare future BP measurements.
2. Compare BP reading with patient's previous baseline and usual BP for patient's age.	Allows you to assess for change in condition. Provides comparison with future BP measurements.
3. **Use Teach-Back:** "I want to be sure I explained why it is important to stand up slowly because you have high BP. Tell me which of your medications might make you dizzy if you stand up too fast." Revise your instruction now or develop a plan for revised patient/family caregiver teaching if patient/family caregiver is not able to teach back correctly.	Determines patient's/family caregiver's level of understanding of instructional topic.

Unexpected Outcomes	Related Interventions
1. Patient's BP is above acceptable range.	• Repeat measurement in other extremity and compare findings. When a clinically significant difference greater than 10 mm Hg exists, use the arm with the higher pressure (AACN, 2016) • Verify correct size and placement of BP cuff. • Have another nurse repeat measurement in 1 to 2 minutes. • Observe for related symptoms that are not apparent unless BP is extremely high, including headache, facial flushing, nosebleed, and fatigue in older patient. • Report BP to nurse in charge or health care provider to initiate appropriate evaluation and treatment. • Administer antihypertensive medications as ordered.
2. Patient's BP is below acceptable range.	• Repeat measurement in other extremity and compare findings. When a clinically significant difference greater than 10 mm Hg exists, use the arm with the higher pressure (AACN, 2016). • Position patient in supine position to enhance circulation and restrict activity that decreases BP further. • Assess for signs and symptoms associated with hypotension, including tachycardia; weak, thready pulse; weakness; dizziness; confusion; and cool, pale, dusky, or cyanotic skin. • Assess for orthostatic (postural) hypotension in a normotensive patient who has symptoms associated with hypotension and a drop in systolic pressure of at least 20 mm Hg or a drop in diastolic pressure by at least 10 mm Hg within 3 minutes of rising to an upright position (Shibao et al., 2013). • Assess for factors that contribute to low BP, including hemorrhage, dilation of blood vessels resulting from hyperthermia, anesthesia, or medication side effects. • Report BP to nurse in charge or health care provider to initiate appropriate evaluation and treatment. • Increase rate of IV infusion or administer vasoconstriction drugs if ordered.
3. Unable to obtain BP reading.	• Determine that no immediate crisis is present by obtaining pulse and respiratory rate. • Assess for signs and symptoms of decreased cardiac output; if present, notify nurse in charge or health care provider immediately. • Use alternative sites or procedures to obtain BP: use Doppler ultrasonic instrument (see Chapter 8); palpate systolic BP.

Recording

- Record blood pressure, extremity assessed, and method of assessment (manual or electronic).
- Record any signs and symptoms of blood pressure alterations.
- Record measurement of blood pressure after administration of specific therapies.
- Document assessment of patient learning.

Hand-Off Reporting

- Report elevated or low blood pressure, a difference of more than 20 mm Hg between extremities, or a drop of more than 20 mm Hg in systolic blood pressure or more than 10 mm Hg in diastolic blood pressure when rising from a supine to a sitting or standing position.

PROCEDURAL GUIDELINE 7.1 *Assessing Blood Pressure Electronically*

Purpose

Electronic blood pressure machines are used when frequent assessment is required, such as in critically ill or potentially unstable patients, during or after invasive procedures, or when therapies require frequent monitoring. Although electronic blood pressure machines are fast, you must consider their advantages and limitations (Box 7.4). Automatic blood pressure measurements are often inaccurate when patients have an irregular heart rate or extremely low or high blood pressure. Always verify an assessment of an abnormal blood pressure by an electronic machine with a sphygmomanometer and stethoscope.

Delegation and Collaboration

The skill of blood pressure measurement using an electronic blood pressure machine can be delegated to nursing assistive personnel (NAP) unless the patient is considered unstable (i.e., hypotensive). The nurse instructs the NAP by:

- Explaining the frequency and extremity to use for measurement
- Reviewing how to select appropriate-size blood pressure cuff for designated extremity and appropriate cuff for the machine
- Reviewing patient's usual blood pressure and reporting significant changes or abnormalities to the nurse

Equipment

Electronic blood pressure machine; blood pressure cuff of appropriate size as recommended by machine manufacturer; pen and vital sign flow sheet in chart or EHR

BOX 7.4

Advantages and Limitations of Assessing Blood Pressure Electronically

Advantages

- Ease of use
- Ability to use a stethoscope not required
- Efficient when frequent repeated measurements are indicated
- Allows blood pressure to be measured frequently, as often as every 15 seconds, with accuracy

Limitations

- Expensive
- Requires source of electricity and space to position machine
- Sensitive to outside motion interference and cannot be used in patients with seizures, tremors, or shivers
- Inaccurate for patients with irregular heart rate or hypotension (blood pressure <90 mm Hg systolic) or in situations of reduced blood flow
- Accuracy standards for electronic blood pressure manufacturers vary
- Vulnerable to error among older-adult and obese patients

Procedural Steps

1. Identify patient using at least two identifiers (e.g., name and birthday or name and medical record number) according to agency policy (TJC, 2019).
2. Assess need to measure blood pressure (see Skill 7.5, Assessment Step 2) and determine patient's baseline blood pressure.
3. Determine appropriateness of using electronic blood pressure measurement. Patients with irregular heart rate, peripheral vascular disease, seizures, tremors, and shivering are not candidates for the device.
4. Perform hand hygiene. Collect and bring appropriate equipment to patient's bedside. Select appropriate cuff size for patient extremity (see Box 7.4) and appropriate cuff for machine. Electronic blood pressure cuff and machine must be matched by manufacturer and are not interchangeable.
5. Determine best site for cuff placement; inspect condition of extremities.
6. Assist patient to comfortable position, either lying or sitting. Plug device into electric outlet and place it near patient, ensuring that connector hose between cuff and machine reaches.
7. Locate on/off switch and turn on machine to enable device to self-test computer systems.
8. Remove constricting clothing to ensure proper cuff application.
9. Prepare blood pressure cuff by manually squeezing all the air out of the cuff and connecting it to connector hose.
10. Wrap flattened cuff snugly around extremity, verifying that only one finger can fit between cuff and patient's skin. Make sure that "artery" arrow marked on outside of cuff is placed correctly (see illustration).

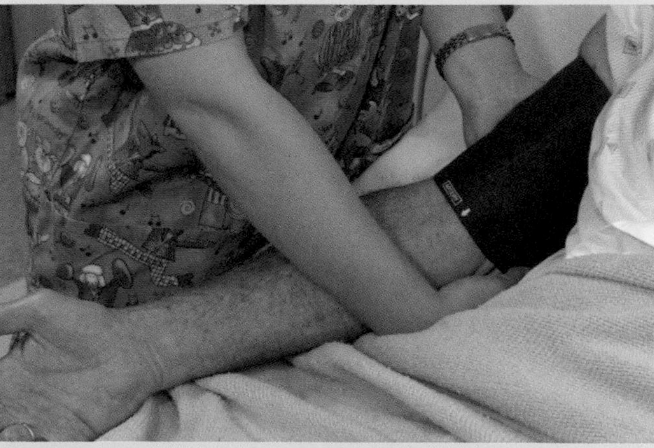

STEP 10 Aligning blood pressure cuff arrow with brachial artery.

PROCEDURAL GUIDELINE 7.1 *Assessing Blood Pressure Electronically—cont'd*

11. Verify that connector hose between cuff and machine is not kinked. Kinking prevents proper inflation and deflation of cuff.
12. Following manufacturer directions, set frequency control for automatic or manual and press the start button. The first blood pressure measurement pumps cuff to a peak pressure of approximately 180 mm Hg. After this pressure is reached, the machine begins a deflation sequence that determines the blood pressure. The first reading determines peak pressure inflation for additional measurements.
13. When deflation is complete, digital display provides most recent values and flash time in minutes that have elapsed since the measurement occurred (see illustration).

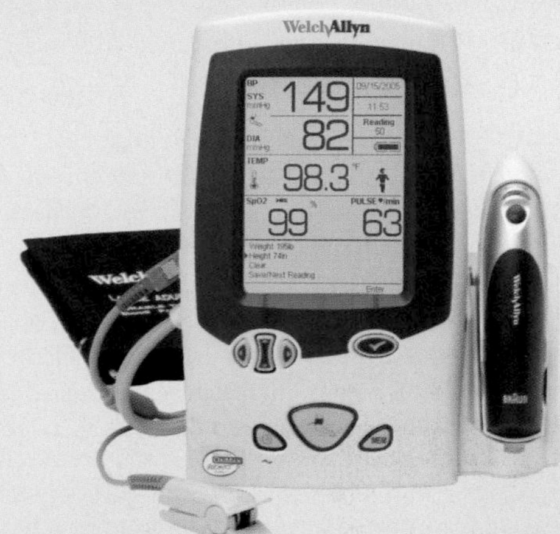

STEP 13 Digital electronic blood pressure display. *(Image courtesy Welch Allyn.)*

Safe Patient Care *If unable to obtain blood pressure with electronic device, verify machine connections (e.g., plugged into working electrical outlet, hose–cuff connections tight, machine on, correct cuff). Repeat electronic blood pressure; if unable to obtain, use auscultatory technique (see Skill 7.5).*

14. Set frequency of measurements and upper and lower alarm limits for systolic, diastolic, and mean blood pressure readings. Intervals between measurements can be set from 1 to 90 minutes. A nurse determines frequency and alarm limits on the basis of patient's acceptable range of blood pressure, nursing judgment, and health care provider order.
15. Obtain additional readings at any time by pressing the start button. Pressing the cancel button immediately deflates the cuff.
16. If frequent measurements are required, the cuff may be left in place. Remove it at least every 2 hours to assess underlying skin integrity and, if possible, alternate measurement sites.

Safe Patient Care *Frequent measurement by electronic blood pressure machines increases the risk of extremity pressure injuries, especially in vulnerable elders. Patients with abnormal bleeding tendencies are at risk for microvascular rupture from repeated inflations. Inspect the skin under the blood pressure cuff at regular intervals depending on the frequency of use.*

17. When patient no longer requires frequent blood pressure monitoring:
    a. Assist patient in return to comfortable position and cover upper arm or leg if previously clothed to restore comfort and provide sense of well-being.
    b. Place nurse call system within reach and instruct patient in use to promote safety and prevent falls.
    c. Raise side rails (as appropriate) and lower bed to lowest position to promote safety and prevent falls.
    d. Wipe cuff with agency-approved disinfectant to reduce transmission of infection. Clean and store electronic blood pressure machine.
18. Perform hand hygiene.
19. Compare electronic blood pressure readings with auscultatory measurements to verify accuracy of electronic device. Electronic measurements can underestimate measurements (Drawz, 2017).

PROCEDURAL GUIDELINE 7.2 *Measuring Oxygen Saturation (Pulse Oximetry)*

Purpose

Pulse oximetry is the noninvasive measurement of arterial blood oxygen saturation, the percentage to which hemoglobin is filled with oxygen. Pulse oximetry is indicated in patients who have an unstable oxygen status or are at risk for impaired gas exchange. A vascular, pulsatile area is needed to detect the change in the transmitted light. In adults you can apply reusable and disposable oximeter probes to the earlobe, finger, toe, bridge of the nose, or forehead.

Delegation and Collaboration

The skill of SpO_2 measurement can be delegated to nursing assistive personnel (NAP). The nurse instructs the NAP by:

- Communicating specific factors related to the patient that can falsely lower SpO_2
- Informing NAP about appropriate sensor site and probe
- Notifying frequency of SpO_2 measurements for a specific patient
- Instructing to notify nurse immediately of any reading lower than SpO_2 of 95% or value for specific patient
- Instructing to refrain from using pulse oximetry to obtain heart rate because oximeter will not detect an irregular pulse

Equipment

Oximeter; oximeter probe appropriate for patient and recommended by oximeter manufacturer; acetone or nail-polish remover if needed; pen and vital sign flow sheet in chart or EHR

Continued

PROCEDURAL GUIDELINE 7.2 *Measuring Oxygen Saturation (Pulse Oximetry)—cont'd*

Procedural Steps

1. Identify patient using at least two identifiers (e.g., name and birthday or name and medical record number) according to agency policy (TJC, 2019).
2. Determine need to measure patient's oxygen saturation. Assess risk factors for decreased oxygen saturation (e.g., acute or chronic compromised respiratory problems, change in oxygen therapy, chest wall injury, recovery from anesthesia).
3. Perform hand hygiene. Assess for signs and symptoms of alterations in oxygen saturation (e.g., altered respiratory rate, depth, or rhythm; adventitious breath sounds [see Chapter 8]; cyanotic nails, lips, mucous membranes, or skin; restlessness; difficulty breathing).
4. Determine if patient has a latex allergy; disposable adhesive sensors are made of latex.
5. Assess for factors that influence measurement of SpO_2 (e.g., oxygen therapy, respiratory therapy such as postural drainage and percussion; hemoglobin level, hypotension, temperature, nail polish, and medications such as bronchodilators).
6. Review patient's electronic health record for health care provider's order or consult agency procedure manual for standard of care for measurement of SpO_2.
7. Determine previous baseline SpO_2 (if available) from patient's record.
8. Perform hand hygiene. Provide privacy and prepare environment. Position patient comfortably. Instruct him or her to breathe normally.
9. Prepare and organize equipment. Determine most appropriate patient-specific site (e.g., finger, earlobe, bridge of nose, forehead) for sensor probe placement by measuring capillary refill (see Chapter 8). If capillary refill is greater than 2 seconds, select alternative site:
   - Site must have adequate local circulation and be free of moisture.
   - A finger free of black or brown nail polish is preferred.
   - If patient has tremors or is likely to move, use earlobe or forehead. Motion artifact is the most common cause of inaccurate readings.
   - If patient's finger is too large for the clip-on probe, as may be the case with obesity or edema, the clip-on probe may not fit properly; obtain a disposable (tape-on) probe.
10. Attach sensor to monitoring site (see illustration). If using finger, remove fingernail polish from digit with acetone or polish remover. Instruct patient that clip-on probe will feel like a clothespin on the finger but will not hurt.

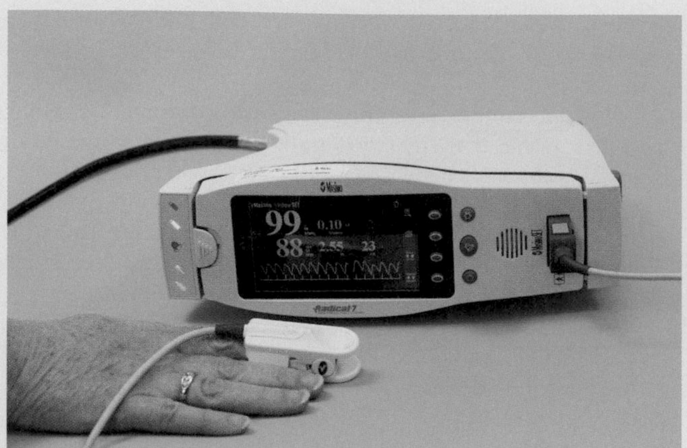

STEP 10 Oximeter sensor attached to finger.

Safe Patient Care *Do not attach probe to finger, ear, or bridge of nose if area is edematous or skin integrity is compromised. Do not use earlobe and bridge of nose sensors for infants and toddlers because of skin fragility. Do not attach sensor to fingers that are hypothermic. Select ear or bridge of nose if adult patient has a history of peripheral vascular disease. Do not use disposable adhesive sensors if patient has a latex allergy. Do not place sensor on same extremity as electronic blood pressure cuff because blood flow to finger will be interrupted temporarily when cuff inflates and cause inaccurate reading that can trigger alarms.*

11. Once sensor is in place, turn on oximeter by activating power. Observe pulse waveform/intensity display and audible beep. Correlate oximeter pulse rate with patient's radial pulse.
12. Leave sensor in place 10 to 30 seconds or until oximeter readout reaches constant value and pulse display reaches full strength during each cardiac cycle. Inform patient that oximeter alarm will sound if sensor falls off or patient moves it. Read SpO_2 on digital display.
13. If you plan to monitor SpO_2 continuously, verify SpO_2 alarm limits preset by manufacturer at a low of 85% and a high of 100%. Determine limits for SpO_2 and pulse rate as indicated by patient's condition. Verify that alarms are on.
14. Assess skin integrity under sensor probe every 2 hours; relocate sensor at least every 4 hours and more frequently if skin integrity is altered or tissue perfusion compromised.
15. If you plan intermittent or spot-checking of SpO_2, remove probe and turn oximeter power off. Clean sensor and store sensor in appropriate location.
16. Assist patient to comfortable position
17. Place nurse call system within reach; instruct patient in use.
18. Perform hand hygiene.
19. Compare SpO_2 with patient's previous baseline and acceptable SpO_2.

SPECIAL CONSIDERATIONS

Patient-Centered Care

- Assess family's financial ability to afford a sphygmomanometer for regular measurement of blood pressure at home.
- Consider an electronic blood pressure cuff with large digital display for home if patient or family caregiver has hearing or vision difficulties.
- Obese individuals have a conical-shaped upper arm, and blood pressure can be underestimated due to poor-fitting cylindrical cuff (Anast et al., 2016).

Patient Education

- Patients taking certain prescribed cardiac or antiarrhythmic medications, or their family caregivers, should learn to assess radial pulse to detect side effects of medications and should understand the impact of certain medications on blood pressure values.

Age-Specific

Pediatric

- For children who cry or become restless, take temperature last, after the other vital signs.
- Axillary temperature cannot be relied on to detect fevers in infants and young children.
- Breath holding in a child affects pulse rate.
- Apical or brachial pulse is the preferred site for assessing pediatric heart rate and rhythm until 2 years of age.
- Assess respiratory rate before other vital signs and before child becomes anxious or fears other procedures.
- Acceptable average respiratory rate for newborns is 30 to 60 breaths/min, for toddlers (2 years) is 24 to 40 breaths/min, and for children is 18 to 30 breaths/min.
- Blood pressure is not a routine part of assessment in children younger than 3 years.

Gerontological

- Older adults without teeth or poor muscle control may be unable to close the mouth tightly to obtain accurate oral temperature readings.
- Older adults are susceptible to subtle body temperature readings; temperatures considered within normal range may reflect a fever in an older adult.
- An elevated pulse rate of an older adult takes longer to return to normal resting rate.
- Older adults have a reduced heart rate with exercise because of a decreased responsiveness to catecholamines.
- A change in lung function with aging results in respiratory rates that are generally higher in older adults, with a normal range of 16 to 25 breaths/min.
- Older adults who have lost upper arm mass, especially a frail elderly adult, require special attention to selection of a smaller blood pressure cuff.

Home Care

- A temperature or blood pressure taken in the home may differ from the measurements assessed in a health care agency because the equipment can differ.
- There is increasing evidence that home blood pressure readings predict cardiovascular events and are particularly useful for monitoring the effects of treatment.

✦ PRACTICE REFLECTIONS

Consider a time in your practice when you cared for an obese patient who required blood pressure measurement. Share any pertinent information you learned that would be beneficial to share with nursing students and/or nurse colleagues who will be performing this skill.

1. What were some of the challenges you faced with this particular patient?
2. Was the outcome what you expected?
3. What did you do to help obtain an accurate measurement?

✦ CLINICAL REVIEW QUESTIONS

1. During a routine office visit, the nurse reports that a patient's blood pressure on her right arm was 134/85. Ten minutes later, the health care provider obtains a blood pressure in the left arm that is 146/80. What could account for the differences in blood pressure measurements? (Select all that apply.)
   1. The patient was talking with the provider during the measurement.
   2. The examination room was too warm.
   3. The blood pressure cuff used by the nurse was larger than that used by the provider.
   4. The patient had just come from a workout at the gym.
   5. The nurse did not support the measurement arm.
   6. The patient had his legs crossed during the first measurement.
   7. The patient has "white coat" blood pressure.
2. You have been assigned to a patient who has just returned from the post-anesthesia care unit following abdominal surgery. Order from first to last how you will complete the following activities.
   1. Assess the patient's abdominal pain.
   2. Repeat the blood pressure the new NAP reported to you as 88/68 when using an electronic blood pressure machine.
   3. Obtain an apical pulse.
   4. Direct the NAP to obtain a temporal temperature.
   5. Obtain a 60-second respiratory rate and rhythm.
3. A patient arrives in the emergency room, and the NAP obtains a SpO_2 of 92%. The nurse observes that the patient is in no distress, and the respiratory rate is 18. What could be the explanation for the low saturation? (Select all that apply.)
   1. The patient's hemoglobin is low.
   2. The patient is hypothermic.
   3. The patient has nail polish on under the oximeter probe.
   4. The patient has cold fingers.
   5. The patient just finished smoking a cigarette.

Answers and rationales for Clinical Review Questions can be found on the Evolve website.

REFERENCES

American Association of Critical-Care Nurses (AACN): Practice alert: obtaining accurate noninvasive blood pressure measurements in adults, *Crit Care Nurse* 36(3):e12–e16, 2016.

Anast N, et al: The impact of blood pressure cuff location on the accuracy of noninvasive blood pressure measurement in obese patients: an observational study, *Can J Anaesth* 63:298–306, 2016.

Boudreaux E, et al: Evaluating and selecting mobile health apps: strategies for healthcare providers and healthcare organizations, *Transl Behav Med* 4(4):363–371, 2014.

Centers for Disease Control and Prevention (CDC): What is health literacy? 2016. https://www.cdc.gov/healthliteracy/learn/index.html.

Coppetti T, et al: Accuracy of smartphone apps for heart rate measurement, *Eur J Prev Cardiol* 24(12):1287–1293, 2017.

Drawz P: Clinical implications of different blood pressure measurement techniques, *Curr Hypertens Rep* 19:54–63, 2017.

Forrest A, et al: Temporal artery and axillary thermometry comparison with rectal thermometry in children presenting to the ED, *Am J Emerg Med* 35:1855–1858, 2017.

Goforth C, Kazman J: Exertional heat stroke in Navy and Marine personnel: a hot topic, *Crit Care Nurse* 35(1):52–59, 2015.

Gunes Ü, Efteli E: Does errors made during indirect blood pressure measurement affect the results? *Int J Caring Sci* 9(2):520–525, 2016.

Hale G, et al: Treatment of primary orthostatic hypotension, *Ann Pharmacother* 51:417–428, 2017.

Hockenberry MJ, et al: *Essentials of pediatric nursing*, ed 10, St. Louis, 2017, Mosby.

Kallioinen N, et al: Sources of inaccuracy in the measurement of adult patients' resting blood pressure in clinical settings: a systematic review, *J Hypertens* 35:421–441, 2017.

Moughrabi S: Nonadherence to hypertension medications in African-American adolescents, *Pediatr Nurs* 43:223–228, 2017.

Opersteny E, et al: Precision, sensitivity and patient preference of non-invasive thermometers in a pediatric surgical acute care setting, *J Pediatr Nurs* 35:36–41, 2017.

Poh M, Poh Y: Validation of a standalone smartphone application for measuring heart rate using imaging photoplethysmography, *Telemed J E Health* 23(8):678–683, 2017.

Ringrose J, et al: The effect of back and feet support on oscillometric blood pressure measurements, *Blood Press Monit* 22(4):213–216, 2017.

Shibao C, et al: Evaluation and treatment of orthostatic hypotension, *J Am Soc Hypertens* 7:317, 2013.

Soyal P, et al: When should orthostatic blood pressure changes be evaluated in elderly: 1st, 3rd or 5th minute? *Arch Gerontol Geriatr* 65:199–203, 2016.

The Joint Commission (TJC): *2019 National Patient Safety Goals*, Oakbrook Terrace, IL, 2019, The Commission. http://www.jointcommission.org/standards_information/npsgs.aspx.

Thomas G, et al: Blood pressure measurement in the diagnosis and management of hypertension in adults, UpToDate, 2017. https://www-uptodate-com./contents/blood-pressure-measurement-in-the-diagnosis-and-management-of-hypertension-in-adults?source=search_result&search=korotokoff%20sounds&selectedTitle=1~150.

Whelton P, et al: ACC/AHA/AAPA/ABC/ACPM/AGS/APhA/ASH/ASPC/NMA/PCNA guideline for the prevention, detection, evaluation, and management of high blood pressure in adults: a report of the American College of Cardiology/American Heart Association Task Force on Clinical Practice Guidelines, *J Am Coll Cardiol* November 2017. doi:10.1016/j.jacc.2017.11.006.

8 Health Assessment

SKILLS AND PROCEDURES

EVOLVE WEBSITE/RESOURCES LIST

http://evolve.elsevier.com/Perry/nursinginterventions
Audio Glossary • Checklists • Clinical Review Questions • Answers and Rationales for Clinical Review Questions • Case Studies • Animations • Video Clips

INTRODUCTION

Nurses perform systematic physical assessments on a regular basis in nearly every health care setting. In acute care settings, you perform a brief physical assessment at the beginning of each shift to identify changes in the patient's status for comparison with the previous assessment. Ongoing, objective, and comprehensive assessments promote continuity in health care. The information that is gathered adds to the patient's database.

PRACTICE STANDARDS

- American Cancer Society (ACS), 2017–2018: Cancer prevention and early detection facts and figures
- The Joint Commission (TJC), 2019: National Patient Safety Goals—Patient identification

EVIDENCE-BASED PRACTICE

Skin Cancer Prevention

The American Cancer Society (ACS) conducts ongoing research and develops practice guidelines regarding prevention and management of certain diseases, such as breast and skin cancer. According to the ACS (2017c), the three main types of skin cancer are melanoma, basal cell carcinoma, and squamous cell carcinoma, which are the most frequently diagnosed and highly curable forms, and melanoma, which is the deadliest form.

Risk factors for skin cancer include the following:

- Fair skin, freckling, light hair
- Presence of more than 50 moles
- Long-term skin conditions from certain treatments and weakened immune system from certain diseases, medical treatments, or medical conditions
- Exposure to high amounts of certain chemicals, including arsenic
- Exposure to ultraviolet (UV) rays, including the use of indoor tanning devices
- Smoking (squamous cell carcinoma only)
- Older age
- Personal or family history of skin cancer, especially melanoma
- History of excessive sun exposure, including sunburns
- Rare inherited conditions

Screening for early detection of skin cancer is very important for all individuals; however, according to the American Academy of Dermatology (AAD, 2018), individuals with red or blond hair, blue or green eyes, or fair skin (with freckles or burn easily) are at higher risk for skin cancer and should have periodic screening by a trained health care provider.

Self-skin examination using the ABCDE rule (see Box 8.4 on p. 142) is also supported by the AAD (2018) to be beneficial for early detection and more treatable stages of melanoma.

Patient education should include the following:

- Informing their health care provider about any new suspicious growths or anything changing, itching, or bleeding on the skin
- Staying in the shade and wearing wraparound sunglasses
- Applying sunscreen
- Wearing a hat with a 2- to 3-inch brim
- Avoiding the use of tanning beds and sunlamps

ASSESSMENT TECHNIQUES

Use assessment techniques during each patient contact, including activities such as bathing, administering medications, administering other therapies, or while talking with a patient. This practice will help you learn to become more observant and better able to identify changes quickly.

Inspection, palpation, percussion, auscultation, and olfaction are the five basic assessment techniques. Each skill allows you to collect a broad range of physical data about patients. Nurses need experience to recognize normal variations among patients and ranges of normal for an individual. Cultural diversity is one factor that influences both normal variations and potential alterations that you may find during an assessment. It is very important to take the time needed to assess each body part carefully. Hurrying can cause you to overlook significant signs and form incorrect conclusions about a patient's condition.

Inspection

Inspection is the visual examination of body parts or areas. An experienced nurse learns to make multiple observations almost simultaneously while becoming very perceptive of any abnormalities. It is important to recognize normal physical characteristics of patients of all ages before trying to distinguish abnormal findings.

Inspection requires adequate lighting and full exposure of body parts. Inspect each area for size, shape, color, symmetry, position, and the presence of abnormalities. If possible, inspect each area compared with the same area on the opposite side of the body. When necessary, use additional light, such as a penlight, to inspect body cavities such as the mouth and throat. *Do not hurry. Pay attention to detail*. Verify and clarify all abnormalities with subjective patient data. In other words, ask the patient for further information about each abnormality or change, such as whether the change is recent.

Palpation

Palpation uses the sense of touch. Through palpation, the hands make delicate and sensitive measurements of specific physical signs. Palpation detects resistance, resilience, roughness, texture, temperature, and mobility. You will often use palpation with or after visual inspection. You will also use different parts of the hand to detect specific characteristics. For example, the dorsum (back) of the hand is sensitive to temperature variations. The pads of the fingertips detect subtle changes in texture, shape, size, consistency, and pulsation of body parts. The palm of the hand is especially sensitive to vibration. You measure position, consistency, and turgor by lightly grasping the body part with the fingertips.

Assist the patient to relax and assume a comfortable position because muscle tension during palpation impairs the ability to palpate correctly. Asking a patient to take slow, deep breaths enhances muscle relaxation. Palpate tender areas last because they could cause a patient to become tense and hinder the assessment. Ask the patient to point out areas that are more sensitive, and note any nonverbal signs of discomfort. Patients appreciate clean, warm hands; short fingernails; and a gentle approach. Palpation is either light or deep and is controlled by the amount of pressure applied with the fingers or hand. Light palpation precedes deep palpation. Consider the patient's condition, the area being palpated, and the reason for using palpation. For example, when a patient is admitted to the emergency department after an automobile accident, consider the factors surrounding the injury, and inspect the chest wall carefully before performing any palpation around the area of the ribs.

For light palpation, apply pressure slowly, gently, and deliberately, depressing about 1 cm (½ inch) (Fig. 8.1A). Check tender areas further, using light, intermittent pressure. After light palpation, you may use deeper palpation to examine the condition of organs. Depress the area being examined approximately 2 cm (0.8 inch) (see Fig. 8.1B). Caution is the rule. Bimanual palpation involves one hand placed over the other while applying pressure. The upper hand exerts downward pressure as the other hand feels the subtle characteristics of underlying organs and masses. Seek the assistance of a qualified instructor before attempting deep palpation.

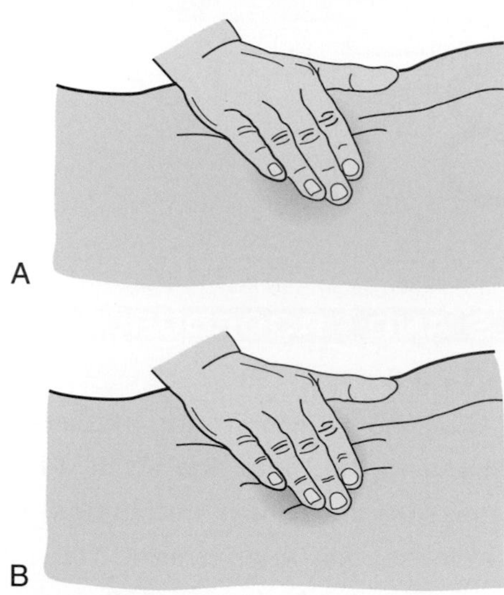

FIG 8.1 (A) During light palpation, gentle pressure against underlying skin and tissues can be used to detect areas of irregularity and tenderness. (B) During deep palpation, depress tissue to assess the condition of underlying organs.

Percussion

Percussion involves tapping the body with the fingertips to vibrate underlying tissues and organs. The vibration travels through body tissues, and the character of the resulting sound reflects the density of underlying tissue. The denser the tissue, the quieter the sound. By knowing various densities of organs and body parts, you learn how to locate organs or masses, map their edges, and determine their size. An abnormal sound suggests a mass or substance, such as air or fluid, in a body cavity. The skill of percussion is used more often by advanced practice nurses (APNs) than by nurses in daily practice at the bedside.

Auscultation

Auscultation is listening with a stethoscope to sounds produced by the body. To auscultate correctly, listen in a quiet environment for both the presence of sound and its characteristics. To be successful in auscultation, you must first recognize normal sounds from each body structure, including the passage of blood through an artery, heart sounds, and movement of air through the lungs. These sounds vary according to the location in which they can most easily be heard. You will also become familiar with areas that do not normally emit sounds. Practice listening to many normal sounds so that you can recognize abnormal sounds when they arise.

To auscultate, you need good hearing acuity, a good stethoscope, and knowledge of how to use the stethoscope properly (see Chapter 7). It is essential to place the stethoscope directly on a patient's skin because clothing obscures and changes sound. There are four characteristics of sound heard through auscultation:

- *Frequency:* Number of sound wave cycles generated per second by a vibrating object. The higher the frequency, the higher the pitch of a sound, and vice versa.
- *Loudness:* Amplitude of a sound wave. Auscultated sounds are either loud or soft.

TABLE 8.1

Assessment of Characteristic Odors

Odor	Site or Source	Potential Causes
Alcohol	Oral cavity	Ingestion of alcohol
Ammonia	Urine	Urinary tract infection, renal failure
Body odor	Skin, particularly in areas where body parts rub together (e.g., underarms, beneath breasts)	Poor hygiene, excess perspiration (hyperhidrosis), foul-smelling perspiration (bromhidrosis)
	Wound site	Wound abscess; infection
	Vomitus	Abdominal irritation, contaminated food
Feces	Rectal area	Fecal incontinence; fistula
	Vomitus/oral cavity (fecal odor)	Bowel obstruction
Fetid, sweet odor	Tracheostomy or mucus secretions	Infection of bronchial tree (*Pseudomonas* bacteria)
Foul-smelling stools in infant	Stool	Malabsorption syndrome
Halitosis	Oral cavity	Poor dental and oral hygiene; gum disease; sinus infection
Musty odor	Casted body part	Infection inside cast
Stale urine	Skin	Uremic acidosis
Sweet, fruity ketones	Oral cavity	Diabetic acidosis
Sweet, heavy, thick odor	Draining wound	*Pseudomonas* (bacterial) infection

- *Quality:* Sounds of similar frequency and loudness from different sources. Terms such as *blowing* or *gurgling* describe quality of sound.
- *Duration:* Length of time that sound vibrations last. Duration of sound is short, medium, or long. Layers of soft tissue dampen the duration of sounds from deep internal organs.

Olfaction

Olfaction uses the sense of smell to detect abnormalities that go unrecognized. Some alterations in body function and certain bacteria create characteristic odors (Table 8.1).

PREPARATION FOR ASSESSMENT

Preparation of the environment, equipment, and patient facilitates a smooth assessment. Provide patients privacy to promote their comfort and the efficiency of the examination. In a health care agency, close the door and pull privacy curtains. In the home, examine the patient in the bedroom. A comfortable environment includes a warm, comfortable temperature; a loose-fitting gown or pajamas for the patient; adequate direct lighting; control of outside noises; and precautions to prevent interruptions by visitors or health care personnel. If possible, place the bed or examination table at waist level so that you can access the patient easily. During an assessment, you must protect patients from falls and injury and return the bed to a safe height after an assessment (TJC, 2019).

BOX 8.1

Patient-Centered Approach to Assessment

- Consider a patient-centered interview to learn about problems from the patient's perspective.
- Show respect to patients and their families in seeking their involvement in the patient's plan of care.
- Have patients explain their symptoms by allowing them to offer details.
- After gathering data, group significant findings into patterns of data (clusters) that reveal actual or potential nursing diagnoses (Table 8.2).
- Be open to constant informing, communicating, and educating patients and family caregivers regarding patient care.
- Integrate health promotion and education into physical assessment activities. It is an ideal time to offer individual patient teaching and to encourage the promotion of health practices such as breast self-examination (Box 8.2).
- A patient should understand any symptoms with which he or she presents and symptoms for which to look in detecting problems. For example, educate patients about the American Cancer Society (ACS, 2017a) recommendations for early detection of breast and genital cancers.
- Ensure the patient is comfortable and free from pain.
- Provide emotional support.
- Provide care that is culturally congruent with patients' values and beliefs when completing a physical assessment (Marion et al., 2016).
- Communicate respect through proper use of distance, attention, eye contact, tone, and loudness of voice.
- Use a professional interpreter familiar with a patient's culture and language.
- Obtain information about health risks common to a cultural group. Certain diseases are prevalent in some groups.
- Use gender-congruent health care providers to perform a physical assessment.
- Ask permission before you touch a patient.
- Drape a patient thoroughly and use the bedside screen or curtains.

Preparing a Patient

Prepare a patient both physically and psychologically for an accurate assessment. A tense, anxious patient may have difficulty understanding, following directions, or cooperating with your instructions. To prepare a patient, take the following steps:

- Provide privacy and use a patient-centered approach (Box 8.1).
- Implement comfort measures (e.g., positioning, hygiene), and provide the opportunity to empty the bowel or bladder (a good time to collect needed specimens).
- Minimize the patient's anxiety and fear by conveying an open, receptive, and professional approach. Using simple terms, thoroughly explain what will be done, what the patient should expect to feel, and how the patient can cooperate. Even if the patient appears unresponsive, it is still important to explain your actions.
- Provide access to body parts while draping areas that are not being examined.
- Reduce distractions. Turn down the volume of or turn off the television or radio.
- Eliminate drafts, control room temperature, and provide warm blankets.
- Help the patient assume positions during the assessment so that body parts are accessible while the patient stays

TABLE 8.2
Development of Individual Nursing Diagnosis

Assessment Method	Findings	Patterns	Nursing Diagnosis
Inspection of skin	Skin along sacral area is intact. There is a 3-cm area of redness around coccyx; skin blanches on palpation. No skin lesions are observed.	There is tissue injury area around coccyx.	Risk for impaired skin integrity
Palpation of skin	Skin is moist from diaphoresis. There is tenderness to palpation at sacral area. Skin turgor is elastic.	Skin moisture promotes maceration.	
Historical data	Patient suffered fractured left leg. Patient is immobilized because of left leg traction.	Continued pressure is exerted over sacrum.	

comfortable. A patient's ability to assume positions depends on physical strength and limitations. Some positions are uncomfortable or embarrassing; keep a patient in such a position no longer than is necessary.
- Pace the assessment according to the patient's physical and emotional tolerance.
- Use a relaxed tone of voice and facial expressions to put the patient at ease.
- Encourage the patient to ask questions and report discomfort felt during the examination.
- Have a third person of the patient's gender in the room during the assessment of genitalia. This prevents the patient from accusing you of behaving in an unethical manner.
- After the assessment, ask the patient if there are any concerns or questions.

PHYSICAL ASSESSMENT OF VARIOUS AGE-GROUPS

Children and Adolescents

- Routine assessment of children focuses on health promotion and illness prevention, particularly for care of well children with competent parenting and no serious health problems (Hockenberry and Wilson, 2017). Focus on growth and development, sensory screening, dental examination, and behavioral assessment.
- Children who are chronically ill, disabled, in foster care, or adopted after birth in a foreign country may require additional assessments because of their unique health risks.
- When obtaining histories of infants and children, gather all or part of the information from parents or guardians.
- Parents may think the examiner is testing or judging them. Offer support during the examination, and do not pass judgment.
- Call children by their preferred name, and address parents as "Mr. and Mrs. Brown" rather than by first names.
- Open-ended questions often allow parents to share more information and describe more of the child's problems.
- Older children and adolescents respond best when treated as adults and individuals and often can provide details about their health history and severity of symptoms.
- The adolescent has a right to confidentiality. After talking with parents about historical information, arrange to be alone with the adolescent to speak privately and perform the examination.

Older Adults

- Do not assume that aging is always accompanied by illness or disability. Most older adults can adapt to change and maintain functional independence (Touhy and Jett, 2018).
- A thorough assessment of an older adult provides critical information that can be used to maximize independence.
- Provide adequate space for an examination, particularly if the patient uses a mobility aid.
- Plan the history and examination, considering the older adult's energy level, physical limitations, pace, and adaptability. You may need more than one session to complete the assessment (Touhy and Jett, 2018).
- Measure performance under the most favorable of conditions. Take advantage of natural opportunities for assessment (e.g., during bathing, grooming, and mealtime) (Touhy and Jett, 2018).
- Be sure that an examination of an older adult includes a review of mental status.

SAFETY GUIDELINES

Nurses must comply with the National Patient Safety Guidelines provided by The Joint Commission (TJC, 2019). These are specific goals regarding patient safety that nurses should follow to improve patient safety, such as the following:

- Prevent skin breakdown by thoroughly assessing the skin, especially in patients who are on prolonged bed rest.
- Consider the possibility of latex allergy. The incidence of serious allergic reaction to latex has increased (Wilson and Giddens, 2017). Use nonlatex gloves if an allergy is present.
- Follow standard precautions for infection control. During an assessment, you may have contact with bodily fluids and discharge. Always wear clean gloves when there are breaks in the skin, lesions, or wounds or having contact with mucous membranes. In some circumstances, you will need to wear a gown and face/eye protection.
- Prioritize the assessment based on a patient's presenting signs and symptoms or health care needs. For example, when a patient develops sudden shortness of breath, first assess the lungs and thorax. If a patient is acutely ill, you may choose to assess only the involved body systems. Use judgment to ensure that an examination is relevant and inclusive.
- Organize the examination. Compare both sides of the body for symmetry. If the patient becomes fatigued, offer rest periods. Perform painful or intrusive procedures near the end of the examination.
- Use a head-to-toe approach following the sequence of inspection, palpation, and auscultation (except for abdominal assessment). This sequence facilitates an effective assessment.

BOX 8.2

Breast Self-Examination

According to the American Cancer Society (ACS, 2017a), screening refers to tests and examinations used to find a disease such as cancer in people who do not have any symptoms. Although research does not support a clear benefit of regular breast self-examination (BSE), it is important for all women to be familiar with their breasts' normal appearance and feel. A BSE is optional for women starting in their 20s (ACS, 2017a). Women should be told about the benefits and limitations of BSE and report any breast changes to their health professional right away.

Breast self-examination plays a small role in finding breast cancer compared with finding a breast lump by chance or simply being aware of what is normal for each woman. Some women feel very comfortable doing BSE regularly (usually monthly after their period), which involves a systematic, step-by-step approach to examining the look and feel of their breasts. Other women are more comfortable simply looking at and feeling their breasts in a less systematic approach (e.g., while showering or getting dressed or doing an occasional thorough examination) (ACS, 2017a). Familiarity makes it easier to notice any changes in the breast from one month to another. Early discovery of a change from what is "normal" is the main idea behind BSE.

For women who menstruate, the best time to do BSE is 2 or 3 days after a period ends, when the breasts are least likely to be tender or swollen. For women who no longer menstruate, pick a day such as the first day of the month to remind yourself to do BSE.

Procedure

1. Stand before a mirror. Inspect both breasts for anything unusual, such as skin redness; any discharge from the nipples; or puckering, dimpling, or scaling of the skin.
2. While in front of the mirror, press hands firmly on hips and look at your breasts, observing for any changes in size, shape, contour, dimpling, or redness or scaliness of the nipple or breast tissue. Pressing down on your hips contracts the chest wall muscles and enhances breast changes.
3. Examine your right breast. Lie down on your back and place your right arm behind your head. When you lie down versus standing, the breast tissue spreads evenly over the chest wall and is as thin as possible, making it much easier to feel all the breast tissue.
4. Use finger pads of the three middle fingers on your left hand to feel for lumps in the right breast. Use overlapping dime-sized circular motions of the finger pads to feel the breast tissue. Use three different types of pressure: light pressure to feel tissue closest to the skin, medium pressure to feel a little deeper, and firm pressure to feel tissue close to the chest and ribs. It is normal to feel a firm ridge in the lower curve of each breast. If you feel anything out of the ordinary, tell your health care provider.
5. Using your finger pads, move around the breast in an up-and-down pattern starting at an imaginary line drawn straight down your side from your underarm and moving across the breast to the middle of the chest bone (sternum or breastbone). Be sure to check the entire breast area, going down until you feel only ribs and up to the neck or collarbone (clavicle).
6. Repeat examination in the left breast, putting your left arm behind your head, and examine the left breast (see Steps 3–5).
7. Instruct patient to call the health care provider if she finds a lump or other abnormality.
8. **Use Teach-Back:** "I want to be sure I explained to you how to do a breast self-examination. Show me how to examine both of your breasts." Document your evaluation of patient learning. Revise your instruction now or develop a plan for revised patient teaching if patient is not able to teach back correctly.

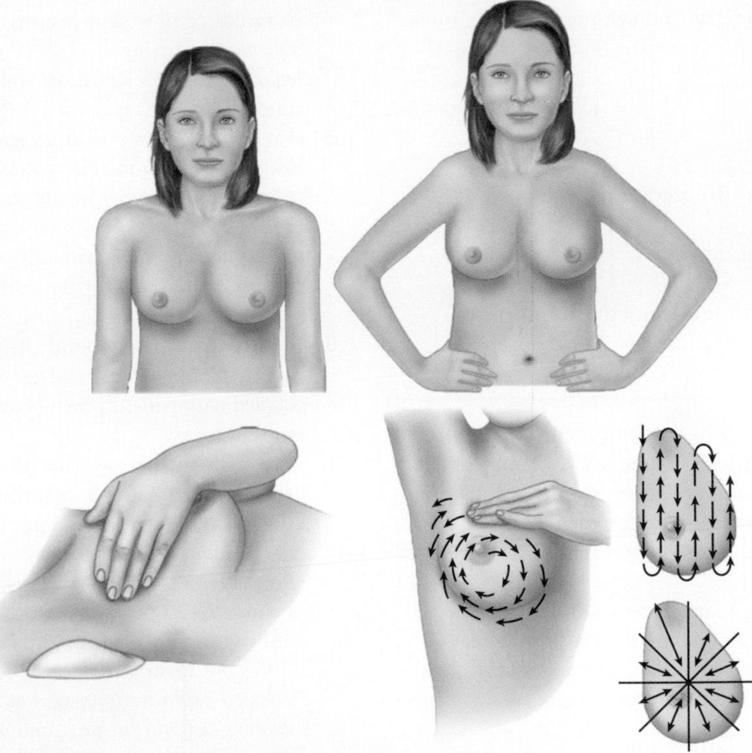

From American Cancer Society (ACS): American Cancer Society recommendations for the early detection of breast cancer, 2017a, https://www.cancer.org/cancer/breast-cancer/screening-tests-and-early-detection/american-cancer-society-recommendations-for-the-early-detection-of-breast-cancer.html. Images from Silvestri LA, Silvestri AE: *Saunders Comprehensive Review for the NCLEX-PN(R) Examination,* ed 7, St Louis, 2019, Elsevier.

- Encourage the patient's active participation. Patients usually know about their physical condition. Often a patient can let you know when certain findings are normal or when there have been changes.
- Always identify a patient using at least two patient identifiers other than the room number. For example, use the patient's name and date of birth, comparing with either the armband or the medical record (TJC, 2019).
- Record quick notes to facilitate accurate documentation. Inform the patient that you will be recording the data.

✦ SKILL 8.1 General Survey

Purpose

The general survey begins with a review of the patient's primary health problems, and it includes assessment of a patient's vital signs, height and weight, general behavior, and appearance. It provides information about the characteristics of an illness and the patient's hygiene, skin condition, body image, emotional state, recent weight changes, and developmental status. The survey reveals important information about a patient's behavior that can influence how you communicate instructions to the patient and continue the assessment.

Delegation and Collaboration

The skill of completing the general survey cannot be delegated to nursing assistive personnel (NAP). The nurse directs the NAP to:

- Measure the patient's height and weight.
- Obtain vital signs (not the initial set, but subsequent measurements if patient is stable).
- Monitor oral intake and urinary output.
- Report a patient's subjective signs and symptoms to the nurse.

Equipment

- Stethoscope
- Sphygmomanometer and cuff
- Thermometer
- Digital watch or wristwatch with second hand
- Tape measure
- Clean gloves (use nonlatex if necessary)
- Tongue blade
- Appropriate electronic record or documentation form

ASSESSMENT

1. When beginning a physical examination, identify patient using at least two identifiers (e.g., name and birthday or name and medical record number) according to agency policy. *Rationale: Ensures correct patient. Complies with The Joint Commission standards and improves patient safety (TJC, 2019).*
2. Note if patient has had any acute distress: difficulty breathing, pain, anxiety. If such signs are present, defer general survey until later and focus immediately on affected body system. *Rationale: Signs establish priorities regarding which part of examination to conduct first.*
3. Review graphic sheet for previous vital signs and consider factors or conditions that may alter values. *Rationale: Provides baseline and historical data about patient's vital signs.*
4. Determine patient's primary language. If you identify need for an interpreter, determine availability of a professional interpreter. It is best to have an interpreter of the same gender who is older and mature. Have interpreter translate verbatim if possible. *Rationale: Facilitates patient understanding and promotes accuracy of information provided by patient.*
5. After reviewing history, confirm primary reason patient has sought health care. *Rationale: Keeps assessment focused on patient to ensure that his or her expectations are addressed.*
6. Identify patient's normal height, weight, and body mass index (BMI). If sudden gain or loss in weight has occurred, determine amount of weight change and period of time in which it occurred. Assess if patient has recently been dieting or following an exercise program. Use growth chart for children under 18 years of age. *Rationale: A BMI of 25 to 29.9 for men and women is overweight, whereas 30 and over is obese (Wilson and Giddens, 2017). Fluid retention is one factor that must be ruled out. A person's weight can fluctuate daily because of fluid loss or retention (1 L of water weighs 1 kg [2.2 lb]).*
7. Ask if patient has noticed any changes in condition of skin (e.g., dryness, changes in color or lack of pigment, changes in moles or new skin lesions). *Rationale: Skin changes can indicate underlying illnesses (e.g., dry skin may be associated with hypothyroidism, changes in moles may indicate early signs of skin cancers; Table 8.3).*
8. Review patient's past fluid intake and output (I&O) records. *Rationale: Fluid and electrolyte balance affects health and function in all body systems. Intake includes all liquids taken orally, by feeding tube, and parenterally. Liquid output includes urine, diarrhea stool, vomitus, drainage from fistulas and gastric suction, and drainage from postsurgical tubes such as chest tubes or Jackson-Pratt drains.*
9. Identify patient's general perceptions about personal health. *Rationale: Assessment of patient's general appearance coupled with patient's own perceptions may reveal specific problem areas.*
10. Assess for history of latex allergy, which may include contact dermatitis or systemic reactions. Ask if patient has risk factors such as food allergies (papaya, avocado, banana, peach, kiwi, or tomato); has high latex exposure (housekeepers, food handlers, health care worker); or must avoid products containing latex (rubber bands, adhesive tape, certain paints or carpets). *Rationale: Gloves are worn during certain aspects of the assessment. Repeated exposure to latex may result in more serious reactions, including asthma, itching, and anaphylaxis (Hockenberry and Wilson, 2017).*
11. Assess patient's/family caregiver's knowledge, experience, and health literacy. *Rationale: Ensures patient/family caregiver has the capacity to obtain, communicate, process, and understand basic health information (Centers for Disease Control and Prevention [CDC], 2016a).*

TABLE 8.3

Skin Color Variations

Color	Condition	Cause	Assessment Location
Bluish (cyanosis)	Related to hypoxia (late sign of decreased oxygen)	Heart or lung disease, cold environment	Nail beds, lips, base of tongue, skin (severe cases)
Pallor (decrease in color)	Reduced amount of oxyhemoglobin Reduced visibility of oxyhemoglobin resulting from decreased blood flow	Anemia Shock	Face, conjunctivae, nail beds, palms of hands Skin, nail beds, conjunctivae, lips
Red (erythema)	Increased visibility of oxyhemoglobin caused by dilation or increased blood flow	Fever, direct trauma, blushing, alcohol intake	Face, area of trauma, and areas at risk of pressure such as sacrum, shoulders, elbows, heels
Yellow-orange (jaundice)	Increased deposit of bilirubin in tissues	Liver disease, destruction of red blood cells	Sclerae, mucous membranes, skin
Loss of pigmentation	Vitiligo	Congenital autoimmune condition causing lack of pigment	Patchy areas on skin over face, hands, arms
Tan-brown	Increased amount of melanin	Suntan, pregnancy	Areas exposed to sun—face, arms; areolas, nipples

BOX 8.3

Characteristics of Dementia

Cognition
- Memory impaired: trouble recalling recent conversations, events, and appointments
- Frequently misplaces objects

Speech/Language
- Struggles to find words
- Conversation possibly incoherent

Activity
- Unchanged from usual behavior
- Difficulty performing tasks that require many steps

Mood and Affect
- Depressed
- Apathetic
- Uninterested

Delusions/Hallucinations
- Can be some delusions
- No hallucinations

Modified from Ball JW, et al.: *Seidel's guide to physical examination*, ed 9, St. Louis, 2019, Elsevier.

STEP	RATIONALE
PLANNING	
1. Expected outcomes following completion of procedure:	
• Patient demonstrates alert, cooperative behavior without evidence of physical or emotional distress during assessment.	You use calm and confident approach during assessment. Patient has no abnormal findings.
• Patient provides appropriate subjective data related to physical condition.	Patient can cooperate with assessment.
2. *Prepare patient:* Tell patient that you will be doing routine process to check for areas of concern. Ask patient to tell you if any area that you examine hurts when touched.	Understanding promotes patient's cooperation. Pain is an important finding during assessment.
3. Perform hand hygiene. Assemble necessary equipment.	Reduces transmission of infection.
4. Provide privacy and prepare environment	Providing privacy and preparing the environment early help the student/nurse think about the need to remove clutter from the over-bed or bedside table.
5. Initially position patient either sitting or lying supine with head of bed elevated.	Promotes efficiency of examination.
IMPLEMENTATION	
1. Throughout assessment, note patient's verbal and nonverbal behaviors. Determine patient's level of consciousness (LOC) and orientation by observing and talking to him or her (Box 8.3).	Behaviors may reflect specific physical abnormalities. Dementia and LOC influence ability to cooperate.

STEP	RATIONALE
2. Obtain temperature, pulse, respirations, and blood pressure unless taken within past 3 hours or if serious potential change is noted (e.g., change in LOC or difficulty breathing). Inform patient of vital signs.	Vital signs provide important information regarding physiological changes related to oxygenation and circulation.
3. Note patient's gender and race and ask his or her age. Note patient's external physical features.	Gender influences type of examination performed and way you make assessments. Different physical characteristics and predisposition to illnesses are related to gender and race.
4. If uncertain whether patient understands a question, rephrase or ask a similar question.	Inappropriate response from a patient may be caused by language barriers or deterioration of mental status, preoccupation with illness, or decreased hearing acuity.
5. If patient's responses are inappropriate, ask short, to-the-point questions regarding information patient should know (e.g., "Tell me your name." "What is the name of this place?" "Tell me where you live." "What day is this?" "What month is this?" or "What season of the year is this?").	Measures patient's orientation to person, place, and time. You may note this in documentation as "Oriented × 3." If disoriented in any way, include subjective and/or objective data rather than just documenting "disoriented."
6. If patient is unable to respond to questions of orientation, offer simple commands (e.g., "Squeeze my fingers." or "Move your toes.").	LOC exists along a continuum ranging from full responsiveness, to inability to consciously initiate meaningful behaviors, to unresponsiveness to stimuli.
7. Assess affect and mood. Note if verbal expressions match nonverbal behavior and if appropriate to situation.	Reflects patient's mental and emotional status, consciousness, and feelings.
8. Watch patient interact with spouse or partner, older-adult child, or caregiver. Be alert for indications of fear, hesitancy to report health status, or willingness to let caregiver control assessment interview. Does partner or caregiver have a history of violence, alcoholism, or drug abuse? Is person unemployed, ill, or frustrated with caring for a patient? Note if patient has any obvious physical injuries.	Suspect abuse in patients who have suffered obvious physical injury or neglect, show signs of malnutrition, or have ecchymosis (bruises) on extremities or trunk. Health care providers are often the first to identify evidence of abuse because patients may not be able to tell family or friends. Partners or caregivers may have history of abusive or addictive behaviors.

Safe Patient Care *Be discreet in how you conduct the interview. Ask direct questions about abuse in private. It is often necessary to delay assessment to a later time when the partner or caregiver is not present. Asking a partner or caregiver to leave during an assessment creates an awkward situation, but inquiring about possible abuse in front of an abuser puts a patient at risk for further abuse. Patients are more likely to reveal any problems when the suspected abuser is absent from the room.*

STEP	RATIONALE
9. Observe for signs of abuse:	
a. *Child:* Blood on underclothing, pain in genital area, difficulty sitting or walking, pain on urination, vaginal or penile discharge, itching or unusual odor in genital area, physical injury inconsistent with parent's or caregiver's account of how injury occurred.	Indicates child sexual abuse (Hockenberry and Wilson, 2017). Suggests child physical abuse.
b. *Female patient:* Fractures, concussions, intraabdominal injuries, bruising or laceration of the perineum, or woman may seem unnaturally calm or withdrawn.	Suggests intimate partner violence (Lewis et al., 2017).
c. *Older adult:* Unexplained bruising or lacerations in unusual places, fractures not consistent with the individual's functional ability, bruises in the breast or genital area, or presence of blood in the undergarments.	Indicates elder abuse/neglect (Touhy and Jett, 2018). Prolonged interval between injury and time patient sought medical care also indicates older adult abuse or neglect.

Safe Patient Care *A pattern of findings indicating abuse usually mandates a report to a social service center (refer to state guidelines). Obtain immediate consultation with health care provider, social worker, and other support staff to facilitate placement in a safer environment.*

STEP	RATIONALE
10. Assess posture and position, noting alignment of shoulders and hips while patient stands and/or sits. Observe whether patient is slumped, erect, or has bent posture (see illustration).	Reveals musculoskeletal problem, mood, or presence of pain.

STEP	RATIONALE

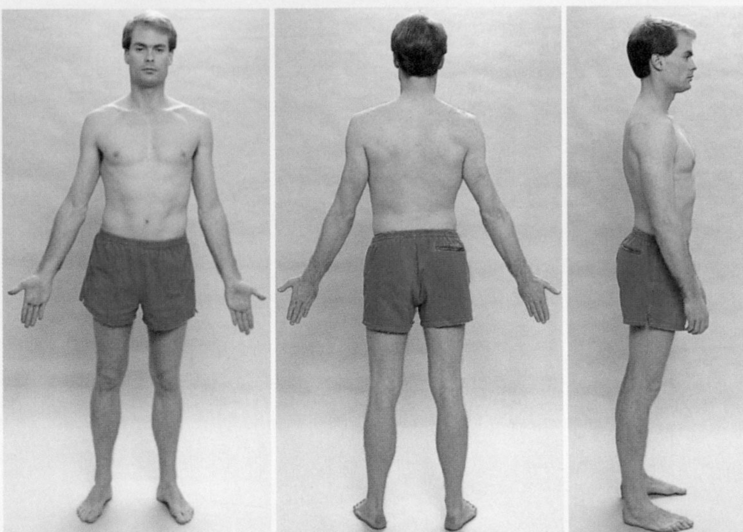

STEP 10 Inspection of overall body posture: anterior view (left); posterior view (middle); right lateral view (right).

STEP	RATIONALE
11. Assess body movements. Are they purposeful? Are there tremors of extremities? Are any body parts immobile? Are movements coordinated or uncoordinated?	May indicate neurological or muscular problem or emotional stress.
12. Assess speech. Is it understandable and moderately paced? Is there association with patient's thoughts?	Alterations reflect neurological impairment, injury or impairment of mouth, improperly fitting dentures, differences in dialect or language, and some mental illnesses.
13. Observe hygiene and grooming for presence or absence of makeup, type of clothes (hospital or personal), and cleanliness. Hair, teeth, and nails are good places to assess hygiene status.	Grooming may reflect activity level before examination, resources available to purchase grooming supplies, patient's mood, and self-care practices. It may also reflect culture, lifestyle, economic status, and personal preferences.
a. Observe color, distribution, quantity, thickness, texture, and lubrication of hair.	Changes in hair may reflect hormonal changes, changes from aging, poor nutrition, or use of certain hair-care products.
b. Inspect condition of nails (hands and feet). Note color, length, symmetry, cleanliness, and shape. Nails are normally transparent, smooth, and well rounded, with smooth, intact cuticle.	Changes indicate inadequate nutrition or grooming practices, nervous habits, or systemic diseases.
c. Assess presence or absence of body odor.	Body odor may result from physical exercise, deficient hygiene, or physical or mental abnormalities. Inadequate oral hygiene or unhealthy teeth cause bad breath.
14. Inspect exposed areas of skin and ask if patient has noted any changes, including the following:	Determines presence of abnormalities and cancerous lesions. Melanoma is an aggressive form of skin cancer; detection and prompt treatment are critical (Box 8.4).
a. Pruritus, oozing, bleeding	Itching could result from dry skin. Oozing could indicate infection, and bleeding may indicate a blood disorder.
b. Appearance of mole (nevus), bump, or nodule; change in sensation; itchiness, tenderness, or pain	These are key indicators that a lesion may be cancerous.
c. Petechiae (pinpoint-size red or purple spots on skin caused by small hemorrhages in skin layers)	Petechiae may indicate serious blood clotting disorder, drug reaction, or liver disease.
15. Inspect skin surfaces. Compare color of symmetrical body parts, including areas unexposed to sun. Look for any patches or areas of skin color variation.	Changes in color can indicate pathological alterations (see Table 8.3).

Safe Patient Care *Be alert for basal cell carcinomas, such as an open sore that does not heal, a shiny nodule, a pink or reddish growth, or scarlike area. These are often seen in sun-exposed areas and frequently occur in sun-damaged skin.*

STEP	RATIONALE
16. Carefully inspect color of face, oral mucosa, lips, conjunctiva, sclera, palms of hands, and nail beds.	Abnormalities are easier to identify in areas of body where melanin production is lowest.

BOX 8.4

Malignant Melanoma Mnemonics

The ABCDE Rule of Melanoma

Here is a simple way to remember the characteristics that should alert you to the possibility of malignant melanoma:

A. *Asymmetry* of lesion: One side different than the other
B. *Borders*: Irregular, ragged, or blurred
C. *Color*: Not the same all over; may have different shades of brown or black; patches of red, white, or blue may be present
D. *Diameter* greater than 6 mm
E. *Evolution*: Change seen in existing pigmented lesions, particularly in an asymmetric pattern

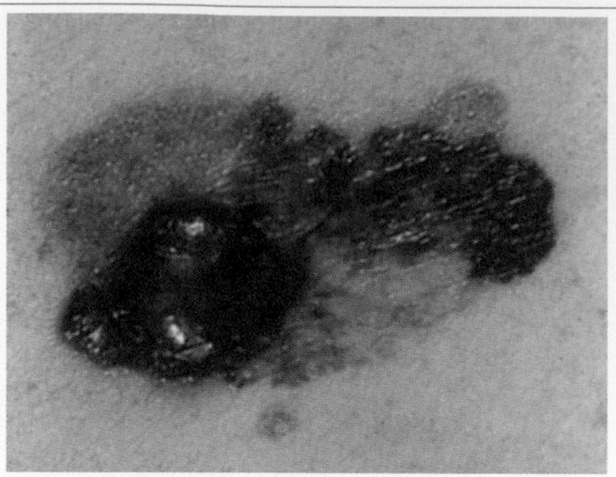

Figure from Ball JW, et al.: *Seidel's guide to physical examination*, ed 9, St. Louis, 2019, Elsevier.

STEP	RATIONALE
Safe Patient Care *When assessing the skin of a patient with bandages, cast, restraints, or other restrictive devices, note report of pain or tingling and areas of pallor, decreased temperature, decreased movement, and impaired sensation, which may indicate impaired circulation. Immediate release of pressure from the restrictive device may be necessary.*	
17. Use ungloved fingertips to palpate skin surfaces to feel texture and moisture of intact skin.	Changes in texture may be first indication of skin rashes in dark-skinned patients. Hydration, body temperature, and environment may affect skin. Older adults are prone to xerosis, presenting as dry, scaly skin (Touhy and Jett, 2018).
a. Stroke skin surfaces lightly with fingertips to detect texture of surface of skin. Note whether skin is smooth or rough, thick or thin, or tight or supple and if localized areas of hardness or lesions are present.	Localized texture changes result from trauma, surgical wounds, or lesions.
b. Palpate any areas that appear irregular in texture.	Allows detection of localized areas of hardness and/or tenderness within subcutaneous skin layers.
c. Using dorsum (back) of hand, palpate for temperature of skin surfaces. Compare symmetrical body parts. Compare upper and lower body parts. Note distinct temperature difference and localized areas of warmth.	Skin on dorsum of hand is thin, which allows detection of subtle temperature changes. Cool skin temperature often indicates decreased blood flow. A stage 1 pressure injury may cause warmth and erythema (redness) of an area. Environmental temperature and anxiety may also affect skin temperature.
Safe Patient Care *In patients who receive routine injections (e.g., insulin, heparin), localized areas of hardness may be palpated over injection sites. Develop a plan to rotate injection sites systematically. Site rotation prevents local skin changes from repeated injections (Lewis et al., 2017).*	
18. Apply clean gloves. Inspect character of any secretions; note color, odor, amount, and consistency (e.g., thin and watery, thick and oily). Remove gloves. Perform hand hygiene.	Description of secretions helps indicate type of lesion, presence of infection, or wound healing.
19. Assess skin turgor by grasping fold of skin on sternum, forearm, or abdomen with fingertips. Release skinfold and note ease and speed with which skin returns to place (see illustration).	With reduced turgor, skin remains suspended or "tented" for a few seconds before slowly returning to place, indicating decreased elasticity and possible dehydration. With altered turgor, provide measures for prevention of pressure injuries.
20. Assess condition of skin for pressure areas, paying attention to regions at risk for pressure (e.g., sacrum, greater trochanter, heels, occipital area, clavicles). If you see areas of redness, place fingertip over area, apply gentle pressure, and release. Look at skin color.	Normal reactive hyperemia (redness) is visible effect of localized vasodilation, the normal response of the body to lack of blood flow to underlying tissue. Affected area of skin normally blanches with fingertip pressure. If area does not blanch, suspect tissue injury.

STEP	RATIONALE

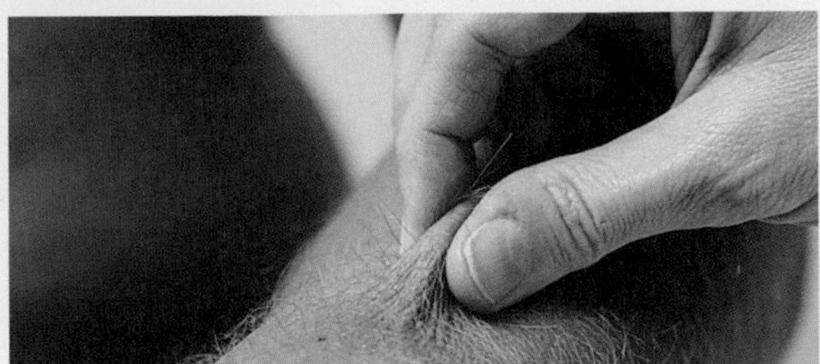

STEP 19 Assessment of skin turgor.

Safe Patient Care *When assessing darkly pigmented skin, visual inspection techniques to identify skin problems are ineffective. Skin inspection techniques for individuals with darkly pigmented skin must include assessment of temperature, edema, and changes in tissue consistency as compared with the surrounding skin (Wound Ostomy and Continence Nurses [WOCN], 2016).*

Safe Patient Care *With evidence of normal reactive hyperemia, reposition patient, and develop a turning schedule if the patient is dependent.*

STEP	RATIONALE
21. When you detect a lesion, use adequate lighting to inspect color, location, texture, size, shape, and type (Box 8.5). Also note grouping (e.g., clustered or linear) and distribution (e.g., localized or generalized).	Observation of skin lesions allows for accurate description and identification.
a. Apply gloves if lesion is moist or draining. Gently palpate any lesion to determine mobility, contour (e.g., flat, raised, or depressed), and consistency (e.g., soft or hard).	Gentle palpation prevents rupture of underlying cysts. Gloves reduce transmission of microorganisms.
b. Note if patient reports tenderness with or without palpation.	Tenderness may indicate inflammation or pressure on body part.
c. Measure size of lesion (height, width, depth) with centimeter ruler.	Provides for baseline to assess changes in lesion over time.
22. Help patient to comfortable position.	Gives patient sense of well-being.
23. Be sure nurse call system is in an accessible location within patient's reach.	Ensures patient can call for assistance if needed.
24. Raise side rails (as appropriate) and lower bed to lowest position.	Ensures patient safety.
25. Remove gloves. Discard used supplies and gloves in proper receptacle. Perform hand hygiene.	Prevents transmission of microorganisms.

EVALUATION

STEP	RATIONALE
1. Observe throughout assessment for evidence of physical or emotional distress, which may alter assessment data.	Interaction during assessment reveals emotional problems. Maneuvers used during physical examination reveal presence of physical problems.
2. Compare assessment findings with previous observations.	Determines if change has occurred.
3. Ask patient if there is information about physical condition that you have not discussed.	Some patients think that they are bothering you by asking questions unless opportunity for questions is provided.
4. **Use Teach-Back:** "I want to be sure I explained everything about the bleeding mole I found on your back during assessment. Tell me why it is important to see a dermatologist." Revise your instruction now or develop a plan for revised patient/family caregiver teaching if patient/family caregiver is not able to teach back correctly.	Determines patient's/family caregiver's level of understanding of instructional topic.

Unexpected Outcomes	Related Interventions
1. Patient demonstrates acute distress (e.g., shortness of breath, acute pain, severe anxiety).	• Respond immediately to identified need (e.g., repositioning, oxygen, or medication as appropriate). • Obtain vital signs. • Notify health care provider.
2. Patient has abnormal skin condition (e.g., change in color of a mole, dry texture, reduced turgor, lesions, or erythema).	• Identify contributing factors and prevent continued irritation or damage as appropriate.
3. Patient is unwilling or unable to provide adequate information relating to identified concerns.	• Seek information from family caregivers if present. • Review patient's record for baseline data.

BOX 8.5

Types of Skin Lesions

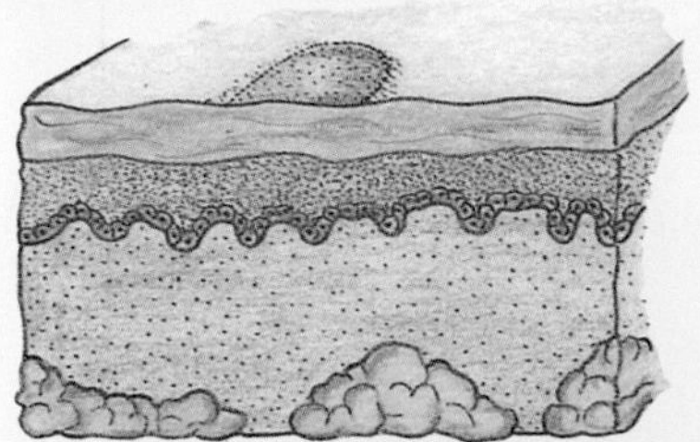

Macule: Flat, nonpalpable change in skin color; <1 cm (0.4 inch) (e.g., freckle, petechia)

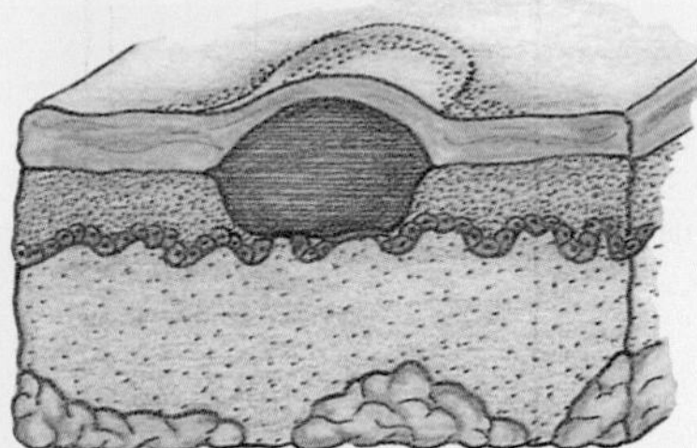

Papule: Palpable, circumscribed, solid elevation in skin; <0.5 cm (0.2 inch) (e.g., elevated nevus)

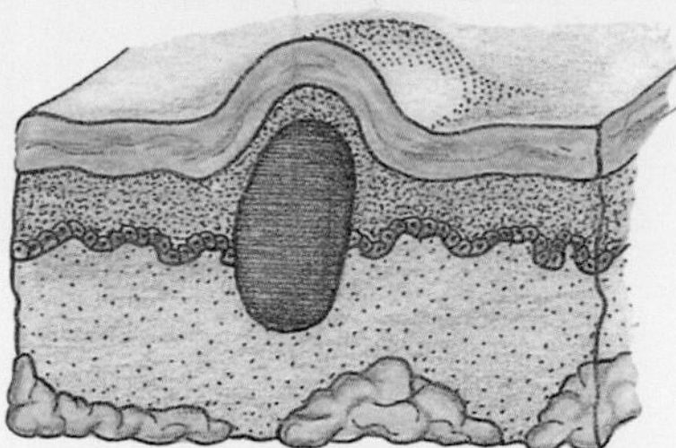

Nodule: Elevated solid mass; deeper and firmer than papule; 0.5 to 2 cm (0.2–0.8 inch) (e.g., wart)

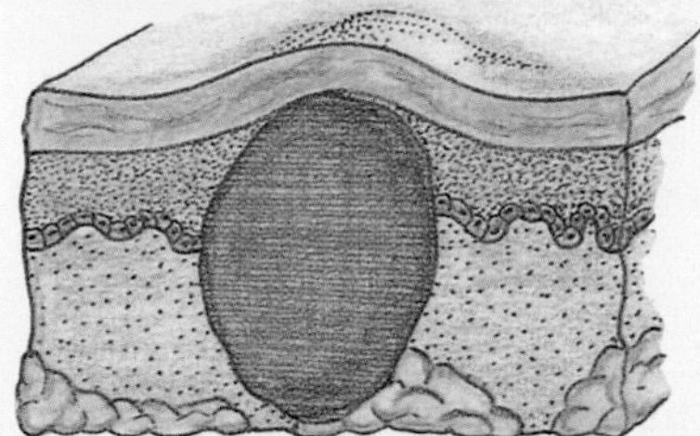

Tumor: Solid mass that may extend deep through subcutaneous tissue; >1 to 2 cm (0.4–0.8 inch) (e.g., epithelioma)

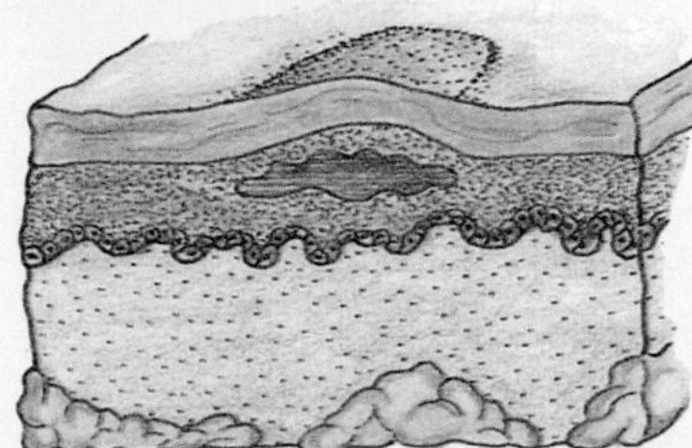

Wheal: Irregularly shaped, elevated area or superficial localized edema; varies in size (e.g., hive, mosquito bite)

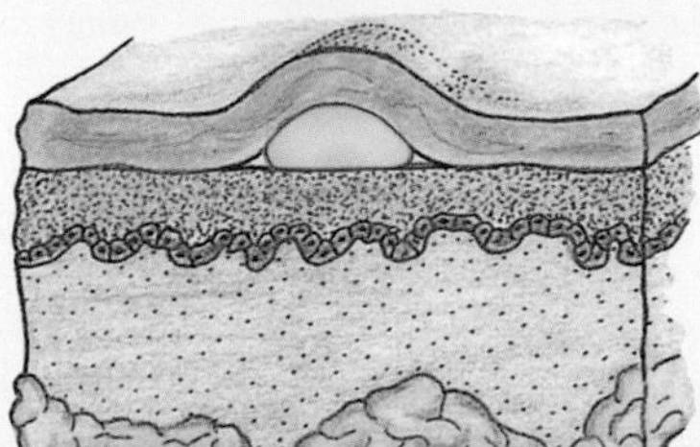

Vesicle: Circumscribed elevation of skin filled with serous fluid; <0.5 cm (0.2 inch) (e.g., herpes simplex, chickenpox)

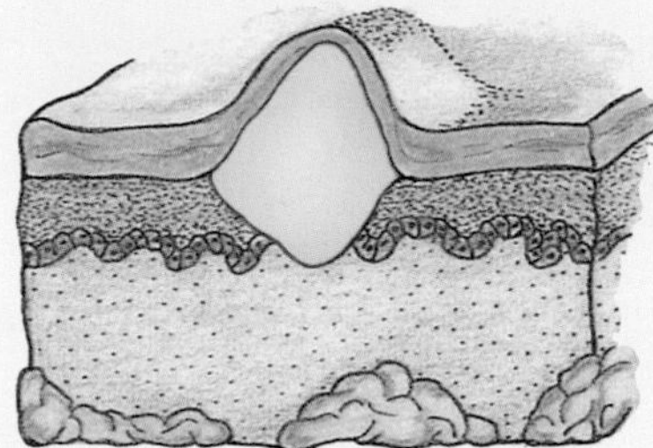

Pustule: Circumscribed elevation of skin similar to vesicle but filled with pus; varies in size (e.g., acne, staphylococcal infection)

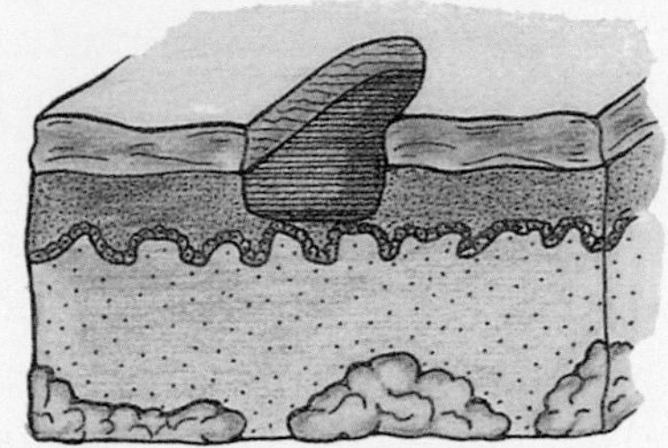

Ulcer: Deep loss of skin surface that may extend to dermis and frequently bleeds and scars; varies in size (e.g., venous stasis ulcer)

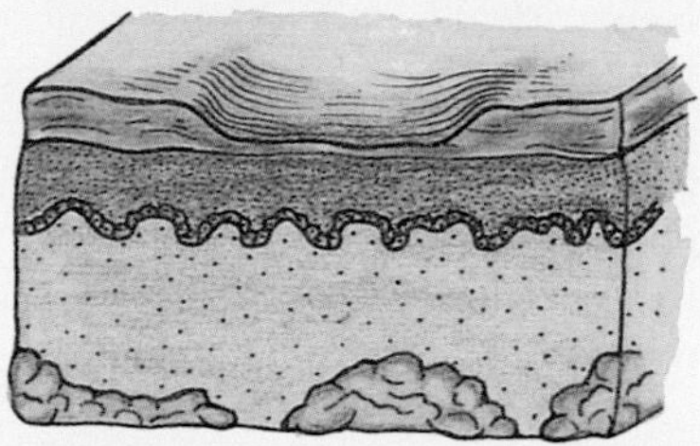

Atrophy: Thinning of skin with loss of normal skin furrow with skin appearing shiny and translucent; varies in size (e.g., arterial insufficiency)

Recording

- Record patient's vital signs. Record description of alterations in patient's general appearance.
- Describe patient's behavior using objective terminology. Include patients' self-report of any signs and symptoms.
- Document your evaluation of patient learning

Hand-Off Reporting

- Report abnormalities and acute symptoms to nurse in charge or health care provider.

PROCEDURAL GUIDELINE 8.1 *Monitoring Intake and Output*

Purpose

Measuring and recording I&O during a 24-hour period is part of the assessment database for fluid and electrolyte balance (Table 8.4). You are responsible for accurate recording of all intake (liquids taken orally, by enteral feedings, and parenterally) and output (urine, diarrhea, vomitus, gastric suction, and drainage from surgical tubes). Monitoring a patient on I&O requires cooperation and help from the patient and family caregivers. Accuracy is critical because health care providers will use findings in the prescription of medications and intravenous (IV) fluids.

PROCEDURAL GUIDELINE 8.1 *Monitoring Intake and Output—cont'd*

TABLE 8.4

Adult Average Daily Fluid Gains and Losses

Fluid Intake	Volume (mL)	Fluid Output	Volume (mL)
Oral fluids	1200	Urine	1500
Solid foods	1000		
Oxidative metabolism	300	Insensible (skin and lungs)	900
Total gains	2500	Gastrointestinal	100
		Total losses	2500

From Lewis S, et al.: *Medical-surgical nursing: assessment and management of clinical problems*, ed 10, St. Louis 2017, Elsevier.

Delegation and Collaboration

The skills of assessing I&O totals at the end of each shift; comparing 24-hour totals over several days; and monitoring and recording IV therapy, wound or chest tube drainage, and tube feedings cannot be delegated to nursing assistive personnel (NAP). The nurse emphasizes maintaining standard precautions related to body fluids, accurately measuring and recording I&O, and using the metric system with standard containers. The nurse directs the NAP to:

- Measure and record oral intake, urinary output, liquid diarrheal stools, vomitus, and wound drainage device output.
- Report changes in patient's condition, such as alteration in intake or changes in color, amount, or odor of output.

Equipment

Sign to alert personnel of I&O measurement; daily I&O record form or computer graphic; graduated measuring container; bedpan, urinal, bedside commode, or urine "hat" (a receptacle that fits under the toilet seat); clean gloves; mask, eye protection, and gown *(optional)*

Procedural Steps

1. Identify patients with conditions that increase fluid loss (e.g., fever, diarrhea, vomiting, surgical wound drainage, chest tube drainage, gastric suction, major burns, or severe trauma).
2. Identify patients with impaired swallowing, unconscious patients, and patients with impaired mobility.
3. Identify patients on medications that influence fluid balance (e.g., diuretics and steroids).
4. Assess signs and symptoms of dehydration and fluid overload (e.g., bradycardia versus tachycardia, hypotension versus hypertension, and reduced skin turgor versus edema).
5. Weigh patients daily using the same scale, at the same time of day, and while wearing comparable clothing.
6. Monitor laboratory reports:
   - Urine specific gravity (normal is 1.010–1.030)
   - Hematocrit (Hct) (normal range is 38%–47% for females and 40%–54% for males).
7. Assess patient's or family caregiver's knowledge, experience, and health literacy level.
8. Assess patient's and family's knowledge of purpose and process of I&O measurement.
9. Explain to patient and family the reasons that I&O measurement is important.
10. Perform hand hygiene.
11. Measure and record all fluid intake:
    a. Liquids with meals, gelatin, custards, ice cream, ice pops, sherbets, ice chips (recorded as 50% of measured volume [e.g., 100 mL of ice chips equals 50 mL of water]). Convert household measures to the metric system: 1 oz equals 30 mL; therefore 12 oz (soda can) equals 360 mL.
    b. Count liquid medicines, such as antacids, and fluids with medications as fluid intake.
    c. Calculate fluid intake from tube feedings.
    d. Calculate fluid intake from parenteral fluids, blood components, and total parenteral nutrition solutions.

Safe Patient Care *Record intake as soon as you measure it to maintain accuracy. If more than one patient is in the same room, each must have urine receptacles labeled with name and bed location.*

12. Instruct patient and family caregiver to call you or the NAP to empty contents of urinal, urine hat, or commode each time patient uses it. Have patient and family monitor incontinence, vomiting, and excessive perspiration and report it to the nurse.
13. Inform patient and family caregiver that Foley catheter drainage bag and wound, gastric, or chest tube drainage are closely monitored, measured, and recorded and who is responsible for this. Each patient must have a graduated container clearly marked with name and bed location and used only for the patient indicated.
14. Apply clean gloves. Measure drainage at the end of the shift or as indicated, using appropriate containers and noting color and characteristics. If splashing is anticipated, wear mask, eye protection, and/or gown.
    a. Measure urine drainage using a urine hat into which patient voids or a graduated container (see illustration).
    b. Observe color and characteristics of urine in Foley tubing and drainage bag. Sometimes a measuring device is part of the drainage bag (see illustration). Otherwise measure with a graduated container.
    c. Measure chest tube drainage by marking and recording the time on the collection chamber at specified intervals (see illustration). Chest tube collection devices are changed when they become full.
    d. Measure Jackson-Pratt/Hemovac drainage with a medicine cup (see illustration).
    e. Measure gastric drainage or larger drainage pouches by opening clamp and pouring into graduated cup with a 240-mL capacity (see illustration).

Continued

PROCEDURAL GUIDELINE 8.1 *Monitoring Intake and Output—cont'd*

15. Remove gloves and dispose of them in appropriate receptacle. Perform hand hygiene.
16. Help patient to a comfortable position.
17. Be sure nurse call system is in an accessible location within patient's reach.
18. Raise side rails (as appropriate) and lower bed to lowest position.
19. Note I&O balance or imbalance and report to health care provider any urine output less than 30 mL/hr or significant changes in daily weight.
20. Document on I&O.

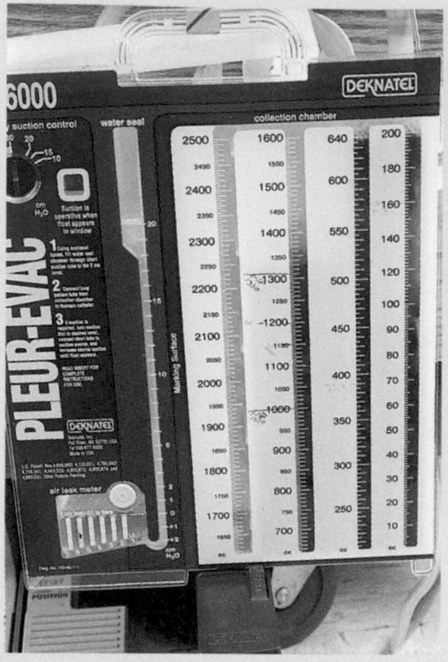

STEP 14c Collection chamber for measuring chest tube drainage.

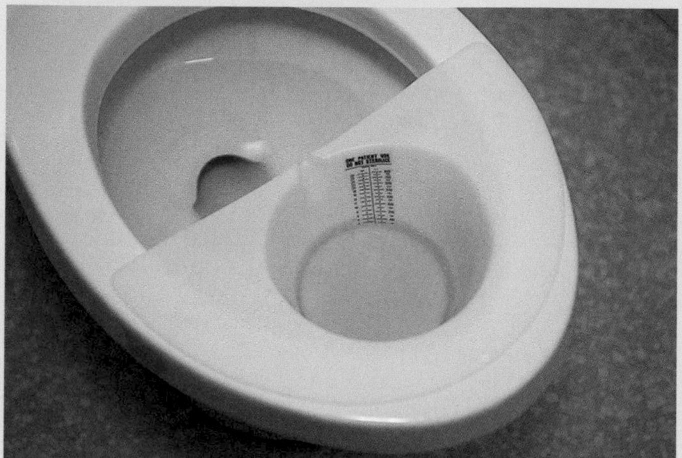

STEP 14a Urine "hat."

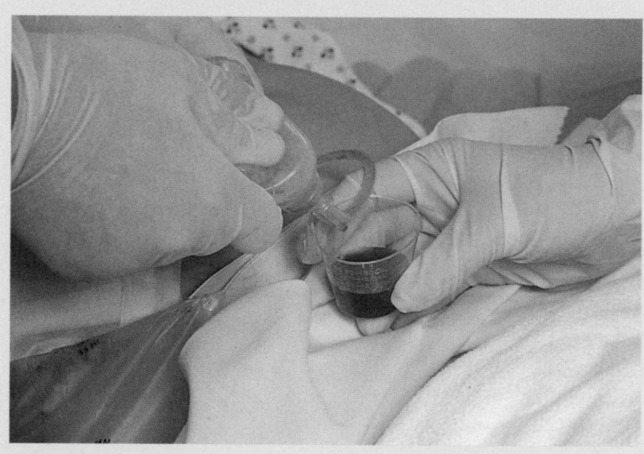

STEP 14d Measuring wound drainage through Jackson-Pratt drain.

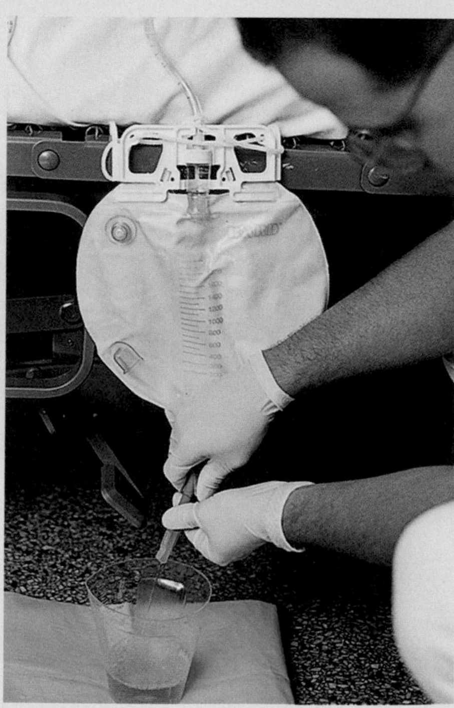

STEP 14b Device for monitoring hourly urine output.

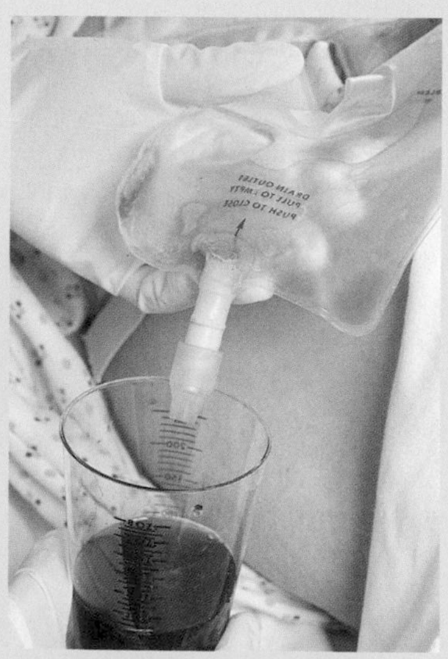

STEP 14e Measuring drainage from large drainage pouch.

✦ SKILL 8.2 Assessing the Head and Neck

Purpose

Examination of the head and neck includes assessment of the head, eyes, ears, nose, mouth, and sinuses. Assessment of the head and neck uses inspection, palpation, and auscultation, with inspection and palpation often used simultaneously.

Delegation and Collaboration

The skill of assessing the head and neck cannot be delegated to nursing assistive personnel (NAP). The nurse directs the NAP to:

- Observe for nasal discharge and nasal bleeding.
- Report any findings found during routine care (e.g., oral care, bathing) to the nurse for further assessment.

Equipment

- Stethoscope
- Clean gloves (use nonlatex if necessary)
- Tongue blade
- Penlight

ASSESSMENT

1. Assess for history of headache, dizziness, pain, or stiffness. *Rationale: Headaches and dizziness are signs of stress, a symptom of another underlying problem such as high blood pressure, or a result of injury.*
2. Determine if patient has history of eye disease, diabetes mellitus, or hypertension. *Rationale: Common conditions predispose patients to visual alterations requiring health care provider referral.*
3. Ask if patient has experienced blurred vision, flashing lights, halos around lights, or reduced visual field. *Rationale: These common symptoms indicate visual problems.*
4. Ask if patient has experienced ear pain, itching, discharge, vertigo, tinnitus (ringing in the ears), or change in hearing. *Rationale: These signs and symptoms indicate infection or hearing loss.*
5. Review patient's occupational history. *Rationale: Patient's occupation can create a risk of injury, potential for eye fatigue, or prolonged noise exposure.*
6. Ask if patient has history of allergies, nasal discharge, epistaxis (nosebleeds), or postnasal drip. *Rationale: History is useful in determining source of nasal and sinus drainage.*
7. Determine if patient smokes or chews tobacco. *Rationale: Tobacco users have greater risk for cancers of the oral cavity and pharynx, larynx, lung, and esophagus (ACS, 2017c).*
8. Assess patient's/family caregiver's knowledge, experience, and health literacy. *Rationale: Ensures patient/family caregiver has the capacity to obtain, communicate, process, and understand basic health information (CDC, 2016a).*

STEP	RATIONALE
PLANNING	
1. Expected outcomes following completion of procedure:	
a. Patient recognizes warning signs and symptoms of eye, ear, sinus, and mouth disease.	Awareness of warning signs improves adherence to reporting problems to health care provider.
b. Patient takes appropriate safety precautions for occupational injury related to head and neck.	Awareness of safety precautions improves adherence to healthful behaviors.
c. Patient exhibits good visual acuity, normal hearing, moist and intact oral mucosa, and head and neck without masses or lesions.	Patient has no abnormal findings.
2. Provide privacy and prepare environment.	Providing privacy and preparing the environment early help the student/nurse think about the need to remove clutter from the over-bed or bedside table.
3. Prepare patient. Tell him or her that you will be completing routine examination of head and neck to check for areas of concerns.	Understanding promotes patient's cooperation.
4. Anticipate teaching topics so that during examination, you can teach patient about common symptoms of eye, ear, sinus, and mouth problems and occupational health safety.	Enables you to incorporate teaching during examination.
IMPLEMENTATION	
1. Perform hand hygiene. Position patient sitting upright if possible.	Provides for more thorough examination of head and neck structures.
2. Inspect head. Note head position and facial features. Look for symmetry.	Head tilting to one side may indicate hearing or visual loss. Neurological disorders such as paralysis often affect facial symmetry.

STEP	RATIONALE
3. Assess eyes (include discussion of signs and symptoms related to eye diseases).	
a. Inspect position of eyes, color, condition of conjunctiva, and movement.	Asymmetrical positioning may reflect trauma or tumor growth. Differences in color are sometimes congenital; changes in color of conjunctiva may be result of local infection or symptomatic of another abnormality (e.g., pale conjunctiva is associated with anemia).
b. Assess patient's near vision (ability to read newspaper or magazines) and far vision (ability to follow movement, read clock, watch television, or read signs at a distance).	Patient with visual acuity or visual field loss indicates need for supporting self-care measures (e.g., feeding, bathing, hygiene, dressing) and teaching.
c. Inspect pupils for size, shape, and equality (see illustration).	Normal pupils are round, regular, and equal in size and shape.
d. Test pupillary reflexes. To test reaction to light, dim room lights. If you cannot dim lights, cup hand over eye to temporarily shield light. As patient looks straight ahead, move penlight from side of patient's face and direct light on pupil. Observe pupillary response of both eyes, noting briskness and equality of reflex (see illustrations *A* and *B*).	Darkened room normally ensures brisk response of pupils to light. Pupil that is illuminated constricts. Pupil in other eye should constrict equally (consensual light reflex).
(1) Test for accommodation by asking patient to focus on distant object, which dilates the pupil. Then have patient shift to near object about 10 to 15 cm (4–6 inches) from nose and observe for pupil constriction and convergence of eyes. **NOTE:** You can also ask patient to follow an object (e.g., finger, pen) with eyes from far to near point.	Absence of constriction, convergence, or an asymmetrical response requires further ophthalmological assessment (Ball et al., 2019; Wilson and Giddens, 2017).
4. Assess hearing. Note patient's response to questions and presence/use of hearing aid. If you suspect patient has hearing loss, ask him or her to repeat random words that you state. Use one- or two-syllable words. Repeat, gradually increasing voice intensity, until patient correctly repeats the words.	Patients normally hear 50% of words clearly when whispered (Wilson and Giddens, 2017). For patient with obvious hearing impairment, speak clearly and concisely, stand so that patient can see your face, stand toward patient's good ear, use low pitch, and avoid yelling.

Safe Patient Care *If hearing deficit is present, have a health care provider inspect patient's ears because impaired hearing may be the result of impacted cerumen, external otitis, or swelling in ear canal because of allergic reactions to materials in hearing aids.*

2 3 4 5 6 7 8 9

STEP 3c Pupil sizes in millimeters.

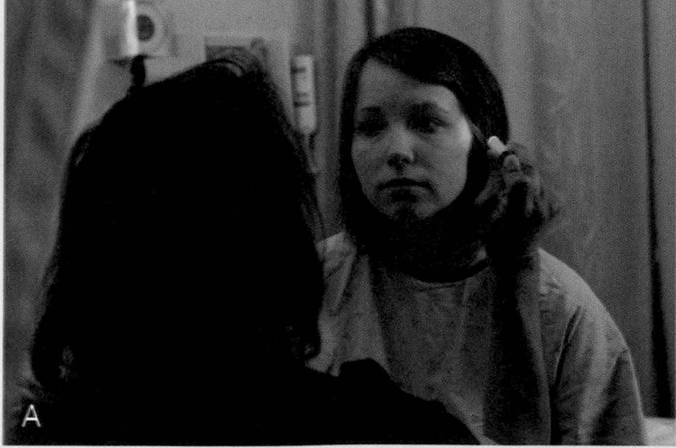

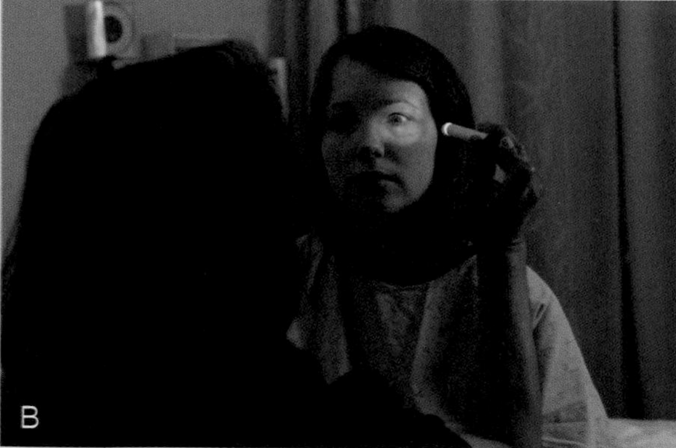

STEP 3d (A) Holding penlight to side of patient's face. (B) Illumination of pupil causes pupillary constriction.

STEP	RATIONALE
5. Inspect nose externally for shape, skin color, alignment, drainage, and presence of deformity or inflammation. Note color of mucosa and any lesions, discharge, swelling, or presence of bleeding. If drainage appears infectious, consult with health care provider about obtaining a specimen.	Character of discharge and inflammation indicate allergy or infection. Perforation and erosion of septum and puffiness and/or increased vascularity of mucosa indicate habitual drug use.
6. In patients with nasogastric (NG), nasointestinal (NI), or nasotracheal tube, inspect nares for excoriation, inflammation, or discharge. Using penlight, look up into each naris. Stabilize tube as needed.	Swallowing or coughing reflex causes movement of tubes against nares, and pressure against tissues and mucosa can result in tissue injury.
7. Inspect sinuses by palpating gently over frontal and maxillary areas. Use thumbs to apply pressure up and under eyebrows to assess frontal sinuses (see illustration). Use thumbs to apply pressure over maxillary sinuses, about 0.4 cm (1 inch) below eyes.	Infection, allergy, or drug use sometimes causes tenderness.
8. Assess mouth (include discussion about signs and symptoms of oral cancer).	
a. Apply clean gloves. Inspect lips for color, texture, hydration, and lesions. Have females remove lipstick.	Normal lips are pink, moist, symmetrical, and smooth.
b. Inspect teeth and note position and alignment. Note color of teeth and presence of dental caries, tartar, and extraction sites.	Reveals quality of hygiene and discoloring effects of cola, coffee, and tobacco. Teeth are normally smooth, white, and shiny.
c. Inspect mucosa and gums. Determine if patient wears dentures or retainers and if they are comfortable. Remove dentures to visualize and palpate gums. Use tongue blade to lightly depress tongue and inspect oral cavity with penlight (see illustration). Inspect oral mucosa, tongue, teeth, and gums for color, hydration, texture, and obvious lesions.	Dentures and retainers can cause chronic irritation. Normal mucosa is glistening, pink, smooth, and moist. Precancerous lesions can go unnoticed and progress rapidly.
d. If oral lesions are present, palpate gently with gloved hand for tenderness, size, and consistency. Remove gloves. Perform hand hygiene.	Cancerous lesions tend to be hard and nontender.
9. Inspect and palpate the neck:	Assesses function of all neck structures, including neck muscles, lymph nodes, thyroid glands, and trachea.
a. Ask patient if there is history of neck pain or difficulty moving neck.	May indicate muscle strain, head injury, local nerve injury, or swollen lymph nodes.

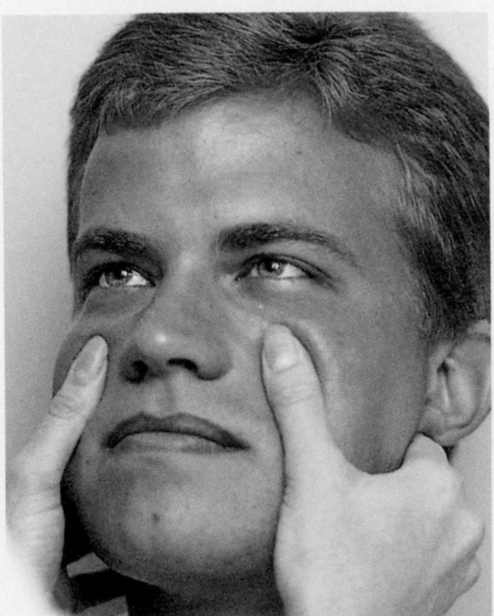

STEP 7 Palpation of maxillary sinuses.

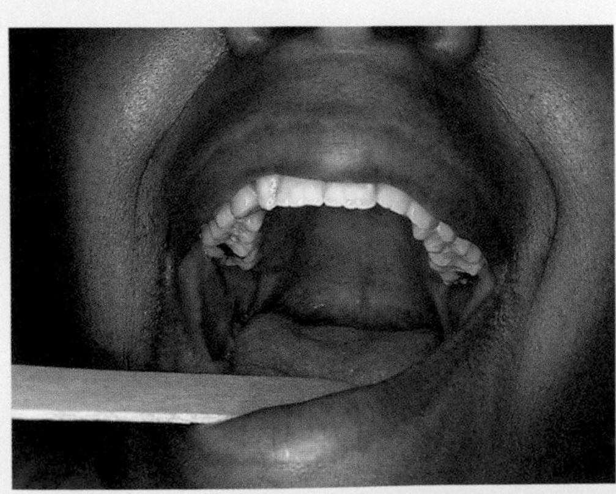

STEP 8c Inspect mouth.

STEP	RATIONALE
b. Neck muscles: Inspect neck for bilateral symmetry of muscles. Ask patient to flex and hyperextend neck and turn head side to side.	Detects muscle weakness, strain, and range of motion (ROM).
c. Lymph nodes:	Lymph nodes are sometimes enlarged from infection or various diseases, such as cancer.
(1) With patient's chin raised and head tilted slightly, inspect area where lymph nodes are distributed and compare both sides (see illustration).	
(2) To examine lymph nodes, have patient relax with neck flexed slightly forward. To palpate, face or stand to side of patient and use pads of middle three fingers of hand (see illustration). Palpate gently in rotary motion for superficial lymph nodes.	This position relaxes tissues and muscles.
(3) Note if lymph nodes are large, fixed, inflamed, or tender.	Large, fixed, inflamed, or tender lymph nodes indicate local infection, systemic disease, or neoplasm.
10. Help patient to comfortable position.	Gives patient sense of well-being.

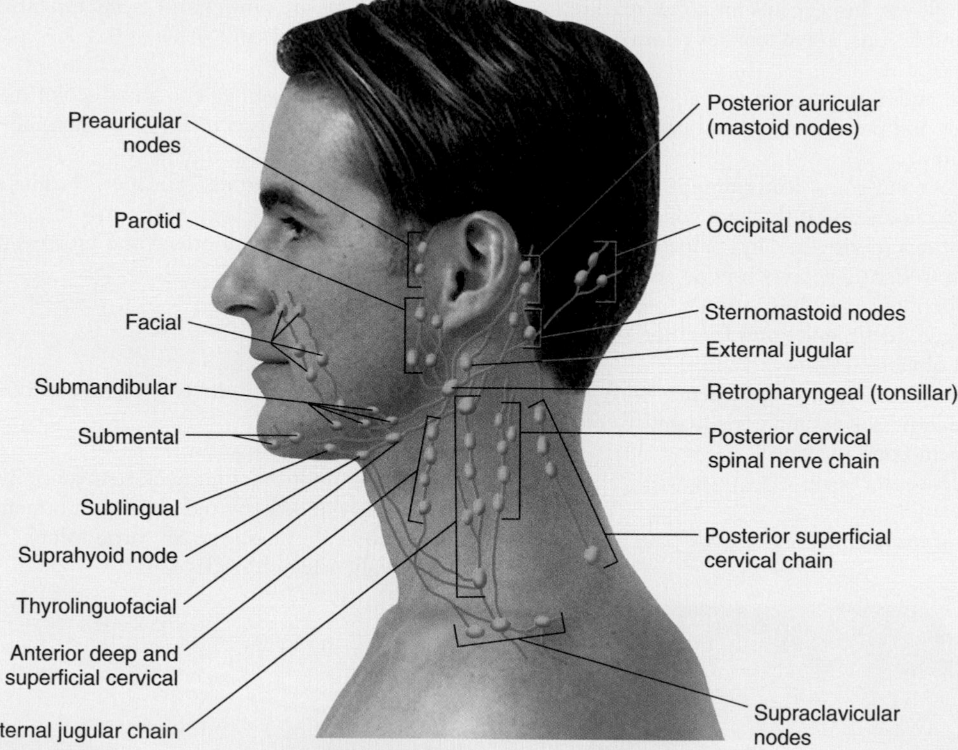

STEP 9c(1) Palpable lymph nodes of head and neck. *(From Ball JW, et al.:* Seidel's guide to physical examination*, ed 9, St. Louis, 2019, Elsevier.)*

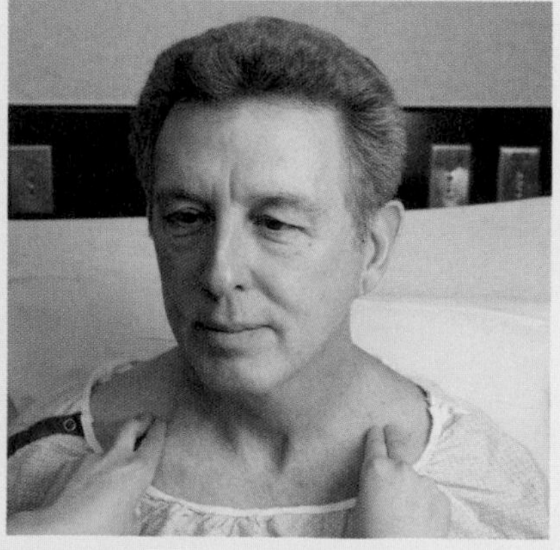

STEP 9c(2) Palpation of cervical lymph nodes.

STEP	RATIONALE

EVALUATION

Step	Rationale
1. Compare assessment findings with previous observations.	Identifies changes in patient's condition.
2. Ask patient to describe common symptoms of eye, ear, sinus, or mouth disease.	Measures patient's ability to recognize abnormalities.
3. Ask patient to list occupational safety precautions.	Knowledge allows patient to take safety precautions.
4. **Use Teach-Back:** "I would like to make sure that you know some of the signs and symptoms of injury to your ears due to your occupation. Tell me what you should do to reduce injury and potential hearing problems." Revise your instruction now or develop a plan for revised patient/family caregiver teaching if patient/family caregiver is not able to teach back correctly.	Determines patient's/family caregiver's level of understanding of instructional topic.

Unexpected Outcomes	Related Interventions
1. Patient has yellow nasal discharge, sneezing, and complaint of sinus pain.	• Reposition into semi-Fowler's or other comfortable position to relieve sinus pain. • Monitor temperature for fever. • Notify health care provider if these are new findings.
2. Patient complains of severe headache and dizziness when standing.	• Respond immediately by obtaining vital signs, especially blood pressure. • Return patient to bed in position of comfort to minimize dizziness and relieve headache. • Identify contributing factors (e.g., stress, pain, or elevated blood pressure). • Notify health care provider.
3. Patient has mouth sore that bleeds easily, lump or thickening in cheek, or white or red patch in mucosa.	• Notify health care provider.

Recording

- Record all findings, including any abnormal findings such as hearing or visual loss, pain and its location, and current infection. Record content of any patient education.
- Document your evaluation of patient learning.

Hand-Off Reporting

- Report increased headache, dizziness, or visual changes immediately to charge nurse or health care provider.

✦ SKILL 8.3 Assessing the Thorax and Lungs

Purpose

Assessment of the thorax and lungs requires review of the ventilatory and respiratory functions of the lungs. It is a critical part of assessment because alterations can be life threatening. Changes in respiration can occur quickly because of immobility, infection, certain analgesic and sedative medications, and fluid overload. Use data from all body systems to determine the nature of pulmonary alterations. You will use inspection, palpation, and auscultation during the examination.

Delegation and Collaboration

The skill of assessing the lungs and thorax cannot be delegated to nursing assistive personnel (NAP). The nurse directs the NAP to:

- Measure the patient's respirations after vital signs and confirm that patient is stable.
- Report respiratory distress, difficulty breathing, and changes in rate and depth.
- Keep head of bed elevated for a patient who has respiratory difficulties.

Equipment

- Stethoscope

ASSESSMENT

1. Before assessing the thorax and lungs, know the landmarks of the chest (Fig. 8.2). *Rationale: These landmarks help you identify findings and use assessment skills correctly.*
   a. A patient's nipples, angle of Louis at the sternum, suprasternal notch, costal angle, clavicles, and vertebrae are key landmarks.
   b. Keep a mental image of the location of the lobes of the lung and the position of each rib (Fig. 8.3).
   c. Locating the position of each rib is critical to visualizing the lobe of the lung being assessed. To begin, locate the angle of Louis on the anterior chest by palpating the "speed bump" at the manubriosternal junction, where the second rib connects with the sternum. The angle is often visible and palpable.

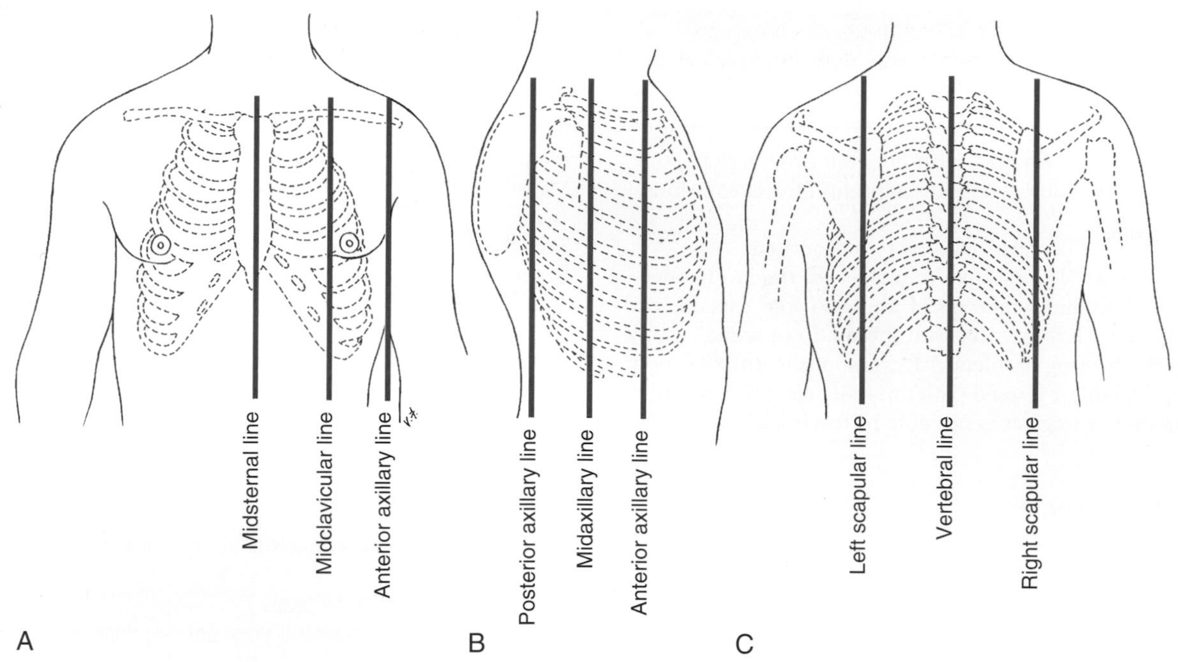

FIG 8.2 Anatomical landmarks and order of progression for examination of the thorax. (A) Anterior thorax. (B) Lateral thorax. (C) Posterior thorax.

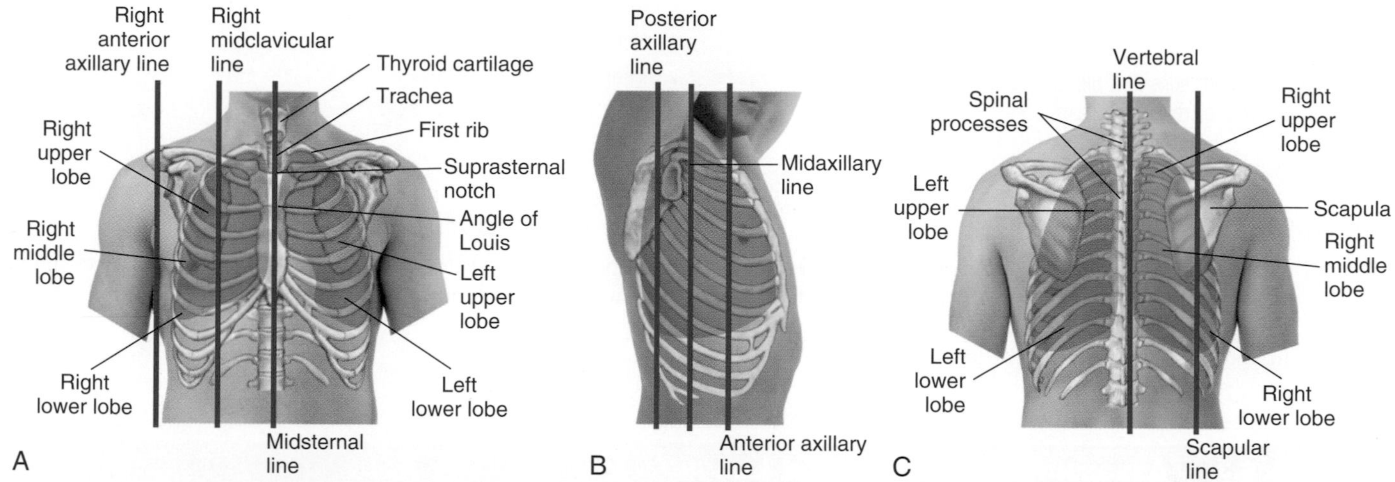

FIG 8.3 Position of lung lobes in relation to anatomical landmarks. (A) Anterior position. (B) Lateral position. (C) Posterior position. *(From Ball JW, et al.:* Seidel's guide to physical examination, *ed 9, St. Louis, 2019, Elsevier.)*

d. Count the ribs and intercostal spaces (between the ribs) from this point. The number of each intercostal space corresponds with that of the rib just above it. The spinous processes of the third thoracic vertebra and the fourth, fifth, and sixth ribs help to locate the lung lobes laterally.
e. The lower lobes project laterally and anteriorly (see Fig. 8.3A-B). Posteriorly, the tip or inferior margin of the scapula lies approximately at the level of the seventh rib (see Fig. 8.3C).

2. Assess history of tobacco or marijuana use, including type of tobacco, duration (number of years), and amount in pack-years. Pack-years equal number of years smoking times number of packs per day (e.g., 4 years × ½ pack per day equals 2 pack-years). If patient has quit, determine length of time since smoking stopped. *Rationale: Smoking is a major cause of lung and tracheal cancers and chronic lung diseases such as emphysema and chronic bronchitis. Risk factors for lung cancer include history of smoking for a greater number of years, exposure to environmental pollution, workplace exposure, family history, HIV infection, and secondhand smoke (National Cancer Institute, 2015).*
3. Ask if patient experiences any of the following: *persistent cough* (productive or nonproductive), sputum production, *blood-streaked sputum, chest pain,* shortness of breath, orthopnea, dyspnea during exertion, activity intolerance, or *recurrent attacks of pneumonia or bronchitis. Rationale: Symptoms of respiratory alterations help to localize objective physical findings. (Warning signals for lung cancer are in italics.)*

4. Determine if patient works in environment containing pollutants (e.g., asbestos, arsenic, coal dust, or chemical irritants) or requiring exposure to radiation. Does patient have exposure to secondhand cigarette smoke? *Rationale: Patients with chronic respiratory disease, particularly asthma, have symptoms aggravated by change in temperature and humidity, irritating fumes or smoke, emotional stress, and physical exertion.*
5. Review history for known or suspected HIV infection, substance abuse, low income, residence or employment in nursing home or shelter, homelessness, recent imprisonment, being a family member of patient with tuberculosis (TB), and immigration to the United States from a country where TB is prevalent (CDC, 2016b). *Rationale: These are known risk factors for exposure to and/or development of TB.*
6. Ask if patient has history of persistent cough, hemoptysis (bloody sputum), unexplained weight loss, fatigue, night sweats, and/or fever. *Rationale: These are signs and symptoms for both TB and HIV infection.*
7. Does patient have history of chronic hoarseness? *Rationale: Hoarseness indicates laryngeal disorder or abuse of cocaine or opioids (sniffing).*
8. Assess for history of allergies to pollen, dust, or other airborne irritants and to any foods, drugs, or chemical substances. *Rationale: Allergic response is associated with wheezing on auscultation, dyspnea, cyanosis, and diaphoresis.*
9. Review family history for cancer, TB, allergies, or chronic obstructive pulmonary disease (COPD). *Rationale: Familial history places patient at risk for lung disease.*
10. Assess patient's/family caregiver's knowledge, experience, and health literacy. *Rationale: Ensures patient/family caregiver has the capacity to obtain, communicate, process, and understand basic health information (CDC, 2016a).*

STEP	RATIONALE
PLANNING	
1. Expected outcomes following completion of procedure:	
• Respirations are passive, diaphragmatic or costal, and regular (12–20/min in adult), with symmetrical expansion.	Characteristics of normal respirations.
• Breath sounds are clear to auscultation and equal bilaterally.	Air flows without interference or obstruction. Corresponding sides should sound the same.
• Patient is able to describe factors that predispose to lung disease.	Awareness of risks can improve patient adherence to healthy behavior.
• Patient assumes appropriate posture for best breathing.	Patient can learn about benefits of good posture as examination maneuvers are performed.
2. Anticipate teaching topics so that during the examination, you can teach patient about any risk factors for lung disease.1	Allows you to incorporate teaching during assessment process.
3. Provide privacy and prepare environment.	Providing privacy and preparing the environment early help the student/nurse think about the need to remove clutter from the over-bed or bedside table.
4. Perform hand hygiene.	Reduces transmission of microorganisms.
IMPLEMENTATION	
1. Position and prepare patient for examination:	
a. Position patient sitting upright. For bedridden patient, elevate head of bed 45 to 90 degrees. If unable to tolerate sitting, use supine and side-lying positions.	Promotes full lung expansion during examination. Patients with chronic respiratory disease may need to sit up throughout examination because of shortness of breath. May require help of another caregiver to position unresponsive patients.
b. Remove gown or drape first from posterior chest, keeping front of chest and legs covered. As examination progresses, remove gown from area being examined.	Avoids unnecessary exposure and provides full visibility of thorax. Allows direct placement of diaphragm or bell on patient's skin, which enhances clarity of sounds.
c. Explain all steps of procedure, encouraging patient to relax and breathe normally through mouth.	Anxiety alters respiratory function. Breathing through mouth decreases extraneous sounds from air passing through nose.
2. Posterior thorax:	
a. If possible, stand behind patient. Inspect thorax for shape and symmetry. Note any deformities, position of spine, slope of ribs, retraction of intercostal spaces (ICSs) during inspiration and bulging of ICSs during expiration, and symmetrical expansion during inspiration. Note anteroposterior (AP) diameter.	Allows for identification of impairment in chest expansion and any symptoms of respiratory distress. Normal chest contour is symmetrical. In a child, the shape of chest is almost circular, with AP diameter in 1:1 ratio. In an adult AP is one-third to one-half of side-to-side diameter. Chronic lung disease causes ribs to be more horizontal and increases AP diameter, resulting in "barrel chest." Patients with breathing problems assume postures that improve ventilation.

STEP	RATIONALE

Safe Patient Care *When a patient holds the chest wall during breathing, it indicates localized chest pain. Assess the nature of pain, including onset, severity, precipitating factors, quality, region, and radiation.*

STEP	RATIONALE
b. Determine rate and rhythm of breathing. Examine thorax as a whole. Have patient relax.	This is a good time to count respirations, with patient relaxed and unaware of inspection. Awareness could alter respirations.
c. Systematically palpate posterior chest wall, costal spaces, and ICSs, noting any masses, pulsations, unusual movement, or areas of localized tenderness (see illustration). If patient voices pain or tenderness, avoid deep palpation. If there is a suspicious mass, palpate lightly for shape, size, and qualities of lesion. Do not palpate painful areas deeply.	Palpation assesses further characteristics and confirms or supplements findings from inspection. Localized swelling or tenderness indicates trauma to ribs or underlying cartilage. A fractured rib fragment could be displaced.
d. Assess chest expansion by standing behind patient and placing thumbs along spinal processes at 10th rib, with palms lightly contacting posterolateral surfaces (see illustration *A*). Keep thumbs about 5 cm (2 inches) apart, with thumbs pointing toward spine and fingers pointing laterally. Press hands toward patient's spine to form small skinfold between thumbs. After exhalation, patient takes deep breath. Note movement of thumbs (see illustration *B*) and symmetry of chest wall movement. Normally, symmetrical separation of thumbs occurs during chest excursion 3 to 5 cm (1½ to 2 inches).	Palpation of chest expansion assesses depth of patient's breathing. This technique is a good measure to evaluate patient's ability to perform deep-breathing exercises. Limited movement on one side indicates that patient is voluntarily splinting during ventilation because of pain. Avoid allowing hands to slide over skin, which gives false measure of excursion.

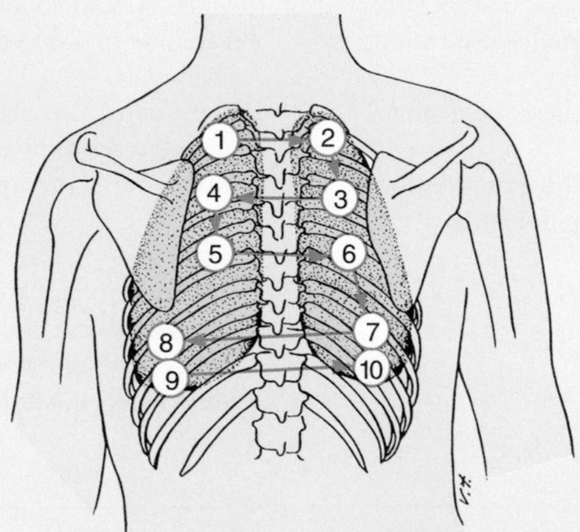

STEP 2c Pattern for assessment of posterior thorax.

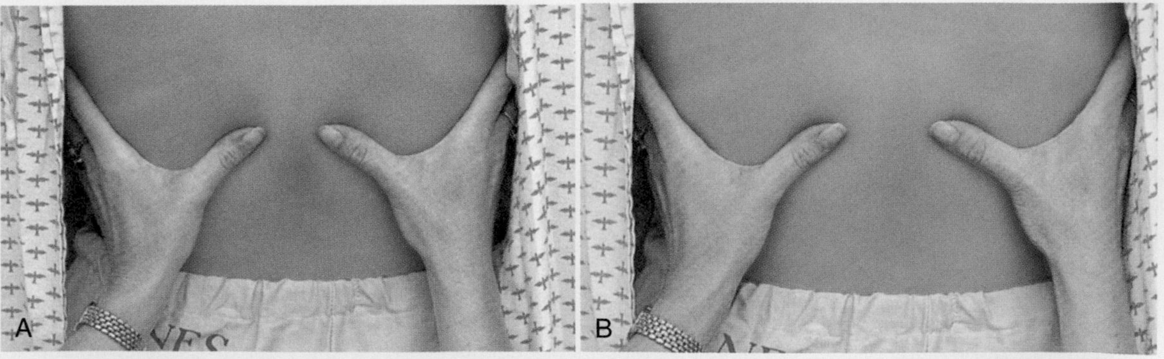

STEP 2d (A) Position of hands for palpation of posterior thorax excursion. (B) As patient inhales, movement of chest excursion separates nurse's thumbs.

STEP	RATIONALE
e. Auscultate breath sounds. Instruct patient to take slow, deep breaths with mouth slightly open. For an adult, place diaphragm of stethoscope firmly on chest wall over intercostal spaces (see illustration). Listen to an entire inspiration and expiration at each stethoscope position (see pattern in Step 2c). If sounds are faint, as in obese patients, ask person to breathe harder and faster temporarily. Systematically compare breath sounds over right and left sides, listening for normal and adventitious sounds.	Assesses movement of air through tracheobronchial tree (Table 8.5). Recognition of normal airflow sounds allows detection of sounds caused by mucus or airway obstruction. Characterize sounds by length of inspiratory and expiratory phases.
f. If you auscultate adventitious sounds, have patient cough. Listen again with stethoscope to determine if sound has cleared with coughing. See Table 8.6 for a description of adventitious breath sounds.	Coughing may clear adventitious sounds. Rhonchi often are eliminated or altered by coughing. Crackles and wheezes are not.
3. Lateral thorax:	
a. Instruct patient to raise arms and inspect chest wall for same characteristics as reviewed for posterior chest.	Improves access to lateral thoracic structures.
b. Extend palpation and auscultation of posterior thorax to lateral sides of chest, except for excursion measurement (see illustration).	Locates abnormalities in lateral lung fields.
4. Anterior thorax:	
a. Inspect accessory muscles while patient is breathing: sternocleidomastoid, trapezius, and abdominal muscles, noting effort to breathe.	Extent to which accessory muscles are used reveals degree of effort to breathe. Accessory muscles move little with normal passive breathing. Patients who require great effort and rely on these muscles may produce a grunting sound.
b. Inspect width or spread of costal angle made by costal margins and tip of sternum. Angle is usually larger than 90 degrees between margins.	Indicates congenital, acquired, or traumatic alterations that may influence patient's chest expansion.
c. Observe patient's breathing pattern, observing symmetry and degree of chest wall and abdominal movement. Respiratory rate and rhythm are more often assessed on anterior chest wall.	Assesses patient's effort to breathe: symmetrical, passive movement indicates no respiratory distress. Male patient's breathing is diaphragmatic, whereas female's is more costal.

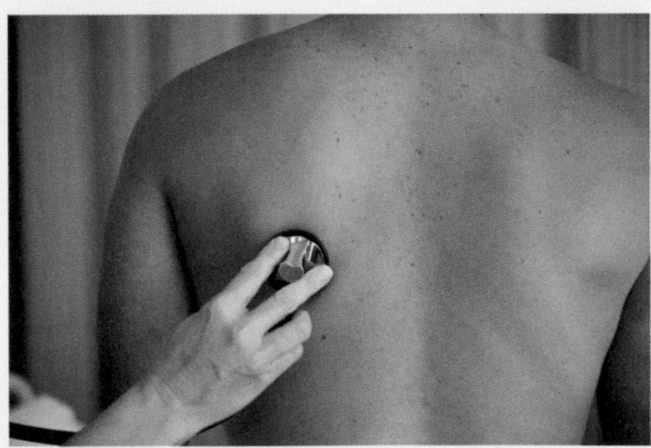

STEP 2e Auscultation with a stethoscope.

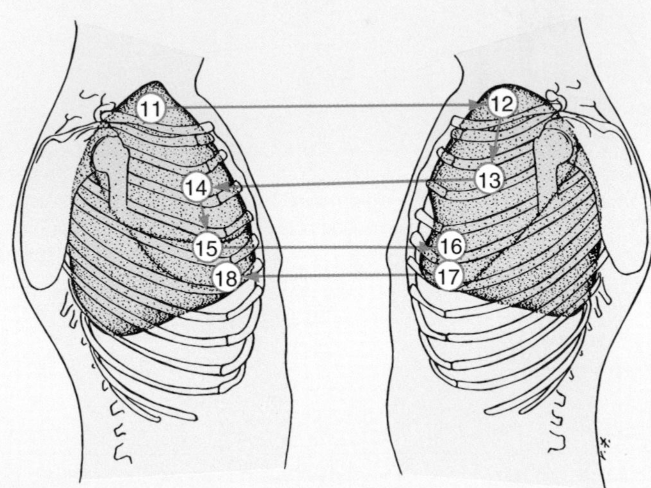

STEP 3b Pattern for assessment of lateral thorax.

TABLE 8.5

Normal Breath Sounds

Type	Description	Location	Origin
Bronchial	Loud and high-pitched sounds with hollow quality; expiration lasts longer than inspiration (3:2 ratio).	Best heard over trachea	Created by air moving through trachea close to chest wall
Bronchovesicular	Medium-pitched and blowing sounds of medium intensity; inspiratory phase is equal to expiratory phase.	Best heard posteriorly between scapulae and anteriorly over bronchioles lateral to sternum at first and second intercostal spaces	Created by air moving through large airways
Vesicular	Soft, breezy, low-pitched sounds; inspiratory phase is 3 times longer than expiratory phase.	Best heard over periphery of lung (except over scapula)	Created by air moving through smaller airways

TABLE 8.6

Adventitious Sounds

Sound	Site Auscultated	Cause	Character
Crackles (formerly called rales) 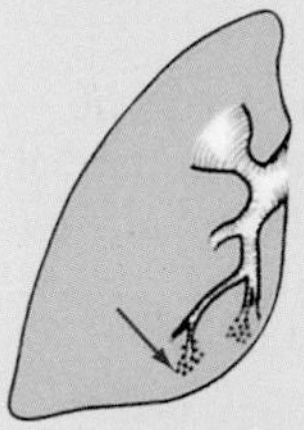	Most common in dependent lobes: right and left lung bases	Random, sudden reinflation of groups of alveoli; also related to increase in fluid in small airways	Fine, short, interrupted crackling sounds heard during end of inspiration; may not change with coughing; medium crackles are lower, more moist sounds heard during middle of inspiration, not cleared with coughing; coarse crackles are loud, bubbly sounds heard during inspiration, not cleared with coughing
Rhonchi (sonorous wheeze) 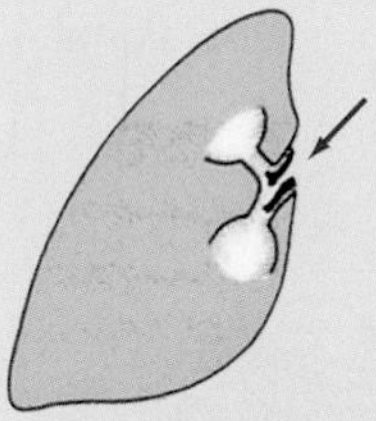	Heard primarily over trachea and bronchi; if loud enough, can be heard over most lung fields	Fluid or mucus in larger airways, causing turbulence; muscular spasm	Loud, low-pitched, continuous sounds heard more during inspiration or expiration; sometimes cleared by coughing; sounds like blowing air through fluid with a straw
Wheezes (sibilant wheeze) 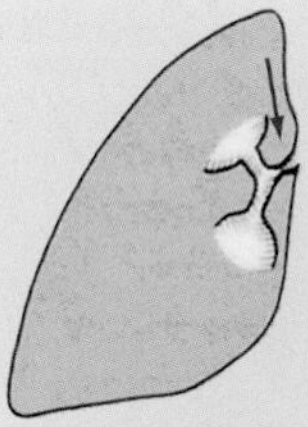	Heard over all lung fields but more distinct over posterior lung fields	High-velocity airflow through severely narrowed or obstructed bronchus	High-pitched, musical sound like a squeak heard continuously during inspiration or expiration; usually louder on expiration; does not clear with coughing
Pleural friction rub 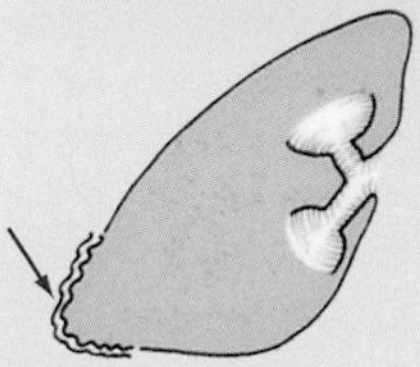	Heard over anterior lateral lung field (if patient is sitting upright)	Inflamed pleura, parietal pleura rubbing against visceral pleura	Has grating quality heard best during inspiration; does not clear with coughing; heard loudest over lower lateral anterior surface

Data from Ball JW, et al.: *Seidel's guide to physical examination,* ed 9, St. Louis, 2019, Elsevier.

STEP	RATIONALE

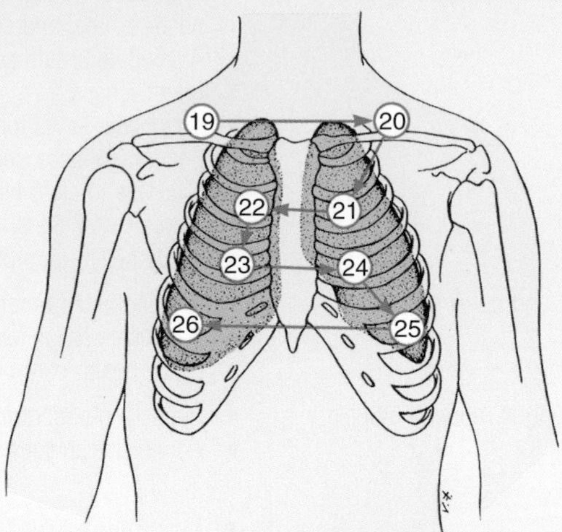

STEP 4d Pattern for assessment of anterior chest.

STEP	RATIONALE
d. Palpate anterior thoracic muscles and ribs for lumps, masses, tenderness, or unusual movement, following a systematic pattern across and down (see illustration).	Localized swelling or tenderness indicates trauma to underlying ribs or cartilage.
e. Palpate anterior chest excursion. Place hands over each lateral rib cage, with thumbs approximately 5 cm (2 inches) apart and angled along each costal margin. As patient inhales deeply, thumbs should symmetrically move apart 3 to 5 cm (1½ to 2 inches), with each side expanding equally.	Assesses depth of patient's breathing and ability to perform deep-breathing exercises. Certain abnormalities are evident if expansion is not symmetrical.
f. With patient sitting, auscultate anterior thorax following same pattern as in Step 4d. Begin above clavicles; move across and then down as during palpation. Compare right and left sides. Give special attention to lower lobes, where mucus commonly gathers.	A systematic pattern of assessment comparing sides helps identify abnormal sounds.
5. Help patient to comfortable position.	Gives patient sense of well-being.
6. Be sure nurse call system is in an accessible location within patient's reach.	Ensures patient can call for assistance if needed.
7. Raise side rails (as appropriate) and lower bed to lowest position.	Ensures patient safety.
8. Clean and store stethoscope. Perform hand hygiene.	Reduces transmission of microorganisms.

EVALUATION

1. Compare respiratory findings with assessment characteristics for thorax and lungs.	Determines presence of abnormalities.
2. Have patient identify factors leading to lung disease.	Demonstrates learning.
3. **Use Teach-Back:** "I would like to make sure that you understand some of the risk factors your occupation poses for lung disease. Tell me what are the specific risks to your lungs from some of the chemical exposure in your hair salon." Revise your instruction now or develop a plan for revised patient/family caregiver teaching if patient/family caregiver is not able to teach back correctly.	Determines patient's/family caregiver's level of understanding of instructional topic.

Unexpected Outcomes	Related Interventions
1. Patient has copious mucus production; audible inspiratory wheezing; or congested cough with thick mucus.	• Help patient cough by splinting chest; teach to inhale slowly through nose, exhale, and cough; encourage expectoration of mucus. • Auscultate breath sounds before and after cough to evaluate cough effectiveness. • Auscultate lungs for adventitious sounds. • Encourage increased oral intake (if permitted). • If unable to clear airway by coughing, suctioning may be indicated. • Monitor vital signs. • Notify health care provider.
2. Respirations are rapid or slow and irregular, and bulging of ICSs is present.	• Position patient more upright if appropriate. • Auscultate lungs for adventitious sounds. • Notify health care provider.
3. Chest excursion is reduced. Depth of breathing is reduced by pain, postural deformity, or fatigue.	• Reposition patient more comfortably. • Administer analgesic if appropriate.

Recording

- Record patient's respiratory rate and character; condition of thorax; character of any mucus; breath sounds, including type, location, and presence on inspiration, expiration, or both; changes noted after coughing; and other physical assessment.
- Document your evaluation of patient and family caregiver learning.

Hand-Off Reporting

- Report any abnormalities immediately to nurse in charge or health care provider.

✦ SKILL 8.4 Cardiovascular Assessment

Purpose

A patient who presents with signs or symptoms of cardiac (heart) problems such as chest pain may have a life-threatening condition that requires immediate attention. In this situation, you must act quickly and perform the parts of the examination that are absolutely necessary. This will reveal baseline heart function and any risks for heart disease. The heart, neck vessels, and peripheral circulation are assessed together because the systems work in unison. You begin assessment of the heart after examining the lungs because the patient is already in a suitable position with the chest exposed. Assessment then proceeds to the neck vessels and ends with evaluating the peripheral circulation. Your assessment can determine the integrity of the circulatory system.

Delegation and Collaboration

The skill of completing a comprehensive cardiovascular assessment cannot be delegated to nursing assistive personnel (NAP). The nurse directs the NAP to:

- Count peripheral pulses after vital signs confirm that patient is stable.
- Recognize skin temperature and color changes of affected extremities and report any changes to the nurse.
- Recognize changes in peripheral pulses and report any changes to the nurse.

Equipment

- Stethoscope
- Doppler stethoscope *(optional)*
- Conducting gel (if a Doppler stethoscope is used)
- Clean gloves (use nonlatex if appropriate)

ASSESSMENT

1. Assess patient for history of smoking, alcohol intake, caffeine intake (e.g., coffee, tea, soft drinks, energy drinks, and chocolate) and use of "recreational" drugs. Determine exercise habits and dietary patterns and intake. *Rationale: These contribute to risk factors for cardiovascular disease. In addition, caffeine and alcohol cause tachycardia. Insufficient exercise and intake of fatty and salty foods increase risk for cardiovascular disease.*
2. Determine if patient is taking medications for cardiovascular function (e.g., antiarrhythmics, antihypertensives, beta blockers, antianginals) and if he or she knows their purpose, dosage, and side effects. *Rationale: Allows you to assess patient's adherence to and understanding of drug therapies. Medications for cardiovascular function cannot be taken intermittently.*
3. Ask if patient has experienced dyspnea, chest pain or discomfort, palpitations, excess fatigue, cough, leg pain or cramps, edema of the feet, cyanosis, fainting, and orthopnea. Ask if symptoms occur at rest or during exercise. *Rationale: These are the cardinal symptoms of heart disease. Cardiovascular function is sometimes adequate during rest but not during exercise.*
4. If patient reports chest pain, determine onset (sudden or gradual), precipitating factors, quality, region, and severity and if it radiates. Anginal pain is usually a deep pressure or ache that is substernal and diffuse, radiating to one or both arms, neck, or jaw. *Rationale: Symptoms reveal acute coronary syndrome or coronary artery disease (CAD).*
5. Assess family history for heart disease, diabetes mellitus, high cholesterol and/or lipid levels, hypertension, stroke, or rheumatic heart disease. *Rationale: Family history of these conditions increases risk for heart and vascular disease.*
6. Ask patient about a history of any preexisting heart conditions (e.g., heart failure, congenital heart disease, CAD, dysrhythmias, or murmurs), heart surgery, or vascular disease (e.g., hypertension, phlebitis, varicose veins). *Rationale: Knowledge reveals patient's level of understanding of*

condition. Preexisting condition influences which examination techniques to use and expected findings.

7. Determine if patient experiences leg cramps; numbness or tingling in extremities; sensation of cold hands or feet; pain in legs; or swelling or cyanosis of feet, ankles, or hand. *Rationale: These are signs and symptoms of vascular disease.*
8. If patient experiences leg pain or cramping in lower extremities, ask if it is relieved by walking or standing for long periods or if it occurs during sleep. *Rationale: Relationship of symptoms to exercise clarifies if problem is vascular or musculoskeletal. Pain caused by vascular condition tends to increase with activity. Musculoskeletal pain is usually not relieved when exercise ends.*
9. Ask women if they wear tight-fitting underwear or hosiery. Ask both men and women if they wear tight-fitting trouser socks and sit or lie in bed with legs crossed. *Rationale: Tight hosiery around lower extremities and crossing legs can impair venous return, promoting clot formation.*
10. Assess patient's/family caregiver's knowledge, experience, and health literacy. *Rationale: Ensures patient/family caregiver has the capacity to obtain, communicate, process, and understand basic health information (CDC, 2016a).*

STEP	RATIONALE

PLANNING

STEP	RATIONALE
1. Expected outcomes following completion of procedure:	
• Heart rate is 60 to 100 beats/min (adolescent through adult), without extra sounds or murmurs.	Indicates normal rate and sinus rhythm.
• Point of maximal impulse (PMI) is palpable at fifth intercostal space at left midclavicular line in children older than 7 years of age and adults (Fig. 8.4).	Indicates normal heart position.
• Patient describes changes in own behavior that could improve cardiovascular function.	Instruction about cardiovascular disease risks may improve patient's health behavior habits.
• Patient describes schedule, dosage, purpose, and benefits of medications being taken for cardiovascular function.	Information related to health benefits may improve adherence to therapy.
• Blood pressure is within normal limits for patient (see Chapter 7).	This is one indicator of normal cardiovascular function.
• Carotid pulse is localized, strong, elastic, and equal bilaterally. No change occurs during inspiration or expiration; without carotid bruit.	This indicates a patent vessel.
• Jugular veins distend when patient lies supine and flatten when patient is in sitting position.	Venous pressure is normal.
• Peripheral pulses are equal and strong (2+); extremities are warm and pink, with capillary refill less than 2 seconds. There is no dependent edema. Peripheral hair growth is symmetrical and evenly distributed, and the skin is free of lesions.	Peripheral circulation is intact.
2. Anticipate teaching topics so that during the examination, you can teach patient about risks for heart and vascular disease.	Allows you to incorporate teaching during examination.
3. Perform hand hygiene. Provide privacy and prepare environment.	Providing privacy and preparing the environment early help the student/nurse think about the need to remove clutter from the over-bed or bedside table.

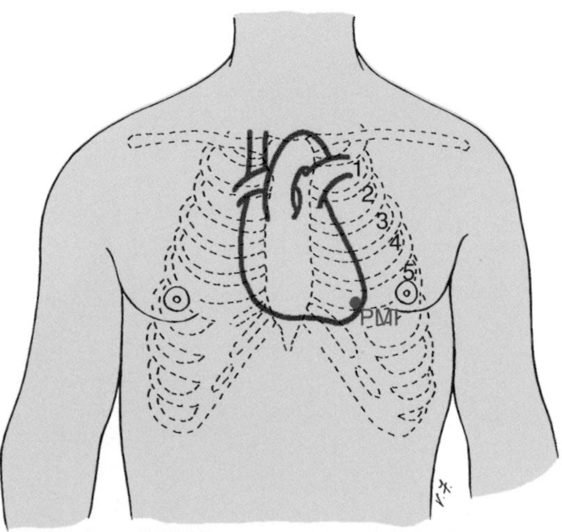

FIG 8.4 Location of point of maximal impulse (PMI) in an adult.

STEP	RATIONALE
4. Explain procedure. Avoid facial gestures reflecting concern.	Patients with previously normal cardiac history may become anxious if you show concern.
5. Help patient be as relaxed and comfortable as possible.	An anxious or uncomfortable patient can have mild tachycardia, which alters findings.
6. Have patient assume semi-Fowler's or supine position.	Provides adequate visibility and access to left thorax and mediastinum. Patient with heart disease often experiences shortness of breath while lying flat.

IMPLEMENTATION

STEP	RATIONALE
1. Be sure that room is quiet.	Subtle, low-pitched heart sounds are difficult to hear.
2. Assess the heart:	
a. Form mental image of exact location of the heart (see illustration). Base of heart is the upper part, and apex is the bottom tip. Surface of right ventricle constitutes most of the anterior surface of the heart.	Visualization improves ability to assess findings accurately and determines possible source of abnormalities.
b. Find angle of Louis, felt as ridge in sternum approximately 5 cm (2 inches) below suprasternal notch (between sternal body and manubrium). Slip fingers down each side of angle to feel adjacent ribs. ICSs are just below each rib.	Provides you with landmarks to locate and assess heart sounds.
c. Find the following anatomical landmarks (see illustration):	Familiarity with landmarks allows you to describe findings more clearly and ultimately may improve assessment.
(1) Aortic area is at second ICS, right of patient's sternum, close to sternal border *(1)*.	Listening to heart sounds from too far away from sternal border decreases ability to hear them clearly.
(2) Pulmonic area is at second ICS, left of patient's sternum, close to sternal border *(2)*.	
(3) Second pulmonic area is found by moving down left side of sternum to third ICS, close to sternal border *(3)*, also referred to as *Erb's point.*	
(4) Tricuspid area *(4)* is located at fourth left ICS along sternum, close to sternal border.	
(5) Mitral area is found by moving fingers laterally to patient's left to locate fifth ICS at left midclavicular line *(5)*.	
(6) Epigastric area *(6)* is at inferior tip of sternum.	
d. Stand to patient's right to inspect and palpate precordium with patient supine. Note any visible pulsations and more exaggerated lifts. Closely inspect area of apex. Palpate for pulsations (placing proximal half of four fingers together and then alternating with ball of hand at all anatomical landmarks).	Reveals size and symmetry of heart. Apical impulse may be visible at midclavicular line in fifth intercostal space. Apical impulse (PMI) may become visible only when patient sits up, bringing heart closer to anterior wall. Obesity obscures ability to visualize PMI. There should be no pulsations or vibrations. A thrill is a continuous palpable sensation, such as purring of a cat. A thrust is the upward lift felt when palpating the chest wall.

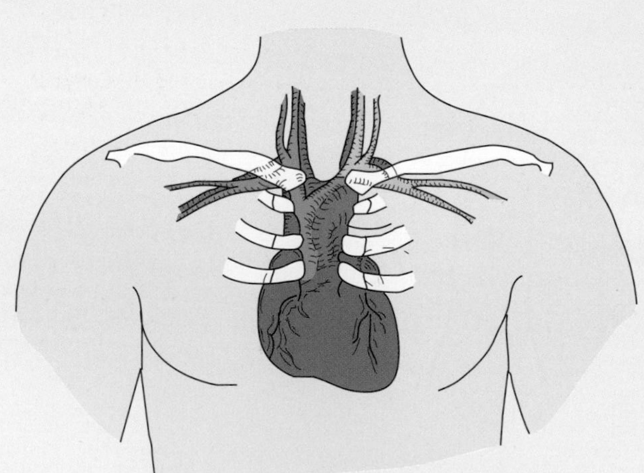

STEP 2a Anatomical position of heart.

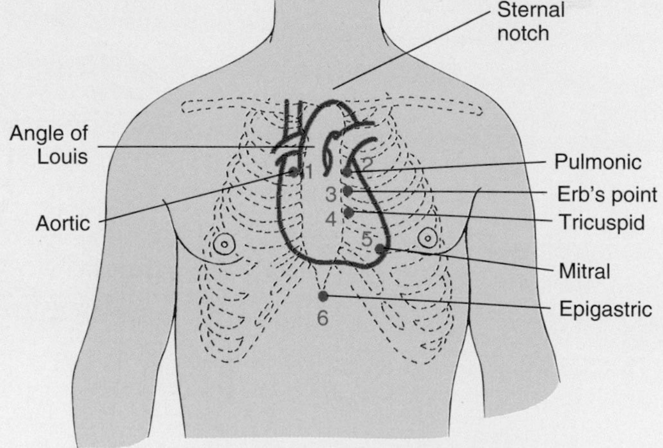

STEP 2c Anatomical sites for assessment of cardiac function.

STEP	RATIONALE
e. Locate PMI by palpating with fingertips along the fifth ICS in midclavicular line (see illustration). Note light, brief pulsation in area 1 to 2 cm (½ to 1 inch) in diameter at the apex.	In presence of serious heart disease, PMI is located to left of midclavicular line related to enlarged left ventricle. In chronic lung disease PMI may be to right of midclavicular line as a result of right ventricular enlargement.

Safe Patient Care *Presence of a palpable thrill is not normal and indicates a disruption of blood flow caused by a defect in closure of a heart valve or atrial septal defect. A stronger-than-expected impulse is a heave or lift, which indicates increased cardiac output or left ventricular hypertrophy. Report to health care provider.*

STEP	RATIONALE
f. If palpating PMI is difficult, turn patient onto left side.	Maneuver moves heart closer to chest wall.
g. Inspect epigastric area and palpate abdominal aorta. NOTE: You should feel a localized strong beat.	Rules out reduced blood flow or diffuse pulse, which indicates abnormality.
h. Auscultate heart sounds:	
(1) Have patient sit up and lean slightly forward; then have him or her lie supine. End examination with patient in left lateral recumbent position (see illustration A to C). In female patient, it may be necessary to lift left breast to hear heart sounds more effectively.	Different positions help to clarify type of sounds heard. Sitting position is best to hear high-pitched murmurs (if present). Supine is common position to hear all sounds. Left lateral recumbent is best position to hear low-pitched sounds.
(2) While auscultating sounds at each anatomical landmark, ask patient not to speak but to breathe comfortably. Begin with diaphragm of stethoscope; alternate with bell. Use very light pressure for bell. Inch stethoscope along; avoid jumping from one area to another. Do not try to hear all heart sounds at once.	Auscultation requires you to isolate each heart sound at all auscultation sites, especially in patients with soft heart sounds.

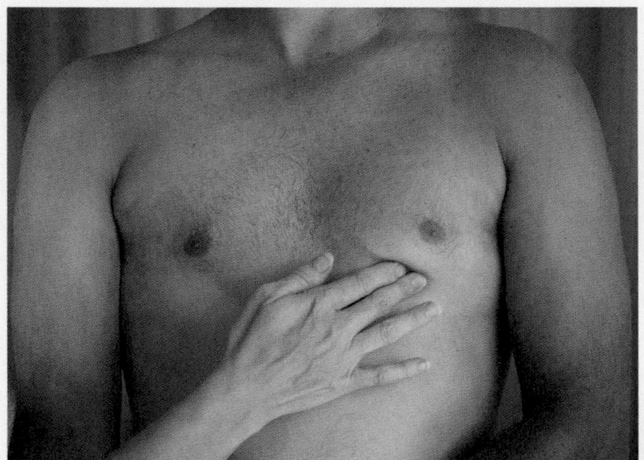

STEP 2e Palpation of point of maximal impulse.

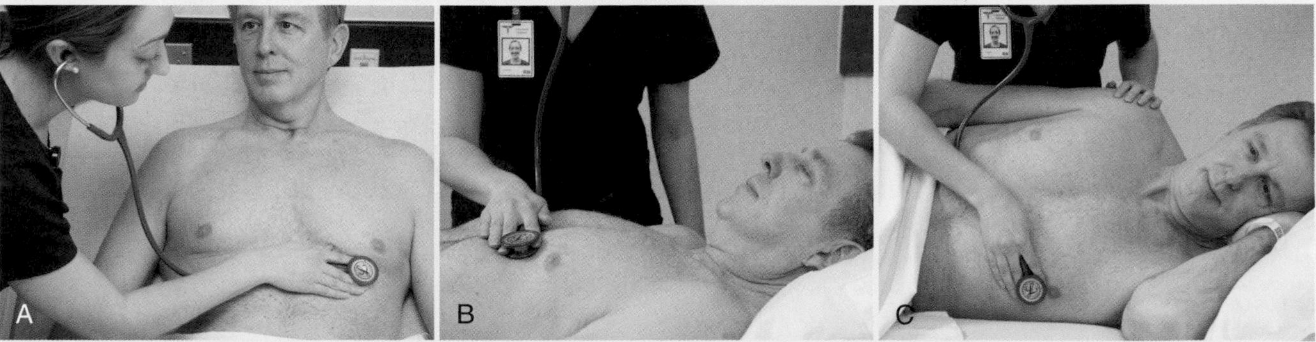

STEP 2h(1) Patient positions for auscultation of heart sounds. (A) Sitting. (B) Supine. (C) Left lateral.

STEP	RATIONALE
(3) Begin at apex or PMI; move systematically to aortic area, pulmonic area, Erb's point, tricuspid area, and mitral area (see illustration in Step 2c). (**NOTE:** Some examiners use reverse sequence.) S_1 is loudest at apex and is simultaneous with carotid pulse. **NOTE:** Helpful mnemonic for remembering heart sound locations: **A P**ig **E**ats **T**oo **M**uch (*A*ortic, *P*ulmonic, *E*rb's point, *T*ricuspid, *M*itral).	At normal slow rates, S_1 is high-pitched and dull in quality and sounds like a "lub." This sound precedes systolic phase of heart contraction.
(4) Listen for S_2 at each site. This sound is loudest at the aortic area. Heart sounds vary in pitch, loudness, and duration, depending on auscultatory site (Table 8.7).	Normal sounds S_1 and S_2 are high-pitched and best heard with diaphragm. S_2 precedes diastolic phase and sounds like "dub."
(5) After both sounds are heard clearly as "lub-dub," count each combination of S_1 and S_2 as one heartbeat. Count number of beats for 1 minute.	Determines apical pulse rate.
(6) Assess heart rhythm by noting time between S_1 and S_2 (systole) and then time between S_2 and the next S_1 (diastole). Listen to full cycle at each auscultation area. Note regular intervals between each sequence of beats. There should be a distinct pause between S_1 and S_2.	Failure of heart to beat at regular intervals is a dysrhythmia, which interferes with ability of heart to pump effectively.
(7) When heart rate is irregular, compare apical and radial pulses (Table 8.8). Auscultate apical pulse and then immediately palpate radial pulse. Also, you can ask a colleague to assess radial pulse while you simultaneously assess apical pulse.	Determines if pulse deficit (radial pulse is slower than apical) exists. Deficit indicates that ineffective contractions of heart fail to send pulse waves to periphery.

TABLE 8.7

Heart Sounds According to Auscultatory Area

	Aortic	Pulmonic	Second Pulmonic	Mitral	Tricuspid
Pitch	$S_1 < S_2$	$S_1 < S_2$	$S_1 < S_2$	$S_1 > S_2$	$S_1 = S_2$
Loudness	$S_1 < S_2$	$S_1 < S_2$	$S_1 < S_2$[a]	$S_1 > S_2$[b]	$S_1 > S_2$
Duration	$S_1 > S_2$	$S_1 > S_2$	$S_1 > S_2$	$S_1 > S_2$	$S_1 > S_2$

[a] S_1 is relatively louder in second pulmonic area than in aortic area.
[b] S_1 may be louder in mitral area than in tricuspid area.
Modified from Ball JW, et al.: *Seidel's guide to physical examination*, ed 9, St. Louis, 2019, Elsevier.

TABLE 8.8

Abnormalities in Rates and Rhythms

Type	Findings	Description
Atrial fibrillation	Rapid, random contractions of atria cause irregular ventricular beats >100 beats/min and atrial beats at 200–350 beats/min.	Atria discharge very rapidly, with some impulses not reaching ventricles. This condition occurs in rheumatic heart disease and mitral stenosis. It causes reduced cardiac output.
Sinus arrhythmia	Pulse rate changes during respiration, increasing at peak of inspiration and decreasing during expiration.	Blood is momentarily trapped in lungs during inspiration, causing a fall in stroke volume of heart.
Sinus bradycardia	Pulse rhythm is regular, but rate is <60 beats/min.	Sinoatrial node fires less frequently. This is common in well-conditioned athletes and with use of antiarrhythmic medications.
Sinus tachycardia	Pulse rhythm is regular, but rate is accelerated to >100 beats/min.	Exercise, emotional stress, and caffeine or alcohol ingestion are common factors that cause increased firing of sinoatrial node.
Premature ventricular contraction	Premature beat occurs before regularly expected heart contraction. Underlying rhythm can be any rate.	Ventricle contracts prematurely because of electrical impulse bypassing normal conduction pathway. It may occur so early that it is difficult to detect as second beat. It may be followed by a pause.

STEP	RATIONALE
i. Auscultate for extra heart sounds at each site. Note pitch, loudness, duration, timing, location on chest wall, and where it is heard in cardiac cycle.	Abnormal sounds include murmurs. Characteristics of murmurs help to identify contributing factors.
(1) Use stethoscope bell and listen for low-pitched extra heart sounds such as S_3 and S_4 gallops, clicks, and rubs. S_3, or a ventricular gallop, occurs just after S_2 at end of ventricular diastole. It sounds like "lub-dub-ee" or "Ken-tuc-ky." S_4, or an atrial gallop, occurs just before S_1 or ventricular systole. It sounds like "dee-lub-dub" or "Ten-nes-see."	Premature rush of blood into a ventricle that is stiff or dilated or an atrial contraction pushing against a ventricle that is not accepting blood causes gallops.
(2) With patient leaning forward or lying on left side, listen for friction rubs as "squeaky" or rubbing sounds.	Rubs result from lungs or inflamed visceral and parietal layers of the pericardium of the heart rubbing against one another.
j. Auscultate for heart murmurs over each auscultation site.	Murmurs are sustained swishing or blowing sounds heard at beginning, middle, or end of systole or diastole. Increased blood flow through a normal valve, forward flow through a stenotic valve or into a dilated vessel or chamber, or backward flow through a valve that fails to close causes murmurs.
(1) When you detect a murmur, listen carefully to note where you hear it best. Note intensity of the murmur.	Intensity is related to rate of blood flow through the heart or amount of blood regurgitated.
(2) Note if murmur is low, medium, or high in pitch, using bell for low-pitched sounds.	Pitch depends on velocity of blood flow through the valves.
3. Assess neck vessels:	
a. To assess carotid arteries, have patient remain in sitting position.	Allows easier mobility of neck to expose artery for inspection and palpation.
b. Inspect neck on both sides for obvious arterial pulsations. Sometimes a pulse wave can be seen.	Carotids are the only sites to assess quality of pulse wave (see illustration). Experience is required to evaluate wave in relation to events of cardiac cycle.
c. Palpate each carotid artery separately with index and middle fingers around medial edge of sternocleidomastoid muscle. Ask patient to raise chin slightly, keeping head straight (see illustration) or slightly away from artery. Note rate and rhythm, strength, and elasticity of artery. Also note if pulse changes as patient inhales and exhales.	If both arteries were occluded simultaneously, patient could lose consciousness from reduced circulation to brain. Turning head improves access to artery. A change indicates a sinus arrhythmia.

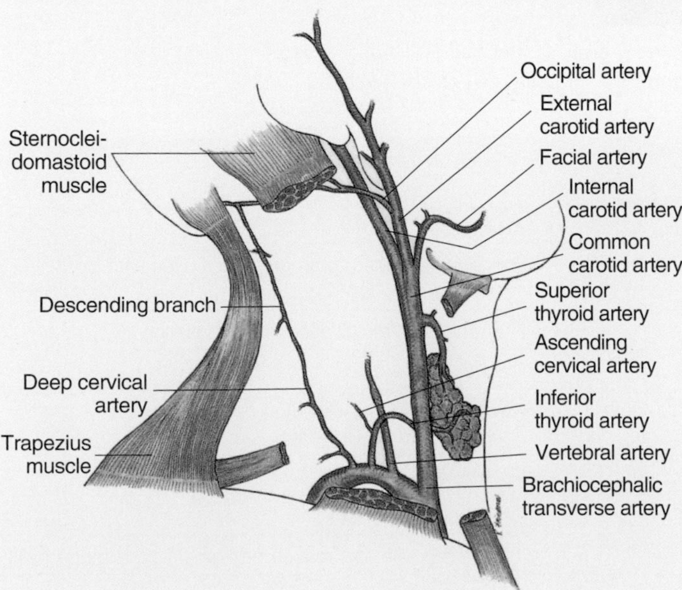

STEP 3b Anatomical position of carotid artery.

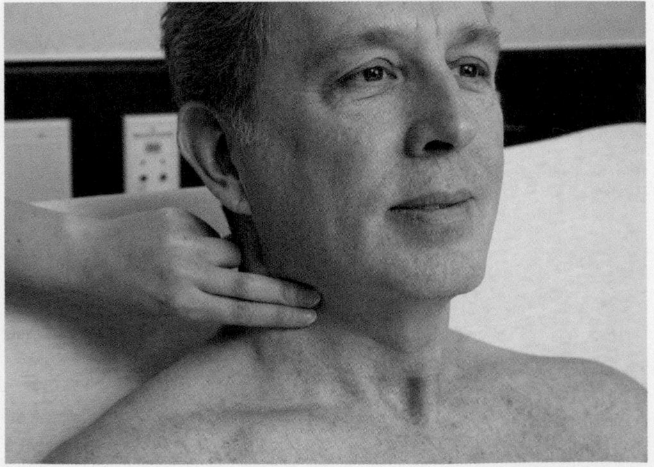

STEP 3c Palpate each carotid artery separately.

STEP	RATIONALE

Safe Patient Care *Do not palpate or massage the carotid artery vigorously. Stimulation of carotid sinus causes a reflex drop in heart rate and blood pressure.*

STEP	RATIONALE
d. Place bell of stethoscope over each carotid artery, auscultating for blowing sound (bruit) (see illustration). Ask patient to exhale and hold breath for a few heartbeats so that respiratory sounds do not interfere with auscultation (Wilson and Giddens, 2017).	Narrowing of lumen of carotid artery by arteriosclerotic plaques causes disturbance in blood flow. Blood passing through narrowed section creates turbulence and emits blowing or swishing sound. Normally you do not hear a bruit.
4. Peripheral vascular assessment:	
a. Inspect lower extremities for changes in color and condition of skin (Table 8.9). Note skin and nail texture, hair distribution, venous patterns, edema, and scars or impaired skin integrity. Compare skin color with patient lying and standing.	Changes may reflect impaired peripheral circulation.
b. Palpate edematous areas, noting mobility, consistency, and tenderness.	Helps determine extent of edema.
c. Assess for pitting edema by pressing area firmly with one finger for 5 seconds and releasing. Depth of indentation determines severity (see illustration): 2 mm: 1+ edema 4 mm: 2+ edema 6 mm: 3+ edema 8 mm: 4+ edema	Limb edema is the most specific sign of deep vein thrombosis (DVT). If DVT is suspected. diagnostic tests must be performed including D-dimer and coagulation studies (Patel et al., 2017).

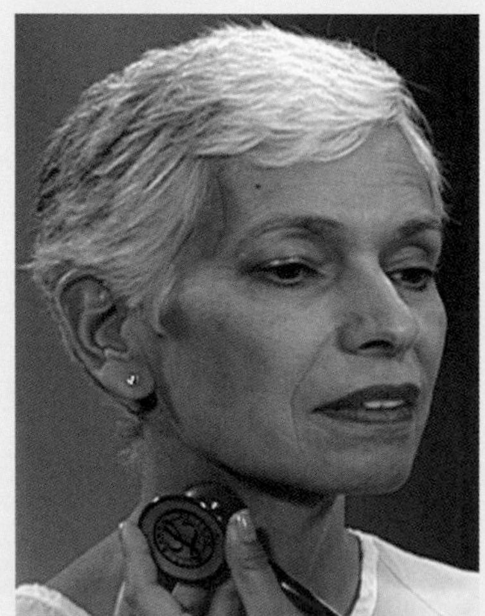

STEP 3d Auscultation for carotid artery bruit. *(From Ball JW et al.:* Seidel's guide to physical examination, *ed 9, St Louis, 2019, Elsevier.)*

TABLE 8.9

Signs of Venous and Arterial Insufficiency

Assessment Criterion	Venous	Arterial
Pain	Aching, increases in evening and with dependent position	Burning, throbbing, cramping, increases with exercise
Paresthesia	None	Numbness, tingling, decreased sensation
Temperature	Normal to touch	Cool to touch
Color	Normal or cyanotic	Pale; worsened by elevation of extremity; dusky red when extremity lowered
Capillary refill	Not applicable	>2 seconds
Pulse	Present	Decreased or absent
Skin changes	Brown pigmentation around ankles	Thin, shiny skin; decreased hair growth; thickened nails
Ulcerations	Shallow ulcers around ankles (chronic venous stasis); edema apparent	Deep, well defined at site of trauma or tips of toes

STEP	RATIONALE
d. Use tape measure to measure circumference of extremity.	Measuring circumference establishes baseline for future comparison.
e. Check capillary refill by grasping patient's fingernail or toenail and noting color of nail bed. Apply gentle, firm pressure to nail bed. Release quickly, watching for color change. Circulation is restored and normally returns to pink color in less than 2 seconds.	Capillary refill is measured in seconds; less than 2 seconds is brisk; whereas greater than 4 seconds is sluggish. Cold environmental temperature with vasoconstriction and vascular disease can delay refill. Local pressure from cast or bandage also slows refill.
f. Ask if patient experiences pain or tenderness and gently palpate for heat, firmness, or localized swelling of calf muscle, all of which are signs of phlebitis or DVT.	The most frequent cause of DVT is immobilization such as in postoperative patients and in individuals after an airplane flight lasting over 8 hours. Other factors that contribute to DVT are chronic illness such as strokes, cancer, and lengthy surgeries (Patel et al., 2017).

Safe Patient Care *Homans' sign (pain in calf on dorsiflexion of foot) is no longer considered a reliable indicator for the presence or absence of DVT (Ball et al., 2019) and should not be considered a reliable test. Trauma to a vein or muscle, reduced mobility, and increased blood clotting are reliable risk factors. If calf is swollen, tender, or red, notify patient's health care provider for further assessment and evaluation. If there is a strong suspicion of DVT, testing for Homans' sign is contraindicated. If a clot is present, it may become dislodged from its original site during this test. This could result in a pulmonary embolism.*

STEP	RATIONALE
g. Palpate peripheral arteries.	
(1) Start at most distal part of each extremity. Palpate each peripheral artery for equality, comparing side to side; elasticity of vessel wall (depress and release artery, noting ease with which it springs back to shape); and strength of pulse (force of blood against arterial wall) using the following rating scale (Ball et al., 2019; Wilson and Giddens, 2017): 0 Absent, not palpable 1+ Diminished, barely palpable, weak and thready, and easy to obliterate 2+ Normal, easy to palpate 3+ Full, easy to palpate, increases 4+ Strong, bounding against fingertips; cannot be obliterated	Comparison of both arteries allows you to determine any localized obstruction or disturbance in blood flow. Pulses should be symmetrical side to side. If asymmetry is noted, look for other factors related to impaired circulation.
(2) Palpate radial pulse by lightly placing tips of first and second fingers in groove formed along radial side of forearm, lateral to flexor tendon of wrist (see illustration).	Pulse is relatively superficial and should not require deep palpation.

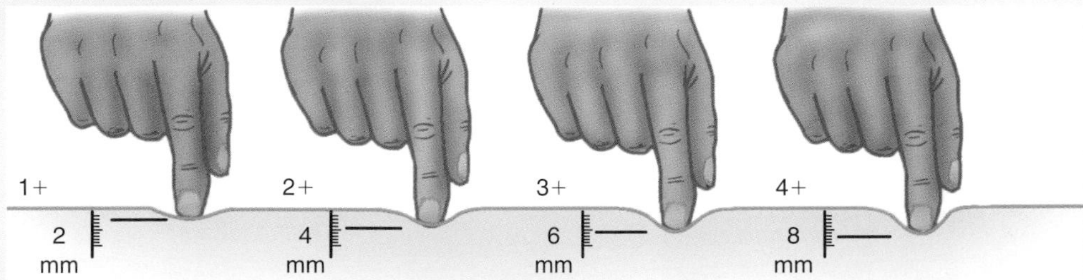

STEP 4c Assessing for pitting edema. *(From Ball JW et al.: Seidel's guide to physical examination, ed 9, St Louis, 2019, Elsevier.)*

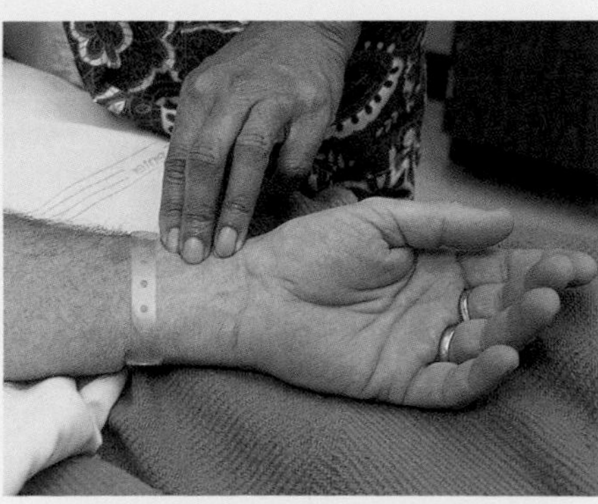

STEP 4g(2) Palpation of radial pulse.

STEP	RATIONALE
(3) Palpate ulnar pulse by placing fingertips along ulnar side of forearm (see illustration).	Palpated when arterial insufficiency to hand is expected or when you assess for radial occlusion (e.g., during arterial blood gas sampling), which may affect circulation to hand.
(4) Palpate brachial pulse by locating groove between biceps and triceps muscles above elbow at antecubital fossa (see illustration). Place tips of first two fingers in muscle groove.	Artery runs along medial side of extended arm, requiring moderate palpation. If difficult to palpate, hyperextend arm to bring pulse site closer to the surface.
(5) Have patient lie supine with feet relaxed and palpate dorsalis pedis pulse. Gently place fingertips between great and first toe; slowly move fingers along groove between extensor tendons of great and first toe until pulse is palpable (see illustration).	Artery lies superficially and does not require deep palpation. Pulse may be congenitally absent.
(6) Palpate posterior tibial pulse by having patient relax and extend feet slightly. Place fingertips behind and below medial malleolus (ankle bone) (see illustration).	Artery is easily palpable with foot relaxed.
(7) Palpate popliteal pulse by having patient slightly flex knee with foot resting on table or bed. Instruct patient to keep leg muscles relaxed. Palpate deeply into popliteal fossa with fingers of both hands placed just lateral to midline. Patient may also lie prone to achieve exposure of artery (see illustration).	Flexion of knee and muscle relaxation improves accessibility of artery. Popliteal pulse is one of the more difficult pulses to palpate.

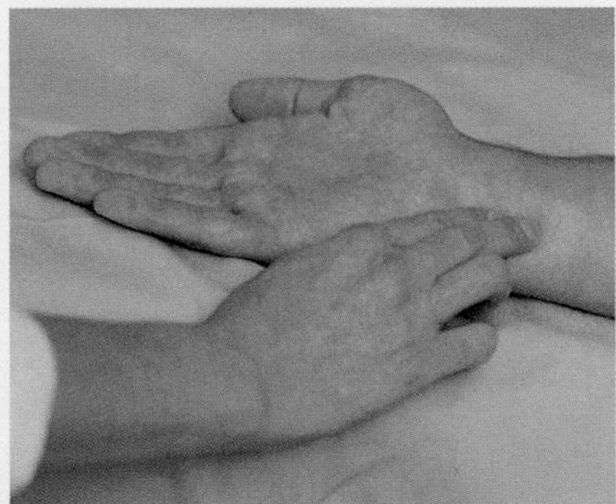

STEP 4g(3) Palpation of ulnar pulse.

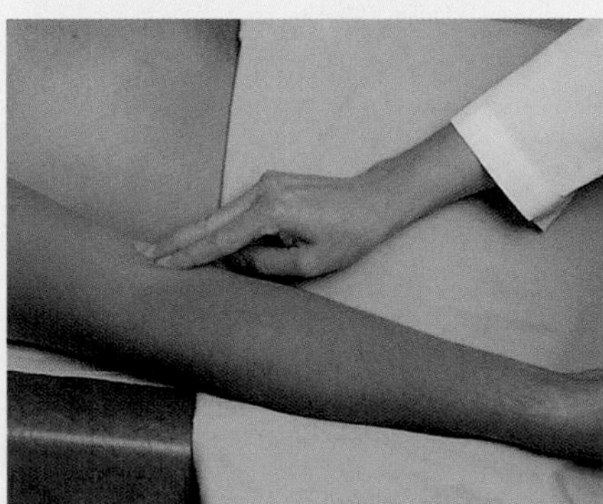

STEP 4g(4) Palpation of brachial pulse.

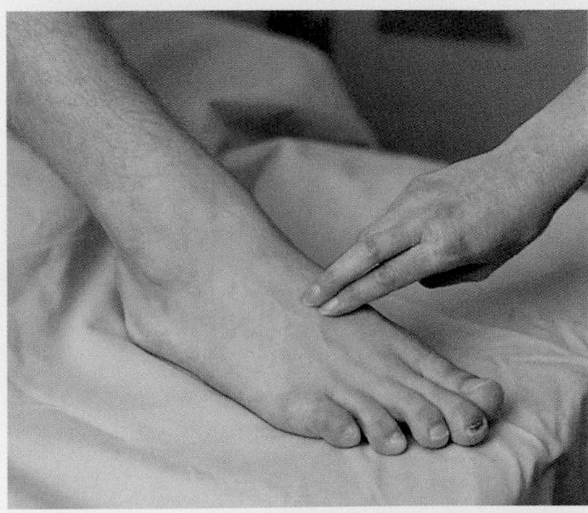

STEP 4g(5) Palpation of dorsalis pedis pulse.

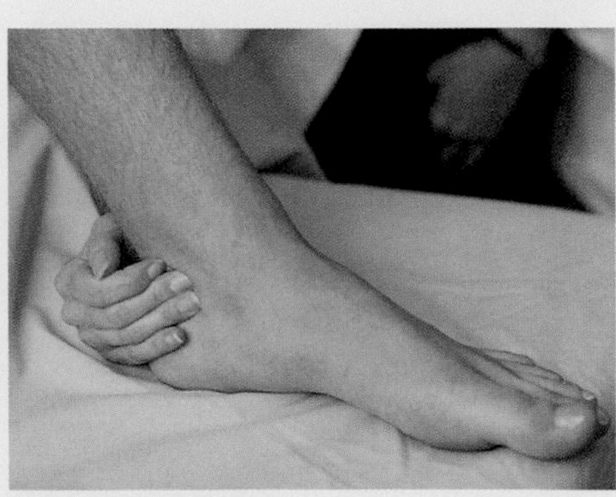

STEP 4g(6) Palpation of posterior tibial pulse.

STEP	RATIONALE
(8) Apply clean gloves. With patient supine, palpate femoral pulse by placing first two fingers over inguinal area below inguinal ligament, midway between pubic symphysis and anterosuperior iliac spine (see illustration). You can locate the anatomy using the mnemonic NAVEL: *N*, nerve; *A*, artery; *V*, vein; *E*, empty space; *L*, lymph nodes (Wilson and Giddens, 2017).	Supine position prevents flexion in groin area, which interferes with artery access.
h. If pulses are difficult to palpate or are not palpable, use a Doppler instrument over pulse site (see illustration).	Doppler amplifies sounds, allowing you to hear low-velocity blood flow through peripheral arteries.
(1) Apply conducting gel to patient's skin over pulse site or onto transducer tip of probe. Turn Doppler on.	
(2) Gently apply ultrasound probe to skin, changing Doppler angle until pulsation is audible. Adjust volume as needed. Wipe off gel from patient and Doppler.	
5. Applying a cardiac monitor:	
a. Clean and prepare chest area for electrode placement with soap and water. Wipe area with rough washcloth or gauze or use edge of electrode to gently scape area. Clip excessive hair from electrode area rather than shaving.	Proper skin preparation before electrodes are placed decreases skin impedance and signal noise, thereby producing a clean and accurate recording. Do not use alcohol to clean area because it is drying to the skin. Roughening the skin helps remove epidermis outer layer to allow electrical signals to travel. Clipping hair reduces the risk for infection.
b. Apply electrodes in correct position for either a three- or five-electrode system (Fig. 8.5).	Proper placement of leads is very important for accurate dysrhythmia interpretation.

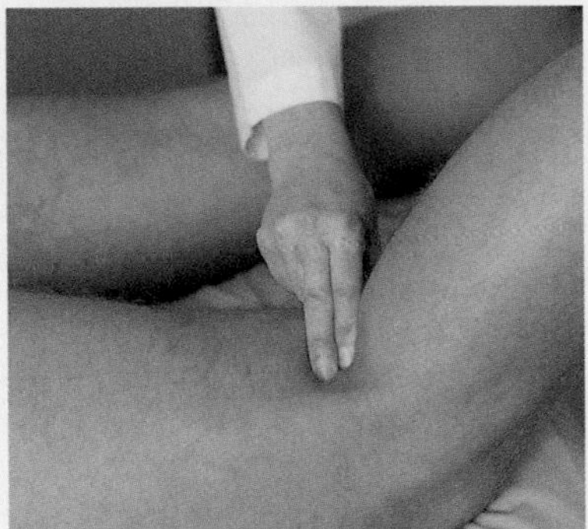

STEP 4g(7) Palpation of popliteal pulse with patient prone.

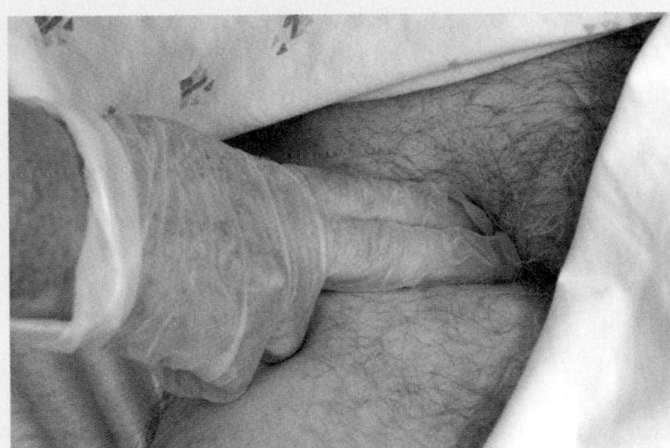

STEP 4g(8) Palpation of femoral pulse.

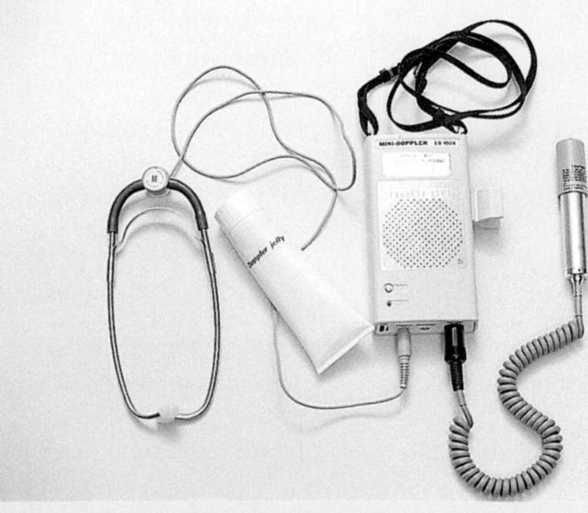

STEP 4h Doppler equipment to assess brachial pulse. *(From Wilson SF, Giddens J:* Health assessment for nursing practice, *ed 6, St. Louis, 2016, Elsevier.)*

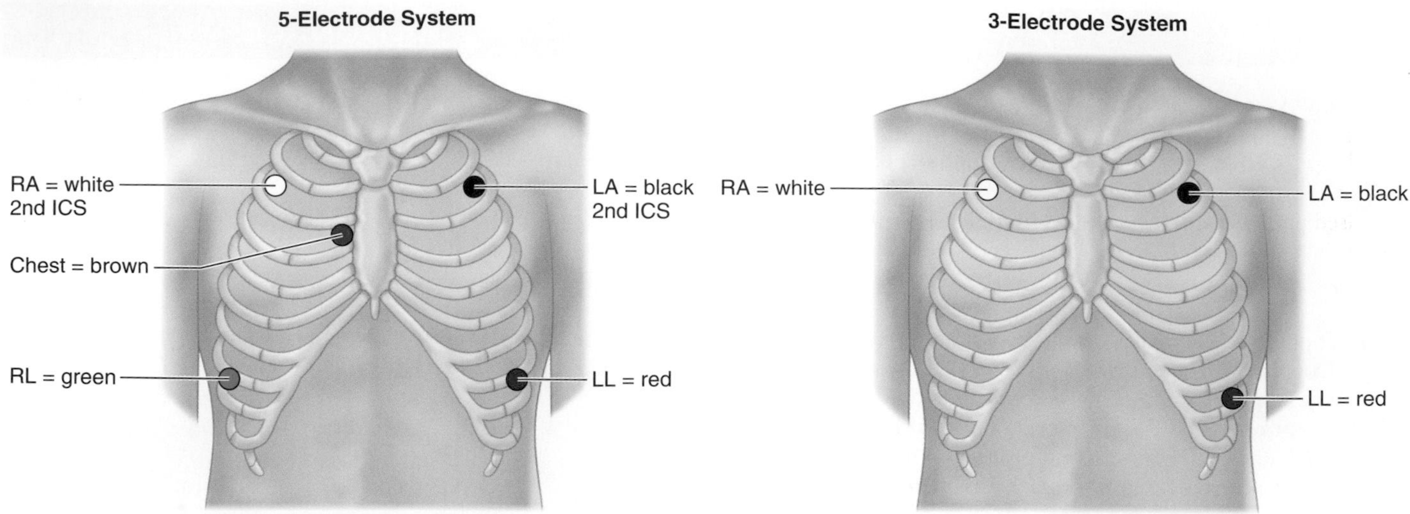

FIG 8.5 Cardiac monitor lead placement: three- or five-electrode system. *ICS*, Intercostal space; *LA*, left arm; *LL*, left leg; *RA*, right arm; *RL*, right leg.

STEP	RATIONALE
c. Attach monitor leads to electrodes. Colors of leads represent their polarity. White is negative. Black is positive. Red is ground or neutral. Two additional leads on five-lead system would include a green lead (positive or negative) and a brown lead (positive), which can be placed at a V lead location on precordial chest.	Coloring system allows for consistent application of leads.
d. Check bedside monitor or telemetry station for any messages indicating electrode or lead issues. Troubleshoot as needed.	Monitoring system itself may detect bad electrode contact with skin or a loose connection.
e. Check that the electrocardiogram rhythm can be visualized on bedside monitor, central station, or remote viewing station.	If monitor is being viewed remotely, communicate with staff before leaving room to correct any connection issues. This call can serve as notification that monitoring has begun.
f. Change electrodes daily or more often if contact to skin is loose.	Changing electrodes decreases the number of false alarms.
g. Customize alarm limits within 1 hour of assuming care of patient and on condition changes. Changes made should be in accordance with agency policies and health care provider's orders.	Customize alarms to individual patient needs to reduce false alarms and focus true alarms on reasons for monitoring.
6. Help patient to comfortable position.	Gives patient sense of well-being.
7. Be sure nurse call system is in an accessible location within patient's reach.	Ensures patient can call for assistance if needed.
8. Raise side rails (as appropriate) and lower bed to lowest position.	Ensures patient safety.
9. Remove gloves and discard used supplies and gloves in proper receptacle. Perform hand hygiene.	Reduces transmission of microorganisms.

EVALUATION

1. Compare findings with normal assessment characteristics of heart and vascular system.	Determines presence of abnormalities.
2. If heart sounds are not audible or pulses are not palpable, ask another nurse to confirm assessment.	Validates abnormal assessment findings.
3. Ask patient to describe behaviors that increase risk for heart and vascular disease.	Demonstrates learning.
4. Compare pulses and capillary refill bilaterally with previous assessment.	Demonstrates change from baseline measures.

STEP	RATIONALE
5. **Use Teach-Back:** "I would like to make sure you understand some of the risks and behaviors that can lead to heart disease. Tell me how your lack of exercise affects your risk for heart disease." Revise your instruction now or develop a plan for revised patient/family caregiver teaching if patient/family caregiver is not able to teach back correctly.	Determines patient's/family caregiver's level of understanding of instructional topic.

Unexpected Outcomes	Related Interventions
1. Findings differ from previous assessments, including: • Pulsations, vibrations, or both are palpable. These are result of valvular problem, murmur, or both. • Extra heart sounds S_3 or S_4 are auscultated. Extra sounds indicate atrial or ventricular gallop. • Murmur is auscultated. Impaired blood flow through heart indicates need for immediate medical attention. Some murmurs are benign. • JVP is elevated. This is sign of right-sided heart failure or fluid overload.	• Prepare to obtain or help with electrocardiogram (ECG).
2. Heart rate is irregular, with rate less than 60 beats/min or more than 100 beats/min.	• Check blood pressure. If low, dysrhythmia is contributing to inadequate cardiac output. • Observe for sensations or reports of dizziness or feeling "faint." • Prepare to obtain ECG.
3. Pulse deficit is noted. There is risk for inadequate cardiac output.	• Obtain vital signs.

Recording

- Record quality (clear or muffled), intensity (weak or pounding), rate, and rhythm (regular, regularly irregular, or irregularly irregular) of heart sounds and peripheral pulses.
- Document additional cardiac findings, jugular venous pressure, and condition of extremities.
- Document activity level and subjective data related to fatigue, shortness of breath, and chest pain.
- Document your evaluation of patient and family caregiver learning.

Hand-Off Reporting

- Report immediately to health care provider any irregularities in heart function and indications of impaired arterial blood flow.
- Report to health care provider any changes in peripheral circulation, which may indicate circulatory compromise, which may result in permanent nerve damage or tissue death if untreated.

✦ SKILL 8.5 Assessing the Abdomen

Purpose

Abdominal assessment is complex because of the multiple organs located within and near the abdominal cavity. Abdominal pain is one of the most common symptoms patients report when seeking medical care. An accurate assessment requires matching a patient's history with a careful assessment of the location of physical symptoms (Table 8.10). To perform an effective abdominal assessment, you need to know the location and function of the underlying structures involved, including the lower pelvis, kidneys, rectum, genitalia, liver, gallbladder, stomach, spleen, pancreas, intestines, and reproductive organs (Fig. 8.6). An abdominal assessment is routine after abdominal surgery, for any patient who has undergone invasive diagnostic tests of the gastrointestinal (GI) tract, and for patients with abnormalities affecting GI function. The order of an abdominal assessment differs from that of other assessments. You begin with inspection and follow with auscultation. It is important to auscultate before palpation and percussion because these maneuvers alter the frequency and character of bowel sounds.

Delegation and Collaboration

The skill of abdominal assessment cannot be delegated to nursing assistive personnel (NAP). The nurse directs the NAP to:

- Report the development of abdominal pain and changes in the patient's bowel habits or dietary intake to the nurse.

Equipment

- Stethoscope
- Tape measure
- Examination light
- Water-based marking pen
- Drapes

TABLE 8.10
Common Causes of Abdominal Pain

Condition	Physical Alteration	Physical Signs and Symptoms
Appendicitis	Obstruction of appendix associated with inflammation, perforation, and peritonitis; patient often lies on back or side with knees flexed to decrease pain	Sharp pain directly over irritated peritoneum 2–12 hours after onset. Often pain localizes in right lower quadrant between anterior iliac crest and umbilicus. Associated with rebound tenderness. Accompanied by anorexia, nausea, and vomiting.
Celiac disease	Damage to small intestinal mucosa from ingestion of barley, oats, rye, and wheat	Foul-smelling diarrhea, abdominal distention, and symptoms of malnutrition may be present.
Cholecystitis	Obstruction of the cystic duct causing inflammation or distention of gallbladder	*Murphy's sign:* Apply gentle pressure below right subcostal arch and below liver margin. Sharp pain and increased respiratory rate occur when patient takes a deep breath (Ball et al., 2019).
Constipation	Disruption in normal bowel pattern that may occur with opioid use or inadequate fiber and fluid intake	Generalized discomfort accompanied by distention and palpation of a hard mass in left lower quadrant. Nausea and vomiting may begin after several days.
Crohn's disease	Chronic inflammatory lesion of the ileum	Steady colicky pain in right lower quadrant, with cramping, tenderness, flatulence, nausea, fever, and diarrhea. Often associated with bloody stools, weight loss, weakness, and fatigue.
Gastroenteritis	Inflammation of stomach and intestinal tract	Generalized abdominal discomfort accompanied by anorexia, nausea, vomiting, diarrhea, and abdominal cramping.
Pancreatitis	Inflammation of pancreas associated with alcoholism and gallbladder disease	Steady severe epigastric pain close to the umbilicus radiates to the back. Associated with abdominal rigidity and vomiting. Pain is unrelieved by vomiting and worsens by lying supine.
Paralytic ileus	Obstruction of small bowel that occurs after abdominal surgery or use of anticholinergic medications	Generalized severe abdominal distention, nausea, and vomiting. Decreased or absent bowel sounds.
Peptic ulcers (gastric and duodenal)	Damage of GI mucosa at any area of GI tract; may be caused by bacterial infection (*Helicobacter pylori*) or nonsteroidal antiinflammatory drugs; thought to be unrelated to stress; aggravated by smoking and excessive alcohol use	*Gastric ulcer:* Dull epigastric pain, localized midline. Early satiety; not usually relieved by food or antacids. *Duodenal ulcer:* Pain is episodic, lasting 30 minutes to 2 hours. Pain is located in midline epigastric region; described as aching, burning, or gnawing. Typically occurs 1–3 hours after meals and at night (12 midnight to 3 AM). Often relieved by food or antacid.

GI, Gastrointestinal.

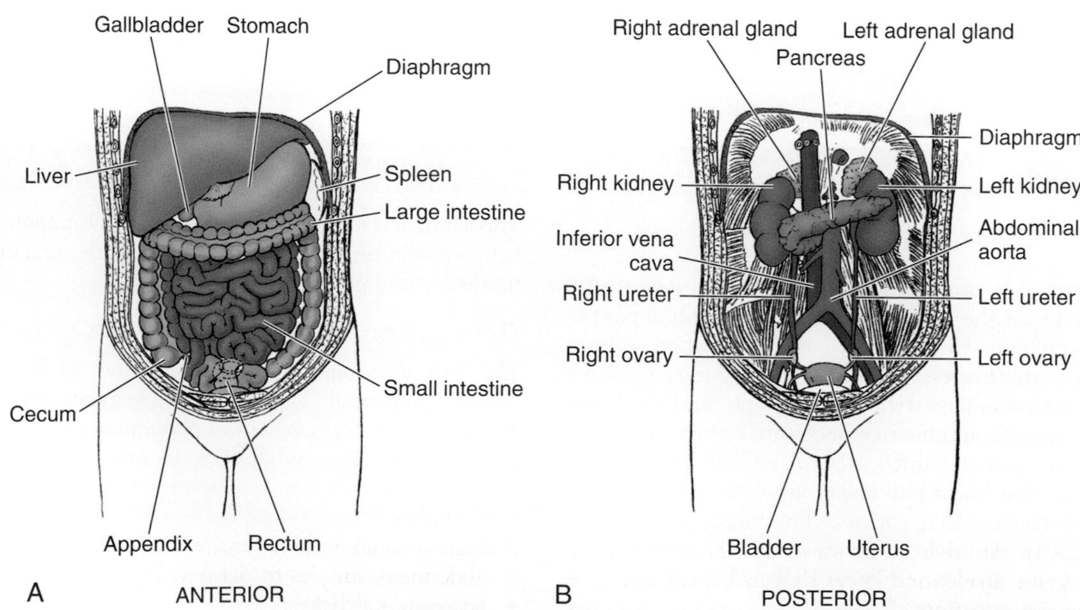

FIG 8.6 Location of organs in the abdomen. (A) Anterior. (B) Posterior. *(Modified from* Mosby's expert 10-minute physical examinations, *ed 2, St. Louis, 2005, Mosby.)*

ASSESSMENT

1. If patient has abdominal or low back pain, assess the character of pain in detail (location, onset, frequency, precipitating factors, aggravating factors, type of pain, severity, length of time). *Rationale: Knowing pattern of characteristics of pain helps determine its source.*
2. Carefully observe patient's movement and position, such as lying still with knees drawn up, moving restlessly to find a comfortable position, or lying on one side or sitting with knees drawn up to chest. *Rationale: Positions assumed by patient reveal nature and source of pain (e.g., peritonitis, kidney stone, appendicitis). Patients with peritonitis lie still because movement aggravates pain. Supine position worsens acute pancreatitis pain; flexed knee, curved-back position brings relief. Patients with appendicitis lie on side or back with knees flexed in attempt to decrease muscle strain on abdominal wall.*
3. Assess patient's normal bowel habits: frequency of stools; character of stools; recent changes in character of stools; measures used to promote elimination such as laxatives, enemas, and dietary intake; and eating and drinking habits. *Rationale: Data compared with information from physical assessment may help identify cause and nature of elimination problems.*
4. Determine if patient has had abdominal surgery, trauma, or diagnostic tests of GI tract. *Rationale: Surgery or trauma to abdomen may result in altered position of underlying organs. Diagnostic tests may change character of stool.*
5. Assess if patient has had recent weight changes or intolerance to diet (nausea, vomiting, cramping, especially in past 24 hours). *Rationale: Changes may indicate alterations in upper GI tract (e.g., stomach or gallbladder) or lower colon.*
6. Assess for difficulty in swallowing, belching, flatulence, bloody emesis (hematemesis), black or tarry stools (melena), heartburn, diarrhea, or constipation. *Rationale: Indicative of GI alterations.*
7. Determine if patient takes antiinflammatory medications (e.g., aspirin, steroids, and nonsteroidal antiinflammatory drugs [NSAIDs]), or antibiotics. *Rationale: These medications may cause GI upset or bleeding.*
8. Review family history of cancer, kidney disease, alcoholism, hypertension, or heart disease. *Rationale: Information may reveal risk for significant abdominal alterations. Chronic alcohol ingestion causes GI and liver problems.*
9. Review patient's history for health care occupation, hemodialysis, intravenous drug use, household or sexual contact with hepatitis B virus (HBV) carrier, sexually active heterosexual person (more than one sex partner in previous 6 months), sexually active homosexual or bisexual man, international traveler in area of high HBV prevalence. *Rationale: These are risk factors for HBV exposure. Abdominal findings for hepatitis include jaundice, hepatomegaly, anorexia, abdominal and gastric discomfort, tea-colored urine, and clay-colored stools (Lewis et al., 2017).*
10. Assess patient's/family caregiver's knowledge, experience, and health literacy. *Rationale: Ensures patient/family caregiver has the capacity to obtain, communicate, process, and understand basic health information (CDC, 2016a).*

STEP	RATIONALE
PLANNING	
1. Expected outcomes following completion of procedure:	
• Abdomen is soft and symmetrical, with smooth and even contour. No mass, distention, or tenderness is palpable. There are no forceful visible pulsations.	These are normal abdominal assessment findings.
• Bowel sounds are active and audible in all four quadrants.	Indicates normal peristaltic activity.
• No costovertebral angle (CVA) tenderness is present.	Indicates no inflammation of kidney.
• Patient denies discomfort or worsening of existing discomfort following examination.	Proper examination procedures have been implemented.
• Patient can list warning signs of colorectal cancer.	Demonstrates learning.
2. Anticipate teaching topics during the examination that you can teach patient about warning signs of colorectal cancer.	Allows you to incorporate instruction during physical assessment.
3. Provide privacy and prepare environment.	Providing privacy and preparing the environment early help the student/nurse think about the need to remove clutter from the over-bed or bedside table.
4. Perform hand hygiene. Prepare patient for abdominal assessment:	
a. Ask if patient needs to empty bladder or defecate.	Palpation of full bladder causes discomfort and feeling of urgency and makes it difficult for patient to relax.
b. Keep upper chest and legs draped.	Maintains patient's comfort during examination, promoting relaxation.
c. Be sure that room is warm.	Promotes patient's comfort. Reduces risk of patient tensing abdominal muscles.
d. Have patient lie supine or in dorsal recumbent position with arms down at sides and knees slightly bent. Place small pillow under patient's knees.	Placing arms under head or keeping knees fully extended causes abdominal muscles to tighten. Tightening of muscles prevents adequate palpation.
e. Move sheet or blanket to expose area from just above xiphoid process down to symphysis pubis.	Provides full visualization of abdomen.

STEP	RATIONALE
f. Maintain conversation during assessment except during auscultation. Explain steps calmly and slowly.	Patient's ability to relax during assessment improves accuracy of findings. Talking interferes with hearing bowel sounds.
g. Ask patient to point to tender areas.	Assess painful areas last. Manipulation of body part increases patient's pain and anxiety and makes remainder of assessment difficult to complete.

IMPLEMENTATION

1. Abdominal assessment:	
a. Identify landmarks that divide abdominal region into quadrants. Boundary begins at tip of xiphoid process to symphysis pubis with line crossing and intersecting umbilicus, dividing abdomen into four equal sections (see illustration).	Location of findings by common reference point helps successive examiners confirm findings and locate abnormalities.
b. Inspect skin of surface of abdomen for color, scars, venous patterns, rashes, lesions, silvery white striae (stretch marks), and artificial openings (stomas). Observe skin lesions for descriptive characteristics described in Skill 8.1.	Scars reveal evidence that patient has had past trauma or surgery. Striae indicate stretching of tissue from growth, obesity, pregnancy, ascites, or edema. Venous patterns reflect liver disease (portal hypertension). Artificial openings indicate bowel or urinary diversion (see Chapters 19, 20, and 21).
c. If you note bruising, ask if patient self-administers injections (e.g., heparin or insulin).	Frequent injections may cause bruising and hardening of underlying tissues.

Safe Patient Care *Bruising may also indicate physical signs of abuse, accidental injury, or bleeding disorder. When bruising is noted, additional information may be needed from the patient.*

d. Inspect contour, symmetry, and surface motion of abdomen. Note any masses, bulging, or distention. (Flat abdomen forms a horizontal plane from xiphoid process to symphysis pubis. Round abdomen protrudes in convex sphere from horizontal plane. Concave abdomen sinks into muscular wall. All are normal.)	Changes in symmetry or contour reveal underlying masses, fluid collection, or gaseous distention. Everted umbilicus (protruding outward) indicates distention. Hernia also causes umbilicus to protrude upward.
e. If abdomen appears distended, note if distention is generalized. Look at flanks on each side.	Distention may be caused by the nine F's (*f*at, *f*latus, *f*eces, *f*luids, *f*ibroid, *f*ull bladder, *f*alse pregnancy, *f*atal tumor, and *f*etus) (Ball et al., 2019). If gas causes distention, flanks do not bulge. If fluid causes distention, flanks bulge. Tumor may cause more unilateral bulging or distention. Pregnancy causes symmetrical bulge in lower abdomen.
f. If you suspect distention, measure size of abdominal girth by placing tape measure under patient and around abdomen at level of umbilicus (see illustration). Use marking pen to indicate where tape measure was applied.	Consecutive measurements show any increase or decrease in abdominal distention. Make all subsequent measurements at same level of umbilicus to provide objective means to evaluate changes. Use water-based pen to make mark on abdomen for subsequent measurements.

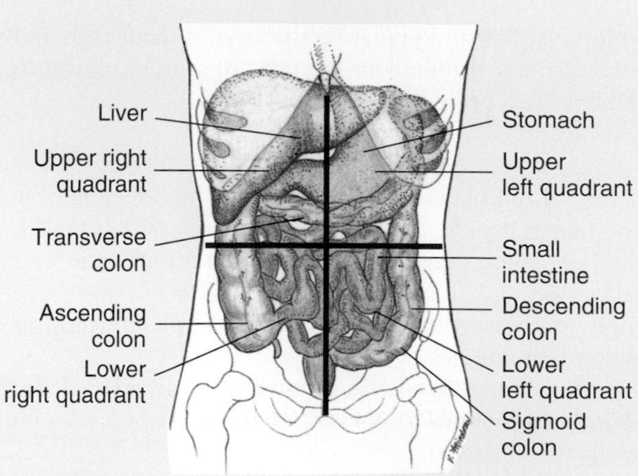

STEP 1a Division of abdomen into quadrants.

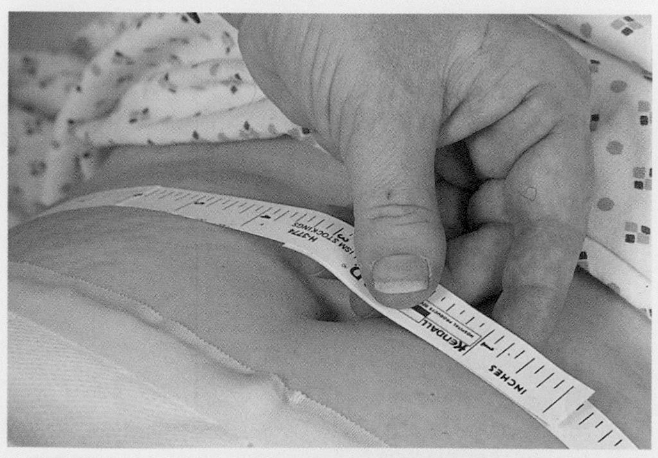

STEP 1f Measuring abdominal girth at level of umbilicus.

STEP	RATIONALE
g. If patient has an NG or NI tube connected to suction, turn off momentarily.	Sound of suction obscures bowel sounds.
h. To auscultate bowel sounds, place diaphragm of stethoscope lightly over each of four abdominal quadrants. Ask patient not to talk. Listen until you hear repeated gurgling or bubbling sounds in each quadrant (minimum of once in 5–20 seconds). Describe sounds as normal, hyperactive, hypoactive, or absent. Listen 5 minutes over each quadrant before deciding that bowel sounds are absent (see illustration).	Normal bowel sounds occur irregularly every 5 to 15 seconds. Absence of sounds indicates cessation of gastric motility. Hyperactive bowel sounds not related to hunger or recent meal may indicate diarrhea or early intestinal obstruction. Hypoactive or absent bowel sounds indicate paralytic ileus or peritonitis. It is common for bowel sounds to be hypoactive after surgery for 24 hours or more, especially following abdominal surgery.

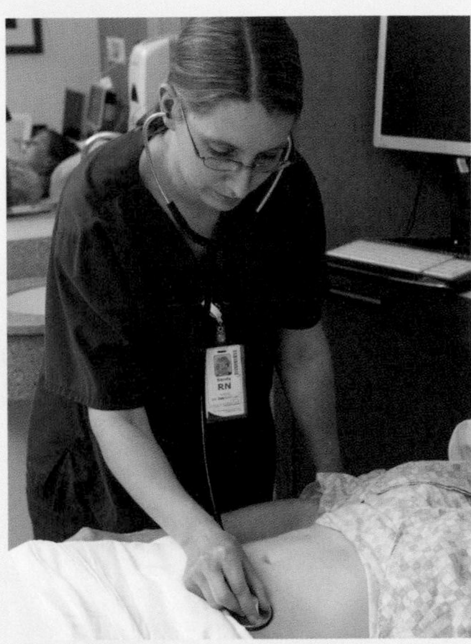

STEP 1h Auscultating bowel sounds.

Safe Patient Care *Nausea and vomiting, increasing distention, and inability to pass flatus may accompany severe paralytic ileus.*

STEP	RATIONALE
i. Place bell of stethoscope over epigastric region of abdomen and each quadrant. Auscultate for vascular (whooshing) sounds.	Determines presence of turbulent blood flow (bruit) through thoracic or abdominal aorta, which may indicate an aneurysm.

Safe Patient Care *If aortic bruit is auscultated, suggesting presence of an aneurysm, stop assessment and notify health care provider immediately. Percussion or palpation over abdominal bruit could cause rupture of an already weakened vessel wall in the presence of an abdominal aneurysm.*

STEP	RATIONALE
j. With patient supine, gently percuss each of four abdominal quadrants systematically. Note areas of tympany and dullness.	Reveals presence of air or fluid in stomach and intestines. Normal percussion is tympanic because of swallowed air in GI tract. Presence of fluid or underlying masses is revealed by dull percussion.
k. Ask patient if abdomen feels unusually tight and determine if this is a recent development.	Continued sensation of fullness helps detect distention. Feeling of fullness after heavy meal causes only temporary distention. Tightness is not felt with obesity.
l. With patient sitting, gently but firmly percuss over each CVA along scapular lines (see illustration *A*). Use ulnar surface of fist indirectly by placing nondominant hand flat against CVA and percussing with dominant hand or percuss directly against patient's skin (see illustration *B*). Note if patient experiences pain.	Determines presence of kidney inflammation.
m. Lightly palpate over each abdominal quadrant, laying palm of hand with fingers extended and approximated lightly on abdomen. Keep palm and forearm horizontal. Pads of fingertips depress skin no more than 1 cm (½ inch) in gentle dipping motion (see illustration). Palpate painful areas last.	Detects areas of localized tenderness, degree of tenderness, and presence and character of underlying masses or fluid. Palpation of sensitive area causes guarding (voluntary tightening of underlying abdominal muscles).

STEP	RATIONALE
(1) Note muscular resistance, distention, tenderness, and superficial masses or organs while observing patient's face for signs of discomfort.	Patient's verbal and nonverbal cues may indicate discomfort from tenderness. Firm abdomen indicates active obstruction with buildup of fluid or gas.
(2) Note if abdomen is firm or soft to touch.	Soft abdomen is normal or reveals that obstruction is resolving.
n. Just below umbilicus and above symphysis pubis, palpate for smooth, rounded mass. While applying light pressure, ask if patient has sensation of need to void.	Detects presence of dome of distended bladder.

Safe Patient Care *Routinely check for distended bladder if patient has been unable to void, patient has been incontinent, or an indwelling Foley catheter is not draining well or has been removed recently.*

STEP	RATIONALE
o. If masses are palpated, note size, location, shape, consistency, tenderness, mobility, and texture.	Descriptive characteristics help to reveal type of mass.
p. When tenderness is present, press one hand slowly and deeply into involved area and let go quickly. Note if pain is aggravated.	Test determines if rebound tenderness is present. Results are positive if pain increases. This indicates peritoneal irritation such as appendicitis (Wilson and Giddens, 2017).
2. Help patient to comfortable position.	Gives patient sense of well-being.

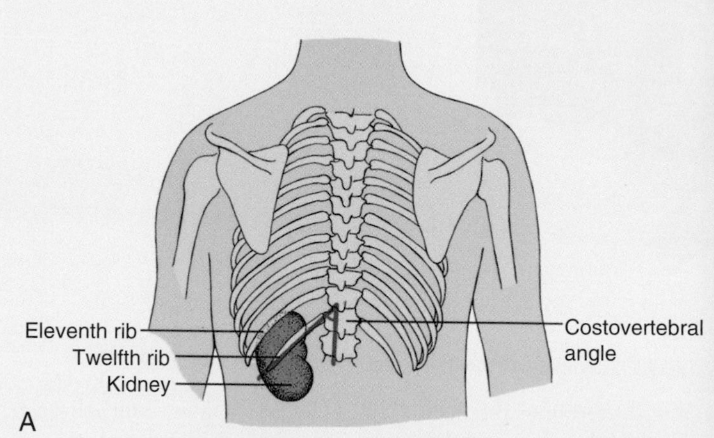

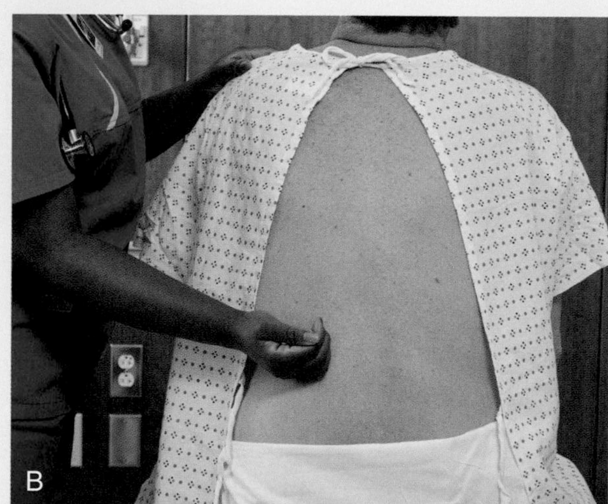

STEP 1l (A) Position of kidney in relation to costovertebral angle. (B) Direct percussion of kidney for costovertebral angle tenderness. *(**A** From Seidel HM, et al.:* Mosby's guide to physical examination, *ed 6, St. Louis, 2006, Mosby.)*

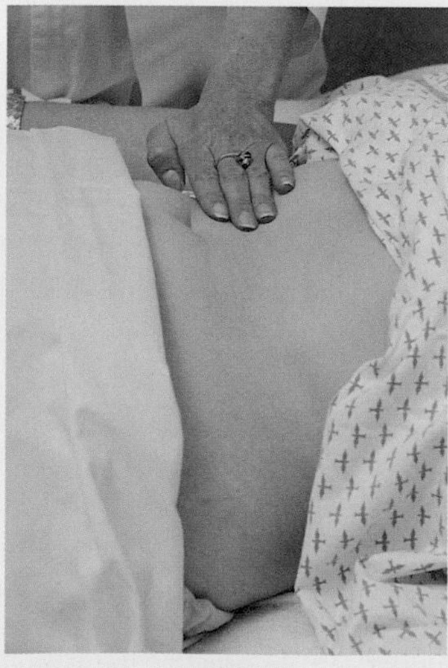

STEP 1m Light palpation of abdomen.

STEP	RATIONALE
3. Be sure nurse call system is in an accessible location within patient's reach.	Ensures patient can call for assistance if needed.
4. Raise side rails (as appropriate) and lower bed to lowest position.	Ensures patient safety.
5. Remove gloves and perform hand hygiene.	Reduces transmission of microorganisms.

EVALUATION

1. Compare assessment findings with previous assessment characteristics to identify changes.	Determines presence of abnormalities.
2. Ask patient to describe signs and symptoms of colorectal cancer.	Demonstrates learning.
3. **Use Teach-Back:** "I would like to make sure that you understand the signs and symptoms of colorectal cancer. Tell me three changes in how your bowel functions that might be signs of colorectal cancer." Revise your instruction now or develop a plan for revised patient/family caregiver teaching if patient/family caregiver is not able to teach back correctly.	Determines patient's/family caregiver's level of understanding of instructional topic.

Unexpected Outcomes	Related Interventions
1. Abdomen protrudes symmetrically with skin taut; patient complains of tightness, and/or bowel sounds are absent. GI motility has ceased. Patient is vomiting. Signs suggest an obstruction.	• Keep patient on nothing by mouth (NPO) status and encourage ambulation. • Notify health care provider. • Gastric decompression following insertion of NG tube sometimes may be necessary.
2. Hyperactive bowel sounds are evident with GI motility. Commonly they result from anxiety, diarrhea, overuse of laxatives, inflammation of bowel, or reaction of intestines to certain foods.	• Patient may need to be NPO. • Contact health care provider to consider ordering antidiarrheal medication.
3. Bladder is palpable over symphysis pubis and distended.	• Facilitate voiding by placing patient in sitting position or encouraging him or her to bear down (if not contraindicated); run water within hearing distance, or have patient place hand in basin of warm water. • Use bladder scan to determine extent of bladder fullness (see Chapter 19). • If unable to void, urinary catheterization is necessary (see Chapter 19).

Recording

- Document appearance of abdomen, quality of bowel sounds, presence of distention, abdominal circumference, and presence of tenderness.
- Record patient's ability to void and defecate, including description of output.
- Document evaluation of patient and family caregiver learning.

Hand-Off Reporting

- Report serious abnormalities, such as absent bowel sounds or presence of mass or acute pain, to nurse in charge and health care provider.

✦ SKILL 8.6 Assessing the Genitalia and Rectum

Purpose

The best time to examine a patient's external genitalia is while performing routine hygiene measures or preparing to insert or care for a urinary catheter. An examination of female and male external genitalia is part of preventive health screenings. Male patients need to learn how to perform self-examinations of the genitalia to detect testicular cancer (ACS, 2018) (Box 8.6). You examine adolescents and young adults because of the growing incidence of sexually transmitted infections (STIs). The average age of menarche among females has declined, and the average age that both males and females become sexually active is 19 (Hockenberry and Wilson, 2017). You can easily combine rectal and anal assessments with this examination

BOX 8.6

Genital Self-Examination

All males 15 years old and older should perform this examination monthly. Perform it after a warm bath or shower when the scrotal sac is relaxed. Call your health care provider if you find a lump or any other abnormality.

Genital Examination

1. Perform the examination after a warm bath or shower when the scrotal skin is less thick.
2. Stand naked in front of a mirror, hold the penis in your hand, and examine the head. Pull back the foreskin if uncircumcised to expose the glans.
3. Inspect and palpate the entire head of the penis in a clockwise motion, looking carefully for any bumps, sores, or blisters.
4. Look for any genital warts.
5. Look at the opening (urethral meatus) at the end of the penis for discharge.
6. Look along the entire shaft of the penis for the same signs.
7. Separate pubic hair at the base of the penis and carefully examine the skin underneath.

Testicular Examination

1. Look for swelling or lumps in the skin of the scrotum while looking in the mirror.
2. Use both hands, placing the index and middle fingers under the testicles and the thumb on top.
3. Gently roll the testicle, feeling for hard lumps; smooth, rounded bumps; or thickening.
4. Find the epididymis (feels like a small "bump" on the upper or middle outer side of the testis).
5. Feel for small, pea-sized lumps on the front and side of the testicle. The lumps are usually painless and are abnormal.
6. Instruct patient to call the health care provider if abnormalities are noted.
7. **Use Teach-Back:** "I want to be sure I explained to you how to do a genital and testicular self-examination. Describe for me the steps you will follow to examine your own genitals for cancer." Document your evaluation of patient learning. Revise your instruction now or develop a plan for revised patient teaching if patient is not able to teach back correctly.

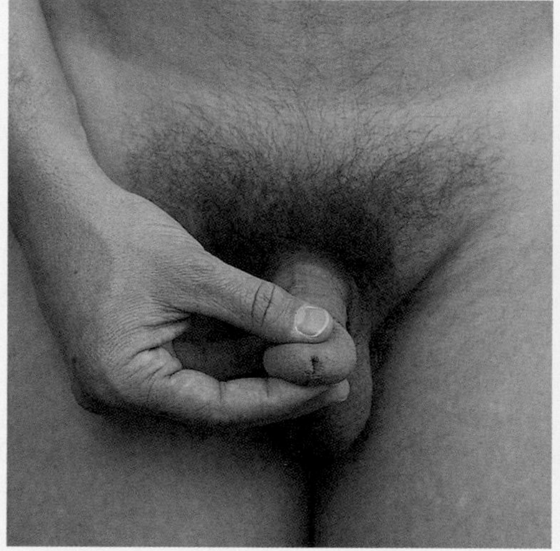

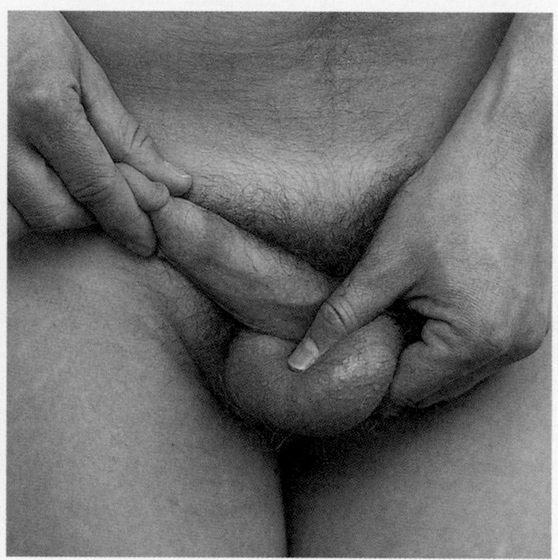

Data from America Cancer Society (ACS): Overview guide for testicular cancer, Atlanta, 2016, The Society. http://www.cancer.org/cancer/testicularcancer/detailedguide/testicular-cancer-detection.
Figures from Ball JW, et al.: *Seidel's guide to physical examination,* ed 9, St. Louis, 2019, Elsevier.

because the patient assumes a lithotomy or dorsal recumbent position.

Delegation and Collaboration

The skill of assessing the genitalia and rectum cannot be delegated to nursing assistive personnel (NAP). The nurse directs the NAP to:

- Report changes in patient's genitourinary function and presence of drainage in the perineal area.

Equipment

- Examination light
- Clean gloves (use nonlatex if necessary)
- Drapes

ASSESSMENT

1. Assessment of female patients:
   a. Determine if patient has signs and symptoms of vaginal discharge, painful or swollen perianal tissues, or genital lesions. *Rationale: These signs and symptoms are consistent with an STI or other pathological condition.*
   b. Determine if patient has symptoms or history of genitourinary problems, including burning during urination (dysuria), frequency, urgency, nocturia, hematuria, or incontinence. *Rationale: Urinary problems are associated with gynecological disorders, including STIs.*
   c. Ask if the patient has had signs of bleeding outside of normal menstrual cycle or after menopause or unusual vaginal discharge. *Rationale: These are warning signs for cervical and endometrial cancer or vaginal infection.*
   d. Determine if patient has received human papillomavirus (HPV) vaccine. *Rationale: Meites et al. (2016) recommend that all 11- or 12-year-old girls get the three doses of HPV vaccine (Gardasil or Cervarix) or the two doses at ages 9–14 years to protect against cervical cancer. Gardasil also protects against most genital warts and some cancers of the vulva, vagina, and anus. The same recommendations for the two-dose*

and the three-dose schedules apply to girls as well as boys. Girls and young women ages 13 through 26 should get HPV vaccine if they have not received any or all doses when they were younger. Gardasil is also recommended for all boys ages 11 or 12 years and for males ages 13 through 21 years who did not get any or all of the three recommended doses when they were younger. All men should confer with their health care provider about vaccination.

e. Determine if patient has history of HPV (condyloma acuminatum, herpes simplex, or cervical dysplasia), had first pregnancy before age of 17, smokes cigarettes, is obese, eats diet low in fruits and vegetables, or has had multiple full-term pregnancies. *Rationale: These are risk factors for cervical cancer. According to the American Cancer Society, cervical cancer is the most common HPV-related cancer in women; hence, women should continue age-appropriate cervical cancer screening (ACS, 2017b).*

f. Determine if patient is older than 63; is obese; has history of ovarian dysfunction, breast or endometrial cancer, or endometriosis; has family history of reproductive cancer; has history of infertility or nulliparity; or uses estrogen (alone) as hormone replacement therapy and use of talcum powder. *Rationale: These are risk factors for ovarian cancer (ACS, 2017b).*

g. Determine if patient is postmenopausal, obese, or infertile; had early menarche or late menopause; has history of hypertension, diabetes mellitus, gallbladder disease, or polycystic ovary disease; has family history of endometrial, breast, or colon cancer; or has a history of estrogen-related exposure (estrogen-replacement therapy, tamoxifen use). *Rationale: These are risk factors for endometrial cancer. Menopausal women should be instructed to report any unexpected bleeding and spotting to their health care provider (ACS, 2017b).*

h. Determine patient's knowledge of risk factors and signs of cervical and other gynecological cancers. *Rationale: Provides baseline for patient education.*

2. Assessment of male patients:

a. Review normal elimination pattern, including frequency of voiding; history of nocturia; character and volume of urine; daily fluid intake; symptoms of burning, urgency, and frequency; difficulty starting stream; and hematuria. *Rationale: Urinary problems are directly associated with genitourinary problems because of anatomical structure of men's reproductive and urinary systems.*

b. Ask if patient has noted penile pain or swelling, genital lesions, or urethral discharge. *Rationale: These are signs and symptoms of STIs.*

c. Determine if patient has noted heaviness, painless enlargement, or irregular lumps of testis. *Rationale: These signs and symptoms are early warning signs for testicular cancer.*

d. Determine if patient reports any enlargement in inguinal area and assess if intermittent or constant, associated with straining or lifting, and painful. Assess whether coughing, lifting, or straining at stool causes pain. *Rationale: Signs and symptoms indicate potential inguinal hernia.*

e. Ask if patient has experienced weak or interrupted urine flow, inability to urinate, difficulty starting or stopping urine flow, polyuria, nocturia, hematuria, or dysuria. Determine if patient has continuing pain in lower back, pelvis, or upper thighs. *Rationale: These are warning signs of prostate cancer. Men at higher risk should have a discussion with their health care provider regarding prostate-specific antigen (PSA) screening at age 40 to 45 depending on individual risk profile (ACS, 2017b). Symptoms also may indicate infection or prostate enlargement.*

f. Assess patient's knowledge of risk factors and signs of prostate and testicular cancer. *Rationale: Provides baseline for patient education.*

3. Assessment of all patients:

a. Determine whether patient has rectal bleeding, black or tarry stools (melena), rectal pain, or change in bowel habits (constipation or diarrhea). *Rationale: These are warning signs of colorectal cancer (ACS, 2017b). These could also be signs of other gastrointestinal (GI) alterations, including ulcerative colitis or Crohn's disease.*

b. Determine whether patient has personal or strong family history of colorectal cancer, polyps, or chronic inflammatory bowel disease. Ask if patient is over age 50. *Rationale: These are risk factors for colorectal cancer (ACS, 2017b).*

c. Inquire about dietary habits, including high fat intake, diet high in processed or red meats, diet high in meats cooked at high temperatures (frying, broiling, grilling), or deficient fiber content (inadequate fruits and vegetables). *Rationale: Research studies have shown strong evidence of links between colon cancer and dietary intake of high-fat and Western diets, which include red meat, processed meats, and insufficient fiber intake (American Institute for Cancer Research, 2017; Cleveland Clinic, 2017).*

d. Determine if patient is obese, physically inactive, smokes, has type 2 diabetes, or consumes alcohol. *Rationale: These are risk factors for colorectal cancer (American Institute for Cancer Research, 2017).*

e. Assess medication history for use of laxatives or cathartic medications. *Rationale: Repeated use causes diarrhea and eventual loss of intestinal muscle tone.*

f. Assess for use of codeine or iron preparations. *Rationale: Codeine causes constipation. Iron turns stool black and tarry.*

g. Assess patient's knowledge of risks and signs of colorectal cancer. *Rationale: Provides baseline for patient education.*

4. Assess patient's/family caregiver's knowledge, experience, and health literacy. *Rationale: Ensures patient/family caregiver has the capacity to obtain, communicate, process, and understand basic health information (CDC, 2016a).*

STEP	RATIONALE

PLANNING

STEP	RATIONALE
1. Expected outcomes following completion of procedure:	
• Patient denies discomfort or worsening of existing discomfort following examination.	Proper examination procedures have been implemented.
• Patient can list warning signs of colorectal cancer: female patient: cervical, endometrial, and ovarian cancer; male patient: testicular and prostate cancer.	Demonstrates learning.
• Patient can discuss guidelines for HPV immunization.	Demonstrates learning.
2. Anticipate teaching topics so that during the examination, you can teach patient about warning signs of colorectal cancer.	Prepares you for incorporating teaching into assessment activities.
3. Provide privacy and prepare environment.	Providing privacy and preparing the environment early help the student/nurse think about the need to remove clutter from the over-bed or bedside table.
4. Perform hand hygiene. Prepare patient for assessment:	
a. Ask if patient needs to empty bladder or defecate.	Palpation of full bladder causes discomfort and feeling of urgency and makes it difficult for patient to relax.
b. Keep upper chest and legs draped and keep room warm.	Maintains patient's comfort during examination, promoting relaxation.
c. Position patient:	
(1) Female should lie in dorsal recumbent position with arms down at sides and knees slightly bent. Place small pillow under her knees.	Placing arms under head or keeping knees fully extended causes tightening of abdominal muscles.
(2) Male should lie supine with chest, abdomen, and lower legs draped; or have him stand during examination.	
d. Apply clean gloves.	

IMPLEMENTATION

STEP	RATIONALE
1. Female genitalia examination. (Use this time to discuss woman's risk for STIs and signs and symptoms of cervical, ovarian, and endometrial cancers.)	
a. Expose perineal area, repositioning sheet as needed.	
b. Inspect surface characteristics of perineum and retract labia majora; observe for inflammation, edema, lesions, or lacerations. Note if there is any vaginal discharge. Presence of discharge may indicate need for a culture.	Skin of perineum is smooth, clean, and slightly darker than other skin. Mucous membranes are dark pink and moist. Labia majora are symmetrical; may be dry or moist. Normally there is no vaginal discharge.
2. Male genitalia examination. (Use this time to discuss man's risk for STIs and signs and symptoms of testicular cancer.)	
a. Expose perineal area. Observe genitalia for rashes, excoriations, or lesions.	Normally skin is clear without lesions.
b. Inspect and palpate penile surfaces (see also Box 8.6).	
(1) Inspect corona, prepuce (foreskin), glans, urethral meatus, and shaft. Retract foreskin in uncircumcised males. Observe for discharge, lesions, edema, and inflammation. Return foreskin to normal position.	Glans should be smooth and pink along all surfaces. Urethral meatus is slitlike and normally positioned at tip of glans. Foreskin should retract easily. Area between foreskin and glans is common site for venereal lesions.
c. Inspect and palpate testicular surfaces.	
(1) Inspect size, color, shape, and symmetry; also, gently palpate for lesions and edema.	Left testicle is normally lower than right. Scrotal skin is usually loose, surface is coarse, and skin color is more deeply pigmented than body skin.
d. Palpate testes (see also Box 8.6).	
(1) Note size, shape, and consistency of tissue.	Testes are normally ovoid and approximately 2 to 4 cm (0.8–1.6 inches) in size, feel smooth and rubbery, and are free from nodules. Most common symptom of testicular cancer is irregular, nontender fixed mass.
(2) Ask if patient experiences tenderness with palpation.	Testes are normally sensitive but not tender.

STEP	RATIONALE
3. Assess rectum.	
a. Female patient remains in dorsal recumbent position or assumes side-lying (Sims') position.	These positions allow for optimum visualization of the rectum.
b. Male patient stands and bends forward with hips flexed and upper body resting across examination table; examine nonambulatory patient in Sims' position.	
c. View perianal and sacrococcygeal areas by gently retracting buttocks with your nondominant hand.	Perianal skin is smooth, more pigmented, and coarser than skin covering buttocks.
d. Inspect anal tissue for skin characteristics, lesions, external hemorrhoids (dilated veins that appear as reddened skin protrusion), inflammation, rashes, and excoriation.	Anal tissues are moist and hairless; voluntary sphincter holds anus closed.
4. Help patient to comfortable position.	Gives patient sense of well-being.
5. Be sure nurse call system is in an accessible location within patient's reach.	Ensures patient can call for assistance if needed.
6. Raise side rails (as appropriate) and lower bed to lowest position.	Ensures patient safety.
7. Remove and discard gloves. Discard disposable supplies. Perform hand hygiene.	Reduces transmission of microorganisms.

EVALUATION

1. Compare assessment findings with previous assessment characteristics to identify changes.	Determines presence of abnormalities.
2. Ask patient to list warning signs of colorectal cancer: female patient: cervical, endometrial, and ovarian cancer; male patient: testicular and prostate cancer.	Demonstrates learning.
3. Ask patient to identify guidelines for HPV vaccination.	Demonstrates learning.
4. **Use Teach-Back:** *Male patient:* "I would like to make sure that you understand the warning signs of colorectal, testicular, and prostate cancer. Tell me some of the signs and symptoms of testicular cancer." Revise your instruction now or develop a plan for revised patient teaching if patient is not able to teach back correctly. *Female patient:* "I would like to make sure that you understand the warning signs of colorectal, cervical, endometrial, and ovarian cancer. Tell me some of the signs and symptoms of cervical cancer." Revise your instruction now or develop a plan for revised patient teaching if patient is not able to teach back correctly.	Determines patient's level of understanding of instructional topic.

Unexpected Outcome	Related Interventions
1. Patient has vaginal/penile drainage and burning sensation during voiding. Women may have vaginal bleeding between menstrual periods. Symptoms may suggest STI.	• Notify health care provider. • Prepare to collect a culture of the discharge. • Provide additional education.

Recording

- Record assessment results, patient's ability to void, including description of output.
- Document your evaluation of patient learning.

Hand-Off Reporting

- Report any abnormalities, such as the presence of mass, drainage, or pain, to nurse in charge or health care provider.

✦ SKILL 8.7 Musculoskeletal and Neurological Assessment

Purpose

You use the skills of inspection and palpation during the musculoskeletal and neurological assessment. During the general survey (see Skill 8.1), you inspect a patient's gait, posture, and body position. A more thorough assessment of major bone, joint, and muscle groups and sensory, motor, and cranial nerve (CN) function is indicated in the presence of abnormalities. The assessment can be performed as you examine other body systems. For example, while assessing head and neck structures, assess neck ROM and examine selected CNs. Integrate assessment into routine activities of care (e.g., while bathing or positioning the patient). Assessment of these systems is important when a patient reports pain, loss of sensation, or impairment of muscle function. Prolonged illness or immobility may result in muscle weakness and atrophy. Neurological assessment is often conducted simultaneously because muscles may be weakened because of nerve involvement.

Delegation and Collaboration

The skill of assessing musculoskeletal and neurological function cannot be delegated to nursing assistive personnel (NAP). The nurse directs the NAP to:

- Report patients' problems with gait, balance, ROM, and muscle strength.
- Be informed of patients at risk for falls (unsteady gait, foot-dragging, weakness of lower extremities).
- Help patients with muscular weakness with transfer and ambulation.

Equipment

- Cotton balls or cotton-tipped applicators
- Penlight
- Tape measure
- Tongue blade
- Tuning fork
- Reflex hammer

ASSESSMENT

1. Review patient history for use of alcohol intake of more than two drinks/day; inadequate intake of protein, vitamin D, or calcium; thin and light body frame; family history of osteoporosis; white or Asian ancestry; sedentary lifestyle; long-term use of certain medications (e.g., corticosteroids, lithium, or heparin); and certain medical conditions (e.g., diabetes, hyperthyroidism) (Ball et al., 2019). *Rationale: These factors increase risk for osteoporosis.*
2. Determine if patient has been screened for osteoporosis. *Rationale: Women age 65 and older need routine screening for osteoporosis. There is insufficient evidence that men require this screening (Kleerekoper et al., 2017).*
3. Ask patient to describe history of changes in bone, muscle, or joint function (e.g., recent fall, trauma, lifting heavy objects, bone or joint disease with sudden or gradual onset) and location of alteration. *Rationale: History helps in assessing nature of musculoskeletal problem. It is estimated that 10 million Americans have osteoporosis. Women with myocardial infarction (MI), stroke, and breast cancer have a higher incidence. For men with prostate cancer, the incidence is also higher (National Osteoporosis Foundation [NOF], 2017).*
4. Assess height and weight. Note if there is a decrease in women older than 50 by subtracting current height from recall of maximum adult height. *Rationale: BMI less than 22 is a risk factor, and loss of height of more than 8.5 cm (3 inches) is one of the first clinical signs of osteoporosis (Touhy and Jett, 2018).*
5. Assess nature and extent of patient's musculoskeletal pain: location, duration, severity, predisposing and aggravating factors, relieving factors, and type of pain. If patient reports pain or cramping in lower extremities, ask if walking relieves or aggravates it. Assess distance walked and characteristics of pain before, during, and after activity. *Rationale: Pain frequently accompanies alterations in bone, joints, or muscle. It has implications for comfort and ability to perform activities of daily living (ADLs). Pain caused by certain vascular conditions tends to increase with activity.*
6. Determine if patient uses analgesics, antipsychotics, antidepressants, nervous system stimulants, or recreational drugs. *Rationale: These medications alter LOC or cause behavioral changes. Abuse sometimes causes tremors, ataxia, and changes in peripheral nerve function.*
7. Determine if patient has recent history of seizures/convulsions: clarify sequence of events (aura, loss of muscle tone, falling, motor activity, loss of consciousness); character of any symptoms; and relationship to time of day, fatigue, or emotional stress. *Rationale: Seizure activity often originates from central nervous system (CNS) alteration. Characteristics of seizure help determine its origin.*
8. Screen patient for headache, tremors, dizziness, vertigo, numbness or tingling of body part; visual changes; weakness; pain; or changes in speech. *Rationale: These symptoms commonly result from CNS dysfunction. Identifying patterns aids in diagnosis.*
9. Discuss with spouse, family member, or friends any recent changes in patient's behavior (e.g., increased irritability, mood swings, memory loss, change in energy level). *Rationale: Behavioral changes may result from intracranial pathology.*
10. Determine if patient has noticed change in vision (cranial nerve I), hearing (cranial nerve VIII), smell, taste (cranial nerve VII), or touch. *Rationale: Major sensory nerves originate from brainstem. These symptoms help to localize nature of problem during cranial nerve examination.*
11. If patient displays sudden acute confusion (delirium), review history for drug toxicity (e.g., anticholinergics, digoxin, antihistamines, antipsychotics, benzodiazepines, opioid analgesics, sedative/hypnotics, steroids); serious infections, metabolic disturbances (e.g., diabetes mellitus); heart failure; and severe anemia. *Rationale: Delirium is one of most common mental disorders in older people (Touhy and Jett, 2018), but it also occurs in children.*
12. Review history for head or spinal cord injury, meningitis, congenital anomalies, neurological disease, or psychiatric counseling. *Rationale: These neurological symptoms or behavioral changes help to focus assessment on possible cause.*
13. Assess patient's/family caregiver's knowledge, experience, and health literacy. *Rationale: Ensures patient/family caregiver has the capacity to obtain, communicate, process, and understand basic health information (CDC, 2016a).*

STEP	RATIONALE

PLANNING

1. Expected outcomes following completion of procedure:
   a. Patient demonstrates erect posture; strong grasp; and steady gait, with arms swinging freely at side. — Indicates normal alignment, gait, and neuromuscular muscle strength.
   b. There is bilateral symmetry of extremities in length, circumference, alignment, position, and skinfolds.
   c. Full active ROM is present in all joints, with good muscle tone and absence of contractures, spasticity, or muscular weakness. — Indicates normal ROM of joints.
   d. Patient is alert and oriented to person, place, and time. Behavior and appearance appropriate for condition/situation. — Indicates normal cerebral function.
   e. Patient demonstrates normal pupil reaction to light and accommodation; external ocular muscles intact; facial sensation intact; symmetrical facial expressions; soft palate and uvula midline and rise on phonation; gag reflex intact; speech clear without hoarseness; no difficulty swallowing. — Indicates normal functioning of CNs III, IV, V, VI, VII, IX, and X.
   f. Patient distinguishes between sharp and dull sensations and light touch on symmetrical areas of extremities. Position sense intact to lower extremities. — Indicates normal function of sensory nerves.
   g. Gait is coordinated, steady with appropriate stance and swing phases. Romberg test negative. — Indicates normal cerebellar and motor system functioning.
2. Provide privacy and prepare environment. — Providing privacy and preparing the environment early help the student/nurse think about the need to remove clutter from the over-bed or bedside table.
3. Perform hand hygiene. Prepare patient:
   a. Integrate musculoskeletal and neurological assessments during other parts of physical assessment or during nursing care (e.g., when patient moves in bed, rises from chair, or walks). — You can conduct assessment as patient performs activities or goes through movements required during complete physical examination. Integration with care conserves patient's energy and allows observation of patient performing more naturally.
   b. Plan time for short rest periods during assessment. — Movement of body parts and various maneuvers may tire patient. Always plan rest periods with older-adult and very ill patients.

IMPLEMENTATION

1. Assess musculoskeletal system. (Discuss any risks patient may have for falls or other injuries.)
   a. Observe ability to use arms and hands for grasping objects (e.g., pen, utensils). — Assesses coordination and muscle strength.
   b. To assess hand grasp strength, cross your hands and have patient grasp index and middle fingers of both of your hands and squeeze them as hard as possible (see illustration). — It is common for patient's dominant hand to be slightly stronger than nondominant hand. By crossing your hands, patient's right hand grasps your right hand. This helps with recall of which is patient's right/left hand.
   c. To assess strength of lower arms or legs, ask patient first to contract the muscle you indicate by extending or flexing the joint. Then have patient resist as you apply force against that muscle contraction. Have patient maintain pressure until told to stop. Compare symmetrical muscle groups. Note weakness and compare right with left. Rate muscle strength on scale of 0 to 5 as follows: — Compares strength of symmetrical muscle groups. Upper and lower extremities on dominant side are usually stronger.
      0 No voluntary contraction
      1 Slight contractility, no movement
      2 Full ROM, passive
      3 Full ROM, active
      4 Full ROM against gravity, some resistance
      5 Full ROM against gravity, full resistance
   d. Observe body alignment for sitting, supine, prone, or standing positions. Muscles and joints should be exposed and free to move to allow for accurate measurement. — Each joint or muscle group requires different position for measurement.

STEP	RATIONALE
e. Inspect gait as patient walks. Have patient use his or her assistive device (e.g., cane, walker) if appropriate. Observe for foot-dragging, shuffling or limping, balance, presence of obvious deformity in lower extremities, and position of trunk in relation to legs.	Gait is more natural if patient is unaware of your observation. Assesses for neuromusculoskeletal disorder.
f. Perform timed "get-up-and-go" (TGUG) test: Have adult wear regular footwear, sit back in comfortable chair, and use normal assist devices, if needed. Have watch with a second hand. On the word "Go," begin timing as you have the patient stand from a sitting position without using chair arms for support, stand still momentarily, walk 10 feet (3 m) in a line, turn around and return to chair, and sit back in chair without using chair arms for support. Observe gait and ability to stand.	The TGUG test is an assessment that should be conducted as part of routine evaluation of older adults. The test helps detect a person's risk for falls. Normally, a person completes the task in less than 10 seconds; over 20 seconds is abnormal.
g. Stand behind patient and observe postural alignment (position of hips relative to shoulders). Look sideways at cervical, thoracic, and lumbar curves (see illustration).	Abnormal curves of posture include kyphosis (hunchback, exaggerated posterior curvature of thoracic spine), lordosis (swayback, increased lumbar curvature), and scoliosis (lateral spinal curvature). Postural changes indicate muscular, bone, or joint deformity; pain; or muscular fatigue. Head should be held erect.

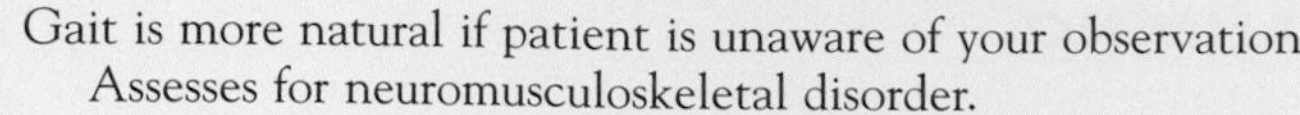

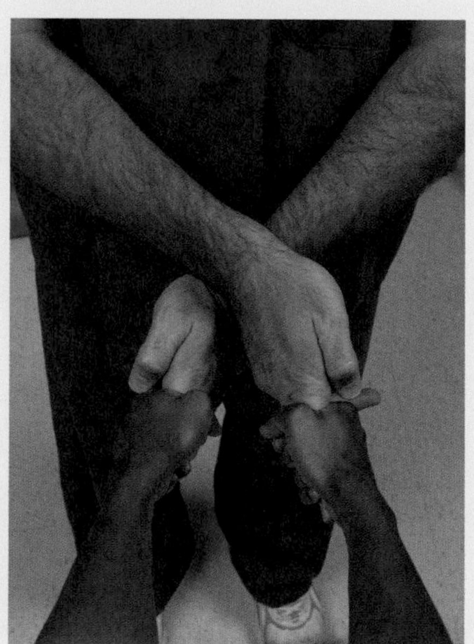

STEP 1b Assessing strength of hand grasps, comparing sides.

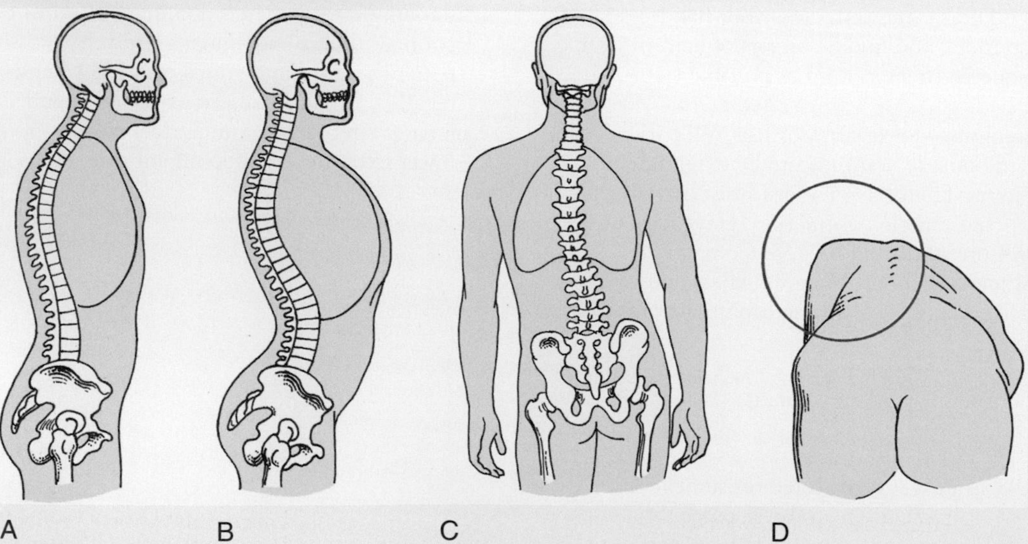

STEP 1g Observe spinal deformities. (A) Kyphosis. (B) Lordosis. (C) Scoliosis. (D) Scoliosis with patient bending forward.

STEP	RATIONALE
h. Make a general observation of extremities. Look at overall size, gross deformity, bony enlargement, alignment, and symmetry.	General review pinpoints areas requiring in-depth assessment.
i. Gently palpate bones, joints, and surrounding tissue in involved areas. Note any heat, tenderness, edema, or resistance to pressure.	Reveals changes resulting from trauma or chronic disease. Do not attempt to move joint when fracture is suspected or joint is apparently "frozen" by lack of movement over a long period of time.
j. Ask patient to put major joint through its full ROM (Table 8.11). Patients with deformities, reduced mobility, joint fixation, or weakness require passive ROM assessment. Observe equality of motion in same body parts:	Assessment of patient's normal ROM provides baseline for assessing later changes after surgery or inactivity.
(1) *Active motion:* (Patient needs no support or help and is able to move joint independently.) Teach patient to move each joint through its normal range. Sometimes it is necessary to demonstrate and ask patient to mimic your movements.	Identifies muscle strength and detects limited ROM.

TABLE 8.11

Assessing Range of Motion[a]

Body Part	Assessment Procedure	ROM
Upper Extremities		
Neck	Bend head forward and then backward. Bend neck side to side. Turn head to look over each shoulder.	Flexion; hyperextension; lateral flexion; rotation
Shoulders	Raise both arms to vertical position level at the sides of the head.	Flexion
	Bring arm across upper chest to touch opposite shoulder.	Adduction
	Place both hands behind the neck, with elbows out to the sides.	External rotation and abduction
	Place both hands behind the small of the back.	Internal rotation
	Have patient make small circles with hands with arms extended at shoulder level.	Circumduction
Elbows	Bend and straighten elbows.	Flexion and extension
	Place hands at waist with elbows flexed.	Internal rotation
Wrists	Flex and extend wrist (bend and straighten).	Flexion and extension
	Bend wrist to radial then ulnar side.	Radial and ulnar deviation
	Turn palm upward and then downward.	Supination and pronation
Hands	Make a fist with both hands; open hand.	Flexion and extension
	Extend and spread fingers and thumb outward; bring back together.	Adduction and abduction
Lower Extremities		
Hips (with patient supine)	With knees extended, raise one leg upward.	Flexion: expect 90 degrees
	Cross leg over other leg.	Abduction: expect 45 degrees
	Swing legs laterally.	Abduction: expect 30 degrees
	With knee flexed, hold ankle and rotate leg inward and outward.	Internal and external rotation: expect 40–45 degrees
Knees (with patient sitting)	Raise foot, keeping knee in place.	Extension: expect full extension and up to 15 degrees hyperextension
Ankles	With foot held off the floor, point toes downward, and then bring toes back toward knee.	Plantar flexion: expect 45 degrees Dorsiflexion: expect 20 degrees
Toes	Turn sole of foot inward and then outward.	Inversion and eversion: expect to reach 5 degrees
	Bend toes down and back.	Flexion and hyperextension: expect to reach 40 degrees

[a]This may be done actively by the patient (active ROM) or passively by the nurse (passive ROM). *ROM,* range of motion.

STEP	RATIONALE
(2) *Passive motion:* (Joint has full ROM, but patient does not have strength to move it independently.) Have patient relax and move same joints passively until end of range is felt. Support extremity at joint. Do not force joint if there is pain or muscle spasm.	Determines ability to perform joint motion in presence of muscle weakness. Forcing joint causes injury and pain.
k. Palpate joint for swelling, stiffness, tenderness, and heat; note any redness.	Indicates acute or chronic inflammation. ROM causes pain or injury.
l. Assess muscle tone in major muscle groups. Normal tone causes mild, even resistance to movement through entire ROM.	If muscle has increased tone (hypertonicity), any sudden movement of joint is met with considerable resistance. Hypotonic muscle moves without resistance. Muscle feels flabby.
2. Neurological assessment:	
a. Assess LOC and orientation by asking patient to identify name, location, day of week, and year; note behavior and appearance. This can be completed during general survey.	A fully conscious patient responds to questions spontaneously. As consciousness declines patient may show irritability, shortened attention span, or unwillingness to cooperate. As consciousness continues to deteriorate patient becomes disoriented to name, time, and place. Behavior and appearance reveal information about patient's mental status.
b. Assess CNs:	
(1) For CNs III (oculomotor), IV (trochlear), and VI (abducens), assess extra-ocular movements (EOMs). Ask patient to look straight ahead without moving head and follow movement of your finger through six cardinal positions of gaze; measure pupillary reaction to light reflex and accommodation using penlight.	These CNs are those most likely to be affected by increasing intracranial pressure (ICP), which causes change in response or size of pupil; pupils may change shape (more oval) or react sluggishly. ICP impairs EOMs. Accommodation is ability of eye to adjust vision from near to far.
(2) For CN V (trigeminal), apply light sensation with cotton ball to symmetrical areas of face.	Sensations should be symmetrical; unilateral decrease or loss of sensation may be caused by CN V lesion.
(3) For CN VII (facial) note facial symmetry. Have patient frown, smile, puff out cheeks, and raise eyebrows.	Expressions should be symmetrical; Bell's palsy causes drooping of upper and lower face; cerebrovascular accident (CVA) causes asymmetry.
(4) For CNs IX (glossopharyngeal) and X (vagus), have patient speak and swallow. Ask him or her to say "ah" while using tongue blade and penlight. Check for midline uvula and symmetrical rise of uvula and soft palate. Use tongue blade and place on posterior tongue to elicit gag reflex.	Damage to CN IX causes impaired swallowing; damage to CN X causes loss of gag reflex, hoarseness, nasal voice. When palate fails to rise and uvula pulls toward normal side, this indicates a unilateral paralysis.
c. Assess extremities for sensation. Perform all sensory testing with patient's eyes closed so that he or she is unable to see when or where a stimulus strikes skin. Use minimal stimulation initially, increasing gradually until patient is aware of it.	For all sensory stimulus testing, patient should note minimal differences side to side, correctly describe the sensation (sharp or dull, hot or cold), and recognize side of the body tested and location.
(1) *Pain:* Ask patient to indicate when sharp or dull sensation is felt as you alternately apply sharp and dull ends of a broken tongue blade to skin surface. Apply in symmetrical areas of extremities.	Patient should be able to distinguish sharp or dull sensations. Impaired sensations indicate disorders of spinal cord or peripheral nerve roots.
(2) *Light touch:* Apply light wisp of cotton to different points along surface of skin in symmetrical areas of extremities.	Patient should be able to distinguish when touched.
(3) *Position:* Grasp finger or toe, holding it by its sides with your thumb and index finger. Alternate moving finger or toe up and down. Ask patient to state when finger is up or down. Repeat with toes.	Patient should be able to distinguish movements of a few millimeters. Decreased/absent position sense may occur in spinal anesthesia, paralysis, or other neurological disorders.
d. Assess motor and cerebellar function:	
(1) *Gait:* Have patient walk across room, turn, and come back. Similarly note use of assistive devices. This is good time to instruct on proper use of assistive devices.	Neurological and musculoskeletal disorders impair gait and balance.

STEP	RATIONALE
(2) *Romberg's test:* Have patient stand with feet together, arms at sides, both with eyes open and eyes closed (for 20–30 seconds). Protect patient's safety by standing at side; observe for swaying.	Romberg's test should be negative; slight swaying is considered normal.
e. Assess deep tendon reflexes (DTRs):	
(1) In patients with back pain or surgery, CVA, or spinal cord compression, it is appropriate to monitor DTRs (Ball et al., 2019). This requires an advanced level of skill. In most settings this is not part of routine physical assessment.	Muscle spasticity and hyperactive reflexes may result from disorders such as stroke and paralysis. Diminished DTRs and muscle weakness may suggest electrolyte abnormalities or lower motor neuron disorders (e.g., amyotrophic lateral sclerosis [ALS] or Guillain-Barré syndrome).
(2) For each reflex tested, compare sides and assign a grade on the following scale: 0 No response 1+ Sluggish or diminished response 2+ Normal, active or expected response 3+ More brisk than expected; slightly hyperactive 4+ Very brisk; hyperactive, with clonus	Grade indicates extent of neuron dysfunction. Clonus is described as repeated spasms of muscular contraction and relaxation.
(3) *Knee reflex:* Palpate patellar tendon just below patella. Tap pointed end of reflex hammer briskly on tendon (see illustration).	Knee reflex is the most common DTR assessment performed. The normal response is knee extension.
(4) *Plantar response (Babinski's reflex):* Using handle end of reflex hammer, stroke lateral aspect of sole from heel to ball of foot.	Toes should flex inward and downward (see illustration).
(5) After stroking soles of feet, if Babinski's reflex is present, great toe dorsiflexes, accompanied by fanning of the other toes.	Indicates CNS dysfunction. Dorsiflexion of great toe and fanning of the others are normal in child younger than age 2 (Hockenberry and Wilson, 2017).
3. Help patient to comfortable position.	Gives patient sense of well-being.
4. Be sure nurse call system is in an accessible location within patient's reach.	Ensures patient can call for assistance if needed.
5. Raise side rails (as appropriate) and lower bed to lowest position.	Ensures patient safety.
6. Dispose of supplies. Remove gloves and perform hand hygiene.	Reduces transmission of microorganisms.

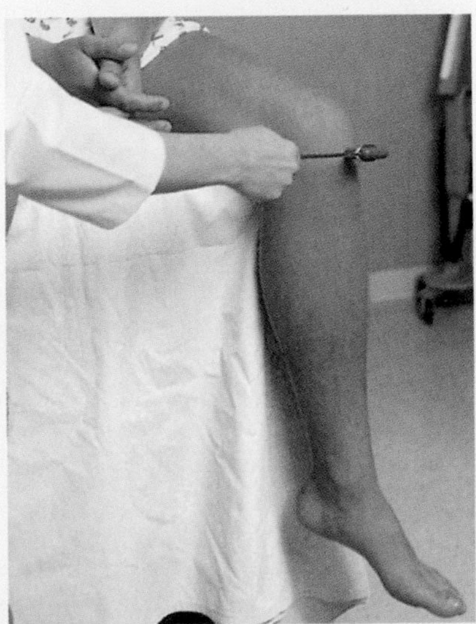

STEP 2e(3) Assessing knee reflex. Knee should extend.

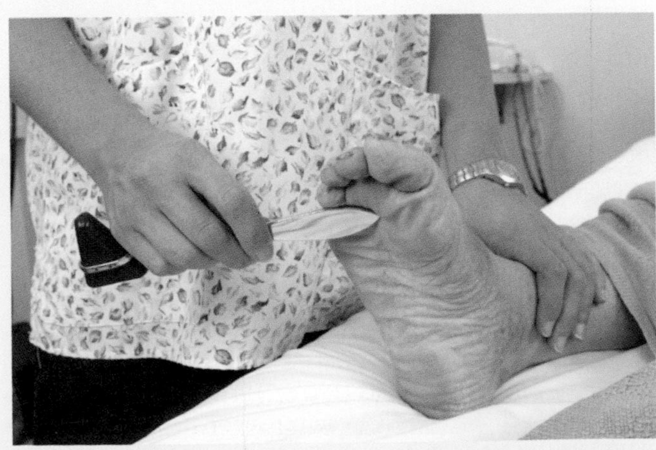

STEP 2e(4) Assessing plantar response. Toes should flex inward and downward.

STEP	RATIONALE
EVALUATION	
1. Compare muscle strength and ROM with previous physical assessment.	Determines presence of abnormalities.
2. Compare neurological status with previous physical assessment.	Determines presence of abnormalities.
3. Evaluate level of patient's discomfort following procedure, using appropriate pain scale.	Determines if manipulation of musculoskeletal structures intensifies patient's discomfort.
4. **Use Teach-Back:** "I want to be sure you understand the reasons why you are at risk for falling that we discussed during your examination. Tell me two reasons why you are at risk for falling." Revise your instruction now or develop a plan for revised patient/family caregiver teaching if patient/family caregiver is not able to teach back correctly.	Determines patient's/family caregiver's level of understanding of instructional topic.

Unexpected Outcomes	Related Interventions
1. Joints are prominent, swollen, and tender, with nodules or overgrowth of bone in distal joints, indicating signs of arthritis.	• Teach patient proper ROM. • Determine patient's knowledge regarding use of antiinflammatory medications and nonpharmacological measures (see Chapter 15).
2. ROM is reduced in one or more major joints: shoulder, elbow, wrist, fingers, knee, hip.	• Assess further for pain during movement with joint unstable, stiff, painful, or swollen or with obvious deformity. • Notify health care provider. • Reduce mobility in extremity until cause of abnormal joint motion is determined.
3. Patient demonstrates weakness in one or more major muscle groups or has difficulty with gait or ability to walk and sit during get-up-and-go test, indicating a fall risk.	• Place patient on fall precautions. • Provide patient safety when ambulating (see Chapter 18). • Notify health care provider.
4. Patient has changes in mental status and pupillary response or other neurological deficits.	• Notify health care provider immediately. • Continue to assess patient's vital signs and LOC closely. • Place on fall precautions.

Recording

- Record posture, gait, muscle strength, ROM, LOC, orientation, pupillary response, CN status, and sensation.
- Record LOC, orientation, pupillary response, sensation, and reflex responses.
- Document your evaluation of patient and family caregiver learning.

Hand-Off Reporting

- Report to nurse in charge or health care provider any acute pain or sudden muscle weakness, change in LOC, or change in size or pupillary reaction, which require immediate treatment.

SPECIAL CONSIDERATIONS

Patient-Centered Care

- Therapeutic communication enables nurses to deliver patient-centered care that is respectful of and responsive to patient preferences, needs, and values (Box 8.7). This ensures that patient values guide clinical decisions and creates positive relationships with health care providers.
- It is important to recognize cultural diversity and demonstrate respect for people as unique individuals.
- Awareness of cultural norms or values enhances understanding of nonverbal cues. Be aware of your own cultural values and expectations and how they may "filter" or direct your care.
- Consider any potential communication barriers with people from other cultures, including cultural perspective, heritage, and health traditions of both the patient and the nurse.
- Adopt an attitude of flexibility, respect, and interest to bridge any communication barriers imposed by cultural differences.
  - Use of language, gestures, and vocal emphasis of words: Taking care to determine if understanding was achieved is important. Avoid overly technical jargon or terms unique to a culture.
  - Eye contact: Direct eye contact is valued in some cultures, whereas other cultures find it improper and intrusive (e.g., it may be improper to make eye contact with an authority figure).
  - Use of touch and personal space: Some cultures are "non-contact" cultures and have needs for clear boundaries; other cultures value close contact, handshakes, and embracing.

Patient Education

- Teach older adults about fall prevention. Make modifications in the home environment to reduce the risk of falls.
- Teach older adults and those with osteoporosis about proper body mechanics, ROM exercises, and moderate weight-bearing exercises (e.g., swimming, walking) to minimize trauma.

BOX 8.7

Therapeutic Communication Techniques

Technique: Listening

Definition: An active process of receiving information and examining one's reaction to messages received

Example: Consider the cultural practices of your patient, maintain appropriate eye contact, and be receptive to nonverbal communications.

Therapeutic Value: Nonverbally communicates your interest and acceptance to a patient

Nontherapeutic Threat: Failure to listen, interrupting patient

Technique: Broad Openings

Definition: Encouraging patient to select topics for discussion

Example: "Can you tell me what you are thinking about?"

Therapeutic Value: Indicates your acceptance valuing of patient's initiative

Nontherapeutic Threat: Domination of interaction by nurse; rejecting responses

Technique: Restating

Definition: Repeating main thought that patient has expressed

Example: "You say that your mother left you when you were 5 years old."

Therapeutic Value: Indicates that you are listening and validates, reinforces, or calls attention to something important that has been said

Nontherapeutic Threat: Lack of validation of your interpretation of message; being judgmental; reassuring; defending

Technique: Clarification

Definition: Attempting to improve your understanding of words, vague ideas, or patient's unclear thoughts or asking patient to explain what he or she means

Example: "I'm not sure what you mean. Could you tell me again?"

Therapeutic Value: Helps clarify patient's feelings, ideas, and perceptions and provide an explicit correlation between them and patient's actions

Nontherapeutic Threat: Failure to probe; assumed understanding

Technique: Reflection

Definition: Directing back to patient ideas, feelings, questions, or content

Example: "You're feeling tense and anxious, and it's related to a conversation you had with your sister last night?"

Therapeutic Value: Validates your understanding of what patient is saying and signifies empathy, interest, and respect for patient

Nontherapeutic Threat: Stereotyping patient's responses, inappropriate timing of reflections; inappropriate depth of feeling of reflections; inappropriate to the cultural experience and educational level of the patient

Technique: Humor

Definition: Discharging energy through comic enjoyment of the imperfect

Example: "This gives a whole new meaning to 'Just relax.'"

Therapeutic Value: Can promote insight by making conscious any repressed material, resolving paradoxes, tempering aggression, and revealing new options; is a socially acceptable form of sublimation

Nontherapeutic Threat: Indiscriminate use; belittling patient; screen to avoid therapeutic intimacy

Technique: Informing

Definition: Demonstrating skills or giving information

Example: "I think it would be helpful for you to know more about how your medication works."

Therapeutic Value: Helpful in patient education about relevant aspects of patient's well-being and self-care

Nontherapeutic Threat: Giving advice

Technique: Focusing

Definition: Asking questions or making statements that help patient expand on a topic of importance

Example: "I think it would be helpful if we talk more about your relationship with your father."

Therapeutic Value: Allows patient to discuss central issues related to problem and keeps communication process goal directed

Nontherapeutic Threat: Allowing abstractions and generalizations; changing topics

Technique: Sharing Perceptions

Definition: Asking patient to verify your understanding of what patient is thinking or feeling

Example: "You're smiling, but I sense that you're really very angry with me."

Therapeutic Value: Conveys your understanding to patient and has potential for clearing up confusing communication

Nontherapeutic Threat: Challenging patient; accepting literal responses; reassuring; testing; defending

Technique: Theme Identification

Definition: Clarifying underlying issues or problems experienced by patient that emerge repeatedly during nurse–patient relationship

Example: "I've noticed that in all the relationships that you've described you've been hurt or rejected by the man. Do you think this is an underlying issue?"

Therapeutic Value: Allows you to best promote patient's exploration and understanding of important problems

Nontherapeutic Threat: Giving advice; reassuring; disapproving

Technique: Silence

Definition: Using silence or nonverbal communication for a therapeutic reason

Example: Sitting with patient and nonverbally communicating interest and involvement

Therapeutic Value: Allows patient time to think and gain insights, slows the pace of the interaction, and encourages patient to initiate conversation while conveying your support, understanding, and acceptance

Nontherapeutic Threat: Questioning patient: asking for "why" responses; failing to break a nontherapeutic silence

Technique: Suggesting

Definition: Presenting alternative ideas for patient's consideration relative to problem solving

Example: "Have you thought about organizing your medications on a daily schedule? For example, you could use a pill organizer that allows you to sort out medicines to be taken each day or over a week."

Therapeutic Value: Increases patient's perceived options or choices

Nontherapeutic Threat: Giving advice, inappropriate timing; being judgmental

Modified from Keltner N, et al.: *Psychiatric nursing*, ed 6, St. Louis, 2011, Mosby.

Female Health Teaching

- Teach patient about purpose and recommended frequency of Papanicolaou (Pap) smears and gynecological examinations.
- Explain warning signs of STIs: pain or burning on urination, pain during sex, pain in pelvic area, bleeding between menstruation, itchy rash around vagina, and abnormal vaginal discharge.
- Teach measures to prevent STIs (e.g., male partner's use of condoms, restricting number of sexual partners, and perineal hygiene measures).
- Reinforce the importance of performing perineal hygiene (as appropriate).

Male Health Teaching

- Explain warning signs of STIs: pain on urination and during sex, abnormal penile discharge, swollen lymph nodes, or rash or ulcer on skin or genitalia.
- Teach measures to prevent STIs: use of condoms, avoiding sex with infected partner, avoiding sex with people who have multiple partners, and using regular perineal hygiene. Tell patients with an STI to inform their sexual partners of the need to have an examination. Instruct patient to seek treatment as soon as possible if partner becomes infected with an STI.
- Teach patient how to perform genital self-examination (see Box 8.6).

Age-Specific

Pediatric

- Measure physical growth, including height, weight, length, and head circumference, which are key elements in evaluation of a child's health status (Hockenberry and Wilson, 2017). Use growth charts specific to child's age and condition.
- Weigh infants nude. Children may be weighed in light underclothes or gown.
- Use the bell of the stethoscope to auscultate lung sounds in children. Breath sounds are louder in children because of their thin chest walls.
- Children younger than 7 years old normally exhibit noticeable abdominal or diaphragmatic movement. Older children and adults exhibit more costal or thoracic movement.
- Capillary refill in infants is usually less than 1 second.
- PMI is at fourth intercostal space at left midclavicular line in children younger than 7 years of age (Hockenberry and Wilson, 2017).
- It is not uncommon for children to have third heart sounds (S_3). Sinus arrhythmia occurs normally in many infants and children (Hockenberry and Wilson, 2017).
- Children have louder, higher-pitched heart sounds because of thin chest walls.
- Have child stand erect and then lie supine during inspection of abdomen. Normal abdomen of infants and young children is cylindrical in erect position and flat in supine position. School-aged children may have a rounded abdomen until 13 years of age when standing.
- Infants and children until 7 years of age are abdominal breathers.
- When examining the testes in a male infant, avoid stimulating the cremasteric reflex, which causes the testes to pull higher into pelvic cavity.
- Examine infants carefully for musculoskeletal anomalies resulting from genetic or fetal insults. An examination includes review of posture; generalized movement, symmetry, and skin creases of the extremities; muscle strength; and hip alignment.
- Normally, the back of a newborn is rounded or C-shaped from the thoracic and pelvic curves.
- Scoliosis, lateral curvature of the spine, is an important childhood problem, especially in girls, apparent at puberty.

Gerontological

- An older adult has a diminished physiological reserve that may mask the usual, or "classic," signs and symptoms of a disease. In older adults, signs and symptoms may be blunted or atypical (Touhy and Jett, 2018).
- Common skin changes with aging include dryness, thinning, decreased elasticity, and prominent small blood vessels. Common lesions include seborrheic keratosis (pigmented, raised, warty lesion); cherry angioma (bright, ruby-red round papules); cutaneous tags (soft pinkish-tan to light-brown pedunculated lesions); and solar lentigines (gray-brown, irregular macular lesions on sun-exposed areas) (Ball et al., 2019).
- Postural hypotension is common in older patients. When dizziness or lightheadedness is reported, check vital signs in lying, sitting, and standing positions.
- Inspection of the feet is critical in the presence of impaired circulation, impaired vision, and diabetes. Common foot conditions include ulceration, fungal infection, calluses, bunions, and plantar warts and hammertoe.
- Older adults commonly have loss of peripheral vision caused by changes in the lens.
- Instruct patients older than age 65 to have regular hearing checks.
- Older adults have a costal angle (anteriorly) of slightly less than 90 degrees. The anteroposterior diameter may be increased from kyphosis.
- In older adults, chest expansion is reduced because of calcification of rib cartilage and partial contraction of inspiratory muscles.
- PMI may be difficult to find in an older adult because the AP diameter of the chest deepens.
- Accidental massage of the carotid sinus during palpation of the carotid artery can be a problem for older adults, causing a sudden decrease in heart rate from vagal nerve stimulation.

Home Care

- The focus may be on the patient's ability to perform basic self-care tasks. Be sure that the assessment builds on all health concerns identified in other settings.

PRACTICE REFLECTIONS

You are caring for a new postoperative patient with an IV infusion, an abdominal dressing, a Foley catheter to gravity, and a Jackson-Pratt surgical drain in place.

1. How might you decide what body systems to assess for this patient?
2. If you assess unilateral lower extremity swelling around the calf, what additional body system should be assessed, and why?
3. After listening for 60 seconds at a site below and to the left of the umbilicus, you are unable to hear bowel sounds. What is the best assessment of this situation? Who might need to be made aware of this finding?

CLINICAL REVIEW QUESTIONS

1. In conducting a general survey of a patient, the nurse knows that the survey should include which of the following? (Select all that apply.)
   1. Appearance
   2. Obtaining peripheral pulses
   3. Measuring chest excursion
   4. Behavior
   5. Posture
2. Which of the following does the nurse document as an abnormal finding during a muscular-neurological assessment? (Select all that apply.)
   1. Grade 1 strength in right arm during flexion
   2. Uses hands to sit down in chair during get-up-and-go test
   3. Negative Romberg's test
   4. Symmetrical rise of uvula
   5. Symmetrical facial expressions
3. Select all the characteristics that can be heard through auscultation.
   1. Adaptability
   2. Quality
   3. Loudness
   4. Duration
   5. Frequency

Answers and Rationales for Clinical Review Questions can be found on the Evolve website.

REFERENCES

American Academy of Dermatology (AAD): Skin cancer, 2018. https://www.aad.org/media/stats/conditions/skin-cancer.

American Cancer Society (ACS): Recommendations for early detection of breast cancer, 2017a. https://www.cancer.org/cancer/breast-cancer/screening-tests-and-early-detection/american-cancer-society-recommendations-for-the-early-detection-of-breast-cancer.html.

American Cancer Society (ACS). Guidelines for the early detection of cancer, 2017b. https://www.cancer.org/healthy/find-cancer-early/cancer-screening-guidelines/american-cancer-society-guidelines-for-the-early-detection-of-cancer.html.

American Cancer Society (ACS): Cancer prevention and early detection facts and figures 2017-2018, Atlanta, 2017c. https://www.cancer.org/content/dam/cancer-org/research/cancer-facts-and-statistics/cancer-prevention-and-early-detection-facts-and-figures/cancer-prevention-and-early-detection-facts-and-figures-2017.pdf.

American Cancer Society (ACS): Can testicular cancer be found early? 2018. https://www.cancer.org/cancer/testicular-cancer/detection-diagnosis-staging/detection.html.

American Institute for Cancer Research: Whole grains decrease colorectal cancer risk, processed meats increase the risk. Science Daily, 2017. www.sciencedaily.com/releases/2017/09/170907093623.htm.

Ball JW, et al: *Seidel's guide to physical examination*, ed 9, St. Louis, 2019, Elsevier.

Centers for Disease Control and Prevention (CDC): What is health literacy, 2016a. https://www.cdc.gov/healthliteracy/learn/index.html.

Centers for Disease Control and Prevention (CDC): Tuberculosis (TB), 2016b. http://www.cdc.gov/mmwr/volumes/66/wr/mm6611a2.htm?s_cid=mm6611a2_w.

Cleveland Clinic: How high-fat impacts colorectal cancer. Science Daily, 2017. www.sciencedaily.com/releases/2017/07/170706121221.htm.

Hockenberry JN, Wilson D: *Wong's essentials of pediatric nursing*, ed 10, St. Louis, 2017, Elsevier.

Kleerekoper M, et al: Screening for osteoporosis, UpToDate, 2017. http://www.uptodate.com/contents/topic.do?topicKey=ENDO/2046.

Lewis S, et al: *Medical-surgical nursing: assessment and management of clinical problems*, ed 10, 2017, Elsevier.

Marion L, et al: Implementing the new ANA standard 8: culturally congruent practice, *Online J Issues Nurs* 22(1):2016.

Meites E, et al: Use of a 2-dose schedule for human papillomavirus vaccination -Updated recommendations of the Advisory Committee on Immunization Practices, *MMWR Morb Mortal Wkly Rep* 65:1405–1408, 2016.

National Cancer Institute: Risk factors for cancer, 2015. https://www.cancer.gov/about-cancer/causes-prevention/risk.

National Osteoporosis Foundation (NOF): The jumping jack challenge to raise awareness about building and maintaining strong bones, Washington, DC, 2017. http://www.nof.org/news/nationalosteoporosismonth/.

Patel K, et al: Deep venous thrombosis (DVT), 2017. http://emedicine.medscape.com/article/1911303-overview.

The Joint Commission (TJC): *2019 National Patient Safety Goals*, Oakbrook Terrace, IL, 2019, The Commission. http://www.jointcommission.org/standards_information/npsgs.aspx.

Touhy T, Jett K: *Ebersole & Hess' toward healthy aging*, ed 10, St. Louis, 2018, Elsevier.

Wilson S, Giddens J: *Health assessment for nursing practice*, ed 6, St. Louis, 2017, Elsevier.

Wound Ostomy and Continence Nurses (WOCN) Society: *Guideline for prevention and management of pressure ulcers, WOCN clinical practice guideline series*, Mt. Laurel, NJ, 2016, The Society.

9 Specimen Collection

SKILLS AND PROCEDURES

EVOLVE WEBSITE/RESOURCES LIST

http://evolve.elsevier.com/Perry/nursinginterventions

Audio Glossary • Checklists • Clinical Review Questions • Answers and Rationales to Clinical Review Questions • Video Clips

INTRODUCTION

Laboratory test results aid in the diagnosis of health care problems, provide information about the stage and activity of diseases, and measure patient responses to therapy. Proficiency and judgment in obtaining specimens minimize patient discomfort, ensure patient safety, and ensure the accuracy and quality of diagnostic procedures. Nurses are accountable for correctly collecting specimens, monitoring patient outcomes, obtaining these specimens in a timely manner, and ensuring that these specimens are delivered to the correct laboratory for analysis.

PRACTICE STANDARDS

- Occupational Safety and Health Administration (OSHA), 2000: Bloodborne pathogens and needlestick prevention
- Occupational Safety and Health Administration (OSHA), 2015: Bloodborne pathogen standards
- The Joint Commission (TJC), 2019: National Patient Safety Goals—Patient identification

EVIDENCE-BASED PRACTICE

Prevention of Hemolysis of Blood Samples

Hemolysis is the breakdown of red blood cells (RBCs) resulting in the leakage of intracellular contents into the plasma, and it affects the accuracy of blood test results. Hemolysis of blood sampling is a leading cause of preanalytical laboratory errors and can result in inaccurate diagnoses, delays in treatment and in monitoring disease progression, and increased cost of care (Makhumula-Nkhoma et al., 2014; McCaughey et al., 2017).

Using a straight needle venipuncture instead of an intravenous (IV) device is effective in reducing hemolysis rates of blood samples collected in emergency departments and is recommended as an evidence-based best practice (Barnaby et al., 2016). When access to IV sites must be used, observed rates of hemolysis may be substantially reduced by placing the IV at the antecubital site. In addition, the use of a butterfly-only protocol cuts hemolysis rates by more than half compared with IV catheter phlebotomy (Barnaby et al., 2016). Second, using plasma collection tubes with smaller volumes and decreased vacuum may reduce hemolysis because of a reduced pressure gradient and less turbulence as the blood moves into the collection tube (McCaughey et al., 2017; Phelan et al., 2015). Best practices that assist in reducing hemolysis rates include the following:

- Venipuncture is recommended over the use of obtaining a blood sample from an IV site (Barnaby et al., 2016).
- Use the antecubital region for optimal blood collection site (McCaughey et al., 2017).
- Avoid vigorous shaking of a blood sample because hemolysis may occur and invalidate test results (Pagana et al., 2017).
- Collect a blood specimen from the arm without an IV device if possible because IV fluids can influence test results (Pagana et al., 2017).
- Use of a butterfly needle reduces the risk of hemolysis (Barnaby et al., 2016; Wollowitz et al., 2013).
- Do not fasten the tourniquet for longer than 1 minute. Prolonged tourniquet application can cause stasis, localized acidemia, and hemoconcentration (McCaughey et al., 2017).
- Because the blood cells continue to live in the collection tubes, they will metabolize some of the components in the blood, which can result in alterations in the concentration

of some blood components before analysis in the laboratory. Blood specimens should be promptly delivered to the laboratory for processing within 1 hour, depending on the test (Pagana et al., 2017).

SAFETY GUIDELINES

When collecting any specimen, know the purpose of the test, how much of the specimen is needed, the appropriate collection technique, and how the specimen is to be transported to the laboratory (Pagana et al., 2017). The *2019 National Patient Safety Goals* by The Joint Commission (TJC, 2019) requires the use of at least two identifiers when providing care, treatment, and services. The intent is to identify the individual reliably as the patient for whom the service or treatment is intended and match the service or treatment to that patient (TJC, 2019).

- Follow standard precautions (see Chapter 5) when collecting specimens of blood or body fluids.
- Everyone who handles body fluids is at risk for exposure to body fluids. The use of hand hygiene and clean gloves are necessary when collecting a specimen.
- Know agency policy regarding infection control practices for transportation of all specimen containers of body substances.
- Use a plastic bag marked "biohazard" to enclose a specimen for delivery to the laboratory (Fig. 9.1).
- A completed laboratory requisition is needed for each specimen to instruct laboratory personnel on the test to be performed and to facilitate accurate reporting of the results.
- After specimen collection and in the presence of the patient, label the container itself (not the lid) with the same two identifiers (e.g., name and birthday or name and account number, according to agency policy), specimen source, collection date and time, series number (if more than one specimen), and anatomical site if appropriate (e.g., wound culture from knee versus abdominal incision).

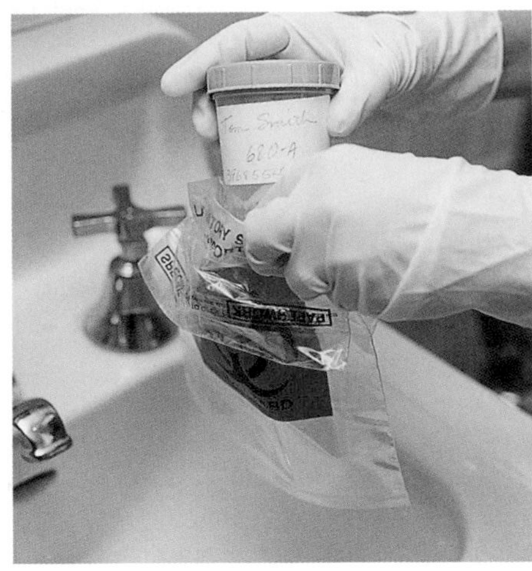

FIG 9.1 Enclose all specimens in a biohazard bag.

- Each requisition includes patient identification (e.g., name and birthday or name and account number, according to agency policy), the date and time the specimen is obtained, the name of the test, and the source of the specimen or culture for each container (TJC, 2019).
- Follow procedures for special conditions (e.g., iced specimens, special containers with preservatives) required for transport of specimens. Specific required prerequisite conditions include fasting and nothing by mouth (NPO) and may need to be completed before the collection of a specimen (Pagana et al., 2017).
- Deliver specimens to the laboratory promptly. Specimens left at room temperature are at risk for additional bacterial growth, altering the results of the test, and so need timely delivery to the laboratory (McCaughey et al., 2017; Pagana et al., 2017).

✦ SKILL 9.1 Urine Specimen Collection—Midstream (Clean-Voided) Urine, Sterile Urinary Catheter

Purpose

Urinalysis provides information about kidney or metabolic function, nutrition, and systemic diseases. Urine collection uses a variety of methods, depending on the purpose of the urinalysis and the presence or absence of a urinary catheter. Routine urinalysis includes measurement of nine or more elements, including urine pH, protein and glucose levels, ketones, blood, specific gravity, white blood cell (WBC) count, and presence of bacteria and casts (Pagana et al., 2017).

Types of Urine Tests and Specimens

- A *random urine specimen for routine urinalysis* in the hospital is usually collected using a specimen "hat" (Fig. 9.2), which you place under a toilet seat to collect voided urine. In an outpatient setting such as a clinic, a patient is instructed to void directly into a specimen container.
- A *culture and sensitivity (C&S) of urine* is performed to identify bacteria causing a urinary tract infection (UTI; culture) and to determine the most effective antibiotic for treatment (sensitivity). Use sterile technique to ensure that any microorganisms present originate in the urine and not from the patient's skin, the hands, or the environment. You collect specimens for C&S either as a clean-voided midstream specimen or under sterile conditions from a urinary catheter.

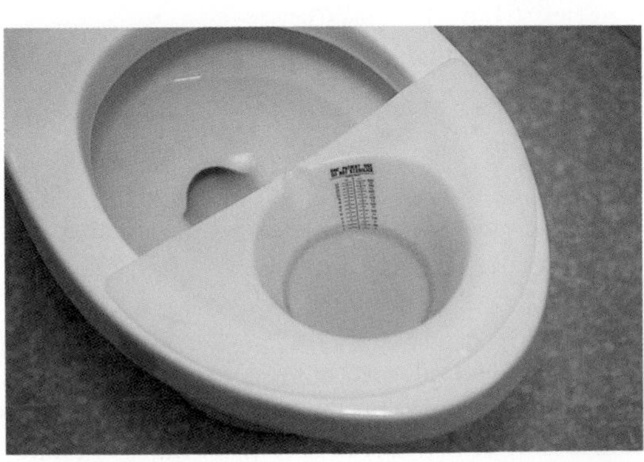

FIG 9.2 Specimen "hat."

- A *timed urine specimen for quantitative analysis* requires urine to be collected over 2 to 72 hours. The 24-hour timed collection is most common and allows for measurement and quantitative analysis of excreted elements (see Procedural Guideline 9.1).
- *Chemical properties* of urine are tested by immersing a specially prepared strip of paper (Chemstrip) in a clean urine specimen (see Procedural Guideline 9.2).

Delegation and Collaboration

The skill of collecting urine specimens can be delegated to nursing assistive personnel (NAP). The nurse instructs the NAP to:

- Obtain the specimens at a specified time when appropriate.
- Position patient as necessary when mobility restrictions are present.
- Report to the nurse if the urine is not clear (e.g., contains blood, cloudiness, or excess sediment).
- Report to the nurse when a patient is unable to initiate a stream or has pain or burning on urination.

Equipment

- Identification labels with name of test
- Completed laboratory requisition, including patient identification, date, time, name of test, and source of culture
- Biohazard bag or container for delivery of specimen to laboratory (as specified by agency)

Clean-Voided Urine Specimen

- Commercial kit for clean-voided urine containing (Fig. 9.3):
    - Sterile cotton balls or antiseptic towelettes
    - Antiseptic solution (chlorhexidine or povidone-iodine solution)
    - Sterile water or normal saline
    - Sterile specimen container
    - Urine cup
- Clean gloves
- Soap, water, washcloth, and towel
- Bedpan (for nonambulatory patient), specimen hat (for ambulatory patient)

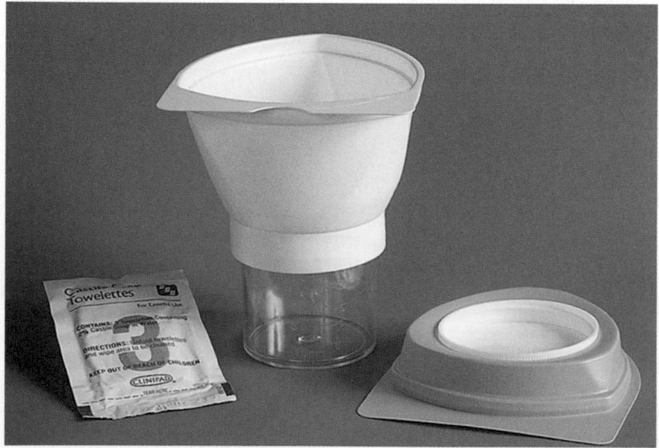

FIG 9.3 Clean-voided urine kit.

Sterile Urine Specimen From Urinary Catheter

- 20-mL Luer-Lok for routine urinalysis or 3-mL safety Luer-Lok syringe for culture
- Alcohol, chlorhexidine, or other disinfectant swab
- Clamp or rubber band
- Specimen container (nonsterile for routine urinalysis; sterile for culture)
- Clean gloves

ASSESSMENT

1. Identify patient using at least two identifiers (e.g., name and birthday or name and medical record number) according to agency policy. Compare identifiers with information on patient's medication administration record (MAR) or medical record. *Rationale: Ensures correct patient. Complies with The Joint Commission standards and improves patient safety (TJC, 2019).*
2. Review health care provider's order. *Rationale: Ensures accurate testing of specimen; order is needed to perform test.*
3. Refer to agency procedures for specimen collection methods. *Rationale: Agency policies may vary regarding collection and/or handling of specimens.*
4. Assess patient's ability to help with urine specimen collection; able to position self and hold container. *Rationale: Determines degree of help patient requires.*
5. Assess for signs and symptoms of UTI (frequency, urgency, dysuria, hematuria, flank pain, fever; cloudy, malodorous urine). *Rationale: May indicate the need for health care provider intervention.*
6. Assess patient's or family caregiver's knowledge, experience, and health literacy. *Rationale: Ensures patient or family caregiver has the capacity to obtain, communicate, process, and understand basic health information (Centers for Disease Control and Prevention [CDC], 2016).*
7. Assess patient's or family caregiver's understanding of purpose of test and method of collection. *Rationale: Allows you to clarify misunderstanding; promotes patient cooperation.*

STEP	RATIONALE
PLANNING	
1. Expected outcomes after completion of procedure:	
• Specimen is free of contaminants.	Proper collection technique prevents substances from changing normal characteristics of urine.
• Patient discusses purpose and benefits and procedure for specimen collection.	Procedure is performed safely. Evaluates patient's learning.
2. Perform hand hygiene. Provide privacy for patient; close curtains around bed or close room door. Allow mobile patients to collect specimen in bathroom.	Reduces transmission of microorganisms. Privacy allows patient to relax and produce specimen more easily.

STEP	RATIONALE
3. Explain the procedure and what is required of the patient.	Patients often prefer to obtain their own clean voided specimen but need appropriate education to correctly collect the sample.

IMPLEMENTATION

STEP	RATIONALE
1. Check labels and verify complete laboratory requisition for specimen container.	Organizes procedure.
2. Perform hand hygiene.	Reduces transmission of microorganisms.
3. **Collect clean-voided urine specimen.**	
a. Apply clean gloves. Give patient cleaning towelette or towel, washcloth, and soap to clean perineum or help with cleaning perineum. Help bedridden patient onto bedpan to facilitate access to perineum. Remove and dispose of gloves and perform hand hygiene.	Patients prefer to wash their own perineal areas when possible. Cleaning prevents contamination of specimen from skin and surface bacteria after urine passes from urethra.
b. Using aseptic technique, open outer package of commercial specimen kit.	Maintains sterility of equipment.
c. Apply clean gloves.	Prevents contact of microorganisms on your hands.
d. Pour antiseptic solution over cotton balls (unless kit contains prepared antiseptic towelettes).	Cotton ball or towelette is used to clean perineum.
e. Open specimen container, maintaining sterility of inside specimen container, and place cap with sterile inside up. Do not touch inside of cap or container.	Contaminated specimen is most frequent reason for inaccurate reporting of urine C&S.
f. Use aseptic technique to help patient or allow patient to independently clean perineum and collect specimen. Amount of help needed varies with each patient. Inform patient that antiseptic solution will feel cold.	Maintains patient's dignity and comfort.
(1) *Male:*	
(a) Hold penis with one hand; using circular motion and antiseptic towelette, clean meatus, moving from center to outside 3 times with different towelettes (see illustration). Have uncircumcised male patient retract foreskin for effective cleaning of urinary meatus and keep retracted during voiding. Return foreskin when done.	Reduces number of microorganisms at urethral meatus and moves from areas of least to most contamination. Return of foreskin prevents stricture of penis.
(b) If agency procedure indicates, rinse area with sterile water and dry with cotton balls or gauze pad.	Prevents contamination of specimen with antiseptic solution.
(c) After patient initiates urine stream into toilet, urinal, or bedpan, have him pass urine specimen container into stream and collect 90–120 mL of urine (Pagana et al., 2017; see illustration).	Initial urine flushes out microorganisms that normally accumulate at urinary meatus and prevents transfer into specimen.

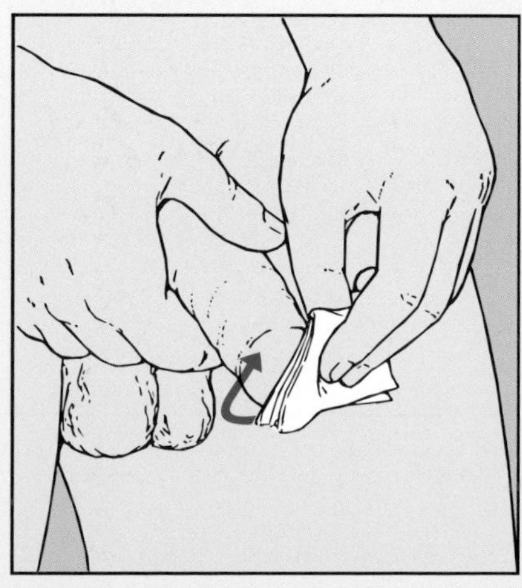

STEP 3f(1)(a) Cleaning technique (male).

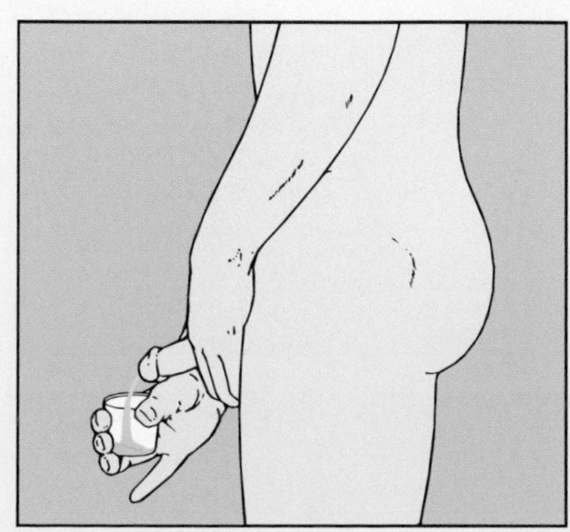

STEP 3f(1)(c) Collecting midstream urine specimen (male).

STEP	RATIONALE
(2) *Female:*	
(a) Either nurse or patient spreads labia minora with fingers of nondominant hand.	Provides access to urethral meatus.
(b) With dominant hand clean urethral area with antiseptic swab (cotton ball or gauze). Move from front (above urethral orifice) to back (toward anus). Use fresh swab each time; clean 3 times; begin with labial fold farthest from you, then labial fold closest, and then down center (see illustration).	Prevents contamination of urinary meatus with fecal material. Cleaning down the center last decreases contamination from labia.
(c) If agency procedure indicates, rinse area with sterile water and dry with cotton ball.	Prevents contamination of specimen with antiseptic solution.
(d) While continuing to hold labia apart, patient initiates urine stream into toilet or bedpan; after stream is achieved, pass specimen container into stream and collect 90–120 mL of urine (Pagana et al., 2017; see illustration).	Initial stream flushes out resident microorganisms that accumulate at urethral meatus and prevents transfer into specimen.
g. Remove specimen container before flow of urine stops and before releasing labia or penis. Patient finishes voiding into bedpan or toilet. Offer to help with personal hygiene as appropriate.	Prevents contamination of specimen with skin flora. Prevents sediment from bladder getting into specimen.
h. Replace cap securely on specimen container, touching only outside.	Retains sterility of inside of container and prevents spillage of urine.
i. Clean urine from exterior surface of container.	Prevents transfer of microorganisms to others.
4. Collect urine from indwelling urinary catheter.	
a. Explain that you will use syringe without needle to remove urine through catheter port and that patient will not experience any discomfort.	Minimizes anxiety when you manipulate catheter and aspirate urine with syringe from catheter port.
b. Explain that you will need to clamp catheter for 10–15 minutes before obtaining urine specimen and that urine cannot be obtained from drainage bag.	Allows urine to accumulate in catheter. Urine in drainage bag is not considered sterile.
c. Apply clean gloves. Clamp drainage tubing with clamp or rubber band for as long as 15 minutes below site chosen for withdrawal (see illustration).	Permits collection of fresh sterile urine in catheter tubing rather than draining into bag.
d. After 15 minutes, position patient so catheter sampling port is easily accessible. Location of port is where catheter attaches to drainage bag tube (see illustration). Clean port for 15 seconds with disinfectant swab and allow to dry.	Prevents entry of microorganisms into catheter.

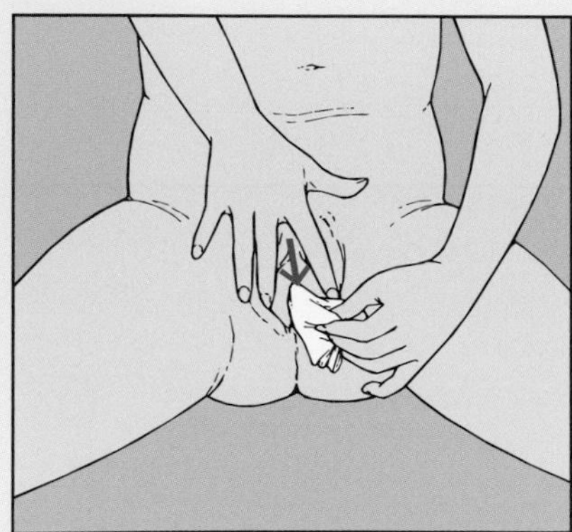

STEP 3f(2)(b) Clean from front to back, holding labia apart.

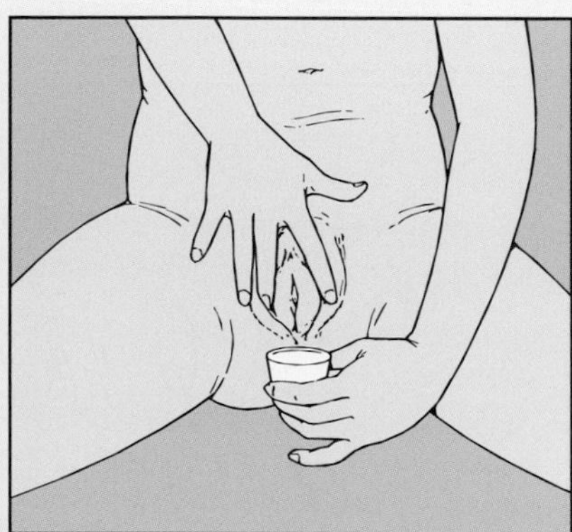

STEP3f(2)(d) Collecting midstream urine specimen (female).

STEP	RATIONALE
e. Attach needleless Luer-Lok syringe to built-in catheter sampling port (see illustration). Some needleless ports use blunt plastic valve or slip-tip syringe inserted into port diaphragm.	Guideline recommends use of Luer-Lok needleless system. Needleless system prevents injury by needlestick.
f. Withdraw 3 mL for culture or 20 mL for routine urinalysis.	Allows collection of urine without contamination. Proper volume is needed to perform test.
g. Transfer urine from syringe into clean urine container for routine urinalysis or into sterile urine container for culture.	Prevents contamination of urine during transfer procedure.
h. Place lid tightly on container.	Prevents contamination of specimen by air and loss by spillage.
i. Unclamp catheter and allow urine to flow into drainage bag. Ensure that urine flows freely.	Allows urine to drain by gravity and prevents stasis of urine in bladder.
5. Securely attach label to container (not lid). If patient is female, indicate if she is menstruating. In presence of patient, complete label (two identifiers, specimen source, collection date and time) and attach to container. Attach completed laboratory requisition to container. Enclose specimen in a biohazard bag and send immediately to laboratory.	Incorrect patient identification could lead to diagnostic or therapeutic error (TJC, 2019). Bacteria multiply quickly. Specimen should be analyzed promptly for accurate results.
6. Dispose of soiled supplies. Remove and dispose of gloves and perform hand hygiene.	Prevents transmission of microorganisms.
7. Offer patient hand hygiene or provide time to wash hands.	Reduces transmission of microorganisms
8. Assist patient to comfortable position	

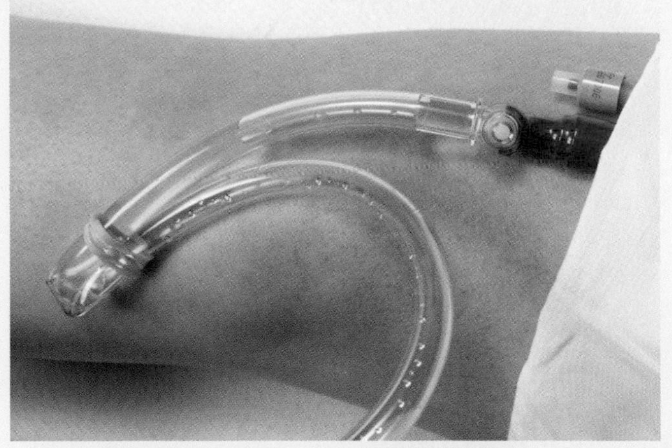

STEP 4c Rubber band used to clamp drainage tube.

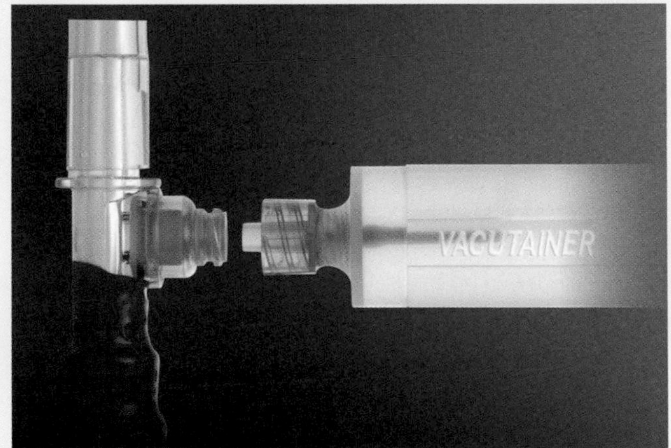

STEP 4d Port with syringe attached.

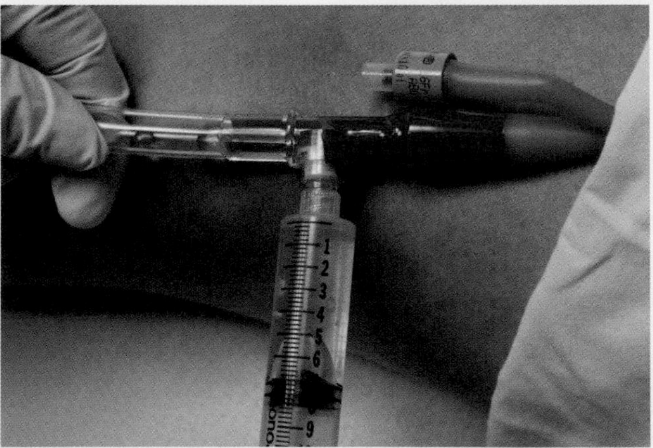

STEP 4e Access urinary catheter port with Luer-Lok syringe or syringe with blunt plastic valve.

STEP	RATIONALE
9. Ensure nurse call system is accessible within reach and instruct patient in its use.	Ensures patient can call for assistance if needed.
10. Raise side rails (as appropriate) and lower bed to lowest position.	Ensures patient safety.
11. Send specimen and completed requisition to laboratory within 20 minutes. Refrigerate specimen if delay cannot be avoided.	Delay of analysis may significantly alter test results (Pagana et al., 2017).

EVALUATION

1. Inspect clean-voided specimen for contamination with toilet paper or stool.	Contaminants prevent specimen from being used.
2. Evaluate patient's urine C&S laboratory report for bacterial growth.	Routine cultures identify organism(s), and sensitivity study identifies antimicrobial medications that may be effective against pathogen.
3. Observe urinary drainage system in catheterized patient to ensure that it is intact and patent.	System must remain closed to remain sterile.
4. **Use Teach-Back:** "I want to be sure I explained the way to obtain a clean-voided specimen. Please repeat the steps back to me." Revise your instruction now or develop a plan for revised patient/family caregiver teaching if patient/family caregiver is not able to teach back correctly.	Determines patient's/family caregiver's level of understanding of instructional topic.

Unexpected Outcomes	Related Interventions
1. Urine specimen is contaminated with stool or toilet paper.	• Repeat patient instruction and specimen collection. If unable to obtain specimen through clean voiding, patient may need catheterization (see Skill 19.2).
2. Patient is unable to void, or urine does not collect in drainage tube.	• Offer fluids if permitted to enhance urine production.
3. Urine culture reveals bacterial growth (determined by colony count of more than 10,000 organisms per milliliter).	• Report findings to health care provider. • Administer medications as ordered. • Monitor patient for fever and dysuria.
4. Lumen leading to balloon that holds catheter in place is punctured.	• Notify health care provider. • Prepare for removal of existing catheter and insertion of new catheter.

Recording

- Record method used to obtain specimen, date and time collected, type of test ordered, laboratory receiving specimen, characteristics of specimen, and patient's tolerance to procedure of specimen collection.
- Document your evaluation of patient learning.

Hand-Off Reporting

- Report the type of urinalysis and when specimen was sent to laboratory.
- Report any abnormal findings to health care provider.

PROCEDURAL GUIDELINE 9.1 *Collecting a Timed Urine Specimen*

Purpose

Some tests of renal function and urine composition require urine to be collected over 2 to 72 hours. The 24-hour timed collection is used most often and measures elements such as amino acids, creatinine, hormones, glucose, and adrenocorticosteroids. To ensure the accuracy of a 24-hour timed urine specimen, the patient and staff must work together to collect all voided urine in a 24-hour period.

Delegation and Collaboration

The skill of collecting a timed urine specimen can be delegated to nursing assistive personnel (NAP). The nurse informs the NAP about:

- When timed collection begins, proper method to store the collected urine, where to place signs that a timed urine collection is in progress, and saving all urine

PROCEDURAL GUIDELINE 9.1 *Collecting a Timed Urine Specimen—cont'd*

- Reporting when blood, mucus, or foul odors are present in the urine specimen or if there is a break in the collection procedure

Equipment

Large collection bottle with cap that usually contains a chemical preservative; bedpan/urinal, specimen hat, bedside commode, or pediatric potty-chair; graduated measuring container for intake and output (I&O) measurement; large basin to hold collection bottle surrounded by ice if immediate refrigeration is required; specimen identification label and completed laboratory requisition (with appropriate patient identifiers and specimen information); instructional signs that remind patient and staff of timed urine collection; clean gloves; biohazard bag or container (as specific by agency)

Procedural Steps

1. Identify patient using at least two identifiers (e.g., name and birthday or name and medical record number) according to agency policy. Compare identifiers with information on patient's MAR or medical record (TJC, 2019).
2. Review health care provider's order.
3. Explain the reason for specimen collection, how patient can help, and that urine must be free of feces and toilet tissue.
4. Label the specimen container with all appropriate identification information and the number of containers sequentially if more than one container is needed.
5. Place specimen container in the bathroom and, if indicated, in pan of ice. Post signs to remind staff, family and visitors, and patient of timed urine collection on patient's door and toileting area. If patient leaves unit, be sure that personnel in receiving area collect and save all urine.
6. If possible, have patient drink two to four glasses of water about 30 minutes before collection start to facilitate ability to void at appropriate time.
7. Perform hand hygiene and apply gloves. Discard first voided specimen as the test begins. Indicate time test began on laboratory requisition. For accurate results the patient must begin the test with an empty bladder. Begin collecting urine for the designated time.
8. Measure volume of each voiding if I&O are to be recorded. Place all voided urine in labeled specimen bottle with appropriate additives/preservatives. **NOTE:** The type of analysis for the 24-hour timed specimen determines the need for any preservative.
9. Unless instructed otherwise, keep specimen bottle in specimen refrigerator or container of ice in bathroom to prevent decomposition of urine.
10. Encourage patient to drink two glasses of water 1 hour before timed urine collection ends. Encourage patient to empty bladder during last 15 minutes of urine collection period.
11. Perform hand hygiene and apply clean gloves. Collect final specimen at end of collection period. Label specimen (two identifiers, specimen source, collection date and time, number of bottle) in patient's presence, attach appropriate requisition, and send to laboratory. Remove gloves and perform hand hygiene.
12. Remove signs. Tell patient that specimen collection period is completed.
13. Assist patient into comfortable position and ensure nurse call system is within reach and patient instructed in its use.
14. Document completion of 24-hour urine and disposition to laboratory in patient's medical record.

PROCEDURAL GUIDELINE 9.2 *Urine Screening for Glucose, Ketones, Protein, Blood, and pH*

Purpose

Tests for chemical properties of urine are part of the routine urinalysis completed in the laboratory or as a point-of-care (POC) test performed at the bedside or in the home. The use of a Multistix reagent test strip may simultaneously assess for up to nine chemical properties: specific gravity, pH, protein, glucose, ketones, blood bilirubin, urobilinogen, leukocytes, and nitrates. This type of screening is used when more detailed laboratory testing is not available (e.g., health care provider's office, clinic, or long-term care setting). The use of urine testing for managing blood glucose is no longer recommended but continues to be useful in detecting the presence of ketones in patients with diabetes (American Diabetes Association [ADA], 2015).

Delegation and Collaboration

The skill of urine screening for chemical properties can be delegated to NAP. The nurse informs the NAP to:

- Obtain the specimen correctly (e.g., before meals, after a "double-voided" specimen).
- Report the results of the test or any odor, blood, or mucus in the urine specimen.

Equipment

Bedpan, urinal, specimen hat, bedside commode, or pediatric potty-chair; container for urine from catheter; watch with second hand or digital counter; reagent test strip (check expiration date on container); test strip color chart; paper towel; clean gloves; biohazard bag or container for delivery of specimen to laboratory (as specified by agency)

Procedural Steps

1. Identify patient using at least two identifiers (e.g., name and birthday or name and medical record number) according to agency policy. Compare identifiers with information on patient's MAR or medical record (TJC, 2019).
2. Review health care provider's order. Determine whether double-voided specimen is needed. If required, ask patient to void, discard, and then drink a glass of water.

Continued

PROCEDURAL GUIDELINE 9.2 *Urine Screening for Glucose, Ketones, Protein, Blood, and pH—cont'd*

3. Perform hand hygiene and apply clean gloves. Ask patient to collect a fresh, random urine specimen. If patient is catheterized, remove a 5-mL specimen from the catheter port (see Skill 9.1).
4. Immerse end of reagent strip into urine container. Remove the strip immediately and tap it gently against the side of the container to remove excess urine.
5. Hold strip in horizontal position to prevent mixing of chemical reagents (see illustration).

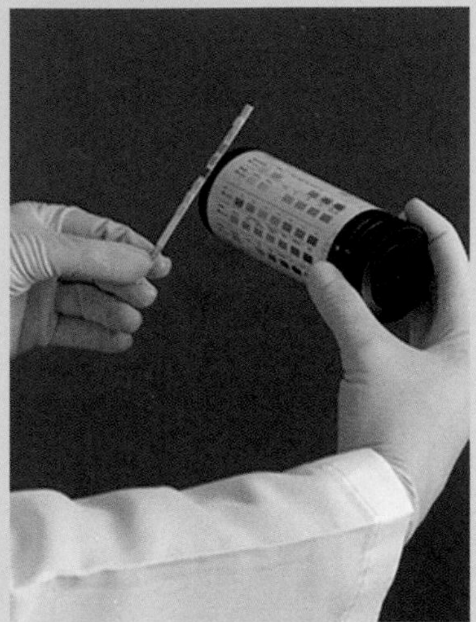

STEP 5 Testing urine using reagent strip.

6. Precisely time the number of seconds specified on container and compare color of strip with color chart on container (Table 9.1).
7. When appropriate, discuss test results with patient. Discard urine. Remove and discard gloves; perform hand hygiene.
8. Record results immediately on appropriate testing flow sheet.
9. Assist patient to comfortable position and ensure nurse call system is within reach and patient instructed in its use.

TABLE 9.1
Color Chart for Reagent Strip

Test	When to Read	Range of Results
pH	Anytime	4.6–8.0
Protein	Anytime	None or up to 8 mg/100 mL
Glucose	10 seconds (qualitative) 30 seconds (quantitative)	(–) to + 4 (–) to + 4 (270)
Ketones	15 seconds	(–) to + 3 (large)
Blood	25 seconds	(–) to + 3 (large)

✦ SKILL 9.2 Testing for Gastrointestinal Alterations—Gastroccult Test, Stool Specimen, and Hemoccult Test

Purpose

The collection of gastric secretions involves obtaining a specimen from an existing nasogastric (NG) or nasointestinal (NI) tube. When a patient has emesis, you test the material for the presence of blood. Analysis of stool or gastric secretions from the gastrointestinal (GI) tract provides useful information about pathological conditions including the presence of occult (not visible) blood in the stool for conditions such as colon cancer, bleeding gastrointestinal ulcers, and localized gastric or intestinal irritation.

Delegation and Collaboration

The skill of testing emesis or stool for occult blood can be delegated to NAP. You cannot delegate the skill of Gastroccult testing if the specimen is collected from an NG or nasoenteral (NE) tube. The nurse informs the NAP to:

- Collect the stool specimen at the specified time.
- Report immediately if blood or coffee-ground emesis is visible in NG or NE tube secretions.
- When blood is detected in stool or emesis, save specimen for repeat testing.

Equipment

- Identification labels and completed laboratory requisitions, including appropriate patient identification, date, time, name of test, and source of specimen
- Small plastic bag for delivery of specimen to laboratory (as specified by agency)
- Clean gloves
- Soap, water, washcloth, and towel

Gastroccult Test

- Facial tissue
- Emesis basin
- Wooden applicator or 3-mL syringe
- 60-mL bulb syringe or catheter tip syringe
- Cardboard Gastroccult slide and developing solution (Fig. 9.4)

Stool Specimen

- "Save stool" signs for 24-hour timed specimen
- Sterile test tube and swabs for culture
- Plastic container with lid
- Two tongue blades
- Paper towel
- Bedpan, specimen hat, or bedside commode

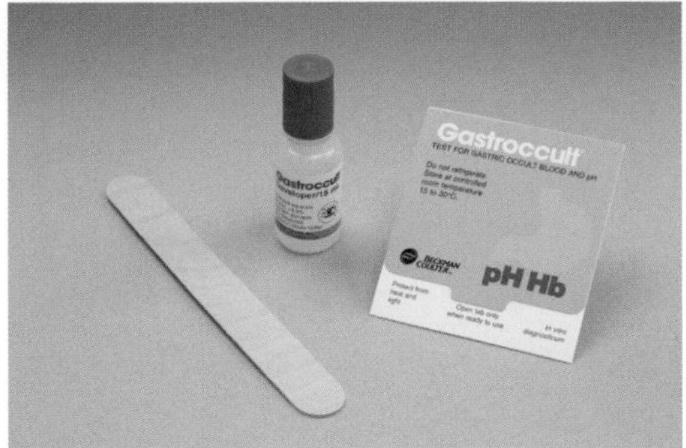

FIG 9.4 Cardboard Gastroccult slide and developing solution.

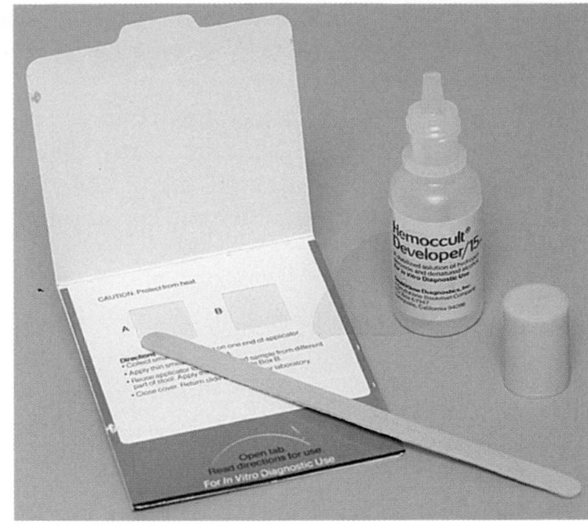

FIG 9.5 Hemoccult slide testing kit for measuring occult blood.

Hemoccult (Guaiac Test)

- Paper towel
- Wooden applicator
- Cardboard Hemoccult slide and Hemoccult developing solution (Fig. 9.5)

ASSESSMENT

1. Identify patient using at least two identifiers (e.g., name and birthday or name and medical record number) according to agency policy. Compare identifiers with information on patient's MAR or medical record. *Rationale: Ensures correct patient. Complies with The Joint Commission standards and improves patient safety (TJC, 2019).*
2. Review health care provider's orders for medication and/or dietary modifications before test. *Rationale: Specimens will be positive if contaminated by menstrual blood, hemorrhoid blood, bleeding gums after dental procedure, ingestion of red meat within 3 days before testing (Pagana et al., 2017).*
3. Assess patient's ability to cooperate with procedure and collect specimen. *Rationale: To avoid embarrassment, patients often prefer to collect their own stool specimen.*
4. Review patient's medical history for GI disorders (e.g., history of bleeding, colitis).
5. Review patient's medications for drugs that contribute to GI bleeding. *Rationale: Anticoagulants increase risk for bleeding in GI tract, even from minor trauma to mucosa. Long-term use of steroids, nonsteroidal antiinflammatory drugs (NSAIDs), and acetylsalicylic acid (aspirin) can irritate mucosa (Pagana et al., 2017).*
6. Assess patient's or family caregiver's knowledge, experience, and health literacy. *Rationale: Ensures patient or family caregiver has the capacity to obtain, communicate, process, and understand basic health information (CDC, 2016).*
7. Assess patient's or family caregiver's understanding of need for test. *Rationale: Provides nurse with information on which to base necessary health teaching.*

STEP	RATIONALE
PLANNING	
1. Expected outcomes after completion of procedure:	
• Test for occult blood is negative.	Patient has only small or no amount of blood in gastric secretions. Test obtained correctly.
• Patient discusses purpose and benefits of testing gastric contents for blood.	Validates learning.
2. Explain procedure to patient and/or family caregiver. Discuss why specimen collection is necessary.	Patient who understands procedure is more likely to be less anxious and more cooperative.
3. Arrange for any dietary or medication restrictions before sample collection	Ensures accuracy of test.
IMPLEMENTATION	
1. Perform hand hygiene and apply clean gloves.	Reduces transmission of microorganisms.
2. Perform point-of-care Gastroccult test.	
a. Verify NG tube placement (see Chapter 13).	Ensures aspiration of gastric contents and not airway or oral secretions.

STEP	RATIONALE
b. Obtain specimen by disconnecting suction or gravity drainage tube from NG or NE tube. Using a bulb or catheter tip syringe, aspirate 5–10 mL of fluid from NG or NE tube. Reconnect tube to drainage tube if appropriate.	Only small amount of specimen is needed for testing.

Safe Patient Care *Observe specimen. If you find red blood or coffee-ground material, save specimen, and report these findings immediately to health care provider.*

STEP	RATIONALE
c. To obtain sample of emesis, use 3-mL syringe or wooden applicator to obtain sample from emesis basin.	Small specimen is sufficient for measuring blood content.
d. Using wooden applicator or syringe, apply 1 drop of gastric sample to Gastroccult blood test slide.	Sample must cover test paper for test reaction to occur.
e. Apply 2 drops of commercial developer solution over sample and 1 drop between positive and negative performance monitors (see illustration).	

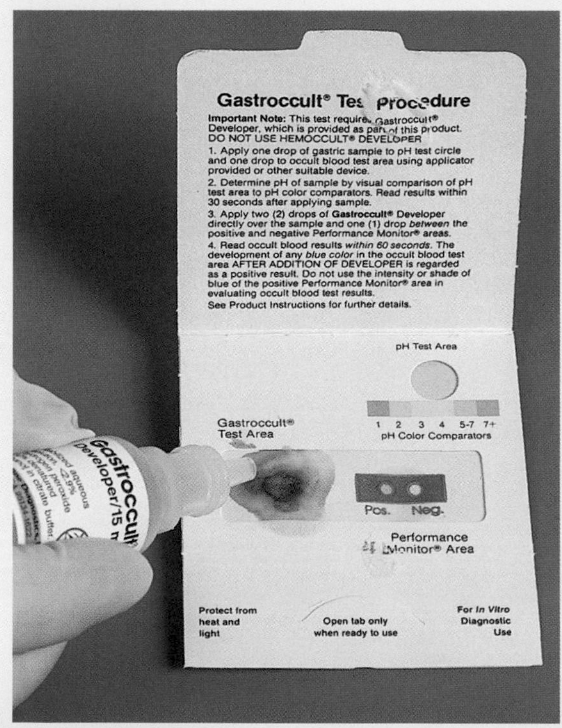

STEP 2e Applying developing solution to Gastroccult test area.

STEP	RATIONALE
f. Verify that performance monitor turns blue in 30 seconds.	Indicates proper function of testing paper.
g. After 60 seconds, compare color of gastric sample with that of performance monitor.	If sample turns blue, test is positive for occult blood. If sample turns green, it is negative for occult blood.
h. Dispose of test slide, wooden applicator, and/or syringe in proper receptacle.	Reduces transmission of microorganisms.
3. Perform stool tests.	
a. Collect stool specimen: Assist patient as needed into bathroom or to commode or bedpan. Instruct patient to void into toilet or urinal before collecting specimen in container. Provide a clean, dry bedpan or specimen hat in which to defecate.	Feces must not be mixed with urine, water, or toilet tissue. Urine inhibits fecal bacterial growth. Toilet tissue contains bismuth, which interferes with test results.

STEP	RATIONALE
b. If needed, assist patient in washing after toileting and leave in a comfortable position.	
c. Take container with stool to bathroom or utility room and place specimen into specimen container.	
(1) Culture:	
(a) Remove swab from sterile test tube, gather bean-size piece of stool, and return swab to tube. If stool is liquid, soak swab in it and return to tube.	Use of sterile swab prevents introduction of bacteria.
(2) Timed stool specimen:	
(a) Place stool from each collection in waxed cardboard container for specific time ordered and keep in specimen refrigerator.	Tests for dietary products and digestive enzymes such as fat content or bile require analysis of all feces over a specific time period.
(b) For timed test, place signs that read "Save all stool" (with appropriate date or time) over patient's bed, on bathroom door, and above toilet.	Helps prevent any accidental disposal of stool.
d. After obtaining the specimen for the laboratory, immediately place lid tightly on container.	Prevents spread of microorganisms by air or contact with other articles.
e. Label specimen (two identifiers, specimen source, collection date and time, number of bottle) in patient's presence, attach appropriate requisition (patient identification, date, time, name of test, and specimen source), and send to laboratory.	Ensures correct patient specimen, correct diagnostic testing, and prompt delivery to laboratory.
f. Remove and discard any soiled supplies into appropriate container.	Reduces transmission of microorganisms.
4. Perform point-of-care Hemoccult test (guaiac).	
a. Collect stool specimen: Assist patient as needed into bathroom or to commode or bedpan. Instruct patient to void into toilet or urinal before collecting specimen in container. Provide a clean, dry bedpan or specimen hat in which to defecate.	Feces must not be mixed with urine, water, or toilet tissue. Urine inhibits fecal bacterial growth. Toilet tissue contains bismuth, which interferes with test results.
b. If needed, assist patient in washing after toileting and leave in a comfortable position.	
c. Take container with stool to bathroom or utility room. Use tip of wooden applicator to obtain small portion of feces.	
d. Open flap of Hemoccult slide. Apply thin smear of stool on paper in first box.	Guaiac paper inside box is sensitive to fecal blood content.
e. Obtain a second fecal specimen from different portion of stool and apply thinly to second box of slide (see illustration).	Occult blood from upper GI tract is not always dispersed equally throughout stool. Findings of occult blood are more conclusive when entire specimen is found to contain blood.
f. Close slide cover and turn slide over to reverse side. Open cardboard flap, and apply 2 drops of Hemoccult developing solution on each box of guaiac paper (see illustration).	Developing solution penetrates underlying fecal specimen. Blood is indicated by change in color of guaiac paper.

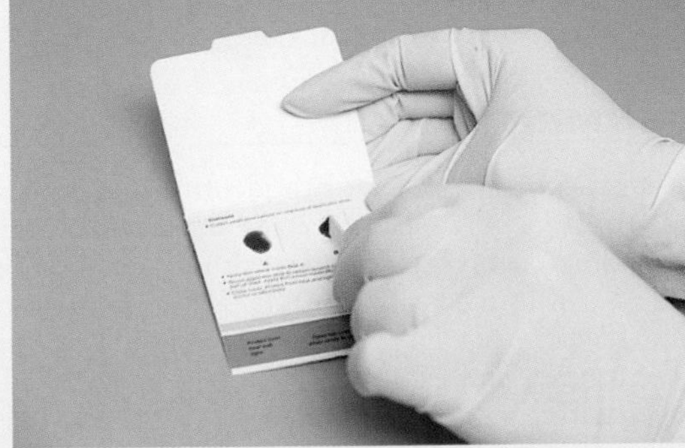

STEP 4e Apply stool to both spots on Hemocccult slide.

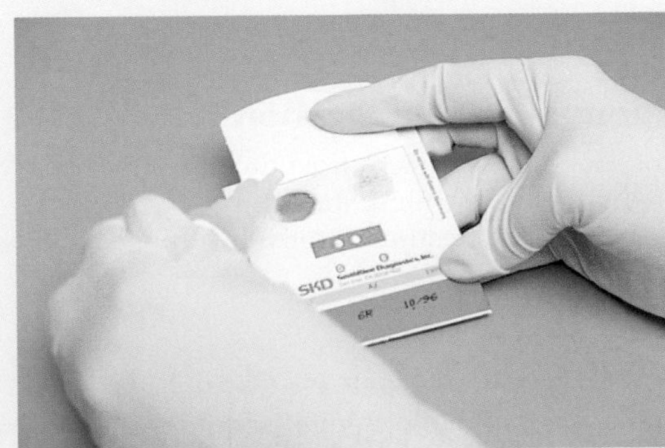

STEP 4f Applying developing solution to Hemoccult slide.

STEP	RATIONALE
g. Read results of test after 30–60 seconds. Note color changes.	Bluish discoloration indicates occult blood (guaiac positive). No change in color of guaiac paper indicates negative results.
h. Dispose of test slide and wooden applicator in appropriate receptacle.	Reduces transmission of microorganisms.
5. Provide or assist with perineal hygiene as needed.	
6. Remove and dispose of gloves. Perform hand hygiene.	Reduces transmission of microorganisms.
7. Assist patient to a comfortable position. Be sure nurse call system is in an accessible location within patient's reach. Instruct patient in its use.	Provides for patient comfort and safety. Ensures patient can call for assistance if needed.
8. Raise side rails (as appropriate) and lower bed to lowest position.	Ensures patient safety.

EVALUATION

1. Note character of stool or gastric secretions.	Blood may be visible, or coffee-ground material denoting blood may be observed.
2. Note color changes in guaiac paper.	Reveals blood in gastric secretions.
3. **Use Teach-Back:** "I want to be sure I explained the purpose and procedure for how to obtain a stool specimen at home. Please state the necessary steps you will use to obtain this specimen." Revise your instruction now or develop a plan for revised patient/family caregiver teaching if patient/family caregiver is not able to teach back correctly.	Determines patient's/family caregiver's level of understanding of instructional topic.

Unexpected Outcome	Related Interventions
1. Test for occult blood is positive.	• Continue to monitor patient. • Notify health care provider.

Recording

- Record results of test in appropriate records (check agency policy); include characteristics of specimen contents in nurses' notes.
- Document your evaluation of patient learning.

Hand-Off Reporting

- Report positive results to health care provider.
- Report whfn timed specimen was transported to laboratory.
- Report any patient discomfort.

✦ SKILL 9.3 Collecting Nose and Throat Specimens

Purpose

Nose and throat cultures are simple diagnostic tools to identify the presence and type of microorganism for patients with signs and symptoms of upper respiratory or sinus infection. Ideally this specimen is collected before antibiotic therapy is begun. If a patient is already on an antibiotic, notify laboratory and identify the specific antibiotics (Pagana et al., 2017).

Delegation and Collaboration

The skill of obtaining specimens from the nose and throat cannot be delegated to NAP. The nurse informs the NAP to:

- Report shortness of breath, difficulty breathing, and other signs of respiratory distress.

Equipment

- Two sterile swabs in sterile culture tubes (flexible wire swab with cotton tip may be used for nose cultures)
- Nasal speculum *(optional)*
- Emesis basin or clean container *(optional)*
- Tongue blades and penlight
- Facial tissues/gauze
- Clean gloves
- Identification labels with name of test
- Completed laboratory requisition (date, time, name of test, patient identification, source of culture)
- Biohazard bag or container for delivery of specimen to laboratory (as specified by agency)

ASSESSMENT

1. Identify patient using at least two identifiers (e.g., name and birthday or name and medical record number) according to agency policy. Compare identifiers with information on patient's MAR or medical record. *Rationale: Ensures correct patient. Complies with The Joint Commission standards and improves patient safety (TJC, 2019).*
2. Review health care provider's orders to determine whether nose, throat, or both cultures are needed. *Rationale: Prevents exposing patient to unnecessary discomfort of repeated cultures.*

3. Determine whether patient experiences postnasal drip, sinus headache or tenderness, nasal congestion, sore throat, or exposure to others with similar symptoms. *Rationale: Possible indicators for testing of nasal secretions.*
4. Assess patient for signs of infection, including fever, chills, and/or fatigue. *Rationale: Infection originating within nasopharynx can become systemic, requiring antibiotic therapy.*
5. Perform hand hygiene and apply clean gloves. Inspect condition of nares and drainage from nasal mucosa and sinuses. *Rationale: Reveals physical signs that indicate infection or allergic irritation. Clear drainage usually indicates allergy. Yellow, green, or brown drainage usually indicates infection.*
6. Assess condition of posterior pharynx (see Chapter 8). Remove and discard gloves. Perform hand hygiene. *Rationale: Reveals local inflammation or lesions of pharynx.*
7. Assess patient's or family caregiver's knowledge, experience, and health literacy. *Rationale: Ensures patient or family caregiver has the capacity to obtain, communicate, process, and understand basic health information (CDC, 2016).*
8. Assess patient's understanding of purpose for procedure and ability to cooperate. *Rationale: Provides basis to determine need for health teaching and assistance.*

STEP	RATIONALE
PLANNING	
1. Expected outcomes after completion of procedure:	
• There is no bacterial growth in specimens.	Absence of bacterial infection.
• Patient does not experience bleeding of nasal mucosa.	Procedure is atraumatic.
• Specimen is not contaminated.	Procedure performed correctly as evidenced by results of laboratory analysis.
• Patient discusses purpose of nose and throat cultures.	Validates learning.
2. Plan to do culture before mealtime or at least 1 hour after eating.	Procedure often induces gagging; timing decreases patient's chances of vomiting.
3. Explain procedure to patient and/or family caregiver. Discuss reason for specimen collection and how patient can help.	Understanding procedure usually decreases anxiety and promotes cooperation.
4. Explain that patient may have tickling sensation or gagging during swabbing of throat. Nasal swab may create urge to sneeze. Each procedure only takes a few seconds to complete.	Helps patient relax.
5. Position patient erect in bed or chair facing you. Acutely ill patient or young child may lie back against bed with head of bed raised to 45-degree angle in semi-Fowler's position.	Provides easy access to nasal or oral structures.
IMPLEMENTATION	
1. Perform hand hygiene. Have swab in tube ready for use. Loosen top so swab can be removed easily.	Reduces transmission of microorganisms. Allows you to grasp swab easily without danger of contamination. Most commercial tubes have tops that fit securely over end of swab. Allows touching outer tops without contaminating swab stick.
2. **Collect throat culture:**	
a. Apply clean gloves.	Reduces transmission of microorganisms.
b. Instruct patient to tilt head backward. For patients in bed, place pillow behind shoulders.	Facilitates visualization of pharynx.
c. Ask patient to open mouth and say "ah." To visualize pharynx, depress tongue with tongue blade and note inflamed areas of pharynx or tonsils. Depress anterior third of tongue only and illuminate with penlight as needed.	Permits exposure of pharynx, relaxes throat muscles, and minimizes gag reflex. Area to be swabbed should be visualized clearly.

Safe Patient Care *Do not attempt throat culture in a pediatric patient if you suspect acute epiglottitis because trauma from swab might increase edema, resulting in occlusion of airway (Hockenberry et al., 2017).*

STEP	RATIONALE
d. Insert swab without touching lips, teeth, tongue, cheeks, or uvula.	Prevents contamination with organisms from oral cavity (Pagana et al., 2017).
e. Gently but quickly swab tonsillar area side to side, contacting inflamed or purulent sites (see illustration).	These areas contain most microorganisms.
f. Carefully withdraw swab without touching oral structures.	Collects microorganisms from throat tissues without contamination from mouth and tongue.

STEP	RATIONALE
3. **Collect nasal culture:**	
a. Apply clean gloves.	Reduces transmission of microorganisms.
b. Encourage patient to blow nose and then check nostrils for patency with penlight. Select nostril with greatest patency.	Clears nasal passages of mucus containing resident bacteria.
c. In sitting position, have patient tilt head backward. Patients in bed should have small pillow behind shoulders.	Provides access to nasal passages and facilitates visualization of nasal septum and sinuses.
d. Gently insert nasal speculum in one nostril *(optional)*.	Allows retraction of mucosa for easier swab insertion.
e. Carefully pass swab into nostril until it reaches that part of mucosa that is inflamed or containing exudate. Rotate swab quickly. **NOTE:** If you need to obtain nasopharyngeal culture, use special swab on flexible wire that can be flexed downward to reach nasopharynx.	Swab should remain sterile until it reaches area to be cultured. Rotating swab covers all surfaces where exudate is present.
f. Remove swab without touching sides of speculum or nasal canal.	Prevents contamination of swab by resident bacteria.
g. Carefully remove nasal speculum (if used) and place in basin. Offer patient facial tissue.	Minimizes period of time that patient experiences discomfort.
4. Insert swab into culture tube. Use gauze to protect your fingers while crushing ampule at bottom of tube to release culture medium (see illustrations).	Placing tip within culture medium maintains life of bacteria for testing.
5. Place tip of swab into liquid medium and place top securely on top of tube.	Preserves specimen for testing.

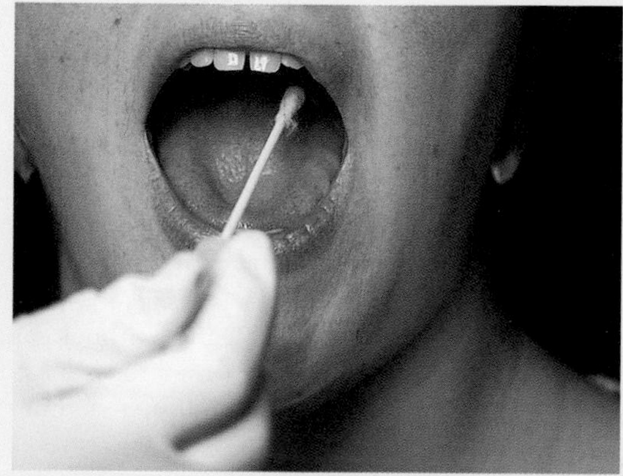

STEP 2e Collecting specimen from posterior pharynx.

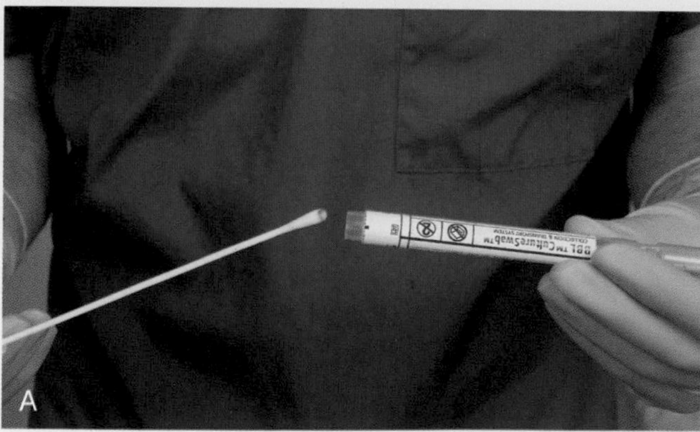

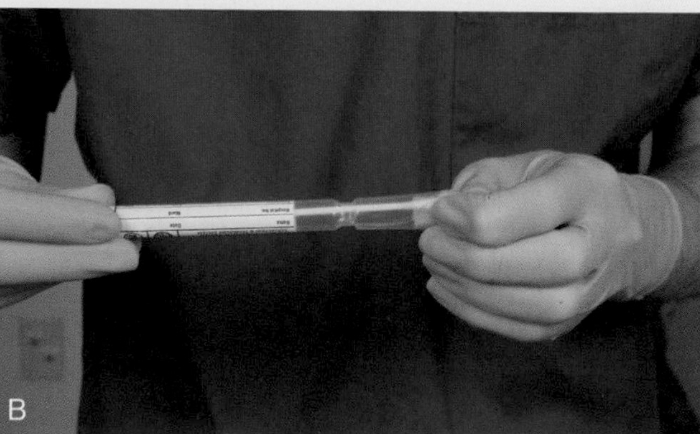

STEP 4 Activating culture tube. (A) Place swab into tube. (B) Crush end of tube to release liquid medium.

STEP	RATIONALE
6. In presence of patient, complete label (two identifiers, specimen source, collection date and time) and attach to container. Attach completed laboratory requisition to container. Enclose specimen in a biohazard bag and send immediately to laboratory.	Incorrect patient identification could lead to diagnostic or therapeutic error (TJC, 2019). Bacteria multiply quickly. Specimen should be analyzed promptly for accurate results.
Safe Patient Care *Mark on laboratory requisition if patient is taking antibiotics or if specific organism is suspected (e.g.,* Bordetella pertussis*).*	
7. Remove and dispose of gloves and perform hand hygiene.	Reduces transmission of microorganisms.
8. Return patient to position of comfort. Ensure nurse call system is in an accessible location within patient's reach. Instruct patient in its use.	Provides for patient comfort. Ensures patient can call for assistance if needed.
9. Raise side rails (as appropriate) and lower bed to lowest position.	Ensures patient safety.

EVALUATION

1. Check laboratory record for results of culture test.	Results reveal type of organisms in nose or pharynx and antibiotics most likely to be effective.
2. **Use Teach-Back:** "I want to be sure I explained the purpose and importance of sitting up straight and tilting your head backward when obtaining a throat culture. Also, please tell me why we are obtaining this culture." Revise your instruction now or develop a plan for revised patient/family caregiver teaching if patient/family caregiver is not able to teach back correctly.	Determines patient's/family caregiver's level of understanding of instructional topic.

Unexpected Outcomes	Related Interventions
1. Nose and throat cultures reveal bacterial growth.	• Notify health care provider of findings. • Administer medications as ordered.
2. Patient experiences minor nasal bleeding.	• Apply mild pressure and ice pack over bridge of nose. • Notify health care provider of patient's condition.
3. Specimen is contaminated.	• Repeat specimen collection.

Recording

- Record type of specimen obtained, source, and time and date sent to laboratory; describe appearance of site and presence or absence of signs of local or systemic infection; note any unusual patient response to procedure.
- Document your evaluation of patient learning.

Hand-Off Reporting

- Report unusual test results to health care provider.
- Report any throat irritation or nasal bleeding or irritation.

✦ SKILL 9.4 Collecting a Sputum Specimen

Purpose

Sputum specimens are obtained to identify cancer cells, to perform culture and sensitivity (C&S) to identify specific pathogens and to determine the antibiotics to which they are most sensitive, and to detect acid-fast bacillus to support the diagnosis of pulmonary tuberculosis. Obtain sputum specimen before antibiotic administration so that C&S analysis is based on a specimen not altered by antibiotic use. The exception to this is when another test is ordered to determine the effectiveness of the current antibiotic order (Pagana et al., 2017).

Delegation and Collaboration

The skill of collecting sputum specimens by suction cannot be delegated to NAP. The nurse instructs the NAP to:

- Notify the nurse if the patient expectorates bloody sputum.

Equipment

- Identification labels with name of test
- Completed laboratory requisition, including patient identification, date, time, name of test, and source of culture

- Biohazard bag or container for delivery of specimen to laboratory (as specified by agency)
- Pulse oximeter

Collecting Sputum Specimen by Expectoration

- Sterile specimen container with cover
- Clean gloves
- Facial tissue
- Emesis basin *(optional)* toothbrush *(optional)*
- Disinfectant wipes

Collecting Specimen by Suctioning

- Suction device (wall or portable)
- Sterile suction catheter (size 14, 16, or 18 Fr [not large enough to cause trauma to nasal mucosa]) or suction catheter with sleeve (see Chapter 16)
- Sterile gloves and clean gloves
- Sterile water in container
- In-line specimen container or sputum trap
- Oxygen therapy equipment if indicated
- Protective eyewear
- Disinfectant wipe

ASSESSMENT

1. Identify patient using at least two identifiers (e.g., name and birthday or name and medical record number) according to agency policy. Compare identifiers with information on patient's MAR or medical record. *Rationale: Ensures correct patient. Complies with The Joint Commission standards and improves patient safety (TJC, 2019).*
2. Review health care provider's orders for type of sputum analysis and specifications (e.g., amount of sputum, number of specimens, time of collection, method to obtain). Specimens for acid-fast bacillus (AFB) require three consecutive morning samples. *Rationale: Specific test dictates when or how frequently specimens are collected. Ideal time to collect sputum is early morning because bronchial secretions tend to accumulate during the night. Bacteria also accumulate in pooled secretions.*
3. Assess when patient last ate meal (or had tube feeding). *Rationale: It is best to obtain specimen 1–2 hours after or 1 hour before meal to minimize gagging, which can cause vomiting and aspiration.*
4. Determine type of help needed by patient to obtain specimen. *Rationale: Positioning, postural drainage, and deep-breathing and coughing exercises may improve ability to cough productively. Suctioning is often indicated when patient is unable to cough and expectorate.*
5. Perform hand hygiene and perform a respiratory assessment, including respiratory rate, depth, and pattern and color of mucous membranes. *Rationale: Respiratory status can depend on amount of sputum in tracheobronchial tree.*
6. Assess patient's or family caregiver's knowledge, experience, and health literacy. *Rationale: Ensures patient or family caregiver has the capacity to obtain, communicate, process, and understand basic health information (CDC, 2016).*
7. Assess patient's level of understanding of procedure and its purpose. *Rationale: Provides baseline to establish teaching plan.*

STEP	RATIONALE
PLANNING	
1. Expected outcomes after completion of procedure:	
• Patient's respirations are same rate and character before and after procedure.	Specimen collection did not alter respiratory status.
• Patient maintains comfort level and experiences minimal anxiety.	Suctioning tends to cause anxiety.
• Sputum is not contaminated by saliva or oropharyngeal flora.	Sputum collected correctly. Must originate from tracheobronchial tree for accurate results.
• Patient discusses purpose and benefit of sputum collection.	Validates learning.
2. Gather and organize equipment at patient's bedside	Ensures an organized approach to obtaining a sputum specimen.
3. Close room door or bedside curtains.	Provides privacy.
4. Explain steps of procedure and purpose. Instruct patient to breathe normally during suctioning to prevent hyperventilation.	Promotes understanding and cooperation.
5. **For obtaining specimen by suction:** Prepare suction machine or device and determine whether it functions properly.	Verifies that equipment is working properly before suctioning procedure.
6. Position patient in high- or semi-Fowler's position.	Promotes full lung expansion and facilitates ability to cough.

Safe Patient Care *If patient has surgical incision or localized area of discomfort, have him or her place pillow or hands firmly over affected area. Splinting of painful area minimizes muscular stretching and discomfort during coughing and thus makes cough more productive.*

IMPLEMENTATION

1. **Collect sputum by expectoration:**

Safe Patient Care *Whenever possible, obtain expectorated sputum specimen when patient awakens, before oral hygiene, eating, or drinking (Pagana et al., 2017).*

STEP	RATIONALE
a. Provide opportunity for patient to clean or rinse mouth with water. Do not allow patient to use toothpaste or mouthwash.	Toothpaste or mouthwash may alter culture results because they contain chemical properties and are not sterile.
b. Perform hand hygiene and apply clean gloves. Provide sputum cup and instruct patient not to touch inside of container.	Decreases contamination, which can alter results.
c. Instruct patient to take three to four deep slow breaths with full exhalation. Then take full inhalation followed immediately by a forceful cough, expectorating sputum directly into specimen container (see illustration). Repeat until 5–10 mL of sputum has been collected.	Sputum must come from tracheobronchial tree, and expectorant must not simply be saliva in mouth.
2. **Collect sputum specimen by suctioning:**	
a. Perform hand hygiene and apply clean glove to nondominant hand.	Adequate amount of suction is necessary to aspirate sputum.
b. Connect suction tube to adapter on sputum trap. Open sterile water (see Chapter 16).	Establishes suction that passes through sputum trap to aspirate specimen.
c. Using sterile technique, apply sterile glove to dominant hand or use clean glove if suction catheter has plastic sleeve.	Tracheobronchial tree is sterile body cavity. Allows you to manipulate suction catheter without contamination.
d. With gloved hand, connect sterile suction catheter to rubber tubing on sputum trap.	Aspirated sputum will go directly to trap instead of to suction tubing.
e. Lubricate suction catheter tip with sterile water *(with suction off)*.	Lubrication allows for easier insertion of catheter.
f. Using dominant hand, gently insert tip of suction catheter through nasopharynx, endotracheal tube, or tracheostomy tube without applying suction (see Chapter 16).	Minimizes trauma to airway as catheter is inserted.
g. Gently and quickly advance catheter into trachea. Warn patient to expect to cough.	Entrance of catheter into larynx and trachea triggers cough reflex.
h. As patient coughs, apply suction for 5–10 seconds, collecting 2–10 mL of sputum.	Ensures collection of sputum from deep within tracheobronchial tree. Suctioning longer than 10 seconds can cause hypoxia and mucosal damage.
i. Release suction and remove catheter; turn off suction.	Suction can damage mucosa if applied during withdrawal.
j. Detach catheter from specimen trap and dispose of catheter in appropriate receptacle.	Decreases risk for spreading microorganisms.
3. Secure top on specimen container tightly. For sputum trap, detach suction tubing and connect rubber tubing on sputum trap to plastic adapter (see illustration).	Contains microorganisms within container, preventing exposure to personnel handling specimen.

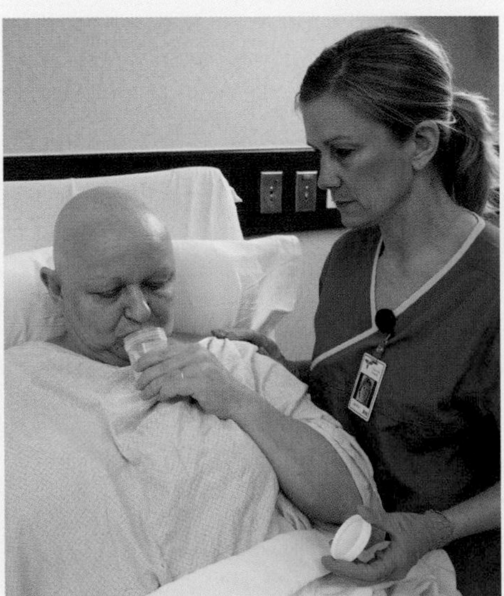
STEP 1c Expectorating sputum.

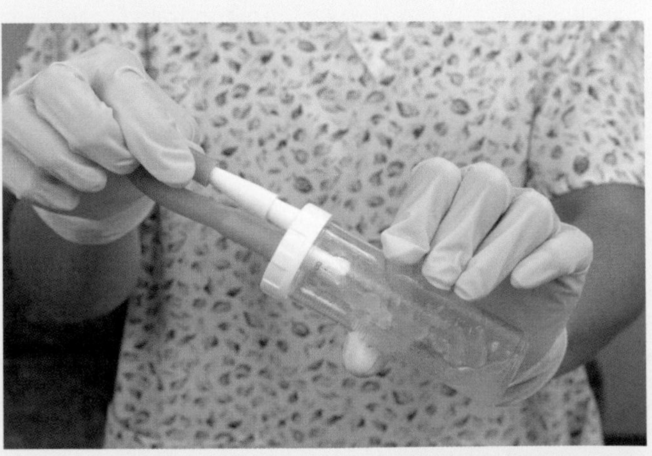
STEP 3 Closing sputum specimen trap.

STEP	RATIONALE
4. If any sputum is present on outside of container, wipe it off with disinfectant.	Prevents spread of infection to people handling specimen.
5 In presence of patient, complete label (two identifiers, specimen source, collection date and time) and attach to container. Attach completed laboratory requisition to container. Enclose specimen in a biohazard bag and send immediately to laboratory.	Incorrect patient identification could lead to diagnostic or therapeutic error (TJC, 2019). Bacteria multiply quickly. Specimen should be analyzed promptly for accurate results.
6. Offer patient tissues after suctioning. Dispose of tissues in emesis basin or appropriate container.	Maintains cleanliness and comfort.
7. Remove and dispose of gloves. Perform hand hygiene.	Reduces transmission of microorganisms.
8. Help patient to comfortable position. Offer patient mouth care if desired.	Promotes comfort.
9. Be sure nurse call system is in an accessible location within patient's reach.	Ensures patient can call for assistance if needed.
10. Raise side rails (as appropriate) and lower bed to lowest position.	Ensures patient safety.
11. Send specimen immediately to laboratory or refrigerate.	Bacteria multiply quickly. Prompt analysis ensures accurate results.

EVALUATION

1. Observe patient's respiratory status throughout procedure, especially during suctioning. If under distress, measure oxygen saturation with pulse oximeter.	Excessive coughing or prolonged suctioning can alter respiratory pattern and cause hypoxia. Determines oxygenation status.
2. Note anxiety or discomfort in patient.	Procedure can be uncomfortable. If patient becomes short of breath, anxiety will develop.
3. Observe character of sputum: color, consistency, odor, volume, viscosity, and/or presence of blood.	Characteristics may indicate disease entities.
4. Refer to laboratory reports for test results.	Indicates if abnormal cells or microorganisms are present in sputum.
5. **Use Teach-Back:** "I want to be sure I explained the purpose and procedure for obtaining a sputum specimen. Please tell me how you will obtain this sputum specimen." Revise your instruction now or develop a plan for revised patient/family caregiver teaching if patient/family caregiver is not able to teach back correctly.	Determines patient's/family caregiver's level of understanding of instructional topic.

Unexpected Outcomes	Related Interventions
1. Patient becomes hypoxic with increased respiratory rate and effort and shortness of breath.	• Discontinue suctioning immediately. • Administer oxygen (if ordered). • Notify health care provider of patient's condition. • Continue to monitor patient's vital signs and pulse oximetry.
2. Patient remains anxious or reports discomfort from suction catheter.	• Discontinue procedure until stable. • Administer oxygen (if ordered). • Notify health care provider of patient's change in condition. • Continue to monitor patient's vital signs and pulse oximetry.
3. Patient reports pain when coughing to produce sputum.	• Encourage patient who is recovering from surgical procedure to splint incision before coughing. • Obtain order for pain medication as needed (prn). • Inform health care provider of changes in patient's condition.

Recording

- Record method used to obtain specimen, date and time collected, type of test ordered, and transport to the laboratory. Describe characteristics of sputum specimen and patient's tolerance of procedure.
- Document your evaluation of patient learning.

Hand-Off Reporting

- Report any unusual findings such as bloody sputum or patient response such as increased dyspnea.
- Report any results of sputum specimen.

✦ SKILL 9.5 Collecting Wound Drainage Specimens

Purpose

A wound drainage specimen identifies the presence of pathogens and specific antibiotics sensitive to the organisms. Infection is best treated with antibiotics after the causative organism or organisms are confirmed from a wound culture. Serial wound cultures (gathered over time) are often necessary to monitor the effectiveness of the treatment (Pagana et al., 2017).

Delegation and Collaboration

The skill of obtaining wound drainage specimens cannot be delegated to NAP. The nurse instructs the NAP to:

- Report foul odor, increase in drainage, and increase in body temperature or patient reports of discomfort.

Equipment

- Culture tube with swab and transport medium for aerobic culture
- Anaerobic culture tube with swab (tubes contain carbon dioxide or nitrogen gas)
- 5- to 10-mL safety syringe and needless access device
- Two pairs of clean gloves and sterile gloves
- Protective eyewear
- Antiseptic swab
- Sterile dressing materials (determined by type of dressing)
- Paper or plastic disposable bag
- Identification label with name of test
- Completed laboratory requisition (date, time, name of test, patient identification, and source of culture)
- Biohazard bag or container for delivery of specimen to laboratory (as specified by agency)

ASSESSMENT

1. Identify patient using at least two identifiers (e.g., name and birthday or name and medical record number) according to agency policy. Compare identifiers and information on patient's MAR or medical record. *Rationale: Ensures correct patient. Complies with The Joint Commission standards and improves patient safety (TJC, 2019).*
2. Review health care provider's orders for aerobic or anaerobic culture. *Rationale: Specimens are taken from different sites and placed in different containers, depending on type of culture.*
3. Assess patient for signs of fever, chills, or excessive thirst. Note in medical record laboratory results if white blood cell (WBC) count is elevated. *Rationale: Signs and symptoms indicate systemic infection.*
4. Ask patient about type of pain at wound site and extent of pain using a scale of 0–10. If patient requires analgesic before dressing changes, give medication 30 minutes before beginning procedure to reach peak effect. *Rationale: Pain at wound site often increases with infection.*
5. Determine when dressing change is scheduled (see Chapter 27). Perform wound assessment as part of actual procedure.
6. Assess patient's or family caregiver's knowledge, experience, and health literacy. *Rationale: Ensures patient or family caregiver has the capacity to obtain, communicate, process, and understand basic health information (CDC, 2016).*
7. Assess patient's understanding of need for wound culture and ability to cooperate with procedure. *Rationale: Use data to develop teaching plan. Wound is painful site. Collection of specimen may cause anxiety or fear.*

STEP	RATIONALE
PLANNING	
1. Expected outcomes after completion of procedure:	
• Wound culture does not reveal bacterial growth.	Wound remains free of pathogenic microorganisms.
• Culture swab is free of contamination from skin bacteria.	Test results indicate type of cells present.
• Patient discusses purpose and procedure for specimen collection.	Validates learning.
2. Explain reason for wound culture and how it will be collected.	Promotes understanding and cooperation and eases anxiety.
3. Explain that patient may feel tickling sensation when wound is swabbed.	Anticipation of expected sensations minimizes anxiety.
4. Close bedside curtains or door to room.	Provides privacy.
5. Position patient so that wound area is accessible for wound assessment and obtaining a culture.	
6. Perform hand hygiene and apply gloves. Remove old dressing and assess wound for swelling, separation of edges, inflammation, and drainage. Palpate gently and note tenderness or drainage. Remove and discard gloves and perform hand hygiene.	Provides baseline for condition of wound. Reduces transmission of microorganisms.
7. Organize supplies at bedside.	Provides for efficient procedure.

STEP	RATIONALE

IMPLEMENTATION

STEP	RATIONALE
1. Apply clean gloves.	Reduces transmission of microorganisms.

Safe Patient Care *If a patient is to undergo wound irrigation, obtain the culture before the wound is irrigated.*

STEP	RATIONALE
2. Clean area around wound edges with antiseptic swab. Wipe from edges outward. Remove old exudate.	Removes skin flora, preventing possible contamination of specimen.

Safe Patient Care *If any antibiotic ointment or solution has been previously applied, remove it with gauze moistened in sterile water or saline, wait several hours, and then obtain the culture (Pagana et al., 2017).*

STEP	RATIONALE
3. Discard swab and remove and dispose of soiled gloves in appropriate receptacle. Perform hand hygiene.	Reduces spread of infection.
4. Open packages containing sterile culture tube and dressing supplies. Apply sterile gloves.	Provides sterile field for picking up and handling sterile supplies.
5. Obtain cultures.	

Safe Patient Care *Cultures of specimens from the skin edge yield much less accurate results than cultures of the suppurative material in the wound (Pagana et al., 2017).*

STEP	RATIONALE
a. Aerobic culture	
(1) Take swab from culture tube, insert tip into wound in area of drainage, and rotate swab gently. Remove swab and return to culture tube (wrap outside of ampule with gauze to prevent injury to your fingers). Crush ampule of medium and push swab into fluid.	Aerobic organisms grow in superficial wounds exposed to the air. Swab should be coated with fresh secretions from within wound. Medium keeps bacteria alive until analysis is complete.
b. Anaerobic culture	
(1) Take swab from special anaerobic culture tube, swab deeply into draining body cavity, and rotate gently. Remove swab and return to culture tube.	Specimen is taken from deep cavity where oxygen is not present. Carbon dioxide or nitrogen gas keeps organisms alive until analysis is complete. Air injected into tube would cause organisms to die.
Or	
(2) Insert tip of syringe (without needle) into wound and aspirate 5–10 mL of exudate. Attach needleless access device, expel all air, and inject drainage into special culture tube.	Sterile large-bore needle (19-gauge) allows exudate to be transferred from sterile syringe into special culture tube without contamination.
6. Remove and dispose of gloves. Perform hand hygiene.	Reduces transfer of microorganisms.
7. In presence of patient, complete label (two identifiers, specimen source, collection date and time) and attach to container. Attach completed laboratory requisition to container. Enclose specimen in a biohazard bag and send immediately to laboratory. NOTE: Indicate if patient is receiving antibiotics and include name of antibiotic.	Incorrect patient identification could lead to diagnostic or therapeutic error (TJC, 2019). Bacteria multiply quickly. Specimen should be analyzed promptly for accurate results.
8. Send specimens to laboratory immediately.	Bacteria multiply rapidly. Prompt analysis ensures accurate results.
9. Clean wound per health care provider's order. Apply new sterile dressing (see Chapter 27) using aseptic technique. Secure dressing with tape or ties.	Protects wound from further contamination; aids in absorbing drainage and debridement of wound.
10. Remove and dispose of gloves and soiled supplies in appropriate receptacle according to agency policy. Perform hand hygiene.	Reduces transmission of microorganisms.
11. Help patient to comfortable position. Be sure nurse call system is in accessible location. Instruct in use.	Promotes patient's ability to relax. Provides for patient safety.
12. Raise side rails (as appropriate) and lower bed to lowest position.	Ensures patient safety.

STEP	RATIONALE
EVALUATION	
1. Obtain laboratory report for results of cultures.	Report indicates if pathogenic organisms are identified.
2. Observe character of wound drainage.	Characteristics can reveal abnormal status and infection.
3. Observe edges of wound for redness and bleeding.	Indicates trauma to healing tissue.
4. Use Teach-Back: "I want to be sure I explained the purpose and procedure for obtaining a wound specimen. In your own words, please tell me why we need to obtain a wound culture." Revise your instruction now or develop a plan for revised patient/family caregiver teaching if patient/family caregiver is not able to teach back correctly.	Determines patient's/family caregiver's level of understanding of instructional topic.

Unexpected Outcomes	Related Interventions
1. Wound cultures reveal bacterial growth.	• Monitor patient for fever, chills, or excessive thirst, which indicate systemic infection. • Inform health care provider of findings.
2. Wound culture is contaminated from superficial skin cells.	• Monitor patient for fever and pain. • Inform health care provider of findings. • Repeat collection of specimen as ordered.
3. Patient reports increased pain.	• Provide analgesia. • Notify health care provider.

Recording

- Record type of specimen obtained, source, and time and date specimen sent to laboratory; describe appearance of wound and characteristics of drainage; describe patient's tolerance to procedure and response to analgesia.
- Document your evaluation of patient learning.

Hand-Off Reporting

- Report any evidence of infection to health care provider.

✦ SKILL 9.6 Blood Glucose Monitoring

Purpose

A blood glucose meter is an effective and efficient method for assessing glucose control in a patient with diabetes mellitus. Blood glucose monitoring (BGM) at the point of care is an effective method to monitor and manage glycemic control in hospital settings (Isbell, 2017). In addition, routine BGM at home is an essential component of any diabetes self-management program (ADA, 2016). The blood glucose meters available today are portable, lightweight, and battery powered (OneTouch [see Fig. 9.6]). They are easy to use and provide fast results, and newer models allow for small, quick skin punctures and a small amount of blood (0.3–1.5 mcL) to obtain results (Diabetes Forecast, 2017).

Delegation and Collaboration

During an acute illness, assessment of a patient's blood glucose cannot be delegated to NAP. When the patient's condition is stable, the skill of obtaining and testing for blood glucose level can be delegated to NAP. The nurse informs the NAP by:

- Explaining appropriate sites to use for puncture and when to obtain glucose levels
- Reviewing expected blood glucose levels and when to report unexpected glucose levels to the nurse

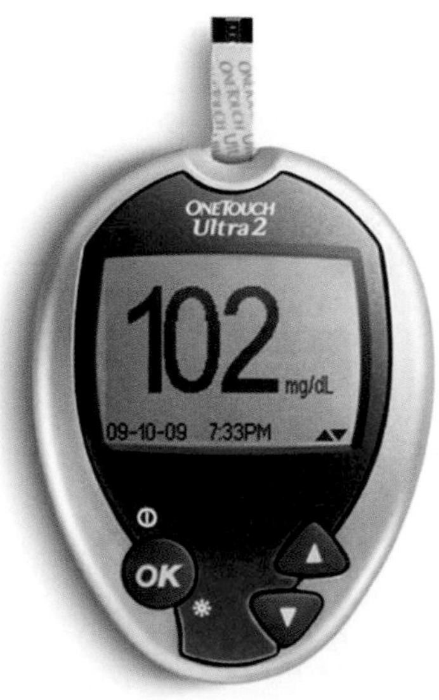

FIG 9.6 Blood glucose monitor. *(Courtesy LifeScan, Milpitas, CA.)*

Equipment

- Antiseptic swab
- Cotton ball
- Lancet device, either self-activating or button activated
- Blood glucose meter (e.g., Accucheck III, OneTouch)
- Blood glucose test strips appropriate for meter brand used
- Clean gloves
- Paper towel

ASSESSMENT

1. Identify patient using at least two identifiers (e.g., name and birthday or name and medical record number) according to agency policy. Compare identifiers with information on patient's MAR or medical record. *Rationale: Ensures correct patient. Complies with The Joint Commission standards and improves patient safety (TJC, 2019).*
2. Review health care provider's order for time or frequency of measurement. *Rationale: Health care provider determines test schedule on basis of patient's physiological status and risk for glucose imbalance.*

Safe Patient Care *For some critically ill patients, handheld point-of-care glucometers yield inconsistent results when the patient has low hematocrit levels or is hypotensive; in the presence of vasopressors, ascorbic acid, or other medications; and with the use of capillary blood specimens as opposed to arterial or venous blood samples. These factors can potentially lead to incorrect insulin dosing (Isbell, 2017).*

3. Determine whether specific conditions need to be met before or after sample collection (e.g., fasting, postprandial, after certain medications, before insulin doses). *Rationale: Dietary intake of carbohydrates and ingestion of concentrated glucose preparations alter blood glucose levels.*
4. Determine whether risks exist for performing skin puncture (e.g., low platelet count, anticoagulant therapy, bleeding disorders). *Rationale: Abnormal clotting mechanisms increase risk for local ecchymosis and bleeding.*
5. Perform hand hygiene. Assess area of skin to be used as puncture site. Inspect fingers or forearms for edema, inflammation, cuts, or sores. Avoid areas of bruising, recently punctured areas, and open lesions. Avoid using hand on side of mastectomy. Sides of fingers are commonly selected because they have fewer nerve endings. *Rationale: Recently punctured areas are avoided because these factors cause increased interstitial fluid and blood to mix and increase risk for infection.*
6. Assess patient's or family caregiver's knowledge, experience, and health literacy. *Rationale: Ensures patient or family caregiver has the capacity to obtain, communicate, process, and understand basic health information (CDC, 2016).*
7. Assess patient's understanding of procedure and purpose of blood glucose monitoring, ability to perform test, and understanding of its importance in glucose control. *Rationale: Provides baseline for developing teaching plan. Patient's physical health may change (e.g., vision disturbance, fatigue, pain, disease process) and affect him or her when performing test.*

STEP	RATIONALE
PLANNING	
1. Expected outcomes after completion of procedure:	
• Puncture site shows no evidence of bleeding or tissue damage.	Hemostasis is achieved. Lancet or needle did not puncture skin too deeply.
• Blood glucose measurements are accurate.	Normal fasting glucose for adults is 74–106 mg/dL, indicating good metabolic control (Pagana et al., 2017). Values may vary slightly; check agency policy.
• Patient can verbalize or demonstrate blood glucose measurement.	Demonstrates psychomotor learning.
• Patient explains test results.	Validates knowledge.
2. Explain procedure and purpose to patient and/or family caregiver. Offer patient and family caregiver opportunity to practice testing procedures. Provide resources/teaching aids for patient and family caregiver.	Promotes understanding and cooperation. Prepares patient and/or family caregiver to correctly perform glucose testing at home.
3. Position patient comfortably in chair or in semi-Fowler's position in bed.	Ensures easy accessibility to puncture site. Patient assumes position when self-testing.
IMPLEMENTATION	
1. Perform hand hygiene. Instruct adult to perform hand hygiene, including forearm (if applicable) with soap and water. Rinse and dry.	Promotes skin cleansing and vasodilation at selected puncture site. Reduces transmission of microorganisms.
2. Remove reagent strip from vial and tightly seal cap. Check code on test strip vial. Use only test strips recommended for glucose meter. Some newer meters do not require code and/or have disk or drum with 10 or more test strips.	Protects strips from accidental discoloration caused by exposure to air or light. Code on test strip vial must match code entered into glucose meter.

STEP	RATIONALE
3. Insert strip into meter (refer to manufacturer directions; see illustration). Do not bend strip. Meter turns on automatically.	Some machines must be calibrated; others require zeroing of timer. Each meter is adjusted differently.
4. Remove unused reagent strip from meter and place on paper towel or clean, dry surface with test pad facing up (see manufacturer's instructions).	Moisture on strip can alter accuracy of final test results.
5. Meter displays code on screen that must match code from test strip vial. Press proper button on meter to confirm matching codes. **Meter is ready for use.**	Codes must match for meter to operate. Meters have different messages that confirm that meter is ready for testing and blood can be applied.
6. Perform hand hygiene and apply clean gloves.	Reduces transmission of microorganisms.
Prepare single-use lancet or multiple-use lancet device. **NOTE:** Some meters recommend that this step be completed before preparing test strip. Remove cap from lancet device; insert new lancet. Some lancet devices have disk or cylinder that rotates to new lancet.	Never reuse a lancet because of risk of infection.
a. Twist off protective cover on tip of lancet.	
b. Cock lancet device, adjusting for proper puncture depth.	Each patient varies as to depth of insertion needed for lancet to produce blood drop.
7. Obtain blood sample.	
a. Wipe patient's finger or forearm lightly with antiseptic swab and allow to dry. Choose vascular area for puncture site. In stable adults, select lateral side of finger. Avoid central tip of finger, which has denser nerve supply (Pagana et al., 2017).	Removes microorganisms from skin surface. Side of finger is less sensitive to pain.
b. Hold area to be punctured in dependent position. Do not milk or massage finger site.	Increases blood flow to area before puncture. Milking may hemolyze specimen and introduce excess tissue fluid (Pagana et al., 2017).
c. Hold tip of lancet device against area of skin chosen for test site (see illustration). Press release button on device. Some devices allow you to see blood sample forming. Remove device.	Placement ensures that lancet enters skin properly.
d. With some devices, a blood sample begins to appear. Otherwise gently squeeze or massage fingertip until round drop of blood forms (see illustration).	Adequate-size blood sample is needed to test glucose.

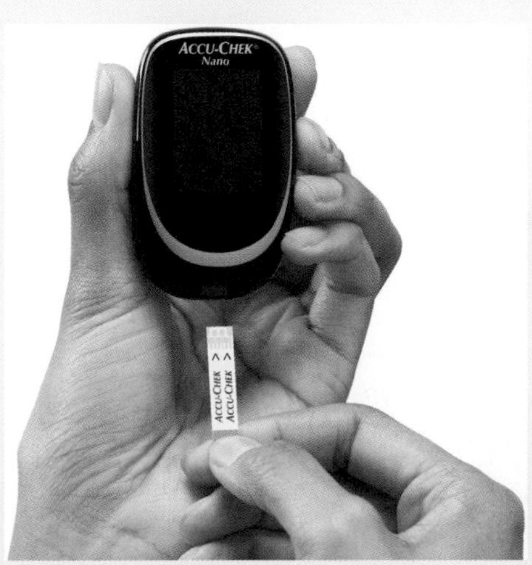

STEP 3 Load test strip into meter. *(Courtesy Accucheck Glucometer.)*

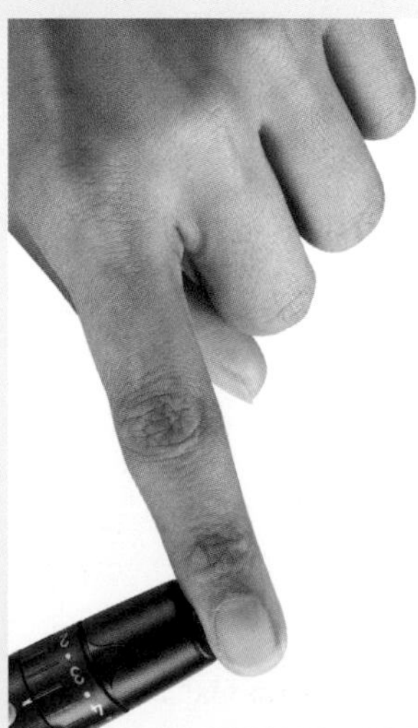

STEP 7c Prick side of finger with lancet. *(Courtesy Accucheck Glucometer.)*

STEP	RATIONALE
8. Obtain test results.	Exposure of blood to test strip for prescribed time ensures proper results.
a. Be sure that meter is still on. Bring test strip in meter to drop of blood. Blood will be wicked onto test strip (see illustration). Follow specific meter instructions to be sure that you obtain adequate sample.	Blood enters strip, and glucose device shows message on screen to signal that enough blood is obtained.

Safe Patient Care *Do not scrape blood onto the test strips or apply it to wrong side of test strip. This results in an inaccurate glucose measurement.*

STEP	RATIONALE
b. Blood glucose test result will appear on screen (see illustration). Some devices "beep" when completed.	
9. Turn meter off. Some meters turn off automatically. Dispose of test strip, lancet, and gloves in proper receptacles.	Meter is battery powered. Proper disposal reduces risk for needlestick injury and spread of infection.

Safe Patient Care *Point-of-care (POC) blood glucose testing meters must be cleaned and disinfected after each patient use (U.S. Food and Drug Administration [FDA], 2015).*

STEP	RATIONALE
10. Perform hand hygiene and remove gloves.	Reduces transmission of microorganisms.
11. Help patient to comfortable position. Be sure nurse call system is in an accessible location within patient's reach.	Ensures patient can call for assistance if needed.
12. Raise side rails (as appropriate) and lower bed to lowest position.	Ensures patient safety.
13. Discuss test results with patient and encourage questions and eventual participation in care if this is a new diabetes mellitus diagnosis.	Promotes participation and adherence to therapy.

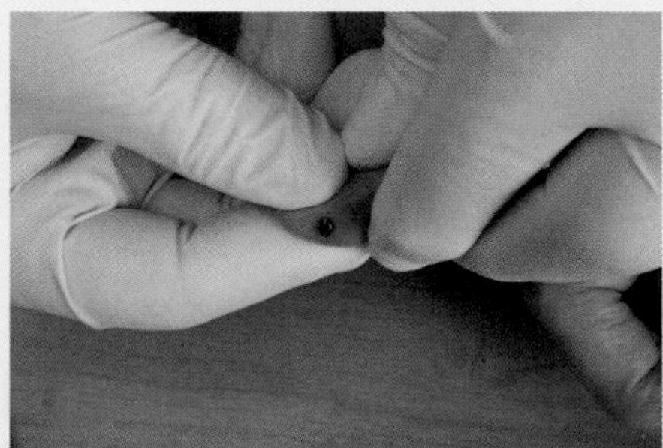

STEP 7d Gently squeeze puncture site until drop of blood forms.

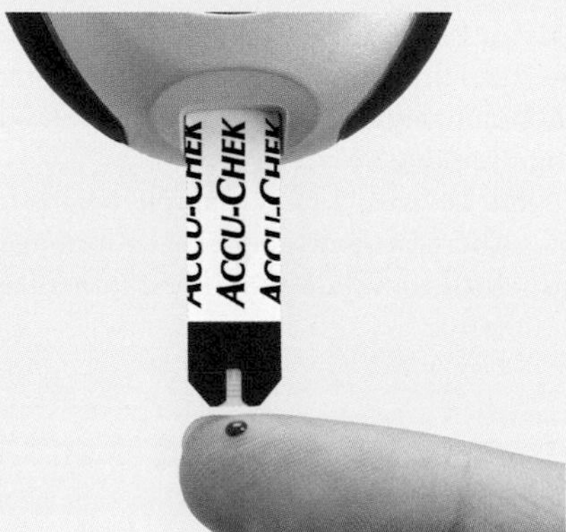

STEP 8a Touch test strip to blood drop. Blood wicks into test strip. *(Courtesy Accucheck Glucometer.)*

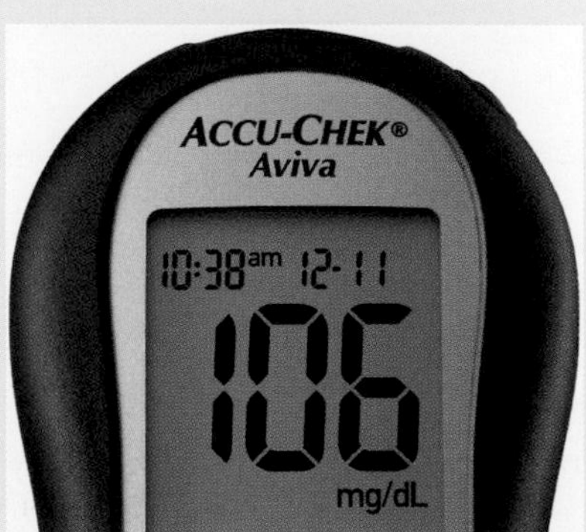

STEP 8b Results appear on meter screen. *(Courtesy Accucheck Glucometer.)*

STEP	RATIONALE

EVALUATION

1. Inspect puncture site for bleeding or tissue injury.	Site can be source of discomfort and infection.
2. Compare glucose meter reading with normal blood glucose levels and previous test results.	Determines whether glucose level is normal.
3. **Use Teach-Back:** "I want to be sure I explained the way to obtain a blood glucose reading. Show me the steps you will use to obtain your blood glucose measurement." Revise your instruction now or develop a plan for revised patient/family caregiver teaching if patient/family caregiver is not able to teach back correctly.	Determines patient's/family caregiver's level of understanding of instructional topic.

Unexpected Outcomes	Related Interventions
1. Puncture site is bruised or continues to bleed.	• Apply pressure. • Notify health care provider if bleeding continues.
2. Blood glucose level is above or below target range.	• Continue to monitor patient. • Check if there are medication orders for deviations in glucose level. • Notify health care provider. • Administer insulin or carbohydrate source as ordered, depending on glucose level.
3. Glucose meter malfunctions.	• Review instructions for troubleshooting glucose meter. • Repeat test.

Recording

- Record glucose results on appropriate flow sheet and describe response, including presence or absence of pain or excessive oozing of blood at puncture site.
- Document your evaluation of patient learning

Hand-Off Reporting

- Report blood glucose levels out of target range and take appropriate action for hypoglycemia or hyperglycemia.
- Report patient response to treatment for out-of-range blood glucose levels.

✦ SKILL 9.7 Collecting Blood and Culture Specimens by Venipuncture (Syringe and Vacutainer Method)

Purpose

Blood and blood culture specimens are collected to assist health care providers to screen patients for early signs of physical illness, monitor changes in acute or chronic diseases, and evaluate responses to therapies. Blood tests are one of the most commonly used diagnostic measures that yield valuable information about a patient's nutritional, hematological, metabolic, immune, and biochemical status.

A blood culture detects bacteria in the blood. Blood cultures are drawn to identify pathogens and document the progress of treatment of the infections. It is important that the culture specimens be drawn from two different sites and are often drawn when symptoms, such as fever and chills, are present (Pagana et al., 2017).

Delegation and Collaboration

The skill of collecting blood specimens by venipuncture can be delegated to specially trained NAP. In some agencies, phlebotomists obtain the venipuncture samples. Agency and government regulations and policies differ regarding personnel who may draw blood specimens. The nurse informs the NAP to:

- Report any patient discomfort or signs of excessive bleeding from the puncture site to the nurse.
- Report changes in vital signs, especially shivering and high fever.

Equipment

All Procedures

- Chlorhexidine or antiseptic swab (check agency policy for use of 70% alcohol or other antiseptic solutions)
- Clean gloves
- Small pillow or folded towel
- Sterile 2 × 2–inch gauze pads
- Tourniquet
- Adhesive bandage or adhesive tape
- Identification labels with name of test
- Completed laboratory requisition (appropriate patient identification, date, time, name of test, and source of culture)
- Biohazard bag or container for delivery of specimen to laboratory (as specified by agency)
- Sharps container

Venipuncture With Syringe

- Sterile safety needles (20- to 21-gauge for adults; 23- to 25-gauge for children)
- Sterile 10- to 20-mL Luer-Lok safety syringes
- Needleless blood transfer device
- Appropriate blood specimen tubes

Venipuncture With Vacutainer

- Vacutainer and safety access device with Luer-Lok adapter
- Sterile double-ended needles (20- to 21-gauge for adults; 23- to 25-gauge for children)
- Appropriate blood specimen tubes

Blood Cultures

- Two sterile needles (20- to 21-gauge for adults; 20- to 25-gauge for children)
- Two 20-mL sterile syringes and two needleless access devices
- Anaerobic and aerobic culture bottles; check agency policy

ASSESSMENT

1. Identify patient using at least two identifiers (e.g., name and birthday or name and medical record number) according to agency policy. Compare identifiers with information on patient's MAR or medical record. *Rationale: Ensures correct patient. Complies with The Joint Commission standards and improves patient safety (TJC, 2019).*
2. Review health care provider's orders for type of tests. *Rationale: Multiple samples are often needed. Health care provider's order is required.*
3. Determine whether special conditions need to be met before specimen collection (e.g., patient allowed nothing by mouth [NPO], specific time for collection in relation to medication given, need to ice specimen). *Rationale: Some tests require meeting specific conditions to obtain accurate measurement of blood elements (e.g., fasting blood sugar, drug peak and trough level, timed endocrine hormone levels).*
4. Assess patient for possible risks associated with venipuncture: anticoagulant therapy, low platelet count, bleeding disorders (history of hemophilia). Review medication history. *Rationale: Patient history may include abnormal clotting abilities caused by low platelet count, hemophilia, or medications that increase risk for bleeding and hematoma formation.*
5. Perform hand hygiene, apply gloves, and assess patient for venipuncture site. Note contraindicated sites for venipuncture: presence of IV infusion, hematoma at potential site, arm on side of mastectomy, or hemodialysis shunt. *Rationale: Drawing specimens from such sites can result in false test results or may injure patient. Samples taken from vein near IV infusion may be diluted or contain concentrations of IV fluids. Postmastectomy patient may have reduced lymphatic drainage in arm on operative side, increasing risk for infection from needlesticks.*

Safe Patient Care *Never use arteriovenous shunt to obtain specimens because of risks for clotting and bleeding. Hematoma indicates existing injury to vessel wall.*

6. Identify presence of tape sensitivities or latex or povidone-iodine (Betadine) allergies. *Rationale: Avoid use of items in presence of allergy.*
7. Before drawing blood cultures, assess for systemic signs and symptoms of bacteremia, including fever and chills. *Rationale: Three blood culture samples should be drawn at least 1 hour apart beginning at the earliest signs of sepsis (Pagana et al., 2017).*
8. Assess patient's or family caregiver's knowledge, experience, and health literacy. *Rationale: Ensures patient or family caregiver has the capacity to obtain, communicate, process, and understand basic health information (CDC, 2016).*
9. Determine whether patient understands purpose of procedure and ability to cooperate. *Rationale: Provides data for you to establish teaching plan and provides emotional support. Some patients' past experiences increase anxiety.*

STEP	RATIONALE
PLANNING	
1. Expected outcomes after completion of procedure:	
• Venipuncture site shows no evidence of continued bleeding or hematoma after specimen collection.	Indicates that hemostasis is achieved.
• Patient denies anxiety or discomfort.	Explanation relieves anxiety; procedure is performed quickly. Removal of painful stimulus lessens anxiety.
• An adequate sample is collected for testing (see agency policy or laboratory manual).	Appropriate laboratory analysis can be conducted.
• Patient discusses purpose, procedure, and benefits of venipuncture.	Validates learning.
2. Explain procedure to patient: describe purpose of tests; explain how sensation of tourniquet, alcohol swab, and needlestick will feel.	Anticipatory guidance helps reduce anxiety.
3. Close room door or bedside curtain.	Provides privacy
4. Perform hand hygiene and bring equipment to bedside and organize.	Facilitates procedure.
5. Help patient to supine or semi-Fowler's position with arms extended to form straight line from shoulders to wrists. Place small pillow or towel under upper arm. (*Optional:* Lower arm briefly so it fills veins in hand and lower arm with blood.)	Helps stabilize extremity because arms are most common sites of venipuncture. Supported position in bed reduces chance of injury to patient if fainting occurs.

STEP	RATIONALE

IMPLEMENTATION

STEP	RATIONALE
1. Raise or lower bed to comfortable working height.	Reduces strain on your back muscles and improves access to venipuncture site.
2. Perform hand hygiene and apply gloves. Apply tourniquet so it can be removed by pulling an end with single motion.	Tourniquet blocks venous return to heart from extremity, causing veins to dilate for easier visibility.
a. Position tourniquet 5–10 cm (2–4 inches) above venipuncture site selected (antecubital fossa site is most often used).	
b. Cross tourniquet over patient's arm (see illustration). May place it over gown sleeve to protect skin.	Older adult's skin is very fragile, and the fabric of the gown can protect the skin.
c. Hold tourniquet between your fingers close to arm. Tuck loop between patient's arm and tourniquet so you can grasp free end easily (see illustration).	Pull free end to release tourniquet after venipuncture.

Safe Patient Care *Palpate distal pulse (e.g., radial) below tourniquet. If pulse is not palpable, remove tourniquet, wait 60 seconds, and reapply it more loosely. If tourniquet is too tight, pressure will impede blood flow.*

Safe Patient Care *Do not keep tourniquet on patient longer than 60 seconds (McCaughey et al., 2017; Pagana et al., 2017). Prolonged tourniquet application causes stasis, localized acidemia, and hemoconcentration and increases risk for hemolysis of blood cells (McCaughey et al., 2017).*

STEP	RATIONALE
3. Quickly reinspect extremity for best venipuncture site, looking for straight, prominent vein without swelling or hematoma. Of three veins located in antecubital area, median cubital vein is preferred (see illustration).	Straight and intact veins are easiest to puncture.

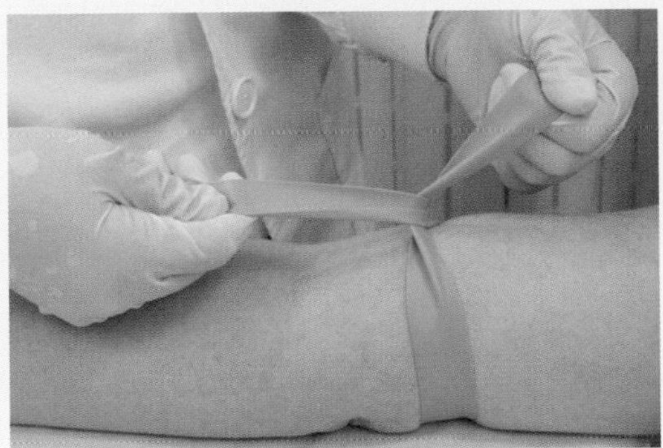

STEP 2b Cross tourniquet over arm.

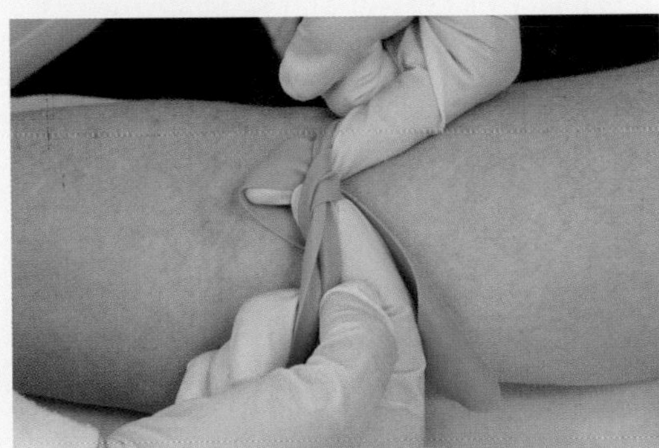

STEP 2c Tuck loop between patient's arm and tourniquet.

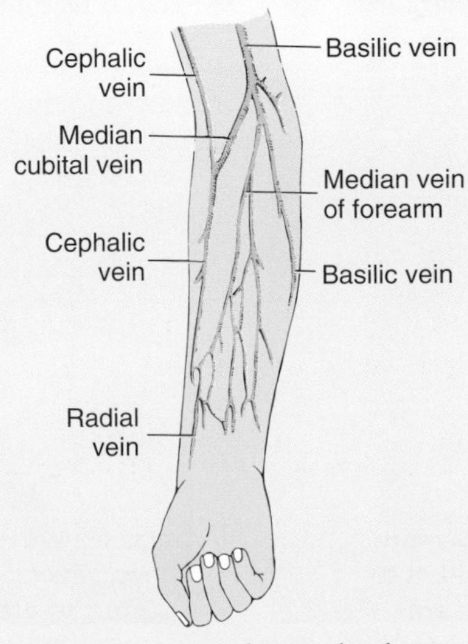

STEP 3 Location of antecubital veins.

STEP	RATIONALE
4. Palpate selected vein with finger (see illustration). Note if vein is firm and rebounds when palpated or if it feels rigid or cordlike and rolls when palpated. Avoid vigorously slapping vein, which can cause vasospasm.	Patent, healthy vein is elastic and rebounds on palpation. Thrombosed vein is rigid, rolls easily, and is difficult to puncture.
5. Obtain blood specimen.	
a. **Syringe method:**	
(1) Have syringe with appropriate needle securely attached.	Needle must not dislodge from syringe during venipuncture.
(2) Clean venipuncture site with antiseptic swab, with first swab moving back and forth on horizontal plane, another swab on vertical plane, and last in circular motion from site outward for about 5 cm (2 inches) for 30 seconds. Allow to dry.	Antimicrobial agent cleans skin surface of resident bacteria so that organisms do not enter puncture site. Allowing antiseptic to dry completes its antimicrobial task and reduces "sting" of venipuncture. Alcohol left on skin can cause hemolysis of sample and retraction of tissue away from puncture site.

Safe Patient Care *When obtaining a sample for blood alcohol level or blood cultures, use only antiseptic swab rather than alcohol swab.*

STEP	RATIONALE
(3) Remove needle cover and inform patient that "stick" lasts only a few seconds.	Patient has better control over anxiety when prepared for what to expect.

Safe Patient Care *Observe needle for defects such as burrs, which can cause increased discomfort and damage to patient's vein (McCall and Tankersley, 2012).*

STEP	RATIONALE
(4) Place thumb or forefinger of nondominant hand 2.5 cm (1 inch) below site and gently pull skin taut. Stretch skin steadily until vein is stabilized.	Stabilizes vein and prevents rolling during needle insertion.
(5) Hold syringe and needle at 15- to 30-degree angle from patient's arm with bevel up.	Reduces chance of penetrating both sides of vein during insertion. Bevel up decreases chance of contamination by not dragging bevel opening over skin and allows point of needle to first puncture skin, reducing trauma.
(6) Slowly insert needle into vein, stopping when "pop" is felt as needle enters vein (see illustration).	Prevents puncture through vein to opposite side.
(7) Hold syringe securely and pull back gently on plunger.	Syringe held securely prevents needle from advancing. Pulling on plunger creates vacuum needed to draw blood into syringe. If plunger is pulled back too quickly, pressure may collapse vein.
(8) Observe for blood return (see illustration).	If blood flow fails to appear, needle may not be in vein.
(9) Obtain desired amount of blood, keeping needle stabilized.	Test results are more accurate when required amount of blood is obtained. You cannot perform some tests without minimal blood requirement. Movement of needle increases discomfort.
(10) After obtaining specimen, release tourniquet.	Reduces bleeding at site when needle is withdrawn.

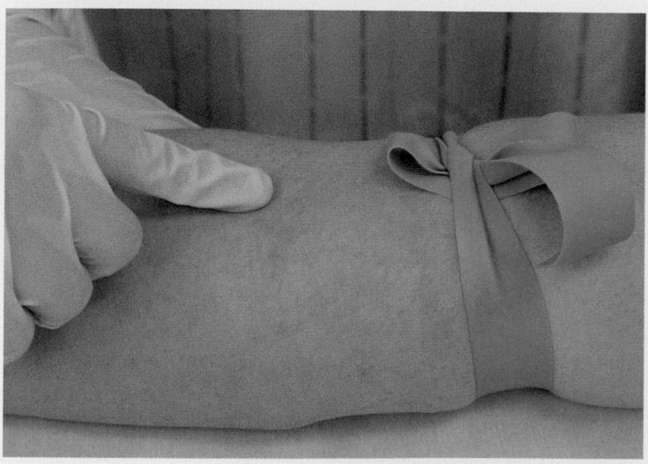

STEP 4 Palpate vein.

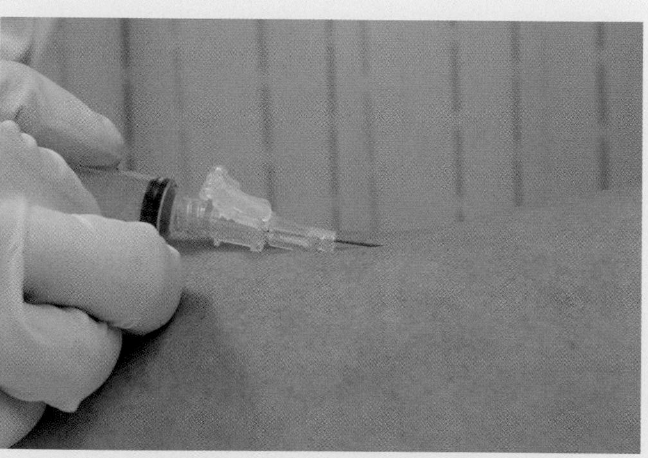

STEP 5a(6) Insert needle into vein.

STEP	RATIONALE
(11) Apply 2 × 2–inch gauze pad without applying pressure. Quickly but carefully withdraw needle from vein and apply pressure after removal of needle (see illustration). Check for hematoma.	Pressure over needle can cause discomfort. Careful removal of needle minimizes discomfort and vein trauma. Hematoma may cause compression injury (Pagana et al., 2017).
(12) Activate safety cover and immediately discard needle in appropriate container.	Prevents needlestick injury.
(13) Attach blood-filled syringe to needle-free blood transfer device. Attach tube and allow vacuum to fill tube to specified level. Remove and fill other tubes as appropriate (see illustration). Gently rotate each tube back and forth 8–10 times.	Additives prevent clotting. Shaking can cause hemolysis of red blood cells (RBCs).
b. **Vacutainer system method:**	
(1) Attach double-ended needle to Vacutainer tube (see illustration).	Long end of needle is used to puncture vein. Short end fits into blood tubes.
(2) Have proper blood specimen tube resting inside Vacutainer device, but do not puncture rubber stopper.	Puncturing causes loss of tube vacuum.
(3) Clean venipuncture site by following Step 5a(2) for antiseptic swab. Allow to dry.	Cleans skin surface of resident bacteria so that organisms do not enter puncture site. Drying maximizes effect of antiseptic.
(4) Remove needle cover and inform patient that "stick" will occur, lasting only a few seconds.	Patient has better control over anxiety when prepared about what to expect.
(5) Place thumb or forefinger of nondominant hand 2.5 cm (1 inch) *below* site and gently pull skin taut. Stretch skin down until vein stabilizes.	Helps stabilize vein and prevent rolling during needle insertion.

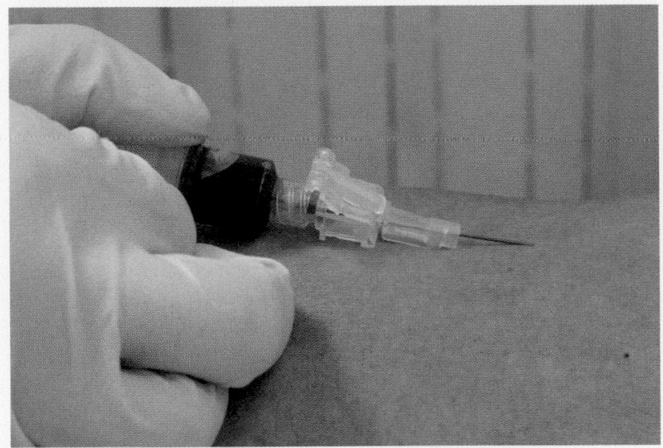

STEP 5a(8) Observe for blood return.

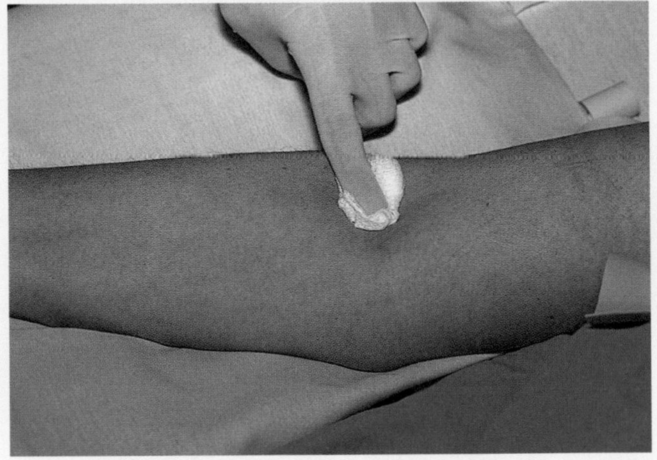

STEP 5a(11) Apply gauze to puncture site.

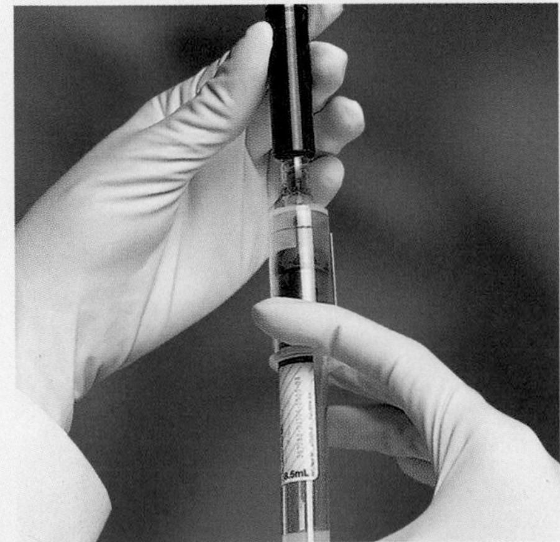

STEP 5a(13) Attach blood-filled syringe to needle-free blood transfer device.

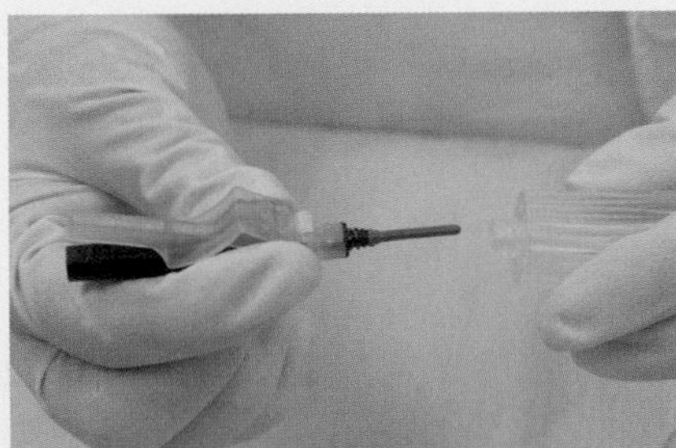

STEP 5b(1) Attach double-ended needle to Vacutainer tube.

STEP	RATIONALE
(6) Hold Vacutainer needle at 15- to 30-degree angle from arm with bevel up.	Smallest and sharpest point of needle will puncture skin first. Reduces chance of penet rating sides of vein during insertion. Keeping bevel up causes less trauma to vein.
(7) Slowly insert Vacutainer needle into vein (see illustration).	Prevents puncture on opposite side.
(8) Grasp Vacutainer securely and advance specimen tube into needle of holder (do not advance needle in vein).	Pushing needle through stopper breaks vacuum and causes flow of blood into tube. If needle in vein advances, vein may become punctured on other side.
(9) Note flow of blood into tube, which should be rapid (see illustration).	Failure of blood to appear indicates that vacuum in tube is lost or needle is not in vein.
(10) After filling specimen tube, grasp Vacutainer firmly and remove tube. Insert additional specimen tubes as needed. Gently rotate each tube back and forth 8–10 times.	Vacuum in tube stops flow at amount to be collected. Grasping prevents needle from advancing or dislodging. Tube should fill completely because additives in certain tubes are measured in proportion to filled tube. Ensures proper mixing with additive to prevent clotting.
(11) After last tube is filled and removed from Vacutainer, release tourniquet.	Reduces bleeding at site when needle is withdrawn.
(12) Apply 2 × 2–inch gauze pad over puncture site without applying pressure and quickly but carefully withdraw needle with Vacutainer from vein.	Pressure over needle can cause discomfort. Careful removal of needle minimizes discomfort and vein trauma.
(13) Immediately apply pressure over venipuncture site with gauze or antiseptic pad for 2–3 minutes or until bleeding stops. Observe for hematoma. Tape gauze dressing securely.	Direct pressure minimizes bleeding and prevents hematoma formation. Hematoma may cause compression and nerve injury. Pressure dressing controls bleeding.
c. **Blood culture:**	
(1) Clean venipuncture site as in Step 5a(2) with antiseptic swab or follow agency policy. Allow to dry.	Antimicrobial agent cleans skin surface so that organisms do not enter puncture site or contaminate culture. Drying ensures complete antimicrobial action and decreases stinging.
(2) Clean bottle tops of culture bottles for 15 seconds with agency-approved cleaning solution. Allow to dry.	Ensures that bottle top is sterile.
(3) Collect 10–15 mL of venous blood using syringe method (see Step 5a) in 20-mL syringe from two different venipuncture sites.	Two blood cultures must be collected from two different sites to confirm culture growth (Pagana et al., 2017).
(4) With each specimen activate safety guard, then remove and discard needle. Replace with needleless access device before injecting each blood sample into culture bottle.	Maintains sterile technique and prevents contamination of specimen.
(5) If both aerobic and anaerobic cultures are needed, fill anaerobic bottle first.	Anaerobic organisms may take longer to grow (Pagana et al., 2017).
(6) Gently mix blood in each culture bottle.	Mixes medium and blood.

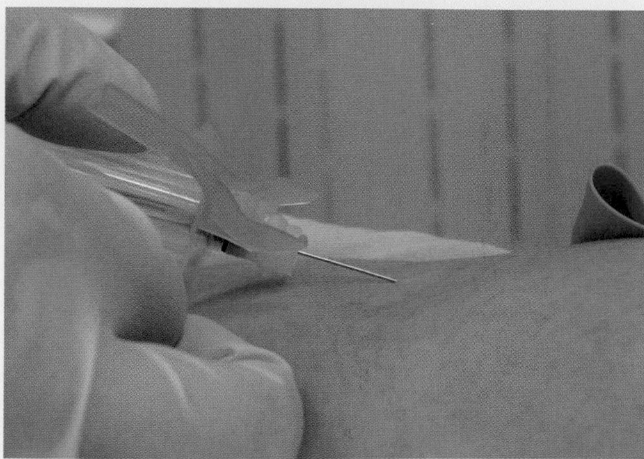

STEP 5b(7) Insert Vacutainer needle into vein.

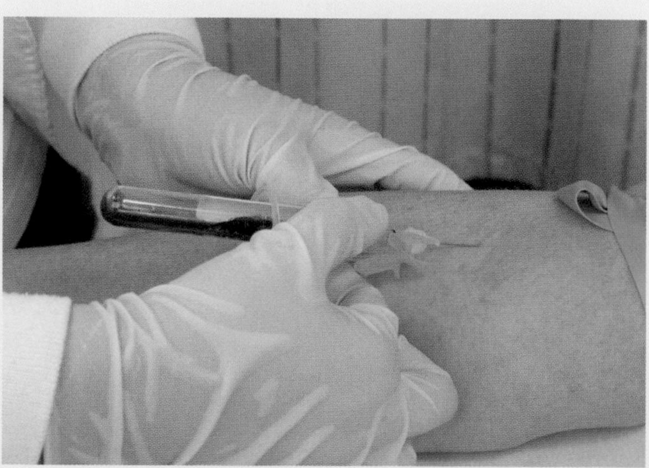

STEP 5b(9) Blood flowing into tube.

STEP	RATIONALE
6. Check tubes for any sign of external contamination with blood. Decontaminate with 70% alcohol if necessary.	Prevents cross-contamination. Reduces risk for exposure to pathogens present in blood.
7. Dispose of syringe, gauze, and other supplies in appropriate containers. Remove and dispose of gloves and perform hand hygiene after specimen is obtained and any spillage is cleaned.	Safe disposal of supplies exposed to body fluids prevents transfer of microorganisms. Reduces risk for exposure to bloodborne pathogens.
8. Help patient to comfortable position. Be sure nurse call system is in an accessible location within patient's reach.	Ensures patient can call for assistance if needed.
9. Raise side rails (as appropriate) and lower bed to lowest position.	Ensures patient safety.
10. In presence of patient, complete label (two identifiers, specimen source, collection date and time) and attach to container. Attach completed laboratory requisition to container.	Incorrect patient identification could lead to diagnostic or therapeutic error (TJC, 2019). Bacteria multiply quickly. Specimen should be analyzed promptly for accurate results.
11. Place specimens in biohazard bag and send to laboratory. Cultures must be sent to laboratory within 30 minutes (Pagana et al., 2017).	Minimizes spread of microorganisms.

EVALUATION

1. Inspect venipuncture site for homeostasis.	Determines whether bleeding has stopped or hematoma has formed.
2. Determine whether patient is anxious or fearful.	Some patients require more blood tests in future. Address concerns and let patient express anxiety.
3. Check laboratory report for test results.	Reveals constituents of blood specimen.
4. **Use Teach-Back:** "I want to be sure I explained the purpose and procedure for obtaining a blood specimen. Tell me why we are collecting this blood specimen." Revise your instruction now or develop a plan for revised patient/family caregiver teaching if patient/family caregiver is not able to teach back correctly.	Determines patient's/family caregiver's level of understanding of instructional topic.

Unexpected Outcomes	Related Interventions
1. Hematoma forms at venipuncture site.	• Apply pressure using 2 × 2–inch gauze dressing. • Continue to monitor patient for pain and discomfort.
2. Bleeding at site continues.	• Apply pressure to site; patient may also apply pressure. • Monitor patient. • Notify health care provider if bleeding continues for 5 minutes.
3. Signs and symptoms of infection at venipuncture site occur.	• Notify health care provider.

Recording

- Record method used to obtain blood specimen, date and time collected, type of test ordered, site (for blood cultures), and laboratory receiving specimen; describe venipuncture site after specimen collection and patient's response to procedure.
- Document your evaluation of patient learning.

Hand-Off Reporting

- Report abnormal results to health care provider.
- Report condition of venipuncture sit.

SPECIAL CONSIDERATIONS

Patient-Centered Care

- Consider both cultural and language barriers when delegating specimen collection to patients and family caregivers. Language and cultural barriers make it difficult to explain the purpose of tests and collection techniques to patients. Incorporate return demonstration in your patient education (Raingruber, 2017).
- Be sensitive to patient embarrassment when obtaining stool and urine specimens.
- When appropriate, ask patients if they prefer a gender-congruent caregiver.

Patient Education

- In the health care setting, POC monitoring of blood glucose might use a monitor different from the type the patient uses at home; provide general principles about the hospital type of monitor.
- Request a family caregiver to bring the meter from home to assess the patient's skill.
- Instruct a patient or family caregiver who will be collecting a sample at home on how to store the sample until it reaches the laboratory to minimize bacterial growth before applying it to a culture medium in a laboratory setting.

Age-Specific

Pediatric

- In some facilities, if you anticipate that the procedure will be painful for the child, perform the procedure in an area other than child's room, keeping the child's room a safe place (Hockenberry et al., 2017).
- Children of school age and older are concrete thinkers, are often curious, and ask many questions about tests. Explain the procedure and answer honestly. Allow child to watch, if desired, while test is performed (Hockenberry et al., 2017).
- It is impossible to obtain a midstream urine collection on a child who has not been toilet-trained; consequently, obtain urine for culture by straight catheterization. Consider age-appropriate fears, especially with preschool- and school-age children (Hockenberry et al., 2017).
- There are several choices to reduce pain from venipuncture, such as acupuncture and topical anesthesia. In a controlled study, nurses preferred the use of acupuncture in reducing venipuncture pain in children 6 to 12 years of age. The acupuncture proved safe, cost-effective, and easy to use (Pour et al., 2017).
- Apply eutectic mixture of local anesthetics (EMLA) cream over planned puncture site 60 minutes before procedure; other local anesthetic cream or vapocoolants may be ordered to reduce pain in infants and young children (Hockenberry and Wilson, 2017).
- Vacutainers are not recommended for children younger than 2 years of age because of possible vein collapse (Hockenberry et al., 2017).

Gerontological

- Older adults may need assistance in positioning to obtain specimen. When patients are confused, the NAP may be necessary to assist the patient in collecting a specimen.
- Older adults who have difficulty seeing the readings on the meter display screen may use a device with a larger display screen and lighted background or an audio blood glucose meter that gives verbal instructions to guide the patient through the procedure and gives an audio result (Touhy and Jett, 2018).
- Older adults with musculoskeletal alterations may not have the fine-motor coordination necessary to manipulate the device and place blood samples on test strips or insert strips in meter. Some models can be loaded with multiple strips.
- Older adults have fragile skin and veins that are easily traumatized during venipuncture. A small-bore needle or catheter may be beneficial.

Home Care

- If a patient must collect Hemoccult specimens at home, drape a piece of plastic wrap over the toilet. If possible, the specimen should not be contaminated with urine. Patient or family caregiver prepares slide with feces, closes cardboard slide, and returns it to the health care provider's office or clinic.
- If patient is to obtain a sputum specimen at home, instruct patient or family caregiver regarding proper technique and importance of having sputum (not saliva) specimen sent to laboratory in timely manner.
- One or more family caregivers should be able to monitor blood glucose levels if the patient is unable to do so independently.
- Risks for wound infections are different in the home setting than in the hospital setting because a patient is less susceptible to infections from microorganisms in the home environment. Careful handwashing and clean technique are usually adequate for performing dressing changes by patients and family caregivers in the home.

✦ PRACTICE REFLECTIONS

A 78-year-old woman was admitted to the medical-surgical unit 3 days ago for uncontrolled diabetes mellitus. Her fasting blood sugar has been decreasing with new medications and moving toward the desired level of 110. At 7:00 AM, the NAP reports that the patient seems confused and is complaining of a constant need to urinate and burning with urination. She also has a productive cough and is expectorating thick sputum. Vital signs are blood pressure (BP) 98/80, pulse 96, respiratory rate 20, temperature 39.4° C (101.2° F), SpO_2 95%, and fasting blood sugar 165. The NAP also saved the patient's recent urine for your assessment. You note that her urine is cloudy, pink-tinged, and foul-smelling.

In addition to blood glucose level, what other laboratory tests might the health care provider order?

Her daughter mentions that her mother has frequent urinary tract infections (UTIs). Reflect on your knowledge about elevated blood glucose and UTI. What further information would you need from the daughter? Would this information lead you to some patient and family caregiver teaching?

The patient is spiking a temperature of unknown origin. Culture and sensitivities on urine and sputum are negative for pathogens; stool sample is negative. The patient doesn't have any rash or skin irritation. The health care provider orders a blood culture when the patient's temperature is elevated. Why is the timing of this sample important? What do you need to do to ensure proper sampling?

✦ CLINICAL REVIEW QUESTIONS

1. The nurse calls the health care provider and receives an order for a urine culture and sensitivity (C&S). The nurse must obtain the urine sample from the needleless port of the catheter. Place the following steps for obtaining a sterile urine specimen in the correct order:
   1. Withdraw 3 to 5 mL of urine and instill into a sterile urine container using sterile technique.
   2. Perform hand hygiene and apply gloves.
   3. Attach completed requisition and send to the laboratory immediately.
   4. Wipe needleless port with antiseptic wipe and attach 3-mL Luer-Lok syringe.
   5. Attach label to sterile urine container and double bag.

2. The nurse is preparing to obtain a throat culture. Which steps would facilitate collecting an accurate specimen? (Select all that apply.)
   1. Place patient in a sitting position or with head elevated at a 45-degree angle.
   2. Have patient lean the head forward.
   3. Depress posterior two-thirds of the tongue.
   4. Swab the tonsillar area.
   5. Swab the uvula.
   6. Have patient blow the nose.

3. The nurse plans to collect a blood specimen. A tourniquet is necessary to obtain the specimen. Which of the following are important interventions when applying a tourniquet? (Select all that apply.)
1. Remove the tourniquet impeding venous blood flow, wait 60 minutes, and then reapply.
2. Position tourniquet 5 to 10 cm (3–4 inches) above venipuncture site.
3. Keep tourniquet in place no more than 60 seconds.
4. Palpate distal pulse (radial artery) below the tourniquet.
5. Release tourniquet after removing needle.

Answers and Rationales for Clinical Review Questions can be found on the Evolve website.

REFERENCES

American Diabetes Association: DKA (Ketoacidosis) and Ketones, 2015. http://www.diabetes.org/living-with-diabetes/complications/ketoacidosis-dka.html.

American Diabetes Association (ADA): Checking your blood glucose, 2016. http://www.diabetes.org/living-with-diabetes/treatment-and-care/blood-glucose-control/checking-your-blood-glucose.html.

Barnaby DP, et al: Generalizability and effectiveness of butterfly phlebotomy in reducing hemolysis, *Acad Emerg Med* 23:204, 2016.

Centers for Disease Control and Prevention: What is Health Literacy, 2016. https://www.cdc.gov/healthliteracy/learn/index.html.

Diabetes Forecast: Everything you need to know about blood glucose meters, 2017. Alexandria, VA, 2017, American Diabetes Association. http://www.diabetesforecast.org/2017/mar-apr/blood-glucose-meters-101.html.

Hockenberry MJ, Wilson D: *Wong's essentials of pediatric nursing*, ed 10, St. Louis, 2017, Mosby.

Isbell TS: Bedside blood glucose testing in critically ill patients, *Med Lib Observ* 49(4):8, 2017.

Makhumula-Nkhoma N, et al: Level of confidence in venepuncture and knowledge in determining causes of blood sample haemolysis among clinical staff and phlebotomists, *J Clin Nurs* 24:370, 2014.

McCall R, Tankersley C: *Phlebotomy essentials*, ed 5, Philadelphia, 2012, Lippincott Williams & Wilkins.

McCaughey EJ, et al: Key factors influencing the incidence of hemolysis: a critical appraisal of current evidence, *Crit Rev Clin Lab Sci* 54(1):59, 2017.

Occupational Safety & Health Administration (OSHA): Bloodborne pathogens and Needlestick Prevention, 29 CFR 1910.1030, 2000. https://www.osha.gov/SLTC/bloodbornepathogens/standards.html.

Occupational Safety & Health Administration (OSHA): Bloodborne pathogen standard 29CFR1910.1030, 2015. https://www.osha.gov/pls/oshaweb/owadisp.show_document?p_table=STANDARDS&p_id=10051.

Pagana KD, et al: *Mosby's diagnostic and laboratory tests reference*, ed 13, St. Louis, 2017, Mosby.

Phelan MP, et al: 66 Use of plasma collection tubes with smaller volumes and decreased vacuum significantly reduces hemolysis in emergence department samples, *Amer Emer Med* 66(4):S23, 2015.

Pour PS, et al: Comparison of effects of local anesthesia and two-point acupuncture on the severity of venipuncture pain among hospitalized 6-12-year-old children, *J Acupunct Meridian Stud* 10(3):187, 2017.

Raingruber B: *Contemporary health promotion in nursing practice*, ed 2, Burlington, MA, 2017, Jones and Bartlett Learning.

The Joint Commission (TJC): *2019 National Patient Safety Goals*, Oakbrook Terrace, IL, 2019. The Commission. http://www.jointcommission.org/standards_information/npsgs.aspx.

Touhy T, Jett K: *Gerontological nursing and healthy aging*, ed 5, St. Louis, 2018, Mosby.

U.S. Food and Drug Administration (FDA): Blood glucose monitoring devices, 2015. http://www.fda.gov/medicaldevices/productsandmedicalprocedures/invitrodiagnostics/glucosetestingdevices/default.htm.

Wollowitz A, et al: Use of butterfly needles to draw blood is independently associated with marked reduction in hemolysis compared to intravenous catheters, *Acad Emerg Med* 20:1151–1155, 2013.

10 Diagnostic Procedures

SKILLS AND PROCEDURES

EVOLVE WEBSITE/RESOURCES LIST

http://evolve.elsevier.com/Perry/nursinginterventions

Audio Glossary • Animations • Checklists • Clinical Review Questions • Answers and Rationales for Clinical Review Questions

INTRODUCTION

Diagnostic procedures are performed at patients' bedsides or in specially equipped rooms within a hospital or outpatient care setting. Before beginning, check the agency protocol specific to the procedure you will be performing or with which you are assisting. As a nurse, you are responsible for assessing a patient's knowledge of a procedure, providing preprocedural and postprocedural assessment and care, preparing the patient, providing a safe environment and emotional support throughout the procedure, documentation, and providing discharge teaching. The health care provider is responsible for providing the patient with an explanation of the test/procedure, risks, benefits, treatment options, and outcomes before the procedure as part of the *informed consent* process.

PRACTICE STANDARDS

- American Society of Anesthesiologists (ASA), 2014: ASA Physical Status Classification System—Intravenous sedation
- American Society of Anesthesiologists (ASA), 2017: Practice guidelines for preoperative fasting and the use of pharmacologic agents to reduce the risk of pulmonary aspiration—Guidelines for preprocedural fasting
- The Joint Commission (TJC), 2019: National Patient Safety Goals—Patient identification

EVIDENCE-BASED PRACTICE

Reducing the Risk of Aspiration

Aspiration of stomach contents during anesthesia is rare but is still a concern to health care providers. The American Society of Anesthesiologists has revised guidelines with the purpose of providing direction for clinical practice related to preoperative/preprocedural fasting and the use of pharmacological agents to reduce the risk of pulmonary aspiration and the severity of complications related to perioperative pulmonary aspiration (ASA, 2017). Clinical practice includes, but is not limited to, withholding liquids and solids for specified time periods before surgery and prescribing pharmacological agents to reduce gastric volume and acidity (ASA, 2017). Follow the suggested guidelines for procedural anesthesia (ASA, 2017; Frank et al., 2017):

- Inform patients of fasting requirements and the reasons for them sufficiently in advance of their procedures.
- Verify patient compliance with fasting requirements at the time of their procedure.
- The guidelines list the same fasting recommendations for patients undergoing procedural sedation and general anesthesia. Clear liquids (not including alcohol) may be ingested for up to 2 hours before procedures that require procedural sedation and analgesia. A light meal or nonhuman milk may be ingested for up to 6 hours before elective procedures.
- The routine preoperative administration of antiemetics to reduce the risk of nausea and vomiting is not recommended for patients with no apparent increased risk for pulmonary aspiration.
- If fasting guidelines cannot be met, the suggestion is to delay the procedure, limit the sedation, or protect the airway with endotracheal intubation.
- In an emergent situation, the guidelines suggest postponing the procedure for patients with severe systemic disease, those who are predisposed to esophageal reflux, and those who are less than 6 months of age or over 70 years of age.

SAFETY GUIDELINES

Guidelines for anesthesia and related procedures are divided into prior to, during, and following the procedure or diagnostic test.

Before a Procedure

- It is essential to be sure that the patient undergoes the correct procedure. Ensure proper identification of a patient by using a minimum of two identifiers, verifying the correct procedure (and site, when applicable). This includes verbal verification and written/computerized documentation of the preceding information on patient arrival, again in the procedure room, and just before starting a procedure (The Joint Commission [TJC], 2019).
- Assess for completion of the relevant documentation (e.g., history and physical, signed procedure consent form, nursing assessment, and preanesthesia assessment) necessary for performing a safe procedure.
- Identify any medications for which uninterrupted dosing is required (e.g., anticonvulsants, antibiotics, and certain cardiac medications). If the procedure requires a patient to have nothing by mouth (NPO), discuss medications with the health care provider to decide if the patient should take any medications before the procedure. When insulin or oral hypoglycemic medications are given to patients before procedures, arrange to have either the patient's meal or other nutritional support available on completion of the procedure.
- Verify that informed consent was obtained before administering any sedatives. The health care provider performing the procedure is responsible for obtaining informed consent from a patient. In some agencies, after the health care provider discusses the procedure and obtains verbal consent, the registered nurse obtains the patient's signature on the consent form. (Check agency policy to determine if a consent form is required and the expectations of the nurse in this process.) *When there is no evidence of informed consent in the patient medical record, hold any preprocedure medications that may alter the patient's level of consciousness, and notify the health care provider performing the procedure and staff in any receiving area.*
- Make sure that emergency equipment (e.g., oxygen, suction, defibrillator) is available in the procedure area and has been checked to ensure function.
- Confirm presence and date of expiration for sedation reversal agents.

During a Procedure

- When a procedure involves the use of radiation:
  - Minimize the amount of radiation exposure by using protective shielding devices such as a lead apron and goggles, radioprotective gloves, and/or thyroid shield.
  - Monitor staff radiation exposure with the use of a dosimeter if necessary.
  - Remain positioned as far away from the radiographic equipment as possible while performing required patient care.
- Monitor physiological parameters indicated by the procedure.
- Position patients carefully to avoid musculoskeletal or neurological injury.
- Label any specimens obtained during a procedure properly.

After a Procedure

- Assess for possible procedural complications and conduct appropriate assessments for early detection.
- Monitor oxygen saturation and vital signs to detect sedation failure and adverse effects (e.g., vomiting, hypoxic events) (American College of Radiology [ACR], 2015; American Society of Anesthesiologists [ASA], 2014b).
- Know the use, side effects, and complications of the sedative and reversal agents to be administered.
- Be able to recognize cardiac dysrhythmias.
- Institute fall precautions until patient has recovered from effects of sedatives.
- Timely and complete neurovascular checks are critical to identify postprocedure limb ischemia or other arterial complications.

✦ SKILL 10.1 Intravenous Moderate Sedation

Purpose

Certain diagnostic or therapeutic procedures require patients to receive intravenous (IV) moderate sedation. Moderate sedation/analgesia produces a minimally depressed level of consciousness induced by the administration of pharmacological agents during which a patient retains a continuous and independent ability to maintain protective reflexes and a patent airway and is aroused by physical or verbal stimulation. Moderate sedation improves a patient's cooperation with a procedure, allows a rapid return to preprocedure status, and minimizes the risk for injury. It often raises a patient's pain threshold and provides amnesia concerning the actual procedural events. In addition, no interventions are required during a procedure to maintain a patent airway, and spontaneous ventilation is adequate (ASA, 2014).

Delegation and Collaboration

The skill of assisting with IV moderate sedation, including the preprocedure assessment, cannot be delegated to nursing assistive personnel (NAP). In most agencies a registered nurse (RN) or health care provider assesses and monitors a patient's level of sedation, airway patency, and level of consciousness. Roles in monitoring depend on scope-of-practice guidelines as determined by state regulations (see agency policy).

Equipment

- Personal protective equipment (PPE): Gloves, mask, head cover, gown, eye protection
- Sedation as prescribed: Benzodiazepines, opiates, propofol, and fentanyl
- Emergency equipment: Crash cart, cardiac monitor/defibrillator, and endotracheal intubation/airway management equipment in various sizes and appropriate for patient's age
- Equipment for insertion of a peripheral IV catheter (see Chapter 28)
- Oxygen and airway supplies: Bag and mask device, oral/nasopharyngeal airways
- Suction equipment (see Chapter 16)
- Sphygmomanometer or noninvasive blood pressure monitor
- Pulse oximeter or end-tidal CO_2 ($ETCO_2$) monitor
- Electrocardiogram (ECG) monitor
- Appropriate reversal drugs (e.g., flumazenil for reversal of benzodiazepines, naloxone for reversal of opiates) and labels for each
- Pain medication (opioids) for procedures anticipated to cause discomfort such as dizziness, disorientation, nausea, vomiting

ASSESSMENT

1. Identify patient using at least two identifiers (e.g., name and birthday or name and medical record number) according to agency policy. Compare identifiers with information in patient's medication administration record (MAR) or medical record. *Rationale: Ensures correct patient. Complies with The Joint Commission standards and improves patient safety (TJC, 2019).*
2. Verify type of procedure scheduled and procedure site with patient. *Rationale: Ensures the correct surgery or procedure is done on the correct patient and at the correct place on the patient's body (TJC, 2019).*
3. Verify that a preprocedure medication reconciliation and history and physical (H&P) examination were completed. *Rationale: Accrediting agencies such as the TJC (2019) require a documented preprocedure medication history and H&P before administration of procedural IV sedation.*
4. Verify that informed consent was obtained before administering any sedatives. *Rationale: Federal regulations, many state laws, and accreditation agencies require informed consent for procedure.*
5. Assess patient's past history of adverse reaction to IV sedation (e.g., hemodynamic instability, nausea or vomiting, airway compromise, altered level of consciousness). *Rationale: Patients with history of these reactions are at higher risk for procedural complications if IV sedation is used.*
6. Verify patient's ASA Physical Status Classification (Box 10.1). *Rationale: ASA recommends that patients receiving classification of III or higher have anesthesia consultation before receiving IV sedation (ASA, 2014).*

Safe Patient Care *Consultation with an anesthesiologist is often required by the agency if a patient has an ASA classification of III to VI or history of or evidence for difficult intubation, sleep apnea, or complications related to sedation/anesthesia.*

7. Assess patient for history of airway abnormalities, liver failure, lung disease, heart failure, hypotonia, morbid obesity, severe gastroesophageal reflux, and history of adverse reaction to sedatives (ACR, 2015). *Rationale: Risk factors that increase likelihood of adverse event.*
8. Assess patient's current or history for substance abuse or liver/kidney disease. *Rationale: A history of substance abuse and/or liver/kidney disease usually requires dose adjustment of sedative agents.*
9. Verify that patient has not ingested food or fluids, except for oral medications, for at least 2 to 6 hours (see agency policy). *Rationale: Because risk of moderate sedation is loss of airway protection, empty stomach reduces risk for aspiration.*
10. Determine if patient is allergic to latex, antiseptic, tape, or anesthetic solutions. If allergy is identified, place allergy alert band on patient's wrist. *Rationale: Allergic reactions to latex or tape range from mild skin reaction to anaphylaxis. Common allergic reactions to local anesthetic agents include central nervous system (CNS) depression, respiratory difficulty, and hypotension.*
11. Assess patient's level of understanding of procedure, including any concerns. *Rationale: Determines extent of instruction or level of support required.*
12. Perform hand hygiene. Assess baseline heart rate, breath sounds, respiratory rate, blood pressure, level of consciousness, pain level, and oxygen saturation (SpO_2). *Rationale: Establishes baseline for comparison during and after procedure.*
13. Determine patient's height and weight. *Rationale: Needed to calculate drug dosages.*
14. Assess patient's baseline status via designated scoring system of agency. A variety of tools are available for scoring, including the "Aldrete score" (Aldrete, 2007; Table 10.1). *Rationale: Establishes baseline for comparison after procedure.*
15. Assess patient's or family caregiver's knowledge, experience, and health literacy. *Rationale: Ensures patient or family caregiver has the capacity to obtain, communicate, process, and understand basic health information (Centers for Disease Control and Prevention [CDC], 2016).*

BOX 10.1

ASA Physical Status Classification System[a]

ASA PS Classification	Definition	Examples, Including, but Not Limited to:
ASA I	A normal healthy patient	Healthy, nonsmoking, no or minimal alcohol use
ASA II	A patient with mild systemic disease	Mild diseases only without substantive functional limitations (e.g., current smoker, social alcohol drinker, pregnancy, obesity [30 < BMI <40], well-controlled DM/HTN, mild lung disease)
ASA III	A patient with severe systemic disease	Substantive functional limitations; one or more moderate to severe diseases (e.g., controlled DM or HTN, COPD, morbid obesity [BMI ≥40], active hepatitis, alcohol dependence or abuse, implanted pacemaker)
ASA IV	A patient with severe systemic disease that is a constant threat to life	Examples include recent (<3 months) MI, CVA, TIA, or CAD/stents, ongoing cardiac ischemia or severe valve dysfunction, sepsis
ASA V	A moribund patient who is not expected to survive without the operation	Examples include ruptured abdominal/thoracic aneurysm, massive trauma, intracranial bleed with mass or multiple organ/system dysfunction
ASA VI	A declared brain-dead patient whose organs are being removed for donor purposes	

[a]The addition of "E" denotes Emergency surgery. (An emergency is defined as existing when delay in treatment of the patient would lead to a significant increase in the threat to life or body part.)

ASA, American Society of Anesthesiologists; *BMI,* body mass index; *CAD,* coronary artery disease; *COPD,* chronic obstructive pulmonary disease; *CVA,* cerebrovascular accident; *DM,* diabetes mellitus; *HTN,* hypertension; *MI,* myocardial infarction; *TIA,* transient ischemic attack.

From American Society of Anesthesiologists: *ASA Physical Status Classification System*, 2014. https://www.asahq.org/resources/clinical-information/asa-physical-status-classification-system.

TABLE 10.1
Aldrete Scoring System

		Score
Activity (moving voluntarily or on command)	4 extremities	2
	2 extremities	1
	Unable to move extremities	0
Respiration	Able to breathe deeply and cough freely	2
	Dyspnea, shallow or limited breathing	1
	Apneic	0
Circulation	BP ± 20 mm Hg of presedation level	2
	BP ± 20–49 mm Hg of presedation level	1
	BP ± 50 mm Hg of presedation level	0
Consciousness	Fully awake	2
	Arousable on having name called	1
	Not responding	0
O_2 saturation	Able to maintain O_2 saturation at 92% or above on room air	2
	Needs O_2 inhalation to maintain O_2 saturation 90% or above	1
	O_2 saturation less than 90 even with O_2 supplement	0

From Aldrete JA: Post-anesthetic recovery score, *J Am Coll Surg* 205(5):3, 2007.

STEP	RATIONALE

PLANNING

STEP	RATIONALE
1. Expected outcomes following completion of procedures:	
• Patient does not experience any procedure or postprocedure complications	Procedure performed safely and successfully.
• Patient's airway remains patent.	Moderate sedation is monitored successfully without progression to deep sedation.
• Patient's level of comfort is equivalent to score of 4 or less on pain scale of 0 to 10.	Procedure managed to minimize patient's pain.
2. Apply a Fall Risk identification band to patient's wrist.	Patients who are to receive procedural sedation are at risk for falls.
3. Explain to patient that IV sedation will cause relaxation and amnesia but that he or she will be awake during procedure. If patient will not be able to verbalize because of nature of procedure, teach him or her agreed-on nonverbal signals such as "yes," "no," and "pain."	Encourages cooperation and minimizes risks and anxiety about procedure.
4. Explain that close monitoring of vital signs and frequent checks to determine that patient is awake are normal and do not mean that there are problems.	Reduces patient anxiety during procedure.
5. Explain to patient major steps of procedure.	Reduces patient anxiety during procedure.
6. Provide privacy and prepare environment. Keep patient warm with blanket.	Promotes patient's comfort and safety.

IMPLEMENTATION

STEP	RATIONALE
1. Perform hand hygiene. Establish peripheral IV access (see Chapter 28).	Provides access for administration of sedation and any emergency medications (as needed).
2. Implement Universal Protocol a second time in presence of appropriate health care team members (as applicable) and in accordance with agency policy (Box 10.2).	Ensures patient safety by correctly identifying correct patient with correct procedure (TJC, 2019).
3. During diagnostic procedure, monitor heart rate and SpO_2 continuously via pulse oximetry equipment. Some agencies also use $ETCO_2$ monitoring (capnography) (Conway et al., 2015). Monitor patient's airway patency, respiratory rate and depth, blood pressure, and level of consciousness and responsiveness every 5 minutes (ACR, 2015). Keep oxygen and suction equipment nearby.	Vital signs, oximetry, and capnography provide comparison with patient's baseline status. Oxygen and suction equipment may be required in an emergent situation.

STEP	RATIONALE
4. Observe for verbal or nonverbal evidence of pain, facial grimacing, and eye opening.	Physical responses indicate level of sedation.
5. Assess level of sedation using Modified Ramsay Sedation Scale (Table 10.2) or other criteria adopted by agency.	Determines patient's level of sedation. Numeric rating scale offers consistent assessment and accurate judgment of patient's changing status and verbal/physical stimulation.

Safe Patient Care *Report a Ramsay sedation score higher than 3 (responsive to commands only) to the health care provider in procedure room.*

STEP	RATIONALE
6. Reposition patient as needed without interrupting diagnostic procedure.	Prevents pressure- and position-related injuries (ACR, 2015).
7. At end of procedure, maintain patient in comfortable position that ensures patent airway. Monitor as consciousness returns.	Ensures safe airway management.
8. Be sure nurse call system is in an accessible location within patient's reach.	Ensures patient can call for assistance if needed.
9. Raise side rails (as appropriate) and lower bed to lowest position.	Ensures patient safety.
10. Remove gloves and perform hand hygiene.	Reduces transmission of microorganisms.

EVALUATION

1. Monitor patient throughout procedure using the Modified Ramsay Sedation Scale (or other criteria adopted by the agency) (see Table 10.2).
   Provides data to verify patient's expected return to baseline status.
2. After procedure: Use Aldrete score (see Table 10.1) and monitor level of consciousness, respiratory rate, SpO_2, blood pressure, heart rate and rhythm, and pain score according to agency policy (ACR, 2015) (e.g., every 5 minutes for at least 30 minutes, then every 15 minutes for an hour, and then every 30 minutes until patient meets discharge criteria).
   Enables prompt detection of any airway compromise or protective reflexes caused by delayed action of medications.
3. Ask patient to repeat back what he or she understands regarding procedure or any postprocedure patient instructions, including medication orders and instructions.
   Verifies patient understanding of procedure or discharge education.
4. Once patient is stable and ready for discharge, have patient's "designated driver" explain any postprocedure education and sign appropriate documents.
   Patients who receive conscious sedation are restricted from driving for 24 to 48 hours, depending on procedure, type of sedation, and postprocedure restrictions.
5. **Use Teach-Back:** "I want to be sure I explained your postprocedure medications to you. Tell me what you know about the medications you will be taking once you are home." Revise your instruction now or develop a plan for revised patient/family caregiver teaching if patient/family caregiver is not able to teach back correctly.
   Determines patient's/family caregiver's level of understanding of instructional topic.

BOX 10.2

The Joint Commission Universal Protocol and Association of PeriOperative Registered Nurses (AORN) Comprehensive Surgical Checklist

- Verification of correct person. Use at least two patient identifiers when providing care, treatment, and services. Acceptable identifiers may be the individual's name, an assigned identification number, telephone number, or other person-specific identifier.
- Verification of correct site, and correct procedure occurs.
- Procedure site is marked before moving to procedure area.
- A "time-out" is performed immediately before starting procedures.

Modified from Association of PeriOperative Nurses (AORN): AORN comprehensive surgical checklist, 2016, http://www.aorn.org/guidelines/clinical-resources/tool-kits/correct-site-surgery-tool-kit/aorn-comprehensive-surgical-checklist; The Joint Commission (TJC): *2019 National Patient Safety Goals,* Oakbrook Terrace, IL, 2019, The Commission. http://www.jointcommission.org/standards_information/npsgs.aspx.

TABLE 10.2

Modified Ramsay Sedation Scale

Minimal sedation (anxiolysis)	1	Anxious and agitated or restless or both
	2	Cooperative, oriented, and tranquil
Moderate sedation/ analgesia (conscious sedation)	3	Responds to commands spoken in a normal voice
Deep sedation/ analgesia	4	Brisk response to a light forehead tap or loud auditory stimulus
	5	Sluggish response to a light forehead tap or loud auditory stimulus
	6	No response to a light forehead tap or loud auditory stimulus

Data modified from Fuchs B, Bellamy C: Sedative-analgesic medications in critically ill adults: selection, initiation, maintenance, and withdrawal, *UpToDate*, 2017. http://www.uptodate.com/contents/sedative-analgesic-medications-in-critically-ill-adults-selection-initiation-maintenance-and-withdrawal.

Unexpected Outcomes	Related Interventions
1. Oversedation, evidenced by decreasing SpO_2 (cyanosis, slow shallow respirations with periods of apnea), tachycardia, or sedation score of 4 (exhibiting brisk response to light glabellar tap or loud auditory stimulus) or higher on Modified Ramsay Sedation Scale or less than 8 on Aldrete scale.	• Support patient's breathing via positioning and manual bagging. • Immediately notify health care provider. • Be prepared to administer reversal agents. Naloxone is for reversal of opioids, and flumazenil is for reversal of benzodiazepines.
2. Patient develops cardiac instability, evidenced by irregular heart rate, change in pulse rate, or change in blood pressure.	• Initiate oxygen therapy as ordered, maintain IV access, and obtain ECG as ordered. • Immediately notify health care provider.

Recording

- Document vital signs, SpO_2, $ETCO_2$, and sedation level at baseline, then every 5 minutes during the procedure, and every 15 minutes for at least 30 minutes after the procedure according to agency policy.
- Record dosage, route, and time of administration for drugs given during and after the procedure, including reversal agents. Record significant patient reactions during the procedure. Include IV fluids and blood products if administered.
- Document discharge teaching, medication reconciliation, discontinuation of IV access, final/discharge assessment, and to whom/how discharged (e.g., designated driver, ambulance/transporter, nursing home).
- Document your evaluation of patient learning.

Hand-Off Reporting

- Immediately report to patient's health care provider any respiratory distress, cardiac compromise, or unexpected altered mental status.

✦ SKILL 10.2 Contrast Media Studies: Arteriogram (Angiogram), Cardiac Catheterization, Intravenous Pyelogram

Purpose

Contrast media studies involve visualization of blood vessel structures of the body by intravascular injection of a radiopaque medium. An arteriogram (angiogram) permits visualization of the vasculature and arterial system of an area of the body or an organ. Arteriography is most frequently performed by an interventional radiologist or cardiologist to diagnose venous or arterial occlusions, stenosis, emboli, thromboses, aneurysms, tumors, congenital malformations, or trauma anywhere in the body.

Cardiac catheterization is a specialized form of angiography. The interventionist inserts a catheter introducer into a femoral artery or vein and threads the tip of a long, thin catheter into the right or left side of the heart (Fig. 10.1). The brachial or radial artery or vein can also be used. A contrast medium is injected through the catheter, allowing for assessment of the structures and functions of the heart, including blood flow. The test studies pressures and blood flow in the heart chambers and large arteries, oxygen levels, cardiac volumes, valve function, and patency of coronary arteries. Cardiac catheterization also allows for collection of blood samples and biopsy of heart muscle. Cardiac catheterizations are performed in specially equipped laboratories.

Intravenous pyelography (IVP) is the examination of the flow of radiopaque contrast medium that shows how the kidneys remove the dye and how it collects in the urine. IVP helps to identify obstruction, hematuria, stones, bladder injury, or renal artery occlusion. Dye is injected via a catheter through a peripheral artery, and serial x-rays are taken over the subsequent 30 minutes.

Delegation and Collaboration

The skill of helping with angiography and IVP can be delegated to nursing assistive personnel (NAP) if the patient is stable and no IV sedation is used. The registered nurse (RN) directs the NAP about:

- When to obtain and report vital signs, urinary output, and weight.
- Which signs and symptoms to report to the nurse.

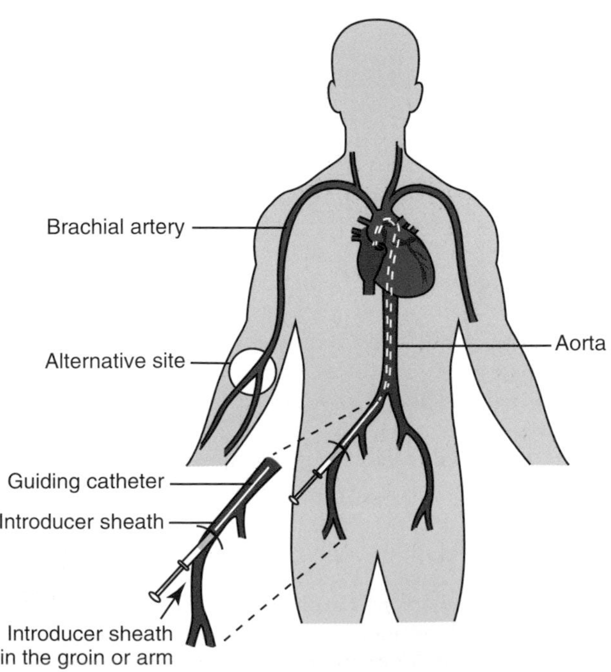

FIG 10.1 A catheter introducer placed into a femoral artery or vein allows for threading the tip of a long, thin catheter into the right or left side of the heart during cardiac catheterization.

- Accompanying the patient to the procedure room and helping specially trained and licensed radiology personnel with the specific angiography procedure.

The skill of assisting with cardiac catheterization can be delegated to specially trained NAP with a nurse continuously present. The nurse provides continuous patient assessment and monitoring for serious complications. The NAP helps with patient transport, positioning, and obtaining supplies.

Equipment

- Personal protective equipment (PPE): Mask, sterile gown, head cover, eye protection, and sterile gloves. Clean gloves optional.
- Sterile packs containing catheters/equipment for performing procedures
- Equipment for peripheral IV access
- Medications, such as sedatives (e.g., diazepam, midazolam, propofol) for IV sedation or analgesics for relaxation and pain control
- Emergency equipment: Oxygen, endotracheal intubation/airway management equipment, emergency cart, cardiac monitor/defibrillator, sedative reversal agents
- Pulse oximeter, end-tidal carbon dioxide ($ETCO_2$) monitor, blood pressure (BP) equipment

ASSESSMENT

1. Identify patient using at least two identifiers (e.g., name and birthday or name and medical record number) according to agency policy. Compare identifiers with information in patient's medication administration record (MAR) or medical record. *Rationale: Ensures correct patient. Complies with The Joint Commission standards and improves patient safety (TJC, 2019).*
2. Verify type of procedure scheduled and procedure site with patient. *Rationale: Ensures correct procedure and patient. Complies with The Joint Commission National Patient Safety Goals (TJC, 2019).*
3. Verify that informed consent was obtained before administering any sedatives. *Rationale: Federal regulations, many state laws, and accreditation agencies require informed consent for procedure.*
4. Determine if patient is taking anticoagulants, aspirin, or any nonsteroidal medication. *Rationale: Some medications increase risk for bleeding and are often stopped before procedure.*
5. Assess patient for history of any allergies to iodine dye, shellfish, or latex and whether patient has had previous reaction to contrast agent (Westermann-Clark et al., 2015). If so, notify cardiologist or radiologist. *Rationale: Allergic individuals may be at a mildly increased risk for developing adverse reactions to radiocontrast media. Hypoallergenic contrast medium is sometimes used.*
6. Review medical record for contraindications:
   a. All contrast media: Contraindicated in pregnancy unless benefits of test outweigh risks to fetus. *Rationale: Radioactive iodinated contrast media crosses blood–placental barrier.*
   b. Angiography: Anticoagulant therapy, bleeding disorders, thrombocytopenia, dehydration, uncontrolled hypertension, renal insufficiency, and pregnancy. *Rationale: Anticoagulants and bleeding disorders interfere with patient's blood-clotting abilities and may cause blood loss. Dehydration and renal insufficiency are contraindications to use of ionic radiographic contrast media because patient has impaired ability to excrete contrast media via kidneys.*
   c. Cardiac catheterization: History of severe cardiomyopathy, severe dysrhythmias, uncontrolled heart failure (HF). *Rationale: Introduction of catheter into myocardium increases risk for dysrhythmias (Van Leeuwen and Bladh, 2017).*
   d. IVP: History of dehydration, known renal insufficiency (with blood urea nitrogen [BUN] level >40 mg/100 mL or creatinine >2 mg/dL) (Van Leeuwen and Bladh, 2017). *Rationale: Iodinated dye is sometimes nephrotoxic and worsens existing renal disease.*
   e. Determine whether patient took metformin hydrochloride within previous 48 hours. If so, notify health care provider immediately. *Rationale: Metformin hydrochloride may or may not be discontinued 1 day before procedure and 2 days after catheterization because of the possibility of causing lactic acidosis and kidney damage (Honicker and Holt, 2016; Maden et al., 2013).*
7. Assess patient's bleeding and coagulation status (e.g., complete blood count [CBC], platelets, prothrombin time [PT], activated partial thromboplastin time [aPTT]/international normalized ratio [INR]) and patient's renal function (e.g., BUN, creatinine levels) before procedure. Assess electrolytes (sodium and potassium). *Rationale: Abnormal laboratory findings may contraindicate procedure because of potential complications of hemorrhage and/or renal failure. Report elevated BUN or creatinine levels to health care provider because such patients are at risk for renal failure induced by contrast media (Van Leeuwen and Bladh, 2017). Abnormal electrolytes may reveal possible electromechanical problems.*
8. Review medical record to determine type of arteriogram scheduled (e.g., carotid, femoral, brachial). For cardiac catheterization, verify if test is for right or left heart or both. For IVP, ask if study is for one or both kidneys. *Rationale: Enables you to anticipate patient teaching needs and postprocedure interventions.*
9. Perform hand hygiene. Obtain vital signs and peripheral pulses. For arterial procedures mark patient's peripheral pulses before procedure. For cardiac catheterization also auscultate heart and lungs and obtain weight. *Rationale: Provides baseline data and locations for comparison with findings during and after procedure.*
10. Assess patient's hydration status, including condition of mucous membranes (clean gloves may be needed) and recent 24-hour intake. *Rationale: Severe dehydration can lead to renal failure (Van Leeuwen and Bladh, 2017).*
11. Determine and document last time of ingested food, drink, or medications. *Rationale: Prevents possible aspiration because patient is sedated. Excessive hydration causes dilution of contrast medium, making structures more difficult to visualize. Patients should be NPO for 2 to 8 hours before procedure (Van Leeuwen and Bladh, 2017).*

Safe Patient Care *Exceptions occur for patients at risk for contrast media–induced renal impairment who are specifically instructed to drink increased fluids in the hours before the procedure or those instructed by the health care provider to take medications before the procedure. Good preprocedure hydration reduces the risk for renal impairment caused by contrast media (Van Leeuwen and Bladh, 2017).*

12. Review health care provider's orders for preprocedure medications, hydration, antihistamines, and IV sedation. *Rationale: Increased sedation is necessary in anxious or confused patients. Increased hydration is often required for renal insufficiency and antihistamines for possible allergic reaction.*
    a. Atropine. *Rationale: Decreases salivary secretions and increases heart rate when bradycardia is present.*
    b. Diphenhydramine. *Rationale: Used prophylactically to block histamine and decrease allergic response.*
    c. Preprocedural sedative. *Rationale: Decreases anxiety and promotes relaxation.*
13. Assess patient's or family caregiver's knowledge, experience, and health literacy. *Rationale: Ensures patient or family caregiver has the capacity to obtain, communicate, process, and understand basic health information (CDC, 2016).*
14. Assess patient's level of understanding of procedure, including any concerns. *Rationale: Determines extent of instruction or level of support required.*

STEP	RATIONALE
PLANNING	
1. Expected outcomes following completion of procedure:	
• Patient does not experience any procedure or postprocedure complications, such as significant changes in vital signs, diminished or absent peripheral pulses, allergic response, or decreased or absent urine output.	Procedure performed without complication.
• Patient's level of comfort is equal to score of 4 or less on pain scale of 0 to 10. Expected discomfort includes soreness at catheter insertion site and possible backache.	Patient tolerates procedure.
• Patient tolerates increased fluid intake and urinates sufficiently (at least 30 mL/hr or 0.5 mL/kg/hr) to excrete radiographic dye.	Adequate renal function.
• Patient recovers from IV sedation without respiratory complications or change in level of consciousness.	Appropriate level of sedation.
2. Explain to patient purpose of and what will happen during procedure.	Helps to minimize patient's anxiety.
3. Remove all of patient's jewelry, metal objects, and body piercings.	Eliminates objects that interfere with radiography visualization of vessels and could be conductive material during electrocautery.
4. Preprocedure preparation:	
a. *For IVP:* Verify that patient has completed necessary bowel preparation of orally administered evacuation preparation 24 hours before test and evacuation enema 8 hours before test (check agency policy).	An evacuated lower intestine and bowel improve visualization of urinary structures.
b. *For cardiac catheterization:* Determine whether hair at site of catheter insertion needs clipping or preparation with antiseptic just before procedure. Allow antiseptic to dry. Do not shave site.	Reduces risk for site-related infection. Drying promotes maximal antibacterial activity. Shaving results in increased chance for infection.
c. For cardiac catheterization it is common to verify availability of emergent cardiac surgery because of risk for complete coronary artery occlusion from dislodged plaque or inadvertent perforation of vasculature. Also verify patient's ASA classification before procedure (see Box 10.1).	Prepares backup plan for possible procedural outcomes that would require emergency surgery.
5. Have patient empty bladder or bowels before procedure.	Ensures that patient will not need to void during procedure.
6. Remove patient's eyeglasses, dentures, or other dental appliances.	Prevents damage to eyeglasses or damage/dislodgement of dental structures during procedure.
7. Provide privacy and prepare environment.	Promotes patient comfort and safety.
IMPLEMENTATION	
1. Prepare cardiac monitor, pulse oximeter, and/or $ETCO_2$ monitor.	Provides easy access to equipment for monitoring patient status during and after procedure.
2. Perform hand hygiene and apply appropriate protective equipment.	Reduces transmission of microorganisms.
3. Provide IV access using large-bore cannula. Remove and dispose of clean gloves.	Provides access for delivery of IV fluids and/or drugs.

STEP	RATIONALE
4. Help patient assume a comfortable supine position on x-ray table. Some patients undergoing IVP may be in supine or in a slight Trendelenburg's position. Immobilize extremity that will be injected. Pad any bony prominences.	For arterial procedures, patient may need to maintain position for 1 to 3 hours. Padding the bony prominences reduces the risk for impaired skin integrity.
5. Take "time-out" to verify patient's name, type of procedure to be performed, and procedure site with patient.	"Time-out" verification just before starting an invasive procedure includes health care provider and all involved personnel and is a safety precaution to prevent wrong patient, wrong site, and wrong procedure errors (TJC, 2019).
6. Monitor vital signs, pulse oximetry (SpO_2), and $ETCO_2$; for arterial procedures, palpate peripheral pulses.	Data provide comparison with baseline to determine patient's response to procedure.
7. Inform patient that during injection of dye, it is common to experience some chest pain and a severe hot flash that is quite uncomfortable but lasts only a few seconds.	Dye causes feeling of warmth, flushing, or metallic taste shortly after injection.
8. Physician cleanses arterial puncture site for catheter insertion (femoral, radial, carotid, or brachial) with antiseptic.	Reduces transmission of microorganisms.
9. All health care team members apply mask and goggles, sterile gown, head cover, and sterile gloves. Drape patient with sterile drapes, leaving puncture site exposed.	Maintains surgical asepsis.
10. Physician anesthetizes skin overlying arterial puncture site.	Provides local anesthetic to area of incision or puncture.
11. For arterial procedures physician does the following:	
a. Punctures artery, inserts introducer (thin plastic tube) into artery, inserts guidewire through introducer and advances, and inserts flexible catheter over guidewire and advances into heart. Introducers allow for use of various procedure catheters, depending on need (e.g., balloon angioplasty, stent placement, ablation).	Permits access to artery and coiling of catheter in artery.
b. Advances catheter to desired artery or cardiac chamber, removes guidewire, and injects contrast medium through catheter.	Permits radiographic visualization of structures, aneurysms, occlusions, or anomalies.
12. During dye injection specialized machinery takes rapid sequence of x-ray films.	Permits radiographic records of visualization of dye through artery and any abnormalities present.
13. If iodinated dye is used, observe patient for signs of anaphylaxis, including respiratory distress, palpitation, itching, and diaphoresis.	Allergic reactions can be life threatening.
14. During cardiac catheterization RN helps with measuring cardiac volumes and pressure.	Provides data related to cardiac output, central venous pressure (CVP), ventricular pressures, and pulmonary artery pressure.

Safe Patient Care *Be prepared to end the cardiac catheterization procedure early in the event of severe unrelieved chest pain, neurological symptoms of a cerebrovascular accident, cardiac dysrhythmias, or hemodynamic changes (Van Leeuwen and Bladh, 2017).*

STEP	RATIONALE
15. Nurse administering IV sedation monitors levels of sedation, level of consciousness, and vital signs continuously.	Proper IV sedation does not cause loss of consciousness.
16. Physician withdraws catheter and applies manual pressure to puncture site until homeostasis occurs (5 to 15 minutes or longer).	Five to fifteen minutes of manual pressure is often enough to stop active site arterial bleeding. However, a certain amount of bed rest is needed to achieve reliable hemostasis. Check agency policy for postprocedure bed rest requirements. This may vary from 2 to 6 hours when no arteriotomy closure device is used.
a. *Option:* Physician may choose to use an arteriotomy closure device (ACD), which can be categorized as either passive-closure device (helps with compression such as clamps/tamping devices, assisted or enhanced coagulation, and sealants) or active-closure device (immediate closure with suture devices, clips, and collagen plug devices).	Use of ACDs is reasonable after invasive cardiovascular procedures performed via femoral artery to achieve faster hemostasis, shorter duration of bed rest, and possibly improved patient comfort. Use of devices should be weighed against risk of complications (Krishnasamy et al., 2015; Schulz-Schüpke et al., 2014).

STEP	RATIONALE

Safe Patient Care *Before removing catheter sheath, check health care provider's orders for instructions for treating a vasovagal reaction. Manual pressure applied to the groin/femoral area can stimulate the baroreceptors and cause a vasovagal reaction in which the patient becomes bradycardic and hypotensive. Vasovagal reactions are usually brief and self-limiting. When applying pressure to the groin after sheath removal, be alert for a vasovagal reaction and prepared to treat it by lowering the head of the bed to the flat position and giving a bolus of IV fluids.*

STEP	RATIONALE
17. If a percutaneous coronary intervention (PCI) such as a percutaneous transluminal coronary angioplasty (PTCA) or directional coronary atherectomy (DCA) was performed during cardiac catheterization, a femoral introducer/sheath is often left in place and removed in several hours.	Postinterventional sheaths provide emergency access to vasculature in event that coronary artery becomes occluded, allowing time for anticoagulants to wear off.
18. Remove and discard gloves. Perform hand hygiene.	Reduces transmission of microorganisms.
19. Help patient to comfortable position.	Gives patient sense of well-being.
20. Be sure nurse call system is in an accessible location within patient's reach.	Ensures patient can call for assistance if needed.
21. Raise side rails (as appropriate) and lower bed to lowest position.	Ensures patient safety.
22. Postprocedure	
a. For arterial procedures:	
(1) Keep affected extremity immobilized for 2 to 6 hours after removal of sheath (see agency policy). Use orthopedic bedpan for female patient as needed for bowel or bladder evacuation while on bed rest.	There is evidence of no benefit relating to bleeding and hematoma formation in patients who have more than 3 hours of bed rest following transfemoral diagnostic cardiac catheterization. There is evidence of benefit relating to decreased incidence and severity of back pain after 3 hours of bed rest. Inconclusive evidence suggests that bed rest for 2 hours following transfemoral cardiac catheterization may be sufficient (Abdollahi et al., 2015).
(2) Emphasize need to lie flat for 6 to 12 hours (and possibly overnight if sheath is left in groin).	Helps to prevent disruption of hemostasis.
b. Encourage patient to drink fluids after procedure.	Facilitates elimination of contrast material and prevents renal damage (Van Leeuwen and Bladh, 2017).

EVALUATION

STEP	RATIONALE
1. Evaluate patient's body position and comfort during procedure.	Position can cause stress on insertion site and patient's musculoskeletal structures.
2. Monitor vital signs and SpO_2 and assess for signs of cardiac complications every 15 minutes for 1 hour, every 30 minutes for 2 hours, or until vital signs are stable.	Verifies patient's physiological status and evaluates effect of procedure. Signs of cardiac complications include chest pain or pressure, new dysrhythmias, and/or shortness of breath.
3. Monitor for complications:	
a. Perform neurovascular checks by palpating peripheral pulses on affected extremity and comparing right and left extremities for skin color, temperature, and sensation (see Chapter 8). Use Doppler ultrasonic stethoscope to locate pulses that are not palpable	Enables prompt detection of circulatory impairment caused by intravascular clotting or bleeding at procedure site. Signs of reduced circulation include diminishing distal pulses and/or coolness, mottling, pallor, pain, numbness, and tingling in affected extremity.
b. With vital signs assess vascular access site for bleeding and hematoma.	Verifies expected sealing of puncture.
c. Auscultate heart and lungs and compare with preprocedure findings.	Evaluates patient response to procedure.
d. Observe patient for possible delayed reaction to iodine dye (if used)—dyspnea, hives, tachycardia, and rash (Van Leeuwen and Bladh, 2017)	Reaction may occur up to 6 hours after injection of dye.
4. Evaluate level of sedation, level of consciousness, and SpO_2. Use Aldrete scale (see Table 10.1).	Determines patient's response to IV sedation.
5. Assess postprocedure laboratory values—CBC, prothrombin time, aPTT, INR, electrolytes, BUN/creatinine.	Detects changes in laboratory values that indicate onset of complications such as bleeding.
6. Have patient rate discomfort on pain scale of 0 to 10.	Pain is early sign of complications.

STEP	RATIONALE
7. **Use Teach-Back:** "I want to be sure I explained what to watch for regarding signs of an allergic reaction after this procedure. Tell me what feelings would make you think you might be having an allergic reaction." Revise your instruction now or develop a plan for revised patient/family caregiver teaching if patient/family caregiver is not able to teach back correctly.	Determines patient's/family caregiver's level of understanding of instructional topic.

Unexpected Outcomes	Related Interventions
1. Vasovagal response occurs (at time of femoral puncture or after procedure with femoral pressure). Symptoms include feeling faint, dizzy, and light-headed and possible momentary loss of consciousness. Bradycardia is caused by stimulation of vagus nerve via baroreceptors.	• Support airway (through positioning). • Lower table or head of bed to flat position or to Trendelenburg's position if ordered. • Be prepared to administer bolus of IV fluid (normal saline).
2. Pedal pulses are nonpalpable bilaterally 2 hours after arteriogram with change in skin color and temperature.	• Assess pulse with Doppler. • Immediately notify health care provider.
3. Hematoma or hemorrhage is present at catheter insertion site.	• Apply pressure over insertion site. • Monitor catheter site every 15 to 30 minutes for 2 to 3 hours; follow agency protocol. • Notify health care provider if interventions do not stop bleeding or if patient has symptoms of acute blood loss (hypotension, tachycardia, decreased level of consciousness).
4. Patient has allergic reaction to contrast medium with symptoms of flushing, itching, and urticaria.	• Monitor vital signs and observe for symptoms of anaphylaxis. • Notify health care provider. • Follow specific postprocedure orders related to findings. • Prepare to administer antihistamine or epinephrine if ordered.

Recording

- Record in medical record patient's condition: Vital signs, pulse oximetry, $ETCO_2$, peripheral pulses for equality and symmetry, blood pressure, temperature and color of catheterized extremity, condition of access/puncture site including any drainage and presence of any VCD, level of consciousness, and status and flow rate of IV.
- Document your evaluation of patient learning.

Hand-Off Reporting

- Report to health care provider immediately: Changes in vital signs, pulse oximetry, $ETCO_2$, arrhythmias, excessive bleeding or increasing hematoma at access/puncture site, decreased or absent peripheral pulses, urine output less than 30 mL per hour (0.5 mL/kg/hr) for adults and 1 mL/kg/hr for children, and decreased level of patient responsiveness.

✦ SKILL 10.3 Care of Patients Undergoing Aspirations: Bone Marrow, Lumbar Puncture, Paracentesis, Thoracentesis

Purpose

Aspirations are sterile invasive procedures involving removal of body fluids or tissue for diagnostic purposes. The nurse assists the health care provider during an aspiration procedure (Table 10.3). *Bone marrow aspiration* is the removal of a small amount of the liquid organic material in the medullary canals of selected bones. A biopsy is the removal of a core of marrow cells for laboratory analysis. A lumbar puncture (LP), called a *spinal puncture* or *tap*, involves the introduction of a needle into the subarachnoid space of the spinal column. The purpose of the test is to measure pressure in the subarachnoid space and obtain cerebrospinal fluid (CSF) for visualization and laboratory testing. LP is also used to inject anesthetic, diagnostic, or therapeutic agents. *Abdominal paracentesis* involves aspiration of peritoneal fluid from the abdomen. The aspirate is analyzed for cell cytology, bacteria, blood, glucose, and protein to help diagnose the causes of an abdominal effusion. *Thoracentesis* is performed to analyze or remove pleural fluid or instill medications intrapleurally.

Delegation and Collaboration

The skill of helping with aspirations can be delegated to nursing assistive personnel (NAP) if the patient is stable (check agency policy). However, assessment of the patient's condition must be completed by the nurse and cannot be delegated. The nurse directs the NAP about:

- Proper positioning of the patient during the procedure.
- When to take and report vital signs.

TABLE 10.3
Summary of Aspiration Procedures

Aspiration Procedure	Preparation/Assessment Specific to Test	Position or Site Prone or Supine Position	Special Considerations
Bone marrow aspiration	Assess complete blood count and clotting studies for abnormalities. For sternal biopsy, place adult patient in supine position. For iliac crest biopsy, place in prone or lateral recumbent position.	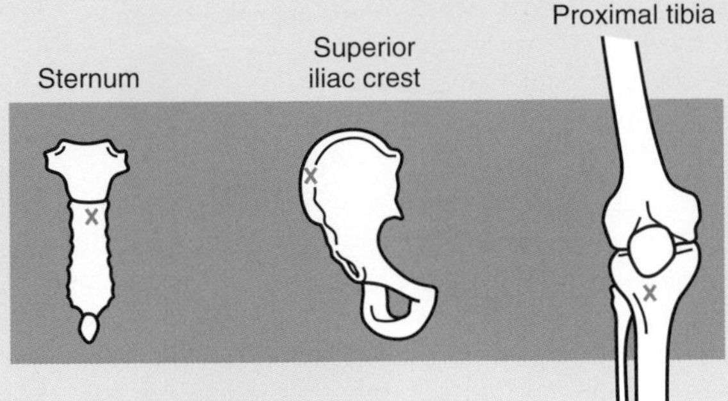	Patients with arthritis or orthopnea may have difficulty assuming the positions. Apply pressure to aspiration site after the procedure.
Lumbar puncture	Assess neurological status, including movement, sensation, and muscle strength of legs to provide a baseline for comparison. Assess bladder for distention and determine last voiding. Allow patient to void before procedure.	Lateral decubitus position 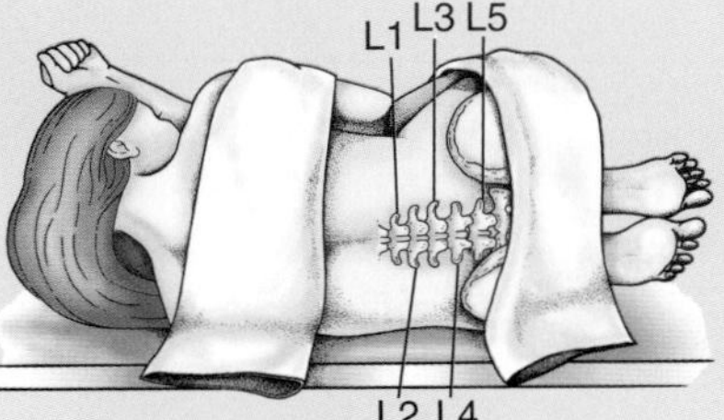 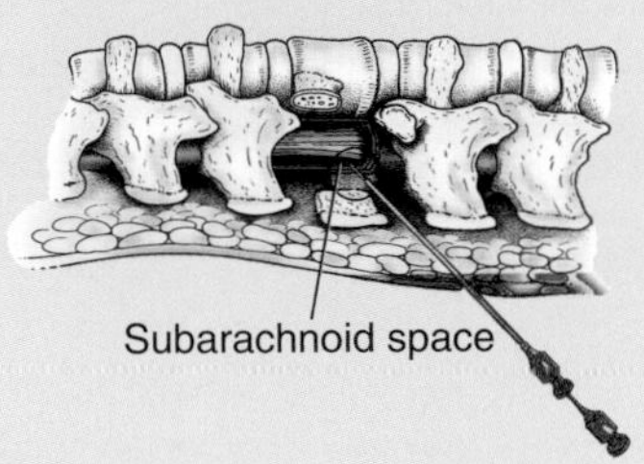 (From Ignatavicius DD, Workman ML: *Medical-surgical nursing: patient-centered collaborative care*, ed 8, Philadelphia, 2016, Elsevier.)	*Risk of spinal headache:* Some physicians still order patients to remain flat and log roll after procedure. Administer NSAIDs or opioids for mild headache and try nonpharmacological relief measures. *Risk of infection:* Observe for excessive drainage at the site.
Paracentesis	Assess bladder for distention and determine last voiding. Weigh patient, assess abdomen, and measure abdominal girth at largest point. Mark location of trocar insertion.	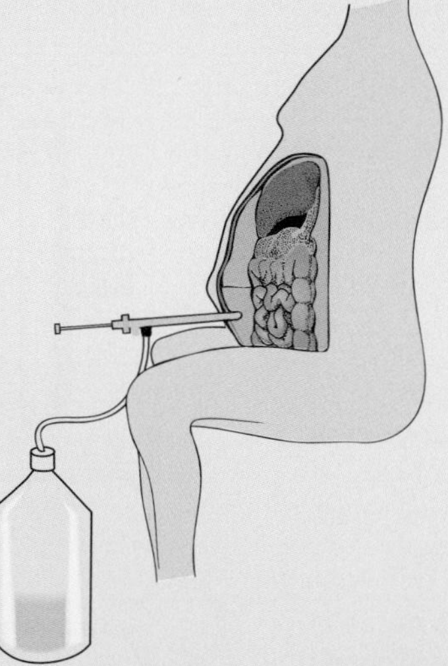 (From Ignatavicius DD, Workman ML: *Medical-surgical nursing: patient-centered collaborative care*, ed 7, Philadelphia, 2012, Saunders.)	After removing fluid, pressure on diaphragm is released, and breathing becomes much easier. *Risk of trauma:* Have patient empty urinary bladder before procedure.

Continued

TABLE 10.3
Summary of Aspiration Procedures—cont'd

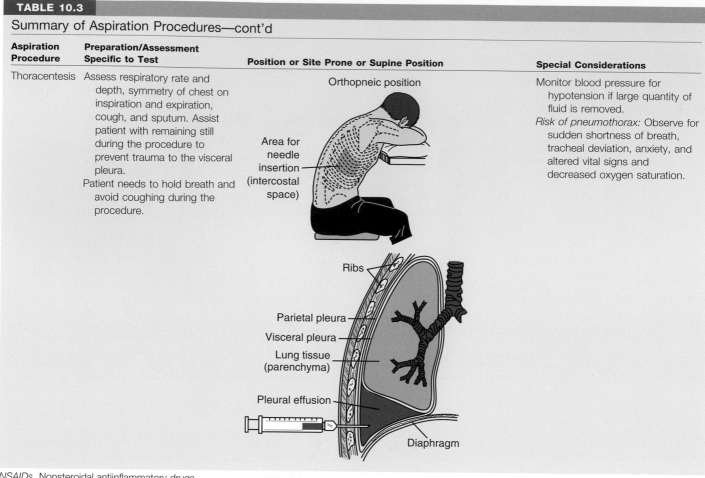

Aspiration Procedure	Preparation/Assessment Specific to Test	Position or Site Prone or Supine Position	Special Considerations
Thoracentesis	Assess respiratory rate and depth, symmetry of chest on inspiration and expiration, cough, and sputum. Assist patient with remaining still during the procedure to prevent trauma to the visceral pleura. Patient needs to hold breath and avoid coughing during the procedure.	Orthopneic position Area for needle insertion (intercostal space) Ribs Parietal pleura Visceral pleura Lung tissue (parenchyma) Pleural effusion Diaphragm	Monitor blood pressure for hypotension if large quantity of fluid is removed. *Risk of pneumothorax:* Observe for sudden shortness of breath, tracheal deviation, anxiety, and altered vital signs and decreased oxygen saturation.

NSAIDs, Nonsteroidal antiinflammatory drugs.

- Which signs and symptoms experienced by the patient would be of immediate concern.

Equipment

- Personal protective equipment: Masks, goggles, gowns, head cover, sterile gloves for all health care personnel performing the procedure
- Test tubes, sterile specimen containers, laboratory requisitions, and labels
- Analgesia (if ordered)
- Antiseptic solution
- 4 × 4–inch sterile gauze pads, tape, Band-Aid
- Sphygmomanometer, pulse oximeter/end-tidal carbon dioxide ($ETCO_2$) monitor
- Aspiration tray: Most agencies provide trays specific to the aspiration procedure. Standard tray includes antiseptic solution (e.g., povidone-iodine; chlorhexidine); gauze sponges (4 × 4–inch); sterile towels; local anesthetic solution (e.g., lidocaine 1%); two 3-mL sterile syringes with 16- to 27-gauge needles.

Additional Equipment for Specific Aspirations

- Bone marrow aspiration: Two bone marrow needles with inner stylet (Fig. 10.2)
- LP: Manometer to measure spinal pressure and at least four test tubes
- Paracentesis: Intravenous (IV) fluids as ordered, vacuum bottles to collect fluid, stopcock with extension tubing, sterile

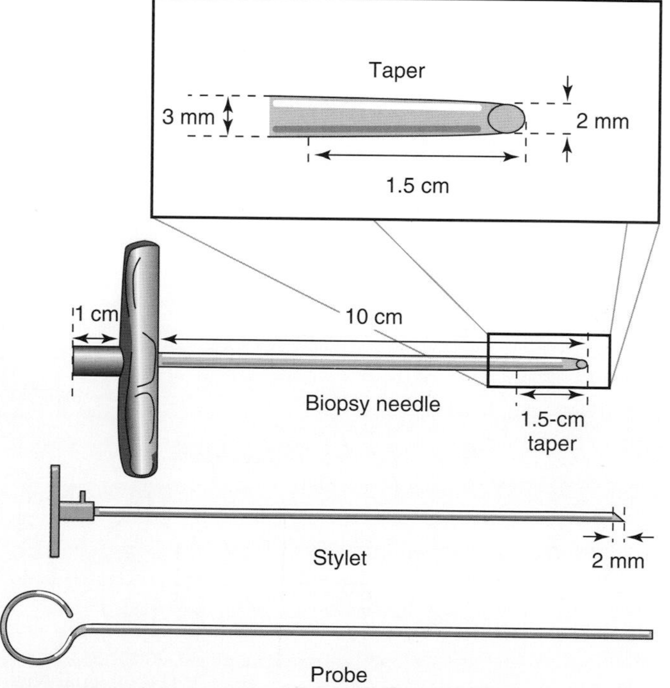

FIG 10.2 Bone marrow biopsy needle showing shape and size. *(From Monahan F, et al: Phipps' medical-surgical nursing: health and illness perspectives, ed 8, St. Louis, 2007, Mosby.)*

collection containers, measuring tape, blunt safety cannula with sharp beveled, hollow needle.
- Thoracentesis: Vacuum bottles to collect fluid, stopcock with extension tubing, blunt safety cannula with sharp beveled, hollow needle.

ASSESSMENT

1. Identify patient using at least two identifiers (e.g., name and birthday or name and medical record number) according to agency policy. Compare identifiers with information in patient's medication administration record (MAR) or medical record. *Rationale: Ensures correct patient. Complies with The Joint Commission standards and improves patient safety (TJC, 2019).*
2. Verify type of procedure scheduled, purpose, and procedure site with patient and medical record. *Rationale: Ensures correct patient and procedure. Complies with The Joint Commission National Patient Safety Goals (TJC, 2019).*
3. Verify that informed consent was obtained before administering any analgesia or antianxiety agents. *Rationale: Federal regulations, many state laws, and accreditation agencies require informed consent for procedures.*
4. Review medical record for contraindications.
   a. Lumbar puncture (LP): Increased intracranial pressure (ICP), spinal deformities, and clotting disorders. *Rationale: Factors can cause hemorrhage, and ICP may cause brainstem herniation.*
   b. Paracentesis: Clotting disorders, intestinal obstructions, and pregnancy. *Rationale: Paracentesis in pregnant woman may injure fetus.*
   c. Bone marrow biopsy: Patient cannot maintain position during procedure.
   d. Thoracentesis: Patient cannot maintain position during procedure.
5. Determine patient's ability to assume position required for procedure and ability to remain still (see Table 10.3). Discuss with health care provider need for premedication for anxious patients. *Rationale: Movement during procedure can cause complications such as bleeding and injury to nerves or tissue. Required position depends on site used for aspiration.*
6. Perform hand hygiene. Before procedure: Obtain vital signs, oxygen saturation (SpO_2)/$ETCO_2$ value, and weight. For paracentesis, obtain abdominal girth measurement. (Use ink pen to mark measurement location for abdominal girth measurement.) For LP, assess lower extremity movement, sensation, and muscle strength. *Rationale: Provides baseline for comparison with vital signs during and after procedure. Patients will have decreased abdominal girth and lose weight after paracentesis.*
7. Assess patient's coagulation status: use of anticoagulants, complete blood count (CBC), platelet count, clotting factors, activated partial thromboplastin time (aPTT)/international normalized ratio (INR), and prothrombin time (PT). *Rationale: Invasive procedures are contraindicated in patients with coagulation disorders because of risk for bleeding (Van Leeuwen and Bladh, 2017).*
8. Determine whether patient is allergic to antiseptic, latex, or anesthetic solutions. If allergy is identified, place allergy band on patient's wrist. *Rationale: Precautions can be taken to decrease chance of allergic reactions.*
9. Assess patient's level of understanding of procedure, including any concerns. *Rationale: Determines extent of instruction and level of support required.*
10. Assess baseline pain level, using scale of 0 to 10. *Rationale: Determines need for preprocedure analgesia. Pain control helps patients maintain proper position and tolerate aspiration procedure.*
11. Assess patient's or family caregiver's knowledge, experience, and health literacy. *Rationale: Ensures patient or family caregiver has the capacity to obtain, communicate, process, and understand basic health information (CDC, 2016).*

STEP	RATIONALE
PLANNING	
1. Expected outcomes following completion of procedure:	
• Patient describes purpose of procedure.	Demonstrates understanding and improves likelihood of cooperation.
• Patient assumes and maintains required position and remains still throughout procedure.	Correct position facilitates safe and timely completion of procedure.
• There is no bleeding at needle insertion site.	Precautions during procedure prevent bleeding.
• Amount of aspirate is sufficient to perform laboratory testing.	
• Patient's level of comfort equals score of 4 or less on pain scale of 0 to 10.	Procedure performed with minimal discomfort to patient.
• Vital signs, SpO_2, and $ETCO_2$ remain within normal limits during and after aspiration procedure.	Removal of abdominal (ascites) or pleural fluid increases lung expansion and improves gas exchange.
• Patient undergoing paracentesis has reduced abdominal girth and improved respirations.	Fluid successfully removed from peritoneal space.
2. Instruct patient to empty bladder.	Reduces risk for bladder trauma during paracentesis. Promotes patient comfort.
3. Explain steps of skin preparation, anesthetic injection, needle insertion, and position required.	Anticipation of expected sensations and procedural activities reduces anxiety.

STEP	RATIONALE
4. If ordered, premedicate for pain 30 minutes before procedure. *Option:* In some cases, patients will receive antianxiety medications.	Pain and anxiety control helps patient to remain in position, minimizes discomfort from needle insertion, and decreases anxiety.
5. Before thoracentesis verify recent chest x-ray film examination.	Provides preprocedure baseline to determine location of pleural fluid.
6. Provide privacy and prepare environment.	Promotes comfort and patient safety.
7. Remove patient's eyeglasses.	Prevents damage to eyeglasses during procedure.

IMPLEMENTATION

STEP	RATIONALE
1. Perform hand hygiene.	Reduces transmission of microorganisms.
2. Set up sterile tray or open supplies to make accessible for health care provider (see Chapter 5).	Maintains integrity of sterile field and promotes prompt completion of procedure.
3. Take "time-out" to verify patient's name, type of procedure scheduled, and procedure site with patient and health care team.	"Time-out" verification just before starting procedure includes physician and all personnel and is a safety precaution to prevent wrong patient, wrong site, and wrong procedure errors. Complies with The Joint Commission National Patient Safety Goals (TJC, 2019).
4. Help patient maintain correct position. Reassure patient while explaining procedure.	Decreases chance of complications occurring during procedure. Explanations increase patient comfort and relaxation.
a. **Bone marrow** • *Adults:* For sternal biopsy, place in supine position. For iliac crest biopsy, place in prone or lateral recumbent position. • *Children:* For iliac crest biopsy place in prone or lateral recumbent position.	Provides best access to bone containing marrow.
b. **LP** Position in lateral recumbent (fetal) position with head and neck flexed (see Table 10.3).	Provides full curvature and flexion of spinal column to allow maximal space between vertebrae.
c. **Paracentesis** Position in bed in semi-Fowler's position or sitting upright on side of bed or in chair with feet supported (see Table 10.3).	Position uses gravity to cause fluid to accumulate in lower abdominal cavity, where it is drained more easily.
d. **Thoracentesis** Place in orthopneic position (upright position with arms and shoulders raised and supported on padded over-bed table) (see Table 10.3). If patient is unable to tolerate, help to side-lying position with affected lung positioned upward.	Expands intercostal space for needle insertions.

Safe Patient Care *Emphasize the importance of remaining immobile during procedure to prevent trauma, especially with the LP. Sudden movement is a risk for spinal cord nerve root damage. Sudden movement during paracentesis or thoracentesis risks damage of the abdominal or pulmonary structures. Also instruct patient not to cough, sneeze, or breathe deeply during the procedures because these actions increase the risk for needle displacement and damage of other structures.*

STEP	RATIONALE
5. Explain to patient that pain may occur when lidocaine (local anesthetic) is injected into tissues. Pressure may also occur when tissue or fluid is aspirated.	Aspiration is painful but lasts for only a few moments. If patient is having bone marrow aspirate, deep pressure feeling is frequently experienced as bone marrow is withdrawn (Van Leeuwen and Bladh, 2017).
6. Physician applies sterile gloves, mask, gown, and goggles; cleans patient's skin with antiseptic solution; and drapes site with sterile drape.	Removes surface bacteria from skin at area of puncture site. Creates sterile field.
7. Physician injects local anesthetic and allows time for anesthesia to occur.	Provides optimal effect of local anesthesia.
8. Physician inserts blunt safety cannula with sharp beveled, hollow needle into spinal space or body cavity involved (see Table 10.3). To aspirate tissue or body fluids for specimen analysis, syringe is attached to needle and aspirate is placed into specimen container.	Success depends on positioning, accurate insertion site, and patient remaining still.

STEP	RATIONALE
9. Nurse assesses patient's condition during procedure, including respiratory status, vital signs if indicated, and any complaints of pain.	Identifies any changes that indicate complication.

Safe Patient Care *Increased or worsening abdominal or thoracic pain is significant in paracentesis and thoracentesis. Severe abdominal pain indicates a possible bowel perforation following a paracentesis. Following a thoracentesis, abdominal pain results from diaphragmatic, liver, or spleen perforation. Inspiratory chest pain results from perforation of the lung.*

STEP	RATIONALE
10. Note characteristics of aspirate:	
a. *Bone marrow aspirate:* Marrow may appear red or yellow.	Normal marrow.
b. *LP:* Record opening pressure; observe fluid for color, cloudiness, or blood.	Normal CSF is clear and colorless. Cloudiness is result of protein, which indicates an infection.
c. *Paracentesis:* Fluid may appear yellow, cloudy, bile-stained green, or blood tinged. Peritoneal lavage fluid may appear bright red.	Blood-tinged fluid is caused by traumatic tap. In patient with abdominal trauma bloody lavage identifies active bleeding.
d. *Thoracentesis:* Pleural fluid may appear clear yellow, puslike, or cloudy.	Clear yellow is normal. Transudate and exudates are typically yellow, straw colored. Blood-tinged fluid indicates malignancy, pulmonary infarction, or severe inflammation. Puslike fluid indicates infection (empyema); milky fluid indicates chylothorax (i.e., leak from thoracic duct resulting in lymphatic drainage in pleural cavity).
11. Properly label specimens in presence of patient and transport to laboratory in proper containers. Label specimens in order of collection.	Ensures that correct laboratory results are assigned to right patient. Test tubes are numbered in sequence of collection (e.g., 1 through 4).
12. Physician removes needle and applies pressure over insertion site until drainage ceases. If necessary, help with direct pressure and application of gauze dressing.	Helps in homeostasis and secures insertion site.
13. All health care team members in procedure remove protective equipment, discard in appropriate receptacle, and perform hand hygiene.	Reduces transmission of infection.
14. Help patient to comfortable position.	Gives patient sense of well-being.
15. Be sure nurse call system is in an accessible location within patient's reach.	Ensures patient can call for assistance if needed.
16. Raise side rails (as appropriate) and lower bed to lowest position.	Ensures patient safety.
17. Perform hand hygiene.	Reduces transmission of microorganisms.

EVALUATION

STEP	RATIONALE
1. Monitor level of consciousness, vital signs, and $SpO_2/ETCO_2$. Check agency policy; sometimes vital signs are obtained every 15 minutes for 2 hours.	Verifies patient's physiological status in response to procedure or any potential complications.
2. Inspect dressing over puncture site for bleeding, swelling, tenderness, and erythema. Inspect area under patient for bleeding. Avoid disrupting healing clot at site if pressure dressing is present.	Determines further blood loss from puncture site. Infection is potential complication, especially if patient is leukopenic (Van Leeuwen and Bladh, 2017).
3. Evaluate pain score to determine if patient's level of comfort is equivalent to a score of 4 or less on pain scale of 0 to 10.	Determines if patient is having increased pain to warrant postprocedure analgesia.
4. Following paracentesis, measure abdominal girth and respirations and compare to preprocedure measurements.	Determines amount of change in abdominal size and ability to ventilate.
5. **Use Teach-Back:** "I want to be sure that I explained what to expect regarding how you may feel after this procedure. Tell me what you know about what to expect." Revise your instruction now or develop a plan for revised patient/family caregiver teaching if patient/family caregiver is not able to teach back correctly.	Demonstrates patient's/family caregiver's level of understanding of instructional topic.

Unexpected Outcomes	Related Interventions
1. Site complications occur:	
a. *Bone marrow:* Tenderness or erythema at site.	• Notify health care provider and obtain further orders. • Administer analgesic as ordered. • Continue to monitor site.
b. *LP:*	
(1) Postprocedure headache (PPH) is evidenced by headache, blurred vision, and tinnitus.	• Monitor fluid loss. • Physician may inject blood patch into epidural space. • Medicate for pain as ordered.
(2) Excess loss of CSF is indicated by decreased level of consciousness, hearing loss, dilated pupils, and decreased ICP.	• Maintain airway. • Transfer to intensive care unit (ICU) per physician order.
c. *Paracentesis:* Leakage of fluid from site and acute abdominal pain occur.	• Reinforce dressing; may also be instructed to place sterile collection bag over site. • Monitor vital signs and SpO_2. • Assess abdomen for bowel sounds.
d. *Thoracentesis:* Pneumothorax is evidenced by sudden dyspnea, tachypnea, and asymmetrical chest excursion.	• Administer oxygen. • Monitor vital signs and SpO_2. • Anticipate chest x-ray film examination and possible chest tube insertion.

Recording

- Record in medical record name of procedure; preprocedure preparation; location of puncture site; amount, consistency, and color of fluid drained or specimen obtained; duration of procedure; patient's tolerance of procedure (e.g., vital signs, SaO_2) and comfort level; laboratory tests ordered; specimen sent; type of dressing; postprocedure activities (e.g., chest x-ray film); and other procedure-specific assessments (e.g., extremity assessment, abdominal girth, level of consciousness [LOC]).
- Document your evaluation of patient learning.

Hand-Off Reporting

- Immediately report to health care provider any unexpected drainage or significant changes in vital signs or SaO_2/$ETCO_2$ status. (For significant changes in vital signs or decrease in SaO_2, call rapid response team if available.)

✦ SKILL 10.4 Care of Patients Undergoing Bronchoscopy

Purpose

Bronchoscopy is the examination of the tracheobronchial tree through a lighted tube containing mirrors (Fig. 10.3). The tube most commonly used is a flexible fiberoptic bronchoscope that allows both visualization and simultaneous administration of oxygen. The fiberoptic bronchoscope has lumens for visualization and for obtaining sputum, foreign bodies, and biopsy specimens.

Bronchoscopy is an emergency or elective procedure performed for diagnostic and therapeutic reasons. The main purposes of this procedure are to aspirate excessive sputum or mucus plugs that airway suctioning cannot remove; to visualize the tracheobronchial tree for assessment of abnormalities of the mucosa, abscesses, aspiration pneumonia, strictures, and tumors; to obtain deep-tissue biopsy and sputum specimens; and to remove foreign bodies.

Delegation and Collaboration

The skill of helping with a bronchoscopy cannot be delegated to nursing assistive personnel (NAP). The nurse directs the NAP to:

- Measure follow-up postprocedure vital signs (after registered nurse's initial assessment).
- Help position the patient appropriately after procedure (based on procedure and patient limitations).
- Immediately report to the nurse if patient has possible respiratory distress or is coughing up blood after the procedure.

Equipment

- Personal protective equipment (PPE): Mask, gown, sterile gloves, head cover, and goggles for all health care providers performing procedure
- Bronchoscopy tray, if available from central supply, which includes flexible fiberoptic bronchoscope; 4 × 4–inch gauze sponges; local anesthetic spray (lidocaine); sterile tracheal suction catheters; diazepam, midazolam, or other sedative for intravenous (IV) sedation
- Oxygen, resuscitative equipment
- Pulse oximeter/end-tidal carbon dioxide ($ETCO_2$) monitor, cardiac monitor
- Sterile gloves

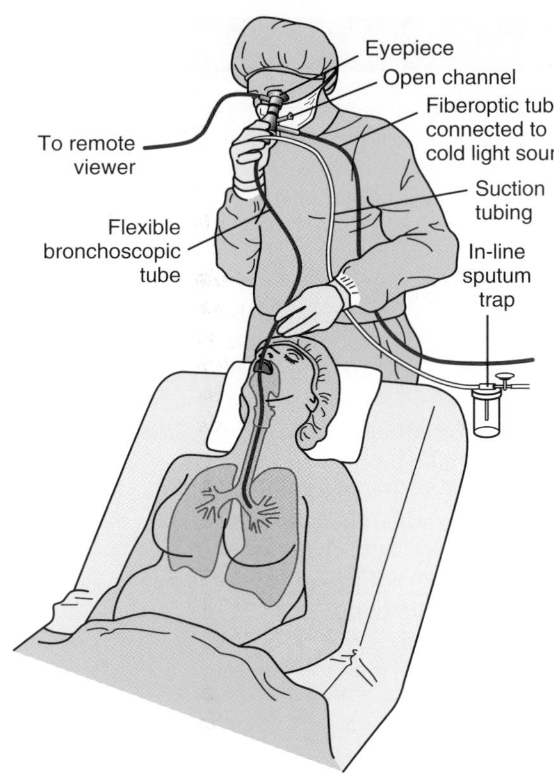

FIG 10.3 Flexible fiberoptic bronchoscopy.

- Sterile water-soluble lubricating jelly (**NOTE:** Petroleum-based lubricants are not used because of the hazard of aspiration and subsequent pneumonia.)
- Emesis basin
- Suction machine and connecting tube
- Blood pressure equipment

ASSESSMENT

1. Identify patient using at least two identifiers (e.g., name and birthday or name and medical record number) according to agency policy. Compare identifiers with information in patient's medication administration record (MAR) or medical record. *Rationale: Ensures correct patient. Complies with The Joint Commission standards and improves patient safety (TJC, 2019).*
2. Verify type of procedure scheduled and procedure site with patient. *Rationale: Ensures procedure and correct patient. Complies with The Joint Commission National Patient Safety Goals (TJC, 2019).*
3. Verify that informed consent was obtained before administration of any sedatives. *Rationale: Federal regulations, many state laws, and accreditation agencies such as The Joint Commission require informed consent for procedure.*
4. Review medical record to determine purpose of procedure: for sputum aspiration, assessment, tissue biopsy, or removal of foreign body. *Rationale: Anticipates equipment needs of physician and type of information to convey to patient during teaching.*
5. Assess patient's history for inability to tolerate interruption of high-flow oxygen unless intubated. *Rationale: Determines need for oxygen administration during procedure.*
6. Perform hand hygiene. Obtain baseline vital signs, pulse oximetry (SpO_2) and $ETCO_2$ values. *Rationale: Baseline data provide for comparison with findings during and after procedure.*
7. Assess type of cough, sputum produced, heart and lung sounds. *Rationale: Provides for comparison with respiratory status during and after procedure.*
8. Determine whether patient is allergic to local anesthetic used for spraying throat (usually lidocaine). *Rationale: Allergy causes laryngeal edema or laryngospasm.*
9. Assess if preprocedure medication (usually atropine and opioid or sedative) has been ordered. *Rationale: Atropine decreases secretions and inhibits vagus nerve stimulation leading to bradycardia; opioids or sedatives relieve anxiety and decrease discomfort.*
10. Assess time patient last ingested food/fluids or medications. Patient must be NPO for at least 2 to 6 hours before a bronchoscopy; however, some medications may be taken before procedure by physician order. *Rationale: Reduces risk for aspiration.*
11. Assess patient's or family caregiver's knowledge, experience, and health literacy. *Rationale: Ensures patient or family caregiver has the capacity to obtain, communicate, process, and understand basic health information (CDC, 2016).*
12. Assess patient's level of understanding of procedure, including any concerns. *Rationale: Determines extent of instruction and level of support required.*

STEP	RATIONALE
PLANNING	
1. Expected outcomes following completion of procedure:	
• Patient recovers from sedation without respiratory complications or change in level of consciousness.	Sedation adequate, and patient tolerates procedure.
• Patient's level of comfort is equivalent to score of 4 or less on pain scale of 0 to 10.	Minimal trauma caused by bronchoscope.
• Physician can observe, suction, and obtain specimens from tracheobronchial tree.	Indicates that purpose of procedure was achieved.
• Patient explains procedure and assumes appropriate position.	Demonstrates patient's understanding.
2. Administer atropine, opioid, or antianxiety agent 30 minutes before procedure.	Ensures that medication takes effect before procedure.

STEP	RATIONALE
3. Explain procedure to patient.	Reduces anxiety and increases cooperation.
4. Remove and safely store patient's dentures and/or eyeglasses.	Minimizes chance of airway obstruction and damage to eyeglasses or dental structures during procedure.
5. Provide privacy and prepare environment.	Promotes patient comfort and safety.

IMPLEMENTATION

STEP	RATIONALE
1. Perform hand hygiene. Assess current IV access or establish new IV access with large-bore cannula (see Chapter 28).	Provides immediate access for IV fluids or medications if emergency occurs.
2. Help patient assume position desired by physician (usually semi-Fowler's).	Provides maximal visualization of lower airway and adequate lung expansion.
3. Take "time-out" to verify patient's name, type of procedure scheduled, and procedure site with patient and health care team.	"Time-out" verification just before starting procedure includes physician and all personnel and is a safety precaution to prevent wrong patient, wrong site, and wrong procedure errors. Complies with The Joint Commission National Patient Safety Goals (TJC, 2019).
4. Perform hand hygiene and apply protective equipment. Position tip of suction catheter for easy access to patient's mouth.	Reduces transmission of microorganisms. Removes secretions to reduce risk for aspiration.
5. Physician usually sprays nasopharynx and oropharynx with topical anesthetic. Lidocaine is commonly used 10 to 15 minutes before procedure. When a patient is intubated or has tracheostomy, anesthetic spray is usually not needed.	Provides swift anesthesia of oropharynx.
6. Instruct patient not to swallow local anesthetic; provide emesis basin for expectorating it.	Reduces unintended anesthesia of esophagus.
7. Another physician or staff member attaches bronchoscope to machine light source.	Enhances visualization during procedure.
8. Physician applies goggles, mask, and sterile gloves; introduces bronchoscope into mouth to pharynx; passes through glottis and into trachea and bronchi (see Fig. 10.3). More anesthetic spray may be used at glottis to prevent cough reflex. For intubated patient's flexible bronchoscope is introduced through their endotracheal tube.	Bronchoscope must be passed through upper airway structures to promote visualization of lower airways. Trachea and bronchi are observed for lesions and obstructions. Adaptor accompanies bronchoscope and is used for bag-valve mask or ventilator use.
9. Physician suctions mucus and performs bronchial washing with cytological specimens taken with wire brush or curette. Biopsy specimens may also be obtained.	Cytological specimens are obtained to diagnose carcinoma.
10. Help patient through procedure by providing explanations, verbal reassurance, and support.	Although premedicated and drowsy, remind patient not to change position and to cooperate. Reinforce that patient will be able to breathe during procedure.
11. Assess patient's pulse, blood pressure, respirations, SpO_2, $ETCO_2$, and breathing capacity during procedure; observe degree of restlessness, capillary refill, and color of nail beds.	Bronchoscope can cause feelings of suffocation and vasovagal response and laryngospasm. Because airway is partially occluded, patient can develop hypoxia during procedure.
12. Note characteristics of suctioned material. Expect small amount of blood mixed with aspirate because of tissue trauma.	Information used to record and report and make further patient observations.
13. Using gloved hand, wipe patient's mouth and nose to remove lubricant after bronchoscope is removed.	Promotes hygiene and comfort.
14. Instruct patient not to eat or drink until tracheobronchial anesthesia has worn off and gag reflex has returned, usually in 2 hours. Use tongue depressor to touch pharynx to test for presence of gag reflex.	Prevents aspiration.
15. Help patient to comfortable position.	Gives patient sense of well-being.
16. Be sure nurse call system is in an accessible location within patient's reach.	Ensures patient can call for assistance if needed.
17. Raise side rails (as appropriate) and lower bed to lowest position.	Ensures patient safety.
18. Remove protective equipment, discard, and perform hand hygiene.	Reduces transmission of microorganisms.

STEP	RATIONALE
EVALUATION	
1. Monitor vital signs, SpO_2, and $ETCO_2$.	Verifies physiological response to procedure.
2. Observe character and amount of sputum. Physician may order serial sputum collection for 24 hours for cytological examination.	Evaluates for complication of bronchial perforation, indicated by severe hemoptysis. Slight blood-tinged sputum is normal after this procedure.
3. Observe respiratory status closely; palpate for facial or neck crepitus.	Detects early sign of bronchial or esophageal perforation.
4. Assess for return of gag reflex. It usually returns in approximately 2 hours.	Helps prevent aspiration pneumonia, which is a risk until gag reflex returns.
5. **Use Teach-Back:** "I want to be sure I explained what are considered postprocedure normal and abnormal symptoms. Tell me what you know about these symptoms." Revise your instruction now or develop a plan for revised patient/family caregiver teaching if patient/family caregiver is not able to teach back correctly.	Demonstrates patient's/family caregiver's level of understanding of instructional topic.

Unexpected Outcomes	Related Interventions
1. Vasovagal response caused by stimulation of baroreceptors during bronchoscope insertion, causing symptoms of: • Feeling nauseous, faint, dizzy, and/or light-headed. • Diaphoresis with slow, steady pulse. • Unconsciousness for few seconds.	• Lower head of table. • Continue vital signs monitoring. • Support airway (positioning/suctioning).
2. Laryngospasm and bronchospasm as evidenced by: • Sudden, severe shortness of breath.	• Call physician immediately. • Support airway with head of table elevated (positioning). • Prepare emergency resuscitation equipment. • Anticipate possible cricothyrotomy.
3. Hypoxemia as evidenced by: • Gradual shortness of breath. • Decreasing level of consciousness.	• Monitor SpO_2. • Maintain airway and breathing. • Notify physician immediately.
4. Hemorrhage as evidenced by: • Acute blood loss • Hypotension and tachycardia • Decreasing level of consciousness	• Notify physician immediately. • Monitor vital signs. • Be prepared to administer IV fluids.

Recording

- Record name of procedure (include biopsy if performed), duration of procedure, patient's tolerance of procedure and any complications, and collection and disposition of specimen. Document return of gag reflex.
- Document your evaluation of patient learning.

Hand-Off Reporting

- Report excessive bleeding, hemoptysis, or respiratory difficulty after procedure or changes in vital signs beyond patient's normal limits to physician immediately. Report results of procedure to appropriate health care personnel.

✦ SKILL 10.5 Care of Patients Undergoing Gastrointestinal Endoscopy

Purpose

Endoscopy allows direct visualization of an internal organ or structure by means of a long, flexible fiberoptic scope. The tip of the scope has a light source and camera lens that allows visualization of the lining of the gastrointestinal (GI) structures on a large display screen (Fig. 10.4, A–C). For visualization of the upper GI tract, esophagoscopy, gastroscopy, gastroduodenojejunoscopy (GDJ), or duodenoscopy is performed or, more frequently, esophagogastroduodenoscopy (EGD), which permits visualization of the esophagus, stomach (Fig. 10.5), and duodenum in one examination. Besides direct observation, endoscopy enables biopsy of suspicious tissue, polyp removal, and performance of many other procedures such as direct visual guidance for fine-needle aspiration biopsies and dilation and stenting of strictures. For visualization of the hepatobiliary tree and pancreatic ducts, an endoscopic retrograde cholangiopancreatography (ERCP) is performed. For visual examination of the lower GI tract, proctoscopy, sigmoidoscopy, or colonoscopy is performed. Typically, these patients receive intravenous (IV) moderate sedation.

Risks of endoscopic procedures include intestinal perforation, hemorrhage, peritonitis, aspiration, respiratory depression, and/or myocardial infarction secondary to vasovagal response. Both upper

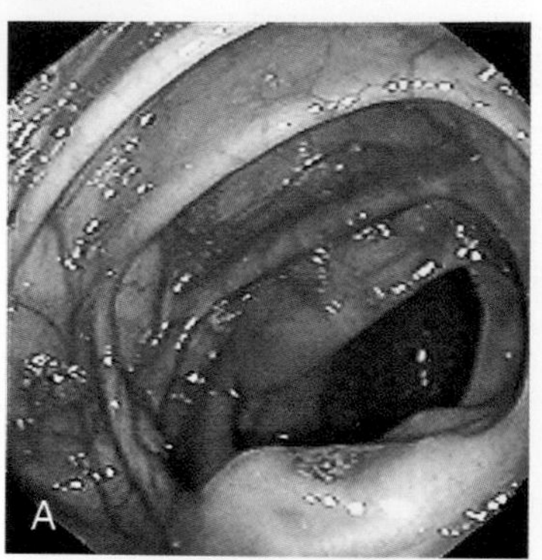

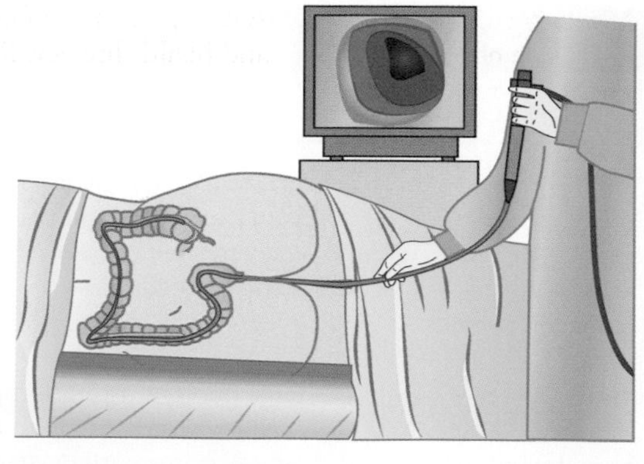

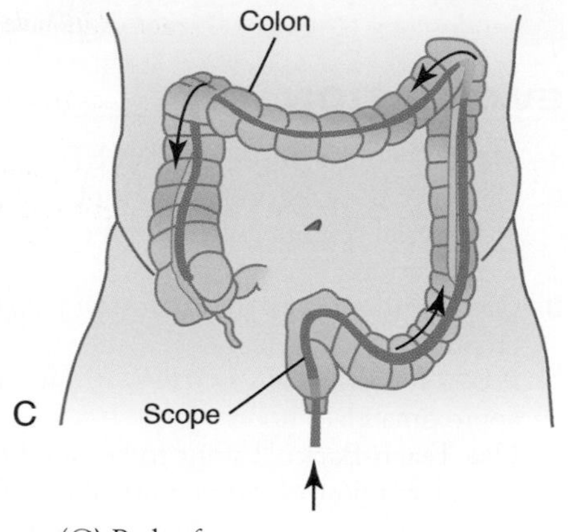

FIG 10.4 (A) Score view of healthy colon. (B) Overview of colonoscopy process. (C) Path of scope through colon.

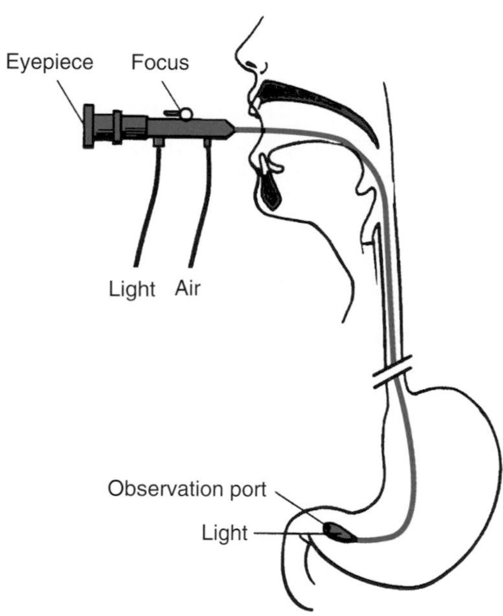

FIG 10.5 Flexible endoscope to visualize stomach.

and lower GI endoscopic examinations may be performed in a specially equipped endoscopic unit or at the patient's bedside.

Delegation and Collaboration

The skill of helping with endoscopy cannot be delegated to nursing assistive personnel (NAP). The nurse directs the NAP about:

- How to help with patient positioning.

Equipment

- Personal protective equipment: Mask, gown, gloves, head cover, goggles for all health care personnel
- Endoscopy tray
- Fiberoptic endoscope and camera
- Solutions for biopsy specimens
- Local anesthetic spray
- Tracheal suction equipment (see Chapter 16)
- Blood pressure equipment
- Sterile water-soluble jelly
- Sterile gloves for physician
- Emesis basin
- IV fluid and equipment for IV start *(optional)*
- Diazepam, midazolam, or other sedative for IV sedation *(optional)*
- Sedative reversal agents
- Carbon dioxide source to inflate colon (for lower GI procedures)
- Oxygen, resuscitative equipment, SpO_2/end-tidal carbon dioxide (CO_2) monitor

ASSESSMENT

1. Identify patient using at least two identifiers (e.g., name and birthday or name and medical record number) according to agency policy. Compare identifiers with information in patient's medication administration record (MAR) or medical record. *Rationale: Ensures correct patient. Complies with The Joint Commission standards and improves patient safety (TJC, 2019).*
2. Verify type of procedure scheduled and procedure site with patient. *Rationale: Ensures correct procedure and patient. Complies with The Joint Commission National Patient Safety Goals (TJC, 2019).*
3. Verify that informed consent was obtained before administering sedation. *Rationale: Federal regulations, many state laws, and accreditation agencies such as The Joint Commission require informed consent for procedure.*
4. Determine purpose of procedure: biopsy, examination, or coagulation of bleeding sites. *Rationale: Anticipates appropriate equipment needs.*
5. Perform hand hygiene. Determine if GI bleeding is present. Observe character of emesis, stool, and nasogastric (NG) tube drainage for frank blood or material that looks like coffee grounds. *Rationale: Test is contraindicated in patients with severe upper GI bleeding because viewing lens becomes covered with blood clots, preventing visualization (Van Leeuwen and Bladh, 2017).*
6. Obtain vital signs and SpO_2/$ETCO_2$ values. *Rationale: Baseline data provide for comparison with findings during and after procedure.*

Safe Patient Care *If patient is bleeding actively, physician may order lavage of the stomach and aspiration to clear clots before procedure is attempted.*

7. Verify that patient was NPO for at least 8 hours for endoscopy of upper GI tract. *Rationale: Introduction of endoscope increases risk for vomiting resulting from stimulation of gag reflex. Empty stomach reduces risk for aspiration of stomach contents.*
8. For lower GI studies (proctoscopy, sigmoidoscopy, or colonoscopy), verify that patient followed clear liquid diet for 2 days and has completed any ordered bowel-cleansing regimen. *Rationale: An empty intestinal tract promotes endoscopic insertion and clear visualization of interior walls.*
9. Assess patient's or family caregiver's knowledge, experience, and health literacy. *Rationale: Ensures patient or family caregiver has the capacity to obtain, communicate, process, and understand basic health information (CDC, 2016).*
10. Assess patient's level of understanding and previous experience with procedure, including any concerns. *Rationale: Determines extent of instruction and level of support required.*

STEP	RATIONALE
PLANNING	
1. Expected outcomes following completion of procedure:	
• Patient does not aspirate and has no postprocedure bleeding.	Indicates absence of complications and tolerance of procedure.
• Patient's level of comfort is equivalent to score of 4 or less on pain scale of 0 to 10.	Provides reliable detection of increasing pain so that postprocedure analgesia is given.
• Patient is without respiratory complications or change in level of consciousness.	Recovers from sedation.
• Patient describes purposes and steps of procedure.	Documents patient understanding.
2. Explain steps of procedure, including sensations to expect.	Relieves anxiety and answers patient's questions.
3. Administer pain medication or preprocedure medication 30 minutes before procedure.	Promotes relaxation and reduces anxiety.
4. Provide privacy and prepare environment.	Promotes patient comfort and safety.
5. Remove patient's eyeglasses, dentures, or other dental appliances.	Prevents damage to eyeglasses or damage to or dislodgement of dental structures during procedure.
IMPLEMENTATION	
1. Perform hand hygiene.	Reduces transmission of microorganisms.
2. Apply protective equipment.	Reduces transmission of microorganisms.
3. Take "time-out" to verify patient's name, type of procedure scheduled, and procedure site with patient and health care team.	"Time-out" verification just before starting procedure includes physician and all personnel and is a safety precaution to prevent wrong patient, wrong site, and wrong procedure errors. Complies with The Joint Commission National Patient Safety Goals (TJC, 2019).
4. Ensure that IV line is patent and administer IV sedation as ordered (see Chapter 28).	Provides route for emergency medications and creates immediate conscious sedation.
5. Help patient assume proper position for procedure and apply appropriate drape.	Improves efficiency of procedure and ability of physician to visualize site. Drape provides comfort and minimizes exposure.
a. *Upper GI procedures:* Help patient maintain left lateral Sims' position.	Sims' position allows easy passage of upper or lower endoscope. Provides airway clearance if patient gags and vomits gastric contents.
b. *Lower GI procedures:* Help patient maintain left lateral decubitus position. Drape patient for privacy.	Left lateral decubitus position provides access to lower GI tract.
6. Physician performs hand hygiene and puts on protective equipment.	Reduces transmission of microorganisms.
7. **Upper GI procedures:**	
a. Help physician spray nasopharynx and oropharynx with local anesthetic.	Topical anesthetic decreases gag reflex caused by passage of endoscope, thus improving safety and comfort.
b. Administer atropine if ordered.	Reduces quantity of secretions, therefore reducing risk for aspiration.
c. Position tip of suction cannula for easy access in patient's mouth.	Drains oral secretions to reduce risk for aspiration.
8. **Lower GI procedures:**	
a. Prepare lubricant for fiberoptic endoscope.	Facilitates passage of tubing.

STEP	RATIONALE
9. Physician slowly passes endoscope into mouth or through anus to view esophagus, stomach, colon, or rectum and advances to desired depth while visualizing lining of structures.	Provides visualization of all structures to detect polyps, cancerous lesions, or areas of inflammation and stricture.
10. Physician insufflates air through endoscope into upper GI tract or carbon dioxide into lower GI tract in case of colonoscopy.	Distends GI structures for better visualization. Carbon dioxide insufflation produces less postprocedure abdominal cramping than air insufflation because it is more readily absorbed.
11. Help patient throughout procedure.	
a. Anticipate needs and promote comfort.	Patient is unable to speak after tube is passed into throat.
b. Tell patient what is happening as each part of procedure is carried out (e.g., abdominal cramping).	Reassures patient about procedure and how long it will last.
c. For upper GI procedures, suction if there are excessive oral secretions or vomitus.	Prevents aspiration of oral secretions or gastric contents.
12. Place tissue specimens in proper laboratory containers or on proper slides. Seal as needed. Date, time, and initial all specimen containers before sending to laboratory.	Ensures proper specimen preservation and labeling and preparation of specimens for microscopic examination.
13. Help patient to comfortable position.	Gives patient sense of well-being.
14. Be sure nurse call system is in an accessible location within patient's reach.	Ensures patient can call for assistance if needed.
15. Raise side rails (as appropriate) and lower bed to lowest position.	Ensures patient safety.
16. Help to dispose of equipment, remove gloves and perform hand hygiene.	Reduces transmission of infection.
17. In recovery, after sedation resolves, inform patient not to eat or drink until gag reflex returns.	Reduces risk for aspiration.

EVALUATION

1. Monitor vital signs and oxygen saturation according to agency policy, which can be every 15 minutes for 2 hours.	Change in vital signs may indicate new bleeding in GI tract or oversedation.
2. Assess for levels of sedation and consciousness.	Determines patient's response to IV sedation.
3. Ask patient to describe level of comfort using pain scale of 0 to 10. Observe for pain.	Monitors for sudden abdominal pain, which can indicate rupture of abdominal organs.
4. Evaluate emesis or aspirate for frank or occult blood.	Monitors for GI bleeding.
5. Assess for return of gag reflex, usually in 2 to 4 hours. Provide oral hygiene when gag reflex returns.	Determines when effects of anesthetic have disappeared. Gag reflex prevents aspiration.
6. **Use Teach-Back:** "I want to be sure I explained your postprocedure diet and activity limitations. Tell me what you can eat and how to limit your activity once you go home." Revise your instruction now or develop a plan for revised patient/family caregiver teaching if patient/family caregiver is not able to teach back correctly.	Determines patient's/family caregiver's level of understanding of instructional topic.

Unexpected Outcomes	Related Interventions
1. Vasovagal response caused by stimulation of baroreceptors during endoscope insertion as evidenced by: • Feeling nauseous, faint, dizzy, and/or light-headed. • Diaphoresis with slow, steady pulse. • Few seconds of unconsciousness.	• Lower head of table. • Support airway.
2. For upper GI procedures: Laryngospasm and bronchospasm as evidenced by: • Sudden, severe shortness of breath.	• Call physician immediately. • Support airway with head of table elevated (positioning). • Prepare emergency resuscitation equipment. • Anticipate possible reintubation.
3. Pulmonary aspiration as evidenced by: • Dyspnea, tachypnea, decreasing levels of oxygen saturation.	• Support airway. • Follow specific postprocedural orders related to findings. • Monitor oxygen saturation.

Reporting

- Record the procedure, duration, patient's tolerance, complications and interventions, and collection and disposition of specimen.
- Document your evaluation of patient learning.

Hand-Off Reporting

- Report onset of difficulty to arouse, bleeding, abdominal pain, dyspnea, and vital sign changes to health care provider.

✦ SKILL 10.6 Obtaining a 12-Lead Electrocardiogram

Purpose

Electrical impulses of the heart are conducted to the body's surface and are detected by electrodes placed on the skin of the limbs and torso. The electrodes carry these impulses to either a continuous monitor or a 12-lead electrocardiogram (ECG) machine. The appearance of the ECG pattern helps diagnose whether there are any abnormalities in the electrical conduction through the heart (Fig. 10.6). The 12-lead ECG provides a snapshot of the waveforms from 12 different angles or views of the heart. One electrode is placed on each of the four extremities, and six electrodes are placed at specific sites on the chest for a total of 10 electrodes on the patient's skin. They are bipolar limb leads I, II, III; augmented limb leads aV_R, aV_L, aV_F; and precordial chest leads V_1 to V_6. The leads view a specific portion of the heart's surface and can help determine which part of the heart has sustained damage, origin, and flow of the impulse.

Delegation and Collaboration

The skill of obtaining a 12-lead ECG can be delegated to nursing assistive personnel (NAP) who are specifically trained in obtaining the measurement. The nurse directs the NAP to:

- Immediately report to the nurse changes in the patient's cardiac status such as complaints of chest pain.

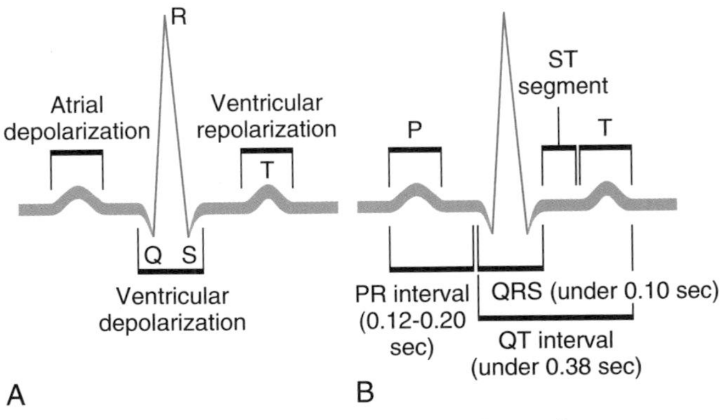

FIG 10.6 (A and B) Normal ECG waveform.

- Immediately deliver the completed 12-lead ECG recording to a health care provider for interpretation.
- Use specific patient precautions related to disease, mobility status, or position restrictions.

Equipment

- 12-lead ECG machine
- 10 ECG leads with alligator clip, suction cup or snap-on attachments
- 10 ECG electrodes (disposable, self-adhesive) or electrode paste
- Clean, dry towel or sponge wipes
- Hair clippers (optional depending on hair at electrode sites)

ASSESSMENT

1. Identify patient using at least two identifiers (e.g., name and birthday or name and medical record number) according to agency policy. *Rationale: Ensures correct patient. Complies with The Joint Commission standards and improves patient safety (TJC, 2019).*
2. Determine indications for obtaining ECG. Assess patient's history and cardiopulmonary status (e.g., heart rate and rhythm, blood pressure, respirations). *Rationale: If 12-lead ECG is ordered for chest pain or other ischemic signs and symptoms, obtain ECG within 10 minutes of patient's pain report.*
3. Assess for chest pain; rate on scale of 0 to 10. *Rationale: Determines level of chest discomfort, which may be a warning for cardiac ischemia.*
4. Assess patient's or family caregiver's knowledge, experience, and health literacy. *Rationale: Ensures patient or family caregiver has the capacity to obtain, communicate, process, and understand basic health information (CDC, 2016).*
5. Assess patient's level of understanding of procedure, including any concerns. *Rationale: Determines extent of instruction and level of support required.*
6. Assess patient's ability to follow directions and remain still in supine position. *Rationale: Provides clear, accurate recording without artifacts.*

STEP	RATIONALE
PLANNING	
1. Expected outcomes following completion of procedure:	
• Patient tolerates procedure without anxiety or discomfort.	Appropriate preparation and education decrease anxiety.
• Clear, accurate recording of ECG waveform is obtained.	Patient relaxes and leads are attached correctly.
2. Provide privacy and prepare environment.	Promotes patient comfort and safety.

STEP	RATIONALE
IMPLEMENTATION	
1. Perform hand hygiene.	Reduces transmission of microorganisms.
2. Prepare patient.	
a. Remove or reposition patient's clothing to expose only patient's chest and arms. Keep abdomen and thighs covered.	Facilitates correct placement of cardiac leads and maintains patient's modesty. Improper lead placement produces artifact, which necessitates repeating test or interpretation errors.
b. Place patient in supine position with head of bed no higher than 30 degrees.	Electrodes must be placed on anterior chest for standard 12-lead ECG.
c. Instruct patient to lie still without talking and not to cross his or her legs.	Body movement or talking produces artifact, which may necessitate repeating test.
3. Turn on machine; enter required demographic information.	Turning machine on first helps you identify electrode and lead issues on application.
4. Clean and prepare skin for isolated electrode placement with soap and water. Wipe area with rough washcloth or gauze or use edge of electrode to gently scrape skin. Clip excessive hair from electrode area.	Proper skin preparation before ECG electrodes are placed decreases skin impedance and signal noise, thereby producing a clean, accurate recording. Do not use alcohol to clean area as it will dry out skin. As per hospital policy, clip hair in the electrode area. Shaving leaves nicks that increase risk for infection (Diaz and Newman, 2015).
5. Apply adhesive backing on electrodes in correct positions. If using leads with suction cups, apply electrode paste to areas before attaching leads.	Proper placement of leads is very important for accurate interpretation of 12-lead ECG. Ensure that correct lead is in correct location. If any leads are misplaced, ECG reading will be inaccurate.
a. Chest (precordial) leads (see illustration)	

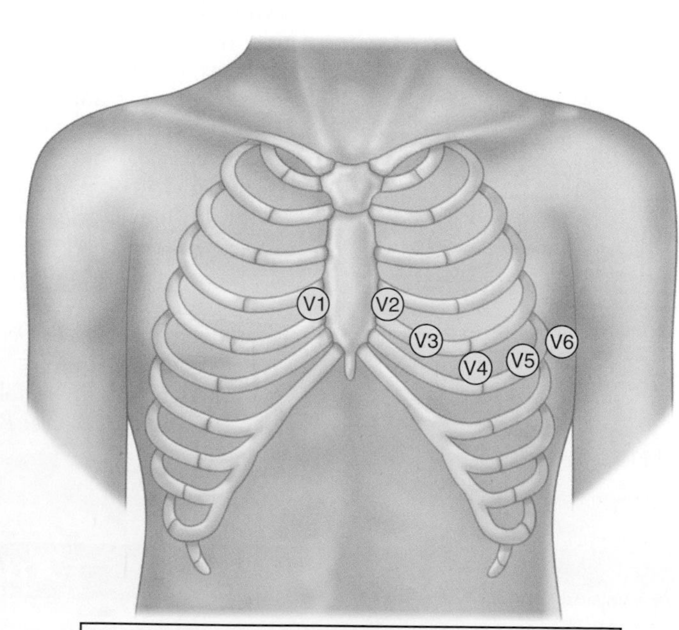

Step 5a Precordial (chest) lead placement for a standard 12-lead ECG.

STEP	RATIONALE
b. Extremities: One lead on each extremity (see illustration); right wrist, left wrist, left ankle, right ankle	

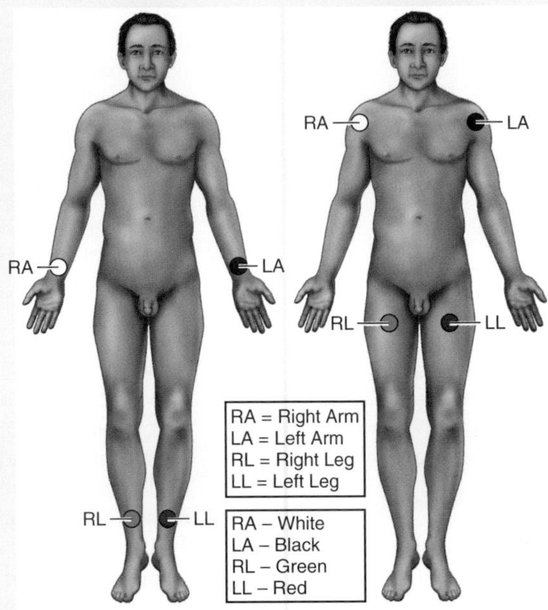

Step 5b Limb lead placement for a standard 12-lead ECG.

STEP	RATIONALE
6. Check 12-lead machine for messages to correct electrode or lead issues. If no messages occur, press button to obtain 12-lead ECG.	Confirms lead placement.
7. If you obtain ECG tracing without artifact, disconnect leads and remove	Promotes comfort and hygiene.
8. If ECG is ordered STAT, immediately deliver ECG tracing (if not computerized) to appropriate health care provider for interpretation.	If non-STAT 12-lead ECG, place in patient's chart or designated area.
9. Help patient to comfortable position.	Gives patient sense of well-being.
10. Be sure nurse call system is in an accessible location within patient's reach.	Ensures patient can call for assistance if needed.
11. Raise side rails (as appropriate) and lower bed to lowest position.	Ensures patient safety.
12. Perform hand hygiene.	Reduces transmission of microorganisms.

EVALUATION

1. Note and document if patient is experiencing any chest discomfort during procedure.	Helps correlate ECG changes to symptoms of chest pain.
2. Discuss findings and results of 12-lead ECG with health care provider to determine next steps in patient's treatment plan.	If myocardial infarction is identified, immediate steps will need to be taken to get patient to cardiac catheterization laboratory or consider use of thrombolytic medications.
3. **Use Teach-Back:** "I want to be sure I explained why you need this ECG. Why are you receiving an ECG?" Revise your instruction now or develop a plan for revised patient teaching if patient is not able to teach back correctly.	Determines patient's level of understanding of instructional topic.

Unexpected Outcomes	Related Interventions
1. ECG cannot be interpreted: • Absence of tracing on one or more leads • Presence of artifact in ECG tracings	• Inspect electrodes for secure placement. • Reposition any wires that move as a result of patient breathing or movement or vibrations in environment. Do not reposition electrodes if in correct position. • Remind patient who is moving that lying still is necessary to obtain good tracing. • If artifact looks like 60-cycle interference (very thick-lined waveform), unplug battery-operated equipment in room one item at a time to see if interference disappears. **NOTE:** 60-cycle interference is rare. • Repeat tracing.
2. Patient has chest pain or anxiety.	• Continue to monitor patient. • Reassess factors contributing to anxiety or distress. • Follow specific orders related to findings. • Notify health care provider.

Recording

- Record date and time ECG was obtained, where tracing was sent, reason for obtaining ECG, and baseline vital signs. Place rhythm strip in patient's chart (if electronic record not available).

Hand-Off Reporting

- Report any arrhythmias or patient chest pain to health care provider immediately.

Special Considerations

Patient-Centered Care

- Diagnostic procedures are often confusing, frightening, and embarrassing. Anticipate that patients will have concerns. Learn about their expectations or fears, and give them the opportunity to ask questions.
- Previous experiences, beliefs about health care (e.g., value of screening or disease prevention), and existing knowledge significantly affect how patients respond to these procedures.
- Learn why a patient is having a diagnostic test and the types of outcomes that are expected. Anxiety commonly develops when a patient does not understand the preparation before a procedure, the procedure itself, or the potential outcome of a test. For example, a colonoscopy is a routine examination to screen for early-stage colon cancer in adults older than age 50. When a patient has had signs and symptoms such as a change in bowel habits or rectal bleeding, the potential of receiving a diagnosis of colon cancer may cause fear and anxiety.
- Family members will have similar concerns, so include them when appropriate in any discussion or instructions, unless patients request that they not be involved. Be aware that a family member or caregiver may be the one to provide postprocedure care or monitoring in the home.

Patient Education

- Educating patients about the purpose of preprocedure activities helps to ensure the procedures will be completed correctly. For example, if a patient does not limit fluid intake before a procedure that requires him or her to "have nothing by mouth" (NPO), the procedure could be canceled. A delay of a test occurs if preprocedure activities are omitted or not performed correctly.
- Explain that it is unlikely for patients to remember the procedure because of the amnesic effect of the sedative(s).
- Before the procedure, instruct patient to arrange for transportation home after the procedure because (at most agencies) patient will not be permitted to drive for 24 hours after receiving sedation.
- Provide patients and family caregivers with discharge instructions that include complications that may occur; how to manage complications; and physical signs and symptoms to report to the health care provider, including contact information and post-procedure medication reconciliation and instructions.
- Teach the patient after-paracentesis symptoms of complications related to liver and spleen perforation that may not be present for several days after procedure and to notify the physician. Instruct patient to report any new abdominal pain to the physician.

Age-Specific

Pediatric

- Children are more likely than adults to sustain a serious complication resulting from anesthesia. Such complications are often linked to either the cardiovascular or respiratory system. For this reason, the American Academy of Pediatrics recommends that personnel who are able to manage a child's airway be present for the procedure (AAP, 2015).
- A preprocedure medical evaluation is required. To safely administer sedation to a pediatric patient, consider anatomical and physiological variations, preprocedure assessments, and pharmacological techniques (AAP, 2015).
- Infants and children are susceptible to the diuretic effects of radiocontrast dyes because of their small body size. Emphasize the importance of fluid intake with the child and parent (Ball et al., 2017).
- Conscious or unconscious sedation is recommended for children because of the risk of injury caused by movement during procedures. Very young children may receive IV moderate sedation or general anesthetic.
- Children are at higher risk of hypoxemia than adults because of their smaller bronchus and because the bronchoscope decreases the available breathing space (Van Leeuwen and Bladh, 2017).

Gerontological

- Closely monitor the effects of medications on patient's respiratory status and pulse. These drugs interfere with breathing or increase or decrease heart rate as a result of reduced drug clearance through the kidneys or liver (Schlitzkus et al., 2015).
- Physical exposure and room temperature contribute to hypothermia in frail adults. Use heated blankets or forced air heat to maintain core temperature at comfortable, safe levels.
- Renal insufficiency contributes to prolonged sedation.

- An older adult with preexisting dehydration or renal insufficiency in combination with NPO status is at risk for dye-induced renal failure. Carefully monitor intake and output.
- During thoracentesis, be aware of ineffective breathing patterns in older adults because of age-related changes, such as reduced elastic lung recoil, declining chest expansion, reduced cough efficiency, and weaker thoracic and diaphragmatic muscles.
- Postprocedure restlessness in the older adult patient often indicates hypoxemia or pain. Thoroughly assess oxygenation status before administration of an opioid analgesic.
- Physical exposure and room temperature contribute to hypothermia in frail older adults, who are unable to communicate that they are cold. Use heated blankets or forced air heat to maintain core temperature at comfortable, safe levels.

Home Care

- Instruct patient to avoid making any legally binding decisions until at least 24 hours after the procedure.
- Instruct patient to contact the physician (or affiliated emergency department) if any of the following occur after cardiac catheterization:
  - Chest pain or shortness of breath.
  - Blood in the urine.
  - Bleeding from the catheterization puncture site: Apply gentle pressure with clean gauze or cloth.
  - Formation of a knot or lump under the skin that increases in size.
  - Worsening of a bruise or its movement down the extremity rather than disappearing.
  - Increased pain at puncture site or in the extremity used for the catheterization.
  - Extremity with arterial puncture that is pale and cool to touch.
  - Appearance of redness, swelling, or warmth of the affected extremity.
  - Although bathing or showering is allowed the day after the catheterization, the leg used as the access site is often stiff, which increases risk of slipping in the bath or shower.

✦ PRACTICE REFLECTIONS

Consider a time when you were caring for a patient who was going to undergo a colonoscopy procedure using conscious sedation. The patient is on blood pressure medication and anticoagulants.

1. How would you educate the patient on this procedure regarding preprocedural management and postprocedure care?
2. How would you manage the medications this patient is on and their possible implications for the procedure?
3. What postprocedure complications might be a consideration?

✦ CLINICAL REVIEW QUESTIONS

1. The nurse is assessing a patient after a cardiac catheterization. What assessments indicate possible bleeding? (Select all that apply.)
   1. Catheter-site pain and loss of distal pulses
   2. Anxiety, backache, and heart rate increase from 90 to 105 beats/min
   3. Atrial fibrillation and drowsiness
   4. Pooling of blood under patient
   5. Fever and bradycardia
2. Place the following steps of bronchoscopy preprocedure care in the correct order.
   1. Perform the preprocedure "time-out."
   2. Instruct patient not to swallow anesthetic.
   3. Establish new IV access.
   4. Verify that informed consent has been obtained.
   5. Remove and store patient's dentures.
3. Following an endoscopy, the patient is nauseated and vomits 200 mL of bright red blood. What are the nurse's correct actions? (Select all that apply.)
   1. Obtain the patient's vital signs.
   2. Notify the health care provider (call Rapid Response Team if available).
   3. Observe and auscultate the abdomen.
   4. Instruct the NAP to obtain next set of vital signs.
   5. Administer oxygen as needed.
   6. Observe the vomitus.

Answers and Rationales for Clinical Review Questions can be found on the Evolve website.

REFERENCES

Abdollahi AA, et al: Effect of positioning and early ambulation on coronary angiography complications: a randomized clinical trial, *J Caring Sci* 4(2):125, 2015.

Aldrete JA: Post-anesthetic recovery score, *J Am Coll Surg* 205(5):3, 2007.

American Academy of Pediatrics (AAP) Section on Anesthesiology and Pain Medicine, Tobias JD, et al: *Procedural sedation for infants, children, and adolescents*, New York, 2015, Bantam.

American College of Radiology (ACR): ACR-SIR practice parameter for sedation/analgesia, 2015. http://www.acr.org/~/media/F194CBB800AB43048B997A75938AB482.pdf.

American Society of Anesthesiologists: ASA Physical Status Classification System, 2014. https://www.asahq.org/quality-and-practice-management/standards-and-guidelines. asa-physical-status-classification-system.pdf.

American Society of Anesthesiologists (ASA): Practice guidelines for preoperative fasting and the use of pharmacologic agents to reduce the risk of pulmonary aspiration: application to healthy patients undergoing elective procedures, *Anesthesiology* 126(3):376, 2017.

Ball J, et al: *Principles of pediatric nursing: caring for children*, ed 7, New York, 2017, Pearson.

Centers for Disease Control and Prevention (CDC): What is health literacy, 2016. https://www.cdc.gov/healthliteracy/learn/index.html.

Conway A, et al: Capnography monitoring during procedural sedation and analgesia: a systematic review protocol, *Syst Rev* 4(92):2015. doi: 10.1186/s13643-015-0085-4.

Diaz V, Newman J: Surgical site infection and prevention guidelines: a primer for certified registered nurse anesthetists, *AANA J* 83(1):63, 2015.

Frank R, et al: Procedural sedation in adults, UpToDate, 2017. http://www.uptodate.com/contents/procedural-sedation-in-adults.

Honicker T, Holt K: Contrast-induced acute kidney injury: comparison of preventive strategies, *Nephrol Nurs J* 43(2):109–117, 2016.

Krishnasamy VP, et al: Vascular closure devices: technical tips, complications, and management, *Tech Vasc Interv Radiol* 18(2):100, 2015.

Maden B, et al: An overview of diabetes and its impact on cath lab care, *Cath Lab Digest*, 2013. http://www.cathlabdigest.com/articles/Overview-Diabetes-Its-Impact-Cath-Lab-Care.

Schlitzkus LL, et al: Perioperative management of elderly patients, *Surg Clin North Am* 95(2):391, 2015.

Schulz-Schüpke S, et al: Comparison of vascular closure devices vs manual compression after femoral artery puncture, *JAMA* 312(19):2014, 1981.

The Joint Commission (TJC): *2019 National Patient Safety Goals*, 2019, Oakbrook Terrace, IL. The Commission. http://www.jointcommission.org/standards_information/npsgs.aspx.

Van Leeuwen AM, Bladh ML: *Davis's comprehensive handbook of laboratory and diagnostic tests*, ed 7, Philadelphia, 2017, FA Davis.

Westermann-Clark E, et al: Debunking myths about "allergy" to radiocontrast media in an academic institution, *Postgrad Med* 127(3):295, 2015.

11 Bathing and Personal Hygiene

SKILLS AND PROCEDURES

EVOLVE WEBSITE/RESOURCES LIST

http://evolve.elsevier.com/Perry/nursinginterventions

Audio Glossary • Case Studies • Checklists • Clinical Review Questions • Answers and Rationales for Clinical Review Questions • Video Clips

INTRODUCTION

Hygiene is important to the health and well-being of patients. Good hygiene supports physical and mental health. Performing hygiene for a patient provides an opportunity for a nurse and patient to discuss health-related concerns and allows the nurse to perform ongoing physical assessment, especially skin assessment. Personal hygiene maintains skin integrity by promoting adequate circulation and hydration. The functions of intact skin include (1) defense against infection, (2) sensory perception, and (3) regulation of body temperature. Bathe the patient and change linens when any body part or linen becomes soiled. Problems such as incontinence, wound drainage, or diaphoresis may require frequent bathing. In addition to cleansing the skin, bathing a patient has benefits such as stimulating circulation, promoting range of motion (ROM), reducing body odors, and improving self-image.

PRACTICE STANDARDS

- Agency for Healthcare Research and Quality (AHRQ), 2013: Universal ICU decolonization: an enhanced protocol—Use of chlorhexidine gluconate for patient baths
- The Joint Commission (TJC), 2019: National Patient Safety Goals—Patient identification
- Wound, Ostomy and Continence Nurses Society (WOCN), 2016: Guideline for prevention and management of pressure ulcers (injuries)

EVIDENCE-BASED PRACTICE

Chlorhexidine Gluconate Bathing and Reduction of Health Care–Associated Infections

Health care–associated infections (HAIs) exist as one of the most common adverse events during hospitalization. Although the critically ill might be most susceptible, all hospitalized patients are at risk (Cassir et al., 2015; Denny and Munro, 2016). Daily bathing with chlorhexidine substantially reduces patients' cutaneous microbial burden (Masuuza et al., 2017), thus reducing a patient's risk for bloodstream HAIs, including methicillin-resistant *Staphylococcus aureus* (MRSA) and vancomycin-resistant *Enterococcus* (VRE) infections (Cassir et al., 2015; Shah et al., 2016). Climo et al. (2013) studied critical care patients and compared chlorhexidine gluconate (CHG) bathing with non-antimicrobial cleansers. The overall rate of multidrug-resistant microorganism acquisition and the overall rate of hospital-acquired bloodstream infections were lower for patients bathed with CHG.

In addition, critically ill patients are at risk for central line–associated bloodstream infections (CLABSIs). The presence of the central line insertion site provides a portal for a pathogen to enter the patient's bloodstream. The use of CHG for whole-body cleansing in critical care patients leads to a reduction in health care–related bloodstream infections, including CLABSI, in patients with central lines (Denny and Munro, 2016; Lin et al., 2017).

Patients with indwelling urinary catheters are also at risk for infections, referred to as catheter-associated urinary tract infections (CAUTIs). CAUTIs occur when pathogens ascend through the external surface of the catheter. The use of CHG for general bathing reduces the incidence of CAUTIs (Denny and Munro, 2016).

Application to Nursing Practice

- For patients with a central line, use a clean CHG-impregnated cloth to cleanse around the vascular access site to reduce the risk for CLABSI (Lin et al., 2017; Shah et al., 2016).
- Develop a policy and procedure to adopt the use of chlorhexidine bathing practice for patients at high risk of developing HAIs (i.e., immunosuppressed patients, older adults, patients with central lines and indwelling urinary catheters; Denny and Munro, 2016; Shah et al., 2016).
- Develop a policy and perineal care procedure for patients with indwelling urinary catheters (Denny and Munro, 2016).
- Provide educational programs for nursing staff on the effectiveness of daily chlorhexidine bathing in the reduction of HAIs in at-risk patients (Musuuza et al., 2017).
- Adopt evidence-based care for central line hubs, including the use of chlorhexidine to cleanse the hubs (Denny and Munro, 2016; Lin et al., 2017) (see Chapter 28).
- To reduce infections, use a clean basin dedicated to bathing only (Martin et al., 2017b)
- Do not use CHG if a patient has an allergy or sensitivity to CHG. Report any sensitivities as an adverse event.

SAFETY GUIDELINES

- Patients who are totally dependent on someone else require assistance with personal hygiene or must learn or adapt new hygiene techniques. When providing personal hygiene, important safety principles to follow are prevention of infection and prevention of patient injury.
- To reduce the risk of infection, always perform hygiene measures moving from cleanest to less clean or dirty areas. (**NOTE**: This often requires you to change gloves and perform hand hygiene during care activities.)
- Use clean gloves when you anticipate contact with nonintact skin or mucous membranes or when there is or may likely be contact with drainage, secretions, excretions, or blood. Additional precautions requiring other personal protective equipment (PPE) may be necessary, depending on the patient's condition (see Chapter 5).
- When using water or solutions for hygiene care, be sure to test the solution temperature to prevent burn injury. This is especially important for patients with reduced sensation, such as those with diabetes, peripheral neuropathy, or spinal cord injury.
- To avoid injury when performing hygiene care, use principles of body mechanics and safe patient handling (see Chapter 17).
- You are responsible and accountable for assessing and evaluating a patient before and after care to detect unexpected outcomes and for giving proper direction to nursing assistive personnel (NAP) when delegating hygiene care.
- To prevent bleeding, monitor laboratory findings, such as coagulation studies, before administering oral care.

✦ SKILL 11.1 Complete or Partial Bed Bath

Purpose

Bathing removes sweat, oil, dirt, and microorganisms from the skin. It also stimulates circulation and provides a refreshed and relaxed feeling. For some patients, a bath is a time for socialization and pleasure, especially for those who are bedridden or seriously disabled. The type of bath, the extent of the bath, and the methods for bathing depend on a patient's ability to participate, the condition of the patient's skin, and in some settings the time of day. Whether you use a basin for bathing, disposable bed bath, tub, or shower often depends on agency policy, availability of the disposable bed bath, patient cooperation and mobility, or type of health care agency. Often the use of a tub or shower is more common in long-term care settings (Box 11.1).

There are two categories of baths: cleansing and therapeutic. Cleansing baths include the bed bath, tub bath, sponge bath at the sink, shower, and prepackaged disposable bed bath (Box 11.2). When

BOX 11.1

Types of Baths

Complete Bed Bath
Bath administered to totally dependent patient in bed.

Partial Bed Bath
Bed bath that consists of bathing only body parts that would cause discomfort if left unbathed, such as the hands, face, axilla, and perineal area. Partial bath also includes washing back and providing back rub. Dependent patients in need of partial hygiene or self-sufficient bedridden patients who are unable to reach all body parts receive a partial bed bath.

Sponge Bath at the Sink
Involves bathing from a bath basin or sink with patient sitting in a chair. Patient is able to perform a portion of the bath independently. Assistance is needed from the nurse for hard-to-reach areas.

Tub Bath
Involves immersion in a tub of water that allows more thorough washing and rinsing than a bed bath. Some patients require the nurse's assistance. Some facilities have tubs equipped with lifting devices or panels that swing open to facilitate entry and positioning of dependent patients in the tub (see Box 11.2).

Shower
Patient sits or stands under a continuous stream of water. Shower provides more thorough washing than a bed bath but can be fatiguing (see Box 11.2).

Bag Bath (Travel Bath)
Bag bath contains several soft, nonwoven cotton cloths that are premoistened in a solution of no-rinse surfactant cleanser and emollient. The bag bath is an appealing alternative because of the ease of use, shorter bathing time, and patient comfort. Several commercial body-cleansing systems are available that contain the same ingredients as the bag bath.

BOX 11.2

Use of Tub or Shower

Although showers are available to patients in acute care, you will see tub and shower bathing more commonly in long-term care settings. When patients use a tub or shower, follow guidelines to maintain patient safety to prevent falls.

Procedural Steps

1. Identify patient using at least two identifiers (e.g., name and birthday or name and medical record number) according to agency policy (TJC, 2019).
2. Assess environment for safety (e.g., check room for spills; make sure that equipment is working properly, and that bed is in locked, low position) and provide privacy.
3. Assess patient's fall risk status; consider patient's physical ability to stand, get into tub, and review orders for precautions concerning his or her movement or positioning. A health care provider's order usually is needed for tub bath or shower.
   a. Schedule use of shower or tub.
   b. Check tub or shower for cleanliness. Use cleaning techniques outlined in agency policy. Place rubber mat on tub or shower bottom. Place skid-proof disposable bath mat or towel on floor in front of tub or shower.
   c. Place hygiene and toiletry items within easy reach of tub or shower. Do not allow patient to use bath oil in tub or shower because this can cause slipping and resultant fall.
   d. Perform hand hygiene and help patient to bathroom if necessary. Have him or her wear robe and skid-proof slippers to bathroom.
   e. Demonstrate how to use nurse call system for help. Place "occupied" sign on bathroom door. Close door.
   f. Fill bathtub halfway with warm water. Check temperature of bath water, have patient test it, and adjust it if it is too warm or too cold. Explain which faucet controls hot water.
   g. If patient is taking shower, turn shower on and adjust water temperature before he or she enters shower stall. Use shower seat or tub chair if available.
   h. Tell patient that you will not allow him or her to remain in tub longer than 20 minutes. Check on patient every 5 minutes.
   i. Apply clean gloves. Return to bathroom when patient signals, and knock before entering.
   j. For patient who is unsteady, drain tub of water before he or she attempts to get out. Place bath towel over patient's shoulders. Help him or her get out of tub as needed and help with drying. If possible, have a shower chair available for patient to sit.
   k. Help patient as needed to don clean gown or pajamas, slippers, and robe. (In home, extended care, or rehabilitation setting, encourage patient to wear regular clothing.)
   l. Help patient assume desired comfortable position. Be sure nurse call system is in an accessible location within patient's reach. Raise side rails (as appropriate) and lower bed to lowest position.
   m. Clean tub or shower according to agency policy. Remove soiled linen and place in dirty laundry bag. Discard disposable equipment in proper receptacle. Place "unoccupied" sign on bathroom door. Return supplies to storage area.
   n. Remove and dispose of gloves. Perform hand hygiene.

a person is unable to perform personal care because of illness or disability, you are responsible for helping with bathing. You can also clean and groom hair, shave a patient, and clean the nails during or immediately after a bath.

Therapeutic baths are ordered for a specific effect, such as soothing the skin, or for promoting the healing process. Types of therapeutic baths include:

- *Sitz bath*: Cleans and reduces pain and inflammation of perineal and anal areas. They are used for patients who have undergone rectal or perineal surgery or childbirth or who have local irritation from hemorrhoids or fissures. A patient sits in a special tub or basin (see Chapter 25).
- *Medicated bath (addition of over-the-counter, herbal, or health care provider–ordered ingredient to bath)*: Relieves skin irritation and creates an antibacterial and drying effect.

Delegation and Collaboration

Assessment of the patient's skin, pain level, and range of motion (ROM) cannot be delegated to nursing assistive personnel (NAP). The skill of bathing can be delegated to NAP. The nurse instructs the NAP about:

- Not massaging reddened skin areas during bathing.
- Contraindications to soaking a patient's feet.
- Reporting any signs of impaired skin integrity to the nurse.
- Proper ways to position male and female patients with musculoskeletal limitations or an indwelling Foley catheter or other equipment (e.g., intravenous [IV] tubing).

Equipment

- Washcloths and bath towels
- Bath blanket
- Bar or liquid soap, or 4-oz bottle of 2% to 4% chlorhexidine gluconate (CHG) (dispensed in a single bath-size bottle)
- Toiletry items (deodorant, lotion)
- Disposable wipes
- Warm water
- Clean hospital gown or patient's own pajamas or gown
- Laundry bag
- Clean gloves
- Washbasin-dedicated for bathing only
- Eye patch/shield and nonallergenic tape (for unconscious patient)

ASSESSMENT

1. Identify patient using at least two identifiers (e.g., name and birthday or name and medical record number) according to agency policy. *Rationale: Ensures patient safety. Complies with The Joint Commission standards and improves patient safety (TJC, 2019).*
2. Review medical record for orders for specific precautions concerning patient's movement or positioning and whether there is an order for a therapeutic bath. Note and confirm with patient any allergies or sensitivities to bath products. *Rationale: Prevents accidental injury to patient during bathing activities. Determines level of help that patient needs. Prevents allergic reactions to hygiene products during bathing.*
3. Perform hand hygiene. Assess room environment for safety (e.g., check room for spills; make sure that equipment is working properly and that bed is in locked, low position). Reduces transmission of microorganisms. *Rationale: Identifies safety hazards in patient environment that when minimized or*

eliminated can reduce risk of harm to patients (Quality and Safety Education for Nurses [QSEN], 2018).

4. Assess patient's fall risk status (if partial bathing out of bed or self-bath is to be performed) (see Chapter 4). *Rationale: Allows you to anticipate needed precautions such as having patient sit on chair in front of basin.*
5. Assess patient's tolerance for bathing: activity tolerance, comfort level, musculoskeletal function, and presence of shortness of breath. *Rationale: Determines patient's ability to perform or tolerate bathing and type of bath to administer (e.g., tub bath, bed bath).*
6. Assess patient's cognitive (Mini-Mental State Examination) and functional status (e.g., Barthel's index or the index of activities of daily living [ADLs] to measure self-care ability). For patients with suspected dementia (Hirschman and Hodgson, 2018; Konno et al., 2014), observe behavior, especially after telling patient it is bath time; does he or she become agitated? *Rationale: Every person entering a long-term care setting should be formally assessed for cognitive and functional status. Functional status assesses a patient's capacity for self-bathing and how much supervision/help is needed to accomplish daily ADL tasks. Every attempt should be made to avoid bathing people against their will (Pinkert et al., 2018).*

Safe Patient Care *Patients with dementia may become agitated. Observe for behaviors such as restlessness, yelling, and fighting with caregivers.*

7. Assess patient's visual status, ability to sit without support, hand grasp, ROM of extremities (see Chapter 8). *Rationale: Further determines degree of help needed for bathing.*
8. Assess for presence and position of external medical device/equipment (e.g., IV line or oxygen tubing). *Rationale: Affects how you will position patient and plan bathing activities.*
9. Assess patient's bathing preferences: How often does the person bathe? What time of day? Is there anything in the past that might affect frequency of bathing (such as growing up without indoor plumbing)? How does the person bathe now (tub, shower, at sink, only with prompting)? Does the person use any special products, robes, towels, or equipment during bathing (e.g., scented soaps, music, back brush, or sponge) to make the experience more enjoyable? Is the person especially modest? *Rationale: Allows patient to participate in plan of care. Promotes patient's comfort and willingness to cooperate. Using a patient's established routine may reduce agitation in a patient with dementia.*
10. Ask if patient has noticed any problems related to condition of skin and genitalia. *Rationale: Provides information to direct physical assessment of skin and genitalia during bathing. Also influences selection of skin-care products.*
11. Before or during bath, assess condition of patient's skin. Note presence of dryness, indicated by flaking, redness, scaling, and cracking or excessive moisture, inflammation, or pressure injuries (see Chapter 26). *Rationale: Provides baseline for comparison of skin integrity over time.*
12. Identify risks for skin impairment: older age, immobilization, reduced sensation, nutrition and hydration, excess skin moisture or drainage, shear or friction on skin, vascular insufficiencies, presence of external devices. Option: Use an agency-approved pressure injury assessment tool (e.g., Braden Scale; see Chapter 26). *Rationale: Risk factors increase the likelihood of injury to the skin because of pressure, impaired tissue synthesis, softening of or friction on tissues, and impaired circulation.*
13. Assess patient's level of comfort on a 0-to-10 pain scale. Bath can soothe and comfort patient. *Rationale: Provides baseline measure.*
14. Assess patient's or family caregiver's knowledge, experience, and health literacy. *Rationale: Ensures patient or family caregiver has the capacity to obtain, communicate, process, and understand basic health information (Centers for Disease Control and Prevention [CDC], 2016).*
15. Assess patient's knowledge and perceptions of the importance of skin hygiene, preventive measures to take, and common skin problems encountered (Table 11.1). *Rationale: Determines patient's willingness to learn and type of instruction required.*

TABLE 11.1

Common Skin Problems and Related Interventions

Problem	Interventions
Dry skin: Flaky, rough texture to skin, which may crack and become infected.	Bathe with warm, not hot, water, and bathe less frequently; use super-fatted soap (e.g., Dove); rinse away all soap, or use a waterless cleanser rather than soap and water; increase fluid intake; use moisturizing lotion.
Acne: Inflammatory papulopustular skin eruption, usually involving bacterial breakdown of sebum, typically on face, neck, shoulders, and back.	Wash hair daily. Wash skin twice daily with warm water and soap to remove oils and cosmetics (if used); cosmetics that can accumulate in pores should be used sparingly. Use prescribed topical antibiotics as directed.
Rashes: Skin eruption from overexposure to sun or moisture or from allergic reaction; may be flat, raised, localized, or systemic; may be associated with pruritus (itching).	Wash and rinse thoroughly; apply antiseptic spray or lotion (as ordered) to prevent further itching and to aid in healing process; warm or cold soaks relieve inflammation.
Contact dermatitis: Inflammation of skin characterized by abrupt onset with erythema, pruritus, pain, and scaly, oozing lesions; usually results from contact with substance difficult to identify and eliminate.	Identify and avoid contributing agents. Apply topical over-the-counter steroids (or prescription steroids as ordered) or calamine lotion. Instruct patient to avoid touching area and then other parts of the skin without washing and rinsing between. Provide rinsed and sterilized linens to minimize irritation.
Abrasion: Scraping or rubbing away of epidermis (e.g., a sheet burn) that results in localized bleeding and later weeping of serous fluid; easily infected.	Wash with mild soap and water; observe dressings for retained moisture, which can increase risk of infection.

STEP	RATIONALE
PLANNING	
1. Expected outcomes following completion of procedure:	
• Skin is free of excretions, drainage, or odor.	Skin is clean.
• Skin shows decreased redness, cracking, flaking, and scaling.	Indicates reduction in skin dryness.
• Joint ROM remains same or improves from previous measurement.	Repeated ROM exercise during bathing helps prevent contractures and promotes joint movement.
• Patient expresses sense of comfort and relaxation.	Bath relaxes patient and removes sources of discomfort.
• Patient tolerates bath without fatigue or chilling.	Fatigue during bathing indicates worsening of chronic cardiopulmonary conditions.
• Patient describes benefits and techniques of proper hygiene and skin care.	Demonstrates learning with ability to repeat back to demonstrate understanding.
2. Adjust room temperature and ventilation, close room doors and windows, and draw room divider curtain.	Warm room that is free of drafts prevents rapid loss of body heat during bathing. Privacy provides for patient's mental and physical comfort.
3. Prepare equipment and place supplies on bedside table. If it is necessary to leave room, be sure that nurse call system is within patient's reach, bed is in low position, and wheels are locked.	Avoids interrupting procedure or leaving patient unattended to retrieve missing equipment. Provides for patient safety.
4. Explain procedure and ask patient for suggestions on how to prepare supplies. If partial bath, ask how much of bath patient wishes to complete.	Promotes patient's cooperation, participation, and promotion of self-care as appropriate.

Safe Patient Care *Never leave the bedside without ensuring that appropriate number of side rails have been raised (see agency policy). The number of side rails depends on the patient's fall risk assessment; however, having all side rails raised is considered a restraint.*

STEP	RATIONALE
IMPLEMENTATION	
1. Offer patient bedpan or urinal. Apply clean gloves to help patient as needed. Provide toilet tissue and dispose of any excrement properly. Dispose of gloves if applied and perform hand hygiene. Provide patient towel and moist washcloth.	Patient feels more comfortable after voiding. Prevents interruption of bath.
2. Perform hand hygiene. If patient has nonintact skin or skin is soiled with drainage, excretions, or body secretions, apply new pair of clean gloves before beginning bath.	Reduces transmission of microorganisms.
3. Raise bed to comfortable working height. Lower side rail closest to you and help patient assume comfortable supine position, maintaining body alignment. Bring patient toward side closest to you (staying supine).	Aids access to patient. Maintains patient's comfort throughout procedure. Uses proper body mechanics, thus minimizing strain on back muscles. If patient is overweight, use other caregiver or lift device for positioning (see Chapter 17).
4. Place bath blanket over patient. Have patient hold top of bath blanket and remove top sheet from under bath blanket without exposing patient. Place soiled linen in laundry bag.	Blanket provides warmth and privacy. Take care to avoid linen contacting uniform.
5. Remove patient's gown or pajamas.	Provides full exposure of body parts during bathing.
a. If gown has snaps on sleeves, simply unsnap and remove gown without pulling IV tubing (if present).	
b. If gown has no snaps and if an extremity is *injured* or has reduced mobility, begin removal from *unaffected* side first.	Undressing unaffected side first allows easier manipulation of gown over body part with reduced ROM.

STEP	RATIONALE
c. If patient has an IV line and gown with no snaps, remove gown from arm *without* IV line first. Then remove gown from arm with IV line (see illustration A). Pause IV fluid infusion by pressing appropriate sensor on IV pump. Remove IV tubing from pump; use regulator to slow IV infusion. Remove IV bag from pole (see illustration B) and slide IV bag and tubing through arm of patient's gown (see illustration C). Rehang IV bag (see illustration D), reconnect tubing to pump, open regulator clamp, and restart IV fluid infusion by pressing appropriate sensor on IV pump. If IV fluids are infusing by gravity, check IV flow rate and regulate if necessary. *Do not disconnect IV tubing to remove gown.*	Manipulation of IV tubing and bag can disrupt IV infusion flow rate.

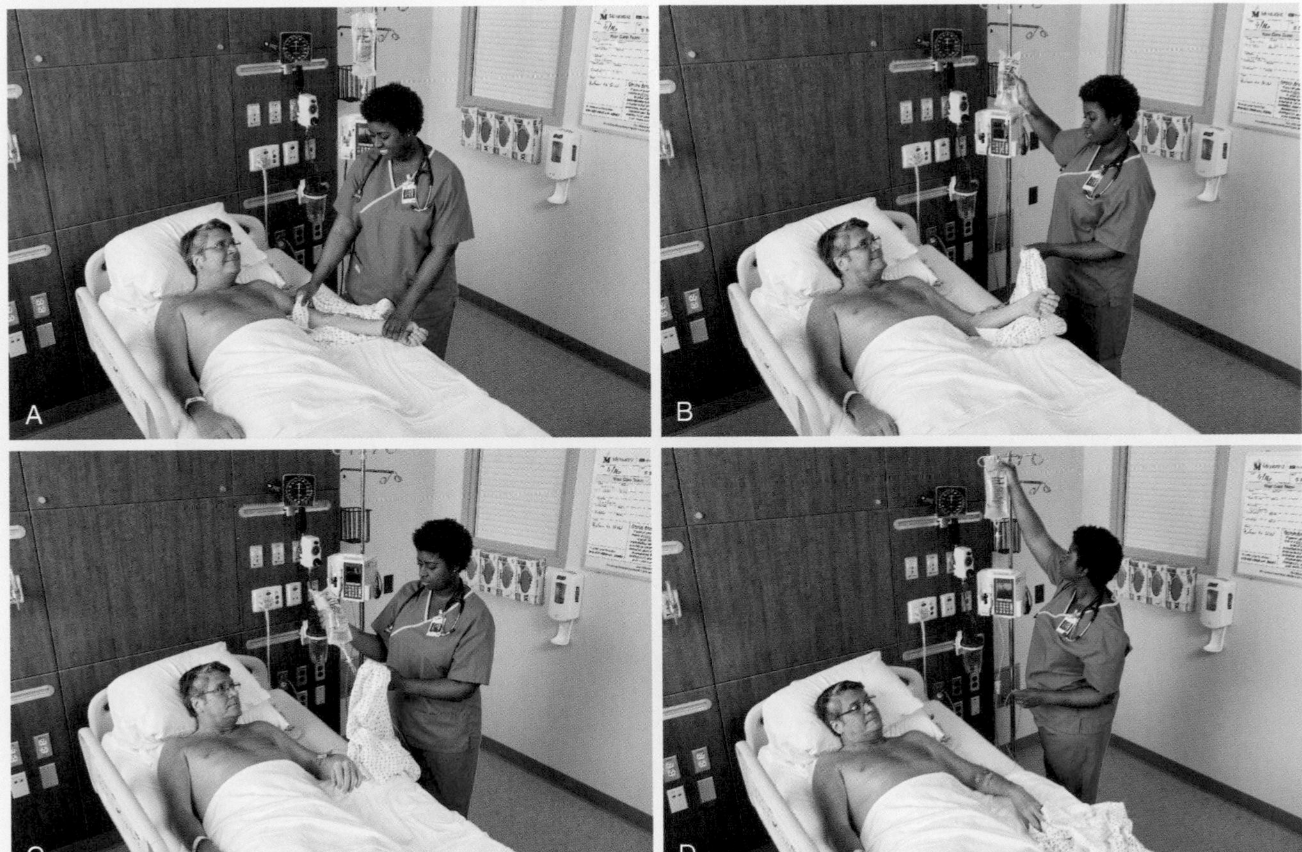

STEP 5c (A) Remove patient's gown. (B) Remove IV bag from pole. (C) Slide IV tubing and bag through arm of patient's gown. (D) Rehang IV bag.

STEP	RATIONALE
6. Raise side rail. Lower bed temporarily to lowest position and raise on return after you fill wash basin two-thirds full with warm water. Place basin along with supplies on over-bed table and position over patient's bed. Check water temperature and have patient place fingers in water.	Raising side rail and lowering bed maintains patient's safety. Warm water promotes comfort, relaxes muscles, and prevents unnecessary chilling. Use of over-bed table allows you to move to opposite side of bed without having to move equipment. Tests water temperature to prevent burns to skin.
7. Lower side rail. Remove pillow (if tolerated). Raise head of bed 30 to 45 degrees if allowed. Place bath towel under patient's head. Place second bath towel over patient's chest.	Removal of pillow makes it easier to wash patient's ears and neck. Placement of towels prevents soiling of bed linen and bath blanket.

STEP	RATIONALE
8. Wash face.	

Safe Patient Care *Do not use bath water with 4% liquid CHG added or 2% CHG bathing cloths (see Procedural Guideline 11.1) on the eyes or face (AHRQ, 2013).*

STEP	RATIONALE
a. Inquire if patient is wearing contact lenses. You may choose to remove them at this time.	Prevents accidental injury to eyes.
b. Form a mitt with washcloth (see illustration); immerse in water and wring thoroughly.	Mitt retains water and heat better than loosely held washcloth; keeps cold edges from brushing against patient and prevents splashing.
c. Wash patient's eyes with plain warm water, using a clean area of cloth for each eye and bathing from inner to outer canthus (see illustrations). Soak any crusts on eyelid for 2 to 3 minutes with warm, damp cloth before attempting removal. Dry around eyes thoroughly but gently.	Soap irritates eyes. Use of separate sections of mitt reduces infection transmission. Bathing eye gently from inner to outer canthus prevents secretions from entering nasolacrimal duct. Pressure causes internal injury.
d. Ask if patient prefers to use soap on face. Otherwise wash, rinse, and dry forehead, cheeks, nose, neck, and ears without using soap. Ask men if they want to be shaved (see Procedural Guideline 11.6).	Soap tends to dry face, which is exposed to air more than other body parts.
e. Provide eye care for unconscious patient.	Patients who are unconscious have lost the normal protective corneal reflex of blinking, increasing the risk for corneal drying, abrasions, and eye infection.
(1) Instill eyedrops or ointment per health care provider's order (see Chapter 23).	

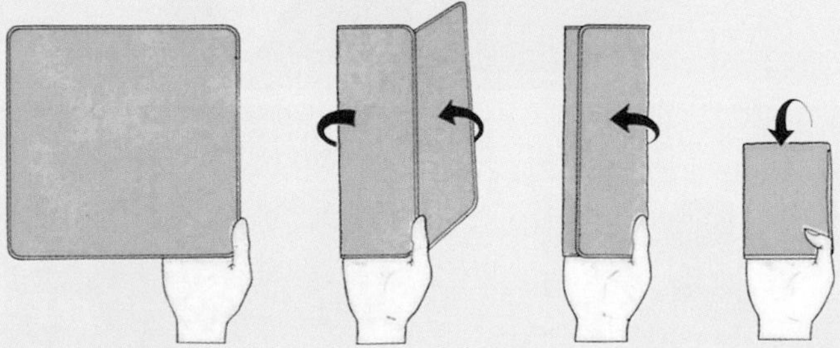

STEP 8b Steps for folding washcloth to form a mitt.

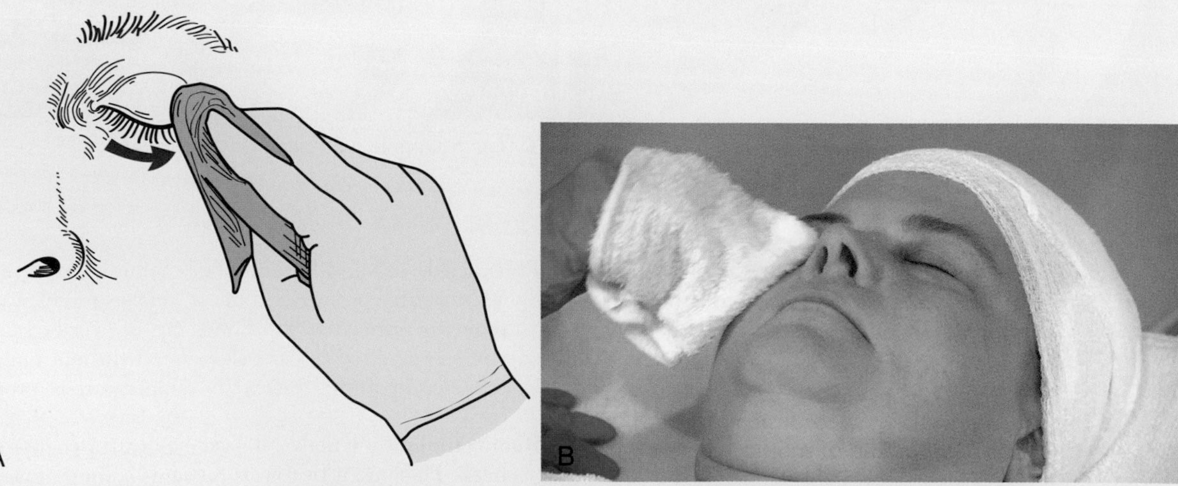

STEP 8c Wash eye from inner to outer canthus. (A) Direction for cleaning eye. (B) Washing eye from inner to outer canthus.

STEP	RATIONALE
(2) In the absence of blink reflex, keep eyelids closed. Close eye gently, using back of your fingertip, before placing eye patch or shield. Place tape over patch or shield. Do not tape eyelid.	When blink reflex is absent, patient loses a protective mechanism. Keeping eyelids closed maintains eye moisture and prevents injury.
9. Wash upper extremities and trunk. *Option:* Change bath water at this time. Obtain new 6-quart basin and mix contents of a 4-ounce bottle of CHG with warm water.	Evidence shows that CHG use in daily bathing can reduce incidence of hospital-acquired infections (Martin et al., 2017b; Petlin et al., 2014; Shah et al., 2016). CHG reduces bacteria for up to 24 hours and prevents infection (AHRQ, 2013).

Safe Patient Care *When using CHG in a bath basin of water, use one washcloth for washing each major body part. Then dispose of cloth and use a new cloth for the next body part (Martin et al., 2017b). Dipping cloth back into basin contaminates solution and makes CHG less effective. Do not rinse after bathing with CHG solution. Allow CHG to dry on the skin to achieve antimicrobial effects.*

STEP	RATIONALE
a. Remove bath blanket from patient's arm that is closest to you. Place bath towel lengthwise under arm using long, firm strokes from distal to proximal (fingers to axilla).	Long, firm strokes promote venous return.
b. Raise and support arm above head (if possible) to wash axilla, rinse, and dry thoroughly (see illustration). Apply deodorant to underarms as needed or desired.	Movement of arm exposes axilla and exercises normal ROM of joint. Deodorant controls body odor.

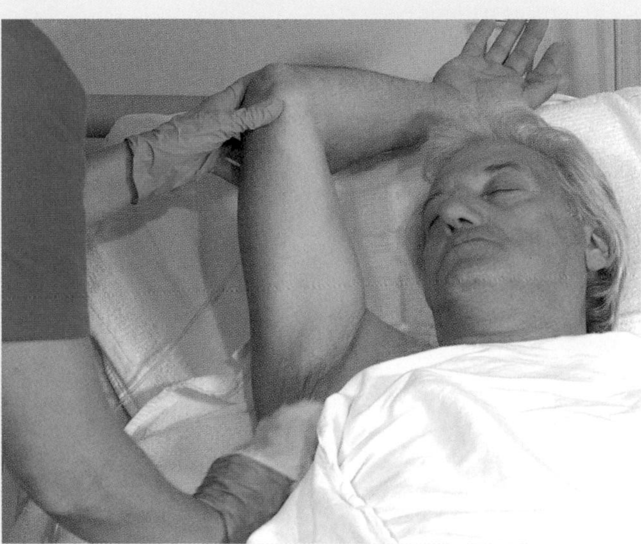

STEP 9b Position of patient's arm for washing axilla.

STEP	RATIONALE
c. Move to other side of bed and repeat steps with other arm.	
d. Cover patient's chest with bath towel and fold bath blanket down to umbilicus. Bathe chest with long, firm strokes. Take special care with skin under female patient's breasts, lifting breast upward if necessary while bathing underneath breast. Rinse if using soap and water and dry well.	Draping prevents unnecessary exposure of body parts. Towel maintains warmth and privacy. Secretions and dirt collect easily in areas of tight skinfolds. Skin under breasts is vulnerable to excoriation if not kept clean and dry.
10. Wash hands and nails.	
a. Fold bath towel in half and lay it on bed beside patient. Place basin on towel. Immerse patient's hand in water. Allow hand to soak for 3 to 5 minutes before cleaning fingernails (see Skill 11.5). Remove basin and dry hand well. Repeat for other hand.	Soaking softens cuticles and calluses of hand, loosens debris beneath nails, and enhances feeling of cleanliness. Thorough drying removes moisture from between fingers. Soaking hands of patient with diabetes mellitus can lead to maceration and risk for infection.

Safe Patient Care *Do not routinely soak fingers of patient with diabetes mellitus.*

STEP	RATIONALE
11. Check temperature of bath water and change water if necessary; otherwise continue. **NOTE:** If using CHG solution in bath water, do not discard water. One bottle of CHG soap is sufficient for a complete bath; you may add warm water.	Warm water maintains patient's comfort.
12. Wash abdomen.	
a. Place bath towel lengthwise over chest and abdomen. (You may need two towels.) Fold bath blanket down to just above pubic region. Bathe, rinse, and dry abdomen with special attention to umbilicus and skinfolds of abdomen and groin. Keep abdomen covered between washing and rinsing. Dry well.	Keeping skinfolds clean and dry helps prevent odor and skin irritation. Moisture and sediment that collects in skinfolds predispose skin to maceration.
b. Apply clean gown or pajama top by dressing affected side first. *Option:* You may omit this step until completion of bath.	Maintains patient's warmth and comfort. Allows easier manipulation of gown over body part with reduced ROM.

Safe Patient Care *If one extremity is injured or immobilized, always dress affected side first.*

STEP	RATIONALE
13. Wash lower extremities.	
a. Cover chest and abdomen with top of bath blanket. Expose near leg by folding blanket toward midline. Be sure that other leg and perineum remain draped. Place bath towel under leg as you support patient's knee and ankle.	Prevents overexposure. Method of placement supports patient's joint.
b. Wash leg using long, firm strokes from ankle to knee and knee to thigh (see illustration). Assess condition of extremities.	Promotes circulation and venous return. Assessment is key to identifying signs and symptoms of venous thrombosis.

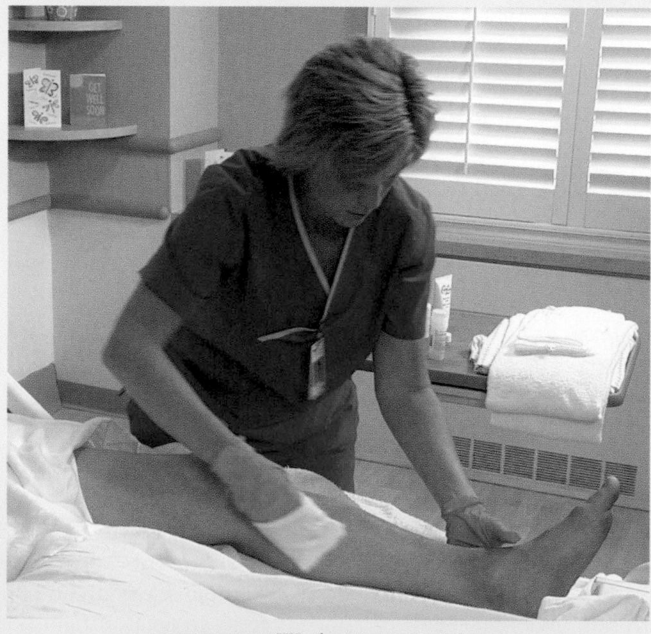

STEP 13b Washing patient's leg.

Safe Patient Care *When bathing the lower extremities, assess for signs of warmth, redness, swelling, tenderness, and pain in the lower extremities because these might be early signs of deep vein thrombosis (DVT).*

STEP	RATIONALE
c. Clean foot, making sure to bathe between toes. Clean and file nails as needed (check agency policy) (see Skill 11.5). Dry toes and feet completely.	Secretions and moisture are often present between toes, predisposing patient to maceration and skin breakdown.
d. Raise side rail; remove towel; move to opposite side of bed, lower side rail, place dry towel under second leg, and repeat Steps 13b and 13c for other leg and foot. Apply light layer of moisturizing lotion to both feet. When finished, remove used towel.	Moisturizers are effective in reducing dry skin; however, in excess they can cause maceration.

STEP	RATIONALE
e. Cover patient with bath blanket, raise side rail, and change bath water (if using plain soap and water).	Decreased bath water temperature causes chilling. Clean water reduces microorganism transmission.
14. Wash back.	
a. Apply clean gloves (if not already applied). Lower side rail. Help patient assume prone or side-lying position, using safe patient-handling techniques (see Chapter 17) (as applicable). Place towel lengthwise along patient's side.	Exposes back and buttocks for bathing.
b. If fecal material is present, enclose in fold of underpad or toilet tissue and remove with disposable wipes.	Skinfolds near buttocks and anus may contain fecal secretions and microorganisms.
c. Keep patient draped by sliding bath blanket over shoulders and thighs during bathing. Wash, rinse, and dry back from neck to buttocks with long, firm strokes. Pay special attention to folds of buttocks and anus.	Maintains warmth and prevents unnecessary exposure.
d. Clean buttocks and anus, washing front to back (see illustration). Clean, rinse, and dry area thoroughly. If needed, place clean, absorbent pad under patient's buttocks.	Cleaning buttocks after back prevents contamination of water.

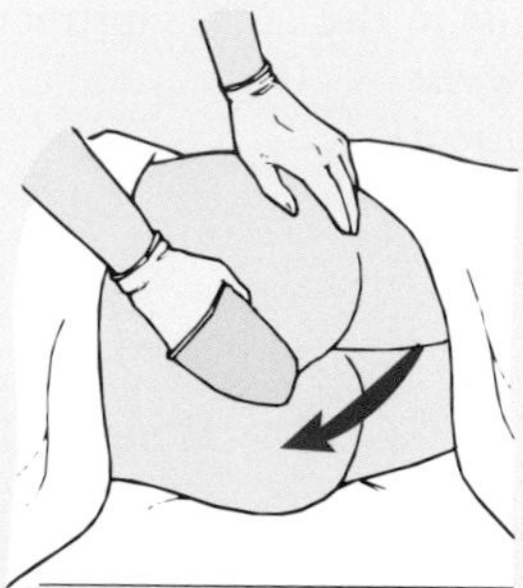

STEP 14d Clean buttocks and anus, washing front to back.

STEP	RATIONALE
15. While patient is supine, provide perineal care (see Procedural Guideline 11.2).	

Safe Patient Care *At end of bath, if you have used 4% CHG solution, skin may feel sticky for a few minutes. Do NOT wipe off. Allow to air dry (AHRQ, 2013).*

STEP	RATIONALE
16. Massage back if patient desires.	Promotes patient relaxation.
17. Apply body lotion to skin and topical moisturizing agents to dry, flaky, reddened, or scaling areas. **NOTE:** If using CHG solution for bathing, only use a product compatible with CHG (AHRQ, 2013).	Dry skin results in reduced pliability and cracking. Moisturizers help to prevent skin breakdown.

Safe Patient Care *Massage is contraindicated in the presence of acute inflammation and where there is the possibility of damaged blood vessels or fragile skin (WOCN, 2016). Massage of the legs is also contraindicated because of the possible presence of a blood clot, which could become dislodged.*

STEP	RATIONALE
18. Remove and dispose of gloves and perform hand hygiene before helping patient complete grooming (e.g., combing hair, shaving).	Reduces transmission of microorganisms. Promotes patient's body image.
19. Check function and position of external devices (e.g., indwelling catheters, nasogastric tubes, IV tubes, braces).	Ensures that bathing activities did not disrupt systems.
20. Replace top bed linen by pulling sheet and bedspread from foot of bed to cover patient before removing bath blanket. Apply gloves if linen is soiled. *Option*: Make occupied bed at this time (see Procedural Guideline 11.6).	Maintains patient warmth and privacy.
21. Place bed in low, locked position and raise appropriate number of side rails so they do not restrain patient from exiting bed safely. Make sure that patient is in comfortable position and personal possessions in reach.	Maintains patient safety. Reaching for nurse call system or personal items can lead to a fall.

STEP	RATIONALE
22. Disinfect/rinse and dry bed basin according to agency policy. This is especially important if using CHG solution. DO NOT use basin for CHG as storage container for supplies.	CHG bathing does reduce contamination of the bath basin (Marchaim et al., 2018; Musuuza et al., 2017; Petlin et al., 2014). Reduces transmission of microorganisms.
23. Place nurse system accessible within reach; instruct patient in use.	Assists patient or family member in calling for assistance.
24. Perform hand hygiene and leave room.	Reduces transmission of microorganisms.

EVALUATION

STEP	RATIONALE
1. Observe skin; pay attention to areas that were previously soiled, reddened, flaking, scaling, or cracking or that showed early signs of breakdown. Inspect areas normally exposed to pressure.	Bathing should leave skin clean and clear. If there are signs of skin irritation (e.g., redness, blistering), take steps to reduce pressure.
2. Observe ROM during bathing.	Measures joint mobility.
3. Ask patient to rate level of comfort (on a scale of 0 to 10).	Determines changes in level of comfort during bathing.
4. Ask if patient feels tired (on a scale of 0 to 10).	Measures tolerance to bathing activity.
5. **Use Teach-Back:** "I want to be sure I explained the importance of keeping your skin clean, especially while in the hospital. Tell me why we want to bathe you daily." Revise your instruction now or develop a plan for revised patient/family caregiver teaching if patient/family caregiver is not able to teach back correctly.	Determines patient's/family caregiver's level of understanding of instructional topic.

Unexpected Outcomes	Related Interventions
1. Areas of excessive dryness, rashes, irritation, or pressure injury appear on skin.	• If using CHG soap, it may become necessary to reduce frequency of bathing. Sensitivity to CHG is rare. • Limit frequency of complete baths. • Complete pressure injury assessment (see Chapter 26). • Institute turning and positioning measures to keep patient off pressure injury. • Obtain special bed surface if patient is at risk for skin breakdown. • Notify health care provider and/or obtain wound consultation.
2. Patient becomes excessively tired and unable to cooperate or participate in bathing.	• Reschedule bathing to a time when patient is more rested. • Patients with cardiopulmonary conditions and breathing difficulties require pillow or elevated head of bed during bathing. • Notify health care provider about changes in patient's fatigue level. • Perform hygiene measures in stages between scheduled rest periods.
3. Patient seems unusually restless or complains of discomfort.	• Use less stressful method of bathing such as a disposable bath (see Procedural Guideline 11.1). • Consider analgesia before bathing. • Schedule rest periods before bathing.

Recording

- Complete flow sheet according to agency policy.
- Record observations made during the bath, which may include type of bath given, patient's ability to assist or cooperate, condition of patient's skin, patient's knowledge of hygiene practices, and any nursing interventions for improving skin integrity.
- Document your evaluation of patient learning.

Hand-Off Reporting

- Use standardized hand-off to communicate patient's response to bathing and any concerns voiced by patient regarding self-care needs.
- Report to health care team any unexpected outcomes, such as increased weakness or fatigue, changes in skin integrity, or changes in wound healing.

PROCEDURAL GUIDELINE 11.1 *Bathing Using Disposable Cloths*

Purpose
While the use of disposable washcloths impregnated with an antiseptic solution such as chlorhexidine gluconate (CHG) is more common now in acute care hospitals, especially critical care settings, they can be used in any setting. CHG cloths should be used for all bathing purposes, including once-a-day full-body bathing, incontinence care, or any other reasons for additional cleaning (AHRQ, 2013; Anderson et al., 2018). CHG replaces soap-and-water baths; thus, the cloths should not be used as a "top coat" after bathing. Rather, CHG cloths clean and remove bacteria, and the antiseptic binds to the skin for persistent antibacterial activity lasting 24 hours (AHRQ, 2013). Disposable cloths reduce the risk of HAIs and contamination of wash basins with multidrug-resistant organisms (MDROs) (Martin et al., 2017b).

Delegation and Collaboration
The skill of bathing using disposable cloths can be delegated to nursing assistive personnel (NAP). The nurse instructs the NAP to:
- Not massage reddened skin areas during bathing.
- Properly position male and female patients with musculoskeletal limitations or an indwelling Foley catheter or other equipment (e.g., intravenous tubing).
- Report changes in skin or perineal area or signs of impaired skin integrity to the nurse.

Equipment
Washcloths and bath towels (for tub or shower), bath blanket, cleaning product, toiletry items (deodorant, lotion), disposable wipes, clean hospital gown or patient's own pajamas or gown, laundry bag; prepackaged, disposable bathing cloths; clean gloves

Procedural Steps
1. Identify patient using at least two identifiers (e.g., name and birthday or name and medical record number) according to agency policy (TJC, 2019).
2. Assess environment for safety (e.g., check room for spills; make sure that any equipment is working properly, and that bed is in locked, low position) and provide privacy.
3. Assess degree of help patient will need for bathing, risk for falling (e.g., ability to stand, walk to sink area), patient's risk for skin breakdown, and presence of allergy or sensitivity to bathing solution (e.g., CHG; see Skill 11.1).
4. Arrange supplies and toiletry items at bedside.
5. Perform hand hygiene and apply clean gloves.
6. **Bathing cloths** (this procedure follows the AHRQ [2013] universal bathing protocol for decolonization, used commonly in critical care and acute care hospitals):
   a. Adjust room temperature and ventilation, close room doors and windows, and draw room divider curtain.
   b. Position patient supine or in a position of comfort. Use a bath blanket to drape areas of body not being cleaned as bath proceeds (see Skill 11.1).
   c. Help patient remove old gown (see Skill 11.1).
   d. *Option:* Warm package of bathing cloths in a microwave, following package directions. Do not use a microwave that is used for food preparation. The cleaning pack contains six premoistened cloths.

Safe Patient Care *Check temperature of cloth after warming and have patient check as well to prevent burns to the skin.*

   e. Wash patient's face and eyes with plain warm water (see Skill 11.1).
   f. Use all six bathing cloths in the following order (see illustration), positioning and using drapes as described in Skill 11.1 (AHRQ, 2013):
      (1) Cloth 1: Neck, shoulders, and chest
      (2) Cloth 2: Both arms, both hands, web spaces, and axilla
      (3) Cloth 3: Abdomen and groin/perineum
      (4) Cloth 4: Right leg, right foot, and web spaces
      (5) Cloth 5: Left leg, left foot, and web spaces
      (6) Cloth 6: Back of neck, back, and buttocks

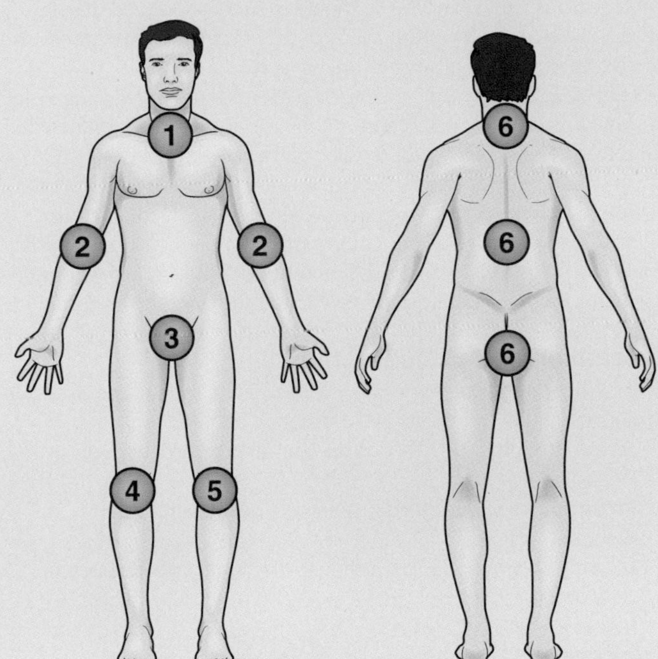

STEP 6f Order for use of six bathing cloths.

   g. Firmly massage skin with CHG cloth. Tell patient that the skin may feel sticky for a few minutes.
   h. Ensure thorough cleaning of soiled areas such as the neck, skinfolds, and perineal areas. CHG is safe to use on perineal areas, including external mucosa. It is also safe for superficial wounds, including stage 1 and stage 2 decubitus pressure injuries (AHRQ, 2013).
   i. Do NOT rinse, wipe off, or dry with another cloth. Allow to air dry (AHRQ, 2013).
   j. CHG cloths have built-in moisturizers, research shows a decrease in skin deterioration when these cloths are used over time (Martin et al., 2017b). Skin may feel sticky for a few minutes.

Continued

PROCEDURAL GUIDELINE 11.1 *Bathing Using Disposable Cloths—cont'd*

k. If additional moisturizer is needed, use only CHG-compatible products.
l. Dispose of leftover cloths and perform hand hygiene
m. Assist patient in applying clean gown. Help patient assume desired comfortable position. Be sure nurse call system is in an accessible location within patient's reach. Raise side rails (as appropriate) and lower bed to lowest position.

7. Evaluate condition of patient's skin. Pay attention to areas that were previously soiled, reddened, blistered, flaking, scaling, or showing signs of breakdown.
8. Ask patient to rate level of fatigue and comfort.

PROCEDURAL GUIDELINE 11.2 *Perineal Care*

Purpose

Perineal care is the thorough cleaning of the patient's external genitalia and surrounding skin. A patient routinely receives perineal care during a complete bed bath (see Skill 11.1). However, patients at risk for acquiring an infection need more frequent perineal care, such as those who have incontinence-associated dermatitis (IAD), have an indwelling Foley catheter, are postpartum, or are recovering from rectal or genital surgery.

This is especially important for patients with indwelling Foley catheters in the effort to reduce catheter-associated urinary tract infection (CAUTI) (Galiczewski, 2016; Meddings et al., 2017). Wear clean gloves during perineal care because of the risk of contact with infectious organisms present in fecal, urinary, or vaginal secretions. To avoid embarrassment, always act in a professional and sensitive manner, ask patient's permission before providing care, and provide patient privacy at all times.

Delegation and Collaboration

The skill of perineal care can be delegated to nursing assistive personnel (NAP). The nurse instructs the NAP to:

- Avoid any physical restriction that affects proper positioning of patient.
- Properly position a patient with an indwelling Foley catheter.
- Inform the nurse of any perineal drainage, excoriation, or rash observed.

Equipment

Washcloths, bath towels, and bath blanket; cleaning product for bath (chlorhexidine gluconate [CHG] cloths can be used for perineal and catheter care; however, some agencies do not use CHG because of concern over risk of mucosal irritation (see agency policy); disposable wipes and wash basin; warm water; laundry bag; waterproof pad or bedpan; clean gloves; additional supplies when perineal care is provided other than during a bath: cotton balls or swabs, solution bottle or container filled with warm water or prescribed rinsing solution, waterproof bag

Procedural Steps

1. Identify patient using at least two identifiers (e.g., name and birthday or name and medical record number) according to agency policy (TJC, 2019).
2. Assess environment for safety (e.g., check room for spills, make sure that any equipment is working properly, and that bed is in locked, low position).
3. Assemble supplies. Provide privacy and explain procedure and importance in preventing infection.
4. Perform hand hygiene. Apply clean gloves. Place basin with warm water and cleansing solution on over-bed table.
5. **Perineal care for a female:**
   a. If patient is able to maneuver and handle washcloth, allow to clean perineum on own.
   b. Help patient assume dorsal recumbent position. Note restrictions or a limitation in patient's positioning. Position waterproof pad under patient's buttocks.
   c. Drape patient with bath blanket placed in shape of a diamond.
   d. Fold both outer corners of bath blanket up around patient's legs onto abdomen and under hip (see illustration). Lift lower tip of bath blanket when you are ready to expose the perineum.

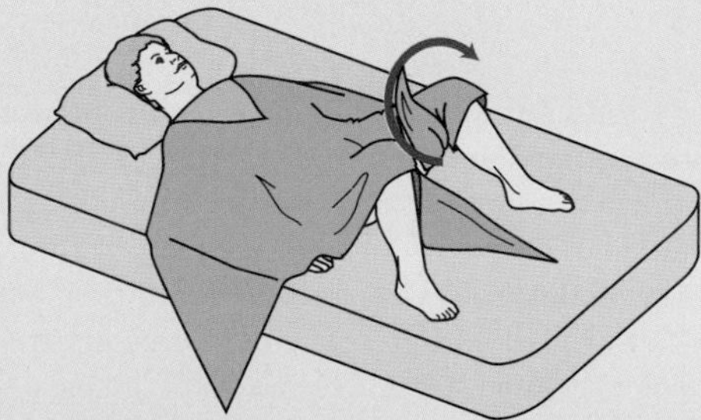

STEP 5d Drape patient for perineal care.

   e. Wash and dry patient's upper thighs. (**NOTE:** If agency uses CHG solution for perineal care, do not rinse; allow to air dry.)
   f. Wash labia majora. Use nondominant hand to gently retract labia from thigh. Use dominant hand to wash carefully in skinfolds. Wipe in direction from perineum to rectum (front to back). Repeat on opposite side using separate section of washcloth or new washcloth. Rinse and dry area thoroughly. Do not rinse if using CHG.

PROCEDURAL GUIDELINE 11.2 *Perineal Care—cont'd*

g. Gently separate labia with nondominant hand to expose urethral meatus and vaginal orifice. With dominant hand wash downward from pubic area toward rectum in one smooth stroke (see illustration). Use separate section of cloth for each stroke. Clean thoroughly over labia minora, clitoris, and vaginal orifice. Rinse and dry thoroughly.

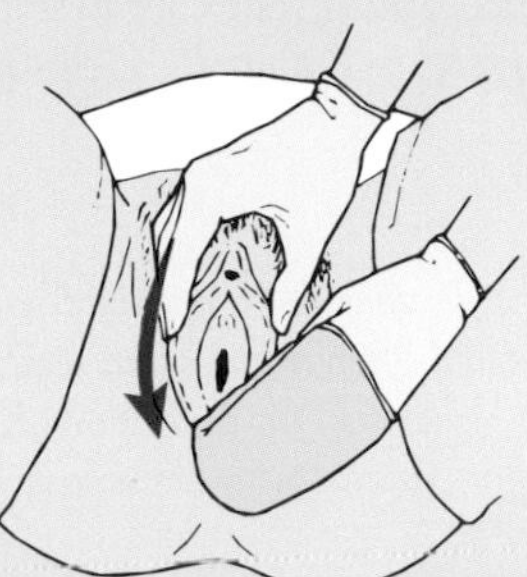

STEP 5g Clean from perineum to rectum (front to back).

Safe Patient Care *Avoid tension on indwelling catheter if present, and clean area around it thoroughly. Follow agency policy regarding perineal care when an indwelling catheter is in place. Currently cleaning periurethral area with antiseptics is not recommended for prevention of CAUTI, but routine perineal care is currently the standard (Martin et al., 2017a; Meddings et al., 2017).*

h. Rinse and dry area thoroughly, using front-to-back method.
i. If patient uses bedpan, pour warm water over perineal area and dry thoroughly. (Exception: Do not rinse if using CHG.)
j. Fold lower corner of bath blanket back between patient's legs and over perineum. Ask patient to lower legs and assume comfortable position.

6. **Perineal care for a male:**
   a. If patient is able to maneuver and handle washcloth, allow him to clean perineum on his own.
   b. Help patient to supine position. Note restriction in mobility.
   c. Fold lower half of bath blanket up to expose upper thighs. Wash, rinse, and dry thighs. Do not rinse if using CHG.
   d. Cover thighs with bath towels. Raise bath blanket to expose genitalia. Gently raise penis and place bath towel underneath. Gently grasp shaft of penis. If patient is uncircumcised, slightly retract foreskin. If patient has an erection, defer procedure until later.
   e. Wash tip of penis at urethral meatus first. Using circular motion, clean from meatus outward (see illustration). Discard washcloth and repeat with clean cloth until penis is clean. Rinse and dry gently and thoroughly. (Exception: Do not rinse if using CHG.)

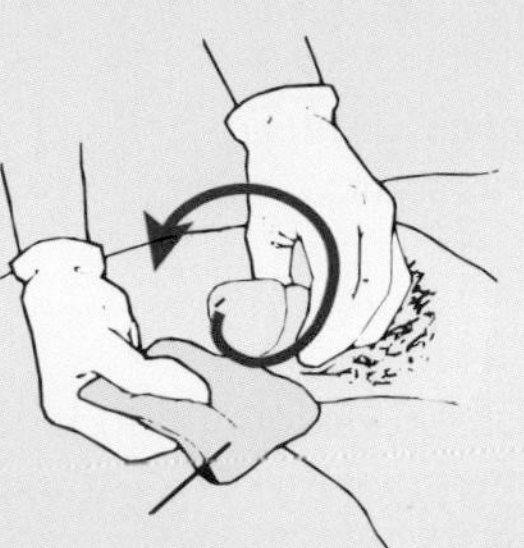

STEP 6e Use circular motion to clean tip of penis.

   f. Return foreskin to its natural position.

Safe Patient Care *After administering male perineal care for uncircumcised males, make sure that foreskin is in its natural position. This is extremely important in patients with decreased sensation in their lower extremities. Tightening foreskin around shaft of penis causes local edema; discomfort; and, if not corrected, may cause permanent urethral damage.*

   g. Take a new washcloth and gently clean shaft of penis and scrotum by having patient abduct legs. Pay special attention to underlying surface of penis. Lift scrotum carefully and wash underlying skinfolds. Rinse and dry thoroughly. (Exception: Do not rinse if using CHG.)
   h. Fold bath blanket back over patient's perineum and help him to comfortable position.
7. For both female and male patient, avoid placing tension on an indwelling catheter, if present, and clean around it thoroughly during procedure.
8. Inspect perineal area for any irritation, redness, or drainage that persists after perineal hygiene.
9. Remove and dispose of gloves and used supplies in proper receptacles and perform hand hygiene.

✦ SKILL 11.2 Performing Mouth Care for an Unconscious or Debilitated Patient

Purpose

Special oral care is needed for unconscious or debilitated patients because they are more susceptible to infection due to the change in the normal flora of the oral cavity, increased plaque formation from the dryness of the mouth, and decreased salivation. Dryness of the oral mucosa is also caused by mouth breathing and oxygen therapy. Respiratory secretions often are thick and place patients at risk for ineffective airway clearance, requiring oral suction (see Chapter 16). The secretions in the oral cavity change very rapidly to gram-negative pneumonia-producing bacteria if aspiration occurs.

Because many debilitated patients have either a reduced or absent gag reflex, providing oral care requires protection of patients from choking and aspiration. The safest technique is to have two nurses provide care. You provide oral care while another nurse or nursing assistive personnel (NAP) suctions oral secretions as necessary with a Yankauer suction tip (see Chapter 16). Evaluate the level and frequency of oral care daily during assessment of the oral cavity.

Delegation and Collaboration

The skill of providing oral hygiene to an unconscious or debilitated patient can be delegated to nursing assistive personnel (NAP). The nurse is responsible for assessing a patient's gag reflex. The nurse instructs the NAP to:

- Have another NAP assist and properly position patient for mouth care.
- Be aware of special precautions such as aspiration precautions.
- Use an oral suction catheter for clearing oral secretions (see Skill 16.3).
- Report signs of impaired integrity of oral mucosa, any bleeding of mucosa or gums, excessive coughing, or choking to the nurse.

Equipment

- Small pediatric, soft-bristled toothbrush, toothette sponges, or suction toothbrushes for patients for whom brushing is contraindicated.
- Antibacterial solution per agency policy (e.g., chlorhexidine gluconate [CHG 0.12%])
- Fluoride toothpaste
- Water-based mouth moisturizer
- Tongue blade
- Penlight
- Oral suction equipment
- Oral airway (uncooperative patient or patient who shows bite reflex)
- Water-soluble lip lubricant
- Water glass with cool water
- Face and bath towel
- Emesis basin
- Clean gloves

ASSESSMENT

1. Identify patient using at least two identifiers (e.g., name and birthday or name and medical record number) according to agency policy. *Rationale: Ensures patient safety. Complies with The Joint Commission standards and improves patient safety (TJC, 2019).*
2. Assess environment for safety (e.g., check the room for spills, make sure that equipment is working properly, and that bed is in locked, low position). *Rationale: Identifies safety hazards in patient environment that could cause or potentially lead to harm (QSEN, 2014).*
3. Assess patient's risk for oral hygiene problems (see Procedural Guideline 11.3). *Rationale: Certain conditions increase likelihood of alterations in integrity of oral cavity mucosa and structures, necessitating more frequent care.*
4. Perform hand hygiene and apply clean gloves. *Rationale: Reduces transmission of microorganisms in blood or saliva.*
5. Assess for presence of gag reflex by placing tongue blade on back half of tongue. *Rationale: Helps in determining aspiration risk.*

Safe Patient Care *Patients with impaired gag reflex are unable to clear airway secretions and often accumulate secretions in the back of the oral cavity and have a higher risk for aspiration. Keep suction equipment available when caring for patients who are at risk for aspiration.*

6. Inspect condition of oral cavity. Inspect lips, teeth, gums, buccal mucosa, palate, and tongue using tongue depressor and penlight if necessary (see Chapter 8). Observe for color, moisture, lesions, injury, or ulcers and condition of teeth or dentures. *Rationale: Determines condition of oral cavity and need for hygiene. Establishes baseline to show improvement following oral care.*

Safe Patient Care *The critically ill patient with an artificial airway who is on mechanical ventilation is at risk for ventilator-associated pneumonia (VAP). Once intubated, the artificial airway causes a bypass of normal airway defenses, which also causes a rapid change in the normal oral flora (CDC, 2018). Some patients require mouth care as often as every 1 to 2 hours until the mucosa returns to normal.*

7. Assess patient's respirations or oxygen saturation. *Rationale: Assists in early recognition of aspiration.*
8. Remove gloves. Perform hand hygiene. *Rationale: Prevents transmission of infection.*

STEP	RATIONALE
PLANNING	
1. Expected outcomes following completion of procedure:	
• Oral cavity structures have normal characteristics: Buccal mucosa and tongue are pink, moist, and intact. Gums are moist and intact. Teeth are clean, smooth, and shiny. Tongue is pink and without coating. Lips are moist, smooth, and without cracks.	Degree of improvement in condition of oral cavity following oral hygiene depends on extent of secretions or changes that existed before care.
• Debilitated patient expresses feeling of mouth cleanliness.	Comfort achieved.
• Oropharynx remains clear of secretions.	Secretions removed, thus avoiding aspiration.
2. Gather equipment and supplies at bedside.	Avoids interrupting procedure or leaving patient unattended to retrieve missing equipment.
3. Explain procedure to patient or family caregiver if present.	Even debilitated or intubated patients are usually able to hear. Explanation can reduce anxiety.

STEP	RATIONALE

IMPLEMENTATION

STEP	RATIONALE
1. Pull curtain around bed or close room door.	Provides privacy.
2. Perform hand hygiene and apply clean gloves.	Reduces transfer of microorganisms.
3. Raise bed to appropriate working height; lower side rail. Unless contraindicated (e.g., head injury, neck trauma), position patient in Sims' or side-lying position. Turn patient's head toward mattress in dependent position with head of bed (HOB) elevated at least 30 degrees.	Position promotes drainage of secretions from mouth instead of collecting in back of pharynx. Prevents aspiration.
4. Place towel on over-bed table and arrange equipment. If needed turn on suction machine and connect tubing to suction catheter.	Prevents soiling of tabletop. Equipment prepared in advance ensures smooth, safe procedure. Supplies within reach create organized workspace.
5. Place towel under patient's head and emesis basin under chin.	Prevents soiling of bed linen.
6. Remove dentures or partial plates if present.	Allows for thorough cleaning of prosthetics later. Provides clearer access to oral cavity.
7. If patient is uncooperative or having difficulty keeping mouth open, insert an oral airway. Insert upside down and turn airway sideways and over tongue to keep teeth apart. Insert when patient is relaxed if possible. Do not use force.	Prevents patient from biting down on nurse's fingers and provides access to oral cavity.

Safe Patient Care *Never place fingers into the mouth of an unconscious or debilitated patient. This could occlude the airway. Also, the normal response is to bite down.*

STEP	RATIONALE
8. Clean mouth using brush moistened in water. Apply toothpaste or use antibacterial solution first to loosen crusts. Hold toothbrush bristles at 45-degree angle to gum line. Be sure that tips of bristles rest against and penetrate under gum line. Brush inner and outer surfaces of upper and lower teeth by brushing from gum to crown of each tooth, then clean biting surfaces of teeth by holding top of bristles parallel with teeth and brushing gently back and forth (see Procedural Guideline 11.3). Brush sides of teeth by moving bristles back and forth. Use a toothette sponge if patient has a bleeding tendency or if use of toothbrush is contraindicated (see illustration). Suction any accumulated secretions. Moisten brush with clear water or CHG solution to rinse. Use brush or toothette to clean roof of mouth, gums, and inside cheeks. Gently brush tongue but avoid stimulating gag reflex (if present). Repeat rinsing several times and use suction to remove secretions. Use towel to dry off lips.	Brushing action removes food particles between teeth, along chewing surfaces and crusts for mucosa. The use of a chlorhexidine gluconate (CHG) oral hygiene protocol as part of daily oral care reduces the incidence of VAP (de Lacerda Vidal et al., 2017; Villar et al., 2015). The Institute for Healthcare Improvement (2017) recommends the use of 0.12% chlorhexidine gluconate (CHG) as part of daily oral care in critically ill patients. Repeated rinsing removes all debris and aids in moistening mucosa. Suction removes secretions and fluids that collect in posterior pharynx, thus reducing aspiration risk.

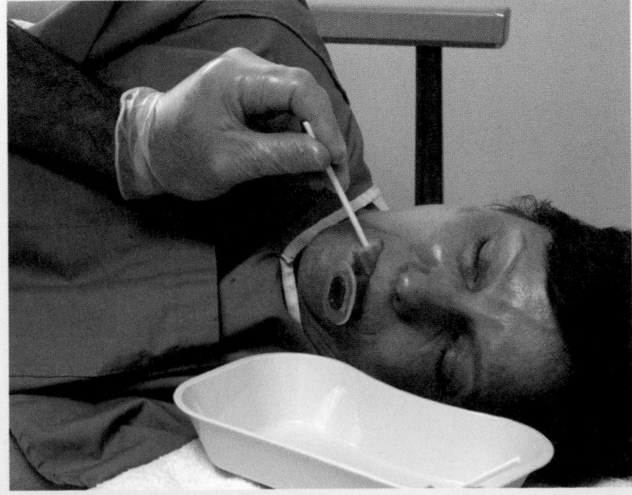

STEP 8 Cleaning lips and mucosa around oral airway with toothette.

STEP	RATIONALE
9. Apply thin layer of water-soluble moisturizer to lips (see illustration).	Lubricates lips to prevent drying and cracking.

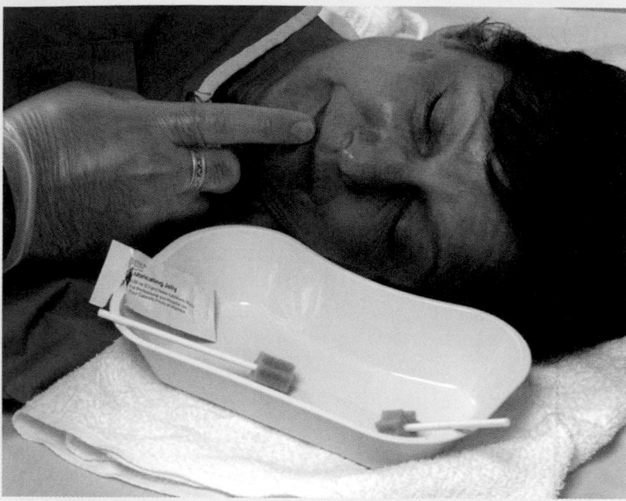

STEP 9 Application of water-soluble moisturizer to lips.

STEP	RATIONALE
10. Inform patient that procedure is completed. Return him or her to comfortable and safe position.	Provides meaningful stimulation to unconscious or less-responsive patient.
11. Raise side rails as appropriate and return bed to locked, low position. Be sure nurse call system is in an accessible location within patient's reach.	Reduces risk of falls from bed.
12. Clean equipment and return to its proper place. Place soiled linen in dirty laundry bag.	Proper disposal of soiled equipment prevents spread of infection.
13. Remove and dispose of gloves in proper receptacle and perform hand hygiene.	Reduces transmission of microorganisms.

EVALUATION

1. Apply clean gloves and use tongue blade and penlight to inspect oral cavity.	Determines efficacy of cleaning. Once thick secretions are removed, underlying inflammation or lesions may be revealed.
2. Ask debilitated patient if mouth feels clean.	Evaluates level of comfort.
3. **Use Teach-Back:** "I explained what is needed to reduce your husband's risk of choking on secretions in his throat. Tell me the ways to prevent him from choking." Revise your instruction now or develop a plan for revised family caregiver teaching if family caregiver is not able to teach back correctly.	Determines family caregiver's level of understanding of instructional topic.

Unexpected Outcomes	Related Interventions
1. Secretions or crusts remain on mucosa, tongue, or gums.	• Provide more frequent oral hygiene.
2. Localized inflammation or bleeding of gums or mucosa is present.	• Provide more frequent oral hygiene with toothette sponges. • Apply a water-based mouth moisturizer to provide moisture and maintain integrity of oral mucosa. • Chemotherapy and radiation can cause mucositis (inflammation of mucous membranes in mouth) because of sloughing of epithelial tissue. Room-temperature saline rinses, bicarbonate and sterile water rinses, and oral care with a soft-bristled toothbrush decrease severity and duration of mucositis.
3. Lips are cracked or inflamed.	• Apply moisturizing gel or water-soluble lubricant to lips more often.
4. Patient aspirates secretions.	• Suction oral airway as secretions accumulate to maintain airway patency (see Chapter 16). • Elevate patient's HOB to facilitate breathing. • If aspiration is suspected, notify health care provider. Prepare patient for chest x-ray examination.

Recording

- Record procedure, appearance of oral cavity, presence of gag reflex, and patient's response to procedure.

Hand-Off Reporting

- Use agency's standardized hand-off communication to communicate specific patient risks for aspiration and dry mouth. Discuss patient-specific interventions taken.
- Report any unusual findings (e.g., bleeding, ulceration, choking response) to nurse in charge or health care provider.
- Report immediately to the health care provider if patient aspirates or there are lesions or irritation in oral cavity.

PROCEDURAL GUIDELINE 11.3 *Oral Hygiene*

Purpose

Daily oral hygiene, including brushing, flossing, and rinsing, is essential for the prevention and control of plaque-associated oral diseases. In addition to preventing inflammation and infection, oral hygiene in general promotes comfort, ease of swallowing for better food intake, and verbal communication. Brushing cleans the teeth of food particles, plaque (the cause of dental caries), and bacteria; massages the gums; and relieves discomfort from unpleasant odors and tastes. Flossing removes tartar that collects at the gum line. Rinsing removes dislodged food particles and excess toothpaste.

Delegation and Collaboration

The skill of oral hygiene (including tooth brushing, flossing, and rinsing) can be delegated to nursing assistive personnel (NAP). However, the nurse is responsible for assessing the patient's gag reflex to determine whether the patient is at risk for aspiration. The nurse instructs the NAP about:

- Types of changes in oral mucosa (e.g., presence of lesions or open sores) to report to the nurse.
- Positioning the patient to avoid aspiration.
- Keeping head of bed (HOB) raised 30 to 45 degrees.
- Explaining the need to immediately report to the nurse excessive patient coughing or choking during or after oral hygiene.
- Reporting bleeding of oral mucosa or gums, patient report of pain, and any changes in oral mucosa (e.g., open areas or lesions).
- Not flossing when the patient has a bleeding tendency.

Equipment

Soft-bristle toothbrush; nonabrasive fluoride toothpaste; dental floss; chlorhexidine gluconate (CHG) solution (*optional*, see agency policy); tongue depressor; water glass with cool water, normal saline, or an antiseptic mouth rinse (*optional*, depending on patient preference); moisturizing lubricant for lips (*optional*); emesis basin; face towel; paper towels; clean gloves; penlight; linen bag or hamper

Procedural Steps

1. Identify patient using at least two identifiers (e.g., name and birthday or name and medical record number) according to agency policy (TJC, 2019).
2. Review medical record and identify presence of common oral hygiene problems.
3. Determine patient's oral hygiene practices, such as frequency of brushing and flossing, type of toothpaste and mouthwash used, last and frequency of dental visits.
4. Perform hand hygiene and apply clean gloves.
5. Using tongue depressor and penlight, inspect integrity of lips, teeth, buccal mucosa, gums, palate, and tongue; also, assess for gag reflex and ability to swallow (see Chapter 8). Note the presence of dental caries—chalky white discoloration of tooth or presence of brown or black discoloration; gingivitis—inflammation of gums; periodontitis—receding gum lines, inflammation, gaps between teeth; halitosis—bad breath; cheilitis—cracked lips; dry, cracked, and coated tongue.
6. Remove gloves and perform hand hygiene.
7. Explain procedure to patient, discussing patient's preferences and assess patient's ability to grasp and manipulate toothbrush and willingness to help with oral care.
8. Place paper towels on over-bed table and arrange other equipment within easy reach.
9. Provide privacy by closing room doors and drawing room divider curtain. Raise bed to comfortable working position. Raise head of bed (if allowed) and lower near side rail. Move patient or help him or her move closer to side. Place patient in side-lying position if needed (if aspiration risk). Place towel over patient's chest.
10. Apply clean gloves. Apply enough toothpaste to brush to cover length of bristles. Hold brush over emesis basin. Pour small amount of water over toothpaste.
11. Patient may help with brushing. Hold toothbrush bristles at 45-degree angle to gum line (see illustration A). Be sure that tips of bristles rest against and penetrate under gum line. Brush inner and outer surfaces of upper and lower teeth by brushing from gum to crown of each tooth. Clean biting surfaces of teeth by holding top of bristles parallel with teeth and brushing gently back and forth (see illustration B). Brush sides of teeth by moving bristles back and forth (see illustration C).

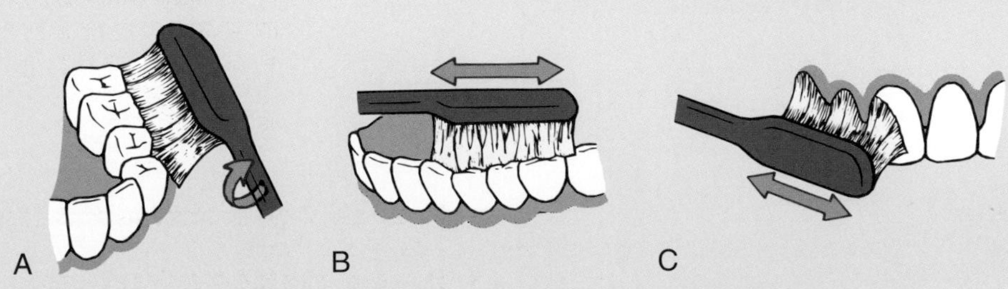

STEP 11 Direction of brushing for tooth brushing

Continued

PROCEDURAL GUIDELINE 11.3 *Oral Hygiene—cont'd*

12. Have patient hold brush at 45-degree angle and lightly brush over surface and sides of tongue (see illustration). Avoid initiating gag reflex.
13. Allow patient to rinse mouth thoroughly by taking several sips of cool water, swishing water across all tooth surfaces, and spitting into emesis basin. Use this time to observe patient's brushing technique and teach importance of regular hygiene.
14. Have patient rinse mouth with antiseptic rinse for 30 seconds. Then have patient spit rinse into emesis basin. Help wipe patient's mouth.
15. Floss or allow patient to floss between all teeth (see illustration).
16. Allow patient to rinse mouth thoroughly with cool water and spit into emesis basin. Help wipe his or her mouth.
17. Inspect oral cavity to determine effectiveness of oral hygiene and rinsing. Ask patient if mouth feels clean or if there are any sore or tender areas. Remove towel and place in linen bag.
18. Remove gloves and perform hand hygiene. Help patient to comfortable position, raise side rail, and lower bed to original position. Be sure nurse call system is within reach.
19. Report bleeding, pain, or presence of lesions to nurse in charge or health care provider.

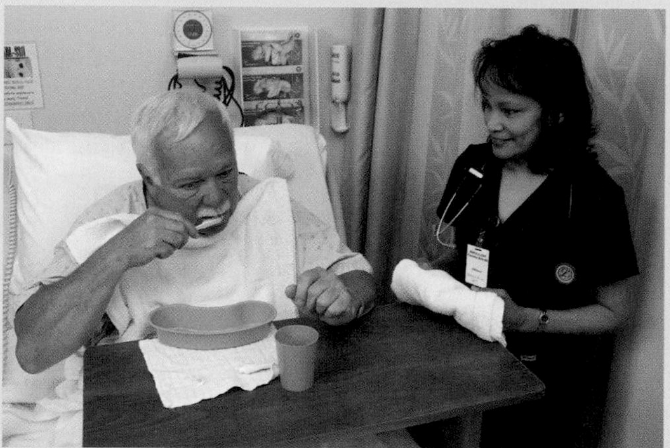

STEP 12 Nurse observes patient's tooth-brushing technique

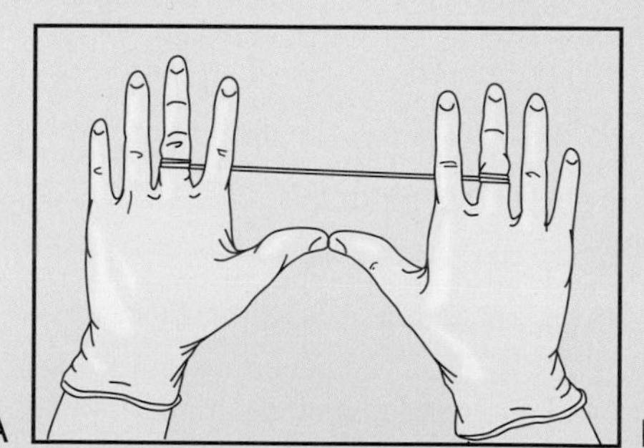

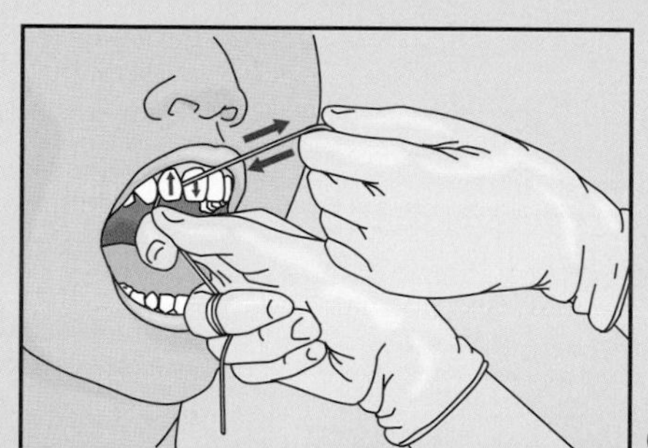

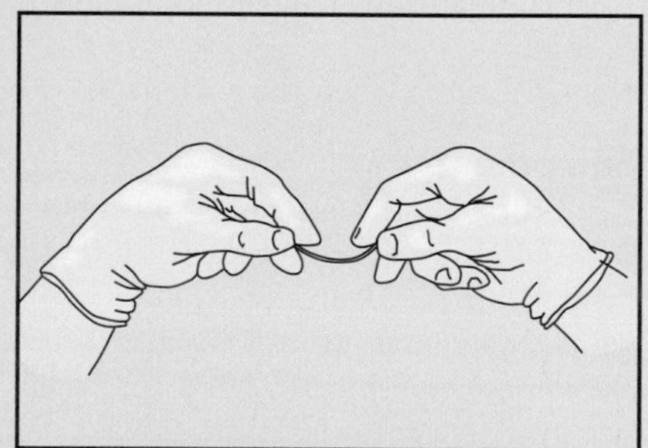

STEP 15 Flossing. (A) Dental floss is held between middle fingers to floss upper teeth. (B) Floss is moved in up-and-down motions between teeth. Floss is moved up and down from crown to gum line. (C) Floss is held with index fingers to floss lower teeth.

PROCEDURAL GUIDELINE 11.4 *Care of Dentures*

Purpose

Denture care removes food and debris from and around dentures. In addition, routine denture care reduces the risk for gingival infection. Denture stomatitis is a common form of candidiasis and is also caused by other oral bacteria (Moosazadeh et al., 2016; Villar et al., 2015). Encourage patients who wear dentures to continue to care for them as frequently as with natural teeth. Loose dentures can cause discomfort and make it difficult for patients to chew food and speak clearly. Offer dental care after every meal and before a patient goes to bed. Some patients are unable to care for their dentures, and nurses become responsible for providing denture and oral care. Dentures are a patient's personal property; thus, be sure to handle them with care because they are easy to break.

Delegation and Collaboration

The skill of denture care can be delegated to nursing assistive personnel (NAP). The nurse instructs the NAP to:

- Not use hot or excessively cold water when caring for dentures.
- Inform the nurse if there are cracks in dentures.
- Inform the nurse if the patient has any oral discomfort and trouble eating.

Equipment

Soft-bristled toothbrush or denture toothbrush; denture dentifrice or toothpaste, denture adhesive *(optional)*; glass of water; emesis basin or sink; 4 × 4–inch gauze; washcloth; denture cup (for storage); clean gloves

Procedural Steps

1. Identify patient using at least two identifiers (e.g., name and birthday or name and medical record number) according to agency policy (TJC, 2019).
2. Assess environment for safety (e.g., check room for spills; make sure that equipment is working properly, and that bed is in locked, low position).
3. Perform hand hygiene.
4. Inspect oral cavity and ask patient if dentures fit and if there is any gum or mucous membrane tenderness or irritation. Ask patient about denture care and product preferences.
5. Determine if patient has necessary dexterity to clean dentures independently or requires help.
6. Position patient comfortably sitting up in bed or help him or her walk from bed to chair placed in front of sink.
7. Fill emesis basin with tepid water. (If using sink, place washcloth in bottom of sink and fill sink with approximately 2.5 cm [1 inch] of water.)
8. Perform hand hygiene again and apply clean gloves.
9. Ask patient to remove dentures. If patient is unable to do this independently, grasp upper plate at front with thumb and index finger wrapped in gauze and pull downward. Gently lift lower denture from jaw and rotate one side downward to remove from patient's mouth. Place dentures in emesis basin or sink lined with washcloth and 2.5 cm (1 inch) of water.
10. Observe oral cavity, paying attention to gums, tongue, and upper palate. Observe for lesions, plaques, and areas of irritation. Palpate areas as needed.

Safe Patient Care *Oral mucosal lesions are common in older adults, especially those with dentures. These lesions are associated with local and systemic factors, and tongue lesions may be the first to appear (Pedersen et al., 2015).*

11. Apply cleaning agent to brush and brush surfaces of dentures (see illustration). Hold dentures close to water. Hold brush horizontally and use back-and-forth motion to clean biting surfaces. Use short strokes from top of denture to biting surfaces to clean outer teeth surfaces. Hold brush vertically and use short strokes to clean inner teeth surfaces. Hold brush horizontally and use back-and-forth motion to clean undersurface of dentures (see Procedural Guideline 11.3).

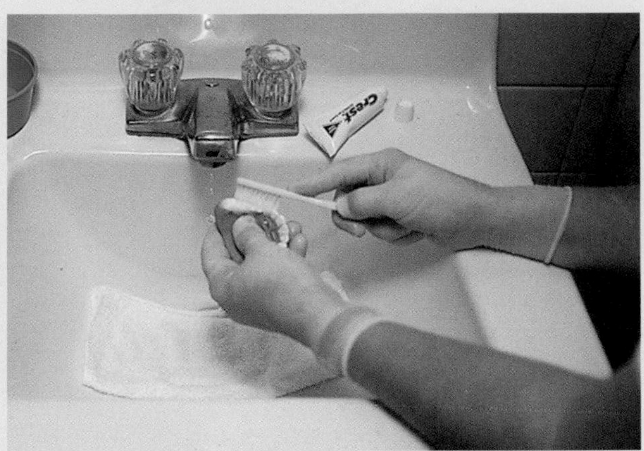

STEP 11 Brushing surface of dentures.

12. Rinse thoroughly in tepid water. If water is too cold, dentures can crack. If it is too hot, dentures can become warped and no longer fit.
13. When necessary apply a thin layer of denture adhesive to undersurface before inserting. Reinsert dentures as soon as possible. If patient needs help with inserting dentures, moisten upper denture and press firmly to seal it in place. Insert moistened lower denture (if applicable). Ask if denture(s) feel comfortable. **NOTE:** It is common for patients to choose to not wear their dentures during an acute illness.
14. Some patients prefer to store their dentures to give gums a rest and reduce risk for infection. Store in tepid water in enclosed, labeled denture cup. Keep denture cup in a secure place labeled with patient's name to prevent loss when not worn (e.g., at night, during surgery).
15. Dispose of supplies. Remove and discard gloves and perform hand hygiene.
16. Help patient assume desired comfortable position. Be sure nurse call system is in an accessible location within patient's reach. Raise side rails (as appropriate) and lower bed to lowest position.

PROCEDURAL GUIDELINE 11.5 *Foot and Nail Care*

Purpose

Care of the nails is important to prevent pain and infections. Nail and foot care should be incorporated into a patient's daily hygiene during a daily bath; however, keep in mind that many agencies require a health care provider's order before you can trim nails. Often people are unaware of foot or nail problems until discomfort or pain occurs (Table 11.2). For proper foot and nail care, instruct patients to protect the feet from injury, keep them clean and dry, and wear appropriate footwear. Instruct patients how to properly inspect the feet for lesions, dryness, or signs of infection.

People with peripheral vascular disease and diabetes develop many types of foot complications associated with nerve damage and poor blood flow to the lower extremities. Foot injuries in these patients can quickly turn into a serious problem with slow healing, infection, and the possibility of amputation. If a patient has diabetes or any other condition affecting peripheral circulation or sensation, recommend a podiatrist for regular examinations and trimming of nails (American Podiatric Medical Association, 2017).

Delegation and Collaboration

The skill of nail and foot care of patients *without diabetes mellitus* or *circulatory compromise* can be delegated to nursing assistive personnel (NAP). The nurse instructs the NAP about:

- Not trimming patient's nails (unless permitted by agency or health care provider).
- Special considerations for patient positioning.
- Reporting any breaks in skin, redness, numbness, swelling, or pain to the nurse.

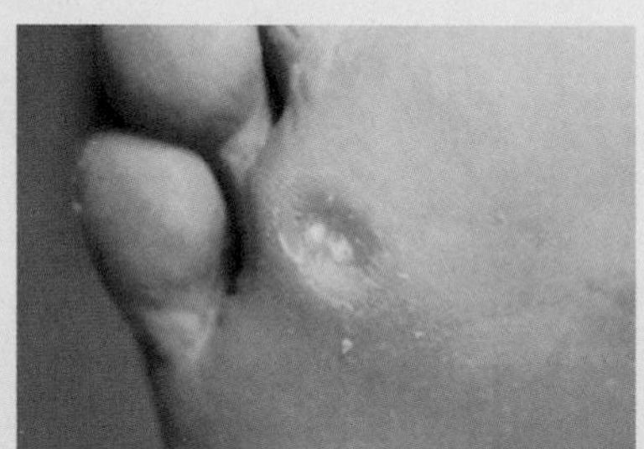

FIG 11.1 Corn. *(From Weston WL, Lane AT:* Color textbook of pediatric dermatology, *ed 4, St. Louis, 2007, Mosby.)*

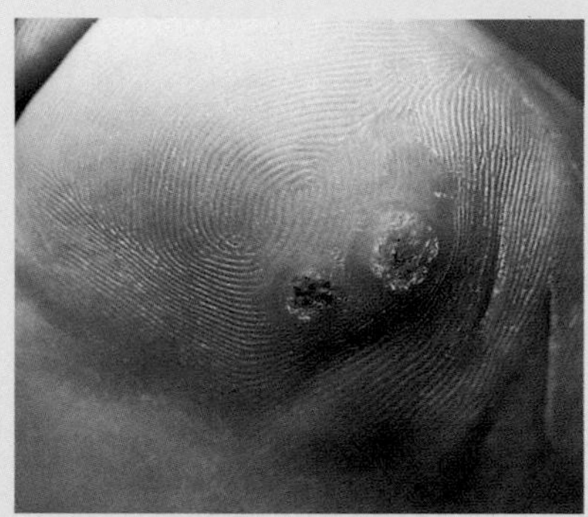

FIG 11.2 Plantar warts. *(From Zitelli BJ, Davis HW:* Atlas of pediatric physical diagnosis, *ed 3, St. Louis, 1997, Mosby.)*

TABLE 11.2

Common Foot and Nail Problems and Related Interventions

Problem	Prevention	Interventions
Callus: Thickened epidermis, usually flat, painless, and on underside of foot; caused by friction or pressure.	Wear proper footwear and always wear clean socks or stockings.	Soak callus in warm water to soften. Creams or lotions can help prevent reformation. Refer patient with diabetes or peripheral vascular disease to a podiatrist.
Corns: Caused by friction and pressure from shoes, mainly on toes, over bony prominence; usually cone-shaped, round, raised, and tender; may affect gait (Fig. 11.1).	Wear proper footwear; pain is aggravated by tight shoes. Always wear clean socks or stockings.	Surgical removal may be necessary. Use oval corn pads carefully because they increase pressure on toes and reduce circulation. Refer patient to podiatrist.
Plantar warts: Fungating lesions on sole of foot caused by papillomavirus (Fig. 11.2).	Warts are contagious. Avoid going barefoot, especially in public places.	Treatment ordered by a podiatrist may include applications of acid, burning, or freezing for removal.
Athlete's foot: Fungal infection of foot; scaling and cracking of skin occur between toes and on soles of feet; may have small blisters containing fluid. Apparently induced by tight footwear (Fig. 11.3).	Feet should be well ventilated. Avoid tight footwear. Dry feet well after bathing; apply powder. Wear clean socks.	Treat with medicated powder or cream. Refer to physician if condition does not improve with medicated products.
Ingrown nails: Toenail or fingernail grows inward into soft tissue around nail; may be painful (Fig. 11.4).	Cut with a nail clipper and file toenails straight across after bathing when they are soft. If nails are thick or vision is poor, have toenails trimmed by a podiatrist.	Treat with frequent warm soaks in antiseptic solution. Surgical removal of portion of nail that has grown into skin may be necessary. Refer patients with diabetes or peripheral vascular disease to podiatrist.
Fungus infection: Thick, discolored nails with yellow streaks.	Keep feet and nails clean and dry. Check feet and nails daily.	Refer to podiatrist.

PROCEDURAL GUIDELINE 11.5 *Foot and Nail Care—cont'd*

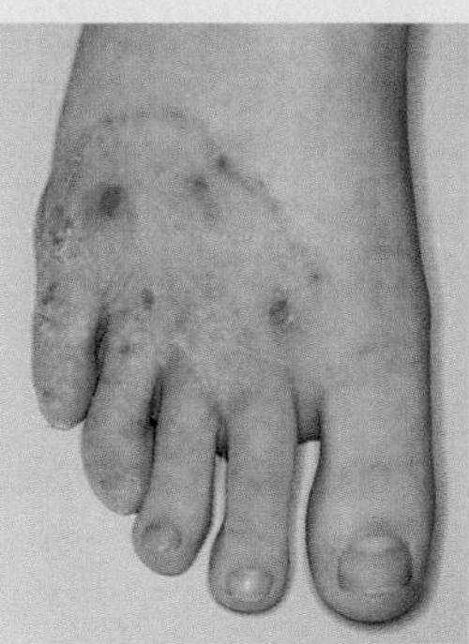

FIG 11.3 Athlete's foot (tinea pedis). *(From Callen J, et al:* Color atlas of dermatology, *ed 2, Philadelphia, 2000, Saunders.)*

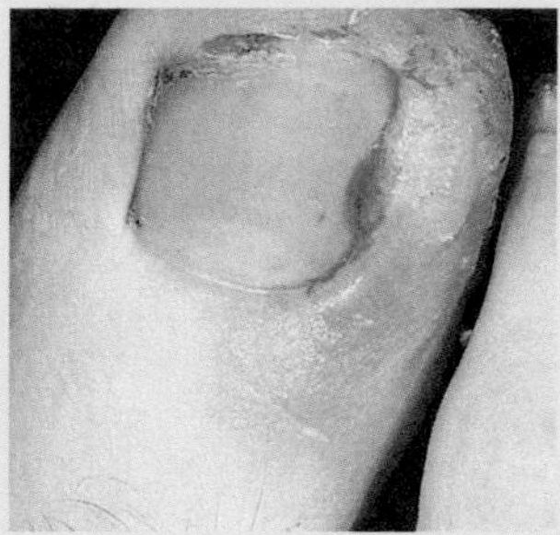

FIG 11.4 Ingrown toenail. *(From Habif TP:* Clinical dermatology: a color guide to diagnosis and therapy, *ed 2, St. Louis, 1990, Mosby.)*

Equipment

Washbasin; emesis basin; washcloth and towel; nail clippers (check agency policy); soft nail or cuticle brush; plastic applicator stick; emery board or nail file; body lotion; disposable bath mat; clean gloves

Procedural Steps

1. Identify patient using at least two identifiers (e.g., name and birthday or name and medical record number, according to agency policy) (TJC, 2019).
2. Verify health care provider's order for cutting nails (check agency policy).
3. Assess environment for safety (e.g., check room for spills; make sure that equipment is working properly, and that bed is in locked, low position).
4. Assess patient's foot and nail care practices for existing foot problems (e.g., home remedies such as cutting corns with razor blade or scissors, applying adhesive tape on foot, or using oval corn pads on toes). Use this time to instruct patients about foot care.
5. Assess type of footwear worn by patients, including type and cleanliness of socks worn, type and fit of shoes, and restrictive garters or knee-high hose.
6. Identify if patient is at risk for foot or nail problems, such as reduced visual acuity, history of diabetes, or history of stroke.
7. Perform hand hygiene and inspect all surfaces of toes, feet, and nails. Pay particular attention to areas of dryness, inflammation, or cracking. Also inspect areas between toes, heels, and soles of feet.
8. Palpate the dorsalis pedis pulse of both feet simultaneously, comparing the strength of pulses (see Chapter 8). Note color and warmth of toes and feet. Observe for capillary refill of nails. (Refill of less than 3 seconds indicates reduced circulation.)
9. Assess sensation in the feet by checking for light touch or discrimination between warm and cold. Perform hand hygiene.
10. Determine patient's ability to perform self-care.
11. Pull curtain around bed or close room door to provide privacy.
12. Prepare to soak feet and fingers:
    a. Explain procedure to patient. Inform patient that proper soaking requires 10 to 20 minutes.
    b. Assist ambulatory patient to sit in chair and place disposable bath mat on floor under patient's feet. Help patient who must stay in bed to supine position with head of bed elevated 45 degrees and place waterproof pad on mattress (keep side rail up until ready to begin).
    c. Fill washbasin with warm water. Test water temperature with back of hand. Place basin on floor or lower side rail and place basin on pad on mattress. Have patient immerse feet.

Safe Patient Care *Patients with diabetes mellitus, peripheral neuropathy, or peripheral vascular disease (PVD) should not soak their feet because of the potential for increased skin dryness and a decreased ability to assess temperature variations related to decreased sensations (ADA, 2014).*

13. Foot and nail care:
    a. Allow patient's feet and fingers to soak for 10 to 20 minutes. If necessary, rewarm water after 10 minutes.
    b. Apply clean gloves. Begin care on fingernails. Clean gently under nails with plastic applicator stick or soft brush while immersing fingers (see illustration).

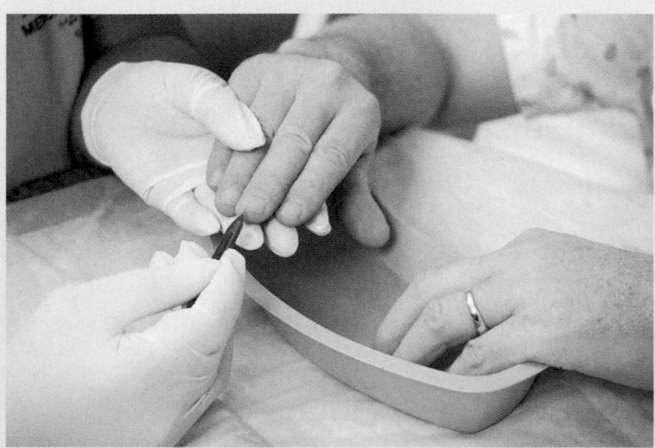

STEP 13b Clean under fingernails.

Continued

PROCEDURAL GUIDELINE 11.5 *Foot and Nail Care—cont'd*

c. Remove hands from basin and dry thoroughly.

d. File fingernails straight across and even with tops of fingers. If permitted by agency policy, use nail clippers and clip fingernails straight across and even with tops of fingers (see illustration) and then smooth nail using file.

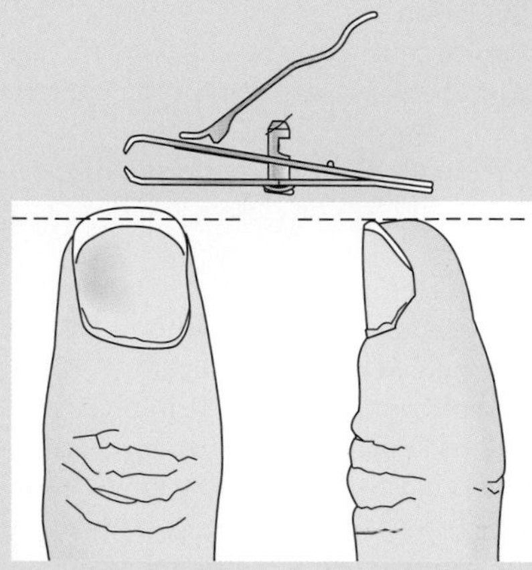

STEP 13d Trim nails straight across when using nail clipper.

e. Use soft cuticle brush or nail brush to clean around cuticles.

14. Move over-bed table away from patient and begin foot care by scrubbing callused areas of feet with washcloth.
    a. Clean between toes with washcloth.
    b. Dry feet thoroughly and trim or cut toenails if permitted by agency policy (see Step 13d).
15. Remove and dispose of gloves. Apply thin layer of lotion to patient's hands and feet. Rub in thoroughly. Do not leave excess lotion between toes.
16. Assist patient back to bed or into a comfortable chair. Be sure nurse call system is within reach. Raise side rails (as appropriate) and lower bed to lowest position.
17. Sanitize equipment according to agency policy. Dispose of used equipment and perform hand hygiene.
18. Inspect nails, cuticles, and areas between fingers and toes and surrounding skin surfaces.

Safe Patient Care *Instruct patients to report any of the following to their health care provider: abnormalities or changes in the nail, including changes in nail shape or color; bleeding around the nails; thinning or thickening of the nails; and redness, swelling, or pain around the nails.*

19. When possible observe patient walk following foot and nail care.
20. Ask patient about any pain or discomfort
21. Return patient to comfortable position. Return bed to locked, low position, and raise side rail (as needed). Be sure nurse call system is within patient's reach.

PROCEDURAL GUIDELINE 11.6 *Hair Care—Combing, Shampooing, and Shaving*

Purpose

A person's comfort, appearance, and sense of well-being are influenced by how the hair looks and feels. Combing, shampooing, and shaving are basic hygiene measures for all patients unable to provide self-care. Many facilities have a beauty shop where patients can go for professional hair care. An immobilized patient's hair soon becomes tangled if not brushed or combed regularly. Dressings may leave sticky adhesive, blood, or antiseptic solutions on the hair. Diaphoresis leaves hair oily and unmanageable. Fever, malnutrition, some medications, emotional stress, and depression affect the condition of hair. Table 11.3 describes common hair and scalp conditions and nursing interventions.

Delegation and Collaboration

The skills of combing, shampooing, and shaving can be delegated to nursing assistive personnel (NAP). The nurse instructs the NAP to:

- Properly position a patient with head or neck mobility restrictions.
- Provide lice care when needed, stressing steps to take to prevent transmission to other patients.
- Report how the patient tolerated the procedure and any concerns (e.g., neck pain).
- Use an electric razor for shaving any patient at risk for bleeding tendencies.

Equipment

Hair Care: Wide-tooth comb and hairbrush

Regular Shampoo: Washcloth; shampoo, hair conditioner *(optional)*, hydrogen peroxide *(optional)*; water pitcher with warm water; plastic shampoo board, wash basin; bath blanket, waterproof pad; hydrogen peroxide and saline *(optional)*

Disposable Shampoo: Disposable shampoo cap product

Shaving With Razor: New disposable or electric razor; clean gloves; bath towel(s), mirror, washcloth, washbasin; shaving cream or soap, aftershave lotion (if patient desires and not contraindicated)

Mustache Care: Scissors, brush or comb; bath towel; gooseneck lamp or overhead light

Procedural Steps

1. Identify patient using at least two identifiers (e.g., name and birthday or name and medical record number) according to agency policy (TJC, 2019).
2. Review medical record to determine that there are no contraindications to procedure. Check agency policy for health care provider order as needed. Certain medical conditions such as head and neck injuries, spinal cord injuries, and arthritis place patient at risk for injury during

PROCEDURAL GUIDELINE 11.6 *Hair Care—Combing, Shampooing, and Shaving—cont'd*

TABLE 11.3

Common Hair and Scalp Conditions and Related Interventions

Problem	Interventions
Alopecia (Hair Loss)	
Chemotherapeutic agents kill cells that rapidly multiply, including both tumor and normal cells.	Some patients wear scarves. Some prefer hairpieces. Referral may be necessary for professional consultation for long-term interventions.
Dandruff	
Scaling of scalp accompanied by itching; if severe, may involve eyebrows.	Shampoo regularly with medicated shampoo.
Pediculosis	
Head lice: Parasites attached to hair strands. Eggs look like oval particles. Bites or pustules may be found behind ears and at hairline. May spread to furniture and other people.	Check the entire scalp. Centers for Disease Control and Prevention recommends treatment for persons diagnosed with an active infection (CDC, 2013). Over-the-counter or prescription treatment may be needed. Machine wash and dry clothing and linens in hot water. Nit combs can be used in combination with medicated shampoo. Change bed linens according to agency policy, and follow agency infection prevention guidelines. Lindane is no longer recommended by American Academy of Pediatrics.
Body lice: Parasites tend to cling to clothing. Patient itches. Hemorrhagic spots may appear on skin where lice are sucking blood. Lice may lay eggs on clothing and furniture.	Have patient bathe or shower thoroughly. Good hygiene and regular changes of clothes, bedding, and towels constitute the only treatment needed for body lice (CDC, 2013). Bag infested clothing or linen until laundered. Follow agency infection prevention policy.
Crab lice: Found in pubic hair. Are grayish white with red legs. May spread via sexual contact.	For pubic lice, shave hair off affected area, cleanse as for body lice, use medicated product for lice, and notify sexual partner of proper treatment.

shampooing because of positioning and manipulation of patient's head and neck.

3. Assess if patient has bleeding tendency. Review medical history, medications, and laboratory values (e.g., platelet count, anticoagulation studies).

Safe Patient Care *Have any patient on anticoagulants or who has low platelets use an electric razor.*

4. Perform hand hygiene. Inspect condition of hair and scalp. This determines if special shampoos or treatments are needed. Inspect for presence of any infestation (e.g., pediculosis). **NOTE:** Apply clean gloves and gown if infestation by lice is suspected (National Pediculosis Association, 2017). Apply clean gloves for inspection if draining head wound suspected. Discard gloves and perform hand hygiene after inspection.
5. Assess patient's hair-care and shaving product preferences (e.g., shampoo, aftershave lotion, skin conditioner).
6. Assess patient's ability to manipulate comb, brush, or razor.
7. Assess environment for safety (e.g., check room for spills; make sure that equipment is working properly, and that bed is in locked, low position) (QSEN, 2014).
8. Gather equipment and supplies at patient's bedside. Explain your intent to provide hair/beard care. Ask patient to explain during procedure steps that he or she uses to comb hair and/or shave. Ask patient to indicate if he or she becomes uncomfortable during procedure.
9. Position patient sitting in chair or up in bed with head elevated 45 to 90 degrees (as tolerated).
10. Provide privacy; close door or pull curtain. Arrange supplies at bedside table and adjust lighting.
11. Perform hand hygiene and apply clean gloves if necessary.
12. **Combing and brushing hair:**
    a. Part hair into two sections and then separate it into two more sections (see illustrations).
    b. Brush or comb from scalp toward hair ends.
    c. Moisten hair lightly with water, conditioner, or alcohol-free detangle product before combing.
    d. Move fingers through hair to loosen any larger tangles.
    e. Using a wide-tooth comb, start on either side of head and insert comb with teeth upward to hair near scalp. Comb through hair in circular motion by turning wrist while lifting up and out. Continue until all hair is combed through and comb into place to shape and style.
13. **Shampooing bed-bound patient with shampoo board:**
    a. Apply clean gloves. Place waterproof pad under patient's shoulders, neck, and head.
    b. Position patient supine with head and shoulders at top edge of bed. Place shampoo board under patient's head and washbasin under end of trough spout (see illustration). Be sure that trough spout extends beyond edge of mattress.
    c. Place rolled towel under patient's neck and bath towel over patient's shoulders.
    d. Brush and comb patient's hair.
    e. Ask patient to hold towel or washcloth over eyes.

Continued

PROCEDURAL GUIDELINE 11.6 *Hair Care—Combing, Shampooing, and Shaving—cont'd*

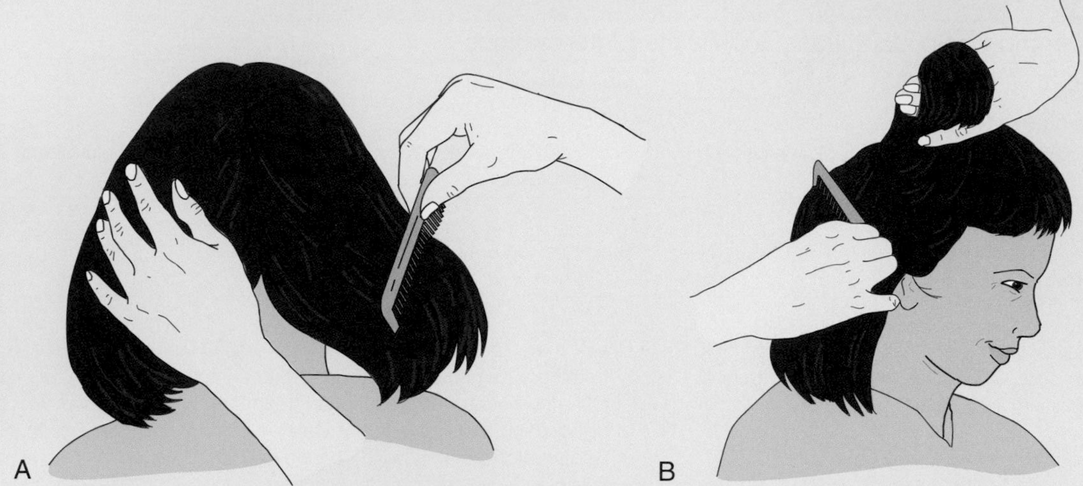

STEP 12a Parting hair. (A) Part hair down the middle and divide it into two main sections. (B) Part main section into two smaller sections.

f. Test water temperature. Slowly pour water from pitcher over hair until it is completely wet (see illustration). If hair contains matted blood, apply hydrogen peroxide to dissolve clots and rinse with saline. Apply small amount of shampoo.

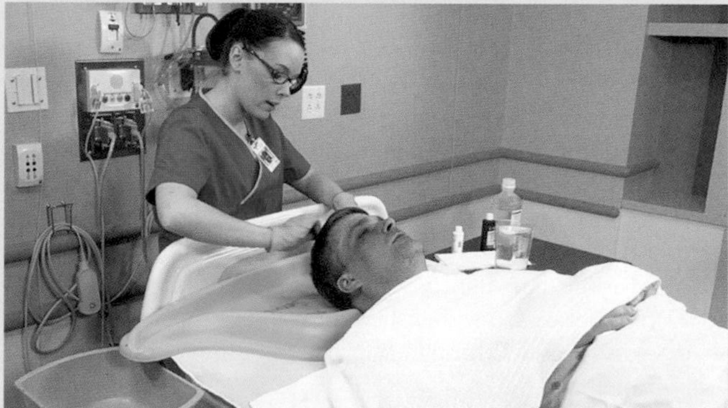

STEP 13b Patient positioned over shampoo board.

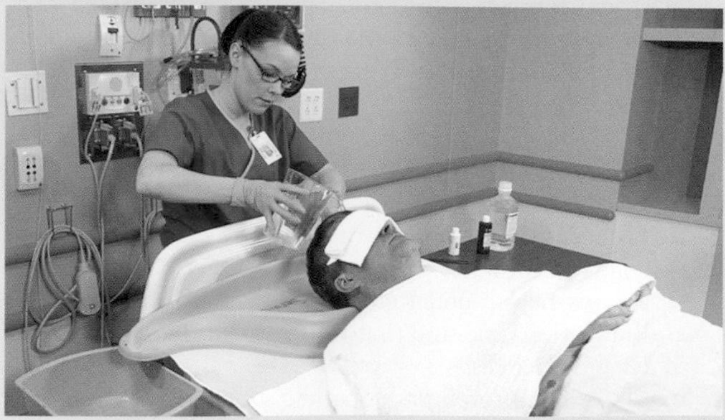

STEP 13f Nurse pouring water over patient's hair

g. Work up lather with both hands. Start at hairline and work toward back of neck. Lift head slightly with one hand to wash back of head. Shampoo sides of head. Massage scalp by applying pressure with fingertips.

h. Rinse hair with water. Make sure that water drains into basin. Repeat rinsing until hair is free of soap. (If you need to refill pitcher, raise side rail when leaving bedside.)

i. Apply conditioner or crème rinse if requested and rinse hair thoroughly.

j. Wrap patient's head in bath towel. Dry face with cloth used to protect eyes. Dry off any moisture along neck or shoulders.

k. Dry patient's hair and scalp. Use second towel if first one becomes saturated.

l. Comb hair to remove tangles and dry with dryer if desired.

m. Apply oil preparation or conditioning product to hair if desired by patient.

n. Variation for patients with coarse, curly hair: Condition hair after washing. To untangle hair, use wide teeth of comb. Beginning at nape of neck, comb small subsections of hair, starting at hair ends. Continue to work through small sections until hair is free of tangles.

o. Help patient to comfortable position and complete styling of hair.

14. Shampooing with disposable shampoo product:

a. Patient can be sitting on chair or in bed. Apply clean gloves.

b. Comb hair to remove any tangles or debris.

PROCEDURAL GUIDELINE 11.6 *Hair Care—Combing, Shampooing, and Shaving—cont'd*

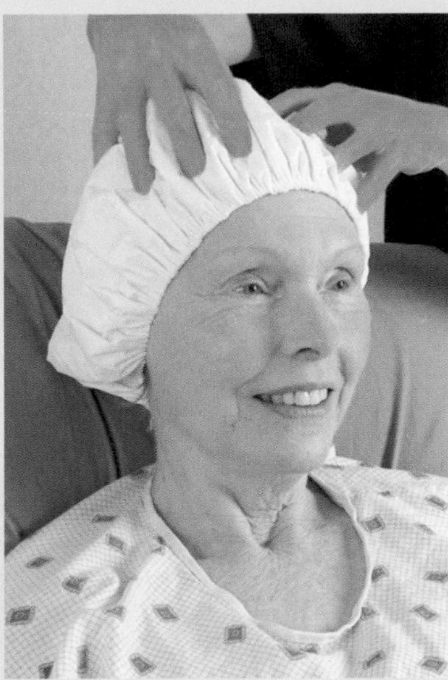

STEP 14c Patient wearing disposable shampoo cap.

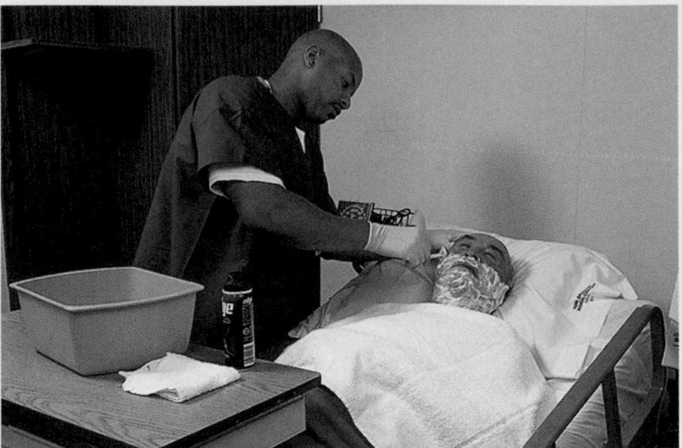

STEP 15e Shaving patient using short, firm strokes.

c. Open package, apply cap, and secure all hair beneath cap (see illustration).
d. Massage head through cap. Check fitting around head to maintain correct fit.
e. Massage 2 to 4 minutes according to directions on package; additional time may be required for longer hair or hair matted with blood.
f. Discard cap in trash; do not dispose of in toilet because it may clog plumbing.
g. If patient desires, towel dry hair. Brush or comb patient's hair.

15. **Shaving with disposable razor:**
    a. Place bath towel over patient's chest and shoulders.
    b. Run warm water in washbasin. Check water temperature.
    c. Place washcloth in basin and wring out thoroughly. Apply cloth over patient's entire face for several seconds.
    d. Apply approximately $\frac{1}{4}$ inch shaving cream or soap to patient's face. Smooth cream evenly over sides of face, on chin, and under nose.
    e. Hold razor in dominant hand at 45-degree angle to patient's skin. Begin by shaving across one side of patient's face using short, firm strokes in direction that hair grows (see illustration). Use nondominant hand to gently pull skin taut while shaving. Ask patient if he feels comfortable.
    f. Dip razor blade in water because shaving cream accumulates on edge of blade.
    g. After all facial hair is shaved, rinse face thoroughly with warm, moistened washcloth.
    h. Dry face thoroughly and apply aftershave lotion if desired. Remove towel.
16. **Shaving with electric razor:**
    a. Place bath towel over patient's chest and shoulders.
    b. Apply skin conditioner or preshave preparation.
    c. Turn razor on and begin by shaving across side of face. Gently hold skin taut while shaving over surface of skin. Use gentle downward stroke of razor in direction of hair growth.
    d. After completing shave, turn razor off, remove towel and apply aftershave lotion as desired unless contraindicated.
17. **Mustache and beard care:**
    a. Place bath towel over patient's chest and shoulders.
    b. If necessary, gently comb mustache or beard.
    c. Allow patient to use mirror and direct areas to trim with scissors.
    d. After completing, remove towel.
18. Help patient assume desired comfortable position. Be sure nurse call system is in an accessible location within patient's reach. Raise side rails (as appropriate) and lower bed to lowest position.
19. Return reusable equipment to proper place. Discard soiled linen in dirty laundry bag. Remove and dispose of gloves (if worn) and perform hand hygiene.
20. Inspect condition of hair and scalp, condition of shaved area and skin underneath beard or mustache. Look for areas of localized bleeding from cuts and areas of dryness.
21. Ask patient if face feels clean and comfortable.

PROCEDURAL GUIDELINE 11.7 *Making an Occupied Bed*

Purpose

Providing clean bed linen is an important part of a patient's personal hygiene. When a patient cannot tolerate being out of bed, you must make an occupied bed. When this is the case, you need to make the bed in a way that conserves time and the patient's energy. The bed is the piece of equipment a patient uses the most. It should be clean, comfortable, safe, and adaptable to various positions. The typical hospital bed consists of a firm mattress on a metal frame that you can raise or lower horizontally. The frame is divided into three sections, so the operator can change bed positions by raising and lowering the head and foot of the bed separately and incline the entire bed with the head up or down (Table 11.4).

A patient's weight, ability to move and turn, pain acuity, and restrictions related to clinical condition or treatment all affect the number of individuals who need to be involved in safely making an occupied bed. Use safe patient-handling techniques when you turn and position a patient over bed linen (see Chapter 17). In cases in which a patient experiences severe pain, an analgesic administered 30 to 60 minutes before making a bed can control pain and maintain comfort.

Delegation and Collaboration

The skill of making an occupied bed can be delegated to nursing assistive personnel (NAP). The nurse instructs the NAP about:

- Any position or activity restrictions that apply.
- Looking for wound drainage or loosened equipment that might be found in the bed linens.
- When to obtain help from other caregivers for positioning a patient during linen change and the importance of using safe patient handling and supporting patient alignment.
- Using special precautions (e.g., aspiration precautions [see Chapter 13] or positioning for tube-feeding infusion [see Chapter 13]) when positioning a patient during bed making.

Equipment

Linen bags: mattress pad (change only when soiled); bottom sheet (flat or fitted); drawsheet *(optional)*; top sheet, blanket, bedspread, pillowcases; waterproof pads *(optional)*; clean gloves (if linen is soiled or there is risk of exposure to body fluids); antiseptic cleanser; washcloth

Procedural Steps

1. Review medical record and assess restrictions in mobility/positioning of patient.
2. Organize supplies and close room door or divider curtain to provide privacy.
3. Assess environment for safety (e.g., check room for spills; make sure that equipment is working properly and that bed is in locked position and appropriate number of side rails are raised).
4. Perform hand hygiene. Apply clean gloves if patient has been incontinent or if drainage is present on linen.
5. Explain procedure to patient, noting that patient will be asked to turn over layers of linen.
6. Raise bed to a comfortable working height; lower head of bed (HOB) as tolerated, keeping patient comfortable. Remove nurse call system.

Safe Patient Care *If patient is on aspiration precautions or receiving tube feeding, keep HOB 30 degrees or higher.*

7. Lower side rail on side where you are standing. Loosen all top linen. Remove bedspread and blanket separately, leaving patient covered with top sheet. If blanket or spread is soiled, place in linen bag. If it is to be reused, fold into square and place over back of chair.
8. Cover patient with clean bath blanket by unfolding it over top sheet. Have patient hold top edge of bath blanket or tuck blanket under shoulders. Grasp top sheet under bath blanket at patient's shoulders and bring sheet down to foot of bed. Remove sheet and discard in dirty laundry bag.
9. Position patient on far side of bed, turned onto side and facing away from you. **NOTE:** This is when another caregiver can help you by standing at bedside across from

TABLE 11.4
Common Bed Positions

Position	Description	Uses
Fowler's	Head of bed raised to angle of 45 degrees or more; semi-sitting position; foot of bed may also be raised at knee	Used during meals, nasogastric tube insertion, and nasotracheal suction; promotes lung expansion
Semi-Fowler's	Head of bed raised approximately 30 degrees; incline is less than Fowler's position; foot of bed may also be raised at knee	Promotes lung expansion; used when patients receive gastric feedings to reduce regurgitation and risk for aspiration
Trendelenburg's	Entire bed tilted with head of bed down	Used for postural drainage; facilitates venous return in patients with poor peripheral venous perfusion
Reverse Trendelenburg's	Entire bedframe tilted with foot of bed down	Used infrequently; promotes gastric emptying; prevents esophageal reflux
Flat/supine	Entire bedframe horizontally parallel with floor	Used for patients with vertebral injuries and in cervical traction; used for patients who are hypotensive; generally preferred by patients for sleeping

PROCEDURAL GUIDELINE 11.7 *Making an Occupied Bed—cont'd*

you. Encourage patient to use side rail to turn. Adjust pillow under patient's head.

10. Assess to make sure that there is no tension on any external medical devices.
11. Loosen bottom linens, moving from head to foot. Fanfold or roll any cloth pads, drawsheet (if present), and bottom sheet (in that order) toward patient. Tuck edges of old linen just under patient's buttocks, back, and shoulders (see illustration). Do not fanfold mattress pad (if it is to be reused). Remove any disposable pads and discard in receptacle.

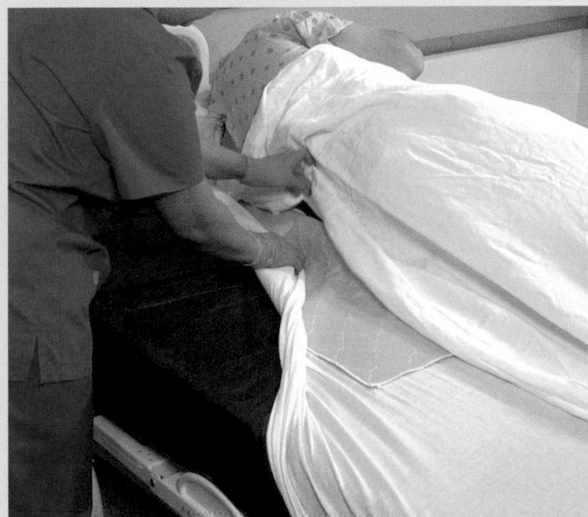

STEP 11 Tuck all soiled linen from one side of bed alongside patient's back.

12. Clean, disinfect, and dry mattress surface if it is soiled or has moisture (see agency policy).
13. Apply clean linens to the exposed half of bed in separate layers. When needed, start with a new mattress pad by placing it lengthwise with center crease in middle of bed. Fanfold pad to center of bed alongside patient. Repeat process with bottom sheet.
14. Pull new fitted sheet smoothly over mattress corner at top and bottom of bed. If using a flat sheet, allow edge of sheet to hang about 25 cm (10 inches) over mattress edge at head of bed. Be sure that lower hem of bottom flat sheet lies seam down and with bottom edge of mattress.
15. If bottom sheet is flat, miter top corner at HOB. Face HOB diagonally. Place hand away from HOB under top corner of mattress, lift, and with other hand tuck edge of bottom sheet smoothly under mattress so side edges of sheet above and below mattress meet when brought together.
16. If bottom sheet is flat, miter top corner at HOB.
    a. Face HOB diagonally. Place hand away from HOB under top corner of mattress, near mattress edge, and lift.
    b. With other hand, tuck top edge of bottom sheet smoothly under mattress so side edges of sheet above and below mattress meet when brought together.
    c. To miter a corner, pick up top edge of sheet at about 45 cm (18 inches) from top end of mattress (see illustration).

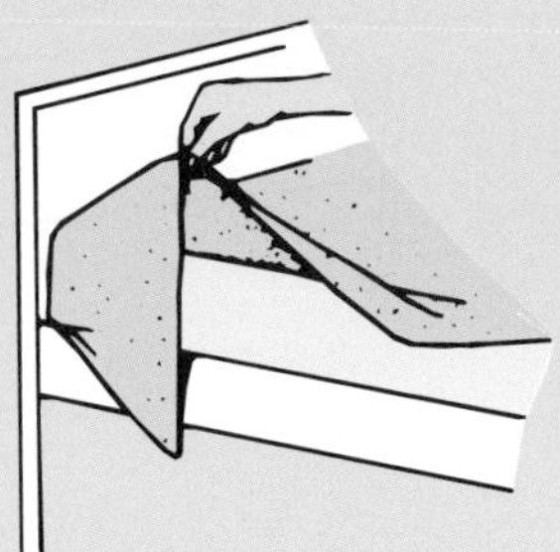

STEP 16c Top edge of sheet picked up.

    d. Lift sheet and lay it on top of mattress to form a neat triangular fold with lower base of triangle even with mattress side edges (see illustration).

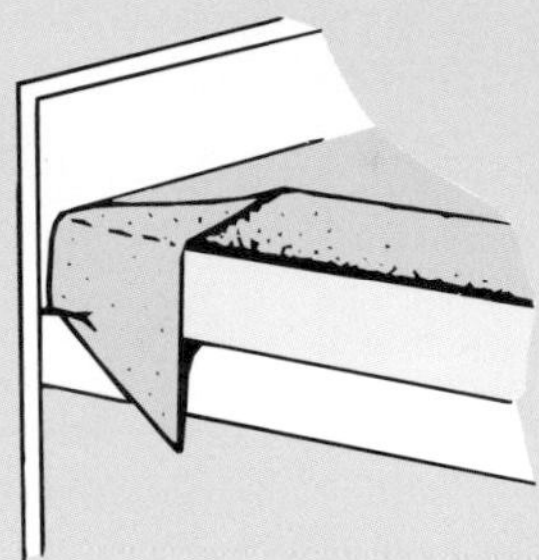

STEP 16d Sheet on top of mattress in a triangular fold.

    e. Tuck lower edge of sheet, which is hanging free below the mattress, under the mattress. Tuck with palms down, without pulling triangular fold.
    f. Hold part of sheet covering side of mattress in place with one hand (see illustrations). With other hand pick up top of triangular linen fold and bring it down over side of mattress. Tuck under mattress with palms down without pulling fold (see illustration).
17. Tuck remaining part of sheet under mattress, moving toward foot of bed. Keep linen smooth.
18. Place new drawsheet along middle of bed lengthwise. Fanfold or roll drawsheet on top of clean bottom sheet. Tuck under patient's buttocks and torso without touching old linen.
19. Add waterproof pad (absorbent side up) over drawsheet with seam side down. Fanfold toward patient. Continue to keep clean and soiled linen separate. Also keep linen under patient as flat as possible because patient will need to roll over old and new layers of linen when you are ready to make other side of bed.
20. Advise patient that he or she will be rolling over a thick layer of linens. Keeping patient covered; ask him or her to roll toward you slowly over layers of linen and to not raise the hips (see illustration). Stress the need to roll while staying aligned.

Continued

PROCEDURAL GUIDELINE 11.7 *Making an Occupied Bed—cont'd*

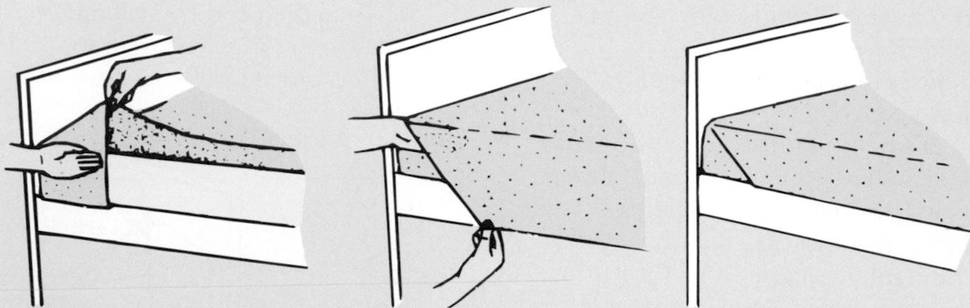

STEP 16f Triangular fold placed over side of mattress; sheet tucked under mattress.

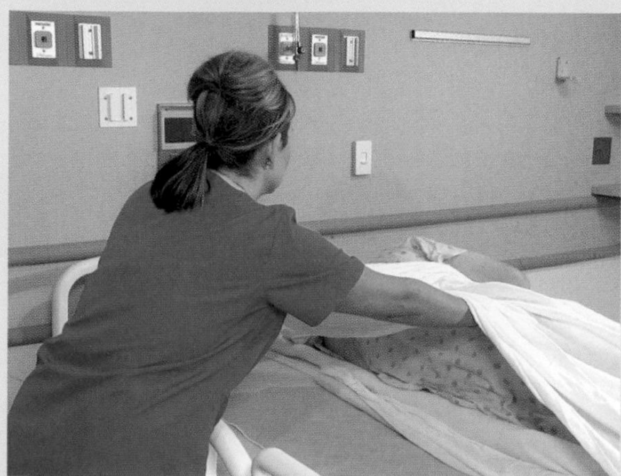

STEP 20 Patient begins rolling over layers of linen.

21. You will now raise side rail and move to opposite side of bed. *Option:* The caregiver helping you will help position patient. Have patient roll away from you toward other side of bed, over all of the folds of linen. Again, have patient keep hips still.
22. Loosen edges of soiled linen from under mattress. Remove soiled linen by folding into a bundle or square.
23. Hold linen away from your body and place it in laundry bag.
24. Clean, disinfect, and dry other half of mattress as needed.
25. Pull clean, fanfolded or rolled mattress pad; sheet; drawsheet; and pad out from beneath patient toward you. Smooth all linen out over mattress from head to foot of bed. Help patient roll back to supine position and reposition pillow.
26. If bottom sheet is fitted, pull corners over mattress edges. If flat sheet is used, miter top corner of bottom flat sheet (see Steps 16a–f).
27. Facing side of bed, grasp remaining edge of bottom flat sheet. Lean back slightly, keep back straight, and pull while tucking excess linen under mattress from HOB to foot of bed. Avoid lifting mattress during tucking.
28. Smooth fanfolded drawsheet over bottom sheet (tucking is optional). Smooth waterproof pads, making sure that bed surface is wrinkle free.
29. Place top sheet over patient with vertical centerfold lengthwise down middle of bed and with seam side of hem facing up. Open sheet out from head to foot and unfold over patient. Be sure that top edge of sheet is even with top edge of mattress.
30. Place clean or reused bed blanket on bed over patient. Make sure that top edge is parallel with top edge of sheet and 15 to 20 cm (6 to 8 inches) from edge of top sheet. Raise side rail.
31. Go to other side of bed. Lower side rail. Spread sheet and blanket out evenly.
32. Have patient hold on to sheet and blanket while you remove bath blanket; discard in linen bag.
33. Make cuff by turning edge of top sheet down over top edge of blanket.
34. Make horizontal toe pleat; stand at foot of bed and fanfold in sheet and blanket 5 to 10 cm (2 to 4 inches) across bed. Pull sheet and blanket up from bottom to make fold approximately 15 cm (6 inches) from bottom edge of mattress.
35. Standing at side of bed, tuck in remaining part of sheet and blanket under foot of mattress. Tuck top sheet and blanket together. Be sure that toe pleats are not pulled out.
36. Make modified mitered corner with top sheet and blanket. Follow Steps 16a–f. After making triangular fold, do not tuck tip of triangle (see illustration).

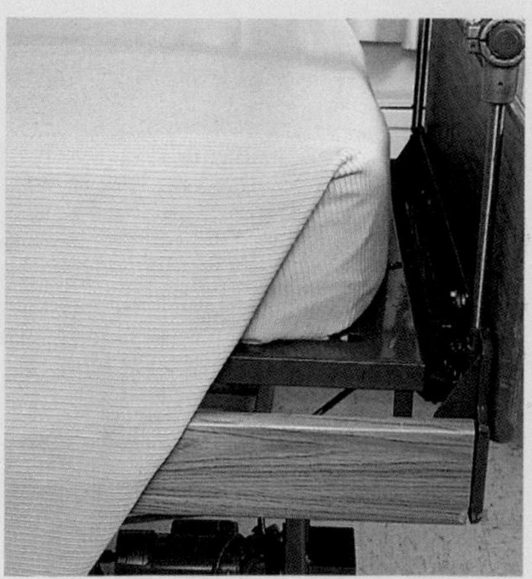

STEP 36 Modified mitered corner.

PROCEDURAL GUIDELINE 11.7 *Making an Occupied Bed—cont'd*

37. Go to other side of bed. Repeat Steps 35 and 36.

38. Change pillowcase. Have patient raise head. While supporting neck with one hand, remove pillow. Allow patient to lower head. Remove soiled case and place in linen bag. Grasp clean pillowcase at center of closed end. Gather case, turning it inside out over the hand holding it. With the same hand, pick up middle of one end of pillow. Pull pillowcase down over pillow with other hand. Do not hold pillow against your uniform. Be sure that pillow corners fit evenly into corners of case. Reposition pillow under patient's head.

39. Help patient assume desired comfortable position. Be sure nurse call system is in an accessible location within patient's reach. Raise side rails (as appropriate) and lower bed to lowest position.

40. Place all linen in dirty laundry bag. Remove and dispose of gloves.

41. Arrange and organize patient's room and perform hand hygiene.

42. During procedure inspect skin for areas of irritation. Observe patient for signs of fatigue, dyspnea, pain, or other sources of discomfort.

SPECIAL CONSIDERATIONS

Patient-Centered Care

- Convey sensitivity and respect for personal beliefs and cultural customs. Take time to talk with patients to identify their personal and cultural preferences for the best methods to perform hygiene.
- Before performing any aspect of hygiene care, inform the patient of the procedure and acknowledge his or her preferences.
- Take the time when performing hygienic care to communicate with patients and assess their physical and psychological conditions.
- Promote independence by encouraging the patient to participate in self-care activities.

Patient Education

- Instruct family caregivers how to perform all aspects of personal hygiene (e.g., how to maintain skin integrity, protect the patient from bathing accidents and falls; and protect patient from aspirating while thoroughly cleaning oral cavity).
- Instruct a patient with diabetes mellitus, peripheral neuropathy, or PVD and family caregiver to use the following foot care practices (American Diabetes Association, 2014):
  - Check your feet every day. Look at your bare feet for red spots, cuts, swelling, and blisters. If you cannot see the bottoms of your feet, use a mirror or ask someone for help.
  - Wash your feet every day. Dry them carefully, especially between the toes. Keep your skin soft and smooth. Rub a thin coat of skin lotion over the tops and bottoms of your feet, but not between your toes.
  - Wear comfortable shoes that fit well and protect your feet. Check inside your shoes before wearing them. Make sure that the lining is smooth and there are no objects inside.
  - Protect your feet from hot and cold. Wear shoes at the beach or on hot pavement.

Age-Specific

- Infants chill easily; keep body covered and work quickly. Use only mild soap for bathing infants and children.
- Older adults with urinary incontinence need meticulous skin care to reduce skin irritation from urine and feces.
- Avoid use of harsh soaps that can increase skin pH, which can cause drying, itching, and breakdown.

Home Care

- Adhesive strips on bottom of tub or shower, handrails, chairs, or stools in tub or shower help protect patients from falls and injury.
- Assess home for grab bars in patient's bathroom.
- Obtain a portable shower seat.

✦ PRACTICE REFLECTIONS

Consider how you would provide bathing and foot care to an older adult woman who has had type 1 diabetes mellitus for 25 years and has a history of skin infections, foot abrasions, and poor wound healing.

1. What evidence-based bathing strategies would you select for the bed bath?
2. How would you monitor her fatigue level and modify the timing of the bathing activities and ensure that she received a complete bath?
3. Tissue injury to the feet of a person with diabetes mellitus can result in major problems. Use the WOCN guidelines (2016) to guide your reflection regarding observing for tissue injuries in this patient's feet.

✦ CLINICAL REVIEW QUESTIONS

1. Which of the following is an appropriate guideline when providing male perineal care? (Select all that apply.)
   1. Leave the foreskin of an uncircumcised male patient retracted.
   2. Cleanse tip of penis at urethral meatus using a circular motion.
   3. Cleanse the shaft and scrotum before cleansing the urethral meatus.
   4. Avoid tension on indwelling catheter if one is present.
   5. Lift scrotum and wash underlying skinfolds.
2. Place the steps for assisting a patient with denture care in the correct order.
   a. Rinse dentures thoroughly in tepid water.
   b. Perform hand hygiene and don clean gloves; remove upper denture plate by applying gentle downward pressure with 4 × 4–inch gauze.

c. Hold dentures over an emesis basin or sink lined with a washcloth and containing 1 inch of water.
d. Gently lift lower denture from jaw and rotate one side downward to remove from patient's mouth.
e. Ask patient about preferences for denture care and products used.
f. Apply cleaning agent to brush, and brush surfaces of dentures.
g. Store dentures in a denture cup with patient's identification label.

3. Which of the following actions are appropriate when providing foot care to a patient with diabetes or peripheral vascular disease? (Select all that apply.)
1. Soak feet for 10 to 20 minutes.
2. Observe for foot problems.
3. Scrub callused areas with a washcloth.
4. Apply alcohol-based lotion to reduce infection.
5. Observe between toes.

Answers and Rationales for Clinical Review Questions can be found on the Evolve website.

REFERENCES

Agency for Healthcare Research and Quality (AHRQ): Universal ICU decolonization: an enhanced protocol, 2013. https://www.ahrq.gov/professionals/systems/hospital/universal_icu_decolonization/index.html.

American Diabetes Association: Foot care, 2014. http://www.diabetes.org/living-with-diabetes/complications/foot-complications/foot-care.html.

American Podiatric Medical Association: Diabetes, 2017. http://www.apma.org/learn/FootHealth.cfm?ItemNumber=980.

Anderson D, et al: Infection prevention: precautions for prevention transmission of infection, *UpToDate*, 2018. https://www.uptodate.com/contents/infection-prevention-precautions-for-preventing-transmission-of-infection.

Cassir N, et al: Chlorhexidine daily bathing: impact on health care-associated infections caused by gram-negative bacteria, *Am J of Infect Control* 43:640, 2015.

Centers for Disease Control and Prevention (CDC): Parasites/lice, 2013. http://www.cdc.gov/parasites/lice/.

Centers for Disease Control and Prevention (CDC): What is health literacy, 2016. https://www.cdc.gov/healthliteracy/learn/index.html.

Centers for Disease Control and Prevention (CDC): Pneumonia (ventilator-associated [VAP] and non-ventilator-associated pneumonia [PNEU] event, 2018. http://6pscvapcurrent.pdf.

Climo MW, et al: Effect of daily chlorhexidine bathing on hospital-acquired infection, *N Engl J Med* 368:533–542, 2013.

de Lacerda Vidal CF, et al: Impact of oral hygiene involving toothbrushing versus chlorhexidine irrigation in the prevention of ventilator-associated pneumonia: a randomized study, *BMC Infect Dis* 17:112, 2017.

Denny J, Munro CL: Chlorhexidine bathing effects on health-care-associated infections, *Biol Res Nurs* 19(2):123, 2016.

Galiczewski JM: Intervention for prevention of catheter associated urinary tract infections in intensive care units: an integrative review, *Intensiv crit care nurs* 32:2016.

Hirschman KB, Hodgson NA: Evidence-based interventions for transitions in care for individuals living with dementia, *Gerontologist* Suppl 58:S129, 2018.

Institute for Healthcare Improvement (IHI): How to guide: prevent ventilator-associated pneumonia, modified 2017. http://www.ihi.org/resources/Pages/Tools/HowtoGuidePreventVAP.aspx.

Konno R, et al: A best-evidence review of intervention studies for minimizing resistance to care behaviours for older adults with dementia in nursing homes, *J Adv Nurs* 70(10):2167, 2014.

Lin SC, et al: Chlorhexidine bed-bath improves CLABSI: a metal analysis, *J Nurs* 64(4):71, 2017.

Marchaim D, et al: Infections and antimicrobial resistance in the intensive care unit: epidemiology and prevention, *UpToDate*, 2018. https://www.uptodate.com/contents/infections-and-antimicrobial-resistance-in-the-intensive-care-unit-epidemiology-and-prevention/contributors.

Martin D, et al: Healthy skin wins: a glowing pressure ulcer prevention program that can guide evidence-based practice, *Worldviews Evid Based Nurs* 14(6):473, 2017a.

Martin ET, et al: Bathing hospitalized dependent patients with prepackaged disposable washcloths instead of traditional bath basins: a case crossover study, *Am J Inf Control* 45(9):990, 2017b.

Masuuza JS, et al: Implementation of daily chlorhexidine bathing to reduce colonization by multidrug-resistant organisms in a critical care unit, *Am J Inf Control* 45:1014, 2017.

Meddings J, et al: Systematic review of intervention to reduce urinary tract infection in nursing home residents, *J Hosp Med* 12(5):356, 2017.

Moosazadeh M, et al: Denture stomatitis and Candida albicans in Iranian population: a systematic review and meta-analysis, *J Dent* 16:283, 2016.

Musuuza JS, et al: Implementation of daily chlorhexidine bathing to reduce colonization by multidrug-resistant organisms in a critical care unit, *Am J Infect Control* 45:1014, 2017.

National Pediculosis Association: Welcome to HeadLice.org, 2017. http://www.headlice.org/index.html.

Pedersen L, et al: Oral mucosal lesions in older people: relation to salivary secretion, systemic diseases and medications, *Oral Dis* 21(6):721, 2015.

Petlin A, et al: Chlorhexidine gluconate bathing to reduce methicillin-resistant *Staphylococcus aureus* acquisition, *Crit Care Nurse* 34(5):17, 2014.

Pinkert C, et al: Experiences of nurses with care of patients with dementia in acute hospitals: a secondary analysis, *J Clin Nurs* 27:163, 2018.

Quality and Safety Education for Nurses (QSEN): Pre-licensure KSAs, 2014. http://qsen.org/competencies/pre-licensure-ksas/.

Shah H, et al: Bathing with 2% chlorhexidine gluconate, *Crit Care Nurs Quarterly* 39:42, 2016.

The Joint Commission (TJC): *2019 National Patient Safety Goals*, Oakbrook Terrace, IL, 2019, The Commission. http://www.jointcommission.org/standards_information/npsgs.aspx.

Villar A, et al: Diagnosis and management of xerostomia and hyposalivation, *Ther Clin Risk Manag* 5(11):45, 2015.

Wound, Ostomy and Continence Nurses Society (WOCN): Guidelines for prevention and management of pressure ulcers (injuries). *WOCN clinical practice guideline series 2.* Mt Laurel, NJ: 2016, Author.

12 Care of the Eye and Ear

SKILLS AND PROCEDURES

EVOLVE WEBSITE/RESOURCES LIST

http://evolve.elsevier.com/Perry/nursinginterventions
Audio Glossary • Checklists • Clinical Review Questions • Answers and Rationales for Clinical Review Questions

INTRODUCTION

Meaningful sensory stimuli help a person learn about the environment. Perceiving and understanding environmental stimuli are necessary for healthy functioning. How well a patient hears also affects health literacy. If a patient is unable to hear clearly, it is difficult to prepare him or her with the knowledge and skill needed to be proactive in health promotion and disease prevention. When there are alterations in vision and hearing, people often seek assistive sensory devices to replace or restore sensory function. These sensory devices are individualized to patients' needs and must fit and work properly for patients to function optimally within their environment. Eyeglasses and contact lenses help to restore visual loss, and hearing aids improve sound reception. Breakage or loss of sensory devices is expensive and may result in serious impairment that places a patient at risk for injury, interferes with communication, socially isolates a patient, and affects patient independence and self-esteem.

PRACTICE STANDARDS

- American Academy of Audiology, 2015: Clinical Practice Guidelines: adult patients with severe to profound unilateral sensorineural hearing loss
- American Optometric Association, 2018a: Comprehensive eye and vision examination
- The Joint Commission, 2019: National Patient Safety Goals—Patient identification

EVIDENCE-BASED PRACTICE

Impact of Dual Sensory Impairment

Vision and hearing impairments occurring together are significant and are referred to as dual sensory impairment (DSI). DSI has the potential to cause a decline in cognitive function or contribute to acute confusion or depression. DSI affects patients in their everyday activities and is often complicated by physical comorbidities, mental health, and social factors (Tiwana et al., 2016). In addition, DSI diminishes communication and well-being and can cause social isolation, depression, reduced independence, cognitive impairment, and mortality (Gopinath et al., 2013). There are risks to safety in patients with DSI; there is an increased likelihood of falls even with best-corrected visual impairment and mild hearing loss (Gopinath et al., 2016). Guidelines for the management of patients with DSI include the following:

- Early identification of sensory loss and prompt interventions to improve vision or hearing loss or both are beneficial in reducing confusion, improving orientation, and increasing patient independence (Roets-Merken et al., 2014).
- Explain to patient and family caregivers that DSI increases a person's risk for falls because patients with DSI may lose their visual and auditory cues regarding obstacles in their environments and sounds such as traffic. Design individualized interventions to teach patient and family caregivers how to reduce this risk (Gopinath et al., 2016).
- There is a risk for cognitive impairment with DSI; however, including the patient in care decisions and the use of frequent clear explanations help maintain independence and a satisfactory quality of life (Mitoku et al., 2016).
- Assist patient and family caregiver with methods to adapt to sensory losses. DSI causes greater impairment in independent activities of daily living (IADLs), such as managing finances, preparing meals, shopping, and using the telephone and computers (Tiwana et al., 2016).
- Encourage family caregivers to help individuals with DSI maintain independence in routine activities of daily living (ADLs), such as grooming and dressing (Tiwana et al., 2016).
- Know the patient's usual method for dealing with sensory loss, what type of hearing aid care is needed, and what type of assistance is required to enhance communication (Tiwana et al., 2016).

SAFETY GUIDELINES

- Health literacy is becoming increasingly more important in preparing patients and caregivers to be proactive in areas of health promotion and disease prevention. Health literacy, which is the capacity to obtain, process, and understand basic health information and services to make appropriate health decisions, is an important aspect of patient care, and it is important to identify resources to improve health literacy (Centers for Disease Control and Prevention [CDC], 2017).
- Sensory impairments make it difficult for patients and family caregivers to communicate health care needs, and these impairments affect health literacy.
- Anticipate how a sensory alteration places a patient at risk for falls or injury (e.g., ability to maneuver through home, climb stairs, and respond to alarms).
- Select safety interventions based on the type of sensory loss and patient preference.
- Orient patient to any new environment or changes within an existing environment to minimize safety hazards. In addition, educate family caregivers, family, and friends about the best way to help the patient adapt to sensory loss.
- When patients have visual impairments, they may have difficulty with tasks requiring visual detail (e.g., reading prescriptions or syringes). This increases the risk of improper administration of medications in the home setting. In addition, certain eye conditions such as cataracts and macular degeneration cause a patient difficulty when adjusting to changes in contrast and brightness.
- When a patient must sign a consent form for a procedure or surgery, be sure to have a method to verify that the patient read, heard, and understood the procedure.

PROCEDURAL GUIDELINE 12.1 *Eye Care for the Comatose Patient*

Purpose

Comatose patients do not have the natural protective mechanisms of blinking and eye lubrication and often develop ocular surface disorders such as exposure keratopathy. Critically ill patients are often sedated, which alters the normal blinking reflex. Left unprotected, damage to the cornea can occur (Demirel et al., 2014). Eye hygiene protocols using moisture chambers, lubrication, and corneal surface protection are the best interventions to decrease the risk for or prevent damage to the cornea (Alansari et al., 2015; Werli-Alvarenga et al., 2013).

Delegation and Collaboration

The skill of providing basic eye care for a comatose patient can be delegated to nursing assistive personnel (NAP). However, it is the nurse's responsibility to assess a patient's eyes and administer the sterile lubricant. The nurse instructs the NAP to:

- Adapt the skill for specific patients (e.g., using skin-sensitive tape to affix eye pads for patients with sensitive skin).
- Immediately report any eye drainage or irritation to the nurse for further assessment.

Equipment

Clean gloves; warm water; normal saline solution; clean washcloth; cotton balls; eye pads or patches; paper tape; eyedropper bulb syringe; sterile lubricant or eye preparations as ordered; *option*: a moisture chamber (e.g., polyethylene covers or polyacrylamide hydrogel dressing that seals off the eye from the environment) may also be used (verify with agency policy).

Procedural Steps

1. Identify patient using at least two identifiers (e.g., name and birthday or name and medical record number) according to agency policy (TJC, 2019).
2. Perform hand hygiene. Apply clean gloves and observe patient's eyes for drainage, irritation, redness, and lesions. Prompt identification of drainage or infections reduces the risk for exposure keratopathy (Demirel et al., 2014).
3. Continually explain each step of the procedure. It is unknown how much a comatose patient can hear; thus it is important to continually orient a patient to any procedure.
4. Assess for blink reflex (see Chapter 8).

Safe Patient Care *The absence of this reflex further increases the risk of visual damage (Guler et al., 2017).*

5. Examine the pupils; determine if pupils are equal and round and react to light and accommodation (PERRLA) (see Chapter 8).
6. Observe patient's eye movements, noting symmetry of movement.
7. Explain procedure to patient and family caregivers.
8. Position patient in supine or side-lying position.
9. Use a clean washcloth or cotton balls moistened with warm water or saline and gently wipe each eye from inner to outer canthus. Use a separate, clean cotton ball or corner of the washcloth for each eye.

Safe Patient Care *Be sure water is warm and not hot to avoid damaging eye.*

10. While holding a clean cotton ball, use an eyedropper to instill the prescribed lubricant (e.g., saline, methylcellulose, liquid tears) as ordered, wiping away any excess lubricant.
11. If the blink reflex is absent, gently close patient's eyes and apply eye patches or pads. Secure patch, being careful not to tape a patient's eyes.
12. Dispose of excess material, remove and dispose of gloves, and perform hand hygiene.
13. Remove eye pads or patches every 4 hours or as ordered and observe condition of patient's eyes for drainage, irritation, redness, and lesions.

PROCEDURAL GUIDELINE 12.1 *Eye Care for the Comatose Patient—cont'd*

14. Assist patient to comfortable position.
15. Be sure nurse call system is in an accessible location within patient's reach.
16. Raise side rails (as appropriate) and lower bed to lowest position.
17. Document eye examination findings, administration of lubricant, and family caregiver learning on flow sheet or in nurses' notes in electronic health record (EHR) or chart.
18. Notify health care provider if signs of irritation or infection are present.

PROCEDURAL GUIDELINE 12.2 *Taking Care of Contact Lenses*

Purpose

Contact lenses correct refractive errors of the eye and are relatively easy to apply and remove. Rigid gas permeable (RGP) and soft contact lens are the most common ones available. RGP lens are smaller than the soft lens, porous, and allow oxygen to pass through to the cornea. An RGP lens is usually removed at the end of the day and can last a year or longer. Daily and extended-wear disposable soft contact lenses are made of a flexible hydrogel plastic and cover the entire cornea and a small rim of the sclera. Silicone hydrogel lenses are an advanced type of soft contact lenses that are more porous than regular hydrogel lenses and allow even more oxygen to reach the cornea. Extended wear soft contacts can be worn overnight, usually for 7 days consecutively without removal (Segre, 2018). Soft lenses are disposed of after a single wear or every 2 weeks, monthly, or quarterly depending on type. Determine whether a patient wears contact lenses; severe corneal injury can result when a seriously ill patient is wearing contact lenses and this fact goes undetected (American Optometric Association, 2017).

Delegation and Collaboration

The skill of taking care of contact lenses can be delegated to nursing assistive personnel (NAP). However, it is the nurse's responsibility to assess a patient's eyes. The nurse directs the NAP to:

- Know a patient's specific type of contact lens, including cleaning solutions and routine, wear schedule, storage, and replacement schedule.
- Report immediately to the nurse any eye pain or discomfort, redness, swelling, tearing, or drainage.
- Carefully handle the lens to prevent damage and injury.

Equipment

Bath towels or waterproof pads; sterile saline solution; sterile lens care solution(s) for cleaning, disinfecting, and rinsing; sterile wetting or conditioning solution (depends on care regimen); sterile enzyme solution (depends on care regimen); flashlight or penlight; clean lens storage container; suction cup (*optional*); powder-free, clean gloves.

Procedural Steps

1. Identify patient using at least two identifiers (e.g., name and birthday or name and medical record number) according to agency policy (TJC, 2019).
2. Perform hand hygiene and inspect patient's eyes or ask patient if contact lens is in place. *Option:* Apply clean gloves if drainage is present. After inspection remove and discard gloves and perform hand hygiene.

Safe Patient Care *If a patient is unconscious or confused, you must assess for presence of contact lenses, which are often difficult to detect if they are colorless (untinted).*

3. Determine if patient can manipulate and hold contact lenses and if glasses are available for periods when contacts are not in use.
4. Determine patient's usual routine for wearing, cleaning, and storing lenses.
5. Assess patient for any unusual visual signs/symptoms (see Chapter 8) (e.g., change in visual acuity, blurred vision, halos, photophobia).
6. Review types of medication prescribed for patient: sedatives, hypnotics, muscle relaxants, antihistamines, or another medication that decreases blink reflex and subsequent lubrication of cornea.
7. Explain procedure to patient.
8. Verify expiration date of all solutions and assemble equipment at bedside.
9. Be sure that your fingernails are short and smooth.
10. Position patient in supine or high-Fowler's position in bed.
11. Perform hand hygiene and apply clean gloves. Place towel just below patient's face.
12. Removing lenses:
    a. Removal of soft lens: Follow Steps 12a(1) through 12a(6) for each eye.
        (1) If you are unable to visualize the lens, shine a penlight or flashlight sideways onto the eye to locate the position of the lens.
        (2) Add 2 or 3 drops of sterile saline solution to patient's eye.
        (3) If possible, ask patient to look straight ahead. Retract lower eyelid and expose lower edge of lens.
        (4) Use pad of index finger to slide lens off cornea down onto lower sclera (white of the eye).
        (5) Pull upper eyelid down gently with thumb of other hand and compress lens slightly between thumb and index finger.
        (6) Gently pinch lens and lift out without allowing edges to stick together. Place lens in storage case.

Safe Patient Care *If lens edges stick together, place lens in palm and soak thoroughly with sterile saline solution. Gently roll lens with index finger in back-and-forth motion. If necessary, soak lens in storage solution, which may return lens to normal shape.*

Continued

PROCEDURAL GUIDELINE 12.2 *Taking Care of Contact Lenses—cont'd*

b. Removal of hard lenses: Follow Steps 12b(1) through 12b(6) for each eye.

(1) Inspect the eye to be sure that lens is positioned directly over the cornea. If you are unable to visualize the lens, shine a penlight or flashlight sideways onto the eye to locate the position of the lens.

Safe Patient Care *If lens is not positioned directly over the cornea, have patient close eyelid, place index and middle fingers of one hand on eyelid just beside the lens and beneath, and gently attempt to massage lens back into place. If lens cannot be repositioned, an immediate referral to an ophthalmologist is needed.*

(2) Place index finger on outer corner of patient's eye and gently draw skin back toward ear.

(3) Ask patient to blink. Do not release pressure until blink is completed.

Safe Patient Care *For patients unable to open eye or blink on command, use a lens suction cup to remove lens from eye. Gently apply suction cup to lens surface and lift out.*

(4) If lens does not dislodge, gently retract eyelid beyond edge of lens. Press lower eyelid gently against lower edge of lens to dislodge lens.

(5) Allow both eyelids to close slightly and grasp lens as it rises from the eye. Cup lens in hand.

(6) Inspect lens to be sure that it is intact. Place it in storage container.

c. After lenses are removed, inspect eye for redness, pain, or swelling of eyelids or conjunctiva; discharge; or excess tearing. Remove and discard gloves, perform hand hygiene.

13. Cleaning and storage: Typical cleaning and disinfecting of contact lenses (verify specific method for lenses):

a. Apply 1 or 2 drops of cleaning solution to lens in palm of hand. Using index finger (soft lenses) or little finger (rigid lenses), rub lens gently but thoroughly on both sides for 20 to 30 seconds.

b. Holding lens over emesis basin, rinse thoroughly with recommended rinsing solution.

Safe Patient Care *Do not use tap water, bottled water, homemade saline, or distilled water for cleaning, rinsing, or storage (Food and Drug Administration [FDA], 2015). Tap water contains microbes and may be absorbed into the lenses, making them uncomfortable to wear. Tap and distilled water have been associated with* Acanthamoeba *keratitis, a corneal infection that is resistant to treatment and cure (FDA, 2015). Periodic cleaning with enzymatic cleaner and/or heat disinfecting may be part of the prescribed regimen. Follow health care provider's instructions and schedules.*

c. Place lens in proper storage case compartment: "R" for right lens and "L" for left. Rigid lenses are placed inside up.

d. Fill with recommended disinfectant or storage solution.

e. Secure cover(s) over storage case. Label case with patient's name, identification number, and room number. Perform hand hygiene.

14. Inserting lenses:

a. Inserting a soft lens: Follow Steps 14a(1) through 14a(5) for each eye.

(1) Remove right lens from storage case and rinse with recommended rinsing solution; inspect lens for foreign materials, tears, and other damage.

(2) Hold lens on tip of index finger of dominant hand with concave side up.

(3) Inspect lens from side at eye level to ensure that it is not inverted (see illustration).

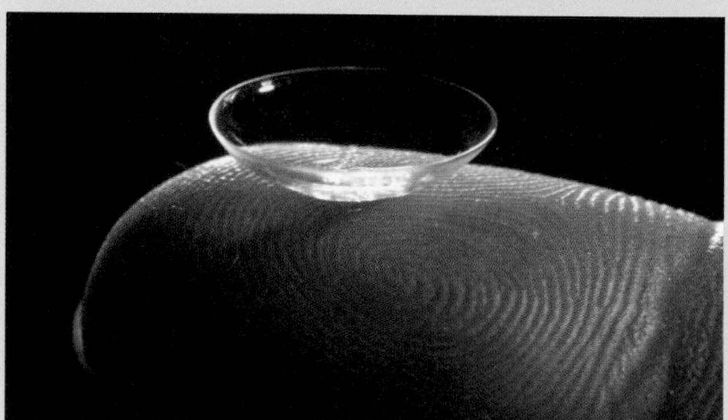

STEP 14a(3) Correct position of soft lens before insertion.

(4) Using middle or index finger of opposite hand, retract upper lid until iris is exposed (see illustration). Using middle finger of hand holding the lens, pull down lower lid.

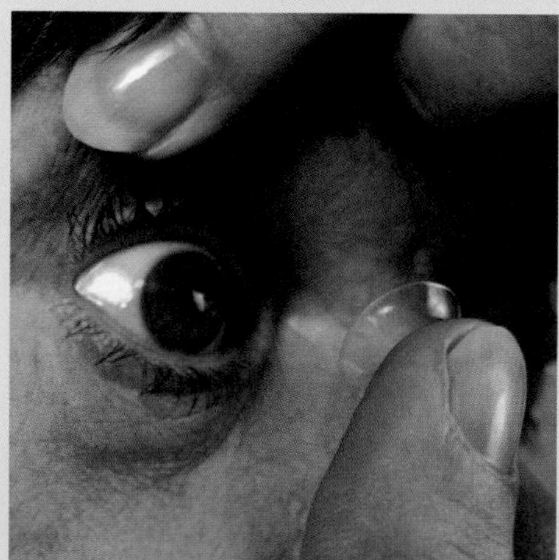

STEP 14a(4) Correct position of hands for soft lens insertion.

(5) Instruct patient to look straight ahead and focus on an object in the distance. Gently place lens directly on cornea and release lids slowly, starting with lower lid.

b. Inserting a rigid lens: Follow Steps 14b(1) through 14b(8) for each eye.

(1) Remove right lens from storage case; attempt to lift lens straight up.

(2) Hold lens on tip of index finger of dominant hand with concave side up.

PROCEDURAL GUIDELINE 12.2 *Taking Care of Contact Lenses—cont'd*

(3) Inspect the lens to ensure that it is moist, clean, clear, and free of chips or cracks.
(4) Wet lens surfaces with a few drops of prescribed wetting solution.
(5) Using middle finger of hand holding lens, pull down lower lid (see illustration).

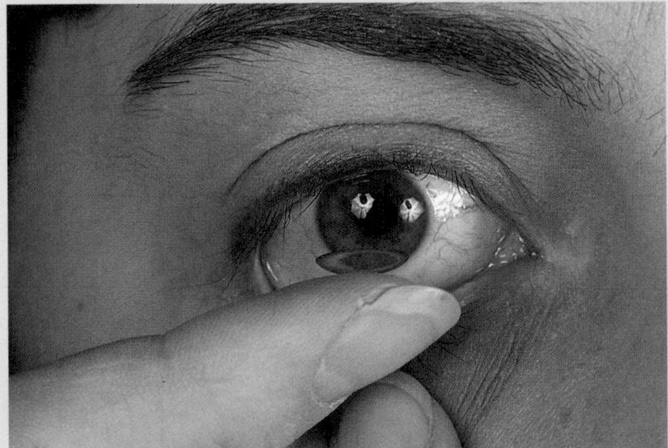

STEP 14b(5) Hand position for rigid lens insertion.

(6) Instruct patient to look straight ahead and focus on an object in the distance (see illustration).

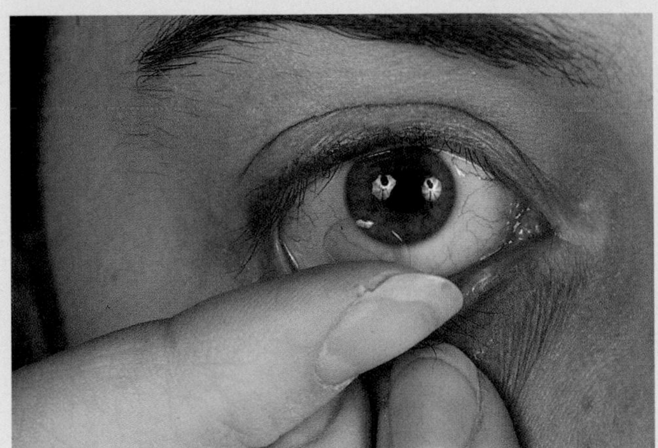

STEP 14b(6) Instruct patient to look straight ahead and focus on an object in the distance.

(7) Gently place lens directly on cornea and release lids slowly, starting with lower lid.
(8) Ask patient to close eyes briefly and avoid blinking.

c. Inspect eye to ensure that lens is on cornea.

Safe Patient Care *If lens is on sclera rather than cornea, ask patient to slowly close eye and look toward the lens. Gentle pressure on the eyelid may help to center the lens on the cornea. Ask patient to blink a few times.*

d. Ask patient to cover other eye with hand and report if vision is clear and lens is comfortable.
e. Repeat procedure to insert lens in other eye.

15. Discard solution from storage case and rinse case thoroughly with sterile lens storage solution. Sterilize or replace case as recommended by manufacturer. Allow case to air dry. Dispose of towel, remove gloves, and perform hand hygiene.
16. Ask patient if lens feels comfortable after removal and reinsertion of lenses.
17. Ask patient if there is blurred vision, pain, or foreign-body sensation.
18. Observe eye for drainage or redness.
19. Assist patient to comfortable position.
20. Be sure nurse call system is in an accessible location within patient's reach.
21. Raise side rails (as appropriate) and lower bed to lowest position.

✦ SKILL 12.1 Eye Irrigation

Purpose

Chemical injuries to the eye may be work related or caused by common household cleaning solutions or other fumes and aerosols. Acids in the eye damage the ocular surface by altering the pH and causing protein denaturation and coagulation (Marsden, 2016; National Library of Medicine [NLM], 2017a). Acid burns, caused by such substances as bleach, toilet cleaners, and battery fluid, cause a haze on the cornea, which often clears, and there is a good chance of recovery. Alkaline burns, such as those caused by lye, ammonia, and dishwasher detergent, often cause permanent injury to the eye (NLM, 2017a).

The priority is to flush the eye with copious amounts of irrigation fluid (Marsden, 2016). Irrigation takes priority over a comprehensive ocular assessment because the sooner the chemical can be diluted and removed, the less likely there is to be damage to the ocular surface (Stevens, 2016). Although irrigating solutions are usually normal saline, cool tap water is effective during the emergent phase. If the person wears contact lens and they did not wash out with the irrigation, have the person try to remove the lens.

Delegation and Collaboration

The skill of eye irrigation cannot be delegated to nursing assistive personnel (NAP). The nurse directs the NAP to:

- Report any patient complaint of discomfort or excess tearing following irrigation.

Equipment

- Emergency: cool tap water
- Prescribed irrigating solution: volume usually 30 to 180 mL at 32° to 38° C (90° to 100° F) (For chemical flushing, use normal saline or lactated Ringer's solution in large volume to provide continuous irrigation over 15 to 30 minutes.)
- pH test strip
- *Option:* local anesthetic eye drops
- Sterile basin or bag of solution
- Curved emesis basin
- Waterproof pad or towel
- 4 × 4–inch gauze pads
- Soft bulb syringe, eyedropper, or intravenous (IV) tubing
- Clean gloves
- Penlight
- Medication administration record (MAR) (electronic or printed)

ASSESSMENT

1. **Acute emergent situations**: Perform hand hygiene and prepare to use copious amounts of clear, cool water (normal saline, or lactated Ringer's if quickly available) to flush eyes for at least 15 minutes; 30 minutes is preferable (Stevens, 2016). Sometimes irrigating volume up to 20 L or more is required to change pH to physiological levels (pH testing should be done; Singh et al., 2013). *Rationale: Minimizes corneal damage (Chau et al., 2012).*
2. Have patient lie supine. Place emesis basin against the cheek on affected side, with head turned toward it. Ask the patient to fix his or her gaze ahead and open the eyelids. *Rationale: Allows easiest access for irrigation of eye.*
3. Use the syringe to direct irrigating fluid laterally from the inner corner of the eye outward (Marsden, 2016). *Rationale: Moves irritant away from and out of the eye.*
4. Maintain a constant flow of the irrigating solution at a low pressure from no more than 5 cm away onto the front surface of the eye, inside the lower eyelid, and under the upper eyelid (Stevens, 2016). *Rationale: Ensures entire surface of eye is flushed.*
5. Ask the patient to move the eye in all directions while the irrigation is maintained. Check and record the visual acuity when the procedure is finished (see Chapter 8). *Rationale: Ensures entire surface of eye is flushed. Provides baseline visual acuity.*

Safe Patient Care *When eye irrigation is an emergency treatment for a chemical burn, follow agency protocol. Irrigation is the immediate treatment; delays in irrigation by as little as 20 seconds have been associated with more severe injury in alkaline burns. Once the acute phase is over, an irrigation solution that buffers alkali or acid chemical is then selected, and further examination of the eye is possible (Serrano et al., 2013).*

6. **Nonemergent situations:** Identify patient using at least two identifiers (e.g., name and birthday or name and medical record number) according to agency policy. *Rationale: Ensures correct patient. Complies with The Joint Commission standards and improves patient safety (TJC, 2019).*
7. Review health care provider's medication order, including solution to be instilled and affected eye(s) (right, left, or both) to receive irrigation. *Rationale: Ensures safe and correct administration of irrigant.*
8. Determine patient's ability to open affected eye. **NOTE:** If patient is unable to open eye, hold eyelids open manually or with an eye speculum (Marsden, 2016). *Rationale: Spasm of the eyelid or pain makes opening the eye difficult. Local anesthetics such as proparacaine or tetracaine cause topical numbness and are used before eye examination procedures.*
9. If time permits, do a complete eye examination, including determining if pupils are equal and round and react to light and accommodation (PERRLA; see Chapter 8). Have patient look in all directions to determine if there are any visible foreign bodies. *Rationale: Provides baseline information and determines presence of any foreign bodies.*
10. Observe eye for redness, excessive tearing, discharge, and swelling. Ask patient about symptoms of itching, burning, pain, blurred vision, or photophobia. *Rationale: Establishes baseline signs and symptoms.*
11. Using a scale of 0 to 10, ask patient to rate level of pain. *Rationale: Establishes baseline for level of pain. Adequate pain control is essential to more complete eye examination by an ophthalmologist (Serrano et al., 2013).*
12. After the acute phase, obtain history of the injury to assess reason for eye irrigation (e.g., type of injury, when it occurred). *Rationale: Determines amount and type of solution and immediacy of need for treatment.*
13. Assess patient's or family caregiver's knowledge, experience, and health literacy. *Rationale: Ensures patient or family caregiver has the capacity to obtain, communicate, process, and understand basic health information (CDC, 2017).*
14. Assess patient's and/or family caregiver's understanding of the procedure and determine patient's ability to cooperate. *Rationale: Determines level of assistance needed.*

STEP	RATIONALE
PLANNING	
1. Expected outcomes following completion of procedure:	
• Patient demonstrates minimal anxiety during and after irrigation.	Potential for anxiety and pain is high during emergency.
• Patient verbalizes reduced pain, burning, or itching and improved visual acuity after irrigation.	Reflects effectiveness of procedure in removing irritant.

STEP	RATIONALE
• Patient maintains normal pupillary reaction and eye movement after irrigation.	Reflects effectiveness of procedure in minimizing exposure to irritant and preventing eye damage.
2. Check accuracy and completeness of each MAR with health care provider's written medication or procedure order. Check patient's name, irrigation solution name and concentration, route of administration, and time for administration. Compare MAR with label of eye irrigation solution.	The order sheet is the most reliable source and only legal record of drugs or procedure that patient is to receive. Ensures that patient receives correct medication.
3. Assemble supplies at bedside.	Provides easy access to supplies.
4. Provide privacy and prepare environment.	Promotes patient's comfort and safety.
5. Explain procedure to patient and family caregiver (if present).	Decreases patient anxiety.

IMPLEMENTATION

STEP	RATIONALE
1. Perform hand hygiene. Apply clean gloves.	Reduces transmission of microorganisms. Protects hands from chemical irritants.
2. Remove any contact lens if possible (see Procedural Guideline 12.2). Remove gloves after contact lens is removed. Reapply new gloves.	Prompt removal of lenses is needed to safely and completely irrigate foreign substances from patient's eyes. Removal of gloves following contact lens removal prevents reintroduction of chemical transferred from lens to glove.

Safe Patient Care *In an emergency such as first aid for a chemical burn, do not delay by removing patient's contact lens before irrigation. Do not remove lens unless rapid swelling is occurring. Flush eye from the inner to outer canthus with cool tap water immediately (Chau et al., 2012; Marsden, 2016; Serrano et al., 2013).*

STEP	RATIONALE
3. Explain to patient that eye can be closed periodically and that no object will touch it.	Informing patients what to expect decreases anxiety and reassures them.
4. With the patient lying down, protect the neck and shoulders with a towel or waterproof pad. Place curved emesis basin just below patient's check on side of affected eye. Turn head toward affected eye. If both eyes are affected, keep patient supine for simultaneous irrigation of both eyes.	Position facilitates flow of solution from inner to outer canthus, preventing contamination of unaffected eye and nasolacrimal duct.
5. Using gauze moistened with prescriber's solution (or normal saline), gently clean visible secretions or foreign material from eyelid margins and eyelashes, wiping from inner to outer canthus.	Minimizes transfer of material into eye during irrigation. Prevents secretions from entering nasolacrimal duct.
6. Explain next steps to patient and encourage relaxation: a. With gloved finger, gently retract upper and lower eyelids to expose conjunctival sacs. b. To hold lids open, apply gentle pressure to lower bony orbit and bony prominence beneath eyebrow. Do not apply pressure over eye.	Retraction minimizes blinking and allows irrigation of conjunctiva.
7. Hold irrigating syringe, dropper, or IV tubing approximately 2.5 to 5 cm (1 to 2 inches) from inner canthus.	Direct contact with irrigation equipment may injure eye. Too far of a distance may not provide adequate flushing (Stevens, 2016).
8. Ask patient to look in all directions while irrigation is maintained (Stevens, 2016). Gently irrigate with steady stream toward lower conjunctival sac, moving from inner to outer canthus (see illustration).	Minimizes force of stream on patient's cornea. Flushes irritant out and away from the other eye and nasolacrimal duct.
9. Reinforce importance of procedure and encourage patient by using calm, confident, soft voice.	Reduces anxiety.
10. Allow patient to blink periodically.	Lid closure moves secretions from upper conjunctival sac.
11. Continue irrigation with prescribed solution volume or time or until secretions are cleared. (**NOTE:** In emergent situation: An irrigation of 15 to 30 minutes or more is needed to flush chemicals.)	Assessment of eye secretion pH may be necessary if eye was exposed to an acidic or basic solution during injury (Chau et al., 2012).

STEP	RATIONALE

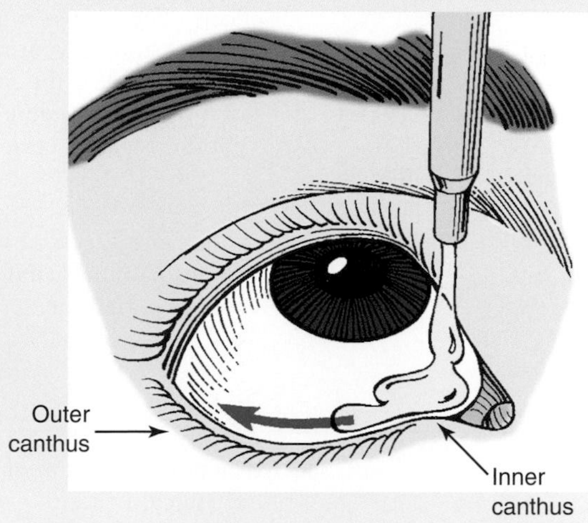

STEP 8 Irrigation of eye from inner to outer canthus.

STEP	RATIONALE
12. Blot excess moisture from eyelids and face with gauze or towel.	
13. Dispose of soiled supplies, remove gloves, and perform hand hygiene.	Reduces transmission of microorganisms.
14. Help patient to comfortable position.	Gives patient sense of well-being.
15. Be sure nurse call system is in an accessible location within patient's reach.	Ensures patient can call for assistance if needed.
16. Raise side rails (as appropriate) and lower bed to lowest position.	Ensures patient safety.

EVALUATION

STEP	RATIONALE
1. Observe for verbal and nonverbal signs of anxiety during irrigation.	Verifies that patient is adequately comforted.
2. Assess patient's comfort level after irrigation.	Verifies effective removal of irritant.
3. Inspect eye for movement and to determine if pupils are equal, round, and react to light and accommodation (PERRLA).	Impaired reaction to light, accommodation, or movement may indicate injury.

Safe Patient Care *Patients who have chemical burns/injury to the eye must have a complete ophthalmologic examination of their eye(s) as part of the evaluation process (Marsden, 2016; Stevens, 2016).*

STEP	RATIONALE
4. Ask patient whether visual acuity has improved. Have patient read written material.	Corneal damage from irritant can result in altered visual acuity (e.g., blurred vision, cloudiness).
5. **Use Teach-Back:** "I want to be sure I explained why it is important to take your eyedrops at home. Tell me the purpose of the drops and when you should use them." Revise your instruction now or develop a plan for revised patient/family caregiver teaching if patient/family caregiver is not able to teach back correctly.	Determines patient's/family caregiver's level of understanding of instructional topic.

Unexpected Outcomes	Related Interventions
1. Patient experiences some anxiety.	• Reinforce rationale for irrigation. • Allow patient to close eye periodically during irrigation. • Instruct patient to take slow, deep breaths.
2. Patient complains of pain or foreign-body sensation in eye.	• Continue irrigating.
3. After irrigation, pain continues or there is excessive tearing or photophobia.	• Advise patient to close eye and avoid eye movement. • Immediately notify health care provider or eye care practitioner.

Recording

- Record in nurses' notes condition of eye and patient's report of pain and visual symptoms.
- Record the type and amount of irrigation solution and length of time irrigation performed.
- Document your evaluation of patient learning.

Hand-Off Reporting

- Use agency's standardized hand-off communication to communicate specific patient tolerance of eye irrigation and risks for changes in vision or pain between caregivers. Discuss patient-specific interventions taken.
- Report immediately to the physician or health care provider if patient complains of increased pain, blurred vision, or other visual changes.

✦ SKILL 12.2 Ear Irrigation

Purpose

Common indications for irrigation of the external ear canal are local inflammation and buildup of cerumen. The greatest danger during ear irrigation is rupture of the tympanic membrane caused by forcing irrigant into the canal under pressure. Damage to the external auditory meatus may also occur by scratching the lining of the canal if the patient suddenly moves or if there is inadequate control of the irrigating syringe (NLM, 2017b). Possible contraindications to ear irrigation include history of diabetes, a ruptured tympanic membrane, myringotomy, skin problems such as eczema in the ear canal, or a weakened immune system (American Academy of Otolaryngology—Head and Neck Surgery, 2018).

Delegation and Collaboration

The skill of administering ear irrigation cannot be delegated to nursing assistive personnel (NAP). The nurse directs the NAP to:

- Immediately report any potential side effects of ear irrigation (e.g., pain, drainage, dizziness).
- Help a patient when ambulating because some light-headedness may be present, which increases a patient's risk for falling.

Equipment

- Clean gloves
- Otoscope *(optional)*
- Irrigation or bulb syringe
- Basin for irrigating solution (Use sterile basin if sterile irrigating solution is used [when tympanic membrane is ruptured].)
- Emesis basin for drainage or irrigating solution exiting the ear
- Towel
- Cotton balls or 4 × 4–inch gauze
- Prescribed irrigating solution warmed to body temperature
- Mineral oil or over-the-counter softener
- Sterile water, saline, or wax-dissolving drops
- Medication administration record (MAR) (print or electronic)

ASSESSMENT

1. Identify patient using at least two identifiers (e.g., name and birthday or name and medical record number) according to agency policy. Compare identifiers with information on patient's MAR or medical record. *Rationale: Ensures correct patient. Complies with The Joint Commission standards and improves patient safety (TJC, 2019).*
2. Review health care provider's medication order, including solution to be instilled and affected ear(s): right (AU), left (AS), or both (AD) to receive irrigation. *Rationale: Ensures safe and correct administration of medication.*
3. Review medical record for history of diabetes, eczema or other skin problem in the ear canal, a weakened immune system, ruptured tympanic membrane, placement of myringotomy tubes, or surgery of the auditory canal (American Academy Otolaryngology—Head and Neck Surgery, 2018). *Rationale: These conditions contradict irrigation.*

Safe Patient Care *Ear emergencies include the presence of foreign bodies, insect bites, or percussion injuries. In addition, the patient can have damage from inside the ear, which includes blood and drainage. Sometimes the cause of bloody drainage may be the result of a head or neck injury. If you suspect a head or neck injury, (1) do not move the patient, (2) cover the outside of the ear with a sterile dressing (if available), (3) get medical help immediately, and (4) do not irrigate the ear (NLM, 2017b).*

4. Perform hand hygiene and inspect pinna and external auditory meatus for redness, swelling, drainage, abrasions, and presence of cerumen or foreign objects. *Rationale: Findings provide baseline to monitor effects of medication or solution.*
   a. Always attempt to remove foreign objects in ear by first simply straightening ear canal. *Rationale: Straightening the ear canal may cause the object to fall out.*

Safe Patient Care *If vegetable matter such as a dried bean or pea is occluded in the canal, do not perform irrigation. The material can swell on contact with water and cause further damage to the canal (Harkin, 2015; Hockenberry et al., 2017).*

5. Use otoscope to inspect deeper parts of auditory canal and tympanic membrane. CAUTION: If you visualize an object, remove otoscope; do not push an object farther into the ear canal. *Rationale: When auditory canal is unobstructed, this inspection verifies if tympanic membrane is intact.*
6. Ask if patient is having earache or fullness in the ear, partial hearing loss, tinnitus, itching or discharge in ear, or coughing. *Rationale: Common symptoms of cerumen impaction. Provides baseline to determine change after irrigation (American Academy Otolaryngology—Head and Neck Surgery, 2018).*
7. Using a scale of 0 to 10, ask if patient is experiencing discomfort. *Rationale: Provides baseline assessment. Pain is symptomatic of external ear infection or inflammation.*

8. Determine patient's ability to hear clearly (see Chapter 8). *Rationale: Occlusion of auditory canal by cerumen or foreign object can impair hearing.*
9. Assess patient's or family caregiver's knowledge, experience, and health literacy level. *Rationale: Ensures patient or family caregiver has the capacity to obtain, communicate, process, and understand basic health information (CDC, 2017).*
10. Determine patient's and family caregiver's knowledge of purpose for irrigation and normal care of ears. *Rationale: May indicate need for instruction regarding ear hygiene.*

STEP	RATIONALE
PLANNING	
1. Expected outcomes following completion of procedure:	
• Patient denies pain during instillation.	Fluid is properly instilled.
• Patient demonstrates hearing conversation more clearly in affected ear.	Obstruction in ear canal is resolved.
• Patient is able to discuss purpose of irrigation and describe correct ear-care techniques.	Feedback reflects patient's learning.
• Patient's canal is clear of cerumen, foreign material, and discharge.	Inflammation, irritation, and occlusion of canal are relieved.
2. Check accuracy and completeness of each MAR with health care provider's written medication or procedure order. Check patient's name, drug name and dosage, route of administration, and time for administration. Compare MAR with label of ear irrigation solution.	The order sheet is the most reliable source and only legal record of drugs or procedure that patient is to receive. Ensures that patient receives correct medication.
3. If patient is found to have impacted cerumen there are two options to prepare for procedure:	Loosens cerumen and ensures easier removal during irrigation.
a. Instill 1 or 2 drops of mineral oil or over-the-counter softener into ear canal twice a day for 2 to 3 days before irrigation.	
b. Instill water, saline, or wax-dissolving drops in the ear canal 15 to 30 minutes before treatment (American Academy Otolaryngology—Head and Neck Surgery, 2018).	
4. Provide privacy and prepare environment.	Promotes patient comfort and safety.
5. Close curtains or room door and assist patient into a sitting or lying position with head turned toward affected ear. Place towel under patient's head and ear. When possible have patient hold emesis basin.	Provides privacy. Positioning minimizes leakage of fluids around neck and facial area. Solution will flow from ear canal to basin.
6. Explain procedure. Inform patient that irrigation may cause sensation of dizziness, ear fullness, and warmth.	Prepares patient to anticipate effects of irrigation and promotes cooperation.
IMPLEMENTATION	
1. Perform hand hygiene. Pour prescribed irrigating solution into basin. Check temperature of solution by pouring small drop on your inner forearm. **NOTE:** If sterile irrigating solution is used, sterile basin is required.	Reduces transmission of microorganisms. Warm liquid avoids vertigo or nausea in some patients.
2. Apply clean gloves. Gently clean auricle and outer ear canal with gauze or cotton balls. Do *not* force drainage or cerumen into ear canal.	Prevents transmission of microorganisms. Prevents infected material from reentering ear canal. Forceful instillation of solution into occluded canal can cause injury to eardrum.
3. Fill irrigating syringe with solution (approximately 50 mL).	Enough fluid is needed to provide a steady irrigating stream.
4. For adults and children over 3 years old, gently pull pinna up and back. In children 3 years or younger, pinna should be pulled down and back (Hockenberry et al., 2017). Adults can lie supine. Place tip of irrigating device just inside external meatus. Leave space around irrigating tip and canal.	Pulling pinna straightens external ear canal. Prevents obstruction of canal with device, which can lead to increased pressure on tympanic membrane.

STEP	RATIONALE
5. Slowly instill irrigating solution by holding tip of syringe 1 cm (½ inch) above opening to ear canal. Direct fluid toward superior aspect of ear canal. Allow it to drain out into basin during instillation (see illustration).	Slow instillation prevents buildup of pressure in ear canal and ensures contact of solution with all canal surfaces.

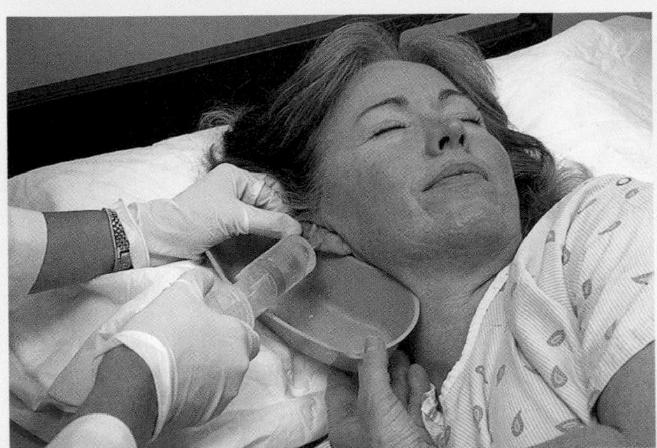

STEP 5 Tip of syringe does not occlude ear canal during irrigation.

STEP	RATIONALE
6. Maintain flow of irrigation in steady stream until pieces of cerumen or exudate flow from canal. Continue until canal is cleaned or solution is used.	Constant flow of fluid loosens cerumen.
7. Periodically ask if patient is experiencing pain, nausea, or vertigo.	Symptoms indicate that irrigating solution is too hot or too cold or instilled with too much pressure.
8. Drain excessive fluid from ear by having patient tilt head toward affected side.	Excess fluid may promote microorganism growth if not drained.
9. Dry outer ear canal gently with cotton ball. Leave cotton ball in place for 5 to 10 minutes.	Improperly drying the ear may lead to acute otitis externa (infection of the outer ear).
10. Help patient to comfortable position.	Gives patient sense of well-being.
11. Be sure nurse call system is in an accessible location within patient's reach.	Ensures patient can call for assistance if needed.
12. Raise side rails (as appropriate) and lower bed to lowest position.	Ensures patient safety.
13. Remove gloves and perform hand hygiene. Dispose of supplies in appropriate receptacle.	Reduces transmission of microorganisms.

EVALUATION

STEP	RATIONALE
1. Ask patient if discomfort is noted during instillation of solution.	Fluid instilled improperly under pressure causes discomfort.
2. Ask patient about sensations of light-headedness or dizziness.	Instillation of fluid into ear can cause some light-headedness or dizziness, which can put patient at risk for falling.
3. Reinspect condition of meatus and canal.	Determines if solution relieves symptoms and removes foreign materials.
4. Assess patient's level of pain and hearing acuity, and assess for presence of preirrigation symptoms.	Determines if cerumen removed and hearing is improved.
5. **Use Teach-Back:** "I want to be sure you understand how I showed you to insert the syringe for an ear irrigation. Show me how you would do this for your mother." Revise your instruction now or develop a plan for revised patient/family caregiver teaching if patient/family caregiver is not able to teach back correctly.	Determines patient's/family caregiver's level of understanding of instructional topic.

Unexpected Outcomes	Related Interventions
1. Patient complains of increased ear pain during irrigation.	• Rupture of eardrum may have occurred. Stop irrigations immediately. • Notify health care provider immediately.
2. Ear canal remains occluded with cerumen.	• Repeat irrigation.
3. Foreign body remains in ear canal.	• Refer patient to otolaryngologist if foreign object remains after irrigation.

Recording

- Document appearance of external ear, symptoms of cerumen buildup, and patient's hearing acuity before and after procedure.
- Record the type and amount of solution, time of administration, and the ear receiving the irrigation.
- Document your evaluation of patient learning.

Hand-Off Reporting

- Report to all health care providers which ear was irrigated and any adverse effects or complaints of pain or discomfort. Note any change in hearing acuity.
- Report patient response to procedure and outcome of irrigation (e.g., cerumen plug removed.)

PROCEDURAL GUIDELINE 12.3 *Caring for a Hearing Aid*

Purpose

Hearing is vital for normal communication and recognition and orientation to sounds in the environment. According to the National Institute on Deafness and other Communication Disorders (NIDCD, 2016), hearing loss affects 36 million people. A proper hearing aid improves the ability to hear and understand spoken words (Table 12.1). People with hearing loss benefit from early identification of the loss and use of hearing aids or other assistive devices (American Academy of Audiology, 2015; World Health Organization [WHO], 2017). Several styles of hearing aids are available, including new programmable aids (Mayo Clinic, 2017; NIDCD, 2017). Hearing aids amplify sound, so it is heard at a more effective level.

Delegation and Collaboration

This skill of caring for a hearing aid can be delegated to nursing assistive personnel (NAP). The nurse directs the NAP to:

- Report ear pain, inflammation, drainage, odor, or changes in hearing.
- Identify alternative ways to communicate with a patient while the aid is not in use.
- Learn how to carefully handle the aid to prevent damage.

Equipment

Soft towel and washcloth; facial tissues; brush or wax loop; storage case; warm water and soap; spare battery, size depends on aid *(optional)*; clean gloves (if drainage present)

Procedural Steps

1. Identify patient using at least two identifiers (e.g., name and birthday or name and medical record number) according to agency policy (TJC, 2019).
2. Ask patient about any unusual physical or auditory signs/symptoms (pain, itching, redness, discharge, odor, tinnitus, decreased acuity). If hearing is reduced, ask: When did this start? Is it present all the time? Does the quality of hearing acuity change with male versus female voices or adult versus children's voices?
3. Assess patient's or family caregiver's knowledge, experience, and health literacy.
4. Determine patient's and family caregiver's knowledge of purpose for cleaning and maintaining hearing aid and plan to incorporate instruction during care.
5. Provide privacy and prepare environment. Place towel over work area.
6. Have patient assume supine, side-lying, or sitting position in bed or chair.
7. Discuss procedure with patient. Explain all steps before removing aid.
8. Perform hand hygiene and apply clean gloves if patient has ear drainage.
9. Removing and cleaning hearing aid(s):
   a. Turn hearing aid(s) volume off, usually by turning volume control to left or toward patient's nose. Then grasp aid securely and gently remove device following natural ear contour.

Safe Patient Care *Some hearing aids, such as the completely-in-canal (CIC) device, do not have a volume control but are turned off by opening the battery door. Other aids have the volume control located on the remote. Be sure that your patient knows the importance of having the volume turned off when the aid is not in use.*

   b. Inspect ear mold for cracks or rough edges, any frays in cords, or accumulation of cerumen around aid, which can block sound (Harkin, 2015; White, 2015).
   c. Hold aid over towel and wipe exterior with tissue to remove cerumen.
   d. Inspect all openings in aid for accumulated cerumen. Carefully remove cerumen with wax loop or other device supplied with hearing aid.

Continued

TABLE 12.1

Types of Hearing Aids

Type	Advantages	Disadvantages	Cautions
In-the-ear (ITE) hearing aids fit completely in the outer ear (illustration A). 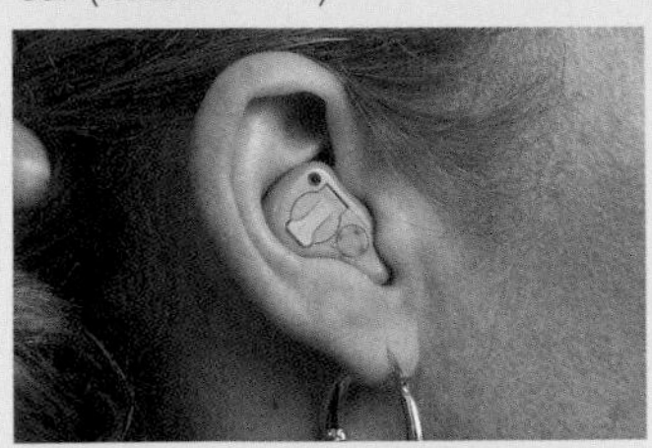 (A) In-the-ear hearing aid.	Used for mild to severe hearing loss. Design of the aid can improve sound transmission through telephone calls. May be easier to handle Uses larger battery with longer life.	Damaged by earwax and ear drainage. May pick up more wind noise. More visible in the ear.	They are not usually worn by children because the casings need to be replaced as the ear grows.
Behind-the-ear (BTE) hearing aids hook over the top of the ear and rest behind the ear. They are connected to a plastic ear mold that fits inside the outer ear (illustration B). 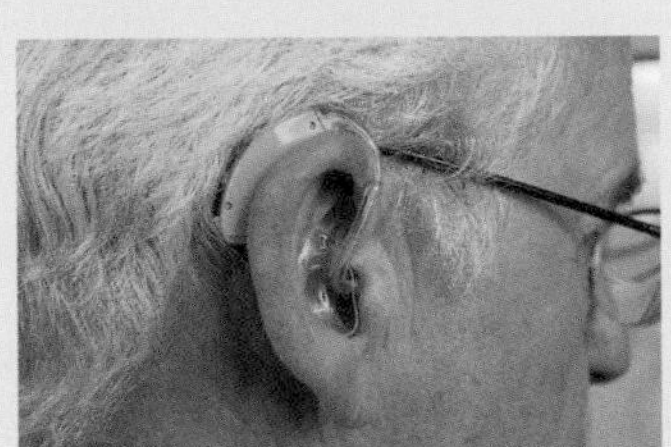 (B) Behind-the-ear hearing aid.	Useful for almost any type of hearing loss. Capable of more amplification.	May pick up more wind noise. Poorly fitting BTE ear molds can cause feedback, a whistling sound caused by the fit of the hearing aid.	May not be appropriate for children or adults who are active in sports because of the potential for damage of the device.
Completely-in canal (CIC) hearing aids are custom molded to fit the size and shape of the ear canal (illustration C). 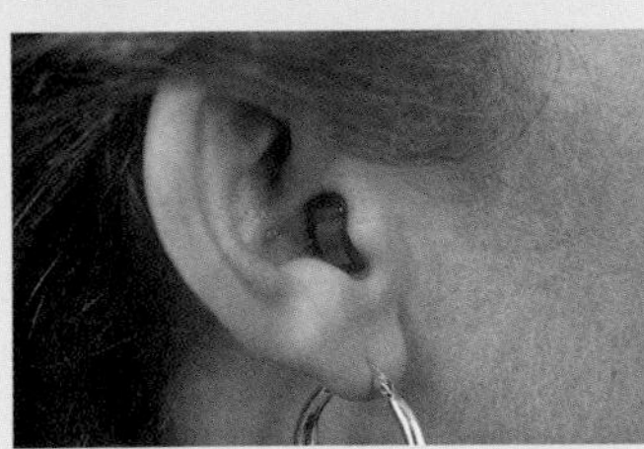 (C) Completely-in-canal hearing aid.	Used for mild to moderate hearing loss in adults. Smallest least visible. Less likely to pick up wind noise. Uses small batteries and directional microphone. Largely concealed in the ear canal.	Smaller batteries have shorter life and can be difficult to handle. Susceptible to earwax clogging the speaker. Doesn't contain extra features, such as volume control.	Expensive and not recommended for children. CIC aids can also be damaged by earwax and ear drainage.
Digital hearing aids (illustration D). 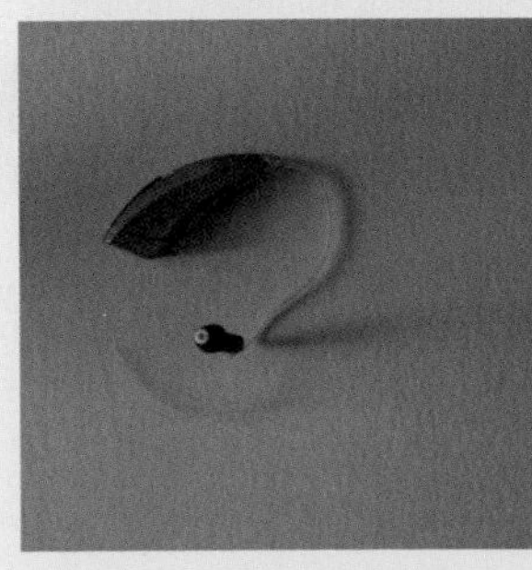 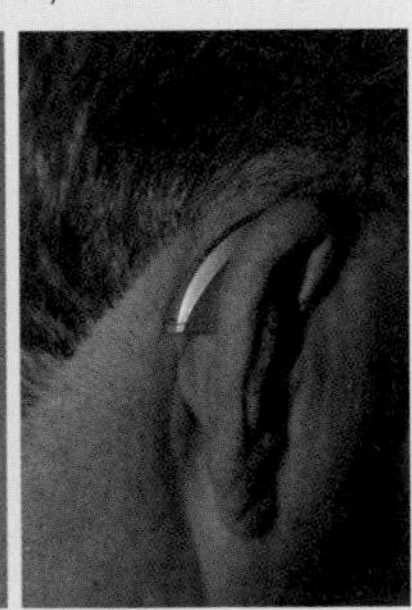 (D) Digital hearing aid.	Analyzes sounds to remove background noise. Programs for low-frequency and high-frequency sounds.	Need to be programmed and adjusted by a licensed audiologist.	Digital aids can be damaged by earwax and ear drainage.

Data from Mayo Clinic: Hearing aids: how to choose the right one, 2017. http://www.mayoclinic.org/diseases-conditions/hearing-loss/in-depth/hearing-aids/art-20044116; National Institute on Deafness and Other Communication Disorders (NIDCD): Hearing Aids, 2017. http://www.nidcd.nih.gov/health/hearing/pages/hearingaid.aspx#hearingaid_01.

PROCEDURAL GUIDELINE 12.3 *Caring for a Hearing Aid—cont'd*

Safe Patient Care *The pressure equalization channel is a tiny hole through the entire length of the ear mold and should be clear for the entire length. The receiver points into the ear through another opening. It is easily damaged. NEVER insert anything into the receiver port!*

e. Open battery door, place hearing aid in labeled storage container, and allow it to air dry.
f. Wash ear canal(s) with washcloth moistened in soap and water. Rinse with moistened cloth and then dry.
g. Dispose of towels, remove and dispose of gloves, and perform hand hygiene.
h. If storing hearing aid(s), place each in dry storage case with desiccant material. Label case with patient's name and room number. If more than one aid, note right or left. Indicate in patient's medical record where aid is stored (see agency policy).

10. Inserting hearing aid(s):
    a. Remove hearing aid(s) from storage case and check battery. Check that volume is off.
    b. Identify hearing aid as either right (marked "R" or red color coded) or left (marked "L" or blue color coded).
    c. When possible, allow patient to insert aid. Otherwise hold hearing aid with thumb and index finger of dominant hand so canal (long part with holes) is at bottom. Insert pointed end of ear mold into ear canal. Follow natural ear contours to guide aid into place.
    d. Anchor any separate pieces, as in case of behind-the-ear (BTE) aid or body aid.
    e. Adjust or have patient adjust volume gradually to comfortable level for talking to patient in regular voice 3 to 4 feet away. Rotate volume control toward nose to increase volume and away from nose to decrease volume.
    f. Close and store case. Remove and dispose of gloves. Perform hand hygiene.
11. Ask patient to rate level of comfort after removal or insertion.
12. Observe patient during normal conversation and in response to environmental sounds.
13. Assist patient to a comfortable position.
14. Be sure nurse call system is in an accessible location within patient's reach.
15. Raise side rails (as appropriate) and lower bed to lowest position.
16. Record that hearing aid is removed and stored if patient is going for surgery or special procedure. Document where or with whom aid is stored. Record patient's preferred communication techniques.
17. Notify health care provider if there are signs of ear canal irritation or infection, injury, or sudden decrease in hearing.

SPECIAL CONSIDERATIONS

Patient-Centered Care

- When a patient is without visual or hearing devices, communication is altered, the patient is isolated socially, and there is an increase in patient dependence (American Academy of Audiology, 2015; Ekberg et al., 2014).
- People who do not wear a hearing aid often say that it is because of the quality of sound that the aid produces (Dawes et al., 2014).
- Understand the cause of a person's sensory loss, and then determine the patient's own perception of the reason for the loss.
- Hospitals, rehabilitation centers, and skilled nursing facilities are environments that make hearing difficult. The hard flooring surfaces, medical equipment, televisions, and constant need to speak with other health care professionals all produce noise.
- Patients with hearing impairments need time to adjust to their hearing aid. In addition, increased background noise makes hearing with an aid even more difficult (Dawes et al., 2014; Mestayer, 2015).
- Sometimes you may use touch to get the attention of a patient with severe visual loss or decreased hearing. Remember to ask patients if touch is permitted. In some cultures, same-sex caregivers are required before touch can be used.
- Some cultures are more comfortable with softly spoken words and silence (Zerwekh and Garneau, 2015). Hearing impairments may force the patient's family and friends to speak louder. In addition, because of the comfort with silence, you can easily mistake a patient's silence as a measure of comfort and never correctly assess what the patient is able to hear or if the information was heard correctly.

Patient Education

- Show patients and family caregivers how to identify potential eye hazards in the home. Instruct them about measures to reduce the risk for eye injuries, such as personal protective eyewear (goggles, face shield, safety glasses). The eye protective device depends on the type of activity and potential for splash or foreign objects entering the eye (AOA, 2018b).
- In the work environment, the type of safety eye protection one should wear depends on the hazards in the workplace (American Optometric Association, 2018b):
  - If a person works in an area that has particles, flying objects, or dust, safety glasses with side protection (side shields) are recommended.
  - If a person is working with chemicals, eye goggles are recommended
  - If a person is working near hazardous radiation (welding, lasers, or fiber optics) special-purpose safety glasses, goggles, face shields, or helmets are designed for that task.
- Warn patients against inserting objects (e.g., cotton swabs, hairpins) into ear canal.
- Instruct patient and family caregiver that hearing aid batteries are toxic when swallowed and to keep them away from pets and children.

- Patient education and postvisit counseling contribute to successful use and care of a hearing aid (American Academy of Audiology, 2015).
- Insert hearing aid after hair is dried and hair spray applied. The heat from the hair dryer or hair spray can damage hearing aid.
- Dogs and cats are attracted to the smell of used hearing aids. Protect aid from pets by properly storing aid out of reach.
  - If an animal ingests the hearing aid, seek veterinary assistance.

Age-Specific

Pediatric

- A child with a foreign body or chemical in the eye may panic. It may be necessary to restrain the child to safely and quickly irrigate the eye.
- When cleaning the ear of a child, be certain that child's head is immobilized to prevent puncturing the eardrum. Obtain assistance from parents or staff as needed (Hockenberry et al., 2017).
- Children are more often fitted with a behind-the-ear (BTE) hearing aid until the ear canal has finished growing.
- Be sure there is no hair caught between the ear mold and canal or lower aid volume to help children reduce acoustic feedback (whistling).

Gerontological

- Store aids and batteries with desiccant or in an electronic dryer to prolong life and reduce repairs.
- The small size of aids is sometimes difficult to manipulate. Encourage patients to work with an audiologist to identify an aid consistent with patient's fine motor skills.
- High-pitched signals associated with consonants (e.g., *f, p, t, k, ch, sh,* and *st*) are more difficult to hear (Touhy and Jett, 2018).

Home Care

- When eye irrigations are necessary at home, instruct the family caregiver about the process.
- Use a clean bulb syringe for ear irrigations. Mineral drops or over-the-counter otic preparations are helpful for softening and removal of cerumen.
- Identify a family caregiver to assist with hearing aid insertion, removal, and cleaning when patient is unable to do it independently.

✦ PRACTICE REFLECTIONS

You are caring for a husband and wife who are both new to wearing hearing aids. Prior to giving care, you want to assess your patients' hearing acuity. In addition, you will need to provide some basic principles of hearing aid care.

1. What are some useful techniques for assessing a patient's hearing acuity?
2. What type of physical assessments of the ear are helpful in a hearing assessment?
3. What advice might you offer someone who has never cared for hearing aids?

✦ CLINICAL REVIEW QUESTIONS

1. Which important nursing interventions pertain to eye care for a comatose patient? (Select all that apply.)
   1. Avoid eye patches when the blink reflex is absent.
   2. Continually explain each step to the patient.
   3. Instill prescribed lubricant.
   4. Remove eye patches once a shift and assess eyes for drainage or irritation.
   5. Gently wipe each eye with a new cotton ball from outer to inner canthus.
2. A young man enters the emergency department with a chemical burn from household bleach. His wife ran tap water over his eyes before bringing him to the emergency department. Which represents the nurse's immediate actions in this situation? (Select all that apply.)
   1. Assess the injured eye.
   2. Determine the patient's level of pain.
   3. Prepare to initiate eye irrigation.
   4. Teach eye safety.
   5. Wait for the health care provider because the patient irrigated the eye at home.
3. Which of the following hazards apply when performing an ear irrigation? (Select all that apply.)
   1. Increased cerumen
   2. Inflammation
   3. Nausea
   4. Rupture of tympanic membrane
   5. Vertigo

Answers and Rationales for Clinical Review Questions can be found on the Evolve website.

REFERENCES

Alansari MA, et al: Making a difference in eye care of the critically ill patients, *J Intensive Care Med* 30(6):311, 2015.

American Academy of Audiology: Clinical Practice Guidelines: adult patients with severe-to profound unilateral sensorineural hearing loss, 2015. http://www.audiology.org/sites/default/files/PractGuidelineAdultsPatientsWithSNHL.pdf.

American Academy of Otolaryngology—Head and Neck Surgery: Earwax and care, 2018. http://www.entnet.org/content/earwax-and-care.

American Optometric Association: Contact lens safety, 2017. http://www.contactlenssafety.org/lenstypes.html.

American Optometric Association: Comprehensive eye and vision examination, 2018a. https://www.aoa.org/patients-and-public/caring-for-your-vision/comprehensive-eye-and-vision-examination.

American Optometric Association: Protecting your eyes at work, 2018b. https://www.aoa.org/patients-and-public/caring-for-your-vision/protecting-your-vision.

Centers for Disease Control and Prevention (CDC): What is health literacy, 2017. https://www.cdc.gov/healthliteracy/learn/index.html.

Chau JP, et al: A systematic review of methods of eye irrigation for adults and children with ocular chemical burns, *Worldviews Evid Based Nurs* 9(3):129, 2012.

Dawes P, et al: "Getting used to" hearing aids from the perspective of adult hearing-aid users, *Int J Audiol* 53:861, 2014.

Demirel S, et al: Effective management of exposure keratopathy developed in intensive care units: the impact of an evidence based eye care education program, *Intensive Care Nurs* 30:38, 2014.

Ekberg K, et al: Addressing patients' psychosocial concerns regarding hearing aids within audiology appointments for older adults, *Am J Audiol* 23:337, 2014.

Food and Drug Administration (FDA): Contact lens risks, 2015. http://www.fda.gov/MedicalDevices/ProductsandMedicalProcedures/HomeHealthandConsumer/ConsumerProducts/ContactLenses/ucm062589.htm.

Gopinath B, et al: Dual sensory impairment in older adults increases the risk of mortality: a population based study, *PLoS ONE* 8(3):e55054, 2013.

Gopinath B, et al: Hearing and vision impairment and the 5-year incidence of falls in older adults, *Age Ageing* 45:409, 2016.

Guler EK, et al: Intensive care nurses' view and practices of eye care: an international comparison, *Clin Nurs Res* 26(4):504, 2017.

Harkin H: Ear care and irrigation with water: an update, *Pract Nurse* 45(7):24, 2015.

Hockenberry MJ, et al: *Wong's essentials of pediatric nursing*, ed 10, St. Louis, 2017, Mosby.

Marsden J: How to perform irrigation of the eye, *Nurs Stand* 30(23):36, 2016.

Mayo Clinic: Hearing aids: how to choose the right one, 2017. http://www.mayoclinic.org/diseases-conditions/hearing-loss/in-depth/hearing-aids/art-20044116.

Mestayer K: Looking for hearing aids? Find the right professional first, *Hearing Health* Spring:34, 2015.

Mitoku K, et al: Vision and hearing impairments, cognitive impairment and mortality among long-term care recipients: a population based-cohort study, *BMC Geriatr* 16:112, 2016.

National Institute on Deafness and Other Communication Disorders (NIDCD): Quick statistics, 2016. Available at http://www.nidcd.nih.gov/health/statistics/Pages/quick.aspx.

National Institute on Deafness and Other Communication Disorders (NIDCD): Hearing aids, 2017. http://www.nidcd.nih.gov/health/hearing/pages/hearingaid.aspx#hearingaid_01.

National Library of Medicine: Medline Plus: Eye emergencies, 2017a. https://www.nlm.nih.gov/medlineplus/ency/article/000054.htm.

National Library of Medicine (NLM): Medline Plus: ear emergencies, 2017b. http://www.nlm.nih.gov/medlineplus/ency/article/000052.htm.

Roets-Merken LM, et al: Screening for hearing, visual and dual sensory impairment in older adults using behavioural cues: a validation study, *Int J Nurs Stud* 51:2014.

Segre L: Contact lens basics, 2018. http://www.allaboutvision.com/contacts/contact_lenses.htm.

Serrano F, et al: Traumatic eye injuries, *JEMS* 38(12):56, 2013.

Singh P, et al: Ocular chemical injuries and their management, *Oman J Ophthalmol* 6(2):83, 2013.

Stevens S: How to irrigate the eye, *Community Eye Health* 29(95):56, 2016.

Tiwana R, et al: Late life acquired dual-sensory impairment: a systematic review of its impact on every day competence, *Br J Vis Impair* 34(3):203, 2016.

The Joint Commission (TJC): *2019 National Patient Safety Goals*, Oakbrook Terrace, IL, 2019, The Commission. http://www.jointcommission.org/standards_information/npsgs.aspx.

Touhy TT, Jett T: *Ebersole and Hess's gerontological nursing and healthy aging*, ed 5, St. Louis, 2018, Mosby.

Werli-Alvarenga A, et al: Nursing interventions for adult intensive care patients with risk for corneal injury: a systematic review, *Int J Nurs Knowl* 24(1):25, 2013.

White S: Practical implementation tips: dual sensory loss, *Guide Pract* 18(6):30, 2015.

World Health Organization (WHO): Deafness and hearing loss, 2017. http://www.who.int/mediacentre/factsheets/fs300/en/.

Zerwekh J, Garneau A: *Nursing today: transitions and trends*, ed 8, St. Louis, 2015, Elsevier.

13 Promoting Nutrition

SKILLS AND PROCEDURES

EVOLVE WEBSITE/RESOURCES LIST

http://evolve.elsevier.com/Perry/nursinginterventions

Audio Glossary • Checklists • Clinical Review Questions • Answers and Rationales for Clinical Review Questions • Video Clips

INTRODUCTION

Nutrition is a basic component of health and plays a major role in disease prevention, recovery from illness, and ongoing good health. Patients suffering from undernutrition or malnutrition have worse outcomes than those with good nutritional status. The role of a nurse is to assess patients' risk for nutritional problems, assist patients with oral feeding when needed, and administer enteral nutritional therapies while protecting patients from the risk of aspiration. Routine identification of malnutrition with screening of patients in a health care setting is required by The Joint Commission (2017). Nurses across the continuum of health care settings should screen their patients' current nutritional status and promote an optimal diet whether for the patient recovering from an acute illness or insult, suffering from a chronic disease, or interested in disease prevention. The optimal route of nutrition is via an oral diet. In some cases, the components or texture of this diet may need to be modified based on the patients' disease state and aspiration risk. Patients who are unable to safely consume an oral diet often require enteral nutrition therapy. In those patients without a functional gastrointestinal (GI) tract, parenteral nutrition may be necessary (see Chapter 14).

PRACTICE STANDARDS

- Boullata J et al., 2017: ASPEN safe practices for enteral nutrition therapy—Guidelines for enteral nutrition administration
- International Dysphagia Diet Standardisation Initiative: IDDSI framework—Dysphagia diet framework
- McClave SA et al., 2016: American College of Gastroenterology (ACG) clinical guidelines: nutrition therapy in the adult hospitalized patient—Guidelines for administration of enteral feedings
- The Joint Commission (TJC), 2019: National Patient Safety Goals—Patient identification
- U.S. Department of Health and Human Services and U.S. Department of Agriculture, 2015: 2015–2020 dietary guidelines for Americans—Guidelines for healthy diet

EVIDENCE-BASED PRACTICE

Malnutrition

The nurse plays a pivotal role in best practices associated with optimal nutrition, including nutrition screening, interventions, monitoring, and documentation (Hakonsen et al., 2018; Smith et al., 2018). As many as 50% of hospitalized patients may be malnourished or at risk of becoming malnourished due to daily patient experiences (Box 13.1), yet malnutrition is often overlooked and undertreated (Meehan et al., 2016). Nursing nutritional screening and interventions (such as use of oral supplements) have been shown to have a positive impact on potential adverse outcomes associated with malnutrition (Box 13.2), which may reduce health care costs (Hand et al., 2016; Hiller et al., 2017; Soderstrom et al., 2017). The Joint Commission (2017) requires nutrition screening for symptoms of chronic or acute malnutrition during the admission process. In addition to an accurate height and weight measurement, a nursing nutrition screen for malnutrition risk should include questions regarding:

- Unplanned weight changes over a specific time period
- Change in appetite and food intake
- Inability to eat certain foods
- Difficulty in swallowing or chewing
- Increased consumption of alcohol or drugs

Beyond the nutrition screen, a nurse should perform a physical examination, noting abnormalities that may be due to malnutrition (Table 13.1) (Hakonsen et al., 2018; Smith et al., 2018). If malnutrition is suspected, a dietitian should be consulted. The Academy of Nutrition and Dietetics and the American Society of Parenteral and Enteral Nutrition (White et al., 2012) have outlined clinical characteristics for a nutrition diagnosis of malnutrition (Box 13.3).

BOX 13.1

Risk Factors for Becoming Malnourished

- Missed meals or enteral nutrition for medical procedures
- Clear-liquid or full-liquid diets for more than 3 days without nutrient supplementation or inappropriate or insufficient nutrient supplementation
- Intravenous feeding (dextrose or saline) or nothing by mouth (NPO) for more than 3 days without supplementation
- Insufficient education of staff regarding the importance of nutrition
- Disease-related barriers to food (anorexia, taste changes, weakness, fatigue, inability to chew or swallow)
- Poor dentition may alter chewing and intake level
- Elderly patient (more prone to disease and disabilities that limit food intake)
- Chronic use of drugs, especially alcohol, which affects nutritional intake

BOX 13.2

Malnutrition-Associated Adverse Events and Outcomes

- Poor wound healing
- More infections
- Increased muscle wasting and weakness
- Higher risk of falling
- Longer hospital stay
- More frequent readmissions
- Greater risk of dying

TABLE 13.1

Physical Signs of Malnutrition

Body Area	Normal Appearance	Indicators of Malnutrition
General appearance and vitality	Alert, responsive, energetic, sleeps well, vigorous	Listless, apathetic, cachectic, easily fatigued, no energy, falls asleep easily, looks tired, apathetic
Weight	Normal for height, age, body build	Overweight, obese, or underweight (special concern for underweight); weight trend, including unintentional weight loss or gain
Muscles and nervous conduction	Well-developed, firm, good tone; some fat under skin	Flaccid, poor tone; weakness and tenderness, "wasted" appearance (temporal, clavicle bone, scapular bone, hand, patella, anterior thigh and calf regions), burning and tingling of hands and feet (paresthesia), impaired ability to walk
Mental status	Good attention span, not irritable or restless	Inattentive, irritable, confused, signs of dementia
Gastrointestinal function	Good appetite and digestion, normal regular elimination, no palpable (perceptible to touch) organs or masses	Anorexia, indigestion, constipation or diarrhea, liver or spleen enlargement; distention, firmness, audible air with percussion
Cardiovascular function	Normal heart rate and rhythm, no murmurs, normal blood pressure for age	Rapid heart rate (>100 beats/min), enlarged heart, abnormal rhythm, elevated blood pressure
Hair	Shiny, lustrous, firm, not easily plucked; healthy scalp	Stringy, dull, brittle, dry, thin and sparse, depigmented; easily plucked
Skin (general)	Smooth, slightly moist, good color and integrity	Rough, dry, scaly, pale, pigmented, irritated, bruises, petechiae, delayed wound healing
Face and neck	Skin color uniform; smooth, healthy appearance; not swollen	Temporal wasting, orbital fat loss, dark circles under the eyes, lumpiness or flakiness of skin around nose and mouth
Lips	Smooth, good color, moist, not chapped or swollen	Dry, scaly, swollen, redness and swelling (cheilosis); angular lesions at corners of the mouth or fissures or scars (stomatitis)
Gums	Good pink color, healthy, red, no swelling or bleeding	Spongy, bleed easily, marginal redness, inflamed, receding
Tongue	Good pink color or deep reddish in appearance, not swollen or smooth, surface papillae present, no lesions	Swelling, scarlet and raw, magenta color, beefy (glossitis), hyperemic and hypertrophic or atrophic papillae
Teeth	No pain, no sensitivity	Missing teeth, broken teeth
Eyes	Bright, clear, shiny; no sores at corner of eyelids, membranes moist and healthy pink color, no prominent blood vessels, no fatigue circles beneath	Eye membranes pale (pale conjunctivae), redness of membranes (conjunctival infection), dryness or infection, redness and fissuring of eyelid corners (angular palpebritis), dryness of eye membrane (conjunctival xerosis), dull appearance of cornea (corneal xerosis)
Neck (glands)	No enlargement	Thyroid or lymph nodes enlarged
Nails	Firm, pink	Spoon-shaped (koilonychia), brittle, ridged
Legs and feet	No tenderness, weakness, or swelling; good color	Edema, tender calf, tingling, weakness, lesions
Skeleton	No malformation	Bowlegs, knock-knees, chest deformity at diaphragm, beaded ribs, prominent scapulae

Adapted from Mahan LK et al., editors: *Krause's food nutrition and the nutrient care process,* ed 14, Philadelphia, 2017, Elsevier.

BOX 13.3

Clinical Characteristics of Malnutrition

No single parameter is definitive for adult malnutrition; thus the identification of two or more of the following six characteristics is recommended for the diagnosis of malnutrition:

- Insufficient energy intake (based on estimated energy requirements over time)
- Weight loss (over time: 1 week, 1 month, 3 months or more)
- Loss of muscle mass
- Loss of subcutaneous fat
- Localized or generalized fluid accumulation that may sometimes mask weight loss
- Diminished functional status as measured by handgrip strength

Adapted from White JV et al: Consensus statement of the Academy of Nutrition and Dietetics/American Society for Parenteral and Enteral Nutrition: characteristics recommended for the identification and documentation of adult malnutrition (undernutrition), *JPEN J ParenterEnteral Nutr* 36(3):275, 2012.

BOX 13.4

Food Safety Tips

- Wash hands, food-preparation surfaces, and utensils with warm soapy water for 20 seconds before touching food. Use separate cutting boards and plates for produce and for meat, poultry, seafood, and eggs.
- Keep meat, poultry, seafood, and eggs separate from all other foods in the grocery bag as well as the refrigerator.
- Wash all fresh fruits and vegetables thoroughly.
- Do not eat raw meats or drink unpasteurized milk or juices.
- Do not use food past the expiration date on a package.
- Keep foods properly refrigerated. Refrigerate perishable foods at 40° F within 2 hours of cooking.
- Never thaw or marinate foods on the counter; thaw frozen foods in the refrigerator.
- Discard food that you suspect is spoiled.
- Do not use wooden cutting boards. Instead use plastic laminate or solid-surface cutting boards that can be disinfected.
- Cook meat, poultry, fish, and eggs until well done (180° F). Use a food thermometer.
- Keep food hot after cooking (at 140° F or above).
- Wash surfaces and utensils after each use. Wash dishcloths, towels, and sponges regularly or run in a dishwasher cycle, or use paper towels.
- Clean the inside of the refrigerator and microwave regularly with bleach or soap.

Adapted from Office of Disease Prevention and Health Promotion: food safety, 2017, https://www.healthypeople.gov/2020/topics-objectives/topic/food-safety; and Nix S: *Williams' basic nutrition and diet therapy,* ed 15, St. Louis, 2017, Elsevier.

SAFETY GUIDELINES

It is important to protect patients from injury when providing any form of nutritional support. When assisting patients with oral or enteral feeding, prevention of accidental aspiration of food into the airway is critical. Based on mealtime observations, follow measures to ensure safety and make any referrals to occupational therapy (specialized feeding utensils), speech therapy (swallowing difficulties), or a dietitian (inadequate intake or diet education). In situations when you educate patients about food safety, infection control should be a focus. Safety guidelines include the following:

- Patients with neurological disorders (e.g., stroke, Parkinson's), dementia, and post-intubation may be at high risk of dysphagia, which involves losing control over the ability to chew, move food into a bolus at the back of mouth, and swallow. Assess a patient's risk for dysphagia (see Skill 13.1) before assisting with a meal by completing a dysphagia screen. Based on findings, either proceed with the oral diet, refer to speech therapy for an instrumental swallow assessment, or discuss the need for enteral nutrition (EN) via enteral access with the medical team (Jiang et al., 2016).
- Ensure delivered meals are consistent with any prescribed diet or texture modifications necessary for patient safety.
- If a patient has dysphagia, use nursing strategies that include safe feeding techniques and aspiration precautions (see Skill 13.2).
- Use clinical standards (see Skills 13.3 and 13.4) for checking the position of the tip of an enteral feeding tube following insertion. Ensure the position of the tip of the tube has been radiographically confirmed in position prior to use.
- Know factors that increase a patient's risk for complications related to feeding tube insertion: altered level of consciousness, abnormal clotting, or impaired gag or cough reflex.
- Use ENFit connectors for all enteral nutrition sets, syringes, and feeding tubes to improve patient safety. The ENFit connector is not compatible with Luer-Lok connections or any other small-bore medical connectors (Institute for Safe Medication Practices [ISMP], 2015). Full conversion to ENFit devices is recommended to reduce the risk of accidental connection of syringes and administration sets meant for other routes of administration. Transition adapters for feeding tubes must be considered a temporary measure only (ISMP, 2015).
- Improper handling, preparation, and storage practices in the home environment may result in foodborne illnesses (Office of Disease Prevention and Health Promotion, 2017). Recommendations for food safety require nurses to educate patients about how to handle and cook food in the home (Box 13.4) while following these guidelines:
  - Determining when certain foods are cooked to appropriate temperatures
  - Separating more risky foods from less risky foods
  - Storing food at safe temperatures
  - Properly cleaning hands and surfaces

✦ SKILL 13.1 Dysphagia Screening and Assisting With Oral Nutrition

Purpose

Patients with severe illness, debility, and/or fatigue may be unable to feed themselves adequately and require assistance with feeding. Some patients have trouble chewing or swallowing, poor vision, or difficulty holding eating utensils. As a nurse, you are responsible for preparing patients and offering the type of assistance needed to help them successfully eat an adequate amount of food at a comfortable pace. Approximately 40% of hospitalized patients will lose weight due in part to decreased intake associated with decreased appetite, increased fatigue, and feeding difficulties, increasing their risk of developing malnutrition (Eglseer et al., 2018; Holst et al., 2015; Simzari et al., 2017). The following interventions improve patient satisfaction and increase caloric intake: improving a patient's eating environment; offering appealing menu offerings, increasing interactions with patients, including inquiring about their normal daily eating patterns and food preferences; providing needed help during meals; and offering diet education (Holst et al., 2017). Involve patients in selecting food preferences that fit their diet specifications when possible, choosing where to eat (bed or chair), and selecting the time to eat (Holst et al., 2015).

Delegation and Collaboration

The skill of assisting a patient with oral nutrition can be delegated to nursing assistive personnel (NAP). However, the nurse must first determine if a patient is able to receive oral nutrition, including swallowing ability and dietary restrictions. The nurse directs the NAP by:

- Explaining any specific swallowing strategies/techniques unique to the patient
- Reviewing when to stop feeding and report immediately to the nurse incidences of coughing, gagging, pocketing of food in the mouth, or difficulty swallowing
- Explaining any specific diet restrictions or tray setup assistance needed by the patient
- Cautioning to not rush the patient during eating

Equipment

- Stethoscope
- Washcloths and towels
- Tongue blade
- Adaptive utensils as needed for self-feeding
- Straw
- Oral hygiene supplies; *optional:* solution for stomatitis care
- Clean gloves

ASSESSMENT

1. Identify patient using at least two identifiers (e.g., name and birthday or name and medical record number) according to agency policy. *Rationale: Ensures correct patient. Complies with The Joint Commission standards and improves patient's safety (TJC, 2019).*
2. Review health care provider's diet order for type of diet and supplements. *Rationale: Ensures that patient will receive proper diet. Order is required for a therapeutic diet.*
3. Review nursing history for any nutritional risk factors (see Box 13.1) and for patient's most recent weight and laboratory values. *Rationale: Data determine if there is need for variation in type of foods offered to patient and level of assistance. Height and weight provide baseline for monitoring patient's nutritional status.*
4. Perform hand hygiene. Assess presence and condition of teeth. (Apply clean gloves if there is risk of exposure to saliva.) Determine if dentures are poorly fitted. If patient has mouth discomfort, measure pain severity on a scale of 0 to 10 on a pain scale. *Rationale: Reduces transmission of microorganisms. Loose, painful teeth or ill-fitting dentures may result in a reduced desire or ability to eat (Pflipsen and Zenchenko, 2017; Razak et al., 2014) and may also influence preparation of food for safe swallowing. Pain can reduce patient's appetite and ability to chew or swallow. These factors increase risk for dysphagia.*
5. Have patient speak and swallow. Watch for laryngeal movement. Ask patient to say "Ah" while using tongue blade and penlight. Check for midline uvula and symmetrical rise of uvula and soft palate. Use tongue blade to elicit gag reflex (see Chapter 8). *Rationale: Patients with chronic neurological disease may have cranial nerve damage that causes impaired swallowing (cranial nerve IX) or loss of gag reflex, hoarseness, and nasal voice (cranial nerve X). These factors increase risk for dysphagia.*
6. Provide patient progressive amounts of water (5 mL, 10 mL, 20 mL, 50 mL) and assess for laryngeal movement, coughing, drooling, and voice change (Christensen and Trapl, 2017). *Rationale: Patients with neurological disease or recently intubated may have cranial nerve damage or laryngeal edema, respectively, that may cause impaired swallowing. These factors are indications of possible dysphagia.*
7. Determine to what extent the patient is able to self-feed. Assess physical motor skills (e.g., ability to grasp utensils, hold cup, and move utensil to mouth). Assess level of consciousness or ability to attend to feeding, visual acuity, and peripheral vision. *Rationale: Assessment of a patient's physical and cognitive limitations alerts you to type of help the patient needs. Visual impairments make it difficult to see food and utensils.*
8. Assess patient's appetite over past week, recent food and fluid intake, cultural and religious preferences for participating in mealtime, and food likes and dislikes. *Rationale: Determines type of foods and size of meals that can potentially improve oral intake.*
9. Assess for presence of generalized fatigue, pain, or shortness of breath. *Rationale: Symptoms affect appetite and ability to participate in feeding. Patients eat better when rested.*
10. Ask if the patient feels nauseated. Also assess recent bowel pattern. Is patient passing flatus? Auscultate for bowel sounds (see Chapter 8). *Rationale: Determines baseline assessment of gastrointestinal function.*
11. Assess the need for toileting, hand hygiene, and oral care (including dentures) before feeding. *Rationale: Reduces interruptions and improves patient's appetite.*
12. Assess patient's or family caregiver's knowledge of patient's prescribed diet and health literacy level. *Rationale: Ensures patient has the capacity to obtain, communicate, process, and understand basic health information (Centers for Disease Control and Prevention [CDC], 2016).*

STEP	RATIONALE
PLANNING	
1. Expected outcomes following completion of procedure:	
• Patient's weight is maintained or trends toward desired level.	Nutritional intake meets daily needs.
• Patient does not demonstrate physical signs of nutrition-related deficiencies.	Physical findings indicate nutritional status.
• Patient demonstrates increased ability to self-feed or open items on tray as appropriate.	Indicates increased strength, improved mental status, and increased well-being.
• Patient coughs appropriately with no indication of respiratory compromise.	Ineffective cough and respiratory compromise are indicators of dysphagia and aspiration.
• Patient completes meal.	Nutritional intake meets daily needs.
• Patient able to describe foods allowed within prescribed diet.	Demonstrates effective learning and comprehension of provided education.
2. Allow patient to rest 30 minutes before mealtime.	Short rest improves patient's energy level and ability to participate in feeding.
3. Administer ordered analgesic 30 minutes before meal if patient has discomfort.	Analgesic reaches peak level during meal, thus improving patient's ability to self-feed.
4. Explain to patient how you plan to set up and help with meal. Allow time for questions and decisions on food choices and approach.	Minimizes any anxiety and engages patient in mealtime participation.
IMPLEMENTATION	
1. Perform hand hygiene	Reduces transmission of microorganisms.
2. Prepare patient for meal.	
a. Help patient with elimination needs and to perform hand hygiene prior to meal.	Increases patient's comfort and enjoyment of meal, which helps increase patient's nutritional intake.
b. Apply clean gloves and offer oral hygiene. If patient has dentures, remove and rinse thoroughly and reinsert. Remove gloves and perform hand hygiene.	Moist, clean oral mucosa and teeth improve taste and appetite.
c. Patients with oral mucositis (inflammation of mucous membranes) benefit from rinsing with solutions such as saline, saline-sodium bicarbonate mouthwash, sodium bicarbonate solution, or topical anesthetics or from using mucosal coating agents (National Cancer Institute [NCI], 2016). Consult with health care provider to best therapy.	Pain of stomatitis causes patients to avoid eating due to difficulty swallowing.
d. Help patient to comfortable sitting position in chair or place bed in high-Fowler's (at least 60 degrees) position. If patient is unable to sit, turn patient on side with head of bed elevated and chin in down position. There are three chin-down positions: head flexion, neck flexion, or both (Kagaya et al., 2011). **NOTE:** Patients with pharynx paralyzed on one side from stroke should turn head toward paralyzed side (Kagaya et al., 2011).	Upright position facilitates swallowing, reducing aspiration risk. Side lying with head turned makes it easier for food bolus to travel down non-rotated side (Kagaya et al., 2011). Conditions such as pressure injury, traction, or spinal surgery prevent positioning with head elevated.

Safe Patient Care *Check agency policy for positioning and feeding spinal surgery or traction patients.*

STEP	RATIONALE
3. Prepare patient's room for mealtime.	
a. Clear over-bed table and arrange any needed supplies.	Prepares room for food tray.
b. Help patient put on eyeglasses or insert contact lenses if used.	Enhances patient's ability to self-feed and makes meal more visually appealing.
c. Limit distractions if possible during feeding. Alert staff to what you are doing. *Option:* If patient enjoys music, play a soothing, low-volume selection	Provides time to provide adequate intake without rushing patient. Promotes patient comfort while enhancing mealtime experience.

STEP	RATIONALE
4. During meal, instruct patient on the guidelines for a healthy eating pattern:	
a. Follow a healthy eating pattern across the life span (U.S. Department of Health and Human Services [USDHHS] and U.S. Department of Agriculture [USDA], 2015).	Food choices are from the *Dietary Guidelines for Americans 2015–2020* (USDHHS and USDA, 2015).
b. Eat a variety of vegetables from all of the subgroups, including dark green, red, orange, legumes (beans and peas), and starchy; fruits, especially whole fruits; grains, at least half of which are whole grains; fat-free or low-fat dairy, including milk, yogurt, cheese, and/or fortified soy beverages; a variety of protein foods, including seafood, lean meats and poultry, eggs, legumes (beans and peas), nuts, seeds, and soy products; and oils. **Limit saturated and trans-fat and added sugar.**	
c. Focus on variety, nutrient density, and amount.	
d. Limit calories from added sugars and saturated fats and reduce sodium intake.	
e. Shift to healthier food and beverage choices.	
f. Support healthy eating patterns for all.	
5. Obtain special assistive devices as needed and instruct on use (see illustration). For example: • Two-handled cup with spout in lid makes it easier to drink and hold and lift a cup. Avoids spills. Cup has wide base that prevents tipping over. • Plate with plate guard and nonskid bottom helps person with limited flexibility of hands or poor motor coordination or who uses only one hand. • Knife, fork, and spoon with large handles or attached splints help patient with limited hand function or a weak grip.	Devices facilitate self-feeding by improving ability to grasp, pick up foods with utensils, and drink liquids.
6. Assess meal tray for completeness and correct diet food options. Use this time (and during actual feeding) to instruct patient about diet, rationale for diet, food options, and dysphagia risks.	Prevents intake of incomplete or incorrect diet. Instruction is more meaningful when applied during real-time activity.
7. Ask in which order patient would like to eat his or her meal. Help to set up meal tray if patient unable to do so: open packages, cut up food, apply seasonings or condiments, place napkin.	Allows patient more independence and control. Small pieces are easier to chew and minimize risk for aspiration.
8. Watch patient successfully swallow first bites of food and drink. If patient is able to eat independently, stop here. Return after 15 or 20 minutes or stay at side for communication and additional teaching.	Aim is to make patient as self-sufficient as possible.

Safe Patient Care *If patient is at risk for aspiration, stay at his or her side during entire feeding.*

STEP	RATIONALE
9. Help patient who cannot eat independently.	
a. If patient is visually impaired, identify food location on plate as if it were a clock (e.g., vegetables at 9 o'clock, meat at 3 o'clock) (see illustration).	Helps patient locate food items; may be able to feed self if given adequate information about food placement on tray.
b. Ask patient in which order he or she would like to eat, and cut food into bite-sized pieces.	Gives patient more independence and control. Small bites reduce risk of aspiration.
c. Provide fluids as requested. Discourage patient from drinking all fluids at beginning of meal.	Promotes swallowing. Prevents patient from filling up on fluids.
d. Pace feeding to avoid patient fatigue. Interact with patient during mealtime. Verbally encourage self-feeding attempts.	Social interaction may improve appetite.

STEP	RATIONALE

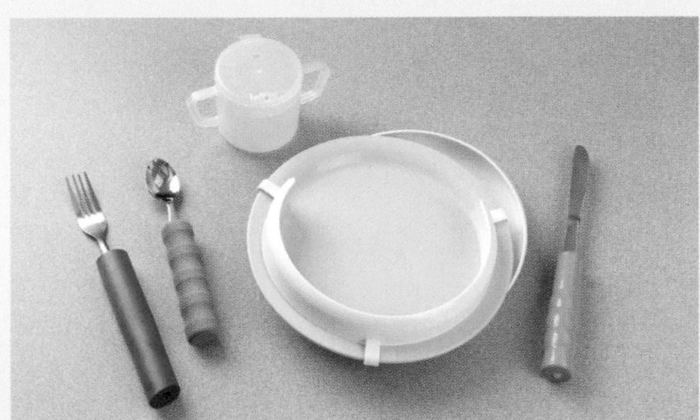

STEP 5 Mealtime adaptive equipment. *Clockwise from upper left:* Two-handled cup with lid, plate with plate guard, utensils with splints, and utensils with enlarged handles.

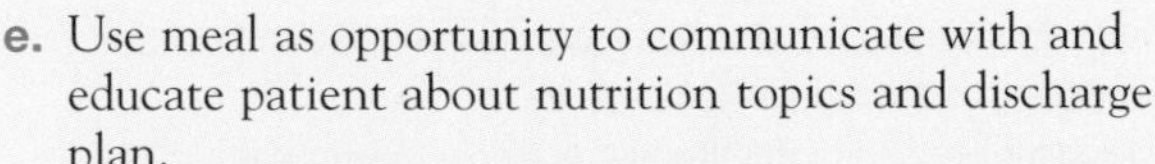

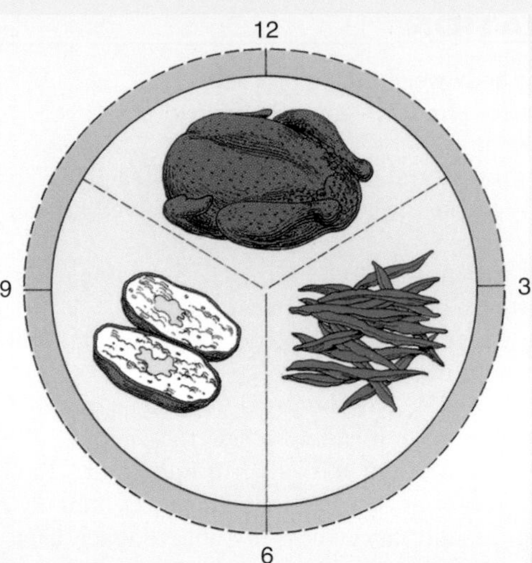

STEP 9a Clock setup to prepare food on a plate for the visually impaired patient.

STEP	RATIONALE
e. Use meal as opportunity to communicate with and educate patient about nutrition topics and discharge plan.	Offers extended time for teaching.
f. Feed patient in manner that facilitates chewing and swallowing. Keep patient's chin down and place food in stronger side of the mouth.	Chin-down position may help to reduce aspiration risk (see Skill 13.3).
10. Use appropriate feeding techniques for patients with special needs:	
a. *Older adult:* Feed small amounts at a time, observing biting, chewing, ability to manipulate tongue to form bolus of food, swallowing, and fatigue between bites. Be sure that patient has swallowed food. Offer variety of foods and frequent rest periods.	Decreased saliva production in older adults impairs swallowing. Aspiration results from decreased or absent gag reflex. Small pieces are easier to chew and minimize risk for aspiration.

Safe Patient Care *If you suspect that patient is aspirating, stop feeding immediately and suction airway (see Chapter 16).*

STEP	RATIONALE
b. *Neurologically impaired patient:* Feed small amounts at a time and observe ability to chew, manipulate tongue to form bolus, and swallow. Have patient open mouth and check for food left inside cheeks (pocketing) after swallowing. Give small amount of thin liquid between bites.	Some patients with limited tongue strength and control are unable to move food to back of mouth for swallowing. Checking for "pocketed" food in mouth prevents aspiration.
c. *Patients with cancer:* Check for food aversions before and during meal. Monitor for fatigue.	Strong, abnormal sense of taste and smell are side effects of chemotherapy. Cancer patients can tire easily.
11. Help patient with hand hygiene and performing mouth care after meal is completed. (Apply gloves as needed.)	Maintains comfort.
12. Help patient to resting position, leave head elevated at least 45 degrees for 30 to 60 minutes after meal. Provide nurse call system to patient and instruct patient to utilize if needed.	Reduces risk of aspiration from regurgitation. Nurse call system summons nurse to patient bedside if assistance is required.
13. Raise side rails (as appropriate) and lower bed to lowest position.	Promotes patient safety.
14. Return patient's tray to appropriate place, remove and discard gloves, and perform hand hygiene.	Reduces transmission of microorganisms.

STEP	RATIONALE
EVALUATION	
1. Monitor body weight daily or weekly.	Determines ongoing nutritional status.
2. Monitor for physical signs of malnutrition.	Physical signs may indicate both micro- and macronutrient deficiencies.
3. Monitor intake and output (I&O) (see Chapter 8) and complete intake measurement (e.g., observed intake, calorie count).	Determines ongoing nutritional status.
4. Observe patient's ability to self-feed, including ability to feed certain items, part, or all of meal.	Helps to determine what help patient needs with feeding.
5. Observe patient for choking, coughing, gagging, or food left in mouth during eating.	Indicates dysphagia and possible aspiration.
6. **Use Teach-Back:** "We discussed ways you can help feed your husband that make it easier for him to swallow. Tell me two ways to help feed him and why it is important." Revise your instruction now or develop a plan for revised family caregiver teaching if family caregiver is not able to teach back correctly.	Determines family caregiver's level of understanding of instructional topic.

Unexpected Outcomes	Related Interventions
1. Patient is unable to eat entire meal or refuses to eat.	• Determine if patient has other food preferences and cultural factors or religious restrictions. • Ask patient what is affecting his or her ability to eat. • Determine if patient's ability or desire to eat is better at other times of the day. • Determine if patient is in pain or nauseated or if he or she has constipation. Implement appropriate interventions (e.g., administering analgesic, antiemetic, or cathartic; offering food or liquid at temperature patient prefers; offering small frequent meals). • Provide more frequent oral care. • If inability to eat meal is a repeated problem, collaborate with health care provider and registered dietitian (RD).
2. Patient chokes on fluids or food.	• Stop feeding immediately; place on side with head forward and pointing down; suction food and secretions from mouth and airway. • Contact health care provider if choking occurs repeatedly. • Suggest appropriate referrals (e.g., speech-language pathologist, RD).

Recording

- Record the patient's type of diet, food and fluids actually consumed (including I&O), extent of patient self-feeds and amount of feeding assistance needed, patient's ability to swallow, tolerance of diet (including any choking that occurs), and calorie count (if ordered).
- Record patient's ability to describe types of food he or she can eat.
- Document your evaluation of patient learning.

Hand-Off Reporting

- Report at end of shift patient's diet type and tolerance.
- Report any swallowing difficulties, food dislikes, or refusal to eat to nurse in charge and the RD.

✦ SKILL 13.2 Aspiration Precautions

Purpose

Aspiration is the misdirection by inhalation of oropharyngeal secretions or gastric contents into the larynx and lower respiratory tract (Metheny, 2018). Dysphagia or impaired swallowing slows eating, resulting in food being left in the mouth, which increases a patient's risk for acute aspiration that may lead to pneumonia and death (Eglseer et al., 2018). Dysphagia results from muscular, nerve, and obstructive causes (Box 13.5) and has a variety of potential symptoms (Box 13.6) (Steele and Cichero, 2014; Tanner

BOX 13.5

Causes and Conditions That Increase Risk for Dysphagia

Myogenic (Muscle)
- Aging
- Muscular dystrophy
- Myasthenia gravis
- Polymyositis

Neurogenic (Nerve)
- Amyotrophic lateral sclerosis (Lou Gehrig's disease)
- Dementia
- Cerebral palsy
- Diabetic neuropathy
- Guillain-Barré syndrome
- Multiple sclerosis
- Parkinson's disease
- Stroke

Obstructive
- Anterior mediastinal masses
- Candidiasis
- Cervical spondylosis
- Benign peptic stricture
- Head and neck cancer
- Inflammatory masses
- Lower esophageal ring
- Trauma/surgical resection

Other
- Medical interventions that compromise the gag reflex (sedation, mechanical ventilation, nasotracheal suctioning, lying flat)
- Connective tissue disorders
- Gastrointestinal or esophageal resection
- Rheumatological disorders
- Vagotomy

BOX 13.6

Symptoms of Dysphagia

Oropharyngeal dysphagia (difficulty moving food or liquid from mouth to upper esophagus):
- Weak voice
- Drooling
- Difficulty initiating swallow
- Choking, coughing, or gagging with food
- Poor tongue control
- Loss of gag reflex
- Nasal regurgitation

Esophageal dysphagia (difficulty moving food from esophagus to stomach):
- Pain with swallowing
- Feeling of food stuck in throat
- Burping
- Chest pressure/heartburn

et al., 2014). Gastric material and secretions in the mouth and pharynx and pathogenic bacteria enter the trachea and lungs, causing an inflammatory response that can lead to pneumonia. Tachypnea (respirations above 26) is an early clue of aspiration, along with signs of cough, dyspnea, and decreased and abnormal breath sounds (see Chapter 8). Common in elderly patients is the decreased urge or ability to cough reflexively, which, when combined with dysphagia, leads to silent aspiration; a patient aspirates without any outward signs of swallowing difficulty (Ebihara et al., 2016). Silent aspiration is most often identified following a chest x-ray film.

Dysphagia management includes dietary modifications by altering the consistency of food and liquids and is most effective when implemented using an interprofessional approach recommended by a speech-language pathologist (SLP) and registered dietitian (RD; Tanner, 2014). Research has shown that thickening agents will not provide the same viscosity for all fluids and that some adjustments may be needed to ensure the proper viscosity is achieved (Liantonio et al., 2014), thus the need for an RD. Early detection of dysphagia and management with swallowing techniques and diet modifications (Table 13.2) and incorporation of aspiration precautions will decrease the risk of a patient developing pneumonia.

Delegation and Collaboration

The skill of following aspiration precautions while feeding a patient can be delegated to nursing assistive personnel (NAP). However, the nurse is responsible for the ongoing assessment of a patient's risk for aspiration and determination of positioning and any special feeding techniques. The nurse directs the NAP to:

- Position patient upright (45–90 degrees preferred) or according to medical restrictions during and after feeding.
- Use aspiration precautions while feeding patients who need help, and explain feeding techniques that are successful for specific patients.
- Immediately report to the nurse any onset of coughing, gagging, or a wet voice or pocketing of food.

Equipment

- Chair or bed that allows patient to sit upright
- Thickening agents as designated by SLP (rice, cereal, yogurt, gelatin, commercial thickener)
- Tongue blade
- Penlight
- Oral hygiene supplies (see Chapter 11)
- Suction equipment (see Chapter 16)
- Clean gloves
- *Option:* Pulse oximeter

ASSESSMENT

1. Identify patient using at least two identifiers (e.g., name and birthday or name and medical record number) according to agency policy. *Rationale: Ensures correct patient. Complies with The Joint Commission standards and improves patient safety (TJC, 2019).*
2. Review patient's medical history, nutritional risks (see Box 13.1), and results of nutritional screening in medical record (see Skill 13.1). Assess for presence of conditions that cause dysphagia (see Box 13.5). Note patient's weight. Consult with SLP and/or RD. *Rationale: Reveals patient risk patterns for altered nutrition and dysphagia. Weight provides baseline for determining change in nutritional status.*
3. Assess patient's current medications for use of sedatives, hypnotics, or other agents that may impair cough or swallowing reflex and for any medications that dry oral secretions (e.g., calcium channel blockers, diuretics; Tan et al., 2018). *Rationale: Medication side effects may increase risk of developing dysphagia.*
4. Perform hand hygiene. Assess patient for signs and symptoms of dysphagia (see Box 13.6). Consult with SLP. *Rationale: Patient symptoms aid in determining if further swallow evaluation is needed and approach to feeding.*
5. Assess patient's mental status: alertness, orientation, and ability to follow simple commands (e.g., open your mouth; stick out your tongue). *Rationale: Disorientation and inability to follow commands present higher risk for dysphagia.*
6. Apply gloves. Assess patient's oral cavity, level of dental hygiene, missing teeth, or poorly fitting dentures. Remove and dispose of gloves. *Rationale: Poorly fitting dentures and absence of teeth can cause chewing and swallowing difficulties, increasing aspiration risk. Poor oral hygiene and periodontal*

TABLE 13.2
Therapeutic Diets

Diet	Description
Texture-Based Therapeutic Diets	
Clear liquid	Foods that are clear and liquid at room or body temperature (e.g., chicken broth, tea, soda, gelatin, and apple or cranberry juice) and that leave little residue and are easily absorbed; commonly ordered for short-term use (24 to 48 hours) after surgery, before diagnostic tests, and after episodes of vomiting or diarrhea
Full liquid	Includes foods on clear-liquid diet plus addition of smooth-textured dairy products (e.g., milk and ice cream), strained soups and custard, refined cooked cereals, vegetable juice, and pureed vegetables; commonly ordered before or after surgery for patients who are acutely ill from infection or for patients who cannot chew or tolerate solid foods; must verify that patients are lactose tolerant before providing dairy products
Pureed	Includes food on clear-liquid and full-liquid diets plus easily swallowed foods that do not require chewing (e.g., scrambled eggs; pureed meats, vegetables, and fruits; mashed potatoes); ordered for patients with head and neck abnormalities or who have had oral surgery; can be modified for low sodium, fat, or calorie count
Mechanical or dental—soft	Includes foods on all previous diets plus addition of lightly seasoned ground or finely diced meats, flaked fish, cottage cheese, cheese, rice, potatoes, pancakes, light breads, cooked vegetables, cooked or canned fruit, bananas, and peanut butter; avoids tough meats, nuts, bacon, and fruits with tough skins or membranes; ordered for patients who have chewing problems or mild gastrointestinal (GI) problems; used as transition diet from liquids to regular
Soft/low residue	Addition of low-fiber, easily digested foods such as pastas, casseroles, moist tender meats, and canned cooked fruits and vegetables; includes foods that are easy to chew and simply cooked; does not permit fatty, rich, and fried foods; is sometimes referred to as low-fiber diet
High fiber	Addition of fresh uncooked fruits, steamed vegetables, bran, oatmeal, and dried fruits; includes sufficient amounts of indigestible carbohydrate to relieve constipation, increase GI motility, and increase stool weight
Regular or diet as tolerated	No restrictions; permits patients' preferences and allows for postoperative diet progression
Disease-Based Therapeutic Diets	
Restricted fluids	Required in severe heart failure and kidney failure, usually limited to 1500 mL or less in 24 hours
Sodium restricted	Allows low levels of sodium and may include a 4-g (no added salt), 2-g (moderate), 1-g (strict), or 500-mg (very strict) diet; may be ordered for patients with heart failure, renal failure, cirrhosis, or hypertension
Fat modified	Low total and saturated fat and low cholesterol; cholesterol intake limited to < 300 mg daily and fat intake to 30% to 35%; eliminates or reduces fatty foods for hypercholesterolemia, malabsorptive disorders, and diarrhea
Diabetic or consistent carbohydrate	Essential treatment for patients with diabetes mellitus; provides patients with a diet recommended by American Diabetes Association, which allows for patients to select set amount of food from basic food groups. Meal-planning tools include carbohydrate counting, the MyPlate method, and glycemic index. It is important that food intake is balanced with patient's exercise and medications for safe management of patient's blood glucose levels.

Modified from Grodner M et al: *Nutritional foundations and clinical applications of nutrition: a nursing approach,* ed 5, St. Louis, 2013, Mosby.

disease can result in growth of bacteria in oropharynx, which, if aspirated, can lead to pneumonia (Liantonio et al., 2014). Findings indicate level of oral hygiene needed and diet selection needed.

7. *Option:* Obtain baseline assessment of oxygen saturation. A decline in SpO_2 2% or higher has been regarded as a possible marker of aspiration (Marian et al., 2017). Perform hand hygiene. *Rationale: Despite its clinical use, research findings question whether oximetry can reliably detect aspiration (American Speech-Language-Hearing Association [ASHA], 2016; Lancaster, 2015; Marian et al., 2017).*
8. Prepare to observe patient during mealtime for signs of dysphagia. Observe patient attempt to feed self; note type of food consistencies and liquids able to swallow. Note during and at end of meal if patient tires. *Rationale: Detects abnormal eating patterns such as frequent clearing of throat or prolonged eating time. Chewing and sitting up for feeding bring on onset of fatigue (Meiner and Yeager, 2019). Provides data for future planning of meal assistance.*
9. Indicate in patient's health record that dysphagia/aspiration risk is present. *Option:* Some agencies use different-colored meal trays to signify patients at risk for aspiration. *Rationale: Identifying patient as dysphagic reduces risk that he or she will receive improperly prepared oral nutrition without supervision.*
10. Assess patient's or family caregiver's knowledge of dysphagia risk and diet options, experience, and health literacy level. *Rationale: Ensures patient has the capacity to obtain, communicate, process, and understand basic health information (CDC, 2016).*

STEP	RATIONALE
PLANNING	
1. Expected outcomes following completion of procedure:	
• Patient does not exhibit signs or symptoms of aspiration.	Interventions for preventing aspiration are successful.
• Patient maintains stable weight.	Patient is able to maintain adequate oral nutrition.
2. Provide patient 30 minutes of rest before a meal.	Fatigue increases risk of aspiration (Liantonio et al., 2014).
3. Explain to patient why you are observing him or her while he or she eats.	Signs or symptoms associated with aspiration indicate need for further swallowing evaluation, such as fluoroscopic examination.
4. Explain to patient and family caregiver techniques to be used to prevent aspiration during feeding.	Increases patient cooperation and prepares family caregiver for being able to help.
5. Provide for patient privacy and organize supplies at bedside.	Promotes patient comfort; reduces distractions during eating. Promotes organized approach.
IMPLEMENTATION	
1. Perform hand hygiene and have patient or family caregiver (if going to help with feeding) perform hand hygiene.	Prevents transmission of microorganisms. Educates patient and family caregiver about need to maintain infection control practices.
2. Apply clean gloves. Provide thorough oral hygiene, including brushing tongue, before meal (see Chapter 11).	Risk for aspiration pneumonia has been associated with poor oral hygiene (Liantonio et al., 2014).
3. Position patient upright (90 degrees) in chair or elevate head of patient's bed to a 90-degree angle or highest position allowed by medical condition during meal.	Position facilitates safe swallowing and enhances esophageal motility (Liantonio et al., 2014; Metheny and Franz, 2013). Side-lying position is an option if patient cannot have head elevated.
4. *Option:* Apply pulse oximeter to patient's finger; monitor during feeding.	Pulse oximetry continues to be used in many agencies in an effort to predict aspiration, but recent research questions its efficacy (ASHA, 2016; Marian et al., 2017).
5. Apply gloves. Use penlight and tongue blade to gently inspect mouth for pockets of food.	Pockets of food found inside cheeks occur when patient has difficulty moving food from mouth into pharynx; may lead to aspiration (Zupec-Kania and O'Flaherty, 2017). Patient is usually unaware of pocketing.
6. Provide appropriate thickness of liquids per SLP and RD assessment (International Dysphagia Diet Standardization Initiative, 2016; Table 13.3). Encourage patient to feed self.	Thin liquids are difficult to control in mouth and pharynx and are more easily aspirated.
7. Have patient assume chin-down position. Remind patient to not tilt head backward when eating or while drinking.	Chin-down position may help reduce aspiration (Kagaya et al., 2011; Liantonio et al., 2014). One study suggests a head-turn-plus-chin-down maneuver may be more successful (Nagy et al., 2016).
8. Adjust the rate of feeding and size of bites to match the patient's tolerance. If patient unable to feed self, place ½ to 1 teaspoon of food on unaffected side of mouth, allowing utensil to touch mouth or tongue (Liantonio et al., 2014).	Small bites help patient swallow (Liantonio et al., 2014). Provides tactile cue to food being eaten; avoids pocketing of food on weaker side.
9. Provide verbal coaching; remind patient to chew and think about swallowing: • "Open your mouth. • Feel the food in your mouth. • Chew and taste the food. • Raise your tongue to the roof of your mouth. • Think about swallowing • Close your mouth and swallow. • Swallow again. • Cough to clear your airway."	Verbal cueing keeps patient focused on normal swallowing (Metheny, 2018). Positive reinforcement enhances patient's confidence in ability to swallow.
10. Avoid mixing food of different textures in same mouthful. Alternate liquids and bites of food (Liantonio et al., 2014). Refer to RD for next meal if patient has difficulty with particular consistency.	Gradual increase in types and textures combined with constant monitoring helps patient to eat more safely. Single textures are easier to swallow than multiple textures. Alternating solids with liquids removes food residue in mouth.

TABLE 13.3

International Dysphagia Diet Framework

Level and Description	Characteristics	Examples
0: Thin liquid	Flows like water, can drink easily from straw *Rationale*: functional ability to safely manage liquids of all types	Coffee, tea, lemonade, juice, water
1: Slightly thick liquid	Thicker than water, requires more effort to drink, still flows through a straw or nipple *Rationale*: primarily used for the pediatric population to reduce speed of flow	Commercially available oral supplements similar in viscosity to an infant "anti-regurgitation" formula, nectar-thick juices
2: Mildly thick liquid	Flows off a spoon, effort required to drink through a straw *Rationale*: suitable if tongue control is slightly reduced	Milkshake
3: Liquidized moderately thick	Can be drunk from a cup, some effort to suck through a straw, cannot be eaten with a fork, will drip between prongs, no oral processing or chewing required, smooth texture with no lumps *Rationale*: Allows more time for oral control, needs some tongue propulsion effort	Runny rice cereal, runny pureed fruit, sauces and gravies, honey-thickened beverages
4: Pureed/extremely thick	Cannot drink from cup, usually eaten with a spoon, cannot suck through a straw, does not require chewing, can be molded, no lumps, not sticky *Rationale*: If tongue control is significantly reduced, requires less propulsion, no biting or chewing is required, missing teeth or poorly fitting dentures	Pureed meat, vegetables, fruits, and thick cereals
5: Minced and moist	Can be eaten with a fork or spoon, soft and moist with no separate thick liquid, small lumps that are easy to squash with tongue *Rationale*: Biting is not required, minimal chewing, tongue force alone can be used to break small soft particles, some missing teeth	Finely minced or ground tender meats served in extremely thick, smooth, non-pouring sauce or gravy, mashed potatoes, mashed fruits, very thick cereals Fluid or milk should NOT separate from items, pre-gelled "soaked" breads
6: Soft and bite-sized	Can be eaten with a fork or spoon; can be mashed/broken down with pressure from utensils; knife is not required to cut; chewing is required before swallowing; soft, tender, and moist throughout *Rationale*: Tongue force and control are required to move the food for chewing and to keep it within the mouth during chewing; tongue force is required to move the bolus for swallowing	Soft cooked meat cut in small pieces, flakey fish, casserole, stews, soft cooked vegetables in bite-sized pieces, mashed fruits
7: Regular	Normal, everyday foods of various textures *Rationale*: Ability to bite hard or soft foods, chew all textures without tiring	No restrictions

STEP	RATIONALE
11. During the meal, explain to patient and family caregiver the techniques being used to promote swallowing.	Enhances patient and family caregiver's ability to use techniques in the home.
12. Monitor swallowing and observe for any respiratory difficulty. Observe for throat clearing, coughing, choking, gagging, and drooling of food; suction airway as needed (see Chapter 16).	These are indications that suggest dysphagia and thus pose risk for aspiration (National Stroke Association, 2017).
13. Minimize distractions, do not talk, and do not rush patient (Liantonio et al., 2014). Allow time for adequate chewing and swallowing. Provide rest periods as needed during meal.	Environmental distractions and conversations during mealtime increase risk for aspiration. Avoiding fatigue reduces aspiration risk.

Safe Patient Care *If patient remains stable without difficulty, this is a good time to delegate continued feeding to NAP so that you can attend to other patients and assigned priorities.*

STEP	RATIONALE
14. Use sauces, condiments, and gravies (if part of dysphagia diet) to facilitate cohesive food bolus formation.	Cohesive food bolus helps to prevent pocketing or small food particles from entering the airway.

STEP	RATIONALE
15. Ask patient to remain sitting upright for at least 30 to 60 minutes after a meal. Provide nurse call system to patient and instruct patient to utilize if needed.	Remaining upright after meals or snack reduces chance of aspiration by allowing food particles remaining in pharynx to clear (Frey and Ramsberger, 2011). Promotes patient safety.
16. Provide thorough oral hygiene after meal (see Chapter 11).	Rigorous oral hygiene reduces plaque and secretions containing bacteria, with studies showing reduction in incidence of pneumonia (Liantonio et al., 2014).
17. Raise side rails (as appropriate) and lower bed to lowest position.	Reduces spread of microorganisms.
18. Return patient's tray to appropriate place. Remove and dispose of gloves, if worn. Perform hand hygiene.	Promotes patient safety. Reduces transmission of microorganisms.

EVALUATION

1. Throughout meal, observe patient's ability to swallow food and fluids of various textures and thicknesses without choking.	Indicates if there is ease with swallowing and absence of signs related to aspiration.
2. Monitor pulse oximetry readings (if ordered) for high-risk patients during eating.	Deteriorating oxygen saturation levels may indicate aspiration, but current research questions predictive ability.
3. Monitor patient's intake and output (I&O), calorie count, and food intake.	Helps to detect malnutrition and dehydration resulting from dysphagia.
4. Weigh patient daily or weekly.	Determines if weight is stable and reflects nutritional status.
5. Observe patient's oral cavity after meal.	Determines presence of food pockets after meal that has included foods of various textures.
6. Use Teach-Back: "We talked about why your husband is at risk to aspirate his food. Tell me the things to observe for that will tell you if he is having trouble swallowing. What should you do if these things happen during a meal?" Revise your instruction now or develop a plan for revised family caregiver teaching if family caregiver is not able to teach back correctly.	Determines family caregiver's level of understanding of instructional topic.

Unexpected Outcomes	Related Interventions
1. Patient coughs, gags, complains of food "stuck in throat," and has wet quality to voice when eating.	• Stop feeding immediately and place patient on nothing-by-mouth (NPO) status. • Notify health care provider and suction as needed (see Chapter 16). • Anticipate consultation with SLP for swallowing exercises and techniques to improve swallowing.
2. Patient experiences weight loss over next several days/weeks.	• Discuss findings with health care provider and RD. Determine if increasing frequency or quality of foods is needed. • Nutritional supplements may be needed.

Recording

- Record patient's diet, tolerance of liquids and food textures, amount of assistance required, response to instruction, position during meal, absence or presence of any symptoms of dysphagia, fluid intake, and amount of food eaten.
- Document your evaluation of patient learning.

Hand-Off Reporting

- Describe patient's tolerance to diet and degree of assistance required during hand-off report.
- Report any coughing, gagging, choking, or swallowing difficulties to nurse in charge or health care provider immediately.

✦ SKILL 13.3 Insertion and Removal of a Small-Bore Feeding Tube

Purpose

Small-bore feeding tubes placed by either the nasal (via the nose) or oral (via the mouth) route may be used to deliver enteral nutrition (EN) directly into the stomach (nasogastric) or small intestine (nasointestinal). These feeding tubes are soft and flexible and therefore may require a removable guidewire or stylet to provide stiffness during insertion. Some evidence suggests post-pyloric feeding (tip of tube placed past pyloric sphincter) may reduce the risk of aspiration and allow for greater delivery of prescribed nutrition (Alkhawaja et al., 2015). Placement of a small-bore tube into the intestine can be technically difficult, and assistive devices (electromagnetic tracing, capnography, etc.) used by nursing, with proven competency, provide improved safety and rate of successful bedside placement (Milsom et al., 2015). However, x-ray confirmation remains the gold standard in confirming tube placement (Milsom et al., 2015). In some instances, the medical provider may order a prokinetic agent such as metoclopramide to assist with advancement of a tube beyond the pylorus. Confirmation of the correct position of a newly inserted tube is mandatory before any feeding or medication administration (see Skill 13.4). Placement of a feeding tube requires a health care provider's order. The patient's coagulation status should be determined prior to placement of a small-bore feeding tube. Anticoagulants and bleeding disorders pose a risk for epistaxis during tube placement. The health care provider may order platelet transfusion or other corrective measures before tube insertion. History of recent nasal surgery and facial trauma are contraindications to placement.

Nasal and oral insertion of feeding tubes is commonly performed at a patient's bedside. Nurses use a variety of bedside tests to determine tube placement. However, the gold standard for confirming correct placement of a blindly inserted enteral tube is a radiographic film that visualizes the entire course of the tube. Assessing the color and pH of gastric aspirate for ongoing monitoring of tube location has been shown to be effective and less costly (Bourgault et al., 2015).

Delegation and Collaboration

The skill of feeding tube insertion cannot be delegated to nursing assistive personnel (NAP). However, NAP may help with patient positioning and comfort measures during tube insertion.

Equipment

Insertion

- Small-bore feeding tube with or without stylet (select the smallest diameter possible to enhance patient comfort)
- 60-mL ENFit syringe
- Stethoscope, pulse oximeter, capnography *(optional)*
- Hypoallergenic tape, semipermeable (transparent) dressing, or tube fixation device
- Tincture of benzoin or other skin barrier protectant
- pH indicator strip (scale 1 to 11)
- Cup of water and straw or ice chips (for patients able to swallow)
- Water-soluble lubricant
- Emesis basin
- Towel or disposable pad
- Facial tissues
- Clean gloves
- Suction equipment in case of aspiration
- Penlight to check placement in nasopharynx
- Tongue blade
- Oral hygiene supplies

Removal

- Disposable pad
- Tissues
- Clean gloves
- Disposable plastic bag
- Towel

ASSESSMENT

1. Verify health care provider's order for type of tube and EN feeding schedule. Also check order to determine if health care provider wants prokinetic agent (e.g., metoclopramide) given before tube placement. *Rationale: Health care provider's order is needed to insert feeding tube. Prokinetic agent given before tube placement may help advance tube into intestine.*
2. Identify patient using at least two identifiers (e.g., name and birthday or name and medical record number) according to agency policy. *Rationale: Ensures correct patient. Complies with The Joint Commission standards and improves patient safety (TJC, 2019).*
3. Review patient's medical history (e.g., for basilar skull fracture, nasal problems, nosebleeds, facial trauma, nasal-facial surgery, deviated septum, anticoagulant therapy, coagulopathy). *Rationale: History of these problems may require you to consult with health care provider to change route of nutritional support. Passage of tube intracranially can cause neurological injury.*

Safe Patient Care *If a patient is at risk for intracranial passage of the tube, avoid the nasal route. Oral placement or placement under medical supervision using fluoroscopic direct visualization is preferable. Insertion of a gastrostomy or jejunostomy tube is another alternative.*

4. Assess patient's height, weight, hydration status, electrolyte balance, caloric needs and intake and output (I&O). *Rationale: Provides baseline information to measure nutritional improvement after enteral feedings.*
5. Perform hand hygiene. Have patient close each nostril alternately and breathe. Examine each naris for patency and skin breakdown (apply clean gloves if drainage present). *Rationale: Reduces transmission of microorganisms. Nares can sometimes be obstructed or irritated, or septal defect or facial fractures are present. Place tube in most patent naris.*
6. Perform physical assessment of abdomen (see Chapter 8). Remove and dispose of gloves (if worn). Perform hand hygiene. *Rationale: Absent bowel sounds, abdominal pain, tenderness, or distention may indicate medical problem contraindicating feedings. Reduces transmission of microorganisms.*
7. Assess patient's mental status (ability to cooperate with procedure, sedation), presence of cough and gag reflex, ability to swallow, critical illness, and presence of artificial airway. *Rationale: These are risk factors for inadvertent tube placement into tracheobronchial tree (Metheny, 2018).*
8. Assess patient's knowledge and experience with procedure. Determine health literacy level. *Rationale: Encourages cooperation and reduces anxiety. Ensures patient has the capacity to obtain, communicate, process, and understand basic health information (CDC, 2016).*

Safe Patient Care *Recognize situations in which blind placement of a feeding tube poses an unacceptable risk for placement. Devices designed to detect pulmonary intubation such as CO_2 sensors or electromagnetic tracking devices enhance patient safety. Alternatively, to avoid insertion complications from blind placement in high-risk situations, clinicians trained in the use of visualization or imaging techniques should place tubes (Metheny and Meert, 2017; Milsom et al., 2015).*

STEP	RATIONALE

PLANNING

STEP	RATIONALE
1. Expected outcomes following completion of procedure:	
• Tube is successfully placed in stomach or small intestine.	Verifying proper position is essential before initiating feeding tube.
• Patient has no respiratory distress (e.g., increased respiratory rate, coughing, poor color) or signs of discomfort or nasal trauma.	Correctly placed tube causes no interference with airway.
2. Provide privacy and prepare environment.	Promotes patient comfort. Removes clutter from over-bed or bedside table.
3. Perform hand hygiene. Prepare supplies at bedside.	Reduces transmission of microorganisms. Ensures organized procedure.
4. Explain procedure to patient, including sensations (e.g., burning in nasal passages) that will be felt during insertion.	Increases patient's cooperation with intubation procedure and helps lessen anxiety.
5. Explain to patient how to communicate during intubation by raising index finger to indicate gagging or discomfort.	Patient must have a way of communicating to alleviate stress and enhance cooperation.

IMPLEMENTATION

STEP	RATIONALE
1. Stand on same side of bed as naris chosen for insertion and position patient upright in high-Fowler's position (unless contraindicated). If patient is comatose, raise head of bed as tolerated in semi-Fowler's position with head tipped forward, using a pillow, chin to chest. If necessary, have an NAP help with positioning of confused or comatose patients. If patient is forced to lie supine, place in reverse Trendelenburg's position.	Allows for easier manipulation of tube. Fowler's position reduces risk of aspiration and promotes effective swallowing. Forward head position helps with closure of airway and passage of tube into esophagus.
2. Apply pulse oximeter/capnograph and measure vital signs. Maintain oximetry or capnography continuously.	Provides baseline for objective assessment of respiratory status during tube insertion and throughout time a tube is in place. Lowered oxygen saturation or increased end-tidal CO_2 can indicate tube being misplaced into the lungs or moving out of the stomach and into lungs (Holland et al., 2013).

Safe Patient Care *If patient has increase in end-tidal CO_2 or decrease in oxygen saturation, tube should not be inserted until you determine patient stability.*

STEP	RATIONALE
3. Place bath towel over patient's chest. Keep facial tissues within reach.	Prevents soiling of gown. Insertion of tube frequently produces tearing.
4. Determine length of tube to be inserted and mark location with tape or indelible ink. *Some tubes have centimeter markings.*	Ensures organized procedure and estimation of the proper length of tube to insert into patient.
a. *Option, Adult:* Measure distance from tip of nose to earlobe to xiphoid process (NEX) of sternum (see illustration). Mark this distance on tube with tape.	Most traditional method. Length approximates distance from nose to stomach. Research has shown this method may be least effective compared with others, although more research is needed (Santos et al., 2016).
b. *Option, Adult:* A nose to earlobe to mid-umbilicus (NEMU) method to estimate appropriate nasogastric tube placement has been recommended.	Promotes placement of the tube end holes in or closer to the gastric fluid pool (Boullata et al., 2017).
c. *Option, Adult:* Measure distance from xiphoid process to earlobe to nose (XEN) + 10 cm (Taylor et al., 2014).	Shown to be more accurate than NEX (Taylor et al., 2014).
d. *Option, Children:* Use NEMU option.	Estimates proper length of tube insertion for pediatric patient.
e. Add 20 to 30 cm (8–12 inches) for post-pyloric tubes.	Length approximates distance from nose to jejunum.

Safe Patient Care *Tip of pre-pyloric tubes must reach stomach to avoid the risk for pulmonary aspiration, which occurs when tubes end instead in the esophagus. Research has mixed findings in regard to the best technique for estimating tube length (Santos et al., 2016). Confirmation of placement via x-ray immediately after completed insertion is still needed.*

STEP	RATIONALE
5. Prepare tube for intubation. **NOTE: Do not ice tubes.**	Iced tube becomes stiff and inflexible, causing trauma to nasal mucosa.

STEP	RATIONALE
a. Obtain order for stylet tube and check agency policy for trained clinician to insert tube.	The practice of inserting a tube requires great care and attention to practice guidelines.
b. If tube has guidewire or stylet, inject 10 mL of water from ENFit syringe into tube.	Aids in guidewire or stylet removal. Activates lubrication of tube for easier passage and ensures that tube is patent. ENFit devices are not compatible with Luer-Lok connection or any other type of small-bore medical connector, thus preventing misadministration of an enteral feeding (ISMP, 2015).
c. If using stylet, make certain that it is positioned securely within tube. Inject 10 mL of water from ENFit syringe into tube.	Promotes smooth passage of tube into gastrointestinal (GI) tract. Improperly positioned stylet can cause tube to kink or injure patient. Ensures that tube is patent and aids in stylet removal. Once tube insertion is confirmed, have trained clinician remove stylet.
6. Prepare tube fixation materials. Cut hypoallergenic tape 10 cm (4 inches) long or prepare membrane dressing or other tube fixation device (e.g., bridle).	Used to secure tubing after insertion. Fixation devices allow tube to float free of nares, thus reducing pressure on nares, preventing device-related pressure injury (DRPI) (see illustration).
7. Apply clean gloves.	Reduces transmission of microorganisms.
8. *Option:* Dip tube with surface lubricant into glass of room-temperature water or apply water-soluble lubricant (see manufacturer directions).	Activates lubricant to facilitate passage of tube into naris and GI tract.
9. Offer an alert patient a cup of water with straw (if able to swallow).	Patient is asked to swallow water to facilitate tube passage.
10. Explain next steps and gently insert tube through nostril to back of throat (posterior nasopharynx). This may cause patient to gag. Aim back and down toward ear (see illustration).	Natural contours facilitate passage of tube into GI tract.

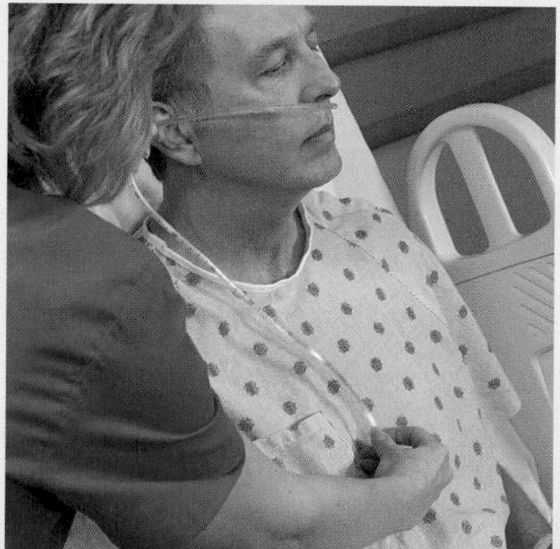

STEP 4a Measure to determine length of tube to insert.

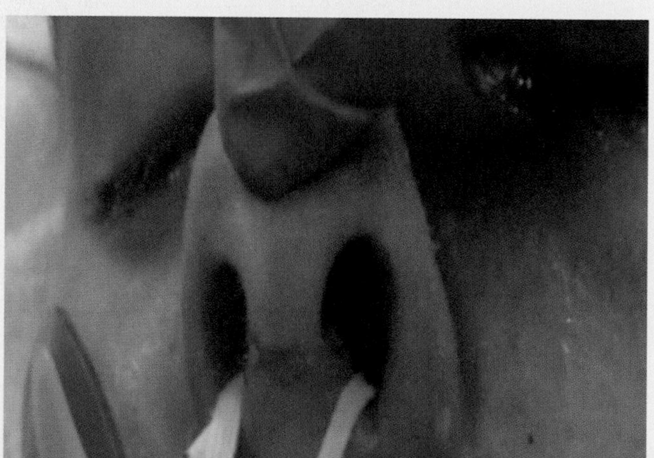

STEP 6 Medical device–related pressure injury under nose.

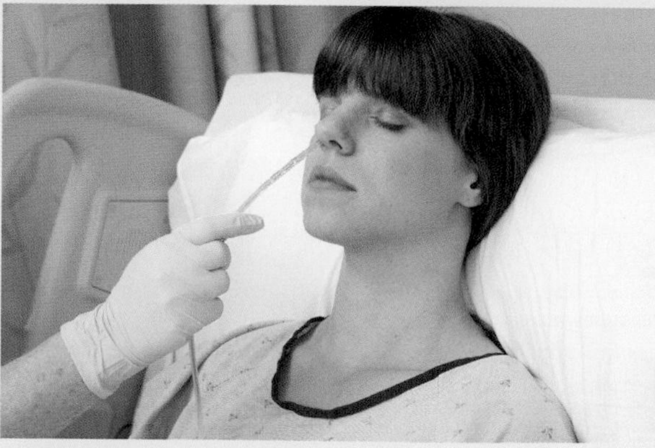

STEP 10 Insert tube through nostril to back of throat.

STEP	RATIONALE
11. Have patient take deep breath, relax, and flex head toward chest after tube has passed through nasopharynx.	Closes off glottis and reduces risk for tube entering trachea.
12. Encourage patient to swallow small sips of water. Advance tube as patient swallows. Rotate tube gently 180 degrees while inserting.	Swallowing water lubricates and facilitates passage of tube past oropharynx. Distinct tug may be felt as patient swallows, indicating that tube is following expected path.
13. Emphasize need to mouth breathe and swallow during insertion.	Helps facilitate passage of tube and alleviates patient's fears during procedure.
14. Do not advance tube during inspiration or coughing because it is more likely to enter respiratory tract. Monitor oximetry and capnography at this time.	Can cause tube to inadvertently enter patient's airway, which will be reflected in changes in oxygen saturation and/or capnography.
15. Advance tube each time patient swallows until desired length has been reached (see illustration).	Reduces discomfort and trauma to patient. Helps facilitate tube passage.

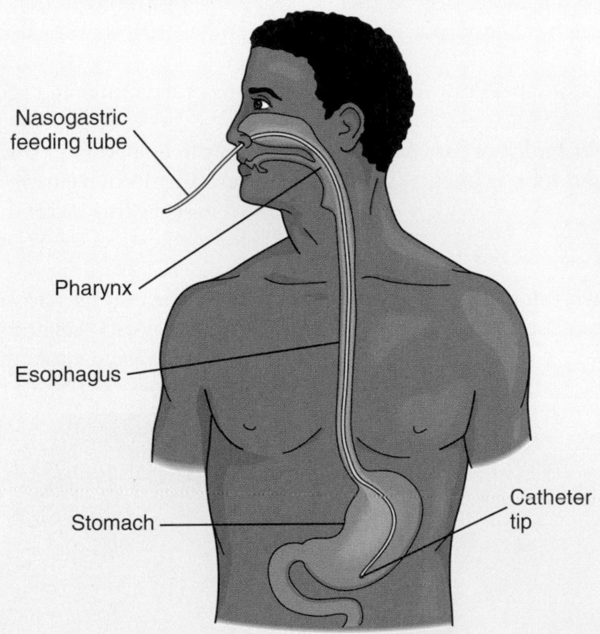

STEP 15 Nasogastric tube inserted through nasopharynx and esophagus into stomach.

Safe Patient Care *Do not force the tube or push against resistance. If patient starts to cough, experiences a drop in oxygen saturation or a rise in end-tidal CO_2, or shows other signs of respiratory distress, withdraw the tube into the posterior nasopharynx until normal breathing resumes.*

STEP	RATIONALE
16. Check for position of tube in back of throat using penlight and tongue blade.	Tube may be coiled, kinked, or entering trachea.
17. Temporarily anchor tube to nose with small piece of tape.	Movement of tube stimulates gagging. Assesses general position before anchoring tube more securely.
18. Keep tube secure and check its placement by aspirating stomach contents to measure gastric pH (see Skill 13.4). Also measure amount, color, and quality of return.	Proper tube position is essential before initiating feeding.

Safe Patient Care *Insufflation of air into tube while auscultating abdomen is not a reliable means to determine position of feeding tube tip (Bourgault et al., 2015).*

STEP	RATIONALE
19. Anchor tube to patient's nose, avoiding pressure on nares. Mark exit site on tube with indelible ink. Select one of the following options for anchoring:	Marking tube can alert nurses to possible displacement of tube. Properly secured tube allows patient more mobility and prevents trauma to nasal mucosa.
a. Apply membrane dressing or tube fixation device:	Permits longer securement without need to change dressing.
(1) Membrane dressing:	Allows membrane to adhere to skin.
(a) Apply tincture of benzoin or other skin protector to patient's cheek and area of tube to be secured.	Used to protect the skin from irritation and infection.

STEP	RATIONALE
(b) Place tube against patient's cheek and secure tube with membrane dressing, out of patient's line of vision.	Eliminates application of tape around naris. Decreases risk for patient's inadvertent extubation.
(2) Tube fixation device:	Secures tube and reduces friction on naris.
(a) Apply wide end of patch to bridge of nose (see illustration).	
(b) Slip connector around feeding tube as it exits nose (see illustration).	
b. Apply tape:	Prevents pulling of tube. May require frequent change if tape becomes soiled.
(1) Apply tincture of benzoin or other skin adhesive on tip of patient's nose and allow it to become "tacky."	Helps tape adhere better. Protects skin from breakdown.
(2) Remove gloves and tear two horizontal slits on each side of tape at ⅓ and ⅔ length. Do not split tape. Fold middle sections forward.	Creates a gap in tape that once secured will allow tube to float and exert less pressure on naris.
(3) Tear vertical strip at bottom of tape. Print date and time on nasal part of tape.	Secures tube firmly and provides date of insertion.
(4) Place intact end of tape over bridge of patient's nose. Wrap each strip around tube as it exits (see illustration).	Tube is free floating in the naris with this taping method, resulting in movement of tube in pharynx. Securing tape to naris in this method reduces pressure on naris and risk for medical device–related pressure injury (Markowitz et al., 2013).
20. Fasten end of tube to patient's gown using clip (see illustration) or piece of tape. Do not use safety pins to secure tube to gown.	Reduces traction on naris if tube moves, which can cause medical device–related pressure injury. Safety pins become unfastened and cause injury to patients.

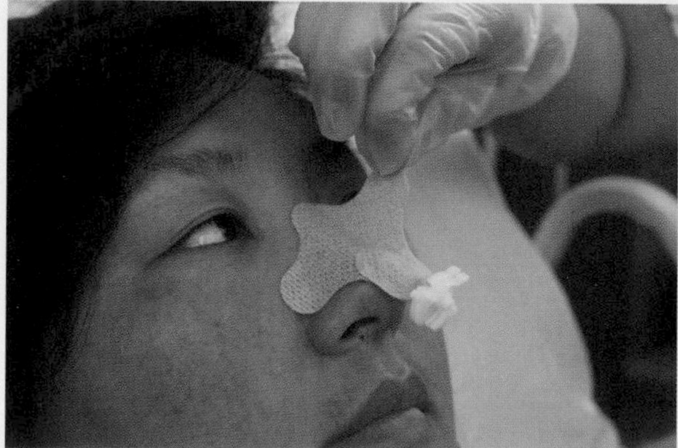

STEP 19a(2)(a) Apply tube fixation device to bridge of nose.

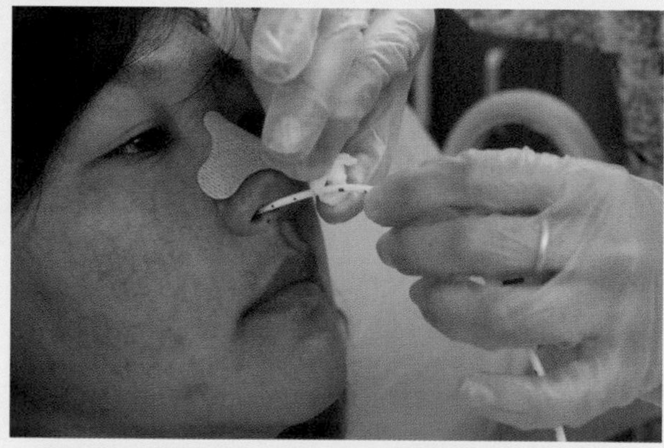

STEP 19a(2)(b) Slip connector around feeding tube.

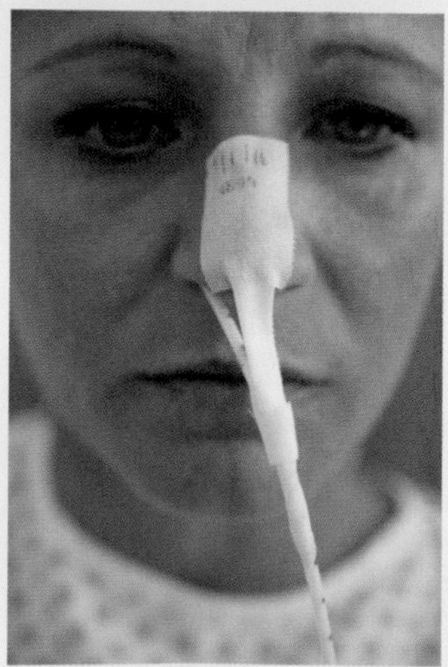

STEP 19b(4) Applying tape to anchor nasoenteral tube.

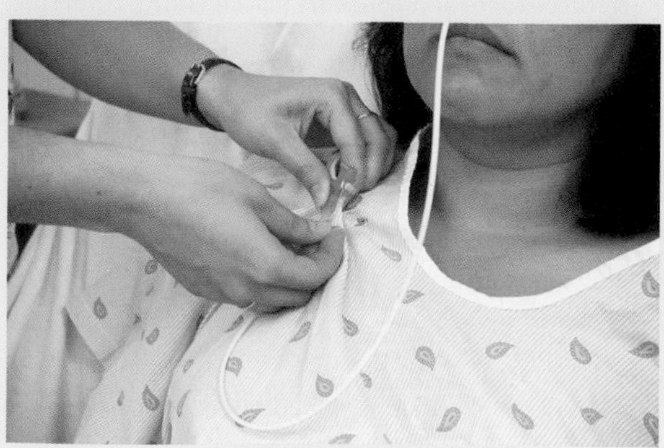

STEP 20 Fasten feeding tube to patient's gown.

STEP	RATIONALE
21. Help patient to comfortable position but keep head of the bed elevated at least 30 degrees (preferably 45 degrees) unless contraindicated (Schallom, 2015).	Promotes patient comfort and lowers risk of aspiration should patient receive tube feeding.
22. Remove gloves and perform hand hygiene.	Reduces transmission of microorganisms.

Safe Patient Care *Leave stylet in place until correct position is verified by x-ray film. Never try to reinsert a partially or fully removed stylet while feeding tube is in place. This can cause perforation of tube and injure patient. Contact the health care provider if problems arise with feeding tube.*

STEP	RATIONALE
23. Contact radiology to obtain x-ray film of chest/abdomen.	Radiographic examination is most accurate method to determine feeding-tube placement (Milsom et al., 2015).
24. Perform hand hygiene. Apply clean gloves and administer oral hygiene (see Chapter 11). Clean tubing at nostril with washcloth dampened in mild soap and water.	Promotes patient comfort and integrity of oral mucous membranes. Reduces transmission of microorganisms.
25. Raise side rails as appropriate and lower bed to lowest position	Promotes patient safety.
26. Remove and dispose of equipment and gloves; perform hand hygiene.	Reduces transmission of microorganisms.
27. Place nurse call system in an accessible location within patient's reach. Instruct patient in its use.	Promotes patient safety.
28. Tube removal:	
a. Verify health care provider's order for tube removal.	Health care provider's order is needed to remove feeding tube.
b. Gather equipment.	Ensures organized procedure.
c. Explain procedure to patient.	Encourages cooperation, reduces anxiety, and minimizes risks. Identifies teaching needs.
d. Perform hand hygiene. Apply clean gloves.	Reduces transmission of microorganisms.
e. Position patient in high-Fowler's position unless contraindicated.	Reduces risk for pulmonary aspiration in event patient should vomit.
f. Place disposable pad or towel over patient's chest.	Prevents mucus and gastric secretions from soiling patient's clothing.
g. Disconnect tube from feeding administration set (if present) and clamp or cap end.	Prevents formula from spilling from tube as it is removed.
h. Remove tape or tube fixation device from patient's nose. Unclip tube from patient's gown.	Allows tube to be removed easily.
i. Instruct patient to take deep breath and hold it. Then as you kink end of tube securely (folding it over on itself), completely withdraw it by pulling it out steadily and smoothly onto towel or disposable bag. Dispose of it into appropriate receptacle.	Prevents inadvertent aspiration of gastric contents while tube is removed. Kinking prevents leakage of fluid from tube. Promotes patient comfort. Reduces transmission of microorganisms.
j. Offer tissues to patient to blow nose.	Clears nasal passages of remaining secretions.
k. Offer mouth care.	Promotes patient's comfort.
l. Remove and dispose of gloves; perform hand hygiene.	Reduces transmission of microorganisms.

EVALUATION

1. Observe patient's response to tube placement. Assess lung sounds; have patient speak; check vital signs; note any coughing, dyspnea, cyanosis, or decrease in oxygen saturation or increase in end-tidal CO_2.	Symptoms may indicate placement in respiratory tract. Auscultation of crackles, wheezes, dyspnea, or fever may be delayed response to aspiration. Lowered oxygen saturation or increased end-tidal CO_2 may detect tip of tube is in trachea or lung.
2. Confirm radiographic film results with health care provider.	Verifies position of tube before initiating enteral feeding.
3. Remove stylet after x-ray film verification of correct placement. Review agency policy regarding requirement of trained clinician for insertion.	If placement needs adjustment, ensure stylet is still in place and contact health care provider.
4. Routinely check condition of nares, location of external exit site marking on tube, and color and pH of fluid aspirated from tube.	Routine evaluation ensures no formation of medical device–related pressure injury and correct placement of tube.
5. After removal, assess patient's level of comfort.	Provides for continued comfort of patient.

STEP	RATIONALE
6. **Use Teach-Back:** "I want to be sure that I explained to you what you can do during insertion of the nasogastric tube so that you can communicate with me. Tell me how you are going to communicate with me during tube insertion." Revise your instruction now or develop a plan for revised patient teaching if patient is not able to teach back correctly.	Determines patient's level of understanding of instructional topic.

Unexpected Outcomes	Related Interventions
1. Aspiration of stomach contents into respiratory tract (delayed response or small-volume aspiration), evidenced by auscultation of crackles or wheezes, dyspnea, or fever.	• Report change in patient condition to health care provider immediately; if there has not been a recent chest x-ray film, suggest ordering one. • Position patient on side to protect airway. • Suction nasotracheally and orotracheally (see Chapter 16). • Prepare for possible initiation of antibiotics.
2. Displacement of feeding tube to another site (e.g., from duodenum to stomach) possibly occurs when patient coughs or vomits.	• Aspirate GI contents and measure pH. • Remove displaced tube and insert and verify placement of new tube. • If there is question of aspiration, obtain chest x-ray film.

Recording

- Tube insertion: Record procedure and report type and size of tube placed, location of distal tip of tube, patient's tolerance of procedure, and confirmation of tube position by x-ray film examination.
- Tube removal: Record procedure and patient's level of comfort and condition of naris.

Hand-Off Reporting

- Report any type of unexpected outcome and the interventions performed to health care provider.
- During hand-off, report tube placement, when confirmation of placement was received, and condition of patient's nares.

✦ SKILL 13.4 Verifying Placement and Irrigating a Feeding Tube

Purpose

Once a feeding tube is inserted (see Skill 13.3), it is essential to routinely check its location and keep the tube patent. It is possible for the tip of a feeding tube to move or migrate into a different location (e.g., from the stomach to the intestine or esophagus, from the intestine into the stomach) without any external evidence that the tube has moved. The risk for aspiration of regurgitated gastric contents into the respiratory tract increases when the tip of the tube accidentally dislocates upward into the esophagus. The nurse is responsible for ensuring that the tube has remained in the intended position before administering formula or medications, by verifying the tube position every 4 to 6 hours. Because it is not practical to take x-ray films every day, other methods of determining placement, including observation for presence of bubbling, pH paper test, use of biochemical markers such as pepsin, capnography, ultrasound, electromagnetic tracing, visualization, and manometer techniques, have been studied and compared, all of which have their own advantages and disadvantages (Fan et al., 2017). Unfortunately, an ideal bedside method remains elusive, causing frustration for nurses. At present, confirming measurement at the naris and pH testing and visualization of gastric aspirate should be used to distinguish between gastric, intestinal, and lung placement (Boullata et al., 2017). Timing of the last enteral feeding and medication administration (especially acid-lowering medications such as proton pump inhibitors) may alter the pH levels (Fan et al., 2017). To ensure a high confirmation rate for a correctly placed pre-pyloric or gastric tube, the pH of gastric aspirate should be less than or equal to 5 (Boullata et al., 2017; Ni et al., 2017). When pH levels are greater than 5, further confirmation of placement should be conducted with an x-ray (Fan et al., 2017; Ni et al., 2017).

A feeding tube is more likely to remain patent through routine irrigation while in place and after the administration of medications and feedings. Plain water is the preferred flush solution. However, sterile water for flushing before and after medication administration and in immunocompromised and critically ill patients has been recommended (Boullata et al., 2017). All types of feeding tubes require routine irrigation, including gastrostomy and jejunostomy tubes (see Skill 13.5). Question the patency of a tube when you cannot instill air or fluid through the tube.

Delegation and Collaboration

The skill of verifying tube placement and irrigating a feeding tube is the responsibility of the nurse and cannot be delegated to nursing assistive personnel (NAP). The nurse directs the NAP to:

- Immediately inform the nurse if patient's respirations change or patient complains of shortness of breath, coughing, or choking.
- Immediately inform the nurse if the patient vomits or the NAP notices vomitus in patient's mouth during oral hygiene.
- Immediately inform the nurse if nasal skin irritation or excoriation is present.
- Immediately inform the nurse if a change in the external length of the tube occurs, which could indicate displacement of the tube.
- Report when a continuous tube feeding stops infusing.

Equipment

- 60-mL ENFit syringe
- Water (tap water or sterile [see agency policy], dated and initialed container at patient's bedside)
- Towel
- Stethoscope
- Clean gloves
- pH indicator strip (scale of 1 to 11)
- Small medication cup
- Pulse oximeter

ASSESSMENT

1. Review agency policy and procedures for frequency of irrigation and frequency and method of checking tube placement. **Do not insufflate air into tube to check placement.** *Rationale: Following agency standards maintains quality of patient care.*
2. Identify patient using at least two identifiers (e.g., name and birthday or name and medical record number) according to agency policy. *Rationale: Ensures correct patient. Complies with The Joint Commission standards and improves patient safety (TJC, 2019).*
3. Review patient's medication record for orders for enteral feeding, a gastric acid inhibitor (e.g., ranitidine, famotidine, nizatidine), or a proton pump inhibitor (e.g., omeprazole). *Rationale: The presence of enteral formula in aspirated secretions diminishes usefulness of pH measurements by buffering pH of stomach. Similarly, H_2 receptor antagonists reduce acid content of secretions, also raising pH value (Fan et al., 2017).*
4. Review patient's medical record for history of prior tube displacement. *Rationale: Patients are at increased risk for repeated tube displacement.*
5. Observe for signs and symptoms of respiratory distress during feeding: coughing, choking, or reduced oxygen saturation. *Rationale: Once a tube has been correctly placed into gastrointestinal (GI) tract, movement into pulmonary system is unlikely. However, a tube that has been pulled back into esophagus can lead to regurgitation and aspiration of formula.*
6. Identify conditions that increase risk for spontaneous tube migration or dislocation: altered level of consciousness, agitation; retching, vomiting; nasotracheal suction. *Rationale: Feeding tubes may become dislocated by increases in intraabdominal pressure or coughing, but most frequently they are displaced when patient moves or during pulls on tube.*
7. Perform hand hygiene. Assess bowel sounds and abdominal examination. *Rationale: Determines if peristalsis is present from increased air or stool. Bowel sounds are not necessary to commence feeding; however, high-pitched or hyperactive sounds may indicate changes in function or obstruction (McClave et al., 2016).*
8. Obtain pulse oximetry reading. *Rationale: Baseline used to compare with oximetry changes in determining if tube has been misplaced into trachea.*
9. Note ease with which previous tube feedings infuse through tubing. Monitor volume of continuous enteral formula administered during shift and compare with ordered amount. *Rationale: Failure of formula to infuse as desired may indicate developing tube obstruction and need for irrigation.*
10. Assess patient's or family caregiver's knowledge, experience and health literacy level. *Rationale: Ensures patient has the capacity to obtain, communicate, process, and understand basic health information (CDC, 2016).*

STEP	RATIONALE
PLANNING	
1. Expected outcomes following completion of procedure:	
• Color, pH, and appearance of gastric aspirate are consistent with initial tube placement.	Indicates that tube has likely remained in correct location, initially confirmed by x-ray film (Boullata et al., 2017; Fan et al., 2017).
• Feeding tube remains patent.	Proper irrigation clears tube of formula and medication residue.
• Patient receives prescribed caloric intake.	Feeding infuses without interruption.
2. Provide privacy and prepare environment.	Provides for patient comfort and prepares environment by reducing clutter on over-bed or bedside table.
3. Perform hand hygiene. Prepare and organize equipment at bedside.	Reduces transmission of microorganisms. Provides for an organized procedure.
4. Help patient assume comfortable position with head of bed (HOB) at least 30 degrees.	Position should be maintained (with turning to sides) when patient receives tube feeding or irrigation as it reduces reflux and risk for pulmonary aspiration. HOB elevation greater than 30 degrees is feasible and preferred to 30 degrees for reducing oral secretion volume, reflux, and aspiration without pressure ulcer development in ventilator patients (Schallom et al., 2015).
5. Explain procedure to patient. Be clear in explaining you are not removing tube.	Relieves anxiety and promotes patient cooperation.

STEP	RATIONALE
IMPLEMENTATION	
1. Perform hand hygiene and apply clean gloves. Be sure pulse oximeter is in place.	Reduces transmission of microorganisms. Used to monitor change in oxygen saturation.
2. Verify tube placement.	

Safe Patient Care *Listening for insufflated air instilled through tube to check tube tip position is unreliable (Boullata et al., 2017; Fan et al., 2017).*

STEP	RATIONALE
a. Check tube placement at following times: (1) For intermittently tube-fed patients, test placement immediately before each feeding (usually a period of at least 4 hours will have elapsed since previous feeding) and before medications.	Each administration of feeding/medication can lead to pulmonary aspiration if tube is displaced. More frequent checking has been associated with increased clogging of small-bore tubes.
(2) For continuous tube-fed patients, test placement following agency policy. AACN (2016a) recommends that if continuous feedings are stopped for greater than 1 hour, a pH test should be done.	Feedings should not be stopped only for the purpose of pH testing. pH testing may be helpful when feedings are interrupted for procedures or diagnostic studies (AACN, 2016a).
(3) Wait to verify placement at least 1 hour after medication administration by tube or mouth.	Premature withdrawal of contents will remove unabsorbed medication, reducing dose delivered to patient.
b. Draw up 30 mL of air into a 60-mL ENFit syringe. Place tip of syringe into end of gastric or small bowel tube and flush with air before attempting to aspirate fluid. Repositioning patient from side to side is helpful. In some cases more than one bolus of air is necessary.	Burst of air helps to aspirate fluid more easily. Smaller syringes generate unnecessarily high pressures inside tube. It is often more difficult to aspirate fluid from small intestine than from stomach or smaller-sized tube (AACN, 2016a).
c. Draw back on syringe slowly and obtain 5 to 10 mL of gastric aspirate (see illustration). Observe appearance of aspirate. Aspirates from gastric tubes of continuously tube-fed patients often look like curdled enteral formula. Gastric aspirates from intermittently tube-fed patients typically are not bile stained (unless intestinal fluid has refluxed into stomach) (AACN, 2016a).	Drawing back quickly or using smaller syringe may cause tube to collapse. Quantity is sufficient for pH testing. Appearance of aspirate helps to assess position of tube.
d. Gently mix aspirate in syringe. Expel a few drops into clean medicine cup. Note color of aspirate. Measure pH of aspirated GI contents by dipping pH strip into fluid or applying a few drops of fluid to strip. Compare color of strip with color on chart (see illustration) provided by manufacturer.	Mixing ensures equal distribution of contents for testing. Most-accurate readings of gastric pH levels are provided by pH paper covering minimal range of from 1 to 11
(1) Gastric fluid from patient who has fasted for at least 4 hours usually has pH range of 5 or less.	A pH value of 5.5 or below will exclude 100% of pulmonary placements in small intestine (Ni et al., 2017).
(2) Fluid from tube in small intestine of fasting patient usually has pH greater than 6 (Bourgault et al., 2015).	Intestinal contents are more basic than stomach contents. A pH greater than 6 indicates intestinal or pulmonary placement (Bourgault et al., 2015).

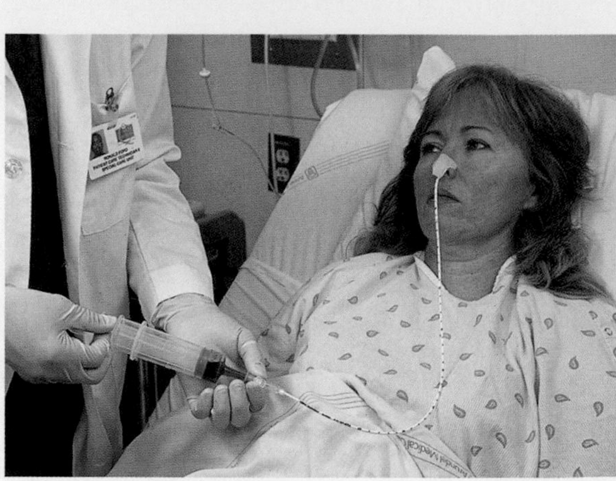

STEP 2c Obtain gastric aspirate.

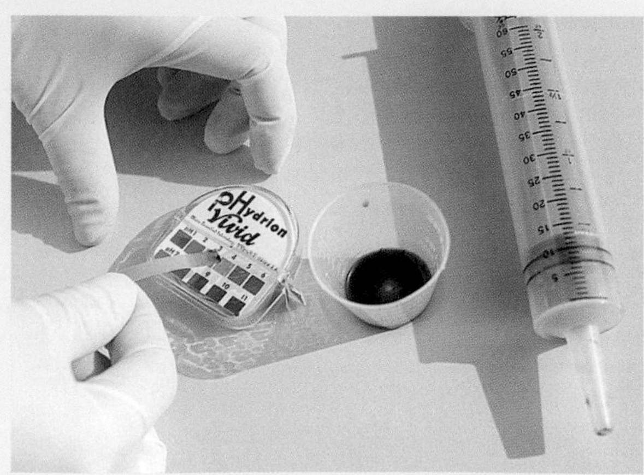

STEP 2d Compare color on test strip with color on pH chart.

STEP	RATIONALE
(3) The pH of pleural fluid from the tracheobronchial tree is generally greater than 6.	pH values of pleural contents are more alkaline and usually greater than 6 (AACN, 2016a).
e. If after repeated attempts it is not possible to aspirate fluid from tube that was confirmed by x-ray film to be in desired position and if (1) there are no risk factors for tube dislocation, (2) tube has remained in original taped position, and (3) patient is not in respiratory distress, assume that tube is correctly placed. Continue with irrigation (AACN, 2016a; Bourgault et al., 2015; Fan et al., 2017).	Reports of routine chest or abdominal x-ray films can monitor tube location. Repeat radiographic confirmation of tube position is indicated if external length of tube changes, tape holding tube comes loose, or patient coughs forcefully or vomits (AACN, 2016a; Fan et al., 2017).
3. Irrigate tube.	Keeps tube patent.
a. Irrigate routinely before, between, and after final medication (before feedings are reinstituted) and before an intermittent feeding is administered.	Certain formulas have properties that predispose to tube clogging. Irrigation prevents mixing of medications in tube, which may cause clogging.
b. Draw up 30 mL of water in ENFit syringe. Do not use irrigation fluids from bottles that are used on other patients. Patient should have individual bottle of solution.	This amount of solution will flush length of tube. Water is most effective agent for preventing tube clogging unless patient is immunocompromised (Boullata et al., 2017).

Safe Patient Care *Do not use cola or fruit juices for flushing tubing because these liquids can clog tube.*

STEP	RATIONALE
c. Change irrigation bottle every 24 hours. Irrigation trays, which hold both irrigation fluid and syringe, are considered open systems and may be more easily contaminated than sterile water bottles. **NOTE:** Be sure that syringe in tray has ENFit adaptor.	Ensures sterile solution. Sterile water is required for neonates and preferred for patients who are immune suppressed or critically ill (Boullata et al., 2017).
d. Continuous feeding: Turn off or place feeding on hold. Clamp or kink infusion tubing and disconnect from feeding tube. **NOTE:** For intermittent feedings, remove plug at end of feeding tube. Kink feeding tube temporarily.	Prevents leakage of formula. Prevents leakage of gastric fluid.
e. Insert tip of ENFit syringe into end of feeding tube. Release kink and slowly instill irrigation solution.	Infusion of fluid clears tubing.
f. If unable to instill fluid, reposition patient on left side and try again.	Tip of tube may be against stomach wall. Changing patient's position may move tip away from stomach wall.
g. When water or sterile saline has been instilled, remove syringe. Reinstitute tube feeding or administer medication as ordered. Then flush each medication completely through tube (see Chapter 23).	Tubing is clear and patent. Ensures that full dose reaches stomach and medications do not mix with formula.
4. Help patient assume comfortable position. Raise side rails as appropriate and lower bed to lowest position.	Promotes patient comfort and safety.
5. Place nurse call system in an accessible location within patient's reach. Instruct patient in its use.	Promotes patient safety.

EVALUATION

STEP	RATIONALE
1. Observe patient for respiratory distress: persistent gagging, paroxysms of coughing, drop in oxygen (O_2) saturation, or respiratory patterns (e.g., rate and depth) that are inconsistent with baseline measures.	Indicates that tube may be displaced in respiratory tract.
2. Verify that external length of tube, pH, and appearance of aspirate are consistent with initial tube placement.	Indicates that tip of tube is likely to be positioned in same place as it was following x-ray film confirmation.
3. Observe ease with which tube feeding instills through tubing.	Successfully irrigated tube is patent, allowing for free flow of solution.
4. Monitor patient's caloric intake.	Total enteral nutrition infuses without difficulty.
5. **Use Teach-Back:** "I want to go over what I explained earlier. Tell me why it is important for me to test the gastric pH and the color of the gastric secretions in your stomach before feedings." Revise your instruction now or develop a plan for revised patient/family caregiver teaching if patient/family caregiver is not able to teach back correctly.	Determines patient's/family caregiver's level of understanding of instructional topic.

Unexpected Outcomes	Related Interventions
1. Red or brown coloring (coffee-grounds appearance) of fluid aspirated from feeding tube indicates new or old blood, respectively, in GI tract.	• If color is not related to medications recently administered, notify health care provider immediately.
2. Patient develops severe respiratory distress (e.g., dyspnea, decreased oxygen saturation, increased pulse rate) as a result of aspiration or tube displacement into lung.	• Stop any enteral feedings immediately. • Notify health care provider immediately. • Obtain chest x-ray film as ordered.
3. Tube cannot be irrigated after testing.	• Reattempt to irrigate tube. Do not force fluid. If unsuccessful, notify health care provider.

Recording

- Record findings of bowel sounds and the pH and appearance of aspirate.
- Record time of irrigation, amount and type of fluid instilled, and patient's tolerance.

Hand-Off Reporting

- Report to health care provider if tubing is clogged or there are indications of tube displacement.
- During change of shift, note most current gastric pH, outcome of irrigations, and status of tube-feeding infusion.

✦ SKILL 13.5 Administering Enteral Nutrition: Nasogastric, Nasointestinal, Gastrostomy, or Jejunostomy Tube

Purpose

Enteral nutrition (EN), or tube feeding, is a method for providing nutrients to patients who are unable to take any or adequate amounts of solid or liquid nutrients orally. The standards for enteral nutrition have largely developed as a result of caring for critically ill patients (McClave et al., 2016; Box 13.7). The goals of EN include maintaining integrity of the gastrointestinal (GI) tract, providing immune regulation, and downregulating inflammatory responses (McClave et al., 2016). The extent to which EN benefits patients depends on disease severity, baseline nutritional status, and the nutrition regimen ordered. Research has shown that early EN (within first 24–36 hours of admission to an intensive care unit [ICU]), versus delayed EN, is associated with reduced infection, hospital length of stay, and mortality (McClave et al., 2016).

Nasally or orally placed feeding tubes are used for short-term feeding (less than 4–6 weeks) and are inserted with tips located in the stomach (nasogastric) or small bowel (nasointestinal). For long-term feeding (more than 4–6 weeks), feeding tubes may be inserted directly through a patient's abdominal wall into the stomach (gastrostomy) or jejunum (jejunostomy). The majority of patients will tolerate feeding into the stomach. Conversion to intestinal feeding should be done only when gastric feeding is poorly tolerated due to ileus (decreased or absent peristalsis of the stomach but not intestine); gastroparesis (delayed gastric emptying); the patient is at high risk for aspiration; or mechanical issues (gastric resection) (McClave et al., 2016). Feeding tubes that end in the stomach are used for gravity bolus or continuous infusion feedings by infusion pump. The small intestine does not have the storage capability of the stomach, and therefore a tube feeding administered into the small intestine is delivered more slowly and continuously with an infusion pump.

BOX 13.7

Clinical Guidelines for Enteral Nutrition

The American College of Gastroenterology released clinical guidelines for the use of enteral nutrition (EN) in adult hospitalized patients (McClave et al., 2016). The scientific evidence guides nutritional support for adult hospitalized patients who are unable to sustain oral intake on their own and are expected to remain in the hospital for more than 3 days (McClave et al., 2016). Recommended best practices include the following:

- Patients with severe malnutrition who are unable to take in adequate amounts of an oral diet should be initiated promptly on EN.
- EN is preferred over parenteral nutrition in patients with a functioning gastrointestinal tract.
- EN is not required for the patient who is well nourished and expected to resume oral intake within 5 to 7 days following hospital admission.
- Oro- or nasogastric feeding is appropriate for the majority of patients starting EN.
- EN delivered into the small bowel should be considered in patients who are intolerant of gastric feeding or at high risk for aspiration.

Delegation and Collaboration

The skill of administration of nasoenteric tube feeding can be delegated to nursing assistive personnel (NAP) (refer to agency policy). A registered nurse (RN) or licensed practical nurse (LPN) must first verify tube placement and patency. The nurse directs the NAP to:

- Elevate head of bed to 30 to 45 degrees or sit patient up in bed or a chair unless contraindicated.
- Not adjust feeding rate; infuse the feeding as ordered.
- Report any difficulty infusing the feeding or any discomfort voiced by patient.
- Report any gagging, paroxysms of coughing, or choking.
- Provide frequent oral hygiene.

Equipment

- Disposable feeding bag, tubing, or ready-to-hang system
- 60-mL or larger ENFit syringe

- Stethoscope
- Enteral infusion pump for continuous feedings
- pH indicator strip (scale 1 to 11)
- Prescribed enteral formula (standard polymeric or high protein; McClave et al., 2016)
- Clean gloves
- ENFit connector

ASSESSMENT

1. Verify health care provider's order for type of tube feeding formula, rate, route, and frequency. *Rationale: Ensures that correct formula will be administered in appropriate volume. Enteral formulas are not interchangeable.*
2. Identify patient using at least two identifiers (e.g., name and birthday or name and medical record number) according to agency policy. *Rationale: Ensures correct patient. Complies with The Joint Commission standards and improves patient safety (TJC, 2019).*
3. Review medical record for risk factors of malnutrition (see Box 13.1) and current clinical characteristics of malnutrition (see Box 13.3). Consult with nutritional support team and health care provider. *Rationale: Determines patient's risk for malnutrition and potential need for early initiation of EN (McClave et al., 2016; Meehan et al., 2016; White et al., 2012).*
4. Assess patient for factors that increase risk for aspiration: sedation, mechanical ventilation, nasotracheal suctioning, neurologic compromise, lying flat, and sepsis (Eglseer et al., 2018). *Rationale: Identifies patients at high risk so that decision may be made based on safety of gastric versus intestinal feeding (McClave et al., 2016).*
5. Perform hand hygiene. Perform physical assessment of abdomen, including auscultation for bowel sounds, before feeding (see Chapter 8). *Rationale: Objective measures for assessing tolerance include changes in bowel sounds, expanding girth, tenderness and firmness on palpation, increasing nasogastric (NG) output, and vomiting (McCarthy and Martindale, 2015). Report findings to health care provider to determine if tube feeding can proceed safely.*
6. Obtain baseline weight and review serum electrolytes and blood glucose measurement (see Chapter 9). Assess patient for fluid volume excess or deficit, electrolyte abnormalities, and metabolic abnormalities (e.g., hyperglycemia). *Rationale: Enteral feedings should restore or maintain patient's nutritional status. Measures provide objective data and baseline to determine selection of formula and measure effectiveness of feedings.*
7. Collaborate with registered dietitian (RD) for determination of patient's caloric and protein requirements. Then set goal for delivery of EN (McClave et al., 2016). *Rationale: Sets objective measure for determining percent of prescribed calories and protein delivered.*
8. Assess patient's or family caregiver's knowledge, experience, and health literacy level. *Rationale: Ensures patient has the capacity to obtain, communicate, process, and understand basic health information (CDC, 2016).*

STEP	RATIONALE
PLANNING	
1. Expected outcomes following completion of procedure:	
• Patient achieves established target for body weight over time.	Indicates that patient's nutritional status is maintained or improved.
• Patient has no sign of respiratory distress.	Feeding tube does not enter airway, and patient does not aspirate feeding.
• Patient achieves established target for calories and protein.	Scheduled feedings are administered as ordered.
• Patient is free of abdominal cramping.	Feeding administered without abdominal distention. Demonstrates tolerance of tube feeding.
2. Provide privacy and prepare environment.	Provides for patient comfort and prepares environment by reducing clutter on over-bed or bedside table.
3. Perform hand hygiene. Prepare and organize equipment at bedside.	Reduces transmission of microorganisms. Provides for an organized procedure.
4. Help patient assume comfortable position with head of bed (HOB) at least 30 degrees (45 degrees preferred). Monitor the patient at least every 4 hours for appropriate positioning (Boullata et al., 2017).	Position should be maintained (with turning to sides) when patient receives tube feeding as it reduces reflux and risk for pulmonary aspiration. HOB elevation greater than 30 degrees is feasible and preferred to 30 degrees for reducing oral secretion volume, reflux, and aspiration without pressure injury to dependent skin areas in ventilator patients (Schallom et al., 2015).
5. Explain procedure to patient and family caregiver.	Decreases patient anxiety. EN may be continued in the home setting.
IMPLEMENTATION	
1. Perform hand hygiene. Apply clean gloves.	Reduces transmission of microorganisms and potential contamination of enteral formula.
2. Re-verify correct formula and check expiration date; note integrity of container and appearance of formula.	Ensures that correct therapy is to be administered and checks integrity of formula.

STEP	RATIONALE
3. Prepare formula for administration, following manufacturer guidelines.	

Safe Patient Care *Discard unused reconstituted and refrigerated formulas within 24 hours of preparation (Boullata et al., 2017).*

STEP	RATIONALE
a. Have formula at room temperature.	Cold formula causes gastric cramping and discomfort because liquid is not warmed by mouth and esophagus.
b. Use aseptic technique to connect administration set tubing to container as needed. Use proper ENFit connecter and avoid handling feeding system or touching can tops, container openings, spike, and spike port.	Bag, connections, and tubing must be free of contamination to prevent bacterial growth. The use of a closed system lowers the risk of infections due to bacterial contamination (Boullata et al., 2017).
c. Shake formula container well. Clean top of canned formula with alcohol swab before opening it.	Ensures integrity of formula; prevents transmission of microorganisms.
d. For closed systems connect administration tubing to container. If using open system, pour formula from brick pack or can into administration bag (see illustration).	Formulas are available in closed-system containers that contain a 24- to 48-hour supply of formula or in an open system, in which formula must be transferred from brick packs or cans to a bag before administration.

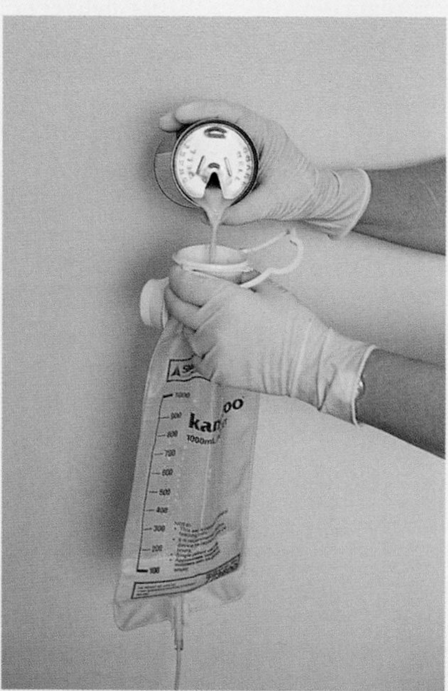

STEP 3d Pour formula into open feeding container.

STEP	RATIONALE
4. Open roller clamp and allow administration tubing to fill. Clamp off tubing with roller clamp. Hang container on intravenous (IV) pole.	Prevents introduction of air into stomach once feeding begins.
5. Keep patient in high-Fowler's position or elevate HOB at least 30 degrees (45 degrees recommended). For patient forced to remain supine, place in reverse Trendelenburg's position, which raises head.	Elevation of HOB helps prevent pulmonary aspiration (Boullata et al., 2017). Researchers recommend HOB elevation of 45 degrees for patients receiving EN who require mechanical ventilation or are heavily sedated, but lowering the head to 30 degrees might be done periodically for patient comfort and in patients at risk of developing pressure injury (AACN, 2016b; Schallom et al., 2015).
6. Verify tube placement (see Skill 13.4). Observe appearance of aspirate and note pH.	Verifies if tip of tube is in stomach, intestine, or lung based on pH value (≤5) (Fan et al., 2017; Ni et al., 2017).
a. *Nasoenteric tube:* Attach ENFit syringe to end of enteral feeding tube and aspirate gastric or intestinal contents. Observe appearance of aspirate and note pH.	Gastric fluid for patient who has fasted for at least 4 hours usually has pH of 1 to 4 (if not receiving gastric acid inhibitor, then pH of ≤5; Fan et al., 2017). If continuous feedings into stomach or intestine, check pH if feedings held for at least one hour for diagnostic reason (stomach pH ≤5; intestinal pH >6; Fan et al., 2017).

STEP	RATIONALE
b. *Gastrostomy tube:* Attach ENFit syringe to end of tube and aspirate gastric contents. Observe appearance of aspirate and note pH.	Same as above.
c. *Jejunostomy tube:* Attach ENFit syringe to end of tube and aspirate intestinal secretions. Observe appearance; if significant amounts are returned or resemble gastric secretions, check pH.	Presence of intestinal fluid at pH greater than 6 indicates that end of tube is in small intestine. If fluid tests acidic on pH test or looks like gastric fluid, tube may be displaced into stomach.
7. Check gastric residual volume (GRV) per agency policy. Routine use is no longer recommended (Boullata et al., 2017) and should not be used as a single measure of tolerance.	GRV has poor correlation with pneumonia, regurgitation, and aspiration. Frequent checking may delay feeding. However, if other signs (e.g., abdominal distention or pain) of intolerance are present, GRV of 250 to 500 mL may indicate the need to take measures to prevent aspiration or hold feeding completely (Boullata et al., 2017). Intestinal residual is usually very small. If residual volume is greater than 10 mL, displacement of intestinal tube into stomach may have occurred.

Safe Patient Care *Limit gastric residual checks to recommended standard intervals because acidic gastric contents may cause protein in enteral formulas to precipitate within the lumen of the tube, creating risk for obstruction (Boullata et al., 2017).*

STEP	RATIONALE
a. Draw up 10 to 30 mL air into ENFit syringe and connect to end of feeding tube. Inject air slowly into tube. Pull back slowly and aspirate total amount of gastric contents you can aspirate.	GRV may not be easy to obtain from small-bore feeding tube. A 60-mL syringe prevents gastric tube collapse.
b. The cut off to return aspirated contents to stomach slowly should be 250 mL or higher (see agency policy) (McCarthy and Martindale, 2015).	Prevents loss of nutrients and electrolytes in discarded fluid. Some questions exist regarding safety of returning high volumes of fluid into stomach.
c. GRVs in range of 200 to 500 mL should raise concern and lead to implementation of measures to reduce risk of aspiration. Automatic cessation of feeding shouldn't occur for GRV less than 500 mL in absence of other signs of intolerance (Boullata et al., 2017; McClave et al., 2016).	Raising cutoff value for GRV from lower number to higher number does not increase risk for regurgitation, aspiration, or pneumonia. Elevated GRV should raise concern and lead to measures to reduce risk of aspiration (McCarthy and Martindale, 2015).
d. Flush feeding tube with 30 mL water (see Skill 13.4).	Prevents clogging of tubing and ensures that complete feeding is administered.

Safe Patient Care *Minimize the use of sedatives in patients receiving continuous feeding because airway clearance is reduced in sedated patients (Boullata et al., 2017).*

STEP	RATIONALE
8. Intermittent feeding (administered at certain times during the day):	
a. Pinch proximal end of feeding tube and remove cap. Connect distal end of administration set tubing to ENFit device on feeding tube and release tubing.	Prevents excessive air from entering patient's stomach and leakage of gastric contents. Ensures that feeding will be administered into correct tubing (Boullata et al., 2017).
b. Set rate by adjusting roller clamp on tubing or attach tubing to feeding pump (see illustration). Allow bag to empty gradually over 30 to 45 minutes (length of time of a comfortable meal). Bag label should include patient identifiers, formula type, enteral delivery site (route and access), administration method and type, and volume and frequency of water flushes (Boullata et al., 2017). Also include a label with date, time, and initials when hanging a feeding.	Gradual emptying of tube feeding reduces risk for abdominal discomfort, vomiting, or diarrhea induced by bolus or too-rapid infusion of tube feedings. Critical elements for an EN order should be on EN label (Boullata et al., 2017). Labeling indicates when to change administration set and confirms that right patient is receiving feeding.

Safe Patient Care *Use pumps designated for tube feeding, not IV fluids.*

STEP	RATIONALE
c. Immediately follow feeding with prescribed amount of water (per health care provider's orders or agency policy). Cover end of feeding tube with cap when not in use. Keep bag as clean as possible. Change administration set every 24 hours.	Prevents tube from clogging. Prevents air from entering stomach between feedings and limits microbial contamination of system.
9. Continuous infusion method:	Method delivers prescribed hourly rate of feeding and reduces risk for abdominal discomfort.
a. Remove cap on tubing and connect distal end of administration set tubing to feeding tube using ENFit connector as in Step 8a.	Prevents excess air from entering patient's stomach and leakage of gastric contents.
b. Thread tubing through feeding pump; set rate on pump and turn on (see illustration).	Delivers continuous feeding at steady rate and pressure. Feeding pump alarms for increased resistance.
c. Advance rate of tube feeding (and concentration of feeding) gradually, as ordered.	Tube feeding can usually begin with full-strength formula. Conservative initiation and advancement of EN nutrition depend on patient's age, medical condition, and nutritional status and expected patient tolerance (Kozeniecki and Fritzshall, 2015).

Safe Patient Care *Limit infusion time for open EN feeding systems to 4 to 8 hours maximum (12 hours in the home setting) (Boullata et al., 2017). Follow the manufacturer's recommendations for duration of infusion through an intact closed delivery device (Boullata et al., 2017).*

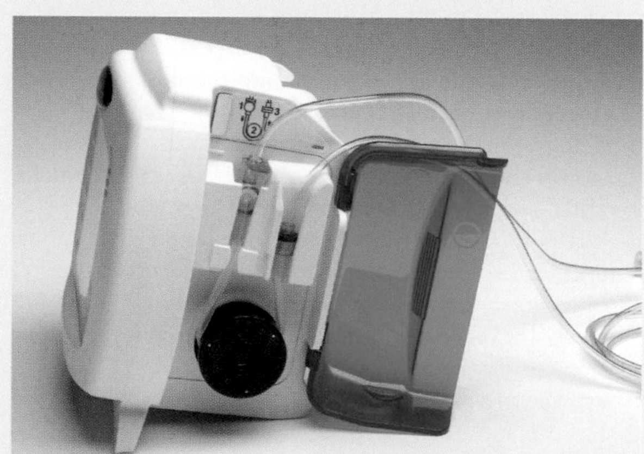

STEP 9b Connect tubing through infusion pump. *(Image used with permission Covidien. All rights reserved.)*

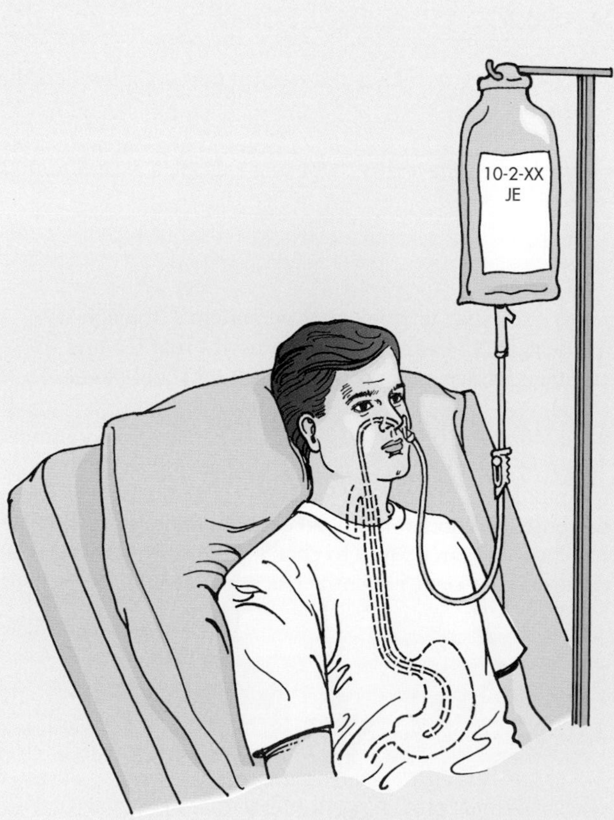

STEP 8b Administer intermittent feeding.

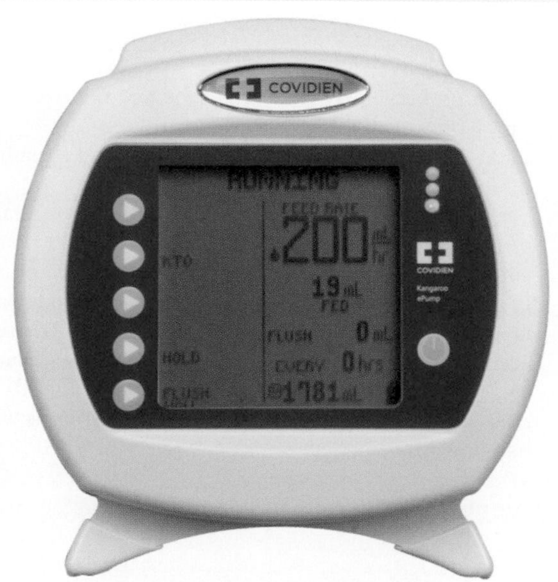

STEP 9c Set pump as ordered. *(Image used with permission of Covidien. All rights reserved.)*

STEP	RATIONALE
10. After feeding, flush tubing with 30 mL water every 4 hours during continuous feeding (see agency policy) or before and after an intermittent feeding. Have registered dietitian (RD) recommend total free-water requirement per day and obtain health care provider's order.	Provides patient with source of water to help maintain fluid and electrolyte balance. Clears tubing of formula.
11. Rinse bag and tubing with warm water whenever feedings are interrupted. Use new administration set every 24 hours.	Rinsing bag and tubing with warm water clears old tube feedings and reduces bacterial growth.
12. Be sure patient is comfortable and remains in position with head of elevated 30 to 45 degrees. Provide nurse call system to patient and instruct patient to utilize if needed.	Reduces risk of aspiration (AACN, 2016b). Call system summons nurse to patient bedside if assistance required.
13. Raise side rails (as appropriate) and lower bed to lowest position.	Promotes patient safety.
14. Dispose of supplies and perform hand hygiene.	Reduces transmission of microorganisms.

EVALUATION

STEP	RATIONALE
1. Monitor patient's tolerance to feeding by assessing for abdominal distention, firmness, feeling of fullness, or nausea (Boullata et al., 2017). GRV checks should be limited and done per policy.	Symptoms are warnings that patient may have gastric reflux, leading to aspiration. Bowel sounds indicate if peristalsis is present.
2. Monitor intake and output at least every 8 hours and calculate daily totals every 24 hours.	Intake and output are indications of fluid balance, which can indicate fluid volume excess or deficit.
3. Weigh patient daily until maximum administration rate is reached and maintained for 24 hours; then weigh patient 3 times per week.	Slow weight gain is indicator of improved nutritional status; however, sudden gain of more than 2 lb (0.9 kg) in 24 hours usually indicates fluid retention.
4. Monitor patient for appropriate feeding tube placement at least every 4 hours or per agency protocol. Monitor visible length of tubing or marking at tube exit site (naris or stoma) and check placement when a deviation is noted (Boullata et al., 2017).	Accidental displacement of tip of tube could lead to aspiration.
5. Monitor laboratory values as ordered by health care provider.	Determines correct administration of formula rate and strength.
6. Observe patient's respiratory status for coughing, dyspnea, tachypnea, change in oxygen saturation, hoarseness, crackles in lungs.	Change in respiratory status may indicate aspiration of tube feeding into respiratory tract.
7. For gastrostomy and jejunostomy tubes, inspect site for signs of impaired skin integrity and symptoms of infection, injury, or tightness of tube (see Procedural Guideline 13.1).	Enteral tubes often cause pressure and excoriation at insertion site.
8. Observe nasoenteral tube insertion site at least daily (see agency policy). Note skin integrity and look for edema under device, excoriation, or presence of injury.	Allows for early detection of excoriation that can progress to a medical device–related pressure injury.
9. **Use Teach-Back:** "I want to be sure that I explained to you what you need to look for that may tell us you're not tolerating your tube feeding. Tell me two things that may tell us that you are not tolerating your tube feedings." Revise your instruction now or develop a plan for revised patient/family caregiver teaching if patient/family caregiver is not able to teach back correctly.	Determines patient's/family caregiver's level of understanding of instructional topic.

Unexpected Outcomes	Related Interventions
1. Feeding tube becomes clogged.	• Attempt to flush tube with water. • Special products are available for unclogging feeding tubes; **do not** use carbonated beverages and juices. • Hold feeding and notify health care provider. • Maintain patient in semi-Fowler's position. • Contact pharmacist to change medications to liquid form and flush before and after intermittent feedings and medications (Kozeniecki and Fritzshall, 2015).

Unexpected Outcomes	Related Interventions
2. Patient develops large amount of diarrhea (more than three loose stools in 24 hours).	• Notify health care provider. • Consult dietitian about need to change formula to prevent malabsorption. • Identify and treat underlying medical/surgical issues and infections (Kozeniecki and Fritzshall, 2015). • Provide perianal skin care after each stool. • Determine other causes of diarrhea (e.g., *Clostridium difficile* infection, contaminated tube feeding, medication containing sorbitol).
3. Patient has an enteral tube misconnection (e.g., connecting an enteral tube to an intravenous [IV] site or ventilator in-line suction catheter).	• Infusion of enteral feeding into vein or directly into lung is a medical emergency. **Call healthcare provider and Rapid Response Team immediately.**
4. Patient aspirates formula, as indicated by sudden appearance of respiratory symptoms (e.g., severe coughing, dyspnea, and cyanosis) associated with eating, drinking, or regurgitation of gastric contents. Auscultation of lungs reveals crackles or wheezes.	• Immediately position patient on side with head of bed elevated. • Report change in condition to health care provider. • Suction nasotracheally or orotracheally.

Safe Patient Care *Small-volume aspirations that produce no overt symptoms are common and are often not discovered until the condition progresses to aspiration pneumonia (Eglseer et al., 2018).*

Recording

- Record amount and type of feeding, infusion rate (continuous feeding) or time for infusion (bolus method), findings on abdominal examination, GRV measures, position of feeding tube, patient's response to tube feeding, patency of tube, and condition of skin at tube site.
- Document your evaluation of patient learning.
- Record volume of formula and any additional water on intake and output (I&O) form.

Hand-Off Reporting

- Report adverse outcomes to health care provider.
- During a hand-off report, note the type of feeding, infusion rate and volume infused during shift, status of feeding tube, and patient's tolerance, and trace the administration set tubing to the enteral tube connection point to ensure the feeding is being infused enterally (Boullata et al., 2017).

PROCEDURAL GUIDELINE 13.1 *Care of a Gastrostomy or Jejunostomy Tube*

Purpose

Patients with long-term needs or who have no easy access to the gastrointestinal (GI) tract through the nose or mouth require more invasive access to the GI tract in the form of gastrostomy, jejunostomy, and gastrojejunostomy tubes. These tubes require endoscopic, radiological, or surgical placement. A gastrostomy tube (also called a G tube) that is surgically placed in the stomach is sutured in place and exits through an incision typically in the upper left quadrant of the abdomen. A jejunostomy (J tube) and gastrojejunostomy (GJ tube) may also be placed surgically. A percutaneous endoscopic gastrostomy tube (PEG tube) is inserted during endoscopic viewing of the stomach. A tube is placed in the stomach and exits through the incision, where an external bumper holds it in place (Fig. 13.1). A jejunostomy tube inserted using the same technique is called a PEJ. A combination GJ tube is threaded through the stomach into the jejunum; it is dual-channeled and has openings in both the stomach and the small-intestine part of the tube. These combination tubes allow simultaneous gastric decompression and intestinal feeding, ideal for patients with impaired gastric emptying or upper GI cancer. Each lumen of a combination tube is clearly labeled to distinguish between the gastric and the jejunal ports (Fig. 13.2). In the case of both combination tubes and PEJ tubes, you must know whether the intended site for formula delivery is gastric or jejunal to ensure safe and effective nutritional care.

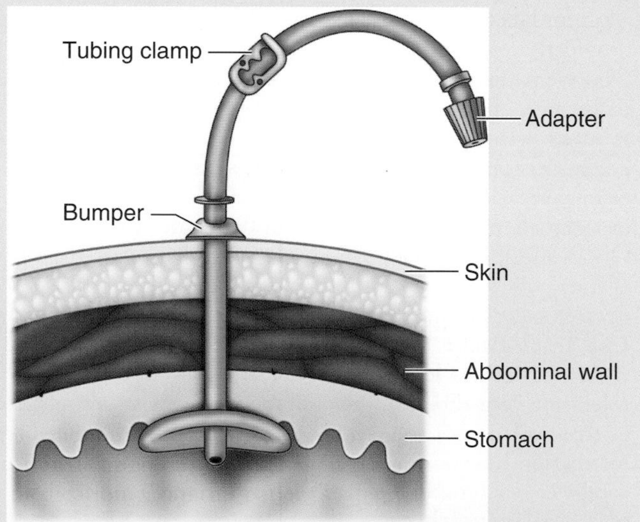

FIG 13.1 Placement of PEG tube into stomach.

Delegation and Collaboration

Care of a new PEG or PEJ tube cannot be delegated to nursing assistive personnel (NAP). However, there may be some exceptions for established tubes (refer to nurse practice acts and agency policy). The nurse directs the NAP to:

- Inform the nurse of any patient complaints of discomfort at the insertion site.
- Inform the nurse of any drainage on the insertion site dressing.

PROCEDURAL GUIDELINE 13.1 *Care of a Gastrostomy or Jejunostomy Tube—cont'd*

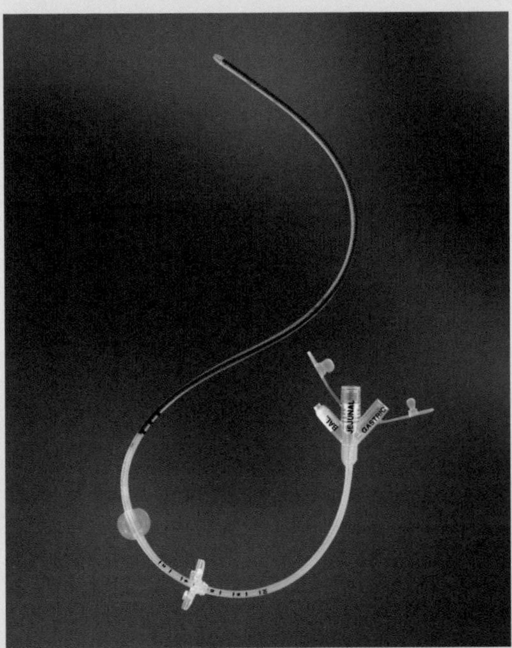

FIG 13.2 Dual lumen "combination tube" to allow jejunal feeding and gastric decompression. *(Image used with permission Kimberly-Clark Health Care. All rights reserved.)*

Equipment

- Normal saline, dated and initialed container at patient's bedside; 4 × 4–inch gauze; prepared drain-gauze dressing; paper tape; clean gloves; warm soapy water (according to agency policy); protective skin barrier (if indicated)

Procedural Steps

1. Identify patient using at least two identifiers (e.g., name and birthday or name and medical record number) according to agency policy (TJC, 2019).
2. Determine whether exit site is to be left open to air or if a dressing is indicated. Check health care provider's order or verify agency policy.
3. Perform hand hygiene. Provide for patient privacy. Organize supplies at bedside.
4. Position patient in comfortable position lying supine or supine with head of bed slightly elevated.
5. Explain procedure to patient and ask patient to lie still.
6. Apply clean gloves.
7. Remove old dressing. Fold dressing with drainage contained inside; remove gloves inside out over dressing. Discard in appropriate container. Perform hand hygiene.
8. Assess exit site for evidence of tenderness, drainage, swelling, excoriation, infection, bleeding, or excessive movement (more than ¼ inch or 6 mm) of the tube in or out of the stomach.
9. Apply new clean gloves. Clean skin around stoma site with warm water and mild soap or saline (according to agency policy) with 4 × 4–inch gauze. (If drainage is present, apply clean gloves.) Clean starting next to the stoma site and work outward using a circular motion.
10. Rinse and dry site completely.
11. Apply thin layer of protective skin barrier to exit site if indicated (e.g., site excoriated).
12. If dressing is ordered, place a drain-gauze dressing over external bar or disk. **NOTE:** Do not place dressing under external bar; this can cause gastric tissue erosion or internal abdominal wall pressure.
13. Secure dressing with paper tape.
14. Place date, time, and initials on new dressing.
15. Dispose of supplies in appropriate receptacle. Remove and dispose of gloves. Perform hand hygiene.
16. Return patient to comfortable position; raise side rails as indicated.
17. Leave nurse call system in accessible location for patient to use.
18. Evaluate condition of site routinely (see agency policy).

SPECIAL CONSIDERATIONS

Patient-Centered Care

- Patients who are unable to feed themselves independently may eat better if other family caregivers participate at mealtimes to avoid social isolation.
- A patient's culture, income, and religious practices all influence what he or she eats and the manner in which he or she plans meals and eats socially.
- Patients who adhere to kosher food preparation methods are prohibited from eating pork, predatory fowl, shellfish (i.e., crab, shrimp), blood, and meat dishes mixed with milk or dairy products. No cooking is done on the Sabbath (sundown Friday through sundown Saturday).
- Collect information on the types of foods that are generally eaten for different disease conditions. Some cultures believe in the hot-and-cold theory of health and illness. Foods are classified as cold or hot based on their characteristics, independent of the temperature at which they are served. There is no universal agreement across cultures about which foods are hot and which foods are cold.
- Vegetarians and vegans prefer meat substitutes.
- Foods are often associated with caring and love, health promotion, maintenance, and restoration. Food preferences are a major factor in patient adherence to a modified diet. A patient must be part of the decision-making process when dietary modifications are made.
- Patients' religious beliefs, quality of life, and goals of care may impact their decision to have long-term enteral access. Patients should be involved in this decision-making process if possible.

Patient Education

- Educate patients on the guidelines for healthy eating.
- Educate patients and family caregivers on the indications for the modified diet or tube feeding.
- Educate patients on the guidelines for safe storage and preparation of tube-feeding products.
- Educate patients and family caregivers on the importance of maintaining the integrity of the patients' feeding access.
- Educate family caregivers on the skills for assisting patients with feeding.

Age-Specific

Pediatric

- Human milk is the most desirable complete diet for infants during first 12 months. Infants who are breastfed or bottle-fed with formula do not require additional fluids (e.g., water or juice) during the first 6 months. Excessive water intake causes water intoxication, failure to thrive, and hyponatremia. Infants usually do not consume solid foods until 6 months. A common sequence for introducing solid food is one new food every 5 to 7 days (American Academy of Pediatrics, 2013).
- An abdominal x-ray is the best practice for verifying the location of a gastric enteral tube.
- Children at high risk for feeding tube displacement include neonates; children with neurological impairment; children in an obtunded neurological state; and children who are encephalopathic, have a decreased gag reflex, or are sedated or critically ill (Boullata et al., 2017).
- Colorimetric carbon dioxide detectors can detect inadvertent tube placement of tubes inserted in the lungs of children at the bedside (Fan et al., 2017). X-ray confirmation is the most accurate method to determine final placement (Metheny and Meert, 2017; Milsom et al., 2015).
- Decrease the amount of air insufflated before gastric aspiration according to the size of the patient (e.g., an infant may need only 1 mL of air; a small child may need 5 mL).
- Sterile liquid formulas or breastmilk for infants are preferred to powdered, reconstituted formulas for tube feeding. Sterile water must be used for reconstitution and all flushes for infants (Boullata et al., 2017).

Gerontological

- Older adults may not consume enough food to prevent unintended weight loss and malnutrition. Therapeutic diets, such as the diabetic diet or the low-sodium diet, can restrict flavors and reduce intake. Collaborate with health care providers and registered dietitians (RDs) to provide optimal nutrition to older adults.
- Changes in taste and smell, oral mucus and saliva production, and dentition with aging may affect the patient's food choices, appetite, and ability to chew or swallow.
- Some older adults have decreased gastric emptying, and formula remains in the stomach longer than for younger patients. These patients may benefit from intestinal feeding.

Home Care

- Homebound older adults may benefit from meal-delivery services that can provide multiple meals per day. Check for other community resources (e.g., food pantries, senior community services).
- Assess the ability of patient or family caregiver to administer feeding and maintain a feeding tube. Then instruct on the following topics:
  - How to administer feedings and monitor for symptoms of discomfort, diarrhea, and aspiration
  - How to monitor intake and output using household measuring devices and what the target intake should be
  - How to provide skin care
  - How to re-secure a feeding tube and check tube placement
  - Signs and symptoms of complications to report to health care provider
- Determine the environmental safety and sanitation of patient's home environment.
- Instruct patient or family caregiver not to proceed with feedings or medication administration via the tube if there is any doubt as to proper placement of the tube or if the tube cannot be irrigated.

✦ PRACTICE REFLECTIONS

A 70-year-old patient with severe Parkinson's is admitted to the hospital with sepsis. Enteral nutrition is ordered within the first 48 hours. The patient is to receive continuous tube feedings via a nasointestinal (NI) tube.

1. What is the likely reason for the patient to have a nasointestinal tube instead of a nasogastric tube?
2. When checking NI tube placement, what pH range do you anticipate?
3. When is it appropriate to irrigate this patient's NI tube?

✦ CLINICAL REVIEW QUESTIONS

1. Which of the following patients has the greatest risk for a complication from a nasogastric tube insertion? (Select all that apply.)
   1. A patient who has an endotracheal tube and is on mechanical ventilation
   2. A patient diagnosed with advanced dementia who has a low platelet count
   3. A patient who is sedated and is restless
   4. A patient who has been NPO (nothing by mouth) for 24 hours
   5. A patient who had recent nasal surgery following a car accident
2. Which of the following feeding techniques are appropriate when assisting a 62-year-old patient who has been diagnosed with a stroke? (Select all that apply.)
   1. Check for food left inside patient's cheeks after swallowing.
   2. Observe patient's ability to chew when providing solid food.
   3. Determine if patient has any food allergies.
   4. Have patient rest 15 minutes between bites.
   5. Offer small bites at a time.
3. Place the following steps in the correct order for irrigation of a feeding tube in which an intermittent infusion is administered.
   1. Complete instilling water.
   2. Remove plug at end of feeding tube and kink tubing temporarily.
   3. Remove syringe.
   4. Insert tip of ENFit syringe into end of feeding tube.
   5. If fluid does not instill easily, turn patient onto left side.
   6. Draw up 30 mL of water in ENFit syringe.
   7. Release kinked feeding tube and slowly instill irrigation solution.

Answers and Rationales for Clinical Review Questions can be found on the Evolve website.

REFERENCES

Alkhawaja S, et al: Post-pyloric versus gastric tube feeding for preventing pneumonia and improving nutritional outcomes in critically ill adults, *Cochrane Database Syst Rev* (8):CD008875, 2015.

American Academy of Pediatrics (AAP): Infant food and feeding, 2013. http://www.aap.org/en-us/advocacy-and-policy/aap-health-initiatives/HALF-Implementation-Guide/Age-Specific-Content/Pages/Infant-Food-and-Feeding.aspx.

American Association of Critical-Care Nurses (AACN): AACN practice alerts: initial and ongoing verification of feeding tube placement in adults, 2016a. https://ccn.aacnjournals.org/content/36/2/e8.full.pdf+html.

American Association of Critical-Care Nurses (AACN): AACN practice alerts: prevention of aspiration in adults, 2016b. http://ccn.aacnjournals.org/content/36/1/e20.full.

American Speech-Language-Hearing Association (ASHA): Pediatric dysphagia: causes, 2016. http://www.asha.org/PRPSpecificTopic.aspx?folderid=8589934965§ion=Causes.

Boullata J, et al: ASPEN safe practices for enteral nutrition therapy, *JPEN J Parenter Enteral Nutr* 41(1):15, 2017.

Bourgault A, et al: Methods used by critical care nurses to verify feeding tube placement in clinical practice, *Crit Care Nurse* 35(1):e1, 2015.

Centers for Disease Control and Prevention (CDC): What is health literacy? 2016. https://www.cdc.gov/healthliteracy/learn/index.html.

Christensen M, Trapl M: Development of a modified swallowing screening tool to manage post-extubation dysphagia, *Nurs Crit Care* 2017. doi:10.1111/nicc.12333. [Epub ahead of print].

Ebihara S, et al: Dysphagia, dystussia, and aspiration pneumonia in elderly people, *J Thorac Dis* 8(3):632, 2016.

Eglseer D, et al: Dysphagia in hospitalized older patients: associated factors and nutritional interventions, *J Nutr Health Aging* 22(1):103, 2018.

Fan EMP, et al: Nasogastric tube placement confirmation: where we are and where we should be heading, *Proc Singapore Healthc* 26(3):189, 2017.

Frey K, Ramsberger G: Comparison of outcomes before and after implementation of a water protocol for patients with cerebrovascular accident and dysphagia, *J Neurosci Nurs* 43(3):165, 2011.

Hakonsen SJ, et al: Nursing minimum data sets for documenting nutritional care for adults in primary healthcare: a scoping review, *JBI Database System Rev Implement Rep* 16(1):117, 2018.

Hand RK, et al: Validation of the Academy/A.S.P.E.N. malnutrition clinical characteristics, *J Acad Nutr Diet* 116(5):856, 2016.

Hiller LD, et al: Difference in composite end point of readmission and death between malnourished and normal nourished veterans assessed using Academy of Nutrition and Dietetics/American Society for Parenteral and Enteral Nutrition clinical characteristics, *JPEN J Parenter Enteral Nutr* 41(8):1316, 2017.

Holland A, et al: Carbon dioxide detection for testing nasogastric tube placement in adults, *Cochrane Database Syst Rev* (10):CD010773, 2013. http://onlinelibrary.wiley.com/doi/10.1002/14651858.CD010773/full.

Holst M, et al: Multi-modal intervention improved oral intake in hospitalized patients: a one year follow-up study, *Clin Nutr* 34:315, 2015.

Holst M, et al: Optimizing protein and energy intake in hospitals by improving individualized meal serving, hosting and the eating environment, *Nutrition* 34:14, 2017.

Institute for Safe Medication Practices (ISMP): ISMP Medication Safety Alert: ENFit enteral devices are on their way…Important safety considerations for hospitals, 2015. http://www.premiersafetyinstitute.org/wp-content/uploads/ismpmsa15-04-09_SC_bill_dang.pdf0_.pdf.

International Dysphagia Diet Standardisation Initiative: IDDSI framework, n.d. http://iddsi.org/resources/framework.

Jiang JL, et al: Validity and reliability of swallowing screening tools used by nurses for dysphagia: a systematic review, *Ci Ji Yi Xue Za Zhi* 28:41, 2016.

Kagaya H, et al: Body positions and functional training to reduce aspiration in patients with dysphagia, *Japan Med Assoc J* 54(1):35–38, 2011.

Kozeniecki M, Fritzshall R: Enteral nutrition for adults in the hospital setting, *Nutr Clin Pract* 30(5):634, 2015.

Lancaster J: Dysphagia: its nature, assessment and management, *Br J Community Nurs* S28, 2015.

Liantonio J, et al: Preventing aspiration pneumonia by addressing three key risk factors: dysphagia, poor oral hygiene, and medication use, *Ann Longterm Care* 22(10):42, 2014.

Marian T, et al: Measurement of oxygen desaturation is not useful for the detection of aspiration in dysphagic stroke patients, *Cerebrovasc Dis Extra* 7(1):44, 2017.

Markowitz J, et al: Device-related pressure ulcers, American Association of Critical Care Nurses (AACN)/Clinical Scene Investigator (CSI) Academy, 2013. http://www.aacn.org/wd/csi/docs/FinalProjects/IU%20Methodist%20ACC%20-%20Power%20Point%20Presentation.pdf.

McCarthy MS, Martindale RG: What's on the menu? Delivering evidence-based nutritional therapy, *Nursing* 45(8):36, 2015.

McClave SA, et al: ACG clinical guidelines: nutrition therapy in the adult hospitalized patient, *Am J Gastroenterol* 111(3):315–334, 2016.

Meehan A, et al: Health system quality improvement: impact of prompt nutrition care on patient outcomes and health care costs, *J Nurs Care Qual* 31(3):217, 2016.

Meiner S, Yeager J: *Gerontologic nursing*, ed 6, St. Louis, 2019, Mosby.

Metheny N: Preventing aspiration in older adults with dysphagia, 2018. *Try This: Best Pract Nurs Care Older Adults* (20), 2018. https://consultgeri.org/try-this/general-assessment/issue-20.pdf.

Metheny NA, Frantz RA: Head-of-bed elevation in critically ill patients: a review, *Crit Care Nurse* 33(3):53, 2013.

Metheny NA, Meert KL: Update on effectiveness of an electromagnetic feeding tube-placement device in detecting respiratory placements, *Am J Crit Care* 26(2):157, 2017.

Milsom SA, et al: Naso-enteric tube placement: a review of methods to confirm tip location, global applicability and requirements, *World J Surg* 39(9):2243, 2015.

Nagy A, et al: The effectiveness of the head-turn-plus-chin-down maneuver for eliminating vallecular residue, *Codas* 28(2):113, 2016.

National Cancer Institute (NCI): Oral complications of chemotherapy and head/neck radiation (PDQ®)–health professional version, 2016. https://www.cancer.gov/about-cancer/treatment/side-effects/mouth-throat/oral-complications-hp-pdq#section/_337.

National Stroke Association: Dysphagia, 2017. http://www.stroke.org/we-can-help/survivors/stroke-recovery/post-stroke-conditions/physical/dysphagia.

Ni MZ, et al: Selecting pH cut-offs for the safe verification of nasogastric feeding tube placement: a decision analytical modelling approach, *BMJ Open* 7(11):e018128, 2017.

Office of Disease Prevention and Health Promotion: Healthy People 2020: Food safety, 2017. https://www.healthypeople.gov/2020/topics-objectives/topic/food-safety.

Pflipsen M, Zenchenko Y: Nutrition for oral health and oral manifestations if poor nutrition and unhealthy habits, *Gen Dent* 65(6):36, 2017.

Razak PA, et al: Geriatric oral health: a review article, *J Int Oral Health* 6(6):110, 2014.

Santos SC, et al: Methods to determine the internal length of nasogastric feeding tubes: an integrative review, *Int J Nurs Stud* 61:95, 2016.

Schallom M, et al: Head-of-bed elevation and early outcomes of gastric reflux, aspiration and pressure ulcers: a feasibility study, *Am J Crit Care* 24(1):57, 2015.

Simzari K, et al: Food intake, plate waste and its association with malnutrition in hospitalized patients, *Nutr Hosp* 34(5):1376, 2017.

Smith L, et al: Nutritional screening, assessment and implementation strategies for adults in an Australian acute tertiary hospital: a best practice implementation report, *JBI Database System Rev Implement Rep* 16(1):233, 2018.

Soderstrom L, et al: Malnutrition is associated with increased mortality in older adults regardless of the cause of death, *Br J Nutr* 117(4):532, 2017.

Steele CM, Cichero J: Physiological factors related to aspiration risk: systematic review, *Dysphagia* 29(3):295, 2014.

Tan ECK, et al: Medications that cause dry mouth as an adverse effect in older people: a systematic review and metaanalysis, *J Am Geriatr Soc* 66(1):76, 2018.

Tanner DC: Avoiding negative dysphagia outcomes, *Online J Issues Nurs* 19(2):6, 2014.

Taylor SJ, et al: Nasogastric tube depth: the 'NEX' guideline is incorrect, *Br J Nurs* 23(12):641, 2014.

The Joint Commission (TJC): *2017 Hospital accreditation standards*, Oakbrook Terrace, IL, 2017, The Commission.

The Joint Commission (TJC): *2019 National Patient Safety Goals*, Oakbrook Terrace, IL, 2019, The Commission. http://www.jointcommission.org/standards_information/npsgs.aspx.

U.S. Department of Health and Human Services and U.S. Department of Agriculture: 2015-2020 dietary guidelines for Americans, ed 8, 2015, https://health.gov/dietaryguidelines/2015/guidelines.

White JW, et al: Consensus statement of the Academy of Nutrition and Dietetics/American Society for Parenteral and Enteral Nutrition: characteristics recommended for the identification and documentation of adult malnutrition, *JPEN J Parenter Enteral Nutr* 112(5):730, 2012.

Zupec-Kania B, O'Flaherty T: Medical nutrition therapy for neurologic disorders. In Mahan LK, Raymond JL, editors: *Krause's food nutrition and the nutrition care process*, ed 14, Philadelphia, 2017, Elsevier.

14 Parenteral Nutrition

SKILLS AND PROCEDURES

EVOLVE WEBSITE/RESOURCES LIST

http://evolve.elsevier.com/Perry/nursinginterventions

Audio Glossary • Checklists • Clinical Review Questions • Answers and Rationales for Clinical Review Questions • Video Clips

INTRODUCTION

Parenteral nutrition (PN) is a lifesaving form of nutritional support that is administered intravenously by an infusion pump to patients with gastrointestinal dysfunction that prevents adequate absorption of oral or enteral nutrition (EN). PN may be provided via the peripheral route (PPN, or peripheral parenteral nutrition) or central route (CPN, indicating central parenteral nutrition). PN may be used to meet nutritional needs with infusions at home if the gastrointestinal dysfunction is expected to be long term (months to years; Box 14.1). PPN or CPN may be provided as a 2-in-1 formulation (a mixture of dextrose and amino acids) or as a total nutrient admixture (TNA), also known as 3-in-1 (a mixture of dextrose, amino acids, and fat). Both formulations may have electrolytes, vitamins, and trace elements (e.g., zinc and manganese needed for enzymatic reactions) added. If only 2-in-1 formulations are provided at an institution, then the intravenous (IV) fat emulsions (IVFEs) are provided separately.

PRACTICE STANDARDS

- Boullata et al., 2014: American Society for Parenteral and Enteral Nutrition (ASPEN) clinical guidelines: parenteral nutrition ordering, order review, compounding, labeling and dispensing—Guidelines for infusions
- Gorski, 2018: Phillip's manual of IV therapeutics: evidence-based practice for infusion therapy—Infusion therapy standards of practice
- Taylor et al., 2016: Guidelines for the provision and assessment of nutrition support therapy in the adult critically ill patient: Society of Critical Care Medicine (SCCM) and American Society for Parenteral and Enteral Nutrition (ASPEN)—Evidence-based practice guidelines
- Worthington et al., 2017: When is parenteral nutrition appropriate?—Standards of care

EVIDENCE-BASED PRACTICE

Peripheral Parenteral Nutrition

Peripheral parenteral nutrition should only be used for the short term (no more than 14 days) as a bridge to EN or other short-term intestinal failure conditions that do not justify the placement of a central catheter. High-quality studies evaluating the benefits of short-term PPN are lacking. This lack of research combined with concerns of maintaining reliable peripheral access has led to infrequent use in the United States. Guidelines for PPN include the following:

- For patients with short-term intestinal failure, the goal of PPN is to prevent nutrition deficits while minimizing PN-related complications until patients can resume full oral diets or meet their needs with enteral tube feedings (Worthington et al., 2017).
- The final osmolarity of an infusion should not exceed 900 mOsm/L to be infused safely (Boullata et al., 2014; Gorski, 2018).
- Patients started on PPN should have acceptable venous integrity to allow for the infusion of a hyperosmolar solution while allowing other intravenous (IV) access for additional drug therapies (Worthington et al., 2017).

Central Parenteral Nutrition

Central parenteral nutrition is the best option for patients with permanent intestinal failure or those expected unable to use the gastrointestinal (GI) tract for feeding for greater than 14 days (Worthington et al., 2017). Guidelines for CPN include the following:

- The type of IV catheter to use for administration of PN depends on patient factors and the expected length of PN therapy. The location of the catheter is defined on the basis of where the distal tip of the catheter lies. The desired tip location is the superior vena cava. Concentrated PN solutions

BOX 14.1

Indications for Parenteral Nutrition

Nonfunctional Gastrointestinal (GI) Tract

- Small bowel resection
- Small bowel surgery or GI bleed
- Paralytic ileus
- Intestinal obstruction
- Trauma to abdomen, head, or neck
- Severe malabsorption
- Intolerant of slow rates of enteral tube feeding
- Chemotherapy, radiation therapy, bone marrow transplantation
- Severely catabolic patients when GI tract is not functioning for more than 7 days

Nonfunctional GI Tract

- Enterocutaneous fistula
- Inflammatory bowel disease
- Severe diarrhea
- Moderate to severe pancreatitis

Preoperative Parenteral Nutrition

- Preoperative bowel rest
- Severe malnutrition before surgery

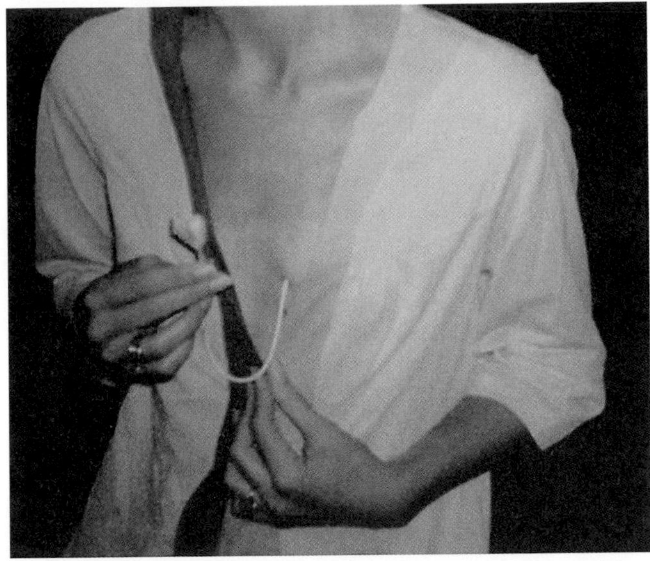

FIG 14.2 Tunneled catheter used for home central parenteral nutrition. *(From Morgan SL, Weinsier RL: Fundamentals of clinical nutrition, ed 2, St. Louis, 1998, Mosby.)*

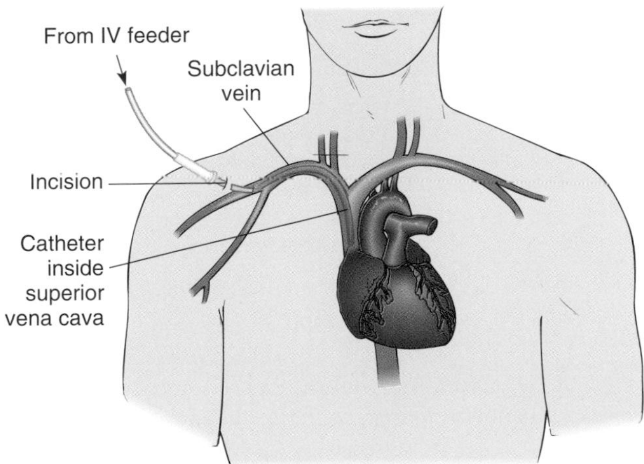

FIG 14.1 Placement of central venous catheter inserted into subclavian vein. *IV*, Intravenous.

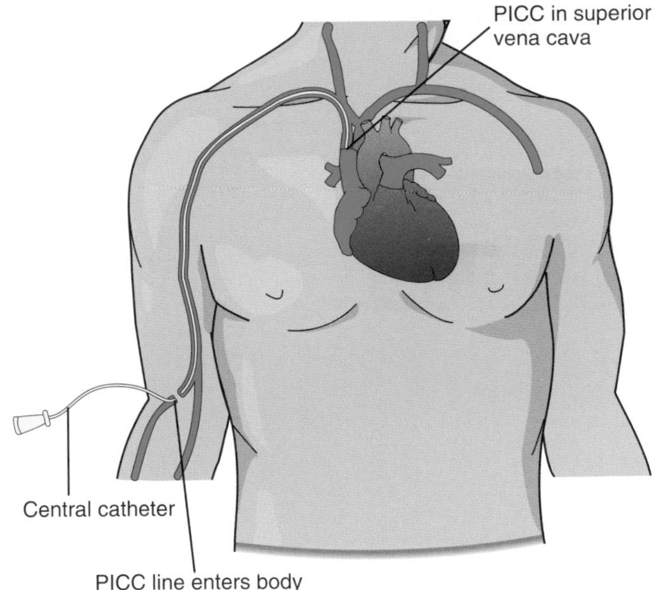

FIG 14.3 Peripherally inserted central catheter (PICC).

are diluted quickly when infused into a large-diameter central vein (Fig. 14.1; see Chapter 28).

- Patients who self-administer their PN solutions at home will require a central catheter, which may be an implanted subcutaneous port, a peripherally inserted central catheter (PICC), or a tunneled central access device (Figs. 14.2 and 14.3). A PICC catheter tip may rest in the superior vena cava or cavoatrial junction. Implanted ports and tunneled central access device tips should rest in the superior vena cava. A higher risk of catheter-related bloodstream infection (CRBSI) in PICC versus a tunneled central access device has been noted in patients requiring home PN for greater than 3 months (Christensen et al., 2016; Gorski, 2018; Table 14.1; see Chapter 28).
- Patients who require PN infusions do so for medical or surgical conditions that are often associated with GI losses (e.g., obstruction, diarrhea, fistula) and organ dysfunction; therefore electrolyte monitoring is paramount. Thus typical laboratory tests relative to PN infusions include a baseline assessment of electrolytes (basic metabolic panel, magnesium, and phosphorus), complete blood count, triglyceride level, and liver function tests (Box 14.2).
- When the goal is to prepare a patient for a cyclic home infusion of PN, it is very important to monitor glucose levels approximately 2 hours after an infusion begins (peak level) and 2 hours after it ends (trough level) to evaluate the need for adjusting regular human insulin in the infusion bag to avoid hyperglycemia or rebound hypoglycemia.
- Because a PN solution is typically provided in response to GI dysfunction and to support nutritional needs, it is important for you to monitor data that describe patient progress (see Box 14.2). Measurement of intake and output is very important to document when a patient's GI function is changing and to provide information regarding the adequacy of fluid intake from the PN solution.

TABLE 14.1

Complications of Parenteral Nutrition

Problem	Cause	Symptoms	Immediate Action	Prevention
Pneumothorax	Tip of catheter enters pleural space during insertion, causing lung to collapse	Sudden chest pain, difficulty breathing, decreased breath sounds, cessation of normal chest movement on affected side, tachycardia	Per health care provider's order, the proper professional (CRNP, PA-C, or MD) may remove the central catheter. Administer oxygen via nasal cannula. Insert chest tube to remove air under water-seal drainage or dry one-way valve system.	Medical personnel should be properly trained to insert central catheters. Researchers suggest use of ultrasound when placing CVCs (Gorski, 2018). Catheter should be secured properly to prevent migration and movement.
Air embolism	IV tubing disconnected; part of catheter system open or removed without being clamped	Sudden respiratory distress: decreased oxygen saturation levels, shortness of breath, coughing, chest pain, decreased blood pressure	Clamp catheter; position patient in left Trendelenburg's position; call health care provider; administer oxygen as needed (Gorski, 2018).	Make sure that all catheter connections are secure; clamp catheter when not in use. Never use a stopcock with a CVC. Unless contraindicated, instruct patient in Valsalva maneuver for tubing changes (Gorski, 2018).
Localized infection (exit site or tunnel)	Poor aseptic technique in removal of skin flora during site preparation and dressing care	*Exit site:* Erythema, tenderness, induration, or purulence within 2 cm (0.8 inch) of skin at exit site *Tunnel:* Same as above but extends beyond 2 cm from exit site	Call health care provider. *Exit:* Apply warm compress, daily care of site, oral antibiotics. *Infection:* Collaborate with health care provider regarding removal of catheter (Gorski, 2018). *Tunnel:* Remove catheter.	Provide catheter site care using aseptic technique, visually inspect site (including cleaning site), apply new stabilization device, and apply sterile dressing (Gorski, 2018). Change transparent dressings at least every 5–7 days and gauze dressings every 48 hours (Gorski, 2018). Change dressing if damp, loosened, or soiled or when inspection of site is necessary (Gorski, 2018). Use chlorhexidine wipes to cleanse site. For adults, consider the use of chlorhexidine-impregnated dressings (Gorski, 2018).
Catheter-related sepsis or bacteremia	Catheter hub contamination; contamination of infusate; spread of bacteria through bloodstream from distant site	*Systemic:* Isolation of same microorganism from blood culture and catheter segment, with patient showing fever, chills, malaise, elevated white blood cell count	*Systemic:* Do not exceed hang time of 24 hours for PN that contains dextrose and amino acids either alone or with fat emulsion added as a 3-in-1 formulation (Gorski, 2018). Administer antibiotics intravenously; remove catheter by proper professional (CRNP, PA-C, or MD).	Use full sterile-barrier precautions during catheter insertion and dressing change. Consider the use of antibiotic-impregnated catheters (Gorski, 2018). Do not disconnect tubing unnecessarily. Replace IV tubing and filter every 24 hours. In some selected situations it is necessary to change administration sets with each new PN container (Gorski, 2018).
Hyperglycemia	Possible blood-draw error; confirm with bedside glucose device; patient receiving too little insulin in PN solution; receiving steroids; new-onset infection	Excessive thirst, urination, blood glucose greater than 160 mg/100 dL, confusion	Call health care provider; may need to slow infusion rate (health care provider order).	Review medical history for blood drawn through central line with PN infusing (repeat peripheral blood draw or obtain fingerstick), glucose intolerance or diabetes, new infection, new medication such as steroids; keep rate as ordered; never increase PN to "catch up." Maintain blood glucose in range ordered by health care provider. Use aseptic technique and routine blood glucose monitoring.
Hypoglycemia	PN abruptly discontinued; too much insulin	Patient shaky, dizzy, nervous, anxious, hungry, blood glucose level less than 80 mg/100 dL	Call health care provider; if PN discontinued abruptly, may need to restart $D_{10}W$ at previous PN rate. If patient has oral intake, give ½ cup fruit juice. Perform blood glucose monitoring; retest in 15 to 30 min.	Decrease PN, "tapering" gradually until discontinued; blood glucose monitoring is used to ensure adequate insulin.

CRNP, Certified registered nurse practitioner; *CVC,* central venous catheter; *IV*, intravenous; *MD,* medical doctor; *PA-C,* physician's assistant–certified; *PN*, parenteral nutrition.

BOX 14.2

Typical Monitoring and Laboratory Orders for Patients With Parenteral Nutrition

Monitor

- Fluid intake, urine and gastrointestinal output every 8 hours
- Vital signs every 4 hours
- Body weight at least 3 times weekly

Initial and Repeated Weekly

- Complete metabolic panel with sodium (Na), potassium (K), chloride (Cl), carbon dioxide (CO_2), glucose, calcium (Ca), phosphate (PO_4), magnesium (Mg), triglycerides, transaminases, liver function
- Complete blood count (CBC) with hemoglobin, hematocrit, white blood count (WBC), red blood cells (RBCs), lymphocyte count
- Serum proteins, often including albumin, transferrin, C-reactive protein, and/or prealbumin

Daily Until Stable

- Electrolyte panel daily until stable; then weekly
- Glucose every 6 hours until within normal limits for 48 hours; then daily
- Glucose in preparation for cyclic home parenteral nutrition (PN); monitor 2 hours after PN begins and 2 hours after PN ends; adjust insulin per orders

Monthly or Biannually

- Trace elements such as zinc, copper, manganese, selenium (depending on underlying condition such as gastrointestinal/malabsorption) and in times of short supply or rationing of trace elements because of national shortages and for long-term home PN
- Selected vitamins for long-term home PN patients

PN Use in Critically Ill Patients

When critically ill patients cannot tolerate enteral nutrition, PN provides an alternative route for nutritional delivery, including a decreased infection rate when it is initiated early versus later in their care. Key evidence-based practice guidelines for management of critically ill patients in intensive care units (ICU) include the following (Patel et al., 2017; Taylor et al., 2016):

- Enteral nutrition is preferred over PN for nutritional support (see Chapter 13).
- If the patient was healthy before this critical illness, with no evidence of protein-calorie malnutrition, use of PN should be reserved and initiated only after the first 7 days of hospitalization, when EN nutrition is not available.
- PN should be initiated only if the duration is anticipated to be greater than or equal to 7 days.
- In patients stabilized on PN, efforts should be made to reintroduce oral or EN.
- PN should not be terminated until greater than or equal to 60% of nutritional needs are being met by the oral or enteral route. However, the calories can be decreased to avoid overfeeding.

SAFETY GUIDELINES

PN is a vital therapeutic modality that allows for the improved care of patients with both short- and long-term intestinal failure. However, PN is a high-alert medication, and as such, bedside safety guidelines should be in place to optimize care and limit medication errors:

- Prior to initiation of PN, the type of vascular access available and the insertion site should be evaluated to ensure safe delivery of the medication and decrease potential complications (Derenski et al., 2016).
- Many health care agencies use PICCs, termed *PICC lines* (see Fig. 14.3), which are placed by specially trained nurses or radiologists.
- Following central venous catheter insertion, do not initiate PN until the placement of the venous catheter tip is confirmed to rest in the superior vena cava or cavoatrial junction by a radiograph or using electrocardiograph (ECG) tip-verification technology (Gorski, 2018).
- PN with an osmolality of 900 mOsm or greater should only be infused in a central line (PICC, percutaneous nontunneled central catheter, tunneled cuffed catheters, or implanted ports). These high-osmolality solutions should not be infused into a peripheral IV, midclavicular, or midline catheter because of the increased risk for phlebitis. If only peripheral lines are available, the orders should clearly state that the administration route should be via a peripheral IV line so that the compounding pharmacy will prepare PPN with a lower osmolarity (Table 14.2), which will require added fluid volume (Boullata et al., 2014; Derenski et al., 2016).
- PN without lipids can be infused using tubing with a 0.20-μm filter, whereas lipid-containing emulsions (3-in-1) must be infused using a larger 1.2-μm filter (Boullata et al., 2014; Gorski, 2018). A filter is necessary because it prevents particulate matter or large droplets of lipid from reaching a patient, which could potentially result in a pulmonary embolism.
- If possible, a lumen of the IV access should be reserved solely for PPN or PN administration. If there is a lack of access, prior to Y-siting any medication into the PPN or PN line, approval should be sought from pharmacy or other nutrition support personnel.
- PPN or PN hang time is 24 hours or less. Intravenous fatty emulsions given separately from the PN solution have a hang time of 12 hours.
- Both hypo- and hyperglycemia have been linked to PPN and PN usage; thus regular monitoring of glucose levels during the infusion is important. If insulin is included with the PN formulation, the amount should be noted. Although hyperglycemia is more common, abrupt withdrawal of PN or increase of insulin in the PN formulation may lead to hypoglycemia. The optimal regimen to maintain euglycemia in patients receiving PN continues to be debated (Vercoza et al., 2017).
- The most frequent complication associated with PN is catheter-related bloodstream infection (CRBSI), a risk that is found in both hospitalized patients and those with PN at home (see Table 14.1). It is critically important that aseptic technique is used when handling the central line, dressings, tubing, and the needleless end cap PN port (see Chapter

TABLE 14.2

Comparison of Central Versus Peripheral Parenteral Nutrition Orders

	Central Parenteral Nutrition	Peripheral Parenteral Nutrition
Osmolality	>900 mOsm	<900 mOsm
Route of administration	Central venous catheter	Small peripheral vein
Usual daily caloric intake	20–35 kcal/kg/day	5–10 kcal/kg/day
Usual daily volume (mL)	1000–2000	2000–3000

28). Regular monitoring of temperature is also important (Gorski, 2018).
- In very malnourished patients, the provision of PN may lead to *refeeding syndrome*, which may have severe consequences. Specific electrolytes (e.g., potassium [K], magnesium [Mg], and phosphorus [P]) may shift intracellularly with glucose provided in the PN, potentially resulting in low serum levels with risk for arrhythmias, pulmonary edema, and heart failure (Derenski et al., 2016). Adequate electrolyte repletion should occur before the initiation of PN, with increased frequency of monitoring during provision of PN until serum levels are stable and within normal limits.

✦ SKILL 14.1 Administering Central Parenteral Nutrition

Purpose

Administration of parenteral nutrition (PN) through a central intravenous (IV) line requires the use of strict aseptic technique (see Chapter 5) and application of critical thinking. Because of the composition of PN fluids, patients can experience changes in metabolic and fluid balance quickly. In addition, the clinical condition of patients receiving PN may be poor, especially when they have alterations in host defenses, severe underlying illnesses, and extremes of age. You will need to anticipate changes in a patient's condition that signal developing complications. Similarly, you need to use good judgment to maintain the IV system and ensure that it is functioning properly.

Delegation and Collaboration

The skill of administering CPN cannot be delegated to nursing assistive personnel (NAP). The nurse directs the NAP to:
- Report when the pump alarms or patient has shortness of breath, headaches, or weakness; feels shaky; or has discomfort or bleeding at IV site.
- Perform fingerstick blood glucose monitoring (see agency policy) as directed and report any abnormal results to the nurse.
- Report vital signs that are out of normal range to nurse.
- Measure urinary output and weigh patient per agency protocol.

Equipment

- PN solution (IV)
- Electronic infusion device (EID) with anti–free-flow control and alarms (INS, 2016)
- IV infusion tubing with Luer-Lok tip
- Appropriate IV filter (1.2-μm filter for 3-in-1 solutions or lipids containing a membrane that is particulate retentive and air eliminating; 0.20-μm filter for solutions that do not contain lipids; INS, 2016)
- 5- to 10-mL syringe with sterile saline flush
- Bedside glucose monitoring kit
- Adhesive tape or tubing label
- Antimicrobial swab
- Clean gloves
- Stethoscope
- Medication administration record (MAR) or computer printout

ASSESSMENT

1. Review medical record and assess for indications of and risks for severe acute protein/calorie malnutrition: weight loss (2% over the past week) from baseline or ideal, decreased intake (50% or less of need for 5 or more days), muscle atrophy/weakness, edema, lethargy, failure to wean from a mechanical ventilator, and chronic illness. Confer with nutritional support team. *Rationale: Clinical indications for PN. These data provide a baseline from which change can be noted (Gorski, 2018; White et al., 2012).*
2. Assess medical record for serum chemistries, liver function tests, triglycerides, complete blood count, international normalized ratio and prothrombin time (see Box 14.2). Check blood glucose level by fingerstick (see Chapter 9). Remove gloves and perform hand hygiene. *Rationale: Provides baseline for measuring patient's metabolic and electrolyte status. In addition, identifies patient's unique requirements so that PN admixture may be tailored to patient's specific needs (Derenski et al., 2016; Gorski, 2018). Serum glucose determines patient's baseline and tolerance to high levels of glucose in PN solution. Reduces transmission of microorganisms.*
3. Assess patient's medical history for factors influenced by PN administration: electrolyte levels; renal, cardiac, and hepatic function. Assess for history of allergies. *Rationale: Some patients require that PN therapy be adapted by composition or volume (requires health care provider order) based on medical history. PN includes constituents (e.g., medications) to which patient may be allergic.*
4. Perform hand hygiene. Apply clean gloves as needed. Inspect condition of central vein access site for presence of inflammation, edema, and tenderness (see Chapter 28). Inspect tubing of access device for patency and kinking. *Rationale: Reduces transmission of infection. Identifies early signs of infection, infiltration, or disruption in system integrity. Development of complication contraindicates infusion of fluids and indicates need to establish new IV site.*
5. Assess vital signs, auscultate patient's lung sounds, inspect for edema of extremities, and measure weight (see Chapter 8). *Rationale: Provides baseline for monitoring patient's response to fluid infusion and nutrients. Crackles in lungs are early indication of fluid volume excess.*
6. Consult with health care provider and dietitian on calculation of calorie, protein, and fluid requirements for patient. *Rationale: Provides interprofessional plan for patient's nutritional support.*
7. Verify health care provider's order for nutrients, minerals, vitamins, trace elements, electrolytes, added medications, and flow rate. Check for compatibility of added medications. *Rationale: PN is often ordered daily in a hospital setting after review of laboratory values. In home setting, orders may be obtained less frequently (e.g., weekly). Pharmacies that prepare PN solutions will check medication compatibility.*
8. Assess patient's and family caregiver's knowledge of PN, including any previous experience with home management and health literacy level. *Rationale: Ensures patient has the capacity to obtain, communicate, process, and understand basic health information (Centers for Disease Control and Prevention [CDC], 2016).*

STEP	RATIONALE

PLANNING

STEP	RATIONALE
1. Expected outcomes following completion of procedure:	
• Patient's ideal weight gain is between 0.5 and 1.5 kg (1 and 3 lb) per week.	Weight may be an indicator of patient's nutritional status or fluid volume in the hospitalized patient. Weight gain greater than 0.5 kg/day (1 lb/day) indicates fluid retention.
• Blood glucose levels are maintained per health care provider's order for desired glucose range.	Glucose levels needed for specific populations differ based on the degree of illness, so a specific health care provider order is needed (Taylor et al., 2016).
• Central venous access device is patent; and site is free of pain, swelling, redness, or inflammation.	Ensures that PN is infusing into vein rather than into surrounding tissues and that there are no signs of an access device infection.
• Patient is afebrile.	Absence of systemic infection.
• Patient and family caregiver can discuss purpose and steps for care of PN.	Proper instruction informs patient and family caregiver and prepares for home care if needed.
2. If PN solution is refrigerated, remove from refrigeration 1 hour before infusion.	Ensures solution will be administered at room temperature for patient comfort.
3. Provide for patient privacy	Provides for patient comfort
4. Organize equipment at bedside and inform colleagues of procedure being performed	Ensures organized approach and avoids interruptions by other staff.
5. Place patient in comfortable position for initiation of infusion.	When patients are comfortable, they tolerate procedures more readily.
6. Explain purpose of PN and procedure to be followed to patient/family caregiver.	Promotes understanding and reduces anxiety.

IMPLEMENTATION

STEP	RATIONALE
1. Perform hand hygiene.	Reduces transmission of microorganisms.
2. Check label on PN bag with health care provider's order on MAR or computer printout and patient's name. Also check any additives and note solution expiration date.	Prevents medication error. ***This is the first check for accuracy.***
3. Inspect 2-in-1 PN solution for particulate matter; inspect 3-in-1 PN solution for separation of fat into top layer (known as creaming) or discoloration throughout (known as cracking).	Presence of particulate matter or fat emulsion separation requires that solution be discarded (Derenski et al., 2016).
4. Before leaving medication room, check IV solution second time using seven rights of medication administration (see Chapter 22). Check label of PN bag against MAR or computer printout.	***This is the second check for accuracy.***
5. Identify patient using at least two identifiers (e.g., name and birthday or name and medical record number) according to agency policy. Compare identifiers with information on patient's MAR or medical record.	Ensures correct patient. Complies with The Joint Commission standards and improves patient safety (TJC, 2019).
6. Take PN solution to patient in advance of previous solution emptying unless patient is receiving cyclic PN. Compare names of solution and additives on label with MAR at bedside.	***This is the third check for accuracy.***
7. Apply clean gloves. Prepare IV tubing for PN solution: a. Attach appropriate filter to IV tubing. b. Prime tubing with PN solution, making sure that no air bubbles remain, and turn off flow with roller clamp (see Chapter 28). Some infusion pumps and IV tubing require that priming be done on pump rather than by gravity. Add sterile capped needle or place sterile cap on end of tubing	Maintains sterility of solution. Air introduced into central circulation could result in air embolus, a fatal IV complication.
8. Wipe end port of central vascular access device (CVAD) with alcohol swab, allow to dry, then attach syringe of 0.9% normal saline (NS) solution to needleless port, aspirate for blood return, and flush saline per agency policy.	Scrubbing hub decreases microorganisms (Gorski, 2018; Infusion Nurses Society [INS], 2016). Determines patency of IV device before infusing PN.

STEP	RATIONALE
9. Remove syringe. Connect Luer-Lok end of PN IV tubing to end port of CVAD; for multilumen lines, label tubing used for PN.	Ensures that tubing is securely connected to IV line. Dedicated line should be used for multilumen devices. Labeling of high-risk catheters prevents connection with inappropriate tube or catheter (TJC, 2019).
10. Place IV tubing in EID. Open roller clamp. Set and regulate flow rate as ordered (see illustration).	PN flow rates are ordered to meet patient's metabolic and electrolyte needs. Maintaining rates prevents electrolyte imbalances.

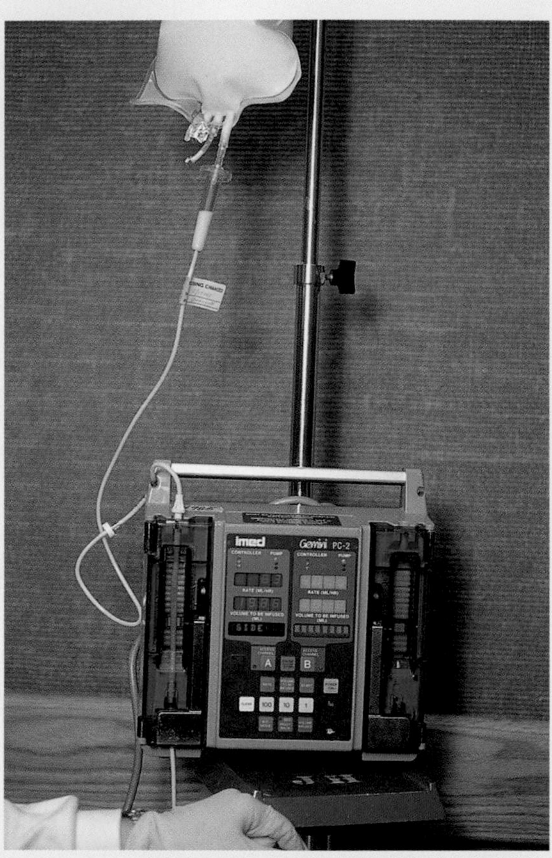

STEP 10 Parenteral nutrition solution infusing via infusion pump.

STEP	RATIONALE
a. *Continuous infusion (optional):* Flow rate is immediately set at ordered rate and given over 24-hour period.	Ensures that blood glucose levels are maintained to prevent hypoglycemia or hyperglycemia (Derenski et al., 2016; Gorski, 2018).
b. *Cycle infusion (optional):* Flow rate may be started at goal unless that patient has difficulty with hyper- or hypoglycemia. In this case, flow rate is initiated at about two-thirds of goal, and the rate is gradually tapered up or down to goal over 1 to 2 hours. The infusion is usually given over a shorter time frame (12–18 hours).	Infusion rates are usually increased and decreased to prevent hypoglycemia or hyperglycemia (Derenski et al., 2016; Gorski, 2018).
11. Infuse all IV medications or blood through alternative IV site or multilumen device. **Do not obtain blood samples or central venous pressure readings through same lumen used for PN.**	Prevents drug incompatibility and IV device occlusion (Boullata et al., 2014; Gorski, 2018).
12. Do not interrupt PN infusion (e.g., during showers, transport to procedure, blood transfusion), and be sure that rate does not exceed ordered rate.	Prevents development of catheter-related bacteremia (Alexander et al., 2014; Gorski, 2018).
13. Change IV administration sets for PN every 24 hours and immediately on suspected contamination. Discard used supplies, remove and dispose of gloves, and perform hand hygiene.	Reduces transmission of infection.

STEP	RATIONALE
14. Assist patient to comfortable position	
15. Raise side rails (as appropriate) and lower bed to lowest position.	Ensures patient safety.
16. Place nurse call system in an accessible location within patient's reach. Instruct patient in its use.	Provides for patient safety.

EVALUATION

STEP	RATIONALE
1. Monitor and document IV flow rate according to agency policy and procedure. If infusion is not running on time, do not attempt to catch up.	Too-rapid or too-slow infusion could result in metabolic disturbances such as hyperglycemia and fluid overload.
2. Monitor fluid intake and urine and gastrointestinal (GI) fluid output every 8 hours.	Prevents fluid imbalance from too-slow or too-rapid infusion.
3. Measure vital signs every 4 hours.	Monitors for fluid overload response.
4. Obtain initial weight and then weigh at least 3 times weekly.	Routine measurement of weights will reflect a gain/loss resulting either from caloric intake or fluid retention. Gradual weight gain, if weight gain is the goal, indicates adequate tolerance.
5. Evaluate for fluid retention; palpate skin of extremities; auscultate lung sounds.	Weight gain in excess of 0.5 kg/day (1 lb/day), dependent edema, lung crackles, and intake greater than output per each 24-hour period indicate fluid retention.
6. Monitor patient's glucose levels every 6 hours or as ordered and other laboratory parameters daily or as ordered.	Maintenance of normal electrolyte levels, satisfactory fluid balance, and acceptable serum glucose levels indicate adequate tolerance to PN.
7. Inspect central venous access site for signs and symptom of swelling, inflammation, drainage, redness, warmth, tenderness, or edema.	Determines IV patency and absence of infection, infiltration, or phlebitis.
8. Monitor for temperature, elevated white blood cell count, and malaise.	Signs of systemic infection.
9. **Teach-Back:** "I want to be sure I explained what can happen with your parenteral nutrition. What signs and symptoms should you report to the nurse or doctor?" Revise your instruction now or develop a plan for revised patient/family caregiver teaching if patient/family caregiver is not able to teach back correctly.	Determines patient's/family caregiver's level of understanding of instructional topic.

Unexpected Outcomes	Related Interventions
1. There is redness, swelling, and tenderness around central venous access site, indicating possible exit site infection.	• Notify health care provider. • Apply warm compress (see Chapter 15) and initiate daily site care as ordered. • Systemic antibiotic therapy may begin.
2. Patient develops fever, malaise, and chills, indicating systemic infection.	• Check exit site for signs of infection. • Notify health care provider and consult about need to obtain cultures of exit site or blood. • Systemic antibiotic therapy may begin.
3. Serum glucose level is greater than 150 mg/dL or target set by health care provider.	• Notify health care provider. • Indicates intolerance to glucose load in PN solution. • May indicate new-onset infection. • Verify that blood was not drawn with PN infusing and that proper procedure to interrupt PN and discard first blood draw was followed. • Possible need for addition to or modification of insulin in PN or sliding-scale insulin coverage.

Recording

- Condition of CVAD, rate and type of infusion, catheter lumen used for infusion, intake and output (I&O), blood glucose levels, vital signs, and weights.
- Signs of infection, occlusion, fluid retention, or infiltration occurring.
- Evaluation of patient and family caregiver learning.

Hand-Off Reporting

- Catheter type and site and infusion rate of PN.
- Most recent blood glucose levels and vital signs.
- Any abnormalities associated with PN noted (e.g., fluid retention, signs of infection, abnormal lab values).
- Report to health care provider immediately signs of IV complications.

✦ SKILL 14.2 Administering Peripheral Parenteral Nutrition With Lipid (Fat) Emulsion

Purpose

The administration of peripheral parenteral nutrition (PPN) requires a lower dextrose content than central parenteral nutrition (CPN) and is more appropriate for short-term use until central access can be achieved or the patient can be fed orally or enterally. Patients with elevated nutritional requirements from hypermetabolic illnesses or conditions and patients with fluid restrictions are not suitable candidates (Worthington et al., 2017). This therapy is usually for 2 weeks or less. The PPN solution uses lower concentrations of dextrose and amino acids to reduce the osmolality (see Table 14.2) and decrease the risk for phlebitis. Adding lipid emulsion provides a source of calories with minimal impact on the osmolality. A lipid emulsion must be administered through vented intravenous (IV) tubing as a primary IV infusion or a piggyback (see Chapter 28). Administration sets (including piggybacks) used for fat emulsions are changed every 24 hours and immediately on suspected contamination (Gorski, 2018). The administration set must have a Luer-Lok design. Indications for PPN include the following (Worthington et al., 2017):

- *Adequate peripheral access:* Despite its lower osmolality, PPN tends to cause phlebitis and often requires frequent changes in the access location. A midline catheter may be an alternative to the typical short-peripheral catheter.
- *Ability to tolerate larger volumes of fluid:* Because of the lower concentration of dextrose in PPN, a larger volume of fluid is required to attain adequate calories. Some patients with impaired renal or cardiac function do not tolerate PPN.
- *Ability to tolerate lipid emulsions:* Lipid is the most calorically dense nutrient. A 1-L amount of 10% dextrose without lipid provides only 340 kcal. A 250-mL amount of 20% lipid solution provides 500 kcal.

Delegation and Collaboration

The skill of administering PPN cannot be delegated to nursing assistive personnel (NAP). The nurse directs the NAP to:

- Report patient complaint of burning, pain, or redness at peripheral IV site.
- Report to nurse infusion pump alarms or moist IV site dressing.
- Report to nurse patient complaints of shortness of breath and change in vital signs.

Equipment

- PPN solution
- Lipid emulsion in glass container or in a separate chamber of the parenteral nutrition (PN) bag
- IV tubing for PPN with 0.20-μm filter for amino acid/dextrose solution
- IV tubing with a 1.2-μm filter for fat emulsion
- Bedside glucose monitoring kit
- Antimicrobial swab
- Electronic infusion pump with anti–free-flow control and alarms (INS, 2016)
- Clean gloves
- Medication administration record (MAR) or computer printout
- Stethoscope

ASSESSMENT

1. Review medical record and assess patient for hypertriglyceridemia. Obtain orders for serum triglyceride level before initiation of PPN and weekly. *Rationale: Determines patient's ability to metabolize lipid.*
2. Assess patient's medical history for factors influenced by PPN administration: electrolyte levels; renal, cardiac, and hepatic function. Assess for history of allergies. *Rationale: PPN includes constituents to which patient may be allergic. PPN requires a larger volume per calorie; therefore patients with medical conditions requiring fluid restriction may not be candidates for PPN.*
3. Perform hand hygiene and apply clean gloves. Select or initiate appropriate functional IV site to administer PPN and lipid emulsion. Assess its patency and function (see Chapter 28). *Rationale: Reduces transmission of microorganisms. PPN may cause phlebitis; therefore appropriate vein selection is important.*
4. Obtain blood glucose level by fingerstick (see Chapter 9). *Rationale: Provides baseline to determine tolerance to glucose infusion.*
5. Assess patient's fluid status by assessing for edema in extremities, lung sounds, and fluid intake greater than fluid output. *Rationale: Fluid intake that is given with PPN may cause fluid overload in elderly patients or those who have impaired renal or cardiac function.*
6. Obtain patient's weight and vital signs. Remove gloves and perform hand hygiene. *Rationale: Provides baseline information to determine effectiveness and tolerance of PPN solution. Reduces transmission of microorganisms.*
7. Check health care provider's order against MAR for volume of fat emulsion, PPN solution, and administration time for fat emulsion. Then check name of solution on label with MAR. *Rationale: Health care provider must order fat emulsions and PPN. Fat emulsions may cause adverse symptoms if infused too rapidly as separate infusion. Infusion time is normally at least 8 hours. Fat emulsions should hang no longer than 12 hours as*

separate infusion from original container. ***This is the first check for accuracy.***

8. Read label of fat emulsion solution. *Rationale: Lipid emulsions are white and opaque; thus be sure to avoid confusing enteral tube-feeding formula with parenteral lipids.*

9. Assess patient's and family caregiver's knowledge of PPN, including any previous experience with home management and health literacy level. *Rationale: Ensures patient has the capacity to obtain, communicate, process, and understand basic health information (CDC, 2016).*

STEP	RATIONALE

PLANNING

STEP	RATIONALE
1. Expected outcomes following completion of procedure:	
• Triglyceride level is less than 400 mg/dL in most patients.	Indicates adequate clearance of lipid (Derenski et al., 2016).
• Blood glucose levels are maintained per health care provider's order for desired glucose range.	Glucose levels needed for specific populations differ based on the degree of illness, so a specific health care provider order is needed (Taylor et al., 2016).
• Venipuncture site is free of phlebitis, pain, swelling, redness, and inflammation.	Ensures proper administration and monitoring of PPN with lipids.
• Patient does not show signs of systemic infection (e.g., elevated temperature).	Temperature is indication of possible systemic infection related to PN.
• Patient does not show signs of allergy to lipids.	Monitoring infusion requires observation for allergic response to infusion.
• Patient and family caregiver are able to explain purpose of PPN and complications to observe for.	Proper instruction informs patient and family caregiver.
2. If PPN solution is refrigerated, remove from refrigeration 1 hour before infusion.	Solution should be removed from refrigeration before administration (Alexander et al., 2014; Gorski, 2018).
3. Provide for patient privacy.	Provides for patient comfort.
4. Explain purposes of PPN and fat emulsion.	Promotes understanding and reduces anxiety.
5. Place patient in comfortable position for insertion of IV line or initiation of infusion.	When patients are comfortable, they tolerate procedures more readily.

IMPLEMENTATION

STEP	RATIONALE
1. Perform hand hygiene.	Reduces transmission of microorganisms.
2. Compare label of PPN bag and lipid emulsion bottle with MAR or computer printout; check for correct additives and solution expiration date. Also check patient's name.	Prevents medication error. ***This is the second check for accuracy.***
3. Examine lipid solution for separation of emulsion into layers or fat globules or presence of froth.	Do not administer if these elements appear.
4. Identify patient using at least two identifiers (e.g., name and birthday or name and medical record number) according to agency policy. Compare identifiers with information on patient's MAR or medical record.	Ensures correct patient. Complies with The Joint Commission standards and improves patient safety (TJC, 2019).
5. Compare identifiers with information on solution bag label and patient's MAR or medical record at the bedside.	Ensures patient receives correct infusion. ***This is the third check for accuracy.***
6. Review patient's recent vital sign levels.	Provides baseline assessment. Immediate allergic reaction can develop once infusion begins.
7. Apply clean gloves. Prepare IV tubing for PPN solution:	
a. Run solution through tubing to remove excess air. Turn roller clamp to "off" position. Some infusion pumps and tubing require priming through infusion pump.	To prevent air from entering vascular system, clear all tubing.
b. Add sterile capped needle or place sterile cap on end of tubing. Follow same procedure with separate infusion set for lipid infusion.	Reduces transmission of microorganisms.
8. Wipe end port of peripheral IV infusion tubing with antimicrobial swab and allow to dry. Connect needleless connector at end of PPN tubing to end port of patient's functional peripheral IV line. Gently disconnect old PPN tubing from IV site and insert adapter of new PPN infusion tubing. Open roller clamp on new tubing. Allow solution to run to ensure that tubing is patent; regulate IV drip rate using electronic infusion pump.	Prevents disruption of existing IV infusion and ensures patent infusion. Pump will deliver infusion at prescribed rate.

STEP	RATIONALE
9. Clean needleless peripheral line tubing injection cap with antimicrobial swab.	Removes surface organisms at injection site and prevents organisms from entering blood system.
10. Attach fat emulsion infusion tubing to injection cap of IV line. Y-connector may be used if patient is receiving separate PPN and lipid infusions. Label tubing.	Fat emulsions cannot infuse through a 0.20-μm IV filter. Refer to agency policy; if larger 1.2-μm filter is used, lipids may be infused using a Y-connector (Alexander et al., 2014; INS, 2016). Labeling high-risk catheters prevents connection with an inappropriate tube or catheter (TJC, 2019).
11. Open roller clamp completely on fat emulsion infusion and check flow rate on infusion pump.	Initial slow infusion allows you to observe for allergic response.
12. Infuse lipids initially at 1 mL/min for adults and 0.1 mL/min for child for first 15 to 30 minutes; increase rate as ordered.	Up to 2.5 g fat/kg per day may be infused, but current practice is generally to give less than 1 g fat/kg body weight per day in adults (Derenski et al., 2016)
13. Begin PPN at ordered rate; 20% fats are infused over at least 8 hours. All lipids can hang for 12 hours as a separate infusion.	Rate of PPN administration does not need to be increased gradually. Lower concentration of dextrose allows most patients to tolerate full administration rate without difficulty.
14. Remove and discard gloves and used supplies and perform hand hygiene.	Reduces transmission of microorganisms.
15. Assist patient to comfortable position.	
16. Raise side rails (as appropriate) and lower bed to lowest position.	Ensures patient safety.
17. Place nurse call system in an accessible location within patient's reach. Instruct patient in its use.	Provides for patient safety.

EVALUATION

STEP	RATIONALE
1. Monitor flow rate routinely hourly or more frequently if necessary.	Too-rapid or too-slow infusion could result in metabolic disturbances such as hyperglycemia.
2. Measure vital signs and patient's general comfort level every 10 minutes for first 30 minutes, then vital signs every 4 hours.	Monitors patient for lipid allergy.
3. Monitor patient's laboratory values (e.g., triglycerides, liver function tests) daily and perform blood glucose monitoring as ordered. Measure serum lipids 4 hours after discontinuing infusion.	Provides objective data to measure response to therapy (e.g., ability of liver to metabolize lipids). Measurement of lipids too soon after infusion will yield incorrect blood values.
4. Monitor temperature every 4 hours and regularly inspect venipuncture site for signs of phlebitis or infiltration.	Determines onset of fever, a complication of intolerance to fat emulsion or sepsis. Determines integrity of IV system.
5. Evaluate patient's weight, intake and output (I&O), condition of peripheral extremities (for edema), and breath sounds.	Weight gain, I&O imbalance, peripheral edema, and crackles in lungs indicate fluid retention.
6. **Teach-Back:** "I want to be sure I explained the purpose of your peripheral parenteral nutrition. In your own words, tell me why you are receiving this type of nutrition." Revise your instruction now or develop a plan for revised patient/family caregiver teaching if patient/family caregiver is not able to teach back correctly.	Determines patient's/family caregiver's level of understanding of instructional topic.

Unexpected Outcomes	Related Interventions
1. There is intolerance to fat emulsion, as evidenced by increased triglyceride levels, increased temperature (3° to 4° F), chills, flushing, headache, nausea and vomiting, diaphoresis, muscle ache, chest and back pain, dyspnea, pressure over eyes, or vertigo.	• Turn PPN infusion off. • Inform health care provider. • Prepare to treat anaphylactic reaction according to health care provider's orders. • Record lipid allergy in patient's medical record.
2. See Unexpected Outcomes and Related Interventions for Skill 14.1.	

Recording

- Condition of IV site, type of solutions, rate and status of infusion, catheter lumen used for infusion, I&O, blood glucose levels, vital signs, and weights.
- Adverse reactions to fat emulsion, such as increased temperature, chills, flushing, headache, nausea and vomiting, diaphoresis, muscle ache, chest and back pain, dyspnea, pressure over eyes, or vertigo.
- Signs of infection, occlusion, fluid retention, or infiltration.
- Evaluation of patient and family caregiver learning.

Hand-Off Reporting

- Report IV site condition and PPN infusion rate, most recent vitals and blood glucose levels, any adverse reactions, and treatment response.
- Report immediately any adverse reactions to health care provider.
- Report patient and family level of understanding.

SPECIAL CONSIDERATIONS

Patient-Centered Care

- Include patient and family caregiver in decisions to maintain patient control, activity level, personal decision making, and socialization with friends and family.
- Nurses collaborate with nutrition support teams and health care providers in administering PN and monitoring patients' response to PN therapy. Although practice patterns vary across agencies, typically dietitians or pharmacists provide advice on nutrition support goals and/or write PN orders in collaboration with the health care provider.
- PN may pose concerns for members of ethnic groups or people with philosophical beliefs that include restriction of animal products. The components of PN are largely synthetic and do not contain pork. The lipid emulsion contains egg phospholipid, a product that may be objectionable to vegan patients.

Patient Education

- Instruct patient and family caregiver in the purpose and goals of PN. Keep them informed about daily care of central line.
- Inform patient of signs of central line infection to report to the nurse.

Age-Specific

Pediatric

- Consider children's developmental needs when they are on long-term PN. Perform regular assessments of development to determine child's progress. Implement interventions to encourage expected milestones (Hockenberry and Wilson, 2017).

Gerontological

- Some older adults have impaired ability to tolerate higher fluid volumes because of cardiac or renal impairment.
- Some older adults may have fragile peripheral veins or poor fluid tolerance because of cardiac or renal dysfunction, making PPN undesirable.

Home Care

- Patients requiring long-term PN benefit from a referral to a home nutrition therapy team.
- Patients should have a home safety (see Chapter 32) and physical, nutritional, and psychological needs assessment (Gorski, 2018).
- Patients receiving home PN may have a PICC line or a tunneled or implanted catheter (see Figs. 14.2 and 14.3) to reduce the possibility of infection. Patients or family caregivers need to learn infection control principles and how to perform catheter site care, dressing changes, techniques for connecting and disconnecting PN solutions, and infusion pump management.
- Some patients receive home PN at night during sleep (cyclic PN) to allow the freedom to leave home during the day. Some patients may also take an oral diet as tolerated, although their impaired GI function limits nutrient absorption. Encourage food/fluid intake for pleasure as prescribed by the home nutrition therapy team but, if patient is eating, monitor for diarrhea or increased output to assess for dehydration.
- Teach patient and family caregiver to monitor patient's temperature, weight, I&O, and serum glucose level and recognize signs and symptoms of PN-related complications.
- Teach patient and family caregiver about actions to take in case of emergency or unexpected outcomes such as telephoning the health care provider or home infusion provider or going to the hospital, depending on the circumstances.
- If home PN patients require insulin in their PN, they will need a home glucose monitoring device and instruction in its use. Teaching should begin in the hospital.
- Patient teaching for home PN administration will be given by home infusion nurses after discharge or may be initiated in the hospital and continued at home.

✦ PRACTICE REFLECTIONS

A 43-year-old patient is admitted to the hospital with worsening of Crohn's disease (chronic inflammatory bowel disease [IBD]). He lost 2% of his body weight in the past week and experiences recurrent abdominal pain, cramping, and loose stools. He is unable to tolerate food orally, becoming easily nauseated. He is admitted for rehydration and central line placement for bowel rest and nutritional support PN. The nutrition support service recommends a 3-in-1 PN via the patient's PICC. The goal is to cycle the PN over 12 hours at night. It is anticipated the patient will go home with PN.

1. Identify four physical parameters that can change quickly and should be part of your baseline assessment before initiating PN.
2. On the third day after central line insertion, the patient develops a fever and fatigue, preferring to stay in bed. What might the fever indicate, and what could be its source?
3. Two days after beginning PN infusion, the patient experiences a 2 kg (5 lb) weight gain. He comments, "I'm gaining back some of the weight I lost." What would be your response? What would you include in a nursing assessment?

✦ CLINICAL REVIEW QUESTIONS

1. A patient is being switched from a standard IV solution to a parenteral nutrition solution with an osmolality of 1040 mOsm. Which of the following venous access devices could be used to infuse this solution? (Select all that apply.)
   1. Midline catheter
   2. Percutaneous nontunneled central catheter
   3. Peripheral catheter
   4. Implanted port
   5. Arterial line

2. A severely malnourished 60-year-old patient with a history of alcohol abuse is admitted for nausea and vomiting. He is found to have severe acute pancreatitis, which is known to cause severe inflammation of the pancreas, often causing outside pressure on the pylorus, where the stomach transitions to the small bowel. In this case, the inflammation is so great that the pylorus is essentially pushed closed, causing a gastric outlet obstruction. The physician orders a PICC placement by IV therapy and PN for nutrition support. What potential metabolic complications could this patient experience within the first 24 hours of PN initiation? (Select all that apply.)
   1. Refeeding syndrome
   2. Diarrhea
   3. Catheter-related bloodstream infection
   4. Hyperglycemia
   5. Phlebitis

3. The hospital policy is to hang the new 24-hour bag of PN at 8 PM nightly. The patient care technician reports to the nurse that one of the six patients receiving PN has a blood glucose level of 564 mg/dL on the 10 PM blood glucose check. The level was obtained by a fingerstick. The registered nurse knows that the patient is on the third bag of PN and that the bag contains insulin. What is the correct order in which the following steps should be taken?
   1. Call the physician and ask how much correctional insulin should be given to the patient or if the PN should be discontinued.
   2. Review the patient's medical record and determine the patient's previous bag order (for calories and insulin) and blood glucose levels with the previous bag of PN.
   3. Go to the patient's room and check the label on the PN bag with the health care provider's order on the MAR or computer printout for the patient's name, calories, and rate of infusion. Recheck the blood glucose level.

Answers and Rationales for Clinical Review Questions can be found on the Evolve website.

REFERENCES

Alexander M, et al: *Core curriculum for infusion nursing*, ed 4, Philadelphia, 2014, Lippincott, Williams & Wilkins.

Boullata JI, et al: American Society for Parenteral and Enteral Nutrition (ASPEN) clinical guidelines: parenteral nutrition ordering, order review, compounding, labeling, and dispensing, *J Parenter Enteral Nutr* 38(3):334, 2014.

Centers for Disease Control and Prevention (CDC): What is health literacy? 2016, https://www.cdc.gov/healthliteracy/learn/index.html.

Christensen LD, et al: Comparison of complications associated with peripherally inserted central catheters and Hickman catheters in patients with intestinal failure receiving home parenteral nutrition: six-year follow up study, *Clin Nutr* 35:912, 2016.

Derenski K, et al: Parenteral nutrition basics for the clinician caring for the adult patient, *Nutr Clin Prac* 31(5):578, 2016.

Gorski L: *Phillip's manual of IV therapeutics: evidence-based practice for infusion therapy*, ed 7, Philadelphia, 2018, Davis.

Hockenberry MJ, Wilson D: *Wong's essentials of pediatric nursing*, ed 10, St. Louis, 2017, Mosby.

Infusion Nurses Society (INS): Infusion therapy standards of practice, *J Intraven Nurs* 39(Suppl 1):S1, 2016.

Patel J, et al: Controversies surround critical care nutrition: an appraisal of permissive underfeeding, protein and outcomes, *J Parenter Enteral Nutr* epub ahead of print, 2017.

Taylor B, et al: Guidelines for the provision and assessment of nutrition support therapy in the adult critically ill patient: Society of Critical Care Medicine (SCCM) and American Society for Parenteral and Enteral Nutrition (ASPEN), *Crit Care Med* 44(2):390, 2016.

The Joint Commission (TJC): *2019 National Patient Safety Goals*, Oakbrook Terrace, IL, 2019, The Commission. http://www.jointcommission.org/standards_information/npsgs.aspx.

Vercoza VM, et al: Insulin regimens to treat hyperglycemia in hospitalized patients on nutritional support: systematic review and meta-analyses, *Ann Nutr Metab* 71(3–4):183, 2017.

White JV, et al: Consensus statement of the Academy of Nutrition and Dietetics/American Society for Parenteral and Enteral Nutrition: characteristics recommended for the identification and documentation of adult malnutrition (undernutrition), *J Acad Nutr Diet* 112:730, 2012.

Worthington PH, et al: When is parenteral nutrition appropriate?, *J Parenter Enteral Nutr* 41(3):374, 2017.

15 Pain Management

SKILLS AND PROCEDURES

EVOLVE WEBSITE/RESOURCES LIST

http://evolve.elsevier.com/Perry/nursinginterventions

Audio Glossary • Case Studies • Checklists • Clinical Review Questions • Answers and Rationales for Clinical Review Questions • Video Clips

INTRODUCTION

Pain is the most common reason a person seeks health care, with an estimated 126 million people in the United States requiring pain-management services (Nahin, 2015). Nurses are at the forefront in evaluating and listening to patients who are experiencing pain, and they have a responsibility to reduce the burden of suffering (ANA, 2018). Several advances in understanding pain and its treatment have occurred since the release of the 2011 Institute of Medicine (IOM) report *Relieving Pain in America,* including advances in precision medicine, which tailors pain management at the level of the individual patient (National Academies of Sciences, Engineering, and Medicine, 2017). Optimal pain control is our goal with every patient, as well as maintaining safety and quality of life. This chapter provides an understanding of acute and chronic pain and pharmacological and nonpharmacological interventions to relieve patients' pain and discomfort.

PRACTICE STANDARDS

- American Nurses Association, 2018: Position Statement: The ethical responsibility to manage pain and the suffering it causes—Pain management
- Chou et al., 2016: Management of postoperative pain: A clinical practice guideline—Pain management
- The Joint Commission, 2017: Prepublication standards—Standards revisions related to pain assessment and management
- The Joint Commission, 2019: National Patient Safety Goals—Patient identification

EVIDENCE-BASED PRACTICE

Pain Management in Older Adults

As the population ages, estimated projections for most major regions of the world show at least a quarter of the population surpassing 60 years of age by 2050 (Savvas and Gibson, 2016). Study findings vary regarding the most common sites and types of pain reported in older adults. In addition, pain management can be difficult due to age-related physiological, psychological, and psychosocial changes (Wickson-Griffiths et al., 2016). Interdisciplinary approaches to managing pain are recommended in practice, given the diverse age-related nature of pain in older adults (Wickson-Griffiths et al., 2016).

Practice Issues/Principles

- A review of current literature emphasizes that nurses need to engage older adults in setting realistic treatment goals and expectations for pain relief and incorporate a surveillance program to monitor goal achievement and possible toxicities (Marcum et al., 2016).
- An overview of later-life pain emphasizes the importance of identifying the presence of cognitive deficits, especially in the domains of memory and language, which limits the use of self-reports for pain identification and assessment (Savvas and Gibson, 2016).
- An integrative review of studies involving the evaluation of digital health technology interventions concluded that there is limited evidence of efficacy in improving pain management with older adults using technological interventions. Such interventions

include virtual pain coaches, Internet self-care and pain report tools, digital diaries, videotaped practitioners, and communication technology. This is an area for further research (Bhattarai and Phillips, 2017).
- It is recommended to initiate opioid therapy for pain in older adults in lower doses than those used with a younger population and titrate subsequent doses slowly under supervision (Greene Naples et al., 2016).

SAFETY GUIDELINES

Pain is unique to each person, which adds to the challenges of assessing pain correctly. Research shows that cross-cultural comparisons differ in defining pain management and perceptions of successful pain control (Botti et al., 2015); therefore it is important for nurses to understand the cultural, spiritual, and religious beliefs of their patients (Burton and Shaw, 2015). Distinct cultural norms also exist for religious; lesbian, gay, bisexual, transgender (LGBT); deaf; disabled; and socioeconomic communities that influence perceptions of health care, including concepts of pain (Narayan, 2017). Safety guidelines include the following:

- Assess a patient's pain using a multidimensional assessment tool in addition to a one-dimensional pain-intensity measure (American Society of Pain Management Nursing [ASPMN], 2016; Topham and Drew, 2017).
- Nonpharmacological therapy and nonopioid pharmacological therapy are preferred for chronic pain and should only be considered if expected benefits for both pain and function are anticipated to outweigh patient risks.
- Monitor a patient's sedation level with pharmacological pain treatment using opioids. The Pasero Opioid Sedation Scale (POSS) is a superior sedation scale for the measurement of opioid sedation and is recommended for use in adult patients during opioid administration for pain management in noncritical care settings (Davis et al., 2017) (Box 15.1). Increased levels of sedation precede opioid-induced respiratory depression. Monitor patients receiving opioids very carefully.

BOX 15.1

The Pasero Opioid Sedation Scale (POSS)[a]

S = Sleep, easy to arouse
1 = Awake and alert
2 = Slightly drowsy, easily aroused
3 = Frequently drowsy, arousable, drifts off to sleep during conversation
4 = Somnolent, minimal-or-no response to physical stimulation

Remember—sedation precedes respiratory depression

[a]Many institutional sedation scales include nursing actions to be taken for each level of sedation.
From Pasero C, McCaffery M: *Pain assessment and pharmacological management*, St. Louis, 2011, Mosby.

- Assist patients receiving opioids with standing, ambulation, and transfers. With kidney and liver disease, drug absorption may be impaired, resulting in overtreatment, making patients more susceptible to falls, fractures, and delirium (Greene Naples et al., 2016).
- Monitor vital signs and assess patients for adverse effects of epidural analgesia, such as hypotension; changes in lower-extremity sensation; decreased bladder tonicity necessitating catheterization; and venous pooling, which may precipitate deep venous thrombosis (National Guideline Clearinghouse, 2016).
- Inspect infusion pumps to ensure proper functioning. Patient readiness for self-management should also be assessed (Chou et al., 2016; Institute for Safe Medication Practices, 2015).
- Know a patient's risk for injury from heat or cold applications. Certain patients are more predisposed to injury than others.
- Be aware of the impact on vital signs with heat application. Vasodilation can decrease blood pressure, causing dizziness and increasing the patient's risk for falls.
- Consider patient age, skin, vital signs, ability to communicate, and ability to sense temperature before applying hot or cold therapies.

✦ SKILL 15.1 Pain Assessment and Basic Comfort Measures

Purpose

An accurate and comprehensive pain assessment is necessary to identify the nature of a patient's pain. A thorough assessment will allow you to arrive at proper nursing diagnoses and select appropriate pain-relief therapies. Effectively managing a patient's pain does not necessarily mean eliminating it, but it is important to reduce pain to a level that is acceptable to the patient. Developing an effective plan of care for pain management requires ongoing education and evaluation of assessment skills and principles of interprofessional pain management (ANA, 2018). Incorporate appropriate pain-assessment tools that reflect your patient's understanding of pain. Nursing education and attitudes about pain management also play an important role in improving the patient experience in successful pain management (Shindul-Rothschild et al., 2017), so it is important to examine your own attitudes of pain and understand how ethnicity, cultural differences, and religious beliefs may reflect on nursing practice (ANA, 2018). Patient-centered care, involving family caregivers and use of appropriate pain-assessment tools, is essential to successful pain-management outcomes. Because pain is subjective, patient report is currently the standard for assessment. Nonverbal observations and the use of a proxy family member to help interpret a patient's behavior should be considered if a patient is unable to self-report pain.

Delegation and Collaboration

The skill of pain assessment cannot be delegated to nursing assistive personnel (NAP); however, the NAP may screen patients for pain and provide selected nonpharmacological strategies (e.g., back rubs, heat or cold application) as instructed by the nurse. The nurse directs the NAP to:

- Eliminate environmental conditions that worsen pain (e.g., an excessively warm, noisy room).
- Provide maximum rest periods for patients; a written schedule for caregivers to follow is ideal.
- Turn and place patients in a position of comfort at least every 2 hours or remind patients to turn themselves. Encourage the patient to use a pillow for splinting if needed.
- Observe for and report to the nurse behavioral signs of pain for patients who are unable to self-report.
- Report in a timely manner to the nurse any patient reports of pain intensity above the predetermined goal and nonverbal behaviors suggestive of pain.

- Screen for pain during patient transfer or other activities that might provoke pain.

Equipment

- Pain rating scales (check agency policy)

ASSESSMENT

1. Identify patient using at least two identifiers (e.g., name and birthday or name and medical record number) according to agency policy. *Rationale: Ensures correct patient. Complies with The Joint Commission standards and improves patient safety (TJC, 2019).*
2. Obtain data from patient's electronic health record: patient demographics, pain history, recent invasive procedures (e.g., tests, surgery), patient condition and co-morbidities, patient's previous response to pain medications, lab test results (e.g., kidney and liver function). *Rationale: Data identify key information to focus your pain assessment and guide safe and effective dosing of pain medication and implementation of nonpharmacological pain-management interventions (Pasero et al., 2016).*
3. Perform hand hygiene and apply gloves. Examine site of patient's pain or discomfort when possible: inspect for discoloration, swelling, or drainage; palpate for change in temperature, area of altered sensation, painful area, or areas that trigger pain; assess range of motion of involved joints. Percussion and auscultation can help to identify abnormalities (e.g., underlying mass or lung crackles) and determine cause of pain (see Chapter 8). ***When assessing abdomen, always auscultate first and then inspect and palpate.*** *Rationale: Reduces transmission of infection. Reveals nature of pain and directs you toward appropriate interventions.*
4. If patient can self-report, ask if the patient is in pain, and assess behavioral and functional impairments. Observe for nonverbal indicators of pain; ask significant others if they believe the patient is in pain (Gélinas, 2016). Pain measures must be selected according to the patient's ability to communicate. Older adults and patients from various cultures may not admit to having pain. Use other terms, such as *hurt* or *discomfort*, or use a professional interpreter if language difference exists. *Rationale: Patient's self-report of pain intensity is helpful and should be accepted from the patient, but when used as the sole assessment, it prohibits a complete pain assessment and the application of critical thinking (Pasero et al., 2016). Cross-cultural comparisons differ in defining pain management and perceptions of successful pain control (Botti et al., 2015).*
5. Assess physical, behavioral, and emotional signs and symptoms of pain. *Rationale: Signs and symptoms may reveal source and nature of pain. Nonverbal responses to pain are useful in assessing pain in patients who are cognitively impaired or unable to self-report (Gallagher et al., 2017). Experiencing pain may decrease opportunities to engage in activities, experiences, or relationships, causing a negative affect that contributes to feelings of depression, hopelessness, anger, fear, and social withdrawal (Hirsch et al., 2016).*
   a. Moaning, crying, whimpering, groaning, vocalizations
   b. Decreased activity
   c. Facial expressions (e.g., grimace, clenched teeth)
   d. Change in usual behavior (e.g., less active, irritable)
   e. Abnormal gait (e.g., shuffling) and posture (e.g., bent, leaning)
   f. Guarding a body part; functional impairment such as decreased range of motion (ROM)
   g. Diaphoresis
   h. Depression, hopelessness, anger, fear, social withdrawal
6. Assess for decreased gastrointestinal (GI) motility, constipation, nausea and vomiting. *Rationale: Constipation can occur with most pain medications; however, it is most common with opioid therapy. Opioid-induced constipation (OIC) develops when GI-tract opioid receptors are activated, resulting in decreased propulsive activity and decreased pancreatic, biliary, and gastric sections (Lacy et al., 2016).*
7. Assess for insomnia, anorexia, and fatigue. *Rationale: Co-occurrence of pain and insomnia or fatigue is common and is strongly associated with reduced functional ability (Baker et al., 2017).*
8. Assess the characteristics of pain (acute or chronic), location(s) of the pain, pain history, pain quality, pain type, pain duration (intermittent, constant, or breakthrough), and pain intensity (Gallagher et al., 2017; Pasero et al., 2016). Follow agency policy regarding frequency of assessment. Use of the PQRSTU pain assessment guides clinicians in collecting complete information about a patient's pain experience.
   a. **P**rovocative/palliative factors (e.g., "What makes your pain better or worse?"): Consider patient's experience with over-the-counter (OTC) drugs (including herbals and topicals) that have helped to reduce pain in the past. *Rationale: Identifies nature and source of pain and what patient uses to reduce discomfort.*
   b. **Q**uality: Use open-ended questions such as, "Tell me what your pain feels like." *Rationale: Helps determine underlying pain mechanism (e.g., nociceptive, inflammatory, or neuropathic pain).*
   c. **R**egion/radiation (e.g., "Show me everywhere your pain is."). Have patient use finger (if possible) to point out areas of pain. *Rationale: Identifies location of pain and possible causative factors for acute/transient pain.*
   d. **S**everity: Use valid pain rating scale appropriate to patient's age, language skills, developmental level, and comprehension (see illustrations). Pain intensity may be determined with a numerical scale, categorical scale, or pictorial scale (e.g., Numerical Rating Scale [NRS], Faces Scale, revised Face Legs Activity Cry Consolability Scale [r-FLACC], Critical Care Pain Observation Tool [CPOT]; National Comprehensive Cancer Network [NCCN], 2017). Ask patient to rate pain at rest, before any intervention, and when he or she is moving or engaged in care activity. In the case of patients with dementia or those who have no verbal skills, use observational pain-assessment scales. *Rationale: An appropriate pain-assessment tool should be multidimensional to capture the complexity of patients' pain experience. An approach to pain-intensity assessment can utilize a numerical scale; however, additional questions should assess the pain experience and how it impacts function (Topham and Drew, 2017).*
   e. **T**iming: Ask patient how long pain has been present and how often it occurs. Is it constant, intermittent, continuous, or a combination? Does pain increase during specific times of day, with particular activities, or in specific locations? *Rationale: Timing of pain may reveal if pain is acute or chronic and source of pain.*
   f. How is pain affecting **U** (patient) regarding activities of daily living (ADLs), work, relationships, and enjoyment of life? *Rationale: Provides baseline information to later gauge effectiveness of interventions.*

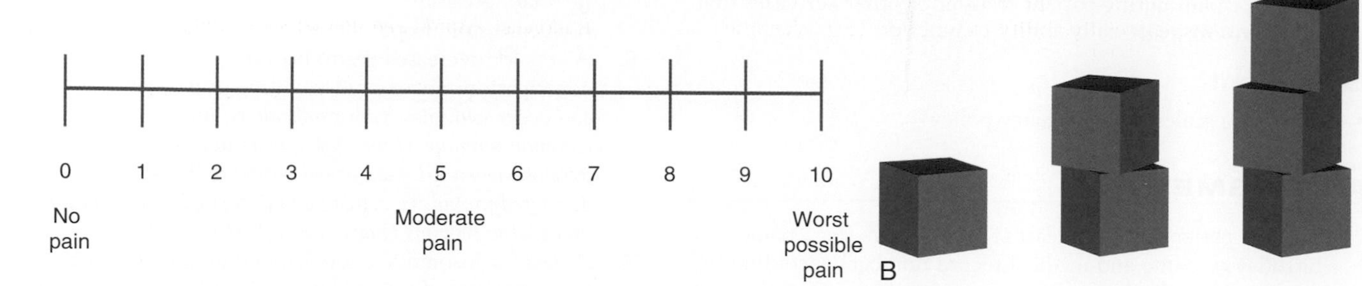

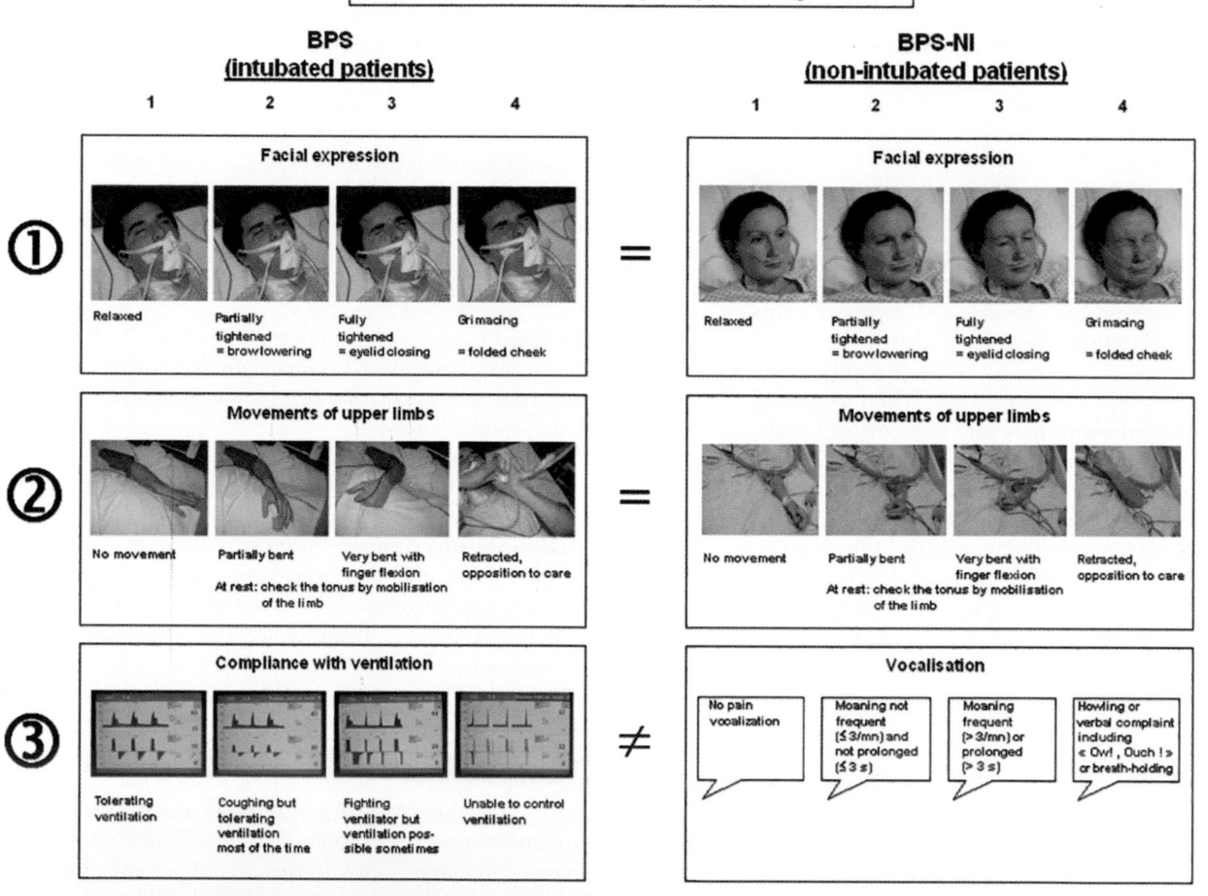

①+②+③ = Total BPS value

C **from 3 (no) to 12 (maximum) pain behavior rated using the BPS**

STEP 8d (A) Pain rating scale. (B) Simplified Concrete Ordinal Scale, S-COS. (C) Behavioral Pain Scale (BPS). [*(A) From McCaffery M, Pasero C: Pain: clinical manual, ed 2, St Louis, 1999, Mosby. (B) From Emmott A et al: Validity of simplified versus standard self-report measures of pain intensity in preschool-aged children undergoing venipuncture,* J Pain *18(5):564, 2017. [C] From Rijkenberg S et al: Pain measurement in mechanically ventilated critically ill patients: behavioral pain scale versus critical-care pain observation tool,* J Crit Care *30(1):167, 2015.)*

9. Assess patient's response to previous pharmacological interventions, especially ability to function (e.g., sleeping, eating, and other ADLs). Determine if any analgesic side effects are likely based on medication and patient's previous responses (e.g., itching or nausea). *Rationale: Determines extent to which therapies have or have not been successful in the past (Pasero et al., 2016). Some side effects, especially itching that can occur with morphine, are often poorly tolerated by the patient and indicate the need to identify another analgesic.*
10. Assess for allergies to medications, with focus on analgesics. *Rationale: Aspirin and nonsteroidal antiinflammatory drugs (NSAIDs) are associated with a wide variety of hypersensitivity reactions (Laidlaw and Cahill, 2017).*
11. Assess patient's and/or family caregiver's knowledge, experience, and health literacy level. *Rationale: Ensures patient has the capacity to obtain, communicate, process, and understand basic health information (Centers for Disease Control and Prevention [CDC], 2016).*

STEP	RATIONALE
PLANNING	
1. Expected outcomes following completion of procedure:	
• Patient verbalizes full or partial relief from pain.	Due to the subjective nature of pain, patient self-report is the most reliable indicator of pain (Pasero et al., 2016).
• Patient displays nonverbal behaviors such as relaxed face and absence of squinting.	When self-report is not possible, validated behavioral pain scales should be used (Gélinas, 2016).
• Patient reports improvement in sleep, nutritional intake, physical activity, and personal relationships.	Adequate pain relief usually permits patient to participate in usual ADLs.
2. Set pain-intensity goal with patient (when able).	Pain is unique to each person and therefore helps the patient set individual goal for tolerable pain severity (ANA, 2018).
3. Provide privacy.	Privacy during conversation and pain-relief measures may enhance pain relief.
4. Prepare patient's environment.	Preparing the environment ensures a clutter-free environment and an organized procedure.
• Temperature suited to patient	Temperature and sound extremes can enhance patient's perception of pain.
• Sound	Loud or sudden noises may contribute to anxiety and exacerbate pain.
• Lighting	Bright or very dim lighting can aggravate pain sensation.
• Eliminate unnecessary interruptions and coordinate care activities; allow for rest.	Fatigue increases pain perception.
5. Explain procedures to be used for pain relief.	Ensures patient understanding.
6. Provide educational materials to patient and family caregiver.	Pain-assessment and pain-relief measures may be needed at home. Education will improve patient and caregiver adherence.
IMPLEMENTATION	
1. Perform hand hygiene and apply clean gloves (if indicated).	Reduces transmission of microorganisms.
2. Teach patient how to use pain rating scale. Explain range of intensity scores and how they relate to measuring pain.	Accurate reporting by patient or family caregiver improves ongoing pain assessment, treatment, and evaluation.
3. Prepare and administer appropriate pain-relieving medications (nonopioids, opioids, co-analgesic or multimodal combination) per health care provider's order (see Chapter 22). Choice of medication depends on patient's condition. For example, postoperative pain is often treated initially with opioids or intravenous acetaminophen, which provides effective nonopioid analgesia for postoperative patients.	Nonopioids are effective for mild to moderate pain. Patients with chronic pain are typically prescribed multimodal therapy (more than one type of analgesic) for pain relief.

STEP	RATIONALE
4. Remove or reduce painful stimuli.	Reduction of pain stimuli and pressure receptors maximizes responses to pain-relieving interventions.
a. Help patient turn and reposition to comfortable position in good body alignment.	Reduces stress on musculoskeletal system.
b. Smooth wrinkles in bed linens.	Reduces pressure and irritation to skin.
c. Loosen constrictive bandages (if appropriate to purpose of bandage) or loosen or remove devices (e.g., blood pressure cuff, elastic hose, or sequential stockings).	Bandage or device encircling extremity can restrict circulation and cause pain (see Chapter 27).
d. Reposition underlying tubes or equipment.	Removes pressure on skin.
e. Use pillows as needed for alignment and positioning support (see illustration)	Helps maintain position that reduces strain on muscles and pressure areas.
5. Teach patient how to splint over painful site using either a pillow or hand.	Splinting reduces pain by minimizing muscle movement at time of stress (e.g., coughing).
a. Explain purpose of splinting.	Promotes patient's cooperation.
b. Place pillow or blanket over site of discomfort and help patient place hands firmly over area of discomfort (see illustration)	Splinting immobilizes painful area.
c. Have patient hold area firmly while coughing, deep breathing, and turning.	Splinting decreases movement and subsequent pain during activity.
6. Reduce or eliminate emotional factors that increase pain experiences (see Skill 15.2). Use biopsychosocial treatments: cognitive-behavioral and/or behavioral therapies.	A variety of mind–body techniques, such as relaxation, guided imagery, and meditation, enhance the mind's ability to lessen pain symptoms (Houzé et al., 2017).
a. Offer information that reduces anxiety (e.g., explaining cause of pain if known).	Increased anxiety has been associated with increased report of chronic pain severity (Curtin and Norris, 2017).
b. Offer patient opportunity to pray (if appropriate).	Serves as form of distraction.
c. Spend time to allow patient to talk about pain and answer questions. Listen attentively.	Conveys a sense of caring and interest in patient's welfare.
7. Before leaving, make sure patient is in a comfortable position.	Positioning is a nonpharmacological intervention for pain relief.
8. Raise side rails (as appropriate) and lower bed to lowest position.	Patient safety measure. However, side rails cannot be used as a restraint.
9. If used, remove and dispose of gloves. Perform hand hygiene.	Reduces transmission of microorganisms.
10. Be sure nurse call system is accessible within patient's reach. Instruct patient in its use.	Patient safety measure.

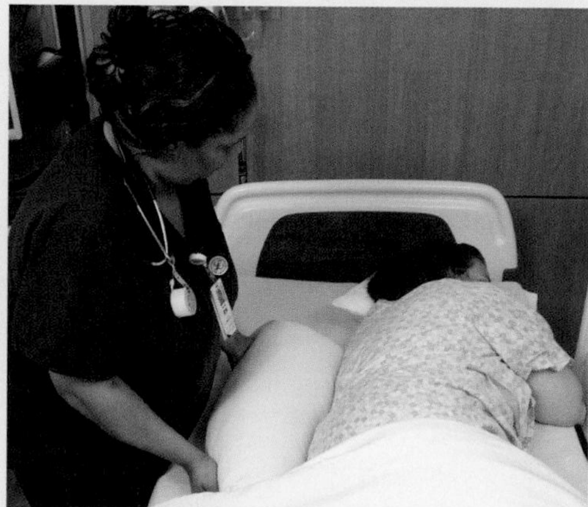

STEP 4e Positioning patient in side-lying lateral position for comfort.

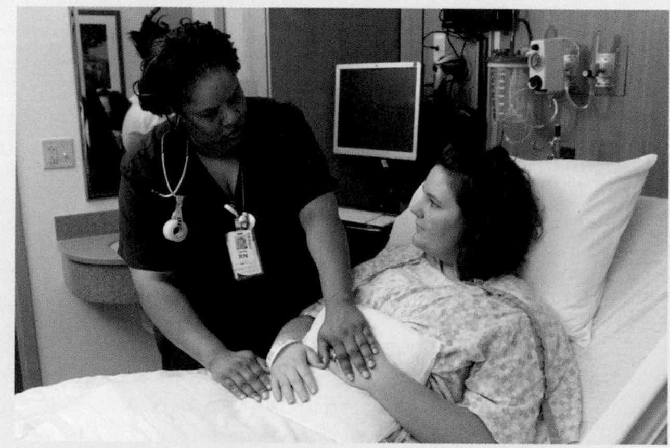

STEP 5b Patient shown how to splint painful area.

STEP	RATIONALE
EVALUATION	
1. Based on agency reassessment criteria (e.g., 30–60 minutes after intervention), reassess patient's pain after nonpharmacological and pharmacological interventions (e.g., repositioning or after a medication reaches its peak effect), using a pain-intensity scale (TJC, 2017).	Evaluates effectiveness of pain-relieving interventions in timely manner (Pasero et al., 2016).
2. Compare patient's current pain with personally set pain-intensity goal.	Helps determine appropriate changes to pain-management plan. Makes patient active participant in care.
3. Compare patient's ability to function and perform ADLs before and after pain interventions. Initiate a nurse–patient dialogue about the effect of pain-relieving interventions on function and ability to perform ADLs.	Pain-intensity ratings aren't necessarily a reflection of pain relief for chronic pain because it is not primarily nociceptive; therefore pre-intervention and postintervention assessment of function should be incorporated to determine effectiveness (Ballantyne and Sullivan, 2015; Chou et al., 2016).
4. Observe patient's nonverbal behaviors. Implement validated observational pain-assessment tool with patients who are unable to self-report (patients who are critically ill and/or intubated, cognitively impaired, or sedated).	Determines effectiveness of pain-relieving interventions and improves pain assessment and management (Varndell et al., 2017).
5. Evaluate for analgesic side effects.	Side effects of analgesics may be controlled by reducing dose, increasing time intervals, or administering other medications.
6. **Use Teach-Back:** "We discussed how splinting, turning on your nonsurgical side, and relaxation can relieve pain. Explain to me when you can use these approaches at home." Revise your instruction now or develop a plan for revised patient/family caregiver teaching if patient/family caregiver is not able to teach back correctly.	Determines patient's/family caregiver's level of understanding of instructional topic.

Unexpected Outcomes	Related Interventions
1. Patient verbalizes continued pain that exceeds pain-intensity goal or displays nonverbal behavior reflecting worsening pain.	• Repeat complete pain assessment. • Implement different nonpharmacological pain-relief measures. • Ask patient and family caregivers which alternatives might be helpful. • Notify health care provider.
2. Patient experiences unexpected or adverse reaction to medication.	• Assess unexpected effects on patient. • Notify health care provider immediately. • Be prepared to administer antidote if indicated (e.g., antiemetic, antihistamine, opioid-reversing agent such as naloxone). • Monitor for effectiveness of antidote; antidote may have shorter half-life than opioid; repeat dose of antidote may be needed. • Complete adverse reaction documentation according to agency policy.

Recording

- Record character of pain before an intervention, the pain-relief therapies used, whether pain relief is achieved, any patient or family education provided, and patient response to interventions
- Document your evaluation of patient learning.

Hand-Off Reporting

- Report inadequate pain relief (not reaching goal), a reduction in patient function, and side effects and adverse effects of both pharmacological and nonpharmacological pain interventions.

✦ SKILL 15.2 Nonpharmacological Pain Management

Purpose

Developing and improving complementary health and integrative treatment strategies for hard-to-manage symptoms such as pain, anxiety, and depression were established as a 2016 strategic plan objective by the National Center for Complementary and Integrative Health (NCCIH, 2016). Whereas complementary therapies are used with Western medicine, alternative therapies are also used in place of Western medicine practices. Mind and body practices (e.g., biofeedback, hypnosis, meditation, music therapy, relaxation techniques) as well as other complementary approaches using acupuncture, massage therapy, deep breathing, and distraction are recommended as nonpharmacological interventions in multimodal approaches to pain management (Chou et al., 2016; Houzé et al., 2017).

Research has established the clinical utility of acupuncture for chronic pain and depression (MacPherson et al., 2017). Massage therapy has been shown to reduce stress and anxiety, leading to decreases in sympathetic activity and increases in parasympathetic activity and subsequent pain reduction (Nelson and Churilla, 2017). A person's full participation and cooperation are necessary for relaxation techniques to be effective. Relaxation and guided imagery provide patients with self-control when pain occurs. Nonpharmacological techniques may diminish the physical effects of pain, alter a patient's perception of pain, and provide a patient with a greater sense of control (Box 15.2).

Delegation and Collaboration

Assessment of a patient's pain cannot be delegated to nursing assistive personnel (NAP). The skill of nonpharmacological pain-management strategies can be delegated to NAP. The nurse directs the NAP by:

- Identifying and explaining which nonpharmacological measures work best for a patient.
- Explaining how to adapt strategies to patient restrictions (e.g., massage in side-lying versus prone position).
- Instructing to report worsening of a patient's pain.

BOX 15.2

Nonpharmacological Measures for Pain[a]

Relaxation and the Power of the Mind
- Progressive muscle relaxation
- Breathing exercises
- Music relaxation
- Visual imagery
- Yoga

Put Your Body to Work
- Exercise
- Pacing
- Conserving energy
- Body mechanics

Spirituality and Reflection
- Engaging in religious practices
- Humor
- Setting aside time to focus on what *is*
- Talking about your stress with others
- Journaling
- Praying

What to Do When Pain Flares
- Cold and hot therapies
- Hand and foot massage
- Herbals[b]

[a]Should be used along with analgesia medications.
[b]Herbals could interact with prescribed analgesics; check with health care provider.

Equipment

- Pain rating scales
- *Distraction:* Patient's (all ages) preference (e.g., reading material, video game, puzzles, music, 3D immersions such as virtual reality, Google Cardboard, smartphone applications).
- *Relaxation*: Patient's music preference for relaxation
- *Massage*: Lotion or oil (consider lavender aromatherapy lotion [non–alcohol-based], sheet, bath towel

ASSESSMENT

1. Identify patient using at least two identifiers (e.g., name and birthday or name and medical record number) according to agency policy. *Rationale: Ensures correct patient. Complies with The Joint Commission standards and improves patient safety (TJC, 2019).*
2. Perform hand hygiene. Perform complete pain assessment (Steps 2–9 in Skill 15.1). *Rationale: Reduces transmission of microorganisms. A complete pain assessment guides safe and effective dosing of pain medication and implementation of nonpharmacological pain-management interventions (Pasero et al., 2016).*
3. Assess patient's language level and values he or she has regarding alternative pain-relief approaches. Identify descriptive terms that you will use when guiding patient through relaxation or guided imagery. *Rationale: Ensures that care is culturally appropriate. Establishes connection with patient to enhance your ability to guide relaxation.*
4. Assess character of patient's respirations. *Rationale: Establishes baseline. Relaxation techniques focus on breathing.*
5. Review health care provider's orders for pain relief (if required by agency). *Rationale: In some acute care settings, a medical order is necessary to perform nonpharmacological therapies.*
6. Assess patient's understanding of pain and willingness to receive nonpharmacological pain-relief measures. *Rationale: Participation increases effectiveness of pain-relief measure. If patient is reluctant to try activity, provide information about suggested therapy.*
7. Assess preferred patient activities (e.g., puzzles, crocheting, game on electronic device, board games, music, or relaxation tape). *Rationale: Improves likelihood of distraction being effective.*
8. Assess type of image patient would prefer to use in guided imagery (e.g., nature scene, interaction with friends, joyful moment). *Rationale: Prevents use of image that could frighten patient.*
9. Review any restrictions in patient's mobility or positioning. *Rationale: Determines whether massage is appropriate and position to have patient assume.*
10. Assess patient's and/or family caregiver's knowledge, experience, and health literacy level. *Rationale: Ensures patient has the capacity to obtain, communicate, process, and understand basic health information (CDC, 2016).*

STEP	RATIONALE
PLANNING	
1. Expected outcomes following completion of procedures:	
• Patient demonstrates and describes pain-relief measures.	Demonstrates patient understanding and learning.
• Patient is relaxed and comfortable after technique as evidenced by slow, deep respirations; calm facial expressions; calm tone of voice; relaxed muscles; relaxed posture.	Nonpharmacological strategies help patient relax and experience less discomfort. Physiological response to relaxation procedures and massage is deep relaxation. The use of complementary and alternative medicine therapies (CAM) may also be added to the patient's pain-management plan of care (NCCIH, 2016).
• Patient reports pain relief on an intensity and behavioral scale.	Patient's subjective report is most reliable indicator of presence of pain.
2. Provide privacy.	Promotes patient's ability to relax.
3. Set up equipment.	Maintains organization.
4. Explain purpose of technique and what you expect of patient during activity. Explain how to use pain rating scale (see Skill 15.1).	Proper explanation of activity enhances patient participation. Accurate reporting of pain by patient improves your evaluation and treatment.
5. Set mutual pain-intensity goal with patient (when able) for rest and during routine care activities.	Patient sets individual goal for tolerable pain severity.
6. Plan time to perform technique when patient can concentrate (e.g., after voiding, awakening from nap).	Increases opportunity for success.
7. Administer an analgesic 30 minutes before implementing a nonpharmacological therapy.	Patient is able to gain a level of comfort needed to perform nonpharmacological therapies.
8. Position the patient and drape if needed.	Promotes comfort.
IMPLEMENTATION	
1. Perform hand hygiene and prepare patient's environment. Make temperature suited to patient. Control level of sound and lighting. Minimize interruptions and coordinate care activities; allow time for rest.	Reduces transmission of microorganisms. Temperature and sound extremes can enhance patient's perception of pain. Bright or very dim lighting can aggravate pain sensation. Fatigue increases pain perception.
2. **Massage:**	
Safe Patient Care *Massage is contraindicated in cases of muscle, bone, or joint injury and bruised, swollen, or inflamed areas.*	
a. Place patient in comfortable position such as prone or side lying. Have patients with difficulty breathing lie on side of bed with head of bed elevated.	Positioning enhances relaxation and exposes areas to be massaged.
b. Adjust bed to comfortable position for you; lower upper side rail on side where you are standing. Drape patient to expose only area that you will massage.	Ensures proper body mechanics and prevents strain on back.
c. Turn on music to patient's preference.	Promotes relaxation.
d. Ensure that patient is not allergic to lotion; warm lotion in hands or in basin of warm water. **NOTE:** If you massage head and scalp, delay use of lotion until completed.	Warm lotion is soothing, and warmth helps produce local muscle relaxation.

STEP	RATIONALE
e. Choose stroke technique based on desired effect or body part.	Ensures fuller relaxation of body part.

Safe Patient Care *Use very gentle massage with patients who are unable to communicate and monitor nonverbal behavior because they cannot tell you if massage becomes uncomfortable.*

STEP	RATIONALE
(1) Effleurage: massaging upward and outward from vertebral column and back again (see illustration)	Light, gliding stroke used without manipulating deep muscles smooths and extends muscles, increases nutrient absorption, and improves lymphatic and venous circulation.
(2) Pétrissage (see illustration)	Kneading tense muscle groups promotes relaxation and stimulates local circulation.
(3) Friction	Strong circular strokes bring blood to surface of skin, increasing local circulation and loosening tight muscle groups.
f. Encourage patient to breathe deeply and relax during massage.	Potentiates effects of massage.
g. Standing behind patient, stimulate scalp and temples.	Position of patient and care provider potentiates effectiveness of massage and facilitates proper body mechanics.
h. Supporting patient's head, use friction to rub muscles at base of head.	Strong circular strokes (friction) stimulate local circulation and relaxation.
i. Reposition if needed. With patient in supine position, massage hands and arms as appropriate.	Hand massage therapy has been reported to contribute to some pain relief in the intensive care unit (ICU) after cardiac surgery, specifically with decreases in muscle tension and pain-intensity levels (Boitor et al., 2015).
(1) Support hand and apply friction to palm using both thumbs.	
(2) Support base of finger and work each finger in corkscrew-like motion.	
(3) Complete hand massage using effleurage strokes from fingertips to wrist.	
(4) Knead muscles of forearm and upper arm between thumb and forefinger.	Encourages relaxation; enhances circulation and venous return.
j. After determining that patient has no neck injury or condition that contraindicates neck manipulation, massage neck as appropriate:	Massage may be contraindicated after spinal cord injuries or surgery to head and neck because of risk for further injury.
(1) Place patient prone unless contraindicated.	Provides access to neck muscles.
(2) Knead each neck muscle between thumb and forefinger.	Reduces tension that often localizes in neck muscles.
(3) Gently stretch neck by placing one hand on top of shoulders and other at base of head. Gently move hands away from one another.	Helps relax muscle body.

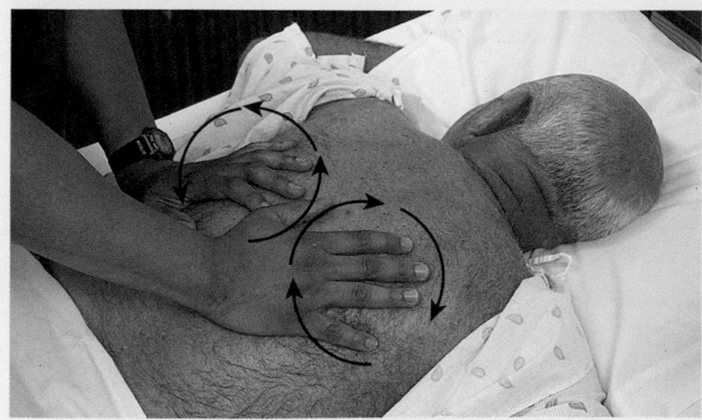

STEP 2e(1) Effleurage.

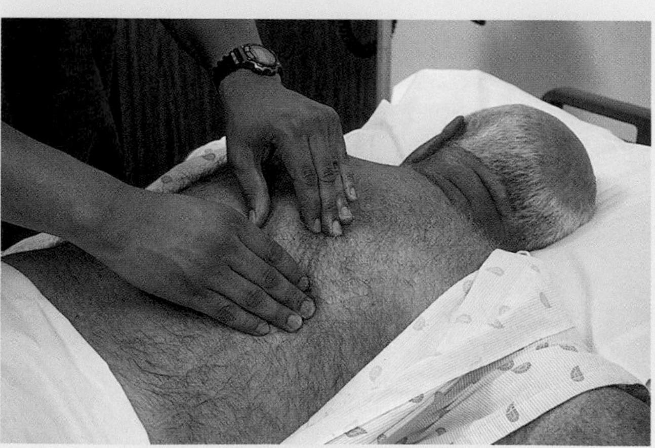

STEP 2e(2) Pétrissage.

STEP	RATIONALE
k. Massage back as appropriate:	Patient with back injury, surgery, or epidural infusion should not receive back massage.
(1) Assist patient to prone position unless contraindicated; side-lying position is option.	Provides access to muscle groups in back.
(2) Do not allow hands to leave patient's skin.	Continuous contact with surface of skin is soothing and stimulates circulation to tissues. Breaking contact with skin can startle patient.
(3) Apply hands first to sacral area; massage in circular motion. Stroke upward from buttocks to shoulders. Massage over scapulae with smooth, firm stroke. Continue in one smooth stroke to upper arms and laterally along sides of back down to iliac crest (see illustration). Continue massage pattern for 3 minutes.	General, firm pressure applied to all muscle groups promotes relaxation.

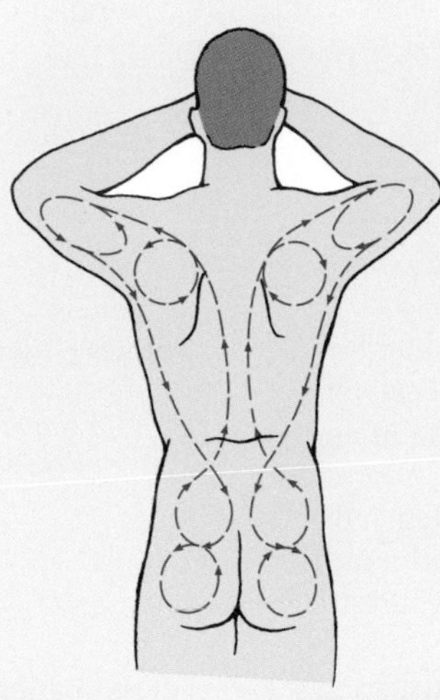

STEP 2k(3) Circular massage of the back.

STEP	RATIONALE
(4) Use effleurage along muscles of spine in upward and outward motion.	Massage follows distribution of major muscle groups.
(5) Use pétrissage on muscles of each shoulder toward front of patient.	Area often tightens because of tension.
(6) Use palms in upward and outward circular motion from lower buttocks to neck.	Brings blood to surface of skin.
(7) Knead muscles of upper back and shoulder between thumb and forefinger.	These muscles are thick and can be massaged vigorously.
(8) Use both hands to knead muscles up one side of back and then the other.	
(9) End massage with long, stroking effleurage movements.	Most soothing of massage movements.
l. Massage feet as appropriate:	
(1) Place patient in supine position.	Returns patient to comfortable anatomical position.
(2) Hold foot firmly. Support ankle with one hand or support sides of foot with each hand while performing massage.	Maintains joint stability during massage (Hatcher, 2017).
(3) Make circular motions with thumb and fingers around bones of ankle and top of foot.	All massage strokes help to relax muscles.
(4) Trace space between tendons with firm finger pressure, moving from toe to ankle.	
(5) Massage sides and top of each toe.	
(6) Use top of fist to make circular motions on bottom of foot.	
(7) Knead sides of foot between index finger and thumb.	
(8) Conclude with firm, sweeping motions over top and bottom of foot.	Too light strokes may tickle.

STEP	RATIONALE
m. Tell patient that you are ending massage.	Informs and prepares patient to inhale and exhale deeply.
n. When procedure is complete, instruct patient to inhale deeply and exhale. Caution him or her to move slowly after resting a few minutes.	Returns patient to more awake and alert state. When deeply relaxed, patient may experience dizziness on arising too rapidly and need time for vessels to redistribute blood supply.
o. Wipe excess lotion or oil from patient's body with bath towel.	Excess lotion or oil can irritate skin and lead to breakdown.
3. Progressive relaxation with deep breathing:	
a. Have patient assume comfortable sitting position: sit with feet uncrossed or lie in supine position with small pillow under head.	Maximizes ability to relax.
b. Instruct patient to take several slow, deep, diaphragmatic breaths. It may help to have patient close his or her eyes.	Increased oxygen lessens anxiety and prevents shortness of breath with relaxation breathing technique. Avoids hyperventilation. Eye closure maintains patient focus on exercise.
c. Explain as follows: "The air coming in through your nose should move downward into your lower belly. Let your belly expand fully. Now breathe out through your mouth (or your nose, if that feels more natural). Alternate normal and deep breaths several times. Pay attention to how you feel when you breathe in and breathe out normally and when you breathe deeply. Shallow breathing feels tense and constricted, while deep breathing helps you relax."	Patient able to focus on exercise with your coaching. Becoming mindful of how body feels can enhance relaxation.
d. Continue the exercise: "To practice, put one hand on your abdomen, just below your belly button. Feel your hand rise about an inch each time you breathe in and fall about an inch each time you breathe out. Your chest will rise slightly, too, along with your belly. Remember to relax your belly so that each time you breathe in, it expands fully. As you breathe out slowly, let yourself sigh out loud."	Allows patient to master slow deep breathing.
e. Observe patient and caution against hyperventilation.	Causes patient to eliminate more carbon dioxide than is produced and consequently results in respiratory alkalosis and an elevated blood pH. Patient becomes dizzy and light-headed.
f. Coach patient to locate any area of muscle tension and alternate tightening and relaxing all muscle groups for 6 to 7 seconds, beginning at feet and working upward toward head.	Relaxation is an integrated response associated with diminished sympathetic nervous system arousal; decreased muscle tension is desired outcome.
(1) Instruct patient to tighten muscles during inhalation and relax muscles during exhalation.	Deep breathing has been reported to reduce resting systolic and pulse pressures in older patients with systolic hypertension (Sangthong et al., 2016) and reduce stress through relaxation (Perciavalle et al., 2017).
(2) As each muscle group relaxes, ask patient to enjoy relaxed feeling and allow mind to drift and think how nice it is to be relaxed. Have patient breathe deeply.	Allows opportunity to enjoy feelings of relaxation.
(3) Calmly explain during exercise that patient may feel sensations of tingling, heaviness, floating, or warmth as relaxation occurs.	Prevents anxiety if sensation occurs without warning.
(4) Have patient continue slow, deep breaths throughout exercise.	
(5) When finished, have patient inhale deeply, exhale, and then initially move about slowly after resting a few minutes.	Returns patient to more awake and alert state. Rising too rapidly can cause dizziness.
4. Guided imagery:	
a. Direct patient through guided imagery exercise while having him or her focus on an image. Example is as follows:	
(1) Instruct patient to imagine that inhaled air is ball of healing energy.	Developing specific images helps remove pain perception.
(2) Imagine that inhaled air travels to area of pain.	Patient's ability to concentrate decreases pain perception.

STEP	RATIONALE
b. Alternatively, you may direct imagery:	
(1) Ask patient to imagine a pleasant place such as beach or mountains. Give examples, but make sure that it is an image and experience that the patient chooses.	Directs imagery after selection of restful place.
(2) Direct patient to experience all sensory aspects of restful place (e.g., for beach: warm breeze, warm sand between toes, warmth of sunshine, rhythmic sound of waves, smell of salt air, gulls gliding and swooping in air).	Helps patient concentrate and relax through stimulation of numerous senses to achieve clinical outcomes of interest (e.g., decrease in pain, anxiety, and stress; Patricolo et al., 2017).
(3) Direct patient to continue deep, slow, rhythmic breathing.	Promotes relaxation through muscle relaxation.
(4) Direct patient to count to three, inhale, and open eyes. Suggest that patient move about slowly initially.	Slowly resuming movement and upright positioning is recommended due to state of relaxation and possible orthostatic changes in blood pressure.
(5) Provide patient time to practice exercise without interruption. Practice relaxation tapes are available almost everywhere; libraries are an excellent source.	Guided imagery requires an intense level of concentration that takes time to achieve.
5. **Distraction:**	
a. Direct patient's attention away from pain by involving him or her in a distraction technique.	Redirection of attention with music therapy has been reported to have a positive effect on pain and anxiety reduction (Li et al., 2017).
b. Music: play selection for approximately 30 minutes in location where patient is comfortable. Set volume or loudness at comfortable level. Use music of patient's choosing. Emphasize listening to rhythm and adjust volume as pain increases or decreases.	A mindfulness-based music therapy intervention has been reported to significantly reduce states of tension, depression, anger, fatigue, and confusion (Lesiuk, 2015).
c. Direct patient to give detailed account of an event or story; describe pleasant memories.	Stress details of event to enhance distraction from painful stimulus.
d. Provide activity (e.g., puzzle, music, virtual reality headset program, video game, reading material) at time when patient is relaxed.	Engagement in activity requires level of comfort for participation.
e. Engage patient in meaningful conversation; encourage participation of family members and visitors.	Visitors can help direct attention away from mild-to-moderate pain. Rarely is someone in severe pain able to use distraction.
6. Return bed to low position and raise side rails (as appropriate) when procedure is finished.	Patient safety measure; however, side rails cannot be used as a restraint.
7. Appropriately dispose of supplies and equipment. Remove and dispose of gloves and perform hand hygiene.	Reduces transmission of microorganisms.
8. Place nurse call system within patient's reach and instruct on its use.	Patient safety measure.

EVALUATION

1. Observe character of respirations, body position, facial expression, tone of voice, mood, mannerisms, and verbalization of discomfort.	Determines effectiveness of procedure, level of relaxation, degree of pain relief achieved, and which procedures were most effective.
2. Ask patient to use pain rating scale to rate comfort level; compare with patient's goal.	Measures change in pain intensity.
3. Observe patient perform pain-control measures.	Confirms learning.
4. **Use Teach-Back:** "I want to be sure I explained some techniques for reducing pain without using medication. Tell me what technique you might want to try." Revise your instruction now or develop a plan for revised patient/family caregiver teaching if patient/family caregiver is not able to teach back correctly.	Determines patient's/family caregiver's level of understanding of instructional topic.

Unexpected Outcome	Related Interventions
1. Patient is not able to concentrate on technique because pain intensity is unchanged or escalating or demonstrates nonverbal behaviors indicative of pain.	• Evaluate character of pain and determine if further analgesia is necessary. • Ensure that environment is conducive to learning and using technique. • Consult with health care provider on increase in dose or alternate medication. • Consider different technique or combination of complementary strategies.

Recording

- Record patient's assessment findings, procedure and technique(s) used, preparation given to patient, patient's response to procedure or technique, change in overall condition, and further comfort needs related to event. Incorporate pain-relief technique into nursing care plan.
- Document your evaluation of patient or family caregiver learning.

Hand-Off Reporting

- Report any unusual responses to techniques (e.g., uncontrolled or aggravated pain or muscle spasms) to nurse in charge or health care provider.
- Report inadequate pain relief (not reaching goal), a reduction in patient function, and side effects or adverse effects from pain interventions to health care provider.
- Report patient's response to nonpharmacological interventions to the staff at change of shift and in care planning meetings.

✦ SKILL 15.3 Pharmacological Pain Management

Purpose

Analgesics are the most common and effective method of pain relief. However, suboptimal pain management often results due to inadequate pain assessment. Health care providers often do not assess pain thoroughly, may access incorrect drug information, and have unjustified concerns about patient addiction. A good assessment requires nursing judgment, critical thinking attitudes, and knowledge of transcultural implications for pain treatment (Drake and Williams, 2017). Undertreatment often occurs in critically ill patients, who may be on ventilators and thus are unable to verbally self-report pain-related symptoms, creating uncertainty with nurses regarding effective pain management (Rababa, 2017).

Older patients who suffer from cognitive impairment or dementia may also have difficulty communicating pain-related symptoms. In addition, many older patients take multiple medications for other co-morbidities, such as cognitive impairment, mobility disorders, diabetes, and cardiovascular disease. This is called *polypharmacy*, and it may contribute to adverse drug-drug interactions (Pasero et al., 2016).

Knowledge of pain and assessment skills are also important in the pediatric population and in patients who experience acute and chronic pain from both noncancer illness and cancer. Nursing judgment is critical to the safe use and management of analgesics for all patients to ensure the best approach for pain management.

Opioids

The growing and unprecedented opioid epidemic in the United States was estimated to have claimed nearly 65,000 American deaths due to drug overdose in 2016, a 21% increase from 2015 (National Academy of Medicine, 2017). The U.S. Department of Health and Human Services (USDHHS, 2017) has targeted three priority initiatives: improving prescribing practices, expanding access to and the use of medication-assisted treatment, and expanding the use of naloxone. Nearly half of opioid overdose deaths are related to legally obtained opioid prescriptions, and although the number of prescriptions has decreased since 2015, health care providers need to **carefully assess for risks for addiction and dependency before prescribing opioids and use multimodal approaches to managing pain** (Fitzgerald, 2017). **It is essential that nurses help educate patients regarding safe use of opioids.**

Patients who receive opioids for chronic pain often require higher doses of analgesics to alleviate new or increased pain; this is tolerance, not an early sign of addiction (Box 15.3). The use of opioids in the perioperative period has increased; therefore opioid-associated morbidity and mortality have increased as well (Nagappa et al., 2017). Nurses must know the signs and symptoms of opioid addiction, as well as the association between opioids and respiratory depression. Sleep-disordered breathing should be assessed as a risk factor for respiratory depression when administering opioids (Nagappa et al., 2017). Assessment and nursing knowledge of interventions in pain management, including the use of opioid-reversing agents (naloxone), are crucial in preventing and acting quickly in life-threatening situations.

Delegation and Collaboration

The skill of analgesic administration cannot be delegated to nursing assistive personnel (NAP). The nurse instructs the NAP by:

- Explaining the behaviors and physical changes associated with pain and to report their occurrence immediately.
- Reviewing comfort measures to use to support pain relief.

BOX 15.3

Terminology Related to the Use of Opioids in Pain Treatment

The American Society for Pain Management Nursing (ASPMN) has released a formal position statement: every patient with pain, including those with substance-use disorders, has the right to be treated with dignity and respect and be provided high-quality pain assessment and management. Failure to identify and treat the concurrent conditions of pain and substance-use disorders will compromise the ability to treat either condition effectively (Oliver et al., 2012). Common conditions involving the use of opioids in pain treatment include the following:

Physical dependence: A state of adaptation that is manifested by a drug class–specific withdrawal syndrome produced by abrupt cessation, rapid dose reduction, decreasing the blood level of an opioid, and/or administration of a drug that can act as an antagonist.

Addiction: A primary, chronic, neurobiological disease with genetic, psychosocial, and environmental factors influencing its development and manifestations. Addictive behaviors include one or more of the following: impaired control over drug use, compulsive use, continued use despite harm, and craving.

Drug tolerance: A state of adaptation in which exposure to a drug induces changes that result in a diminution of one or more of the effects of the drug over time.

Approved by the Boards of Directors of the American Academy of Pain Medicine, The American Pain Society, and American Society of Addiction Medicine, February 2011, American Pain Society, 2011.

Equipment

- Prescribed medication
- Pain scales (numerical or visual and behavioral)
- Necessary medication administration device (see Chapters 22 and 23)
- Medication administration record (MAR) or computer printout
- Controlled substance record (for opioids only)
- Clean gloves (optional depending on dose form of medication administered)
- Stethoscope, sphygmomanometer, pulse oximeter

ASSESSMENT

1. Check accuracy and completeness of each MAR or computer printout with health care provider's written medication order. Check patient's name, medication name and dosage, route of administration, and method of delivery (e.g., bolus). Recopy or reprint any portion of MAR that is difficult to read. *Rationale: The order sheet is the most reliable source and only record of medications that patient is to receive. Ensures that patient receives the correct medications (Mandrack et al., 2012). Illegible MARs are a source of medication errors.*
2. Assess patient's medical and medication history, including history of allergies. *Rationale: Determines need for medication or possible contraindications for medication administration. Screens patient for risk for allergic reaction.*
3. Perform hand hygiene and complete a pain assessment (see Skill 15.1, Steps 2–9), including patient's previous response to ordered analgesic. *Rationale: Provides baseline for type and nature of pain condition to determine efficacy of analgesic. Assists in selection of type of analgesic to administer and assists in choosing amount of medication to give within a range order.*
4. Assess the anticipated time of onset, time to peak effect, duration of action, and side effects of the analgesic to be administered (review pharmacology reference). For example, intravenous (IV) medications act quickly and can relieve severe acute pain within 1 hour; oral extended-release preparations may take 2 hours to be effective. *Rationale: Allows for planning pain-relief measures with patient activities, anticipating peak and duration of analgesic, and evaluating effectiveness of analgesic.*
5. Consider the type of activities patient is scheduled to undergo (e.g., rehabilitation, scheduled tests, ambulation). *Rationale: Allows you to time administration of analgesic early enough to gain maximal pain relief during the time of the activity.*
6. Check last time medication was administered (including dose and route) and degree of relief experienced. Verify the appropriateness of the dose and the dosing interval for the current situation. Consult with health care provider about an around-the-clock (ATC) dose. ATC administration with multimodal use of pain medications (opioids and nonopioids) should be incorporated into the pain-management nursing care plan (Chou et al., 2016; Coluzzi et al., 2017). *Rationale: Determines if next dose can be administered and whether dose adjustment is necessary. ATC maintains medication at therapeutic blood level.*
7. Assess patient's risk for using nonsteroidal antiinflammatory drugs (NSAIDs; e.g., history of gastrointestinal [GI] bleeding or renal insufficiency) or opioids (e.g., history of obstructive or central sleep apnea). *Rationale: Presence of risk factors contraindicates NSAID use.*
8. Know the comparative potencies of analgesics in oral and injectable form. Refer to an equianalgesic chart (ClinCalc .com, 2018) or pharmacist. *Rationale: If nurses on succeeding shifts choose different routes for the same doses, a patient will not receive the same level of pain control.*
9. Talk with patient and determine an individualized pain-management strategy that is agreeable to the patient (ANA, 2018). Use the wipe-off whiteboard in patient's room to write the plan for administration times. Identify strategies such as staggering prn acetaminophen (Tylenol) and ibuprofen between doses of prn opioids (Chou et al., 2016). *Rationale: Gives patient a sense of ownership and control of drug schedule without need to rely on memory. Teaches patient how to make medication choices effectively after discharge or independently at home.*
10. Assess patient's and family caregiver's knowledge, experience, and health literacy level. *Rationale: Ensures patient has the capacity to obtain, communicate, process, and understand basic health information (CDC, 2016).*

STEP	RATIONALE
PLANNING	
1. Expected outcomes following completion of procedure:	
• Patient sets mutually agreeable pain-intensity goal with health care providers.	Gives patient a sense of ownership and control in managing and reporting pain.
• Patient achieves a self-report of pain intensity at or below pain-intensity goal.	Patient achieves acceptable level of comfort.
• Patient experiences a reduction in pain behaviors (e.g., guarding, moaning, restlessness).	
• Patient is able to function adequately and perform ADLs (e.g., walking, working, eating, sleeping, interacting).	A return to performing ADLs has a positive impact on reducing psychological and physiological stress (Ostby and Armer, 2015)
• Patient does not experience intolerable or unmanageable drug side effects.	Safe effective dose of medication administered.
• Patient understands the pain-management plan and actively participates in the decision-making process.	Teaches patient how to make medication choices effectively after discharge or independently at home.
2. Provide privacy.	Promotes sense of comfort.
3. Set up equipment.	Organizes the work area in preparation for the procedure.
4. Position and drape patient if needed.	Ensures patient's comfort.
5. Explain medication to be administered, anticipated effects, and what patient should report.	Proper explanation enhances patient participation. Accurate reporting of pain by patient improves your evaluation and treatment.
6. Provide educational information to patient and family caregiver. If the patient will need opioid therapy at home, education and a prescription for naloxone and training in the administration of naloxone should be given. Naloxone is available as a nasal spray. This is particularly important with patients who have a history of opioid addiction (Kampman and Jarvis, 2015).	Pain-management education may be needed when managing symptoms at home, including information about adverse reactions. Nasal spray administration of naloxone provides an easy route of administration if the patient is able.
IMPLEMENTATION	
1. Check accuracy and completeness of each MAR or computer printout with health care provider's written medication order. Check patient's name, medication name and dosage, route of administration, and frequency (e.g., one time, range order, prn) or time of administration. Recopy or reprint any portion of MAR that is difficult to read.	The order sheet is the most reliable source and only legal record of medications that patient is to receive. Ensures that patient receives the correct medications (Mandrack et al., 2012). Illegible MARs are a source of medication errors.
2. Perform hand hygiene. Prepare selected analgesic, following the "seven rights" for medication administration (see Chapter 22).	Reduces transmission of microorganisms. Ensures safe and appropriate medication administration. *This is the first and second check for accuracy.*
3. Identify patient using two identifiers (e.g., name and birthday or name and account number) according to agency policy. Compare identifiers with information on the patient's MAR or medical record.	Ensures correct patient. Complies with The Joint Commission standards and improves patient safety (TJC, 2019).
4. At the bedside, compare MAR or computer printout with the name of the medication on the medication label and patient name (armband). Ask patient if he or she has allergies.	Timely administration improves pain management. Final check of medication ensures that right patient receives right medication. Confirms patient's allergy history. *This is the third check for accuracy.*
5. Reassess patient's pain/sedation level and respiratory status before administering the medication.	Ensures appropriateness of medication administration. Safe patient monitoring requires assessing a patient's level of sedation and respiratory status at baseline and ongoing interval assessments (Pasero et al., 2016).

STEP	RATIONALE
6. Perform hand hygiene and apply gloves (if needed based on route of medication). Administer analgesic (see Chapters 22 and 23) following these guidelines:	Reduces transmission of infection. Ensures safe medication administration.

Safe Patient Care *If a patient is unable to swallow or has a gastrostomy or jejunostomy tube in place, remember that, with the exception of methadone, the extended-release opioid formulations may not be crushed for administration. Some capsules may be opened, and the contents mixed in applesauce or other soft food, but they may not be crushed.*

STEP	RATIONALE
a. Administer as soon as pain occurs or ATC as ordered.	Pain is easier to prevent than to treat. The ATC schedule avoids the low plasma concentrations that permit breakthrough pain. This is especially important the first 24 to 48 hours postoperatively to control pain.
b. Administer prn or one-time dose 30 to 60 minutes before pain-producing procedures or activities.	Reduces or blocks pain transmission in the central nervous system (CNS), allowing procedure to be completed with less discomfort.
7. Provide basic and nonpharmacological comfort measures in addition to analgesics (see Skills 15.1 and 15.2).	Increases effectiveness of pharmacological agents; treats nonphysiological aspects of pain.
8. Administer nursing care measures during times of peak effects of analgesics. Explain after giving medication (for example): "I will return in 30 minutes after the medicine reduces your pain to do the dressing change." Consider duration of action of analgesics when planning activities.	Effects vary depending on the type of medication used; allows for anticipation of next dose; permits evaluation of analgesic effects; maximizes effectiveness of nursing measures to prevent complications.
9. Assist patient to comfortable position.	Promotes patient's comfort.
10. Raise side rails (as appropriate) and lower bed to lowest position.	Patient safety precaution.
11. Remove gloves (if used) and perform hand hygiene.	Prevents spread of microorganisms.
12. Be sure nurse call system is in an accessible location with patient's reach. Instruct patient is its use.	Patient safety precaution.

Safe Patient Care *Patients receiving ATC opioids should also receive stimulant laxatives. Opioids decrease intestinal propulsion (peristalsis) but not intestinal motility (churning), so stool softeners alone are ineffective. Recommend stimulant laxatives (Argoff et al., 2015).*

EVALUATION

STEP	RATIONALE
1. Have patient self-report pain intensity using appropriate pain scales both at rest and with activity.	Evaluates effectiveness of pain-management regimen.
2. Monitor for adverse medication effect and perform vital sign measurement, note signs of opioid-induced sedation and respiratory depression (OSRD).	Use a valid sedation scale (Pasero Opioid Sedation Scale [POSS]) to detect early opioid-induced respiratory depression (see Box 15.1). Monitoring sedation levels may be more effective for detection than a decreased respiratory rate because hypoxemic episodes may occur in the absence of a low respiratory rate; therefore the use of both pulse oximetry and capnography is recommended (Meisenberg et al., 2017; Nagappa et al., 2017; Pasero et al., 2016).
3. Evaluate PQRSTU aspects of pain; use nonverbal assessment if patient unable to respond (see Skill 15.1, Step 8).	Provides for thorough evaluation of pain characteristics to determine if pain was relieved.

STEP	RATIONALE
4. Observe patient's position; mobility; relaxation; and ability to rest, sleep, eat, and participate in usual activities.	Provides nonverbal and behavioral information for evaluation of patient response to analgesic.
5. When opioids are used, evaluate for opioid-induced constipation (OIC). A recommended tool is the Bowel Function Index (BFI). Patients are asked to score the following three parameters on a scale of 1 to 100 over the previous 7-day period (Argoff et al., 2015; Yoon and Bruner, 2017): • Ease of defecation • Feeling of incomplete defecation • Personal judgment of patient regarding constipation during the past 7 days	For patients using first-line therapies for constipation (e.g., fiber, OTC laxatives, enemas, dietary changes, exercise) a BFI score of 30 or higher might indicate benefit from a new emerging class of prescription medication for OIC, such as naloxegol (Argoff et al., 2015; Yoon and Bruner, 2017).
6. Use Teach-Back: "I want to be sure you understand when to ask for medication to treat your pain. Can you give me an example?" Revise your instruction now or develop a plan for revised patient/family caregiver teaching to be implemented at an appropriate time if patient/family caregiver is not able to teach back correctly.	Determines patient's/family caregiver's level of understanding of instructional topic.

Unexpected Outcomes	Related Interventions
1. Patient reports that pain intensity is greater than desired or shows nonverbal behaviors reflecting pain.	• Discuss current pain-control regimen with the patient. • Determine what has worked best to provide relief. If the medication has failed, document the result and inform the patient that you will notify the health care provider that the treatment is not effective, and options will be discussed. • Evaluate the dose of medication administered with the health care provider and consider an alternative dose or an adjuvant. • Try alternative nonpharmacological interventions. • Reassure patient you will do everything you can to solve the problem of inadequate pain control. Discomfort that is unrelieved or worse may indicate need for additional diagnostic, medical, or surgical intervention or a change in pain management.
2. Patient develops respiratory depression.	• Give no additional dose of analgesic. Stay with patient and protect airway. • Notify health care provider and be prepared to administer an opioid-reversing agent per health care provider order, such as naloxone. Naloxone is an opioid antagonist that can reverse severe respiratory depression and should be administered immediately per health care provider's order (American Society of Addiction Medicine, 2015; Kampman and Jarvis, 2015). • Continue to monitor vital signs, including pulse oximetry.

Recording

- Record patient's pain rating (15 to 30 minutes after IV medication and 30 to 60 minutes after per os [PO] medication), behavioral and physiological response to analgesic, and additional comfort measures given in nurses' notes. Incorporate pain-relief techniques in nursing care plan.
- Record medication, dose, route, and time given in MAR or computer printout.
- Document your evaluation of patient learning.

Hand-Off Reporting

- Report unsuccessful or untoward patient response to analgesics to health care provider.

✦ SKILL 15.4 Patient-Controlled Analgesia

Purpose

Patient-controlled analgesia (PCA) is an interactive method of pain management that gives patients pain control through self-administration of analgesics. Routes for PCA administration include subcutaneous, intravenous (IV; the most common), and epidural. PCA is a safe method of analgesic administration for acute and chronic pain, including postoperative and pain related to trauma, labor and delivery, sickle cell crisis, myocardial infarction, cancer, and end of life (American Society of Clinical Oncology [ASCO], 2016). Patients receive analgesic doses as they need them by using a small, computerized pump to deliver a prescribed dose of medication with a push of a button. The three most common medications used in PCA are the opioids morphine, hydromorphone, and fentanyl.

Patient safety is critical during PCA administration. Risk factors for oversedation and respiratory depression when using PCA include opioid-naïve status; obesity; age (infants and small children or older adults); confusion; obstructive sleep apnea syndrome (OSAS); multiple co-morbid conditions, such as lung, renal, and hepatic diseases; smoking; and use of medications (e.g., opioids, muscle relaxants, sleeping medications) (Meisenberg et al., 2017). Because patients depress a button on a PCA device to deliver a regulated dose of analgesic, they must be able to understand how, why, and when to self-administer medication and be able to depress the device physically. Family members must understand the purpose of PCA and why they cannot push the PCA button for a patient. The exception is in the care of children, where some hospitals allow parents to press the device; this is called authorized agent-controlled analgesia (AACA) (American Society of Pain Management Nursing, 2016; Cooney, 2016; Pasero, 2015). An agency must have a policy describing clear guidelines for the use of AACA. Nurses must advise patients, family, and other visitors that PCA is for patient use only. PCA is not recommended in situations in which oral analgesics could easily manage pain.

Delegation and Collaboration

The skill of PCA administration cannot be delegated to nursing assistive personnel (NAP). The nurse directs the NAP to:

- Notify the nurse if the patient complains of change in status, including unrelieved pain or difficulty awaking.
- Notify the nurse if the patient has questions about the PCA process or equipment.
- Never administer a PCA dose for the patient and notify the nurse if anyone other than the patient is observed administering a dose for the patient.

Equipment

- PCA pump system and tubing
- Analgesic cartridge or syringe with identification label and time tape (may already be attached and completed by pharmacy)
- Needleless connector
- Antiseptic swab
- Adhesive tape
- Clean gloves (when applicable)
- Opioid-reversal agent (e.g., naloxone)
- Equipment for vital signs, pulse oximetry, and capnography
- Medication administration record (MAR)

ASSESSMENT

1. Check accuracy and completeness of each MAR or computer printout with health care provider's written medication order. Check patient's name, medication name and dosage, route of administration, lockout period, and frequency of medication (demand, continuous, or both). Recopy or reprint any portion of MAR that is difficult to read. *Rationale: The order sheet is the most reliable source and only legal record of medications that patient is to receive. Ensures that patient receives the correct medications (Mandrack et al., 2012). Illegible MARs are a source of medication errors.*
2. Assess patient's medical and medication history, including drug allergies. *Rationale: Determines need for medication or possible contraindications for medication administration.*

Safe Patient Care *When assessing allergies, be aware that nausea is not an allergic reaction, and it can be treated; pruritus alone is not an allergic reaction and is common to opioid use. Pruritus is treatable and does not contraindicate the use of PCA (Masato et al., 2017).*

3. Perform hand hygiene. Perform a complete assessment of character of pain (see Skill 15.1, Steps 2–9) and measure vital signs. *Rationale: Provides baseline for type and nature of pain condition for determination of efficacy of PCA.*
4. Review medication information in drug reference manual or consult with pharmacist if uncertain about any PCA medications to be administered. *Rationale: Understanding medications before administering them prevents medication errors (Pasero et al., 2016).*
5. Also assess patient's ability to manipulate PCA control and cognitive status for ability to understand purpose of PCA and how to use control device. *Rationale: Determines patient's ability to use PCA safely and correctly.*
6. Assess environment for factors that could contribute to pain (e.g., noise, room temperature). *Rationale: Elimination of irritating stimuli may help to reduce pain perception.*
7. Assess for conditions that predispose patients to unwanted effects from opioids. Known, untreated, or unknown obstructive sleep apnea syndrome (OSAS) poses a significant risk for respiratory depression (Gokay et al., 2016). Use the STOP-BANG questionnaire to assess for OSAS (see agency policy; Gokay et al., 2016). *Rationale: Assessment should be completed before surgery by anesthesia. Identification allows treatment teams (surgeon, respiratory therapy, anesthesia) to take appropriate precautions, such as making continuous positive airway pressure (CPAP) or bi-level positive airway pressure (BiPAP) ventilation devices available.*
8. Apply clean gloves. Assess patency of intravenous (IV) access and surrounding tissue for inflammation or swelling (see Chapter 28). *Rationale: IV line needs to be patent for safe administration of pain medication. Confirmation of placement of IV catheter and integrity of surrounding tissues ensures that medication is safely administered.*

9. If patient has had surgery, inspect incision, continuing to wear clean gloves. Gently palpate around area for tenderness. Use sterile gloves if necessary to place hand directly on incision. Remove and dispose of gloves and perform hand hygiene. *Rationale: Unusual incisional pain, swelling, redness, and/or discharge may indicate infection. Reduces transmission of infection.*
10. Assess patient's knowledge and perceived effectiveness of previous pain-management strategies, especially previous PCA use. *Rationale: Response to pain-control strategies helps identify learning needs and affects patient's willingness to try therapy.*
11. Assess patient's or family caregiver's knowledge, experience, and health literacy level. *Rationale: Ensures patient has the capacity to obtain, communicate, process, and understand basic health information (CDC, 2016).*

STEP	RATIONALE
PLANNING	
1. Expected outcomes following completion of procedure:	
• Patient verbalizes pain relief.	Subjective measure of pain relief.
• Patient rates pain lower on pain scale.	Objective measure of pain relief.
• Patient exhibits relaxed facial expression and body position.	Nonverbal cues of pain relief.
• Patient remains alert and oriented.	Indicates freedom from overly sedating effects of opioids. Sleepiness is usually from fatigue and not necessarily a sign of oversedation.
• Patient increasingly participates in self-care activities.	Suggests successful pain relief.
• Patient correctly operates PCA device.	Demonstrates safe and appropriate use of PCA.
2. Provide privacy.	Promotes patient's comfort.
3. Set up equipment.	Organizes the work area in preparation for the procedure.
4. Position and drape patient if needed.	Ensures patient's comfort.
5. Provide patient and family caregiver with individually tailored education, including information on procedure for administration and treatment options for management of postoperative pain with PCA. If the patient will need opioid therapy at home, education and a prescription for naloxone and training in the administration of naloxone should be given. Naloxone is available as a nasal spray. This is particularly important with patients who have a history of opioid addiction (Kampman and Jarvis, 2015).	It is important that the patient and family caregiver understand pain management with PCA and establish realistic pain-control goals.
IMPLEMENTATION	
1. Perform hand hygiene.	Reduces transmission of microorganisms.
2. Follow the "seven rights" for medication administration (see Chapter 22). Obtain PCA analgesic in module prepared by pharmacy. Check label of medication two times: when removed from storage and when preparing for assembly.	Ensures safe and appropriate medication administration. *This is the first and second check for accuracy.*
3. Identify patient using at least two identifiers (e.g., name and birthday or name and medical record number) according to agency policy. Compare identifiers with information on patient's MAR or medical record.	Ensures correct patient. Complies with The Joint Commission standards and improves patient safety (TJC, 2019).
4. At bedside, compare MAR or computer printout with name of medication on drug cartridge. Have second registered nurse (RN) confirm health care provider's order and correct setup of PCA. Second RN should check order and the device independently and not just look at existing setup.	Ensures that correct patient receives right medication. *This is the third check for accuracy.*

STEP	RATIONALE
5. Before initiating analgesia, explain purpose and demonstrate function of PCA to patient and family caregiver. This includes education about the use of PCA and verbal and written instruction warning against anyone other than the patient pressing the PCA button (Cooney et al., 2016; Pasero, 2015)	It is important that the patient and family members understand how to use PCA safely. Allows for patient-centered care and improved patient outcomes with pain control (Shindul-Rothschild, 2017).
a. Explain type of medication in device.	Informs patient of therapy to be received.

Safe Patient Care *Background basal infusion of opioids has been associated with increased risk of nausea, vomiting, and respiratory depression. However, in opioid-tolerant patients, a background basal infusion may be necessary due to the potential for undertreatment and possible opioid withdrawal (Chou et al., 2016).*

STEP	RATIONALE
b. If a background basal rate is used, explain that device safely administers continuous medication, but self-initiated small but frequent amounts of medication can be administered for unrelieved pain by using the PCA button.	A background basal infusion delivers a continuous dose of analgesic medication. The PCA pump is programmed to allow additional patient-controlled doses for pain that is not relieved by the continuous infusion (breakthrough pain; Pasero, 2015).
c. Explain that self-dosing aids in repositioning, walking, and coughing or deep breathing.	Promotes patient's participation in care.
d. Explain that device is programmed to deliver ordered type and dose of pain medication, lockout interval, and 1- to 4-hour dosage limits. Explain how lockout time prevents overdose.	Relieves anxiety in patients who might be concerned about overdosing.
e. Demonstrate to patient how to push medication demand button (see illustration). Instruct family caregiver to not push PCA button to give medication.	Administration by proxy is not recommended in adults (Chou et al., 2016; TJC, 2017).
f. Instruct patient to notify nurse for possible side effects, problems in gaining pain relief, changes in severity or location of pain, alarm sounding, or questions.	Engages patient as partner in care.
6. Apply clean gloves. Check infuser and patient-control module for accurate labeling or evidence of leaking.	Avoids medication error and injury to patient.
7. Position patient comfortably to be sure that venipuncture or central-line site is accessible.	Ensures unimpeded flow of infusion.
8. Insert drug cartridge into infusion device (see illustration) and prime tubing.	Locks system and prevents air from infusing into IV tubing.

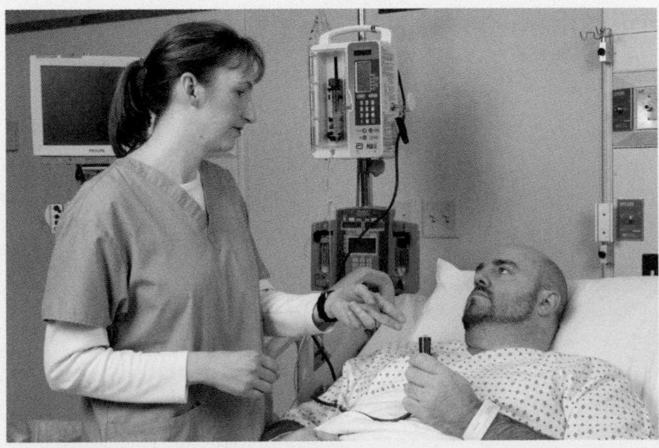

STEP 5e Patient learns how to press PCA device button.

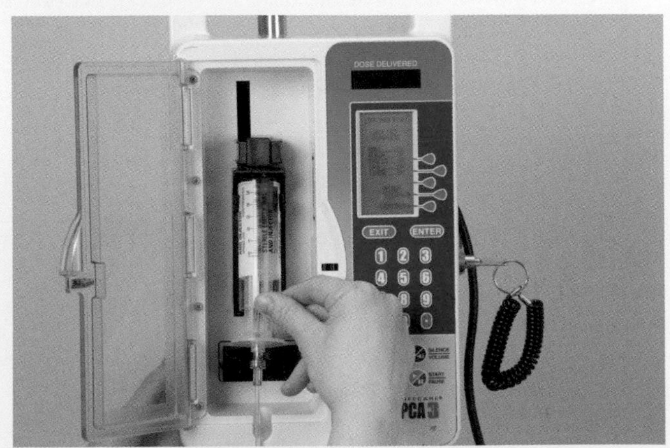

STEP 8 Nurse inserting drug cartridge into PCA device.

STEP	RATIONALE
9. Attach needleless adapter to tubing adapter of patient-controlled module.	Needed to connect with IV line.
10. Wipe injection port of maintenance IV line vigorously with antiseptic swab for 15 seconds and allow to dry.	Minimizes entry of surface microorganisms during needle insertion, reducing risk of catheter-related bloodstream infection.
11. Insert needleless adapter into injection port nearest patient (at Y-site of peripheral IV or central line or connect to its own IV site). There should not be a chance to use PCA tubing for administering IV push with another drug.	Establishes route for medication to enter main IV line. Needleless systems prevent needlestick injuries. Prevents medication interaction and incompatibility.
12. Secure connection and anchor PCA tubing with tape. Label PCA tubing.	Prevents dislodging of needleless adapter from port. Facilitates patient's ability to ambulate. Label prevents error from connecting tubing from different device to PCA.
13. Program computerized PCA pump as ordered to deliver prescribed medication dose and lockout interval. Have second nurse check setting. (**NOTE:** Recheck with oncoming RN during shift hand-off to ensure line reconciliation.)	Ensures safe, therapeutic drug administration. With appropriate dose intervals (e.g., 10 minutes), usually an appreciable analgesic effect and/or mild sedation is achieved before patient can access the next dose; thus there is lower chance for oversedation and respiratory depression. A second nurse check reduces risk for medication error (Kane-Gill et al., 2017).
14. Administer loading dose of analgesia as prescribed. Manually give one-time dose or turn on pump and program dose into pump.	Establishes initial level of analgesia.
15. Remove and discard gloves and supplies in appropriate containers. Dispose of empty cassette or syringe in compliance with institutional policy. Perform hand hygiene.	Reduces transmission of microorganisms. The Federal Controlled Substances Act regulates control and dispensation of opioids for all institutions.
16. If experiencing pain, have patient demonstrate use of PCA system; if not, have patient repeat instructions given earlier.	Repeating instructions reinforces learning. Checking patient's understanding through return demonstration helps you determine patient's level of understanding and ability to manipulate device.
17. Be sure that venipuncture or central-line site is protected, and recheck infusion rate before leaving patient.	Ensures patency of IV line.
18. Assist patient into comfortable position.	Patient comfort.
19. Raise side rails (as appropriate) and lower bed to lowest position.	Patient safety precaution.
20. Place nurse call system within patient's reach and instruct patient in its use.	Patient safety precaution.
21. To discontinue PCA:	
a. Check health care provider order for discontinuation. Obtain necessary PCA information from pump for documentation; note date, time, amount infused and amount of drug wasted and reason for wastage.	Ensures correct documentation of a schedule II drug. Two RNs must witness wastage of opioids (narcotics) and sign record to meet requirements of the Controlled Substances Act for scheduled drugs.
b. Perform hand hygiene and apply clean gloves. Turn off pump. Disconnect PCA tubing from primary IV line but maintain IV access.	Reduces transmission of microorganisms. Follow health care provider order for maintenance of IV site.
c. Dispose of empty cartridge, tubing, and gloves according to agency policy. Remove and dispose of gloves and perform hand hygiene.	Reduces transmission of microorganisms.
d. Place patient in comfortable position.	Promotes patient comfort.
e. Raise side rails (as appropriate) and lower bed to lowest position.	Patient safety precaution.
f. Be sure nurse call system is within patient's reach and instruct on its use.	Patient safety precaution.

STEP	RATIONALE

EVALUATION

STEP	RATIONALE
1. Use pain rating scale to evaluate patient's pain intensity following treatments and procedures according to agency policy (see Skill 15.1).	Determines response to PCA dosing. Documenting "PCA in use" or "PCA effective" is not an adequate record of patient's pain level.
2. Observe patient for nausea or pruritus.	Common treatable side effects of opioids.
3. Monitor patient's level of sedation. It is recommended that the Pasero Opioid Sedation Scale (POSS) (see Box 15.1) be used to monitor for unintended patient sedation (Davis et al., 2017; TJC, 2017). Vital signs, pulse oximetry, and capnography should be used for monitoring; however, study findings report nurse observation and administration of the POSS as superior in earlier identification of respiratory depression and oversedation (Chou et al., 2016). Monitoring should be frequent per agency policy and health care provider order (e.g., every 1 to 2 hours for first 12 hours for the first 24-hour period after surgery). Monitor more often at start, during first 24 hours, and at night when hypoventilation and hypoxia tend to occur during sleep.	Patient is at highest risk for oversedation and respiratory distress (OSRD) during the first 24 hours of PCA administration. Although there is low sensitivity for detecting hypoventilation with pulse oximetry when supplemental oxygen is used, and evidence is insufficient to firmly recommend capnography (Chou et al., 2016), these interventions are used in monitoring for OSRD and provide important clinical information in your assessment. Excess sedation (difficult to arouse) precedes respiratory depression. Differences in ventilation are observed between wakefulness and sleep, which correlates with states of brain arousal. Opioid-induced respiratory depression is also regulated by sleep-wake mechanisms (Nagappa et al., 2017).
4. Have patient demonstrate dose delivery.	Evaluates skill in use of PCA.
5. According to agency policy, evaluate number of attempts (number of times patient pushed button), delivery of demand doses (number of times drug actually given and total amount of medication delivered in particular time frame), and basal dose if ordered.	Helps evaluate effectiveness of PCA dose and frequency in relieving pain. Maintains compliance with Controlled Substances Act.
6. Observe patient initiate self-care.	Demonstrates pain relief.
7. **Use Teach-Back:** "I want to be sure I explained how PCA will help with your pain and how you should use the device. Tell me the steps you will use to activate the PCA." Revise your instruction now or develop a plan for revised patient/family caregiver teaching if patient/family caregiver is not able to teach back correctly.	Determines patient's/family caregiver's level of understanding of instructional topic.

Unexpected Outcomes	Related Interventions
1. Patient verbalizes continued or worsening discomfort or displays nonverbal behaviors indicative of pain.	• Perform complete pain reassessment. • Assess for possible complications other than pain. • Inspect IV site for possible catheter occlusion or infiltration. • Evaluate number of attempts and deliveries initiated by patient. • Check that maintenance of IV fluid is running continuously. • Evaluate pump for operational problems. • Consult with health care provider.
2. Patient is sedated and not easily aroused.	• Stop PCA. • Notify health care provider immediately. • Elevate head of bed 30 degrees unless contraindicated. • Instruct patient to take deep breaths. • Apply oxygen at 2 L/min per nasal cannula (if ordered). • Assess vital signs, oxygen saturation, and/or capnography. • Evaluate amount of opioid delivered within past 4 to 8 hours. • Ask family members if they pressed button without patient's knowledge. • Review MAR for other possible sedating drugs. • Prepare to administer an opioid-reversing agent (e.g., naloxone). • Observe patient frequently (Association of periOperative Registered Nurses, 2017).
3. Patient unable to manipulate PCA device to maintain pain control.	• Consult with health care provider regarding alternative medication route or possibly a basal (continuous) dose.

Recording

- Record appropriate MAR drug, concentration, dose (basal and demand), time started, lockout time, and amount of solution infused and remaining per agency policy. Many facilities have a separate flow sheet for PCA documentation.
- Record assessment of patient's response to analgesic on PCA medication form, narrative notes, or patient assessment flow sheet (see agency policy), including vital signs, oximetry and capnography results, sedation status, pain rating, and status of vascular access device.
- Calculate infused dose: add demand and continuous dose together.
- Document your evaluation of patient learning.

Hand-Off Reporting

- During hand-off report, the oncoming and outgoing nurse should inspect and agree with PCA pump programming as a means of medication reconciliation (Kane-Gill et al., 2017).
- Hand-off report should include detailed information regarding vital signs, pulse oximetry and capnography, pain-assessment scores, STOP-BANG score for OSAS if done, POSS sedation scores, level of consciousness, anxiety level, and activity level (Chou et al., 2016; Cooney, 2016; Meisenberg et al., 2017).
- Nursing research has been reported on the benefit of "safety priming" during hand-off reporting, such as using words to activate a mental construct, prompting nursing safety-oriented behavior (Groves et al., 2017). An example of safety priming during hand-off reporting may include the nurse's words to express concerns of what may happen (e.g., excess opioid infusion) because of certain behaviors, instead of reporting only factual information.

✦ SKILL 15.5 Epidural Analgesia

Purpose

The administration of analgesics into the epidural space is an efficient intervention to manage acute pain during labor (Sng and Sia, 2017); pain after surgery (Roeb et al., 2017; Solanki et al., 2017); pain following trauma to the chest, abdomen, pelvis, or lower limbs (Bouzat et al., 2017); and chronic cancer pain (ASCO, 2016; He et al., 2015). The epidural space is a potential space that contains a network of vessels, nerves, and fat located between the vertebral column and the dura mater, the outermost meninges covering the spinal cord (Fig. 15.1). An anesthesia provider, using sterile technique, typically places a catheter into the epidural space below the second lumbar vertebra, where the spinal cord ends (Fig. 15.2). Temporary short-term and long-term catheters are inserted. Opioids and local anesthetics, separately or in combination, are delivered into the epidural space, creating a blockade of pain transmission through the spinal cord. Reported benefits of epidural analgesia include higher patient satisfaction (Sng and Sia, 2017) and a reduction in complications such as oversedation, nausea and vomiting, and respiratory depression (Bouzat et al., 2017). Common opioids given epidurally include morphine, hydromorphone (Dilaudid), fentanyl, and sufentanil, which require safe, effective management using a coordinated interprofessional approach.

Delegation and Collaboration

The skill of epidural analgesia administration cannot be delegated to nursing assistive personnel (NAP). The nurse directs the NAP to:

- Observe the dressing over the insertion site when repositioning or ambulating patients to prevent catheter disruption.
- Avoid pulling patient up in bed while he or she is lying flat on the back, which can dislodge the epidural catheter.
- Report any catheter disconnection or leakage from dressing immediately.
- Immediately report to the nurse any change in patient status, comfort level, or loss of sensation or movement.

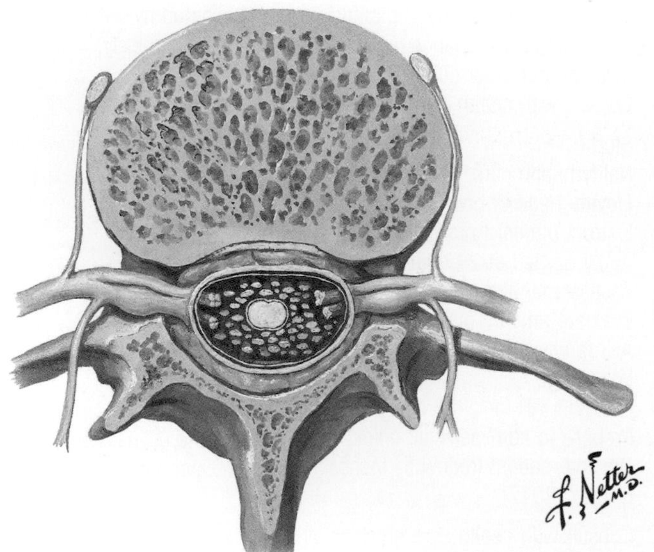

FIG 15.1 Anatomical drawing of epidural space. *(Reprinted from* www.netterimages.com *© Elsevier Inc. All rights reserved.)*

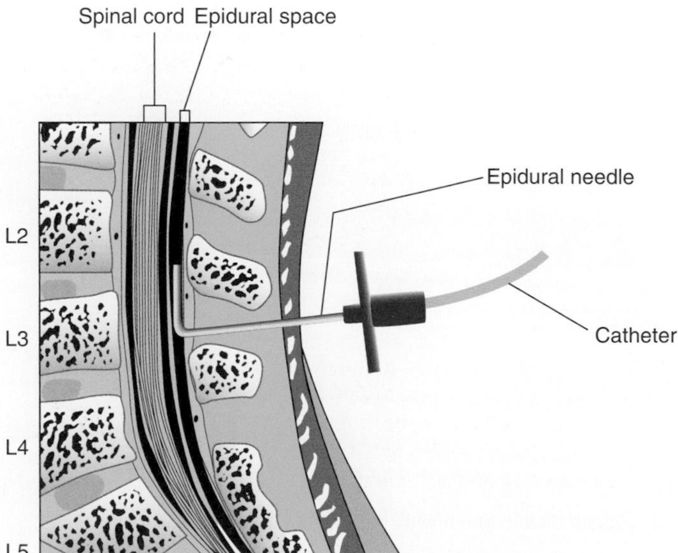

FIG 15.2 Placement of epidural catheter.

Equipment

- Clean gloves
- Sterile gloves (if removing epidural dressing)
- Prediluted preservative-free opioid as prescribed by health care provider for use in intravenous (IV) infusion pump (This is prepared by pharmacy.)
- Infusion pump and compatible International Organization for Standardization (ISO) tubing. (Do not use Y-ports for infusions; some infusion pumps have color-coded tubing for intraspinal use.)
- Antibacterial filter
- Tape
- Label (for injection port)
- Equipment for vital signs and pulse oximetry or capnography (see agency policy)
- Medication administration record (MAR) or computer printout

ASSESSMENT

1. Verify health care provider's order against MAR for name of medication, dosage, route, infusion method (bolus, continuous, or demand), and lockout settings. Recopy or reprint any portion of MAR that is difficult to read. *Rationale: The provider's order is the most reliable source and the only legal record of medications that patient is to receive. Ensures that right drug is administered to patient.*
2. Assess if patient has completed informed consent and is aware of risk and benefits of epidural analgesia (see agency policy; Schatz et al., 2017). *Rationale: Epidural analgesia is a significant procedure that poses risks of complications ranging from adverse medication reactions to serious neurologic damage (Lourens, 2016).*
3. Check medical record to see if patient recently received anticoagulants. *Rationale: Recent anticoagulation may contraindicate the placement of epidural catheter because of inability to apply pressure at insertion site and risk for bleeding (Lourens, 2016; Schreiber, 2015).*
4. Assess if patient routinely takes herbal medications; document complete list. *Rationale: Some herbal medications interfere with the clotting mechanism (e.g., ginkgo biloba, ginseng, ginger). Currently there is no contraindication to their use when receiving epidural medication (Liperoti et al., 2017).*

Safe Patient Care *Contraindications to epidural analgesia include allergies to anesthetic, hypovolemia, increased intracranial pressure, insertion-site infection or sepsis, thrombocytopenia (<100,000 μl), prior spinal surgery, spinal instability/abnormalities, and lack of staff trained in essential competencies for managing epidural analgesia (Schreiber, 2015).*

5. Perform hand hygiene and a complete pain assessment (see Skill 15.1, Steps 2–9). *Rationale: Reduces transmission of microorganisms. Assessment data guide safe and effective dosing of pain medication and establish baseline to evaluate epidural efficacy and patient response.*
6. Assess patient's sedation level by assessing level of wakefulness or alertness, ability to follow commands, and drowsiness (see Box 15.1). *Rationale: Establishes baseline before first dose. Assessment of sedation level is more reliable for detecting early opioid-induced respiratory depression than decreased respiratory rate. Sedation always precedes respiratory depression from opioids.*
7. Assess rate, pattern, and depth of respirations; pulse oximetry or capnography; blood pressure; and temperature (see Chapter 7). *Rationale: Establishes baseline of circulatory and oxygenation status. Opioids can cause hypotension. Infection is a complication of an epidural, reflected by fever.*
8. Assess initial motor and sensory function of lower extremities (see Chapter 8). Test sensation to touch in lower extremities. Have patient flex both feet and knees and raise each leg off bed. Pay special attention to patients with preexisting sensory or motor abnormalities. *Rationale: Establishes baseline. Ongoing monitoring of motor and sensory status ensures that neural blockage is not affecting function (Lourens, 2016).*

Safe Patient Care *For all patients on patient-controlled epidural anesthesia (PCEA), assess for sensory and motor function before ambulation or transfer (Goldberg et al., 2017).*

9. Perform hand hygiene and apply clean gloves. Inspect catheter insertion site for redness, warmth, tenderness, swelling, and drainage. Apply sterile gloves when removing occlusive dressing. *Rationale: Catheter sites are at risk for local infections. Purulent drainage is sign of infection. Clear drainage may indicate cerebrospinal fluid (CSF) leaking from punctured dura. Bloody drainage may indicate that catheter entered blood vessel (Lourens, 2016).*
10. Follow catheter tubing and check connection site with IV tubing. Verify that catheter is secured to patient's skin from back, side, or front. Be sure that catheter is connected securely to IV tubing with ISO connector. Remove and dispose of gloves and perform hand hygiene. *Rationale: Prevents catheter dislodgement or migration. Incidents with catastrophic consequences have been reported due to inappropriate medication, enteral feeding liquid, or air being mistakenly administered into epidural space (ISO, 2016; Mattox, 2017). The ISO tubing and connectors were developed to prevent misconnections between small-bore catheters used for different applications (ISO, 2016).*

Safe Patient Care *Note that pharmacies in most health care settings prepare and provide the medication/infusion bag.*

11. Check patency of IV tubing. Check infusion pump flow rate for proper calibration and operation. *Rationale: Kinked or clamped tubing interrupts analgesic infusion; may cause clotting at end of IV catheter and require replacement. A patent IV line allows IV access in case medications are needed to counteract adverse reactions.*

Safe Patient Care *Infusion pumps should be configured specifically for epidural analgesia with preset limits for maximum infusion rate and bolus size; lock-out time should be standardized if used for PCEA (Mattox, 2017).*

12. Assess patient's or caregiver's knowledge, experience, and health literacy level. *Rationale: Ensures patient has the capacity to obtain, communicate, process, and understand basic health information (CDC, 2016).*

STEP	RATIONALE
PLANNING	
1. Expected outcomes following completion of procedure:	
• Patient verbalizes pain relief within 30 to 60 minutes of initiating epidural infusion.	Indicates that drug and dose are effective in relieving pain.
• Patient has no headache during epidural infusion or after discontinuation.	Indicates that catheter is positioned correctly in the epidural space. Headache is an indication of a postdural puncture headache in which there is CSF leakage from the puncture site and usually occurs between 12 and 72 hours after catheter insertion (Lourens, 2016).
• Patient remains normotensive, and heart rate remains at or above baseline.	Indicates absence of circulatory side effects of epidural opioids.
• Patient is alert, oriented, and easily aroused.	Indicates absence of excessive sedation/oversedation (see Box 15.1).
• Patient's respirations are regular, of adequate depth, and equal to or greater than 8 breaths/min. Pulse oximetry SpO_2 95% or greater; capnography end-tidal CO_2 5% or 35 to 37 mm Hg.	Indicates adequate ventilation and reduced risk for respiratory depression from opioids.
• Patient voids without difficulty; averages a minimum of 30 mL/h.	Indicates absence of urinary retention (potential opioid side effect).
• Patient has no or minimal pruritus and no paresthesia of lower extremities.	Indicates absence of potential side effect of epidural medications.
• Epidural system remains intact and functioning.	Infusion system is patent; no interruption in medication delivery to epidural space.
2. Provide privacy.	Promotes patient comfort.
3. Set up equipment.	Organizes the work area in preparation for the procedure.
4. Position and drape patient as needed.	Ensures patient's comfort.
5. Place patients receiving epidural analgesia close to the nurses' station.	Ensures close supervision during infusion.
6. Clinicians should provide patient and family caregiver with individually tailored education, including information on treatment options for management of postoperative pain with PCEA. If the patient will need opioid therapy at home, education and a prescription for naloxone and training in the administration of naloxone should be given. Naloxone is available as a nasal spray. This is particularly important with patients who have a history of opioid addiction (Kampman and Jarvis, 2015).	It is important that the patient and family caregiver understand pain management with PCEA and establish pain-control goals.
IMPLEMENTATION	
1. Perform hand hygiene.	Reduces transmission of microorganisms.
2. Follow the "seven rights" for medication administration (see Chapter 22). **NOTE:** *Pharmacy prepares medication for pump*. Check label of medication carefully with MAR or computer printout two times.	Ensures safe and appropriate medication administration. *This is the first and second check for accuracy*.
3. Identify patient using at least two identifiers (e.g., name and birthday or name and medical record number) according to agency policy if you are preparing infusion. Compare identifiers with information on patient's MAR or medical record.	Ensures correct patient. Complies with The Joint Commission standards and improves patient safety (TJC, 2019).
4. At the bedside, compare MAR or computer printout with name of medication on drug container.	*This is the third check for accuracy* and ensures that right patient receives right medication.
5. Before initiating analgesia, explain purpose and demonstrate function of epidural analgesia to patient and family caregiver (Cooney et al., 2016; Pasero, 2015).	Proper explanation enhances patient cooperation and helps with effective results.
6. Apply clean gloves. Administer infusion: Anesthesia provider typically starts or administers first dose. Thereafter, nurse maintains infusion.	Prevents transmission of infection.

STEP	RATIONALE
a. **Continuous infusion:**	
(1) Attach container of diluted preservative-free medication to infusion pump tubing and prime tubing.	Tubing filled with solution and free of air bubbles avoids air embolus.
(2) Insert tubing into infusion pump and attach distal end of tubing to antibacterial filter; then connect to epidural catheter using aseptic technique.	Pump propels fluid through tubing. Filter reduces entrance of microorganisms into infusion line.
(3) Check infusion pump for proper calibration, setting, and operation. Many facilities have two nurses independently check settings.	Ensures that patient is receiving proper dosing.
(4) Tape all connections using ISO tubing/connectors. Epidural infusion system between pump and patient should be considered closed, with no injection or Y ports. Epidural infusions should be labeled "For Epidural Use Only." Start infusion.	Taping maintains secure closed system to prevent infection. Labeling helps ensure that analgesic is administered into correct line and the epidural space (Mattox, 2017).
b. Bolus dose via infusion pump.	
(1) While helping anesthesia provider, perform Steps 6a(1) to(4) above. Adjust infusion pump setting for preset limit for maximum bolus size. Initiate pump to deliver ordered bolus.	Prevents accidental infusion of an overdose.
c. Dose on demand	
(1) While helping anesthesia provider, perform Steps 6a(1) to (4) above. Set pump for lockout time (as ordered).	Gives patient control over administration of analgesia.
(2) Have patient initiate demand dose as needed.	
7. Explain that nurses will monitor patient's response to epidural analgesic routinely. Also instruct patient on signs or problems to report to nurse (e.g., pru ritus, inability to pass urine, change in sensation).	Builds trust to encourage patient to be partner in care.
8. Assist patient to a comfortable position.	Promotes patient comfort.
9. Raise side rails (as appropriate) and lower bed to lowest position.	Patient safety precaution.
10. Appropriately dispose of supplies and equipment.	Maintains clean and organized workspace.
11. Remove and dispose of gloves. Perform hand hygiene.	Reduces transmission of microorganisms.
12. Be sure nurse call system is in an accessible location within patient's reach. Instruct patient on its use.	Patient safety precaution.
13. Postanalgesia:	
a. Keep an IV line patent for 24 hours after epidural analgesia has ended.	Provides route for any emergency medications.
b. Before removal of epidural catheter, check for presence of therapeutic anticoagulation. Check agency policy for removal of epidural catheter and extra precautions if patient is receiving anticoagulation therapy.	Removal of epidural catheter while patient is anticoagulated increases risk for spinal hematoma because of anticoagulation and inability to compress vessels.

EVALUATION

1. Evaluate patient's pain severity using a pain rating scale of 0 to 10 and evaluate character of pain.	Evaluates effectiveness of epidural analgesia.
2. Evaluate blood pressure and heart rate; respiratory rate, rhythm, depth, and pattern; pulse oximetry or capnography; and sedation level based on patient's clinical condition. Generally measured more frequently in first 12 hours of infusions (e.g., hourly; see agency policy), after bolus infusions or changes of infusion rate, and in periods of cardiovascular or respiratory instability (Nagappa et al., 2017).	Oversedation occurs before respiratory depression and should be monitored closely to prevent respiratory depression. Postural hypotension, vasodilation, and heart-rate changes may occur from pain or medication side effects (Mattox, 2017).

Safe Patient Care *Help patient when changing positions. Protects patient who is at risk for postural hypotension.*

3. Evaluate catheter insertion site every 2 to 4 hours for redness, warmth, tenderness, swelling, or drainage. Note character of drainage (e.g., bloody, clear, or purulent).	Bloody drainage may occur if catheter has migrated into a vessel. Report immediately and treat as emergency (Lourens, 2016).

STEP	RATIONALE
4. Inspect epidural site for disruption or displacement of catheter.	Could lead to infusion of medication into higher level of spinal cord.
5. Observe for pruritus, especially of face, head, neck, and torso. Inform patient that this is a side effect but is often not an allergic response.	Pruritus *alone* is rarely an allergy to opioids (Masato et al., 2017).
6. Observe for nausea and vomiting and presence of headache. Note any nonverbal signs of headache (grimacing, massaging head).	Nausea from epidural analgesia worsens by movement. Headache and cerebrospinal fluid (CSF) fluid leakage may occur from a dural puncture.
7. Monitor intake and output. Evaluate for bladder distention and urinary frequency or urgency. Consult with health care provider for possible need for intermittent catheterization.	Prevents urinary retention.
8. Evaluate for motor weakness or numbness and tingling of lower extremities (paresthesias).	Reducing epidural dose (per order) may help eliminate unwanted motor and sensory deficits (Goldberg et al., 2017).
9. **Use Teach-Back:** "We discussed the side effects or problems that you might have from the epidural medicine that you are receiving. Which effects should you tell me about?" Revise your instruction now or develop a plan for revised patient/family caregiver teaching if patient/family caregiver is not able to teach back correctly.	Determines patient's/family caregiver's level of understanding of instructional topic.

Unexpected Outcomes	Related Interventions
1. Patient states that pain is still present or has increased. Primary causes are insufficient drug dose or catheter blockage, breakage, or improper position.	• Check all tubing, connections, medication doses, and pump settings. • Confer with health care provider on adequacy of medication dose.
2. Patient is sedated or not easily aroused and/or experiences periods of apnea or respirations less than 8 breaths/min.	• Stop epidural infusion immediately and elevate patient's head of bed 30 degrees (unless contraindicated). *Stay with patient and call for help.* • Notify health care provider and prepare to administer opioid-reversing agent (e.g., naloxone) per health care provider's order (agency procedure manual may have protocol). • Monitor all vital signs, pulse oximetry, capnography, and sedation level continuously until patient is easily aroused and respiratory rate is 8 to 10 breaths/min with adequate depth for 2 hours.
3. Patient reports sudden headache. Clear drainage is present on epidural dressing, or more than 1 mL of fluid is aspirated from catheter.	• Stop infusion or bolus dosing. Stay with patient and call for help. • Notify health care provider.
4. Patient experiences minimal urinary output, urinary frequency or urgency, bladder distention, pruritus, or nausea and vomiting.	• Consult with health care provider about reducing dose of opioid and discuss treatment for side effects.

Recording

- Record drug name, dose, method of infusion (bolus, demand, or continuous), and time given (if bolus) or time begun and ended (if continuous or demand infusion) on appropriate MAR. Specify concentration and diluent.
- With continuous or demand infusion, obtain and record pump readout hourly for first 24 hours after infusion begins and then every 4 hours.
- Record regular periodic assessments of patient's status including vital signs, SpO_2 or end-tidal carbon dioxide, intake and output, sedation level, pain-severity score, neurological status, appearance of epidural site, presence or absence of side effects or adverse reactions to medication, and presence or absence of complications resulting from placement and maintenance of epidural catheter.
- Document your evaluation of patient learning.

Hand-Off Reporting

- Report the patient's pain-management plan, changes, responses, and most recent doses to aid in reducing medication errors (Sadule-Rios, 2017).
- The oncoming and outgoing nurse should inspect and agree with PCEA infusion pump programming/settings as a means of medication reconciliation (Kane-Gill et al., 2017).
- Include detailed information regarding vital signs, pulse oximetry and capnography, pain-assessment scores, STOP-BANG score for obstructive sleep apnea syndrome (OSAS) if done, Pasero Opioid Sedation Scale (POSS) sedation scores, level of consciousness, anxiety level, and activity level (Chou et al., 2016; Cooney, 2016; Meisenberg et al., 2017).

✦ SKILL 15.6 Local Anesthetic Infusion Pump for Analgesia

Purpose

The insertion of a small one-way catheter into a surgical site may be used for delivering a local anesthetic to maintain analgesia during and after surgery (Rawal, 2016). The catheter is usually secured to the skin with a surgical dressing such as Tegaderm and then attached to a portable infusion system (Fig. 15.3). The system delivers a local anesthetic agent (e.g., bupivacaine [Marcaine], lidocaine, ropivacaine [Naropin], or mepivacaine) so that it constantly "bathes" the specific nerve or nerve plexus responsible for pain at the surgical site. There are a variety of infusion pump systems, with most offering targeted pain relief (e.g., up to 5 days), with variable flow-rate settings and/or a patient-controlled bolus device (e.g., flow rate of 1–14 mL/hr and up to 5-mL on-demand bolus). Use of local anesthetic pumps can significantly decrease the amount of early postoperative pain; however, patients may still require oral analgesics, but the total oral dosage is often reduced (Chou et al., 2016; Cooney, 2016). Local infusion pumps are for one-time use only and usually remain in for a few days, allowing patients to control their postoperative pain at home. Patients and their family caregivers learn how to remove the catheter at home. The elastomeric pumps used for local anesthetic analgesia do not have alarms and should be monitored closely for failure such as early emptying of medication. All staff and patient and family caregivers should be given education on signs and symptoms and emergency management of local anesthetic toxicity (Chou et al., 2016). Nursing care also involves assessment of catheter site and connections and evaluation of local anesthetic side effects.

Delegation and Collaboration

The skill of managing local anesthetic infusion pump analgesia cannot be delegated to nursing assistive personnel (NAP). The nurse directs the NAP to:

- Pay close attention to the insertion site when providing care to avoid dislocation.
- Report if the dressing becomes moist; report any catheter disconnection immediately.
- Notify nurse immediately of a change in patient's status or level of comfort.

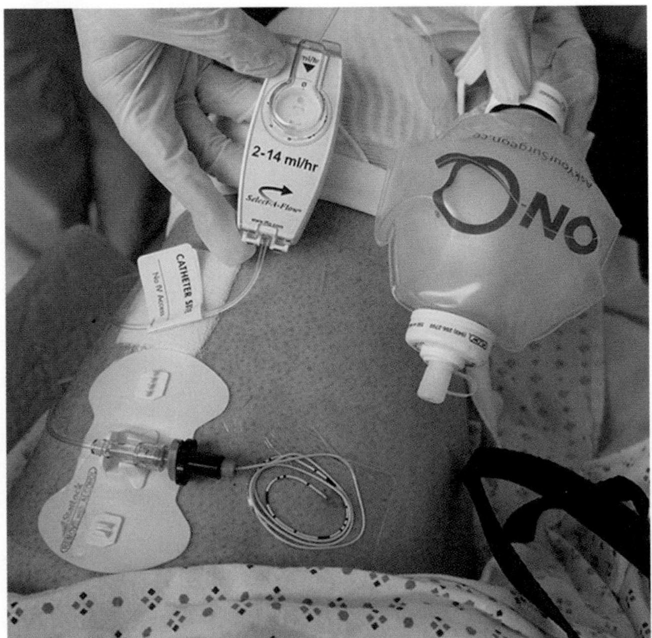

FIG 15.3 External epidural catheter attached to ambulatory infusion pump.

Equipment

- Pump in place from surgery

Home Catheter Removal

- Clean gloves
- Sterile 4 × 4–inch gauze pads
- Band-Aid
- Tape
- Plastic bag

ASSESSMENT

1. Identify patient using two identifiers (e.g., name and birthday or name and medical record number) according to agency policy. Compare identifiers with information on the patient's medication administration record (MAR) or medical record. *Rationale: Ensures correct patient. Complies with The Joint Commission standards and improves patient safety (TJC, 2019).*
2. Review surgeon's operative report for position of catheter. *Rationale: Confirms catheter location with your own observation.*
3. Perform hand hygiene, apply clean gloves, and assess surgical dressing and site of catheter insertion. Dressing should be dry and intact. *Rationale: Determines if catheter is placed properly.*
4. Be sure that catheter tubing is correctly labeled; then assess catheter connection. Be sure that it is secure. If catheter becomes detached, do *not* reattach or reinsert; instead notify surgeon immediately. *Rationale: Reattachment could lead to infection. Tubing misconnections could lead to infusion of inappropriate agents into surgical wound site.*
5. Perform a complete pain assessment (see Skill 15.1, Steps 2–9). *Rationale: Provides baseline to determine efficacy of analgesia.*
6. Read medication label on device and compare to MAR or health care provider's order. *Rationale: Provides information regarding type of anesthetic, concentration, volume, flow rate, and date and time prepared.*
7. Assess for presence of blood backing up in tubing. If blood is present, stop infusion and notify health care provider. Remove gloves and perform hand hygiene. *Rationale: Indicates possible displacement of catheter into blood vessel. Reduces transmission of microorganisms.*
8. Determine level of activity that patient can perform per health care provider's orders. *Rationale: Excessive activity can cause catheter displacement.*
9. Confirm patient's allergies (should be initially completed preoperatively and intraoperatively). Assess for signs of local anesthetic toxicity: central nervous system (CNS) excitement (e.g., oral numbness, metallic taste, dizziness or lightheadedness, drowsiness or disorientation, visual or auditory disturbances); cardiovascular signs and symptoms such as hypertension, tachycardia, bradycardia, cardiac arrhythmias, and asystole (Wadlund, 2017). *Rationale: Early*

identification of toxicity prevents or lessens possibility of complications. Although local anesthetic systemic toxicities are rare, systemic toxicity can occur in five categories: CNS, cardiovascular, hematologic, allergic, and local tissue responses. Signs and symptoms of toxicity usually involves the CNS or the cardiovascular system and can be potentially fatal (Wadlund, 2017).

10. Assess patient's or family caregiver's knowledge, experience, and health literacy level. *Rationale: Ensures patient has the capacity to obtain, communicate, process, and understand basic health information (CDC, 2016).*
11. Assess patient's and family caregiver's knowledge regarding purpose and duration of infusion. *Rationale: Determines extent of instruction required.*

STEP	RATIONALE
PLANNING	
1. Expected outcomes following completion of procedure:	
• Patient verbalizes full or partial relief from pain at surgical site.	Patient's self-report of pain is single most reliable indicator of pain.
• Patient achieves reduction of nonverbal behaviors indicative of pain, such as grimacing, clenching teeth, and rocking.	Nonverbal behaviors are valid and reliable indicators of pain in absence of self-report (Gallagher et al., 2017; Gélinas, 2016).
• Patient moves about in bed, sleeps and eats better, is more active, and communicates easily with family and friends.	Adequate pain relief allows patient to participate in activities of daily living (ADLs).
• Catheter is removed without injury to patient.	Patient and family caregiver correctly follow instructions for catheter removal.
2. Provide privacy.	Promotes patient comfort.
3. Set up equipment.	Organizes the work area in preparation for the procedure.
4. Position and drape patient as needed.	Ensures patient's comfort.
IMPLEMENTATION	
1. Perform hand hygiene. When repositioning or ambulating patient, use caution.	Avoids catheter dislodgement.
2. **Prepare patient for discharge**: Depending on type of pump, it may be necessary for you to connect the catheter to a smaller pump for use at home. One example is a pump about the size of a baby bottle. When pump is connected, balloon inside pump is full of medication, and plunger is all the way to the top. As medication infuses, balloon inside pump shrinks, and plunger goes down.	Easier pump management and visualization of medication infusion; smaller pumps are used when smaller drug reservoirs are sufficient in the home setting.
3. Teach the patient or family caregiver what to observe and how to remove catheter at home (may also be done by home health nurse). Provide educational materials (e.g., printed brochures, DVD, phone app accessibility). It is rare that the catheter and pump are removed in the hospital. Instructions for removal are as follows:	Visual and auditory materials help with comprehension and retention and serve as a review for patient and family caregiver when providing catheter care and monitoring for local anesthetic toxicity.
a. Explain how to perform hand hygiene and apply clean gloves.	Decreases transmission of microorganisms.
b. Have patient assume relaxed position in bed or chair with lower extremity in normal alignment.	Relaxes joint muscles, reducing traction from muscle tension, and provides distraction.
c. Apply clean gloves. Have patient or family caregiver gently lift adhesive dressing covering catheter insertion site and remove any remaining tape.	Exposes catheter insertion site.
d. Direct the patient or family caregiver to place 4 × 4–inch gauze over site, grasp catheter as close as possible to where it enters skin, and gently pull it out with steady motion. This will cause little discomfort or resistance, and a small amount of blood or fluid drainage is normal.	Prevents breakage of catheter.
e. Have patient or family caregiver look for mark on end of catheter tip. Hold new sterile gauze using pressure over the site for at least 2 minutes.	Indicates complete removal of catheter. Achieves hemostasis.
f. Wash skin to remove any surgical soap or adhesive near the site. Apply Band-Aid.	Cleanses insertion site.

STEP	RATIONALE
g. Place catheter in plastic bag using standard precautions. Remind patient to bring to health care provider's office at first follow-up visit. Remove and dispose of gloves; perform hand hygiene.	Catheter will be inspected by surgeon to ensure that no breakage occurred. Reduces transmission of microorganisms.
h. Explain to patient that any remaining numbness should go away within 24 hours after catheter is removed.	Allows patient and caregiver to anticipate progress and recognize problems.
4. Remind patient or family caregiver of follow-up appointment with surgeon.	Increases patient adherence.
5. Discharge per health care provider order and agency policy.	Verifies that all discharge planning steps were completed and that there is appropriate equipment for the patient at home.

EVALUATION

STEP	RATIONALE
1. Ask patient to rate pain intensity using appropriate scale at both rest and with activity.	Determines patient response to local infusion of medication.
2. Observe for signs of adverse drug reaction and report any signs immediately.	Local analgesics can result in systemic adverse effects if absorbed by veins (Wadlund, 2017).
3. Observe patient's position, mobility, relaxation, participation in ADLs, and any nonverbal behaviors.	Indicates successful pain management.
4. Inspect condition of surgical dressing.	Wet dressing indicates possible catheter migration out of wound, especially if drainage is clear.
5. During follow-up visit inspect catheter exit site.	Determines if area has healed without infection.
6. **Use Teach-Back:** "It is important for you to remove the catheter at home correctly. Explain to me the steps to take to remove the catheter." Revise your instruction now or develop a plan for revised patient/family caregiver teaching if patient/family caregiver is not able to teach back correctly.	Determines patient's/family caregiver's level of understanding of instructional topic.

Unexpected Outcomes	Related Interventions
1. Patient verbalizes pain intensity greater than previously determined goal or demonstrates nonverbal behaviors indicative of pain.	• Check reservoir for presence of medication. • Check patency of tubing. • Notify health care provider.
2. Patient reports symptoms of local anesthetic adverse reaction (bleeding, arrhythmias, weakness or numbness of affected area, seizure, confusion, infection, drowsiness, ringing in ears), possible hypersensitivity to local anesthetic, displacement of catheter into vein, or pump failure (releasing too much drug into site).	• Stop infusion (Wadlund, 2017). • Notify health care provider.

Recording

- Record drug, concentration, dose administered, type of demand feature (continuous or demand), additional analgesics needed to control pain, and any side effects or adverse reactions to local anesthetic.
- Record location of catheter, date catheter inserted, patient's pain rating, response to anesthetic, and additional comfort measures.
- Document your evaluation of patient learning.

Hand-Off Reporting

- Report damp dressing or displaced catheter to surgeon.
- Report the location of catheter, type of pump, type of medication, concentration, dose and time local analgesia initiated, patient bolus administration history, patient response, and any side effects or adverse reactions to local anesthetic (Wadlund, 2017).
- Report patient's pain-management plan, including additional comfort measures.
- The oncoming and outgoing nurse should inspect infusion pump programming as a means of medication reconciliation (Kane-Gill et al., 2017).
- Report patient's pain rating scores, vital signs, pulse oximetry and capnography, level of consciousness, anxiety level, and activity level (Chou et al., 2016; Cooney, 2016; Meisenberg et al., 2017).

✦ SKILL 15.7 Moist and Dry Heat Application

Purpose

Heat and cold therapies can be beneficial in promoting healing of wounds and soft tissue injuries. Moist heat is beneficial in increasing muscle and ligament flexibility; promoting relaxation and healing; and relieving spasm, joint stiffness, and pain (Table 15.1). Moist heat has many indications; however, it is most commonly used following the acute phase of a musculoskeletal injury and during and after childbirth, surgery, and superficial thrombophlebitis (Petrofsky et al., 2017a; Szekeres et al., 2017). Moist heat applications include warm compresses and commercial moist heat packs (Fig. 15.4), warm baths, soaks, and Sitz baths (Fig. 15.5). Dry heat is also used to reduce pain and increase healing by increasing blood flow in tissues and can be used at a low level for a longer period with little chance of tissue injury (Petrofsky et al., 2016). A water-flow pad (e.g., aquathermia pad), electric heating pads, and commercial dry heat packs (Fig. 15.6) are common forms of dry heat therapy. Both types of heat applications are advantageous to patients in relieving pain, improving range of motion (ROM), and facilitating healing. A nurse's primary responsibility is to know if a patient is at risk for injury from a heat application and how to apply heat safely (Table 15.2).

Delegation and Collaboration

The skill of applying dry or moist heat can be delegated to nursing assistive personnel (NAP). However, in most settings the nurse applies any sterile applications. The nurse must assess and evaluate the condition of the skin and tissues in the area that is treated and explain the purpose of the treatment. If there are risks or expected

TABLE 15.1
Temperature Ranges for Hot and Cold Applications

Temperature	Celsius Range	Fahrenheit Range
Warm	34°–37°	93°–98°
Tepid	26°–34°	80°–92°
Cool	18°–26°	65°–79°
Cold	10°–18°	50°–64°

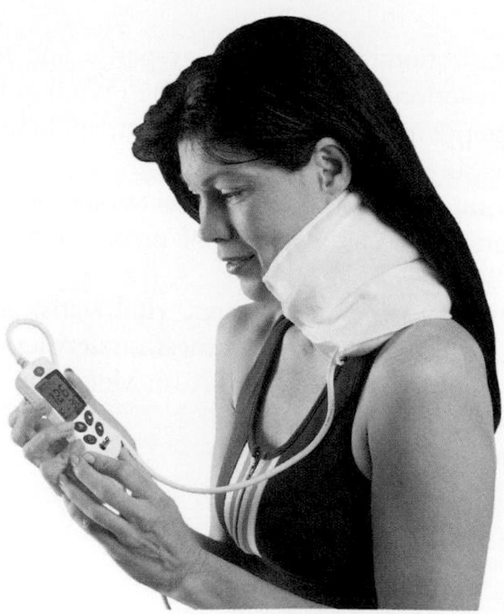

FIG 15.4 Digital moist heat pack. *(Image used with permission from Theratherm, Chattanooga, a DJO Company. All rights reserved.)*

TABLE 15.2
Pathophysiological Effects of Hot and Cold Applications

	Cold	Hot
Pain	↓	↓
Spasm	↓	↓
Metabolism	↓	↑
Blood flow	↓	↑
Inflammation	↓	↑
Edema	↓	↑
Extensibility	↓	↑

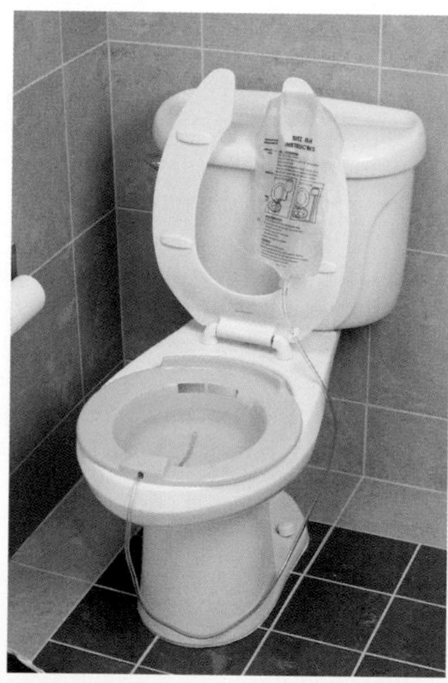

FIG 15.5 Disposable Sitz bath. *(Used with permission, Briggs Corporation.)*

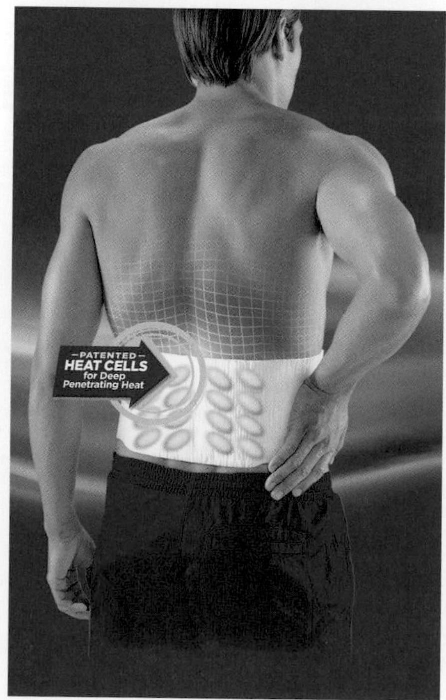

FIG 15.6 Dry heat wrap. *(Image used with permission, ThermaWrap, Pfizer Consumer Healthcare. All rights reserved.)*

complications, this skill cannot be delegated. The nurse instructs the NAP about:

- Proper temperature of the application.
- Skin changes to immediately report to the nurse (e.g., burning, blistering, or excessive redness).
- Specific patient complaints and changes in vital signs to immediately report to the nurse (e.g., pain, dizziness or light-headedness, increased or decreased pulse, decreased blood pressure).
- Specific requirements for positioning and application time based on agency policy and manufacturer instructions.
- Reporting when treatment is complete so that an evaluation of the patient's response can be made.

Equipment

All Moist Heat Applications

- Prescribed analgesia (if ordered)
- Dry bath towel, bath blanket
- Warmed prescribed solution (i.e., normal saline) or commercially prepared compress
- Biohazard waste bag
- Clean gloves
- Compress
- Clean basin
- Waterproof pad
- Ties or cloth tape
- Clean gauze or towel
- Options for moist heat application, depending on health care provider's order:
  - Sterile compress, sterile basin, sterile gauze, and sterile gloves
  - Disposable Sitz bath: prescribed solution and any topical medication after the soak

Dry Heat Applications

- Aquathermia pad and control unit or commercial chemical heat pack
- Distilled water (for aquathermia pad)
- Bath towel or pillowcase
- Ties, tape, or gauze roll

ASSESSMENT

1. Identify patient using at least two identifiers (e.g., name and birthday or name and medical record number) according to agency policy. *Rationale: Ensures correct patient. Complies with The Joint Commission standards and improves patient safety (TJC, 2019).*
2. Refer to health care provider's order for type of heat application, location and duration of application, and desired temperature (see Table 15.1) and agency policies regarding temperature. *Rationale: Ensures safe practice by verifying specific location for therapy and type and duration of heat application. Agency policy usually sets recommended temperature for aquathermia pad.*
3. Refer to patient's medical record to identify any contraindications to moist or dry heat application: unstable cardiac conditions, active bleeding, nitroglycerin or other therapeutic medicinal patch, acute inflammatory reactions, recent (less than 72 hours) musculoskeletal injury, and skin conditions such as eczema (see Table 15.2). *Rationale: Patients with certain cardiovascular conditions and who exhibit side effects of certain medications such as cardiac, hypertensive, and vasoactive medications may be at risk for sudden changes in blood pressure and blood flow caused by vasodilation. Heat causes vasodilation, which aggravates active bleeding, which can increase hemorrhage or bleeding into soft tissues adjacent to musculoskeletal injury (Cheung, 2017; Petrofsky et al., 2017b). Vasodilation increases rate of medication absorption when direct heat is applied over a medication patch.*
4. Perform hand hygiene, apply gloves, and assess condition of skin around area to be treated. Perform neurovascular assessments for sensitivity to temperature and pain by measuring light touch, pinprick, and temperature sensation (see Chapter 8). *Rationale: Certain conditions alter conduction of sensory impulses that transmit temperature and pain, predisposing patients to injury from heat applications. Patients with diminished sensation to heat or cold must be monitored closely during treatment.*

Safe Patient Care *Patients who are elderly or have diabetes mellitus, vascular diseases, paralysis, peripheral neuropathy, or rheumatoid arthritis or who are taking certain cardiovascular medications are at greater risk for thermal injury (Ratliff, 2017).*

5. When treating a wound, assess it for size, color, drainage volume, pain (using pain scale), and odor (this assessment may be deferred until dressing is removed and heat is applied). Remove and discard gloves; perform hand hygiene. *Rationale: Provides baseline to determine change in wound following heat application. Provides baseline for patient's comfort level.*
6. Ask patient to describe pain intensity on pain scale of 0 to 10. Assess ROM if patient is being treated for muscle sprain. *Rationale: Provides baseline to determine if pain relief or improved ROM is achieved following heat therapy.*
7. Assess patient's blood pressure and pulse. *Rationale: Establishes baseline to determine response to therapy.*
8. Assess patient's mobility: ability to align extremity for aquathermia pad application and ability to position self in Sitz bath and sit up from bath. *Rationale: Determines level of help needed to position patient for treatment.*
9. Assess patient's level of consciousness and responsiveness (e.g., confusion, disorientation, dementia). *Rationale: Patients with reduced level of consciousness are unable to sense or report reduced sensation or discomfort.*
10. Check electrical plugs and cords of aquathermia pad for obvious fraying or cracking. *Rationale: Prevents injury from accidental electrical shock.*
11. Assess patient's or family caregiver's knowledge, experience, and health literacy level. *Rationale: Ensures patient has the capacity to obtain, communicate, process, and understand basic health information (CDC, 2016).*

STEP	RATIONALE

PLANNING

1. Expected outcomes following completion of procedure:
   - Affected area is pink and warm to touch immediately after heat application. — Vasodilation increases blood flow to site.
   - After multiple moist heat applications, wound shows signs of healing (e.g., tissue granulation; reduced edema, inflammation, drainage). — Moist heat increases blood flow, enhances white blood cell infiltration, and removes waste products from cells (Chatterjee, 2017).
   - Patient denies burning sensation. — Indicates temperature applied appropriately.

Safe Patient Care *Note that in some situations heat applications cause pain signals to be overridden and decrease pain perception in cerebral cortex (Wu et al., 2017).*

   - Patient reports measurable increased mobility and ROM and decrease in pain in affected region. — Superficial heat increases joint mobility by increasing connective tissue extensibility and reducing pain and tissue viscosity (Petrofsky et al., 2017a; Szekeres et al., 2017). Heat used in conjunction with physical therapy and/or exercise improves function and mobility (Szekeres et al., 2017).
   - Blood pressure and pulse are within patient's normal range. — No systemic vascular changes occur. Goal of therapy is to achieve localized vascular response.
   - Patient is able to self-apply therapy safely. — Measures level of learning; necessary for home care.
2. Provide privacy. — Promotes patient comfort.
3. Prepare and organize equipment. — Prevents unnecessary delays in procedure.
4. Position patient in bed, keeping affected body part in proper alignment. Expose body part to be covered with heat application and drape patient with bath blanket or towel as need. — Limited mobility in uncomfortable position causes muscular stress. Draping prevents cooling.
5. Place waterproof pad under patient (exception: do not do this with Sitz bath or commercial heat pad). — Protects bed linen from moisture and soiling.
6. Explain steps of procedure and purpose to patient. Describe sensation that patient will feel, such as warmth and wetness. Explain precautions to prevent burning. — Minimizes patient's anxiety and promotes relaxation during procedure.
7. Provide patient and family caregiver education materials regarding heat therapy. — Educational materials guide patients and family caregivers when using heat therapy at home.

IMPLEMENTATION

1. Perform hand hygiene and apply clean gloves. — Reduces transmission of microorganisms.
2. **Apply moist sterile compress:**
   a. Heat prescribed solution to desired temperature by immersing closed bottle of solution in basin of very warm water. **DO NOT USE A MICROWAVE TO WARM SOLUTION.** — Prevents burns by ensuring proper temperature of solution.
   b. Prepare aquathermia pad if it is to be placed over compress. Temperature is usually preset by manufacturer or bioengineering. — Prevents burning by using proper temperature.
   c. Remove any present existing dressing covering wound. Inspect condition of wound and surrounding skin. Inflamed wound appears reddened, but surrounding skin is less red in color. Remove and place gloves and soiled dressing in biohazard bag and dispose per agency policy. — Reduces transmission of microorganisms. Provides baseline to measure wound healing.

Safe Patient Care *If skin surrounding wound is inflamed or reddened or has active bleeding or drainage, moist heat application may be contraindicated. Verify with health care provider.*

   d. Perform hand hygiene. — Reduces transmission of microorganisms.
   e. Prepare compress. — Use of appropriate aseptic technique keeps gauze compress clean or sterile. Sterile compress is needed when applied to open wound.
      (1) Pour warmed solution into container. **If sterile asepsis is required**, use sterile technique (see Chapter 5) to add sterile gauze into warmed sterile solution.

STEP	RATIONALE
(2) Open gauze. **If applying sterile compress,** open sterile supplies using sterile technique.	Sterile compress is needed when applied to open wound.
(3) **If sterile technique is NOT required,** immerse gauze into container of solution using clean aseptic technique.	
(4) If using commercially prepared compress, follow manufacturer instructions for warming.	Reduces chance of accidental burning.

Safe Patient Care *To avoid injury to a patient, test temperature of sterile solution by applying a drop to your forearm (without contaminating solution). It should feel warm to the skin without burning.*

STEP	RATIONALE
f. Apply sterile gloves if compress is sterile; otherwise apply clean gloves.	Allows you to manipulate sterile dressing and touch open wound.
g. Pick up one layer of immersed gauze, wring out any excess solution, and apply it lightly to wound; avoid surrounding unaffected skin. *Option:* Apply commercial compress or heat pack over wound only; only use with clean wounds.	Excess moisture macerates skin and increases risk for burns and infection. Skin is sensitive to sudden change in temperature.
h. After a few seconds, lift edge of gauze to assess for skin redness.	Increased redness indicates burn. Burns and injuries from hot therapies are preventable events.
i. If patient tolerates compress, pack gauze snugly against wound. Be sure to cover all wound surfaces with warm compress.	Packing compress prevents rapid cooling from ambient air currents.
j. Cover moist compress with dry sterile dressing and bath towel. If necessary, pin or tie in place. Remove and dispose of gloves and perform hand hygiene.	Dry sterile dressing prevents transfer of microorganisms to wound via capillary action caused by moist compress. Towel insulates compress to prevent heat loss.
k. *Option:* Apply aquathermia, commercial heat pack, or waterproof heating pad over towel. Keep it in place for desired duration of application. (See Step 4.)	Provides constant temperature to compress.
l. Leave compress in place for 20 minutes or less (per order or agency policy) and change warm compress using sterile technique every 5 to 10 minutes or as ordered during duration of therapy.	Maintains constant temperature for best therapeutic benefit. Moist heat promotes transfer of heat to underlying subcutaneous tissues, which helps reduce thermal injury to skin (Petrofsky et al., 2017b). Time limits with higher temperatures prevent risk of overexposure and injury to underlying skin.
m. After prescribed time, perform hand hygiene and apply clean gloves. Remove pad, towel, and compress. Evaluate wound and condition of skin and replace dry sterile dressing (using sterile gloves) as ordered.	Continued exposure to moisture macerates skin. Prevents entrance of microorganisms into wound site.
3. **Sitz bath or warm soak to intact skin or wound:**	
a. Remove any existing dressing covering wound. Remove and dispose of gloves and dressings in proper receptacle and perform hand hygiene.	Reduces transmission of microorganisms.
b. Inspect condition of wound and surrounding skin. Pay particular attention to suture line.	Provides baseline to determine response to warm soak.
c. When exudate or drainage is present, apply a new pair of clean gloves and clean intact skin around open area with clean cloth and soap and water. Sterile gloves and gauze may be needed to clean open wound (check agency policy). Dispose of gloves and perform hand hygiene.	Cleaning removes organisms so that bath solution does not spread infection.
d. Fill Sitz bath or bathtub in bathroom with warmed solution (see Fig. 15.5). Check temperature (check agency policy). *Option:* If using bag of normal saline, warm per agency policy.	Ensures proper temperature and reduces risk for burns.
e. Assist patient to bathroom to immerse body part in Sitz bath, bathtub, or basin. Cover patient with bath blanket or towel once position is achieved.	Prevents falls. Covering patient prevents heat loss through evaporation and maintains constant temperature.
f. Assess heart rate. Make sure that patient does not feel light-headed or dizzy and that nurse call system is within reach.	Provides baseline to determine if vascular response to vasodilation occurs during treatment.

STEP	RATIONALE
g. After 15 to 20 minutes remove patient from soak or bath; dry body parts thoroughly. (Wear clean gloves.)	Avoids chilling. Enhances patient's comfort.
h. Assist patient to preferred comfortable position.	Maintains patient's comfort.
i. Drain solution from basin or tub. Clean and place in proper storage area according to agency policy. Dispose of soiled linen.	Reduces transmission of microorganisms.
4. Aquathermia heating pad:	
a. Cover or wrap area to be treated with single layer of bath towel or enclose pad with pillowcase.	Prevents heated surface from touching patient's skin directly and increasing risk for injury to patient's skin.

Safe Patient Care *Do not pin wrap to pad because this may cause a leak in the device.*

STEP	RATIONALE
b. Place pad over affected area and secure with tape, tie, or gauze as needed (see illustration).	Pad delivers dry, warm heat to injured tissues. Pad should not slip onto different body part.

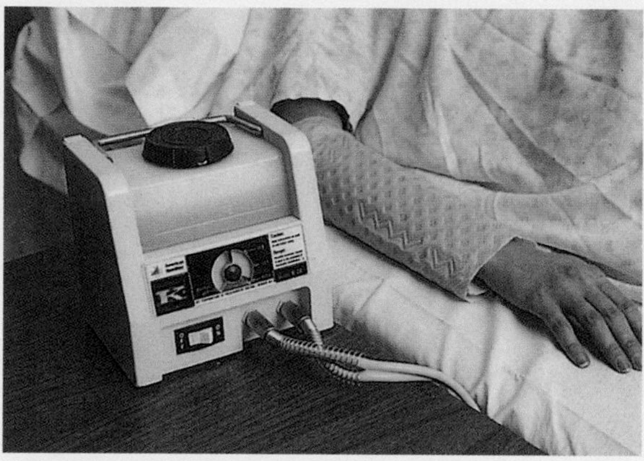

STEP 4b Aquathermia pad.

STEP	RATIONALE
c. Turn on aquathermia unit and check temperature setting. **NOTE:** Temperature of unit is usually set by agency's bioengineering department.	Prevents exposure of patient to temperature extremes.
d. Monitor condition of skin over site every 5 minutes and ask patient about sensation of burning.	Determines if heat exposure is causing any burn, blistering, or injury to underlying skin.
e. After no more than 20 minutes (or time ordered by health care provider), perform hand hygiene, apply clean gloves, and remove pad and store.	Heat therapy may reduce pain and spasm and increase blood flow and compliance of soft tissue structures (Petrofsky et al., 2017a).
5. Apply commercially prepared heat pack.	
a. Break pouch inside larger pack (follow manufacturer guidelines).	Activates chemicals within pack to warm outer surface.

Safe Patient Care *Never position patient so that he or she is lying directly on heating device. This position prevents dissipation of heat and increases risk for burns.*

STEP	RATIONALE
b. Monitor condition of skin over site every 5 minutes and ask patient about sensation of burning.	Determines if heat exposure is causing any burn, blistering, or injury to underlying skin.
c. After no more than 20 minutes (or time ordered by health care provider), perform hand hygiene, apply clean gloves, and remove pad and store.	Heat therapy may reduce pain and spasm and increase blood flow and compliance of soft tissue structures (Petrofsky et al., 2017a).
6. Remove and dispose of any remaining equipment and gloves; perform hand hygiene.	Reduces transmission of microorganisms.
7. Help patient return to preferred comfortable position.	Promotes patient comfort.
8. Raise side rails (as appropriate) and lower to lowest position. Place nurse call system within easy access.	Patient safety precautions.

STEP	RATIONALE

EVALUATION

1. Inspect condition of body part or wound; observe skin integrity, color, and temperature, and note any dryness, edema, blistering, or sensitivity to touch.	Evaluates effectiveness of heat application and whether there is presence of injury.
2. Obtain blood pressure and pulse; compare with baseline.	Determines if systemic vascular response to vasodilation has occurred.
3. Ask patient to describe level of comfort on pain scale of 0 to 10. Ask about any sensation of burning following treatment.	Determines if patient was exposed to temperature extreme, resulting in burn. Evaluates patient's subjective response to therapy.
4. Evaluate ROM of affected body part.	Determines if edema or muscle spasm is relieved.

Safe Patient Care *Do not have patient actively exercise muscle to evaluate results of therapy. Active exercise can aggravate muscle strain.*

5. **Use Teach-Back:** "I want to be sure you understand how to apply a warm moist compress so that you can do this at home. Show me how you would apply this compress at home." Revise your instruction now or develop a plan for revised patient/family caregiver teaching if patient/family caregiver is not able to teach back correctly.	Determines patient's/family caregiver's level of understanding of instructional topic.

Unexpected Outcomes	Related Interventions
1. Patient's skin is reddened and sensitive to touch during/after moist heat application, or patient complains of burning.	• Discontinue moist application immediately. • Verify proper temperature or check aquathermia device for proper functioning. • Notify health care provider and, if there is a burn, complete an incident or adverse event report (see agency policy).
2. Body part remains painful to move after dry heat application.	• Discontinue aquathermia pad or heat pack use. • Observe for localized swelling. • Notify health care provider.
3. Patient complains of increased discomfort.	• Reduce temperature of warm compress. • Assess for skin breakdown. • Notify health care provider.
4. Patient or family caregiver applies heat incorrectly or is unable to explain precautions.	• Reinstruct patient or family caregiver as necessary. Consider possible home health referral (if patient is eligible).

Recording

- Record and report type of application (solution, pad, or pack); location and duration of application; condition of body part, wound, or skin before and after treatment; and patient's response to therapy.
- Document your evaluation of patient learning.

Hand-Off Reporting

- Report the location and type of heat therapy, medication used (if ordered), duration and time of therapy, skin assessment, vital signs, pain assessment before and after therapy, patient response to therapy, and any adverse reactions.
- Report patient's heat therapy management plan.

✦ SKILL 15.8 Cold Application

Purpose

Cold therapy treats the localized inflammatory response of an injured body part that presents as edema, hemorrhage, muscle spasm, or pain (see Table 15.2). Improvement to joint mobility following cold therapy is related to reducing pain and swelling, inhibiting muscle spasm, and reducing muscle tension (Chatterjee, 2017; Quinlan et al., 2017). Cold therapy most commonly is used immediately after soft tissue and musculoskeletal injuries such as sprains or strains; however, it has been used in the postoperative setting with patients who have undergone orthopedic surgeries, spinal fusion, and lumbar discectomy (Quinlan et al., 2017). The most common cold therapy modalities used include cold compresses, ice packs, electrically controlled continuous-flow devices, and cold-water immersion athletic therapy (Chatterjee, 2017; Lindsay et al., 2016; Rigby and Dye, 2017). The most important nursing responsibilities in providing cold therapy include knowing a patient's risk for injury, understanding normal body responses to cold, assessing the integrity

TABLE 15.3

Characteristics of Heat and Cold Application

	Examples of Conditions	Precautions	Adverse Outcomes
Cold application	Immediately after direct trauma such as a sprain, strains, fractures, muscle spasms; after superficial lacerations or puncture wounds; after minor burns; chronic pain from arthritis, joint trauma; delayed-onset muscle soreness; inflammation	Circulatory insufficiency Cold allergy Diabetes mellitus	Cardiovascular effects (bradycardia) Raynaud's phenomenon Cold urticaria Nerve and tissue damage Slow wound healing Frostbite
Heat application	Inflamed or edematous body part; new surgical wound; infected wound; arthritis; degenerative joint disease; localized joint pain, muscle pain, muscle strains; low back pain; menstrual cramping; hemorrhoid, perianal, and vaginal inflammation; local abscess	Pregnancy Laminectomy sites Spinal cord Malignancy Vascular insufficiency Eyes, testes, heart	Burns Infections Increased pain Increased inflammation

of the body part to be treated, determining a patient's ability to sense temperature variations, and ensuring proper function of equipment (see Table 15.2).

Delegation and Collaboration

The skill of applying cold applications can be delegated to nursing assistive personnel (NAP) in special situations (see agency policy). The nurse must assess and evaluate the patient and explain the purpose of the treatment. If there are risks or possible complications, this skill is not delegated. The nurse instructs the NAP to:

- Keep the application in place for only the length of time specified in the health care provider's order.
- Immediately report to the nurse any excessive redness of the skin, increase in pain, or decrease in sensation.
- Report when treatment is complete so that a nurse can evaluate the patient's response.

Equipment

All Compresses, Bags, and Packs

- Clean gloves (if blood or body fluids are present)
- Cloth tape or ties or elastic wrap bandage
- Soft cloth cover: towel, pillowcase, or stockinette
- Bath towel or blanket and waterproof absorbent pad

Cold Compress

- Absorbent gauze (clean or sterile) folded to desired size
- Basin
- Prescribed solution at desired temperature

Ice Bag or Gel Pack

- Ice bag
- Ice chips and water or
- Reusable commercial gel pack (cold pack)
- Disposable commercial chemical cold pack

Electronically Controlled Cooling Device

- Cool-water flow pad or cooling pad and electrical pump
- Gauze roll or elastic wrap

ASSESSMENT

1. Identify patient using at least two identifiers (e.g., name and birthday or name and medical record number) according to agency policy. *Rationale: Ensures correct patient. Complies with The Joint Commission standards and improves patient safety (TJC, 2019).*
2. Refer to health care provider's order for type, location, and duration of application. Temperature of cooling pad will be ordered or preset (Table 15.3). *Rationale: Health care provider's order is required for all cold applications.*
3. Review medical history for conditions that contraindicate use of cold therapy: peripheral vascular diseases (e.g., Raynaud's disease, Buerger's disease), diabetic neuropathy, rheumatoid arthritis, frostbite. *Rationale: These conditions increase risk for skin and tissue injury when exposed to cold.*
4. Perform hand hygiene and inspect condition of injured or affected part. Gently palpate area for edema (apply clean gloves if there is risk of exposure to body fluids). *Rationale: Provides baseline for determining change in condition of injured tissues. Reduces transmission of microorganisms.*

Safe Patient Care *Keep injured part in alignment and immobilized. Movement can cause further injury to strains, sprains, or fractures.*

5. Assess patient's level of consciousness and responsiveness. *Rationale: Patients with reduced level of consciousness are unable to sense or report reduced sensation or discomfort.*
6. Perform neurovascular check and inspect surrounding skin for integrity, circulation (presence of pulses), color, temperature, and sensitivity to touch (see Chapter 8). *Rationale: Determines if patient is insensitive to cold extremes, which increases risk for injury.*
7. Consider time elapsed since injury occurred. *Rationale: Apply cold therapy as soon as possible after injury to reduce swelling, inflammation, tissue bleeding, and pain (Chatterjee, 2017; Quinlan et al., 2017).*
8. Ask patient to describe character of pain and rate severity on scale of 0 to 10 (or other pain scale when applicable) if able. Assess ROM of affected part if muscle sprain is involved. *Rationale: Provides baseline for determining pain relief and ROM with therapy.*
9. Assess patient's or family caregiver's knowledge, experience, and health literacy level. *Rationale: Ensures patient has the capacity to obtain, communicate, process, and understand basic health information (CDC, 2016).*

STEP	RATIONALE

PLANNING

STEP	RATIONALE
1. Expected outcomes following completion of procedure:	
• Affected area is slightly pale and cool to touch.	Result of vasoconstriction.
• There is decreased edema and/or bleeding in tissues at site of injury.	Cold reduces blood flow to affected part by reducing protein extravasation from vasculature and subsequent edema formation (Quinlan et al., 2017).
• Patient reports decreased pain as measured on scale of 0 to 10.	Cold decreases local swelling, reduces inflammatory response, and decreases nerve conduction and subsequent pain, creating localized analgesic effect (Codding and Getz, 2017).
• Patient's ROM increases.	Cold reduces swelling.
• Patient or family caregiver correctly states how to apply cold and provides demonstration.	Documents learning for home care.
2. Provide privacy and prepare environment.	Promotes comfort.
3. Position patient in bed, keeping affected body part in proper alignment. Expose body part to be covered with cold application and drape patient with bath blanket or towel as need.	Limited mobility in uncomfortable position causes muscular stress. Draping avoids unnecessary exposure of body parts, maintaining patient's comfort and privacy.
4. Explain procedure and precautions.	Improves likelihood of patient's adherence to therapy.
5. Provide patient and family caregiver education materials regarding cold therapy at home.	Educational materials guide patients and family caregivers when using cold therapy at home.

IMPLEMENTATION

STEP	RATIONALE
1. Perform hand hygiene and apply clean gloves.	Reduces transmission of microorganisms.
2. Place towel or absorbent pad under area that you will treat.	Prevents soiling of bed linen.
3. Apply cold compress:	
a. Place ice and water in basin and test temperature on inner aspect of your arm.	Extreme temperature can cause tissue damage.
b. Submerge gauze into basin filled with cold solution; wring out excess moisture.	Dripping gauze is uncomfortable to patient.
c. Apply compress to affected area, molding it gently over site.	Ensures that cold is directed over site of injury.
d. Remove, remoisten, and reapply to maintain temperature as needed.	
4. Apply ice pack or bag:	
a. Fill bag with water, secure cap, and invert.	Ensures that there are no leaks.
b. Empty water and fill bag two-thirds full with small ice chips and water.	Bag is easier to mold over body part when it is not full.
c. Express excess air from bag, secure bag closure, and wipe bag dry.	Excess air interferes with cold conduction. Allows bag to conform to area and promotes maximum contact.
d. Squeeze or knead commercial ice pack according to manufacturer's directions.	Releases alcohol-based solution to create cold temperature.
e. Wrap pack or bag with single layer of towel, pillowcase, or stockinette. Apply over injury. Secure with tape as needed. Always place a barrier (e.g., towel, pillowcase, ice pack covering) between cooling device and the patient's skin to avoid tissue injury.	Protects patient's tissue and absorbs condensation. Prevents direct exposure of cold against patient's skin.
5. Apply commercial gel pack:	
a. Remove from freezer.	
b. Wrap pack with towel, pillowcase, or stockinette. Apply pack directly over injury.	Protects patient's tissue and absorbs condensation. Prevents direct exposure of cold against patient's skin.
c. Secure with gauze, cloth tape, or ties as needed.	

Safe Patient Care *Do not reapply ice pack to red or bluish areas; continual use of ice pack makes ischemia worse.*

STEP	RATIONALE
6. Apply electrically controlled cooling device:	
a. Prepare device following manufacturer's directions. Some devices are gravity-fed and require you to manually fill with iced water. Motorized units circulate chilled water.	

STEP	RATIONALE
b. Make sure that all connections are intact and temperature, if adjustable, is set (see agency policy).	Ensures safe temperature application.
c. Wrap cool-water flow pad in single layer of towel or pillowcase.	Prevents adverse reactions from cold such as burn or frostbite.
d. Wrap cool pad around body part.	Ensures even application of cold temperature.
e. Turn device on and check correct temperature. (**NOTE:** Temperature is usually preset in health care settings [check agency policy].)	Ensures effective therapy. Preset temperature reduces risk of skin and tissue injury.
f. Secure with elastic wrap bandage, gauze roll, or ties.	Ensures cold is distributed to correct body part.
7. Remove and dispose of gloves in proper container. Perform hand hygiene.	Reduces transmission of microorganisms.
8. Check condition of skin every 5 minutes for duration of application.	Determines if there are adverse reactions to cold (e.g., mottling, redness, burning, blistering, numbness).
a. If area is edematous, sensation may be reduced; use extra caution during cold therapy and assess site more often.	
b. Numbness and tingling are common sensations with cold applications and indicate adverse reactions only when severe and coupled with other symptoms. Stop treatment when patient complains of burning sensation or skin begins to feel numb.	When applying cold, skin will initially feel cold, followed by relief of pain. As cryotherapy continues, patient will feel burning sensation, then pain in skin, and finally numbness.
9. After 20 minutes (or as ordered by health care provider), perform hand hygiene, apply clean gloves, remove compress or pad, and gently dry off any moisture.	Drying prevents maceration of skin.

Safe Patient Care *Areas with little body fat (e.g., knee, ankle, and elbow) do not tolerate cold as well as fatty areas (e.g., thigh and buttocks) do. For bony areas, decrease time of cold application to lower range.*

STEP	RATIONALE
10. Assist patient to comfortable position.	Maintains relaxing environment.
11. Raise side rails (as appropriate) and lower bed to lowest position.	Patient safety precaution.
12. Dispose of soiled linen, supplies, and equipment.	Reduces transmission of microorganisms.
13. Remove gloves and perform hand hygiene.	Reduces transmission of microorganisms.
14. Place nurse call system within reach and instruct patient in its use.	Patient safety precaution.

EVALUATION

STEP	RATIONALE
1. Inspect affected area for integrity, color, temperature, and sensitivity to touch. Reevaluate 30 minutes after procedure.	Determines reaction to cold application.
2. Palpate affected area gently and note any edema, bruising, and bleeding (apply gloves if there is risk of exposure to body fluids).	Determines level of improvement.
3. Ask patient to report pain level on scale of 0 to 10.	Determines if pain has been relieved.
4. Measure ROM of affected body part.	Determines if edema or muscle spasm is relieved.
5. **Use Teach-Back:** "I want to be sure you know how to apply an ice pack to your ankle. Show me how to apply an ice pack." Revise your instruction now or develop a plan for revised patient/family caregiver teaching if patient/family caregiver is not able to teach back correctly.	Determines patient's/family caregiver's level of understanding of instructional topic.

Unexpected Outcomes	Related Interventions
1. Skin appears mottled, reddened, or bluish as a result of exposure to cold.	Stop treatment. Notify health care provider.
2. Patient complains of burning pain and numbness.	Stop therapy. Notify health care provider.
3. Patient or family caregiver is unable to describe or demonstrate therapy.	Provide further instruction and/or demonstration.

Recording

- Record appearance and condition of skin and affected body part; type, location, and duration of application; and patient's response to therapy (including pain level assessment scores).
- Document your evaluation of patient and family caregiver learning.

Hand-Off Reporting

- Report any sensations of burning, numbness, or unrelieved pain or skin-color changes to health care provider.
- During hand-off to next shift, report the location and type of cold therapy, medication used (if ordered), duration and time of therapy, skin assessment, vital signs, pain assessment before and after therapy, patient response to therapy, and any adverse reactions.
- Report patient's cold therapy management plan and patient and family caregiver's understanding of therapy.

SPECIAL CONSIDERATIONS

Patient-Centered Care

- If patient is not English speaking, have a professional interpreter present or available.
- Family members or "ad hoc" interpreters may be helpful; however, the accuracy of medical information may be lower than what a professional interpreter can offer (Terui, 2017).
- Use a behavioral pain-assessment tool and input from family caregiver for a patient unable to self-report (Chou et al., 2016).
- The involvement of family caregivers and the use of appropriate pain-assessment tools are essential to successful pain-management outcomes in the home setting.
- Provide effective, equitable, understandable, and respectful quality care and services that are responsive to diverse cultural health beliefs and practices, preferred languages, health literacy, and other communication needs (Narayan, 2017).
- Knowledge and attitudes about pain management play an important role in improving the patient experience in successful pain management (Shindul-Rothschild et al., 2017). Knowledge of pain-management principles also facilitates patient-centered care by empowering patients to engage in their plan to achieve maximum pain relief. It is critical that you assess each patient with open-mindedness, without incorporating personal cultural norms.

Patient Education

- Choose pain-assessment scales that are consistent with the educational and health literacy levels of the patient and family caregiver (Chang et al., 2017).
- Explain to patient and family caregiver the behavioral changes that may result from pain (e.g., change in activity level, splinting a body part, decreased social interaction).
- Ask patient and family caregiver about fear of addiction, a common primary concern, or other misconceptions that could undermine the patient's pain relief.
- Teach patients and family caregivers the purpose, action, and signs and symptoms of adverse reactions to opioids or local anesthetics and when to report to a nurse.
- Provide patients and family caregivers information about non-pharmacological pain-management strategies that supplement or enhance pharmacological intervention. Information should include purpose, rationale for how pain is relieved, how to use therapy, and how patient can maximize benefits.

Age-Specific

Pediatric

- Adapt distraction strategies to a child's developmental level (e.g., use a pacifier for an infant; offer reading or playing a recording of a favorite story for a preschooler; and use breathing techniques [e.g., Hey Hu technique], music, virtual reality games, and books with earphones for a teenager; Bukola and Paula, 2017).
- Infants have an unstable temperature-control mechanism; mottling of extremities is common and does not always indicate an adverse reaction to cold. Monitor any cold application carefully every 5 minutes (Hockenberry, 2017).
- It may be difficult for younger children (aged 3–4 years) to use self-report scales effectively because they may lack developmental skills associated with awareness of internal states, processing and matching, estimating quantity and quality, and the ability to talk to a stranger (Emmott et al., 2017).
- Studies report that when using a faces pain-rating scale, younger children between the ages of 4 and 7 find it easier to distinguish between two to three faces to report their pain intensity instead of six (Emmott et al., 2017; Quinn et al., 2014).

Gerontological

- Visual, auditory, mobility impairments; emotional disorders; and behavioral changes affect the ability of older adults to use pain-intensity tools (Booker and Herr, 2016; Chang et al., 2017). Ensure that glasses, hearing aids, and other assistive devices are in place.
- Reminiscence (e.g., sharing stories from the past) is an effective form of distraction in older adults.
- Older-adult patients are at a higher risk for local anesthetic systemic toxicity (LAST) because of co-morbidities such as decreased systemic blood flow and liver function, cardiovascular disease, and renal insufficiency. Signs and symptoms of LAST may appear 30 seconds to 60 minutes after injection, but they typically appear within 1 to 5 minutes (Wadlund, 2017).
- It is important to monitor for tissue damage with hot and cold applications. Absorption of topical medications can be affected as well due to dryness and thinning of the older adult's epidermal layer (Marcum et al., 2016).
- Because of renal and liver decline, maximum daily dosages of acetaminophen (Tylenol) may need to be lower.
- If an older adult is cognitively impaired and had a procedure that usually causes pain, consult with the health care provider about ordering an appropriate analgesic ATC instead of prn.

Home Care

- Consider patient's home living conditions, such as the type of bed and environmental stimuli. A supportive bed and quiet environment enhance sleep and promote pain management.
- Assess the physical environment of the home (see Chapter 32) to determine the adequacy of facilities for the use of heat therapy.
- Assess the availability of a family caregiver to help patient in application of hot or cold therapy as well as his or her willingness to remain with patient. Provide instruction and evaluate understanding of the procedure.
- Teach and provide information to patients and family caregivers about the skills involved in pain assessment, nonpharmacological management, hot and cold therapy, and pharmacological management that will be performed at home.
- Teach patient and family caregiver to reassess pain after a medication is given at predetermined times: (1) at the onset of action of pain relief, (2) during the peak analgesic effect, and (3) at

the time when medication levels are lowest (i.e., generally 4–6 hours after administration; Booker and Herr, 2016). Family caregivers need to know how to observe and recognize pain in the person they care for and to accept and acknowledge the patient's report of pain.

- If patients need opioid therapy at home, teach signs and symptoms of adverse effects, such as respiratory depression, and give written instructions on the use of an opioid-reversing agent (e.g., naloxone) in the case of respiratory depression, especially with patients who have a history of opioid addiction (Kampman and Jarvis, 2015).
- Provide written instructions regarding possible adverse reactions to the local anesthetic bupivacaine (Marcaine) that patient should report to surgeon immediately: (e.g., CNS: oral numbness, metallic taste, dizziness or light-headedness, drowsiness or disorientation, visual or auditory disturbances; cardiovascular: hypertension, tachycardia, bradycardia, cardiac arrhythmias; Wadlund, 2017).
- When PCA is administered at home, teach patient and family caregiver aseptic technique for medication administration and for all catheter care procedures, including dressing changes. Instruct them to change dressing every week (see home health agency policy). Teach signs and symptoms of infection and what to report and when to the nurse or health care provider.
- Provide a list of all supplies needed for procedures, where to purchase them, and phone numbers of health care providers to contact in emergency.
- *If patient has pruritus from anesthetic agent:* Advise patient to wear clean, lightweight cotton clothing; keep room cool; use cool moist compresses; and lubricate skin.
- If an older adult is frail and has a cardiac condition, monitor vital signs throughout a heat application.

✦ PRACTICE REFLECTIONS

Imagine yourself in a busy urgent care clinic. The patient you are admitting is an older-adult female who is confused to time and place and incoherent in her speech. She is accompanied by her husband, who is her family caregiver. He states that he found her lying on the kitchen floor. She is distraught and appears to be in pain, and she is stooped over, with her hand guarding the left lower quadrant of her abdomen.

1. What are some of the challenges faced in caring for this patient?
2. What do you feel is the best way to start your assessment to find the origin of her pain?
3. What types of pain-assessment tools do you think you should choose in this situation?

✦ CLINICAL REVIEW QUESTIONS

1. A patient with a patient-controlled analgesia (PCA) pump tells the nurse that he must be allergic to the pain medication because he is itching and feels nauseated. Which statement made by the nurse is correct? (Select all that apply.)
   1. "This is not an allergic reaction, but I will assess you further to be sure you have no other symptoms of concern."
   2. "Itching and nausea are not an allergic reaction but are side effects of your pain medication."
   3. "The itching and nausea will subside as the pain medicine reaches the adequate blood level to control your pain."
   4. "The machine is set to deliver medication only if you need it, so your itching and nausea must be related to another cause."
   5. "It's important not to scratch, because that will make the itching worse."
2. A client with chronic pain is being treated with opioid administration via the epidural route. The nurse checks the patient to find him sedated and not easily aroused. The nurse knows that oversedation occurs before respiratory depression. Given the situation, prioritize the following list of initial nursing interventions that should be taken:
   - _____ a. Assess vital signs, oxygen saturation, and/or capnography.
   - _____ b. Evaluate the amount of opioid delivered within the past 4 to 6 hours.
   - _____ c. Stop the PCA.
   - _____ d. Prepare to administer the opioid-reversing agent naloxone (Narcan).
   - _____ e. Notify health care provider.
   - _____ f. Elevate head of bed 30 degrees unless contraindicated.
   - _____ g. If able, instruct patient to take deep breaths.
   - _____ h. Apply oxygen at 2 L/min per nasal cannula (if ordered).
3. A patient with musculoskeletal pain has been ordered to receive dry heat therapy. Read the following statement and answer whether it is true or false: The application of heat to an affected body part allows for pain relief, reduces muscle spasms, and facilitates healing through vasoconstriction of the vessels.
   1. True
   2. False

Answers and Rationales for Clinical Review Questions can be found on the Evolve website.

REFERENCES

American Nurses' Association: Position statement: the ethical responsibility to manage pain and the suffering it causes, 2018. https:/www.nursingworld.org/~495e9b/globalassets/docs/ana/ethics/theethicalresponsibilitytomanagepainandthesufferingitcauses2018.pdf.

American Society of Addiction Medicine: National practice guideline for the use of medications in the treatment of addiction involving opioid use, 2015. https://www.asam.org/docs/default-source/practice-support/guidelines-and-consensus-docs/asam-national-practice-guideline-supplement.pdf.

American Society of Clinical Oncology (ASCO): ASCO issues new guideline on chronic pain management in adult cancer survivors, 2016. https://www.asco.org/about-asco/press-center/news-releases/asco-issues-new-guideline-chronic-pain-management-adult-cancer.

American Society of Pain Management Nursing: Position statement: prescribing and administering opioid doses based solely on pain intensity, 2016. http://www.aspmn.org/Pages/ASPMNPositionStatements.aspx.

Argoff CE, et al: Consensus recommendations on initiating prescription therapies for opioid-induced constipation, *Pain Med* 16(12):2324, 2015.

Association of periOperative Registered Nurses: AORN guideline at a glance: moderate sedation/analgesia, *AORN J* 105(6):638, 2017.

Baker S, et al: Musculoskeletal pain and co-morbid insomnia in adults: a population study of the prevalence and impact on restricted social participation, *BMC Fam Pract* 18(1):17, 2017.

Ballantyne JC, Sullivan MD: Intensity of chronic pain: the wrong metric?, *N Engl J Med* 373(22):2098, 2015.

Bhattarai P, Phillips JL: The role of digital health technologies in management of pain in older people: an integrative review, *Arch Gerontol Geriatr* 68:14, 2017.

Boitor M, et al: Evaluation of the preliminary effectiveness of hand massage therapy on postoperative pain of adults in the intensive care unit after cardiac surgery: a pilot randomized controlled trial, *Pain Manage Nurs* 16(3):354, 2015.

Booker SQ, Herr KA: Assessment and measurement of pain in adults in later life, *Geriatr Pain Manage* 3(4):677, 2016.

Botti M, et al: Cross-cultural examination of the structure of the revised American Pain Society Patient Outcome Questionnaire (APS-POQ-R), *J Pain* 16(8):727, 2015.

Bouzat P, et al: Chest trauma: first 48hours management, *Anaesth Crit Care Pain Med* 36(2):135, 2017.

Bukola I, Paula D: The effectiveness of distraction as procedural pain management technique in pediatric oncology patients: a meta-analysis and systematic review, *J Pain Symptom Manage* 54(4):589, 2017.

Burton A, Shaw R: Pain management programmes for non-English-speaking black and minority ethnic groups with long-term or chronic pain, *Musculoskeletal Care* 13(4):187, 2015.

Centers for Disease Control and Prevention (CDC): What is health literacy?, 2016. https://www.cdc.gov/healthliteracy/learn/index.html.

Chang HC, et al: Evaluation of pain intensity assessment tools among elderly patients with cancer in Taiwan, *Cancer Nurs* 40(4):269, 2017.

Chatterjee R: Elbow pain: the 10-minute assessment, *Co-Kinetic J* 73:18, 2017.

Chou R, et al: Management of postoperative pain: a clinical practice guideline from the American Pain Society, the American Society of Regional Anesthesia and Pain Medicine, and the American Society of Anesthesiologists' Committee on Regional Anesthesia, Executive Committee, and Administrative Council, *J Pain* 17(2):131, 2016.

ClinCalc.com: Equivalent opioid calculator, 2018. http://clincalc.com/Opioids/.

Codding J, Getz C: Pain management strategies in shoulder arthroplasty, *Orthop Clin North Am* 49:81, 2017.

Coluzzi F, et al: The challenge of perioperative pain management in opioid-tolerant patients, *Ther Clin Risk Manag* 13:1163, 2017.

Cooney MF: Postoperative pain management: clinical practice guidelines, *J Perianesth Nurs* 31(5):445, 2016.

Curtin KB, Norris D: The relationship between chronic musculoskeletal pain, anxiety and mindfulness: adjustments to the Fear-Avoidance Model of Chronic Pain, *Scand J Pain* 17:156, 2017.

Davis C, et al: A multisite retrospective study evaluating the implementation of the Pasero Opioid-Induced Sedation Scale (POSS) and its effect on patient safety outcomes, *Pain Manage Nurs* 18(4):193, 2017.

Drake G, Williams AC: Nursing education interventions for managing acute pain in hospital settings: a systematic review of clinical outcomes and teaching methods, *Pain Manage Nurs* 18(1):3, 2017.

Emmott A, et al: Validity of simplified versus standard self-report measures of pain intensity in preschool-aged children undergoing venipuncture, *J Pain* 18(5):564, 2017.

Fitzgerald S: CDC report: opioid prescribing declined but not nearly enough alternative pain management strategies are needed, experts say, *Neurol Today* 17(15):1, 2017.

Gallagher E, et al: Cancer-related pain assessment: monitoring the effectiveness of interventions, *Clin J Oncol Nurs* 21(3):8, 2017.

Gélinas C: Pain assessment in the critically ill adult: recent evidence and new trends, *Intensive Crit Care Nurs* 34:1, 2016.

Gokay P, et al: Is there a difference between the STOP-BANG and the Berlin Obstructive Sleep Apnoea Syndrome questionnaires for determining respiratory complications during the perioperative period?, *J Clin Nurs* 25(9–10):1238, 2016.

Goldberg S, et al: Practical management of a regional anesthesia-driven acute pain service, *Adv Anesth* 35:191, 2017.

Greene Naples J, et al: The role of opioid analgesics in geriatric pain management, *Clin Geriatr Med* 32(4):725, 2016.

Groves PS, et al: Priming patient safety through nursing handoff communication: a simulation pilot study, *West J Nurs Res* 39(11):1394, 2017.

Hatcher J: Manual therapy student handbook: assessment and treatment of the ankle and foot, *Co-Kinetic Journal* 71:34, 2017.

He Q, et al: Impact of epidural analgesia on quality of life and pain in advanced cancer patients, *Pain Manage Nurs* 16(3):307, 2015.

Hirsch J, et al: Pain and depressive symptoms in primary care: moderating role of positive and negative affect, *Clin J Pain* 32(7):562, 2016.

Hockenberry MJ: *Wong's essentials of pediatric nursing*, ed 10, St. Louis, 2017, Mosby.

Houzé B, et al: Efficacy, tolerability, and safety of non-pharmacological therapies for chronic pain: an umbrella review on various CAM approaches, *Prog Neuropsychopharmacol Biol Psychiatry* 79(Pt b):192, 2017.

Institute for Safe Medication Practices: Accidental overdoses involving fluorouracil infusions, 2015. https://www.ismp.org/resources/accidental-overdoses-involving-fluorouracil-infusions.

Institute of Medicine: Relieving pain in America: a blueprint for transforming prevention, care, education, and research, 2011. http://nationalacademies.org/hmd/reports/2011/relieving-pain-in-america-a-blueprint-for-transforming-prevention-care-education-research.aspx.

International Organization for Standardization (ISO): Small bore connectors for liquids and gases in healthcare applications—part 6: connectors for neuraxial applications, ISO 80369-6:2016. https://www.iso.org/standard/50734.html.

Kampman K, Jarvis M: American Society of Addiction Medicine (ASAM) national practice guideline for the use of medications in the treatment of addiction involving opioid use, *J Addict Med* 5:358, 2015.

Kane-Gill S, et al: Clinical practice guideline: safe medication use in the ICU, *Crit Care Med* 45(9):e877, 2017.

Lacy BE, et al: Bowel disorders, *Gastroenterology* 150(6):1393, 2016.

Laidlaw TM, Cahill KN: Current knowledge and management of hypersensitivity to aspirin and NSAIDs, *J Allergy Clin Immunol Pract* 5(3):537, 2017.

Lesiuk T: The effect of mindfulness-based music therapy on attention and mood in women receiving adjuvant chemotherapy for breast cancer: a pilot study, *Ocol Nurs Forum* 42(3):276, 2015.

Li J, et al: The effects of music intervention on burn patients during treatment procedures: a systematic review and meta-analysis of randomized controlled trials, *BMC Complement Altern Med* 17(1):158, 2017.

Lindsay A, et al: Repetitive cryotherapy attenuates the in vitro and in vivo mononuclear cell activation response, *Exp Physiol* 101:851, 2016.

Liperoti R, et al: The present and future: herbal medications in cardiovascular medicine, *J Am Coll Cardiol* 69:1188, 2017.

Lourens GB: Complications associated with epidural catheter analgesia, *Nurse Pract* 41(10):12, 2016.

MacPherson H, et al: Acupuncture for chronic pain and depression in primary care: a programme of research, 2017. Southampton, UK, NIHR Journals Library (Programme Grants for Applied Research No. 5.3.), https://www.ncbi.nlm.nih.gov/books/NBK409491.

Mandrack M, et al: Nursing best practices using automated dispensing cabinets: nurses' key role in improving medication safety, *Medsurg Nurs* 21(3):134, 2012.

Marcum ZA, et al: Pharmacotherapies in geriatric chronic pain management, *Clin Geriatr Med* 32(4):705, 2016.

Masato H, et al: Prophylactic pentazocine reduces the incidence of pruritus after cesarean delivery under spinal anesthesia with opioids: a prospective randomized clinical trial, *Anesth Analg* 124(6):1930, 2017.

Mattox E: Complications of peripheral venous access devices: prevention, detection, and recovery strategies, *Crit Care Nurse* 37(2):e1, 2017.

Meisenberg B, et al: Implementation of solutions to reduce opioid-induced oversedation and respiratory depression, *Am J Health Syst Pharm* 74(3):162, 2017.

Nagappa M, et al: Opioids, respiratory depression and sleep-disordered breathing, *Best Pract Res Clin Anaesthesiol* 2017. http://www.sciencedirect.com/science/article/pii/S1521689617300216. published online.

Nahin RL: Estimates of pain prevalence and severity in adults: United States, 2012, *J Pain* 16(8):769, 2015.

Narayan MC: Strategies for implementing the national standards for culturally and linguistically appropriate services (CLAS) in home health care, *Health Care Manage Pract* 29(3):168, 2017.

National Academies of Sciences, Engineering, and Medicine: Pain management and the opioid epidemic: balancing societal and individual benefits and risks of prescription opioid use, 2017. https://www.nap.edu/resource/24781/Highlights_071317_Opioids.pdf.

National Academy of Medicine (NAM): *First do no harm: marshaling clinician leadership to counter the opioid epidemic*, Washington DC, 2017, Author.

National Center for Complementary and Integrative Health (NCCIH): 2016 strategic plan, 2016. https://nccih.nih.gov/sites/nccam.nih.gov/files/NCCIH_2016_Strategic_Plan.pdf.

National Comprehensive Cancer Network (NCCN): NCCN guidelines, version 2.2017: adult cancer pain, 2017. https://www.nccn.org/professionals/physician_gls/pdf/pain.pdf.

National Guideline Clearinghouse: Pain management for blunt thoracic trauma: a joint practice management guideline from the Eastern Association for the Surgery of Trauma and Trauma Anesthesiology Society, 2016. Rockville, MD, Agency for Healthcare Research and Quality, https://www.guideline.gov.

Nelson NL, Churilla JR: Massage therapy for pain and function in patients with arthritis: a systematic review of randomized controlled trials, *Am J Phys Med Rehabil* 96(9):665, 2017.

Ostby PL, Armer JM: Complexities of adherence and post-cancer lymphedema management, *J Pers Med* 5(4):370, 2015.

Pasero C: Unconventional use of a PCA pump: nurse-activated dosing, *J Perianesth Nurs* 30(1):68, 2015.

Pasero C, et al: American Society for Pain Management Nursing position statement: prescribing and administering opioid doses based solely on pain intensity, *Pain Manage Nurs* 17(3):170, 2016.

Patricolo EG, et al: Beneficial effects of guided imagery or clinical massage on the status of patients in a progressive care unit, *Crit Care Nurse* 37(1):62, 2017.

Perciavalle V, et al: The role of deep breathing on stress, *Neurol Sci* 38:451, 2017.

Petrofsky J, et al: Use of low level of continuous heat as an adjunct to physical therapy improves knee pain recovery and the compliance for home exercise in patients with chronic knee pain: a randomized controlled trial, *J Strength Cond Res* 30(11):3107, 2016.

Petrofsky J, et al: The efficacy of sustained heat treatment on delayed-onset muscle soreness, *Clin J Sport Med* 27(4):329, 2017a.

Petrofsky JS, et al: Use of low level of continuous heat and ibuprofen as an adjunct to physical therapy improves pain relief, range of motion and the compliance for home exercise in patients with nonspecific neck pain: a randomized controlled trial, *J Back Musculoskelet Rehabil* 30(4):889, 2017b.

Quinlan P, et al: Effects of localized cold therapy on pain in postoperative spinal fusion patients: a randomized control trial, *Orthop Nurs* 36(5):344, 2017.
Quinn BL, et al: Pediatric pain assessment by drawn faces scales: a review, *Pain Manage Nurs* 15(4):909, 2014.
Rababa M: The association of nurses' assessment and certainty to pain management and outcomes for nursing home residents in Jordan, *Geriatr Nurs* 39(1):66, 2017.
Ratliff CR: Descriptive study of the frequency of medical adhesive–related skin injuries in a vascular clinic, *J Vasc Nurs* 35(2):86, 2017.
Rawal N: Current issues in postoperative pain management, *Eur J Anaesthesiol* 33(3):160, 2016.
Rigby J, Dye S: Effectiveness of various cryotherapy systems at decreasing ankle skin temperatures and applying compression, *Int J Athl Ther Train* 22(6):32, 2017.
Roeb M, et al: Epidural against systemic analgesia: an international registry analysis on postoperative pain and related perceptions after abdominal surgery, *Clin J Pain* 33(3):189, 2017.
Sadule-Rios: Off to a good start: bedside report, *Medsurg Nurs* 26(5):343, 2017.
Sangthong B, et al: Breathing training for older patients with controlled isolated systolic hypertension, *Med Sci Sports Exerc* 48(9):1641, 2016.
Savvas SM, Gibson SJ: Overview of pain management in older adults, *Clin Geriatr Med* 32(4):635, 2016.
Schatz T, et al: Improving comprehension in written medical informed consent procedures, *Geropsych* 30(3):97, 2017.
Schreiber M: Nursing care considerations: the epidural catheter, *Medsurg Nurs* 24(4):273, 2015.
Shindul-Rothschild J, et al: Beyond the pain scale: provider communication and staffing predictive of patients' satisfaction with pain control, pain management nursing, *Pain Manage Nurs* 18(6):401, 2017.
Sng B, Sia A: Maintenance of epidural labour analgesia: the old, the new and the future, *Best Pract Res Clin Anaesthesiol* 31:15, 2017.
Solanki NM, et al: Comparison of epidural versus systemic analgesia for major surgeries in neonates and infants, *J Clin Neonatol* 6(1):23, 2017.
Szekeres M, et al: The short-term effects of hot packs vs therapeutic whirlpool on active wrist range of motion for patients with distal radius fracture: a randomized controlled trial, *J Hand Ther* 2017. published online.
Terui S: Conceptualizing the pathways and processes between language barriers and health disparities: review, synthesis, and extension, *J Immigr Minor Health* 19:215, 2017.
The Joint Commission (TJC): *Prepublication standards—standards revisions related to pain assessment and management*, Oakbrook Terrace, IL, 2017, Author. https://www.jointcommission.org/standards_information/prepublication_standards.aspx.
The Joint Commission (TJC): *2019 National Patient Safety Goals*. Oakbrook Terrace, IL, 2019, The Commission. http://www.jointcommission.org/standards_information/npsgs.aspx.
Topham D, Drew D: Quality improvement project: replacing the numeric rating scale with a clinically aligned pain assessment (CAPA) tool, *Pain Manage Nurs* 18(6):363, 2017.
U.S. Department of Health and Human Services (USDHHS): The opioid epidemic by the numbers, 2017. Washington DC, https://www.hhs.gov/sites/default/files/Factsheet-opioids-061516.pdf.
U.S. Department of Health and Human Services (USDHHS), Office of Minority Health: National standards for culturally and linguistically appropriate services (CLAS) in health and health care, 2013. https://www.thinkculturalhealth.hhs.gov/pdfs/enhancednationalclasstandards.pdf.
Varndell W, et al: A systematic review of observational pain assessment instruments for use with nonverbal intubated critically ill adult patients in the emergency department: an assessment of their suitability and psychometric properties, *J Clin Nurs* 26(1–2):7, 2017.
Wadlund D: Local anesthetic systemic toxicity, *AORN J* 106(5):367, 2017.
Wickson-Griffiths A, et al: Interdisciplinary approaches to managing pain in older adults, *Clin Geriatr Med* 32(4):693, 2016.
Wu Y, et al: Characterizing human skin blood flow regulation in response to different local skin temperature perturbations, *Microvasc Res* 111:96, 2017.
Yoon SC, Bruner HC: Naloxegol in opioid-induced constipation: a new paradigm in the treatment of a common problem, *Patient Prefer Adherence* 11:1265, 2017.

16 Promoting Oxygenation

SKILLS AND PROCEDURES

EVOLVE WEBSITE/RESOURCES LIST

http://evolve.elsevier.com/Perry/nursinginterventions

Audio Glossary • Checklists • Clinical Review Questions • Answers and Rationales for Clinical Review Questions • Video Clips

INTRODUCTION

Oxygen is necessary for the body's organs and tissues to function properly. When oxygen levels decrease due to reasons such as ineffective breathing patterns, obstructed airways, or excess mucus, patients show signs of hypoxia or hypoxemia, such as dyspnea, tachypnea, tachycardia, anxiety, or confusion. Interventions to treat the cause of decreased oxygenation need to be completed quickly to prevent permanent tissue or organ damage (Lewis et al., 2017).

PRACTICE STANDARDS

- American Association for Respiratory Care (AARC), 2010: AARC clinical practice guidelines: endotracheal suctioning of mechanically ventilated patients with artificial airways
- Institute for Healthcare Improvement (IHI), 2012: How-to guide: prevent ventilator-associated pneumonia—Guidelines for preventing the development of VAP in patients with artificial airways
- Intensive Care Society (ICS), 2014: ICS tracheostomy standards—Comprehensive multidisciplinary care of a patient requiring tracheostomy
- The Joint Commission (TJC), 2019: National Patient Safety Goals—Patient identification and infection prevention

EVIDENCE-BASED PRACTICE

Ventilator-Associated Pneumonia

Ventilator-associated pneumonia (VAP) is defined as a pneumonia that occurs 48 hours or more after endotracheal intubation (Institute for Healthcare Improvement [IHI], 2016; Letchford and Bench, 2018). It is the most frequent nosocomial infection seen in patients in intensive care settings (Li et al., 2017). It has a mortality rate between 4.4% and 13%, with each instance of infection increasing patient costs by $20,000 to $40,000 (American Association of Critical Care Nurses [AACN], 2017b; Larrow and Klich-Heartt, 2016). IHI (2012) developed the set of bundled guidelines for the prevention of VAP.

Detailed interventions for the prevention of VAP include the following:

- Elevating the head of the bed between 30 and 45 degrees
- Daily sedative interruption with daily assessment of the patient's readiness to extubate
- Peptic ulcer disease prophylaxis
- Deep venous thrombosis prophylaxis
- Daily oral care with chlorhexidine
- Continuous subglottic suctioning
- Closed-system suctioning (for late-onset VAP)
- Continuous control of cuff pressure on endotracheal and tracheostomy tubes (Letchford and Bench, 2018; Li et al., 2017; Rouzé et al., 2017)

Future research is ongoing to attempt to identify the best method to perform oral care (toothbrush versus oral swabs) and different tracheostomy tube designs (AACN, 2017a; Chacko et al., 2017; Rouzé et al., 2017). Additional interventions are provided in Box 16.1.

SAFETY GUIDELINES

Oxygen is a medication, requiring the seven rights of medication administration, and should be treated with care (Table 16.1). Patients

BOX 16.1

Care Bundle for Ventilator-Associated Pneumonia

- Practice good hand hygiene.
- Check internal endotracheal cuff pressure at 25 to 30 cm H_2O every 2 hours.
- Maintain head of bed at 30 to 45 degrees.
- Provide prophylaxis for deep vein thrombosis and peptic ulcer disease.
- Provide daily interruptions of sedation to assess accurately for readiness to extubate.
- Provide oral care with chlorhexidine 0.12% every 12 hours and general oral care every 2 hours secondary to microbial colonization within the mouth.
- Perform complete subglottal suctioning to decrease risk of oral fluid aspiration.
- Maintain timely ventilator circuit changes and removal of condensation.
- Provide for mobility through turning and repositioning every 2 hours.

Data from American Association of Critical Care Nurses (AACN): AACN practice alert: prevention of ventilator-associated pneumonia in adults, 2017b. https://www.aacn.org/clinical-resources/practice-alerts/ventilator-associated-pneumonia-vap; Chacko R et al: Oral decontamination techniques and ventilator-associated pneumonia, *Br J Nurs* 26(11):594, 2017; Institute for Healthcare Improvement (IHI): How-to guide: prevent ventilator-associated pneumonia, 2012. http://www.ihi.org/resources/Pages/Tools/HowtoGuidePreventVAP.aspx; Larrow V, Klich-Heartt EI: Prevention of ventilator-associated pneumonia in the intensive care unit: beyond the basics, *J Neurosci Nurs* 48(3):160, 2016; Letchford E, Bench S: Ventilator-associated pneumonia and suction: a review of the literature, *Br J Nurs* 27(1):13, 2018; Li J et al: Evaluation of the safety and effectiveness of the rapid flow expulsion maneuver to clear subglottic secretions in vitro and in vivo, *Respr Care* 62(8):1007, 2017; and Wiegand D: *AACN procedure manual for high acuity, progressive, and critical care,* ed 7, St. Louis, 2017, Elsevier.

who require oxygen therapy should have a thorough assessment with appropriate diagnostic testing performed before the administration of oxygen. Patients who require more invasive measures for assistance with their oxygenation needs, such as mechanical ventilation or artificial airways, have additional safety needs:

- Know a patient's normal range of vital signs, pulse oximetry (SpO_2) values, most recent hemoglobin values, and past and current arterial blood gas (ABG) values, when available.
- Review a patient's previous respiratory assessment and perform a systematic respiratory assessment, noting rate, pattern, accessory muscle use, breath sounds, ability to cough, and integrity of the rib cage.
- Assess patient's cognitive level of function and medical and surgical history.
- Document a patient's smoking history. Smoking damages the mucociliary clearance mechanism of the lungs, resulting in a decreased ability to clear mucus from the airways.
- A home environmental assessment must be performed for patients who receive home oxygen therapy.
    - Be aware of environmental conditions. Patients with chronic respiratory diseases have difficulty maintaining optimal oxygen levels in polluted environments or in the presence of allergens.
- Suction equipment should be available to help clear airway secretions, particularly in patients with artificial airways such as an endotracheal tube (ETT) or a tracheostomy.
    - Use caution when suctioning patients with head injuries. The procedure causes an elevation in intracranial pressure (Galbiati and Paola, 2015).
- Most health care agencies require that a self-inflating resuscitation bag and appropriate-size mask be available in patient rooms, particularly for patients requiring mechanical ventilation.

TABLE 16.1

Oxygen Safety Guidelines

Guideline	Explanation
Treat oxygen as a medication.	Follow seven rights of medication administration; do not adjust oxygen-delivery system without a health care provider's order.
"Oxygen in use" sign is on patient's door.	Notifies all personnel of oxygen in patient's room.
Ensure that oxygen is set at prescribed rate.	Oxygen is a medication, and you should not adjust it without a health care provider's order.
Smoking is not permitted. Avoid electrical equipment that may result in sparks.	Oxygen supports combustion. Delivery systems and cylinders must be kept 10 feet from open flames and at least 5 feet from electrical equipment or heat source.
Store oxygen cylinders upright. Secure with chain or holder.	Prevents tipping and falling while stationary or when patient is being transported.
Check oxygen available in portable cylinders before transporting or ambulating patients.	Gauge on cylinder should register in green range, indicating that oxygen is available. Have backup supply available if level is low.
Tubing extensions should not be added if patient is ambulatory.	Added tubing length increases fall hazard and also decreases amount of delivered oxygen.
Check for tight seal when delivering oxygen via mask.	When using a mask, a tight seal around the mouth is necessary to prevent room air from entering and decreasing the FiO_2. If a tight seal is required, a nasal cannula cannot be added.

FiO_2, Fraction of inspired oxygen concentration.

✦ SKILL 16.1 Oxygen Administration

Purpose

The purpose of supplemental oxygen therapy is to prevent or treat hypoxia (a state in which the supply of oxygen is insufficient for normal life functions) or hypoxemia (a lower-than-normal concentration of oxygen in arterial blood). Routes of administration include, but are not limited to, nasal cannula, face masks, noninvasive ventilation, and positive-pressure ventilators. Special care is required for each of these types of delivery devices (Table 16.2).

Delegation and Collaboration

The skill of applying a nasal cannula or oxygen mask (but not adjusting oxygen flow) can be delegated to nursing assistive personnel (NAP). The nurse is responsible for assessing the patient's respiratory system and the response to oxygen therapy. The nurse, in some agencies, may collaborate with the respiratory therapist in the setup of oxygen therapy, including adjustment of oxygen flow rate. The nurse directs the NAP by:

- Informing how to safely adjust the device (e.g., loosening the strap on the oxygen cannula or mask) and clarifying its correct placement and positioning.
- Instructing to inform the nurse immediately about any changes in vital signs; changes in pulse oximetry (SpO_2); changes in level of consciousness (LOC); skin irritation from the cannula, mask, or straps; or patient complaints of pain or shortness of breath.
- Instructing personnel to provide extra skin care around patient's ears and nose or other parts of the patient's body that might be irritated by the device.

TABLE 16.2

Oxygen-Delivery Systems

Delivery System	FiO_2 Delivered*	Advantages	Disadvantages
Low-Flow Delivery Devices			
Nasal cannula	1–6 L/min: 24%–44%	Safe and simple Easily tolerated Effective for low concentrations Does not impede eating or talking Inexpensive, disposable	Unable to use with nasal obstruction Drying to mucous membranes Can dislodge easily May cause skin irritation or breakdown around ears or nares Patient's breathing pattern (mouth or nasal) affects exact FiO_2
Oxygen-conserving cannula (Oxymizer)	8 L/min; 30%–50%	Indicated for long-term O_2 use in the home Allows increased O_2 concentration and lower flow	Cannula cannot be cleaned More expensive than standard cannula
Simple face mask	6–12 L/min: 35%–50%	Useful for short periods such as patient transportation	Contraindicated for patients who retain CO_2 May induce feelings of claustrophobia Therapy interrupted with eating and drinking Increased risk of aspiration
Partial nonrebreather mask (**NOTE:** Reservoir bag should always remain partially inflated.)	10–15 L/min: 60%–90%	Useful for short periods Delivers increased FiO_2 Easily humidifies O_2 Does not dry mucous membranes	Hot and confining; may irritate skin; tight seal necessary Interferes with eating and talking Bag may twist or kink; should not totally deflate
High-Flow Delivery Devices			
Venturi mask	24%–50%	Provides specific amount of O_2 with humidity added Administers low, constant O_2	Mask and added humidity may irritate skin Therapy interrupted with eating and drinking Specific flow rate must be followed
High-flow nasal cannula	Adjustable FiO_2 (21%–100%) with modifiable low flow (up to 60 L/min)	Wide range of FiO_2 Can use on infants, children, and adults Shown to have similar and, in some cases, superior clinical efficacy compared with conventional low-flow oxygen (Drake, 2018)	FiO_2 dependent on patient respiratory pattern and input flow Risk for infection (Messika et al., 2015; Urden et al., 2016).
Noninvasive Ventilation			
Continuous positive airway pressure (CPAP) and bilevel positive airway pressure (BiPAP)	21%–100%	Avoids the use of an artificial airway in some patients with acute respiratory distress, postextubation respiratory failure, or neuromuscular disorders Successfully treats obstructive sleep apnea	Nasal pillows/face masks can cause skin breakdown May cause claustrophobia in some patients

CO_2, Carbon dioxide; *FiO_2*, fraction of inspired oxygen concentration.
*FiO_2 delivered may differ by manufacturer. Check manufacturer's guidelines.
Source for high-flow nasal cannula: Walsh BK, Smallwood CD: Pediatric oxygen therapy: a review and update, *Respir Care* 62(6):645, 2017.
Source for noninvasive ventilation: Wiegand D: *AACN procedure manual for high acuity, progressive, and critical care,* ed 7 St. Louis, 2017, Elsevier.

Equipment

- Oxygen-delivery device as ordered by health care provider
- Oxygen tubing (consider extension tubing as needed)
- Humidifier, if indicated
- Sterile water for humidifier
- Oxygen source
- Oxygen flowmeter
- "Oxygen in use" sign
- Pulse oximeter
- Stethoscope
- Clean gloves
- Face shield, if risk of splash from secretions is present

BOX 16.2

Signs and Symptoms of Hypoxia

- Apprehension
- Restlessness
- Irritability
- Confusion
- Lethargy
- Tachypnea
- Dyspnea
- Accessory muscle use
- Inability to speak in complete sentences
- Tachycardia
- Mild hypertension
- Diaphoresis
- Fatigue
- Dysrhythmias

From Lewis SL et al: *Medical-surgical nursing: assessment and management of clinical problems,* ed. 10, St. Louis, 2017, Elsevier.

ASSESSMENT

1. Identify patient using at least two identifiers (e.g., name and birthday or name and medical record number) according to agency policy. *Rationale: Ensures correct patient. Complies with The Joint Commission standards and improves patient safety (TJC, 2019).*
2. Review accuracy of health care provider's order for oxygen, noting delivery method, flow rate, duration of oxygen therapy, and parameters for titration of oxygen settings. *Rationale: Ensures safe and accurate oxygen administration. Safe oxygen delivery includes the seven rights of medication administration (see Chapter 22).*
3. Obtain data from patient's electronic health record (vital signs, pulse oximetry, arterial blood gas values). *Rationale: Need to know patient baseline values to accurately evaluate effectiveness.*
4. Perform hand hygiene and apply clean gloves. Perform respiratory assessment, including symmetry of chest wall expansion, chest wall abnormalities (e.g., kyphosis), temporary conditions affecting ventilation (e.g., pregnancy, trauma), respiratory rate and depth, sputum production, and lung sounds and for signs and symptoms associated with hypoxia (Box 16.2). *Rationale: Reduces transmission of microorganisms. Changes in ventilation and gas exchange resulting in hypoxia require oxygen therapy.*
5. Observe for cognitive and/or behavioral changes (e.g., apprehension, anxiety, confusion, decreased ability to concentrate, decreased LOC, fatigue, and dizziness). *Rationale: Decreased levels of oxygen (hypoxia) or increased levels of carbon dioxide (hypercapnia) affect a person's cognitive abilities, interpersonal interactions, and mood (Lewis et al., 2017).*

Safe Patient Care *Patients with sudden changes in their vital signs, LOC, or behavior may be experiencing profound hypoxia. Patients who demonstrate subtle changes over time may have worsening of a chronic or existing condition or a new medical condition (Lewis et al., 2017).*

6. Assess airway patency and remove airway secretions by having patient cough and expectorate mucus or by suctioning (see Skill 16.3). **NOTE:** Perform additional hand hygiene and change gloves if there is contact with mucus. *Rationale: Secretions plug the airway, decreasing amount of oxygen that is available for gas exchange in lungs.*

Safe Patient Care *Excessive amounts of secretions, signs of respiratory distress (increased work of breathing, increased respiratory rate), presence of rhonchi on auscultation, excessive coughing, or decrease in patient pulse oximeter can indicate need for suctioning.*

7. Inspect condition of skin around nose and ears. *Rationale: Provides baseline for monitoring development of skin breakdown from medical device irritation.*
8. Assess patient's or family caregiver's knowledge, experience, and health literacy level. *Rationale: Ensures patient has the capacity to obtain, communicate, process, and understand basic health information (Centers for Disease Control and Prevention [CDC], 2016).*

STEP	RATIONALE
PLANNING	
1. Expected outcomes following completion of procedure:	
• Patient's SpO_2 (peripheral capillary oxygen saturation) and/or arterial blood gases (ABGs) return to or remain within normal limits or baseline levels.	Objective determinants of stable or improved arterial oxygenation.
• Patient's vital signs remain stable or return to baseline.	When there is no underlying cardiovascular disease, patients adapt to decreased oxygen levels by increasing pulse and blood pressure. This is a short-term adaptive response. Once signs of hypoxia are reduced or controlled, patient's vital signs usually return to normal.
• Patient's work of breathing decreases.	Pulmonary conditions such as pneumonia or asthma cause varying degrees of airway narrowing. With improved oxygenation, patient's airways are open, and work of breathing decreases.

STEP	RATIONALE
• Patient experiences increased lung expansion.	Improved oxygenation helps resolve collapsed and constricted airways, improves work of breathing, and thus improves lung expansion.
• Patient's LOC returns to baseline.	Improvement in oxygenation relieves hypoxia and improves patient's mental status.
• Patient verbalizes improved levels of comfort, and subjective sensations of anxiety, fatigue, and breathlessness decrease.	Increased oxygen levels in the blood reduce patient's anxiety, fatigue, and breathlessness.
• Patient's ears, nares, and nasal mucosa remain intact.	Intact skin indicates no device-related pressure to underlying skin and mucous membrane (Pittman et al., 2015; Schallom et al., 2015).
2. Close room door or curtains around bed and prepare equipment and environment.	Provides privacy and facilitates a smooth and organized procedure.
3. Adjust bed to appropriate height. Check locks on bed.	Minimizes caregiver muscle strain and prevents injury. Prevents bed from moving.
4. Instruct patient and/or family caregiver about need for oxygen. If the oxygen is for home use, educate the patient about oxygen safety in the home (see Table 16.1) and the equipment that will be utilized.	Education helps reduce patient and caregiver anxiety. Proper education about the use of and need for the oxygen equipment will help to ensure the safe and proper use of the equipment.

IMPLEMENTATION

STEP	RATIONALE
1. Perform hand hygiene. Apply face shield if risk of exposure to splashing mucus exists. Apply clean gloves if patient has oral or nasal secretions.	Reduces transmission of microorganisms.
2. Attach oxygen-delivery device (e.g., nasal cannula, face mask) to oxygen tubing and attach end of tubing to humidified oxygen source adjusted to prescribed flow rate (see illustration).	Humidity prevents drying of nasal and oral mucous membranes and airway secretions. Flowmeters with smaller calibrations may be required for patients requiring low-dose oxygen such as pediatric patients (Hockenberry et al., 2017).
3. Apply oxygen device:	
a. Place tips of the nasal cannula into patient's nares. If tips are curved, they should point downward inside nostrils. Then loop cannula tubing up and over patient's ears. Adjust lanyard so that cannula fits snugly but not too tight, without pressure to patient nares and ears (see illustration).	Tips of nasal cannula direct flow of oxygen into patient's upper respiratory tract.
b. Apply a face mask by placing it over patient's mouth and nose. Then bring straps over patient's head and adjust to form a comfortable but tight seal.	A properly fitting device that does not create pressure on nares or ears is comfortable, and patient is more likely to keep it in place; reduces risk for skin breakdown (Schallom et al., 2015).
c. Maintain sufficient slack on oxygen tubing and secure to patient's clothes.	Allows patient to turn head without causing mask to shift position or dislodge nasal cannula.

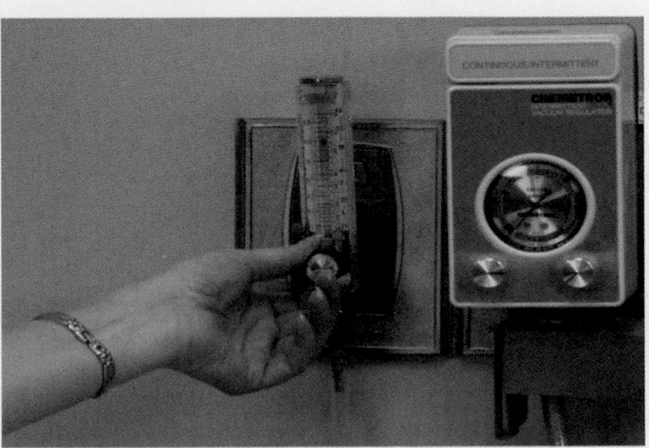

STEP 2 Flowmeter attached to oxygen source.

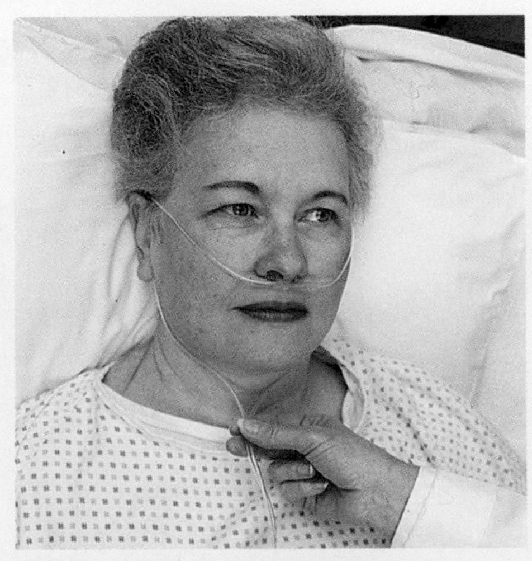

STEP 3a Nasal cannula adjusted for proper fit.

STEP	RATIONALE
4. Observe for proper function of oxygen-delivery device:	Ensures patency of delivery device and accuracy of prescribed oxygen flow rate (see Table 16.2).
a. *Nasal cannula:* Cannula is positioned properly in nares; oxygen flows through tips.	Provides prescribed oxygen rate and reduces pressure on tips of nares.
b. *Partial nonrebreather mask:* Mask seals tightly around mouth. Reservoir fills on exhalation and almost collapses on inspiration. Reservoir should not collapse completely (see illustration).	Easily humidifies oxygen and does not dry mucous membranes. Useful for short-term therapy of 24 hours or less.
c. *Oxygen-conserving cannula (Oxymizer):* Fit as for nasal cannula. Reservoir is located under patient's nose or worn as a pendant.	Delivers higher flow of oxygen with nasal cannula. Delivers 2 : 1 ratio (e.g., 6 L/min nasal cannula is approximately equivalent to 3.5 L/min with Oxymizer device).
d. *Nonrebreather mask:* Apply as regular mask. Contains one-way valves with reservoir; exhaled air does not enter reservoir bag. Can be combined with nasal cannula to provide higher inspired oxygen concentration (FiO_2).	Device of choice for short-term high FiO_2 delivery. Valves on mask side ports permit exhalation but close during inhalation to prevent inhaling room air.
e. *Simple face mask:* Select appropriate flow rate (see illustration).	Used for short-term oxygen therapy.
f. *Venturi mask* (see illustration): Apply as regular mask. Select appropriate flow rate (see Table 16.2).	Used when high-flow device is desired.
g. *Face tent:* Apply tent under patient's chin and over mouth and nose. It will be loose, and a mist is always present (see illustration).	Excellent source of humidification; however, you cannot control oxygen concentrations, and patient who requires high oxygen cannot use this device.
h. *High-flow nasal cannula* (see illustration).	Provides adjustable O_2 delivery and flow-dependent CO_2 clearance to reduce work of breathing and better match inspiratory demand during respiratory distress (Drake, 2018).
5. Verify setting on flowmeter and oxygen source for proper setup and prescribed flow rate.	Ensures delivery of prescribed oxygen therapy in conjunction with specific cannula/mask.
6. Check nasal cannula/face mask every 8 hours or as agency policy indicates. Keep humidification container filled at all times.	Ensures patency of cannula and oxygen flow. Oxygen is a dry gas; when it is administered via nasal cannula of 4 L/min or more, or administered to pediatric patients, you must add humidification to prevent thickening of secretions, minimize atelectasis, and prevent heat loss (Walsh and Smallwood, 2017).
7. Post "Oxygen in use" signs on wall behind bed and at entrance to room.	Alerts visitors and care providers that oxygen is in use.

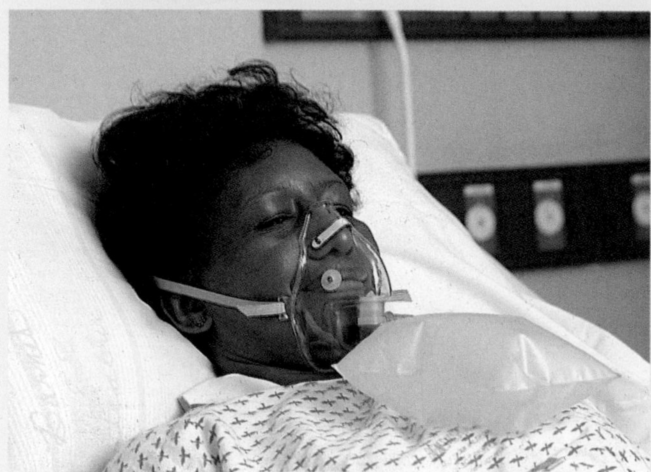

STEP 4b Plastic face mask with reservoir bad.

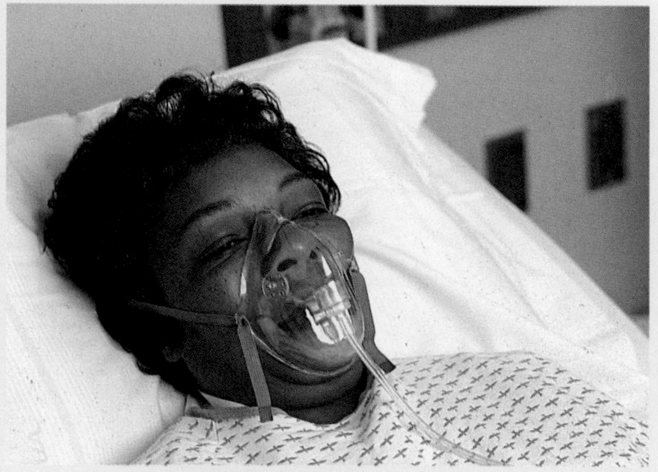

STEP 4e Simple face mask.

STEP	RATIONALE

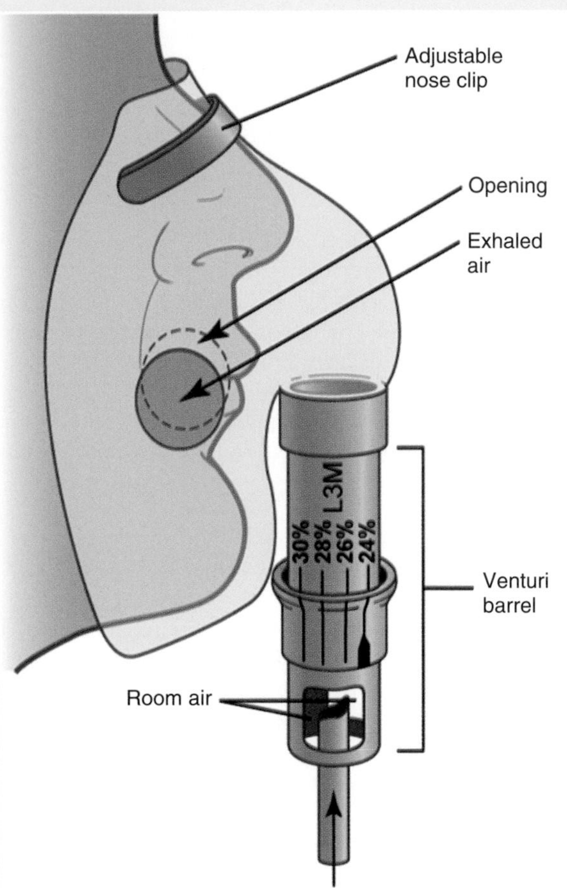

STEP 4f Venturi mask.

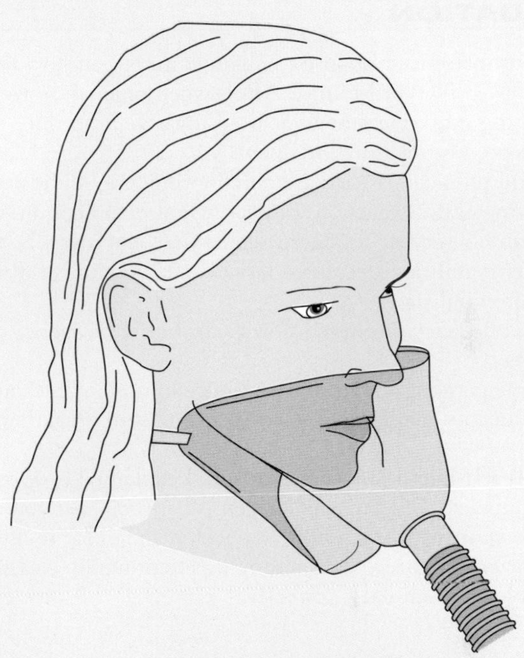

STEP 4g Face tent for oxygen delivery. *(From Hockenberry MJ, Wilson D: Wong's nursing care of infants and children, ed 10, St. Louis, 2015, Mosby.)*

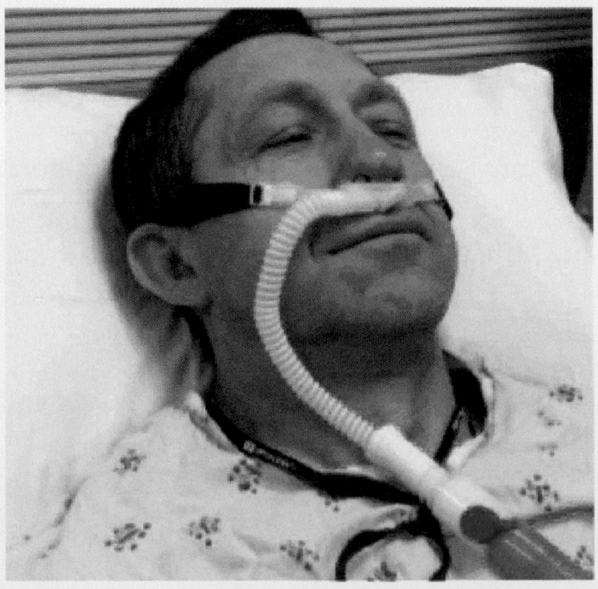

STEP 4h High-flow nasal cannula. *(Courtesy Fischer & Paykel Healthcare.)*

STEP	RATIONALE
8. Properly dispose of gloves (if used) and perform hand hygiene.	Reduces transmission of microorganisms.
9. Raise side rails (as appropriate) and lower bed to lowest position.	Ensures patient safety.
10. Be sure nurse call system is accessible and within patient's reach. Instruct the patient on its use.	Helps decrease incidence of falls; alerts the nurse when the patient needs assistance.

EVALUATION

1. Monitor patient's response to changes in oxygen flow rate with SpO_2. **NOTE:** Monitor ABGs when ordered; however, obtaining ABG measurement is an invasive procedure, and ABGs are not measured frequently.	Continual monitoring with SpO_2 is required for patients on oxygen therapy. Base changes in supplemental oxygen on individual patient's oxygen saturation levels.
2. Perform physical assessment, auscultating lung sounds; palpating chest excursion; inspecting color and condition of skin; and observing for decreased anxiety, improved LOC and cognitive abilities, decreased fatigue, and absence of dizziness. Measure vital signs.	Evaluates patient's response to supplemental oxygen. As patient's oxygen level improves, physical signs and symptoms improve.
3. Assess adequacy of oxygen flow each shift or as agency policy dictates.	Ensures patency of oxygen-delivery device.
4. Observe patient's external ears, bridge of nose, nares, and nasal mucous membranes for evidence of skin breakdown.	Oxygen therapy sometimes causes drying of nasal mucosa. The delivery device can cause skin breakdown where device comes in contact with face, neck, and ears (Schallom et al., 2015).
5. **Use Teach-Back:** "I want to be sure I explained how oxygen will help you. Tell me why oxygen is beneficial for you." Revise your instruction now or develop a plan for revised patient/family caregiver teaching if patient/family caregiver is not able to teach back correctly.	Determines patient's/family caregiver's level of understanding of instructional topic.

Unexpected Outcomes	Related Interventions
1. Patient experiences skin irritation or breakdown (e.g., at ears, bridge of nose, nares, other pressure areas).	• Provide appropriate skin care. Do not use petroleum-based gel around oxygen because it is flammable (American Lung Association, 2018).
2. Patient experiences continued hypoxia.	• Notify health care provider. • Obtain health care provider's orders for follow-up SpO_2 monitoring or ABG determinations. • Consider measures to improve airway patency, including but not limited to coughing techniques and oropharyngeal or orotracheal suctioning.
3. Patient experiences nasal and upper airway mucosa drying.	• If oxygen flow rate is greater than 4 L/min, use humidification. At rates greater than 5 L/min, nasal mucous membranes dry, and pain in frontal sinuses may develop (Lewis et al., 2017). • Assess patient's fluid status and increase fluids if appropriate. • Provide frequent oral care.

Recording

- Record the respiratory assessment findings, method of oxygen delivery and flow rate, patient vital signs and pulse oximetry values, and patient's response and any adverse reactions.
- Document evaluation of patient learning.

Hand-Off Reporting

- Report patient status, including recent assessment findings, vital signs, and SpO_2 before oxygen administration.
- Report the type of oxygen-delivery device initiated and utilized, the initial flow rates, and if any adjustments to the flow rates were made during the shift. Include the patient response to the flow-rate adjustments and what interventions were successful.
- Report any unexpected outcomes, such as the development of reddened areas on ears or nose.

✦ SKILL 16.2 Airway Management: Noninvasive Positive-Pressure Ventilation

Purpose

Noninvasive positive-pressure ventilation (NIPPV or NPPV) treats a variety of conditions, including obstructive sleep apnea (OSA), chronic obstructive pulmonary disease (COPD), and neuromuscular disorders (see Table 16.2). There are two types of NIPPV: continuous positive airway pressure (CPAP) and bi-level positive airway pressure (BiPAP). NIPPV has fewer complications than invasive ventilation strategies, and it allows patients an increased ability to communicate with family caregivers.

Delegation and Collaboration

The skill of caring for a patient receiving noninvasive ventilation cannot be delegated to nursing assistive personnel (NAP). The nurse collaborates with the respiratory therapist when providing care for the patient. However, the skills of patient positioning and mask application can be delegated to NAP. The nurse directs the NAP by:

- Informing about the need to immediately report to the nurse any changes in patient's vital signs; oxygen saturation; mental status; skin color; or skin abrasions, bruising, or blistering around mask area.
- Informing about the need to immediately report to the nurse any ventilator or CPAP/BiPAP machine alarms or patient monitor alarms.
- Instructing on how to modify care, such as for how long the mask can be removed, oral care, or any special skin-care needs.
- Informing about the prescribed settings on the NIPPV equipment and instructing personnel to immediately notify the nurse of any change in settings or patient comfort.

Equipment

- Nasal mask/full face mask (with quick release straps) or nasal pillows
- Oxygen source and tubing
- BiPAP and/or CPAP machine/ventilator as per health care provider order
- Humidification source
- Delivery tubing
- Pulse oximeter
- Clean gloves
- Personal protective equipment as appropriate
- Stethoscope
- Suction equipment
- Self-inflating manual resuscitation bag-valve-mask device
- Appropriate signs for in-use oxygen

ASSESSMENT

1. Identify patient using at least two identifiers (e.g., name and birthday or name and medical record number) according to agency policy. *Rationale: Ensures correct patient. Complies with The Joint Commission standards and improves patient safety (TJC, 2019).*
2. Review accuracy of health care provider's order. *Rationale: Health care provider's order is necessary for this therapy.*
3. Perform hand hygiene and apply clean gloves, and assess patient's respiratory status, including symmetry of chest wall expansion, respiratory rate and depth, sputum production, and lung sounds (see Chapters 7 and 8). When possible, ask patient about dyspnea and observe for signs and symptoms associated with hypoxia (see Box 16.2). *Rationale: Decreased chest wall movement, crackles or decreased lung sounds, increased respiratory rate, increased sputum production, or signs of worsening hypoxia may make patient a candidate for noninvasive positive-pressure ventilation or changes in NIPPV settings.*
4. Observe patient's skin over bridge of nose, around external ears, back of head. *Rationale: The mask can place pressure on skin and increase risk for skin breakdown (Schallom et al., 2015).*
5. Observe patient's ability to clear and remove airway secretions by coughing. *Rationale: Secretions plug the airway, decreasing amount of oxygen that is available for gas exchange in the lung.*
6. Assess patient's vital signs and pulse oximetry; when available, note patient's most recent arterial blood gas (ABG) results. *Rationale: Objectively documents patient's pH, arterial oxygen, arterial carbon dioxide, or arterial oxygen saturation. Identifies need for NIPPV.*
7. Assess patient's level of consciousness, behaviors, and ability to maintain and protect airway. Remove and dispose of gloves. Perform hand hygiene. *Rationale: Patients who cannot maintain their own airway or who are uncooperative are not candidates for NIPPV.*

Safe Patient Care *NIPPV is contraindicated in patients in cardiac or respiratory arrest or with facial deformities, hemodynamic instability, inability to protect airway, severe agitation, excessive secretions, or high inspired oxygen concentration (FiO_2) requirements (Wiegand, 2017). Its use in palliative care and end-of-life care is still being investigated (Gale et al., 2015).*

8. Assess patient's or family caregiver's knowledge, experience, and health literacy level. *Rationale: Ensures patient or caregiver has the capacity to obtain, communicate, process, and understand basic health information (CDC, 2016).*

STEP	RATIONALE
PLANNING	
1. Expected outcomes following completion of procedure:	
• Patient has increased lung expansion.	Patient experiences improved gas exchange when lungs are expanded from constant pressure of NIPPV.
• Patient maintains ABG levels and/or pulse oximetry (SpO_2) readings improve or remain normal.	NIPPV delivered is appropriately based on patient assessment data.

STEP	RATIONALE

Safe Patient Care *When first initiating CPAP/BiPAP, it is important to monitor gas exchange, especially in patients with COPD, cardiogenic pulmonary edema, or acute respiratory failure. You do this to observe for carbon dioxide retention. If patient has "do not resuscitate" orders or is receiving palliative care services, careful consideration is given before starting noninvasive ventilation (Wiegand, 2017).*

STEP	RATIONALE
• Patient experiences reduction in feelings of dyspnea and work of breathing.	In patients with acute conditions, dyspnea usually improves. Patients with chronic pulmonary diseases often require nocturnal CPAP/BiPAP indefinitely to achieve long-term benefits.
• Patient's vital signs and respiratory assessment parameters improve.	Reduced pulse and respiratory rate, improved mental status, improved skin color, and decreased use of accessory and abdominal muscles occur because patient's work of breathing decreases as level of oxygenation improves.
• Patient's skin around bridge of nose, ears, and back of head remains clear, without breakdown.	Mask applied properly and monitored for pressure occurrence.
• Patient able to teach back how to use CPAP/BiPAP in the home setting.	Demonstrates learning.
2. Close room door or curtains around bed and prepare equipment and environment.	Provides privacy and facilitates a smooth and organized procedure.
3. Collaborate with the respiratory therapist to prepare and organize equipment, including the mask, oxygen source, ventilator/CPAP machine, and suction equipment.	Provides organized implementation of the noninvasive ventilation.
4. Explain to patient and family the purpose and reasons for CPAP/BiPAP.	Helps reduce sense of claustrophobia from mask. In addition, information reduces anxiety and increases cooperation and adherence to therapy.

IMPLEMENTATION

STEP	RATIONALE
1. Perform hand hygiene; apply clean gloves. Apply mask, gown, and goggles/face shield if secretions are projectile or if patient is in isolation (see Chapter 5).	Reduces transmission of infection and exposure to pulmonary secretions.
2. Adjust bed to appropriate height and lower side rail on side nearest you. Raise head of bed. Check locks on bed wheel.	Minimizes caregiver's muscle strain and prevents injury. Raising head of bed eases ventilatory effort. Prevents bed from moving.
3. Determine correct mask size. Use masking chart to determine correct size (S, M, L, XL). **NOTE:** *It is imperative that masks have quick-release straps.*	Mask should fit snugly over patient's nose (CPAP) or nose and/or mouth (BiPAP) to create a tight seal for delivering positive pressure. In case of emergency (e.g., vomiting, respiratory arrest), quick-release straps allow mask to be removed quickly. This system also allows patient to remove mask quickly as needed (Urden et al., 2016).

Safe Patient Care *A patient receiving NIPPV via a full-face mask should never be restrained. The patient must be able to remove the mask if he or she begins to vomit, needs to remove excess secretions, or needs to reposition a mask that has moved. A displaced mask can force the patient's jaw inward, which can obstruct the patient's airway (Urden et al., 2016).*

STEP	RATIONALE
4. Connect CPAP/BiPAP device-delivery tubing to pressure generator or ventilator.	Ensures that patient is receiving proper NIPPV as ordered.
5. Connect patient to pulse oximetry.	It is important to continually monitor patient's level of oxygenation when initiating NIPPV.
6. Set CPAP/BiPAP initial settings per health care provider order:	These settings allow the health care team to determine initial patient response.
a. CPAP: 5 to 15 cm H_2O is the typically prescribed pressure range (Pooboni et al., 2015)	CPAP provides single positive pressure throughout breathing cycle, which helps keep alveoli open at end-expiration.
b. BiPAP: Inspiratory pressure is usually set at 10 to 12 cm H_2O initially and can be titrated up to 15 to 20 cm H_2O as patient condition dictates; expiratory pressure is usually set at 5 to 7 cm H_2O initially and can be titrated up as patient condition warrants (Pooboni et al., 2015).	BiPAP supplies pressure at both inhalation and exhalation. The inhalation pressure is set according to health care provider's order and helps prevent airway closure. Expiratory pressure is set according to health care provider's order and keeps alveoli open at end-expiration (Wiegand, 2017).
7. Select FiO_2 level as indicated and per prescriber order.	Patients on NIPPV may also need supplemental oxygen to decrease signs and symptoms of hypoxia (Hill and Kramer, 2018).

STEP	RATIONALE
8. Ensure that humidification and heating appliances are connected and on.	Humidification of gas is thought to improve comfort in patients receiving NIPPV (Elliott and Elliott, 2018).
9. Ensure that mask is tight fitting, no air leak is present, and there are no excessive pressure points.	An ill-fitting mask leads to loss of pressure getting into airways or desynchrony with ventilator. It also can lead to air blowing into eyes, which can cause patient discomfort (Wiegand, 2017). Pressure points around mask area can cause device-related pressure injuries (Schallom et al., 2015).
10. If patient is to use CPAP at home, have patient or family caregiver demonstrate mask placement and adjustment of settings.	Return demonstration indicates learning.
11. Dispose of supplies as appropriate, remove gloves and other personal protective equipment, and perform hand hygiene.	Reduces transmission of microorganisms.
12. Raise side rails (as appropriate) and lower bed to lowest position.	Ensures patient safety.
13. Ensure that the patient is in a comfortable position and that the nurse call system is in an accessible location with the patient's reach. Instruct the patient on its use.	Increase patient's comfort level. Allows the patient to alert the nurse when they need assistance.
14. Continuous care of patient:	
a. Ensure that all alarms are on and active and that ventilator circuit is intact and properly functioning.	Ensures patient safety.
b. Ensure that emergency resuscitation equipment is at bedside.	Allows for quick resuscitation in case of worsening patient condition (Wiegand, 2017).
c. Investigate all alarms that come with ventilator/CPAP machine and/or patient monitor.	Alarms can alert health care team to problems with patient or with circuit that adversely affects patient status.
d. Change patient's position every 2 hours or encourage patient to change position every 2 hours.	Reduces incidence of atelectasis or pneumonia secondary to stasis of secretions.
15. Weaning patient from NIPPV:	
a. Ensure that all alarms are on and properly functioning.	Amount of positive airway pressure is being reduced, and alarms alert if patient status declines (Hyzy et al., 2018a)
b. Begin ambulating patient when he or she has been disconnected from NIPPV.	Weaning allows the patient to be disconnected for longer periods (Hyzy et al., 2018a).

EVALUATION

STEP	RATIONALE
1. Observe for decreased anxiety, improved level of consciousness and cognitive abilities, decreased fatigue, and absence of dizziness.	Determines patient's response to NIPPV. As hypoxia and hypercapnia are reduced or corrected, patient's behavioral assessment parameters improve.
2. Measure vital signs, perform respiratory assessment, and observe skin color, and ask patient to describe sense of dyspnea.	Physical assessment parameters reveal oxygenation status.
3. Monitor pulse oximetry.	Documents patient's level of oxygenation. When first initiating NIPPV, it is important to also obtain ABG levels in patients in whom abnormal gas exchange is suspected, after the first hour, and per agency protocol.
4. Observe skin integrity over bridge of patient's nose every 2 hours. Ask patient about level of comfort.	Mask that is too tight causes skin breakdown, and frequent skin assessment is necessary (Pittman et al., 2015; Schallom et al., 2015).
5. If NIPPV is planned for use in home, observe and monitor patient's and family's ability to manipulate CPAP or BiPAP machine/ventilator and face mask.	Determines patient's ability to perform self-care and adhere to CPAP/BiPAP plan. Success of noninvasive ventilation depends largely on patient acceptance and adherence (Gale et al., 2015).
6. Monitor patient's response to weaning from NIPPV.	Monitor for a minimum of the first 8 hours. Review blood gas measurements and notify health care provider if pH or $PaCO_2$ rises, indicating failure to wean from NIPPV (Hyzy et al., 2018a).
7. **Use Teach-Back:** "I want to be sure I explained how NIPPV works and why you are receiving this therapy. Explain to me why this therapy is necessary." Revise your instruction now or develop a plan for revised patient/family caregiver teaching if patient/family caregiver is not able to teach back correctly.	Determines patient's/family caregiver's level of understanding of instructional topic.

Unexpected Outcomes	Related Interventions
1. Patient experiences hypoxia, hypercapnia, or other signs of worsening respiratory function.	• Notify health care provider. • Reassess patient. • Determine correct settings and integrity of NIPPV.
2. Patient develops skin breakdown at mask sites or sites where mask straps are located, such as bridge of nose, nasal septum, or ears.	• Notify health care provider. • Place protective synthetic coverings on nasal bridge or areas of irritation/possible irritation to protect skin. • Fit mask so that it is tight enough to not cause air leak but loose enough to not cause skin breakdown. • Reassess patient (Pooboni et al., 2015).
3. Patient states sense of smothering or claustrophobia.	• Explain system to patient again. • Demonstrate use of quick-release straps. • Have patient demonstrate use of quick-release straps.
4. Patient develops stomach distention secondary to positive-pressure air being forced into esophagus and trachea (Pooboni et al., 2015).	• Notify health care provider. • Be prepared for possible insertion of nasogastric tube (see Chapter 20).

Recording

- Record type of NIV, including pressure and oxygen flow rates, assistance needed with positioning, coughing effectiveness, and respiratory assessment findings.
- Record patient adherence and tolerance, mask fit and skin assessment beneath mask, effectiveness of therapy, witnessed periods of apnea, and status of daytime hypersomnolence.
- Document evaluation of patient learning.

Hand-Off Reporting

- Report patient status, including respiratory assessment findings, before initiation of noninvasive ventilation.
- Report the type of noninvasive ventilation initiated and utilized, the initial pressure and oxygen flow rates, and if any adjustments to the pressures and flow rates were made during the course of the shift. Include the patient response to the flow-rate adjustments and what other interventions were successful.
- Report any unexpected outcomes, such as development of reddened areas on ears or nose.

PROCEDURAL GUIDELINE 16.1 *Use of a Peak Flowmeter*

Purpose

Peak expiratory flow rate (PEFR) measurements are useful for patients with asthma who have measurable changes in the flow of air through the airways. The PEFR is the maximum flow that a patient forces out during one quick, forced expiration and is measured in liters per minute. These measurements are used as an objective indicator of a patient's status or to evaluate the effectiveness of treatment (e.g., bronchodilators) (Gerald et al., 2018).

Delegation and Collaboration

Initial assessment of the patient's condition is a nursing responsibility and cannot be delegated. The skills of follow-up PEFR measurements in a stable patient can be delegated to nursing assistive personnel (NAP). The nurse directs the NAP to:

- Report immediately to the nurse patient's difficulty breathing or decrease in PEFR measurement.

Equipment

Peak flowmeter (Fig. 16.1); patient diary/action plan (if appropriate); writing utensil to record value; clean gloves

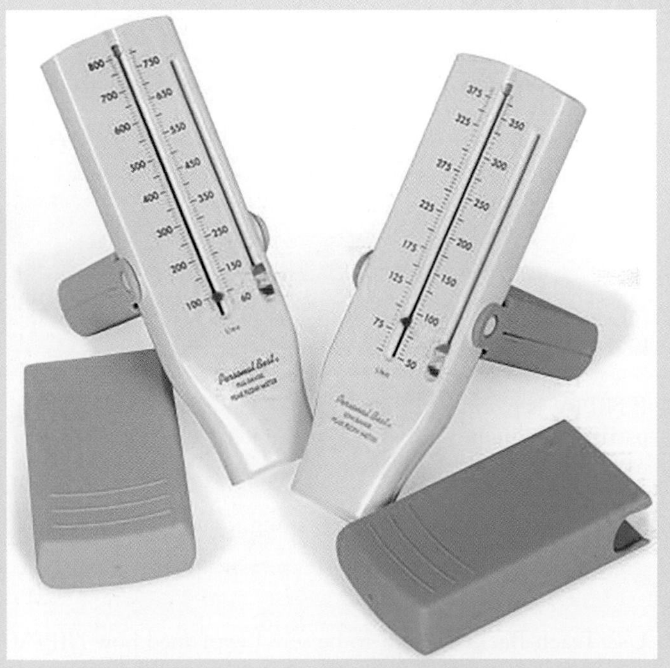

FIG 16.1 Peak flowmeter. *(Courtesy Phillips Respironics.)*

Procedural Steps

1. Identify patient using at least two identifiers (e.g., name and birthday or name and medical record number) according to agency policy (TJC, 2019).

PROCEDURAL GUIDELINE 16.1 *Use of a Peak Flowmeter—cont'd*

2. Assess previous PEFR readings from patient's electronic health record (EHR) and the target set by patient's health care provider.
3. Assess patient's and family caregiver's baseline knowledge of when and how to use PEFR and correct response to results.
4. Assist patient to a standing or a high-Fowler's position, as able, to promote optimum lung expansion.
5. Instruct patient to remove any food or gum from mouth.
6. Perform hand hygiene and apply clean gloves.
7. Slide clean mouthpiece into base of the numbered scale or clean the mouthpiece of the flowmeter if it permanently attached.
8. Instruct patient to take a deep breath through nose and slowly blow out through mouth. Take second deep breath.
9. Have patient place metered mouthpiece in mouth and close lips, making a firm seal.
10. Have patient blow out as hard and fast as possible through mouth only.
11. Record the number or mark it on the flowmeter with the attached marker.
12. Repeat Steps 8 to 11 two more times.
13. Record the highest number of the three attempts.
14. If patient is to record PEFR at home, have him or her demonstrate how to record it accurately on chart using "traffic light" pattern that is often located on the patient's asthma action plan as set by the health care provider. A system of asthma zones—green, yellow, and red—is commonly used (DeVrieze and Bhimji, 2017).
    - Green indicates that the PEFR is 80% to 100% of patient's personal best value and means that he or she should continue with the currently prescribed treatment regimen.
    - Yellow indicates that the PEFR is 50% to 90% of the personal best and that the person should add the prescribed quick-relief medication to the treatment regimen and continue with his or her daily long-term control medications.
    - Red indicates that the PEFR is less than 50% of the patient's personal best and that the person should take the prescribed quick-relief medication and seek medical attention.
15. Remove gloves and dispose in appropriate receptacle, perform hand hygiene.
16. Instruct patient to clean unit following the manufacturer instructions.
17. Document procedure, PEFR target achieved, and patient's tolerance.

PROCEDURAL GUIDELINE 16.2 *Using an Acapella Device*

Purpose
The Acapella device is a handheld airway clearance device for patients who have cystic fibrosis, COPD, asthma, and lung diseases with secretory problems, as well as for patients with atelectasis (Fig. 16.2). It utilizes positive expiratory pressure to open the airways and mobilize secretions (Naswa et al., 2017)

Delegation and Collaboration
The skill of using an Acapella device can be delegated to nursing assistive personnel (NAP). The nurse is responsible for performing respiratory assessment, determining that the procedure is appropriate and that a patient can tolerate it, and evaluating a patient's response to it. The nurse instructs the NAP to:

- Be alert for patient's tolerance of procedure, such as comfort level and changes in breathing pattern, and immediately report changes to the nurse.
- Use specific patient precautions such as positioning restrictions related to disease or treatment.

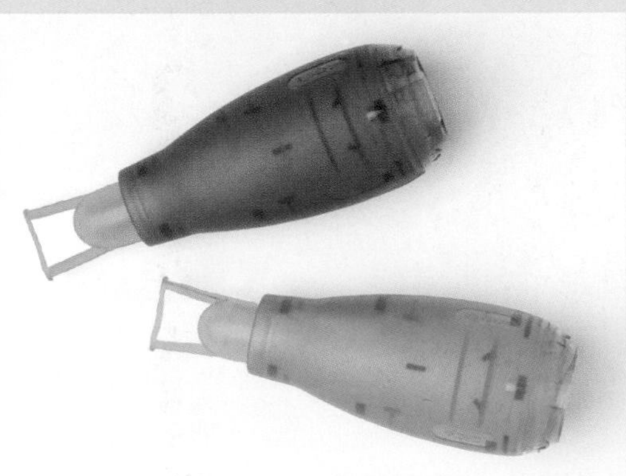

FIG 16.2 Acapella device. (*Used with permission*, Smithsmedical.com.)

Equipment
Stethoscope; pulse oximeter; glass of water; chair; tissues and paper bag; clear graduated screw-top container; suction equipment (if patient unable to cough and clear own secretions); Acapella device (see Fig. 16.2); clean gloves; patient education materials

Procedural Steps
1. Identify patient using at least two identifiers (e.g., name and birthday or name and medical record number) according to agency policy (TJC, 2019).
2. Verify the need for a health care provider's order per agency policy.
3. Perform hand hygiene and complete a respiratory assessment (including lung auscultation, inspection of mucus, and oxygen saturation) to determine oxygenation status and lung segments requiring percussion and/or vibration.
4. Assess patient's and family's understanding of the device and procedure and explain and clarify procedure as needed (CDC, 2016).
5. Prepare prescribed Acapella device:

Continued

PROCEDURAL GUIDELINE 16.2 *Using an Acapella Device—cont'd*

Safe Patient Care *Verify that the correct device is used to match patient's expiratory flow rate. Blue: patients who cannot maintain their expiratory flow above 15 L/min for greater than 3 seconds. Green: patients who can maintain expiratory flow above or equal to 15 L/min for at least 3 seconds.*

a. Initial setting: turn Acapella frequency adjustment dial counterclockwise to lowest resistance setting.
b. As patient improves or is more proficient, adjust the proper resistance level upward by turning the dial clockwise. This initial setting helps patient adjust to the device.

Safe Patient Care *Determine if aerosol drug therapy is ordered. If so, attach a nebulizer to the end of the Acapella valve, or administer medication before using the Acapella.*

6. Instruct patient to:
   a. Sit comfortably.
   b. Take in a breath that is larger than normal but not to fill lungs completely. Instruct patient to inhale to about 75% of inspiratory capacity.
   c. Place mouthpiece into mouth, maintaining a tight seal.
   d. Hold breath for 2 to 3 seconds.
   e. Try not to cough and to exhale slowly for 3 to 4 seconds through the device while it vibrates.

Safe Patient Care *If patient cannot maintain an exhalation for this length of time, adjust the dial clockwise. Clockwise adjustment increases the resistance of the vibrating opening, which allows the patient to exhale at a lower flow rate. Or it may be necessary to change from the blue to green device.*

   f. Repeat cycle for 5 to 10 breaths as tolerated.
   g. Remove mouthpiece and perform one or two forceful exhalations and "huff" coughs.
   h. Repeat Steps 6b through 6e, as ordered.
7. Auscultate lung fields.
8. Obtain vital signs, SpO_2.
9. Inspect color, character, and amount of sputum.
10. Perform hand hygiene and assist patient with oral hygiene as needed.
11. Document procedure and patient's tolerance.

PROCEDURAL GUIDELINE 16.3 *Performing Percussion and Vibration (Chest Physical Therapy)*

Purpose

The purpose of percussion and vibration overlying the rib cage is to to help loosen and remove mucus from the lung airways. Percussion is the manual external clapping of a patient's chest wall, with cupped hands or with a mechanical device, in a rhythmic fashion to loosen secretions from the bronchial walls. Vibration augments the natural movement of the rib cage during exhalation and helps with secretion clearance. Apply vibration to a patient's external chest wall by placing both hands (one over the other) over the areas to be vibrated (Strickland et al., 2015).

High-Frequency Chest Wall Compression

An additional method for perfusion and vibration is high-frequency chest wall compression (HFCWC). The purpose of HFCWC is to deliver high-frequency, small-volume expiratory pulses to a patient's external chest wall; one example is the vest airway clearance system, which helps loosen and remove secretions from the airways (Fig. 16.3). This mechanical action helps loosen and mobilize airway secretions (Chatwin et al., 2018). It is beneficial for selected patients with neuromuscular diseases, cystic fibrosis, and ineffective coughing and airway clearance.

Delegation and Collaboration

The skill of performing percussion and vibration can be delegated to trained nursing assistive personnel (NAP; see agency policy). The nurse is responsible for the respiratory assessment and review of the patient's chest x-ray film (with a health care provider) to determine patient stability, which areas of the lungs are affected, and specific positions for the patient to assume. The nurse instructs the NAP about:

- Any patient precautions related to disease or treatment.
- Reporting to the nurse any problems with tolerance of the procedure, pain, dyspnea, or changes in vital signs.

In some health care agencies, the respiratory therapist is responsible for performing percussion and vibration. The nurse must collaborate with the respiratory therapist when planning care for the patient in the acute care setting.

Equipment

Stethoscope; hospital bed (tilt table placed in Trendelenburg's position is optional; check agency policy); chair (for upper lobes); 1 to 4 pillows; water pitcher (with water) and glass; tissues and paper bag; clear graduated screw-top container; mechanical vibrator or percussor *(optional)*; HFCWC device such as the vest airway

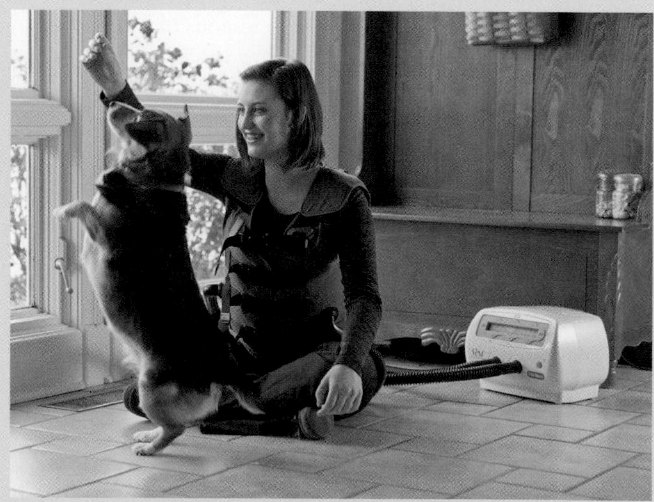

FIG 16.3 High-frequency chest wall oscillation vest for home use. *(Copyright ©2012 Hill-Rom Services, Inc. Reprinted with permission. All rights reserved.)*

PROCEDURAL GUIDELINE 16.3 *Performing Percussion and Vibration (Chest Physical Therapy)—cont'd*

clearance system; single layer of clothing; clean gloves; oral hygiene care items (toothbrush, toothpaste, mouthwash, or chlorhexidine oral rinse if ordered); suction equipment *(optional)*; pulse oximeter

Procedural Steps

1. Identify patient using at least two identifiers (e.g., name and birthday or name and medical record number) according to agency policy (TJC, 2019).
2. Assess patient and review medical record for x-ray findings and signs, symptoms, and conditions that indicate need to perform percussion and vibration (see Skill 16.1).
3. Review medical record for risks (e.g., use of steroids) and contraindications for percussion and vibration.

Safe Patient Care *Percussion and/or vibration can cause rib fractures and are contraindicated with rib fracture, fracture of other rib-cage structures such as clavicle or sternum, pain, severe dyspnea, and severe osteoporosis. Thin, frail patients with osteoporosis are most susceptible to injury and are taught other secretion-control measures (e.g., forceful coughing, humidification).*

4. Perform hand hygiene and perform respiratory assessment (including vital signs, pulse oximetry, and chest inspection and palpation) to assess breathing pattern, including muscles used for breathing, respiratory rate and depth, extent of excursion, chest wall movement, and oxygen saturation.
5. Auscultate lung sounds over lung segments drained during postural drainage.
6. Inspect and gently palpate rib cage over affected bronchial segment(s) for pain, tenderness, abnormal configuration, abnormal excursion or chest wall movement during breathing, and muscle tension. Percussion or vibration is contraindicated if one of these assessment findings is present because the treatment has the potential to cause further injury and impair chest wall motion. Remove gloves and perform hand hygiene.
7. Determine patient's understanding and assess ability to cooperate with therapy, both in health care agency and at home.
8. Explain procedure in detail: patient's positioning, sensations to be felt, how it will be done, how long it will take, use of vest (if applicable), and any discomforts or side effects.
9. Help patient relax and deep breathe during procedure. Have him or her practice exhaling slowly throu gh pursed lips while relaxing chest wall muscles and blow out using abdominal muscles, not rib-cage muscles.
10. Perform hand hygiene and apply clean gloves (only if risk of contacting mucus secretions).
11. Elevate bed to comfortable working height and stand close to bed with arms directly in front and knees slightly bent.
12. Use findings from physical assessment and chest x-ray film to select congested areas of lung. Position patient in appropriate drainage position (Table 16.3) and place pillows for support and comfort.
13. Perform percussion and vibration.
    a. Percussion and vibration with hands:
        (1) Perform percussion for 3 to 5 minutes in each position as tolerated. Begin on appropriate part of chest wall over draining area (see Table 16.3). Always ask if patient is experiencing any discomfort such as undue pressure or stinging of the skin.
        (2) Place hands side by side on chest wall over area to be drained. Cup hands with fingers and thumbs held tightly together. Make sure that entire outer part of hand makes contact with chest wall to avoid air leaks (see illustration).

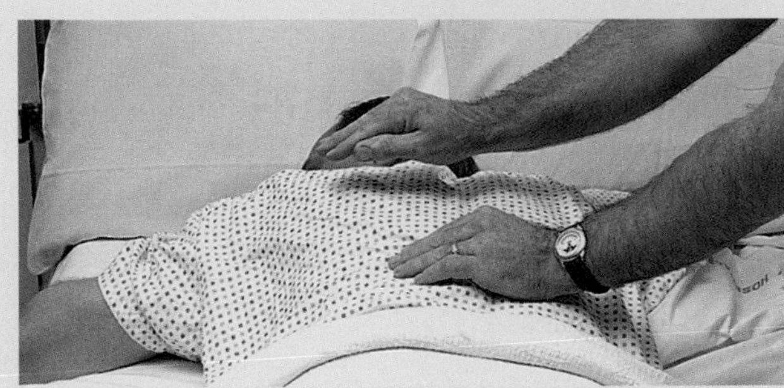

STEP 13a(2) Chest wall percussion, alternating hand clapping against patient's chest wall.

        (3) When clapping, most arm movement comes from the elbow and wrist joints. Clapping is often done for 5 minutes without stopping or for 2 to 3 minutes, alternating with vibration.
        (4) Alternately clap chest with cupped hands to create rhythmic popping sound resembling galloping horse. Perform clapping at moderate or fast speed, whichever is most comfortable and effective.
        (5) Perform chest wall vibration over each affected area (see Table 16.3).
            (a) Place flat part of hand over area and have patient take a slow, deep breath through nose.
            (b) Gently resist chest wall as it rises during inhalation.
            (c) Have patient hold breath for 2 to 3 seconds and exhale through pursed lips while contracting abdominal muscles and relaxing chest wall muscles. Chest wall relaxes and falls.
            (d) While patient is exhaling, gently push down and vibrate chest wall with flat part of hand (Volsko, 2013).
            (e) Repeat vibration three times and have patient cascade cough by taking deep breath and doing series of small coughs until end of breath. Instruct patient not to inhale between coughs. Vibrate chest wall as patient coughs. When applying pressure to ribs, always follow natural movement of rib cage. Allow patient to sit up and cough as needed.

Continued

TABLE 16.3

Positions and Procedures for Drainage, Percussion, Vibration, and Shaking

Area and Procedure	Anatomical Area	Position of Patient
Left and Right Upper Lobe Anterior Apical Bronchi Position patient in chair, or high-Fowler's, leaning back. Percuss and vibrate with heel of hands at shoulders and fingers over collarbones (clavicles) in front; do both sides at same time. Note body posture and arm position of nurse. Nurse's back is kept straight, and elbows and knees are slightly flexed.	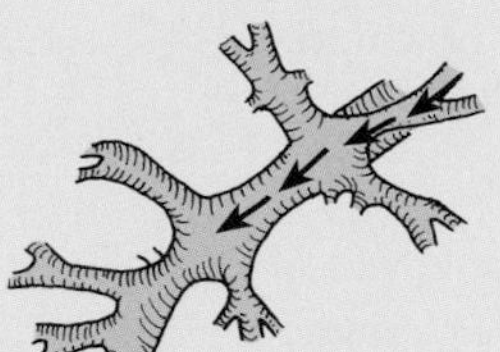	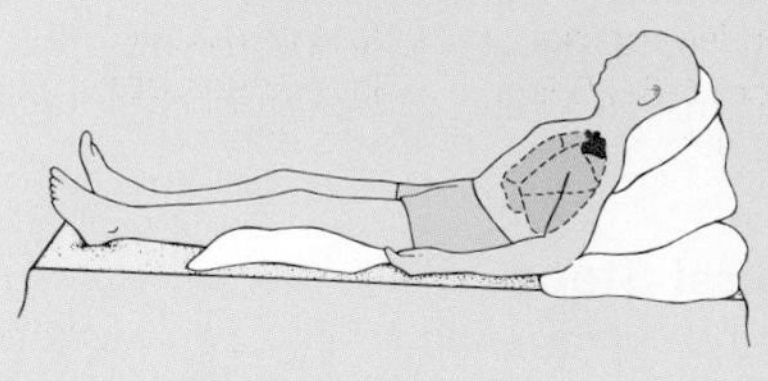 Anterior apical segments
Direction of mucus flow through upper lobe anterior apical bronchi.	Position hands for chest physiotherapy over left and right upper anterior apical bronchi.	
Left and Right Upper Lobe Posterior Apical Bronchi Position patient in chair, leaning forward on pillow or table. Percuss and vibrate with hands on either side of upper spine. Do both sides at same time.	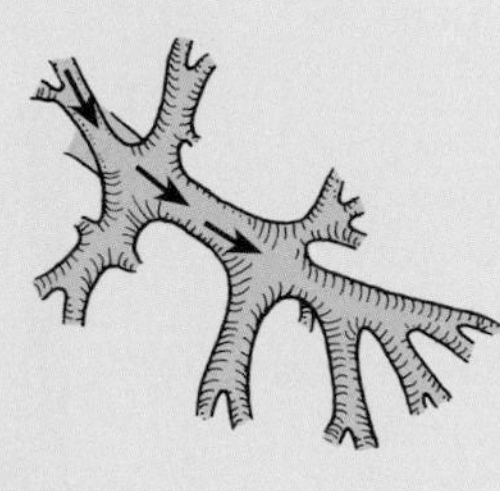	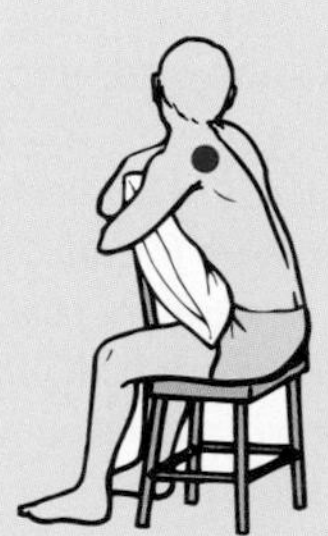 Posterior apical segments
Direction of mucus flow through upper lobe posterior apical bronchi.	Position hands for chest physiotherapy over left and right upper lobe posterior apical bronchi.	
Right and Left Anterior Upper Lobe Bronchi Position patient flat on back with small pillow under knees. Percuss and vibrate just below clavicle on either side of sternum.	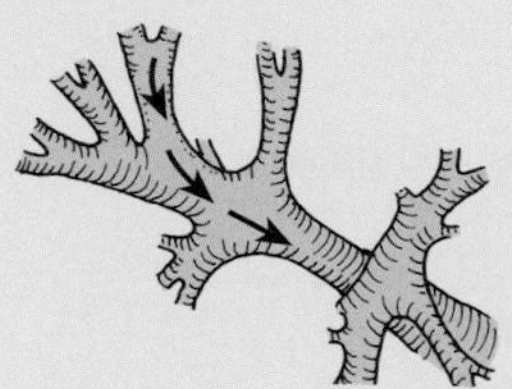	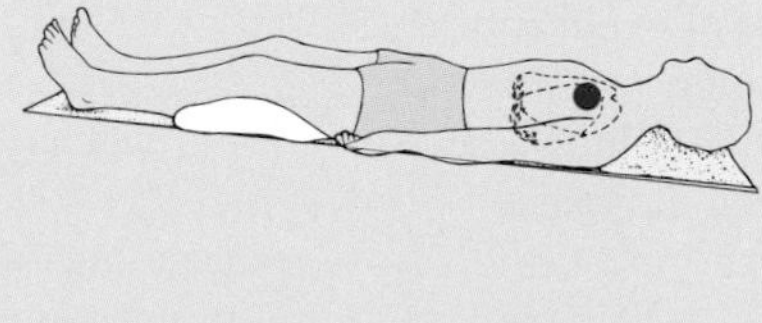 Left and right anterior upper lobe segments
Direction of mucus flow through anterior upper bronchi.	Position hands for chest physiotherapy over right and left anterior upper lobe bronchi.	
Left Upper Lobe Lingular Bronchus Position patient on right side with arm overhead in Trendelenburg's position, with foot of bed raised 30 cm (12 inches), as tolerated.* Place pillow behind back and roll patient one-quarter turn onto pillow. Percuss and vibrate lateral to left nipple below axilla.	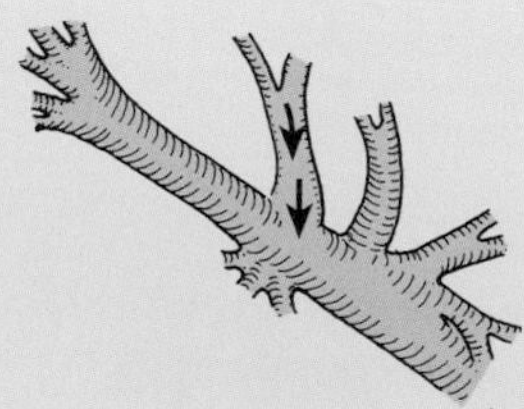	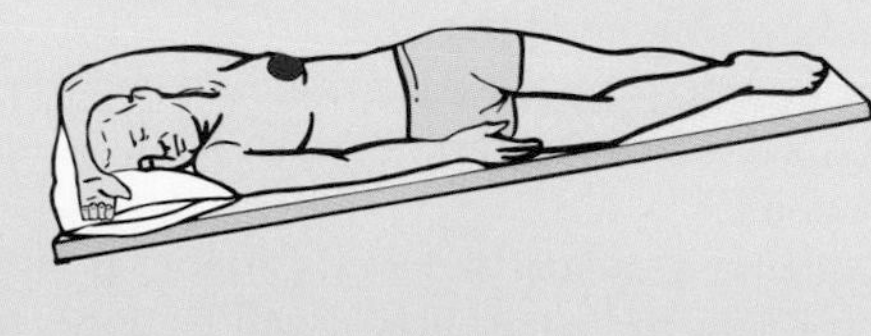 Left upper lobe lingular segment
Direction of mucus flow through left upper lobe lingular bronchus.	Position hands for chest physiotherapy over left upper lobe lingular bronchus.	
Right Middle Lobe Bronchus Position patient on left side or abdomen. Place pillow behind back and roll patient one-quarter turn onto pillow. Percuss and vibrate to right nipple below axilla.	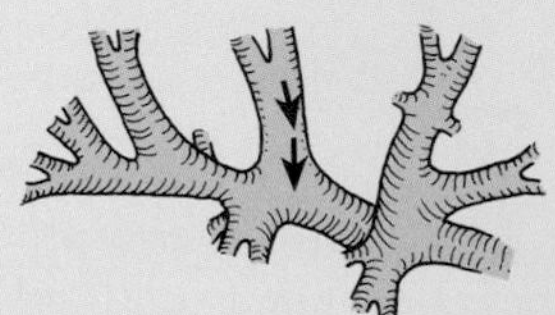	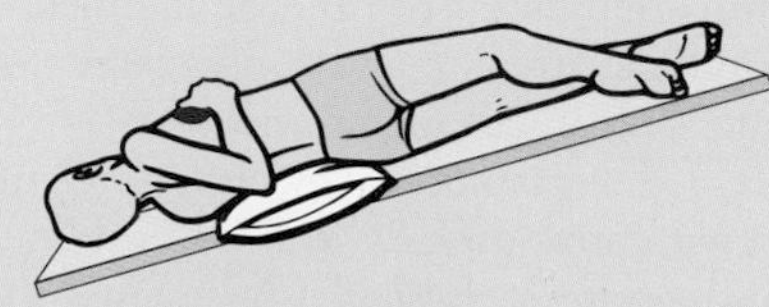 Right middle lobe segment
Direction of mucus flow through right middle lobe bronchus.	Position hands for chest physiotherapy over right middle lobe bronchus.	

TABLE 16.3

Positions and Procedures for Drainage, Percussion, Vibration, and Shaking—cont'd

Area and Procedure	Anatomical Area	Position of Patient
Left and Right Anterior Lower Lobe Bronchi Position patient on back, with foot of bed elevated to 45–50 cm (18–20 inches). Have knees bent on pillow. Percuss and vibrate over lower anterior ribs on both sides. Direction of mucus flow through anterior lower lobe bronchi.	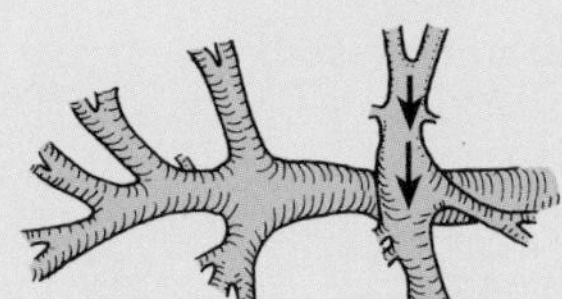	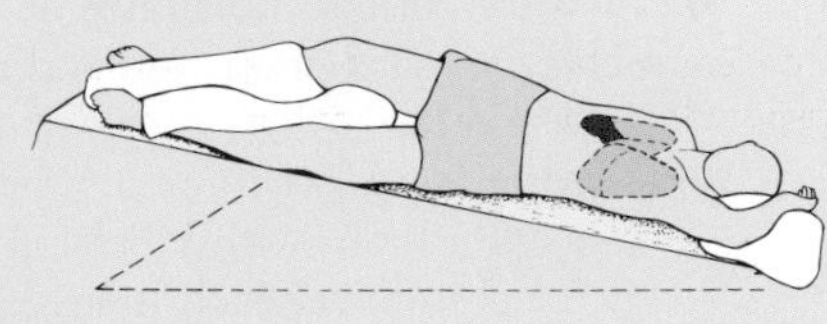 Left and right anterior lower lobe segments Position hands for chest physiotherapy over left and right anterior lower lobe bronchi.
Right Lower Lobe Lateral Bronchus Position patient on abdomen in Trendelenburg's position with foot of bed raised 45–50 cm (18–20 inches), as tolerated. Percuss and vibrate on left and right sides of chest below shoulder blades (scapulas) posterior to midaxillary line. Direction of mucus flow through right lower lobe lateral bronchus.	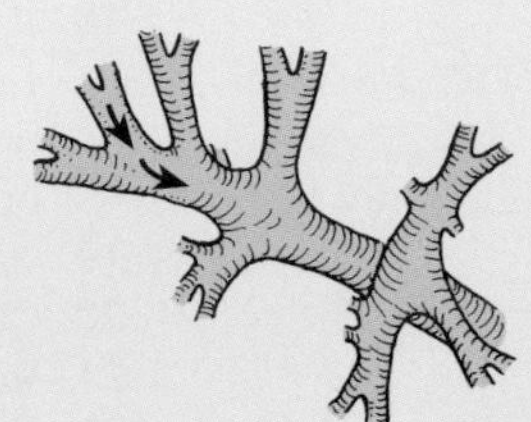	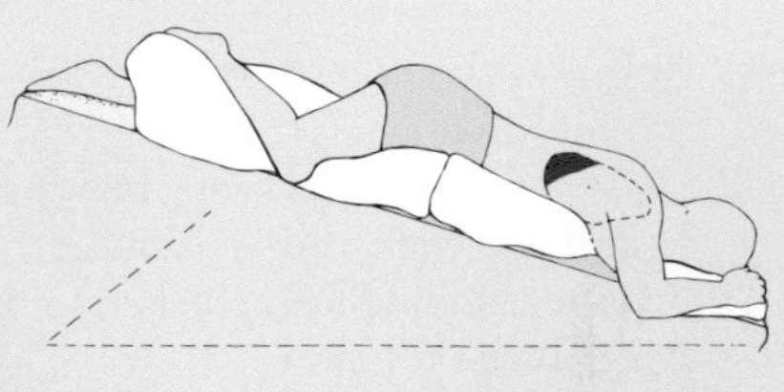 Right lower lateral lobe segment Position hands for chest physiotherapy over right lower lobe lateral bronchus.
Left Lower Lobe Lateral Bronchus Position patient on right side in Trendelenburg's position with foot of bed raised 45–50 cm (18–20 inches), as tolerated. Percuss and vibrate on left side of chest below scapulas posterior to midaxillary line. Direction of mucus flow through left lower lobe lateral bronchus.	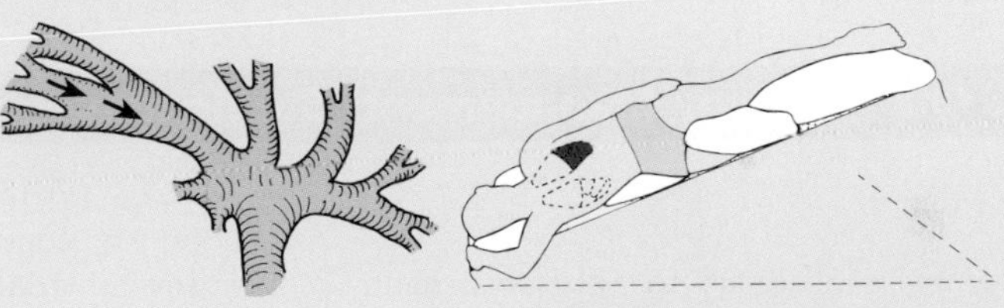	Left lower lobe lateral segment Position hands for chest physiotherapy over left lower lobe lateral bronchus.
Right and Left Lower Lobe Superior Bronchi Position patient flat on stomach with pillow under stomach. Percuss and vibrate below scapula on either side of spine. Direction of mucus flow through lower lobe superior bronchi.	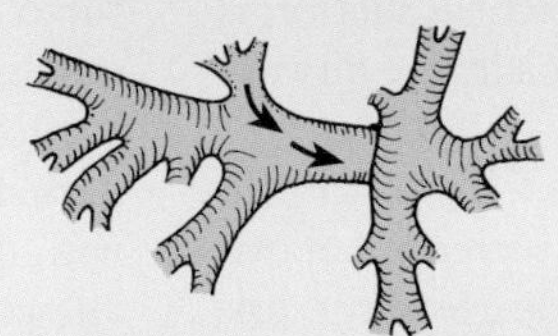	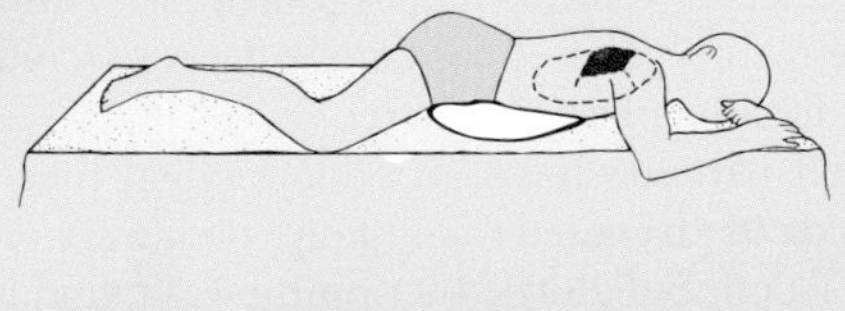 Right and left lower lobe superior segments Position hands for chest physiotherapy over right and left lower lobe superior bronchi.
Right and Left Posterior Basal Bronchi Position patient on stomach in Trendelenburg's position with foot of bed raised 45–50 cm (18–20 inches), as tolerated. Percuss and vibrate over low posterior ribs on either side of spine. Direction of mucus flow through posterior basal bronchi.	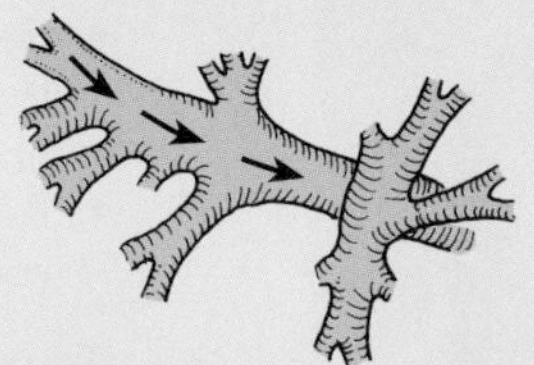	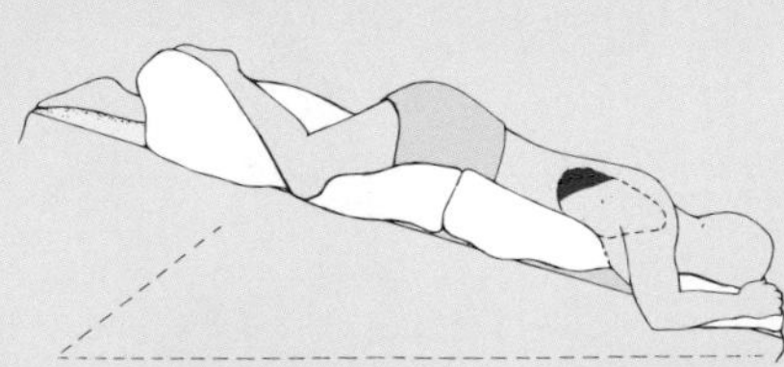 Right and left posterior segments Position hands for chest physiotherapy over right and left posterior lower lobe bronchi.

*In adult settings, Trendelenburg's position is not used as frequently. Verify use with agency policy and health care provider's order.

PROCEDURAL GUIDELINE 16.3 *Performing Percussion and Vibration (Chest Physical Therapy)—cont'd*

(f) Monitor patient's tolerance of vibration and ability to relax chest wall and breathe properly as instructed.
(g) Perform a total of three or four sets of three vibrations with vibration followed by coughing over each lung segment as tolerated. Strength and frequency of vibration will vary.

b. HFCWC device:
(1) Place vest on patient and assess for proper fit.
(a) With vest deflated, adjust closures so that it fits comfortably.
(b) Vest should rest on shoulder and extend to top of hip bone.
(2) Assess chest wall motion. Breathing should not be restricted when vest is deflated.
(3) Connect tubing to the generator and ports of the vest. Turn on power.
(4) Adjust pressure control as ordered; usually pressure is between 5 and 6.
(5) Adjust frequency; usually set between 10 and 15 Hz (Ntoumenopoulos, 2012; Clinkscale et al., 2012).
(6) Administer any aerosol therapy as prescribed.
(7) Depress and maintain pressure on the hand/foot control to initiate vest therapy.
(8) After 5 to 10 minutes, release hand/foot control.

14. Instruct patient to cough or suction if he or she is unable to cough up mucus (see Skill 16.3).
15. Continue with treatment; usually 15 to 30 minutes.
16. Assist patient with oral hygiene.
17. Remove gloves and perform hand hygiene.
18. If long-term therapy is needed, teach patient and significant others the procedure for home use for Acapella or HFCWC devices. If they cannot learn or use, refer for outpatient or home care follow-up.
19. Auscultate lung fields.
20. Obtain vital signs, pulse oximetry.
21. Inspect color, character, and amount of sputum.
22. Document procedure and patient's response.

✦ SKILL 16.3 Airway Management: Suctioning

Purpose

Airway suctioning is necessary to assist with removal of airway secretions. For some patients, coughing, chest PT, nebulization, and medications are insufficient to remove secretions and maintain a patent airway. Suctioning oropharyngeal secretions is done with a rigid plastic catheter (e.g., *Yankauer*) with one large and several small eyelets to remove mucus (Fig. 16.4). Nasotracheal suction is a sterile technique used to remove deeper secretions in the airways using a flexible plastic catheter.

When patients have an endotracheal tube (ETT), subglottic suctioning is advocated to minimize pooling of oral secretions above the ETT cuff. Subglottic suctioning was found to decrease the risk of ventilator-associated pneumonia (VAP) (Letchford and Bench, 2018). Suctioning of the lower airway is needed when patients cannot cough forcefully enough to clear secretions and requires the use of sterile technique. ETTs (Fig. 16.5) and tracheostomy tubes (TTs; Fig. 16.6) allow direct access to the lower airways for suctioning.

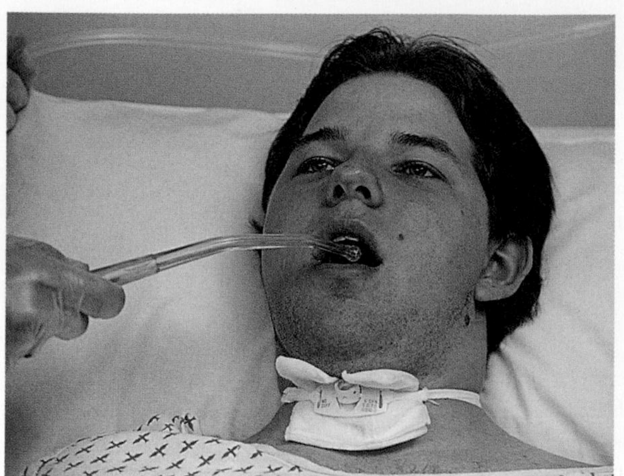

FIG 16.4 Oropharyngeal suctioning with a Yankauer catheter.

Delegation and Collaboration

The skill of suctioning endotracheal (ET) or nasotracheal (NT) tubes or newly inserted tracheostomy tubes cannot be delegated to nursing assistive personnel (NAP). In some agencies the NAP may suction a patient with a well-established tracheostomy that the nurse has determined to be stable. The nurse may need to collaborate with the respiratory therapist because respiratory therapists are also allowed to perform this procedure at certain health care agencies. The nurse directs the NAP about:

- Any modifications of the skill, such as the need for supplemental oxygen.
- Appropriate suction limits for suctioning ETTs and TTs and risks of applying excessive or inadequate suction pressure.
- Reporting any changes in patient's respiratory status, level of consciousness, restlessness, secretion color and amount, and unresolved coughing or gagging.
- Reporting any changes in patient's color, vital signs, or complaints of pain.

Equipment

Oropharyngeal Suctioning

- Clean, nonsterile suction catheter or Yankauer suction tip catheter
- Clean gloves
- Clean towel or paper drape
- Mask, goggles, or face shield if indicated; gown if required by isolation procedures

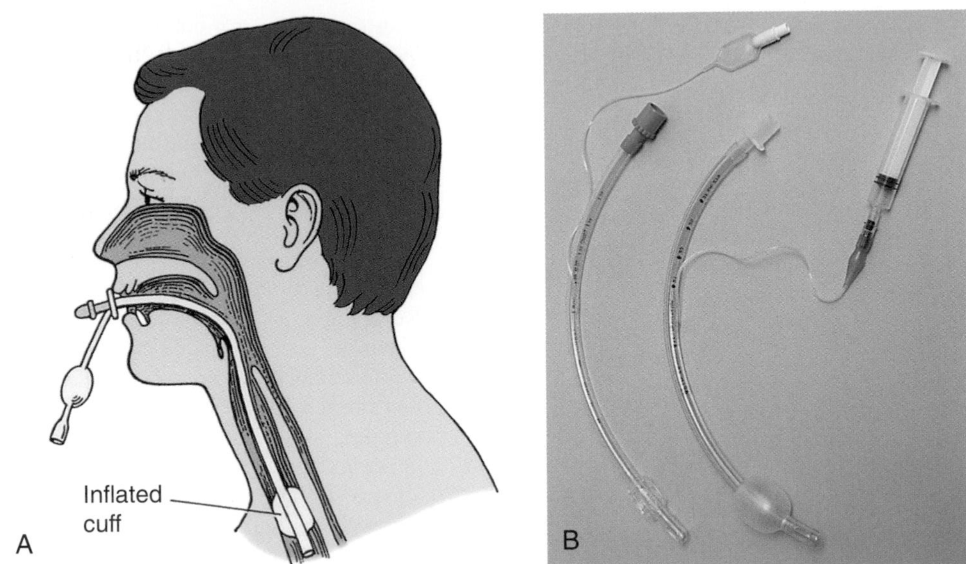

FIG 16.5 (A) Endotracheal tube with inflated cuff. (B) Endotracheal tubes with uninflated and inflated cuffs with syringe for inflation.

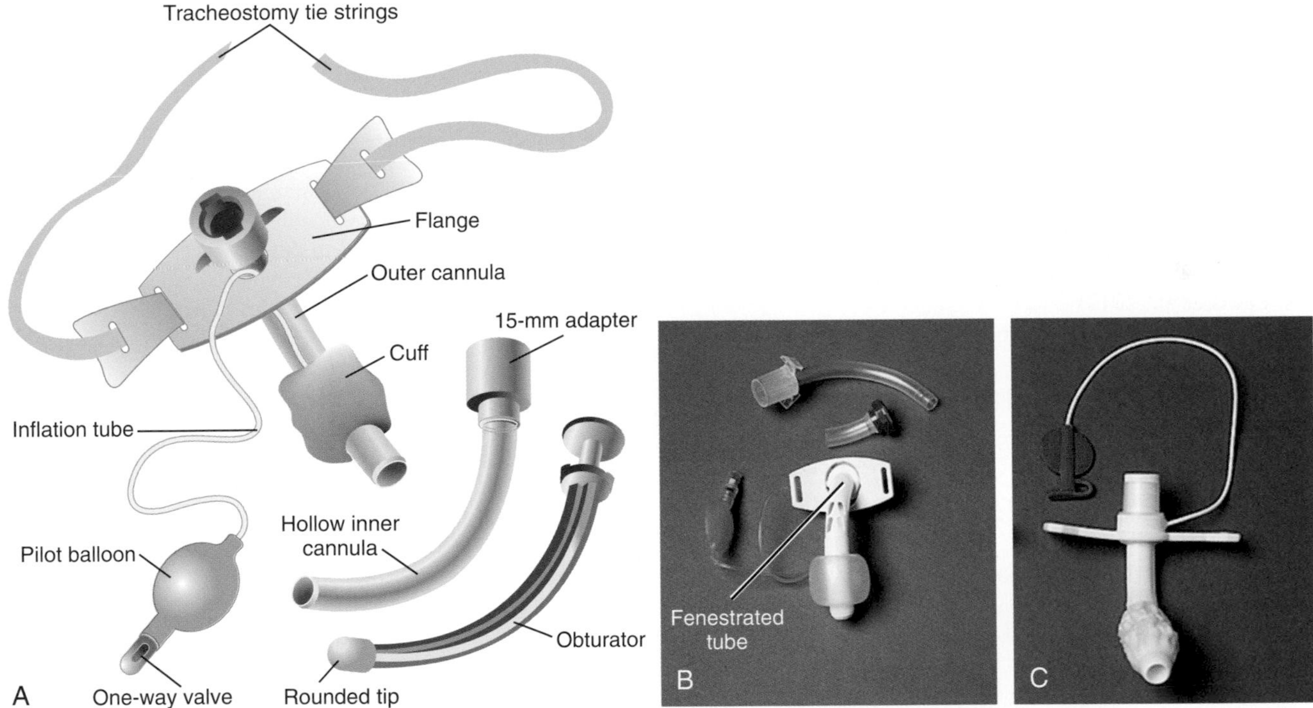

FIG 16.6 (A) Parts of a tracheostomy tube. (B) Fenestrated tracheostomy tube with cuff, inner cannula, decannulation plug, and pilot balloon. (C) Tracheostomy tube with foam cuff and obturator. *(From Lewis SL et al:* Medical-surgical nursing: assessment and management of clinical problems, *ed 9, St. Louis, 2014, Mosby.)*

- Disposable cup or basin
- Tap water or normal saline (about 100 mL)
- Suction machine or wall suction device with regulator
- Connecting tubing (6 feet)
- Stethoscope
- Pulse oximeter
- Oral airway (if indicated)
- Washcloth
- Manual self-inflating resuscitation bag (bag-valve-mask) with oxygen connecting tubing

Nasotracheal Suctioning

- Sterile suction catheter (12–16 Fr; smallest diameter that effectively removes secretions)
- Two sterile gloves or one sterile and one clean glove
- Sterile basin (e.g., sterile disposable cup)
- Sterile water or normal saline (about 100 mL)
- Clean towel or paper drape
- Mask, goggles, or face shield if indicated; gown if isolation procedures dictate
- Stethoscope

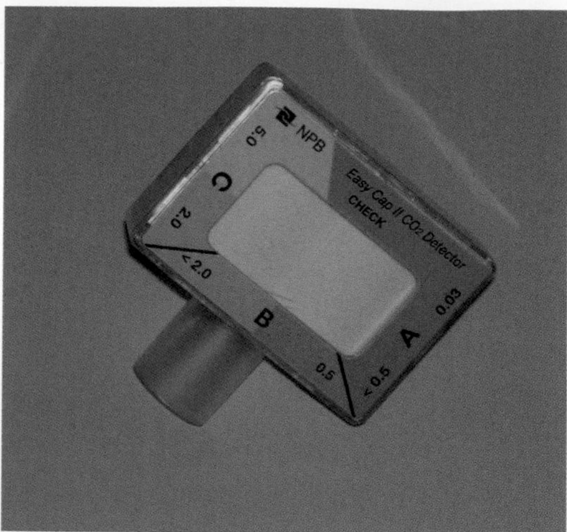

FIG 16.7 End-tidal CO_2 detector

- Pulse oximeter
- Suction machine or wall suction device with regulator
- Connecting tubing (6 feet)
- Manual self-inflating resuscitation bag (bag-valve-mask) with oxygen connecting tubing
- Bedside table

Endotracheal or Tracheostomy Suctioning

- Appropriate-size suction catheter, usually 12 to 16 Fr (smallest diameter that effectively removes secretions, preferably one that is no more than half of the internal diameter of the artificial airway to minimize decrease in PaO_2 (Branson et al., 2014; Lewis et al., 2017)
- Suction machine or wall suction device with regulator
- Bedside table
- Two sterile gloves or one sterile and one clean glove
- Sterile basin
- Sterile normal saline (about 100 mL)
- Clean towel or sterile drape
- Mask, goggles, or face shield, if indicated; gown if isolation procedures dictate
- Small Y-adapter (if catheter does not have a suction control port)
- Pulse oximeter, stethoscope and end-tidal CO_2 detector (Fig. 16.7)
- Manual self-inflating resuscitation bag (bag-valve-mask) with oxygen connecting tubing
- Positive end-expiratory pressure (PEEP) valve for resuscitation bag

ASSESSMENT

1. Identify patient using at least two identifiers (e.g., name and birthday or name and medical record number) according to agency policy. *Rationale: Ensures correct patient. Complies with The Joint Commission standards and improves patient safety* (TJC, 2019).
2. Review medical record for contraindications to nasotracheal suctioning: occluded nasal passages; nasal bleeding; epiglottis or croup; acute head, facial, or neck injury or surgery; coagulopathy or bleeding disorder; irritable airway; laryngospasm or bronchospasm; gastric surgery with high anastomosis; myocardial infarction (AARC, 2004). *Rationale: These conditions contraindicate suctioning because passage of suction catheter through nasal route causes trauma to existing facial trauma/surgery, increases nasal bleeding, or causes severe bleeding in presence of coagulopathy or bleeding disorders. In presence of epiglottis or croup, laryngospasm, or irritable airway, passage of suction catheter through nose causes intractable coughing, hypoxemia, and severe bronchospasm, necessitating emergency intubation or tracheostomy. Hypoxemia could worsen cardiac damage in myocardial infarction (AARC, 2004).*
3. Review sputum microbiology data in laboratory report. *Rationale: Certain bacteria are easier to transmit or require isolation because of virulence or antibiotic resistance.*
4. Perform hand hygiene and apply clean gloves if risk of exposing self to secretions. Assess for signs and symptoms of upper and lower airway obstruction requiring suctioning: abnormal respiratory rate, adventitious lung sounds, nasal secretions, gurgling, drooling, restlessness, gastric secretions or vomitus in mouth, and coughing without clearing airway secretions and/or improving adventitious lung sounds. *Rationale: Physical signs and symptoms result from secretions in upper and lower airways that decrease oxygen delivery to the tissues. Presuction assessment provides baseline data to identify need for suctioning and measures the effectiveness of suction procedures (Branson et al., 2014; Lewis et al., 2017).*
5. Assess vital signs, pulse oximetry, and signs and symptoms associated with hypoxia and hypercapnia: decreased SpO_2, increased pulse and blood pressure, apprehension, anxiety, lack of concentration, lethargy, decreased level of consciousness, confusion, dizziness, behavioral changes (e.g., irritability), irregular heart pulse, pallor, and cyanosis (a very late sign of hypoxia). Keep pulse oximeter on patient. *Rationale: Physical signs and symptoms resulting from decreased tissue oxygenation. Provides presuction baseline to measure patient tolerance to suctioning and effectiveness of suctioning on* SpO_2 *levels.*
6. Assess for risk factors for upper and lower airway obstruction, including chronic obstructive pulmonary disease, impaired mobility, decreased level of consciousness, nasal feeding tube, decreased cough or gag reflex, and decreased swallowing ability. *Rationale: Risk factors can impair patient's ability to clear secretions from airway, increase risk for retaining secretions, and necessitate nasopharyngeal or nasotracheal suctioning (Urden et al., 2016).*
7. Identify patients with an increased risk for ineffective airway clearance (e.g., patients with decreased level of consciousness, neuromuscular or neurological impairment, or anatomical factors that influence upper or lower airway function such as recent surgery head chest or neck tumors). *Rationale: Changes in neurological status and neuromuscular impairment increase likelihood that patient is unable to clear respiratory secretions. Abnormal anatomy or head and neck surgery/trauma and tumors in and around lower airway impair normal secretion clearance. Accumulating pulmonary secretions impede patient's ability to effectively clear airway through cough mechanism (Urden et al., 2016).*
8. Assess for excessive amounts of secretions or secretions visible in the oral cavity or artificial airway, signs of respiratory distress (increased work of breathing, increased respiratory rate), presence of rhonchi on auscultation, excessive coughing, increased peak inspiratory pressures (if on mechanical ventilator), saw-tooth pattern on ventilator monitor, or changes in capnography waveform (if patient on

mechanical ventilator) or decrease in patient pulse oximeter (Branson et al., 2014). *Rationale: Suctioning should only be performed as patient condition indicates and not in a scheduled fashion such as hourly (Lewis et al., 2017; Myatt, 2015).*

9. Assess patency of ETT (if present) with capnography/end-tidal carbon dioxide (CO_2) detector. *Rationale: ETT may become displaced or blocked by secretions. Capnography measures the amount of carbon dioxide (CO2) in exhaled air, which assesses ventilation and is visualized by the sawtooth pattern on the capnography monitor (Sole et al., 2015).*
10. Assess factors that may affect volume and consistency of secretions. *Rationale: Thickened or copious secretions increase risk for airway obstruction.*
    a. Fluid balance. *Rationale: Fluid overload increases amount of secretions. Dehydration can cause thicker secretions.*
    b. Lack of humidity. *Rationale: Environment influences secretion formation and gas exchange. Lack of humidity, particularly in patients with artificial airways, can lead to atelectasis or airway obstruction (Restepro and Walsh, 2012).*
    c. Infection (e.g., pneumonia). *Rationale: Patients with respiratory infections are prone to increased secretions that are thicker and sometimes more difficult to expectorate.*
11. For endotracheal suctioning, assess patient's peak inspiratory pressure when on volume-controlled ventilation or tidal volume during pressure-controlled ventilation. *Rationale: Increased peak inspiratory pressure or decreased tidal volume may indicate airway obstruction (Urden et al., 2016).*

Safe Patient Care *The patient's vital signs, pulse oximetry, end-tidal CO_2, and respiratory status will be assessed before and continuously throughout the procedure (Wiegand, 2017).*

12. Determine presence of apprehension, anxiety, decreased ability to concentrate, lethargy, decreased level of consciousness (especially acute), increased fatigue, dizziness, behavioral changes (especially irritability), pallor, cyanosis, dyspnea, or use of accessory muscles. Remove and dispose of gloves and perform hand hygiene. *Rationale: These are signs and symptoms of hypoxia and/or hypercapnia, which can indicate need for suction. These signs can also help to identify patient's ability to cooperate with procedure.*
13. Assess patient's or family caregiver's knowledge, experience, and health literacy. *Rationale: Ensures patient or family caregiver has the capacity to obtain, communicate, process, and understand basic health information (CDC, 2016).*
14. Assess for patient's understanding of procedure and presence of any apprehension. *Rationale: Reveals need for instruction or psychosocial support.*

STEP	RATIONALE

PLANNING

1. Expected outcomes following completion of procedure:	
• Upper and lower airways demonstrate absent or diminished gurgles, crackles, rhonchi, and wheezes on inspiration and expiration.	Absent or diminished adventitious sounds indicates that airways are cleared of secretions and are patent.
• Heart rate, blood pressure, respiratory rate, and effort are within normal range for patient.	When airway secretions are removed, and oxygenation improves, patient's vital signs and respiratory assessment findings improve.
• Patient's SpO_2 is at or above baseline, whereas end-tidal carbon dioxide ($ETCO_2$) concentration, if being monitored, is at or below baseline.	Demonstrates improvement in gas exchange (Branson et al., 2014; Wiegand, 2017).

Safe Patient Care *Although normal $ETCO_2$ ranges from 35 to 45 mm Hg, it is important to ensure that the patient's value is below the normal baseline. Persons with pulmonary diseases often have abnormal CO_2 values.*

• Patient's peak inspiratory pressure decreases back to baseline, and exhaled tidal volume increases back to baseline.	Demonstrates removal of secretions (Wiegand, 2017).
2. Provide privacy and assist patient to comfortable position, typically semi-Fowler's or high Fowler's.	Reduces stimulation of gag reflex, promotes patient comfort and secretion drainage, and prevents aspiration.
3. If not already present, place pulse oximeter on patient's finger. Take reading and leave oximeter in place.	Provides continuous SpO_2 value to determine patient's response to suctioning.
4. Prepare and organize equipment. Place towel across patient's chest.	Ensures that you have the necessary equipment in place to complete procedure.
5. Explain to patient how procedure will help clear airway and relieve breathing difficulty. Explain that temporary coughing, sneezing, gagging, or shortness of breath is normal during procedure.	Encourages cooperation and minimizes risks, anxiety, and pain of procedure.

IMPLEMENTATION

1. Perform hand hygiene and apply appropriate personal protective equipment (mask with face shield or goggles; gown if necessary).	Reduces transmission of microorganisms.

STEP	RATIONALE
2. Adjust bed to appropriate height (if not already done) and lower side rail on side nearest you. Check locks on bed wheel.	Minimizes caregiver's muscle strain and prevents injury. Prevents bed from moving.
3. Connect one end of connecting tubing to wall suction device and place other end in convenient location near patient. Turn suction device on and set suction pressure to as low a level as possible and yet able to effectively clear secretions. This value is typically between 100 and 150 mm Hg in adults (between 60 and 100 mm Hg in neonates) (AARC, 2010). Suction pressure should not exceed 180 mm Hg (Branson et al., 2014). Occlude end of suction tubing to check pressure.	Ensures equipment function. Excessive negative pressure damages tracheal mucosa and induces greater hypoxia (Wiegand, 2017).
4. Prepare suction catheter for all types of open suctioning.	
a. One-time use catheter (open suction technique):	
(1) Using aseptic technique, open suction kit or catheter package. If sterile drape is available, place it across patient's chest or on bedside table. Do not allow suction catheter to touch any nonsterile surfaces.	Prepares catheter, maintains asepsis, and reduces transmission of microorganisms. Provides sterile surface on which to lay catheter between passes.
(2) Unwrap or open sterile basin or disposable cup and place on bedside table. Be careful not to touch inside of basin or cup. Fill with about 100 mL sterile normal saline solution or tap water for oral suctioning (see illustration).	Saline or water is used to clean tubing after each suction pass.
(3) If performing nasotracheal suctioning, open packet of water-soluble lubricant and apply small amount to catheter. **NOTE:** *Lubricant is not necessary for artificial airway suctioning.*	Water-soluble lubricant eases passage of nasotracheal tube and helps avoid lipid aspiration pneumonia. Excessive amount of lubricant occludes catheter.
5. Apply gloves: Note that oropharyngeal suctioning is a clean technique, and clean gloves are appropriate. For nasotracheal tube, endotracheal tube, or tracheal tube suctioning, sterile gloves are required. When this is the case, apply sterile gloves to each hand or nonsterile glove to nondominant hand and sterile glove to dominant hand.	Reduces transmission of microorganisms and maintains sterility of suction catheter.
6. Pick up suction catheter with dominant hand without touching nonsterile surfaces. Pick up connecting tubing with nondominant hand. Secure catheter to tubing (see illustration).	Maintains catheter sterility. Connects catheter to suction.
7. Place tip of catheter into sterile basin or disposable cup and suction small amount of normal saline/tap water solution from basin by occluding suction vent.	Ensures equipment function. Lubricates internal catheter and tubing.

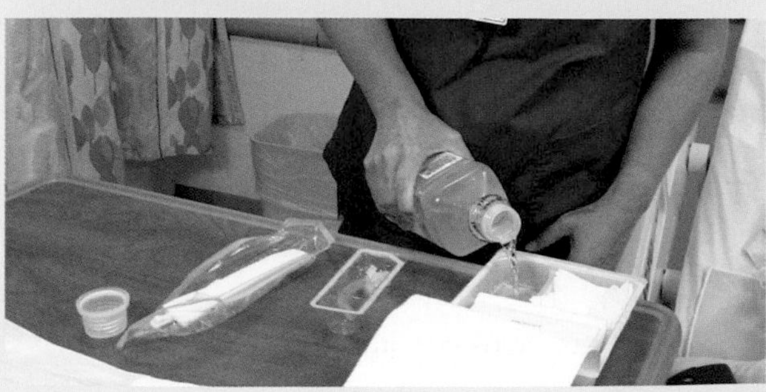

STEP 4a(2) Pouring sterile saline into tray.

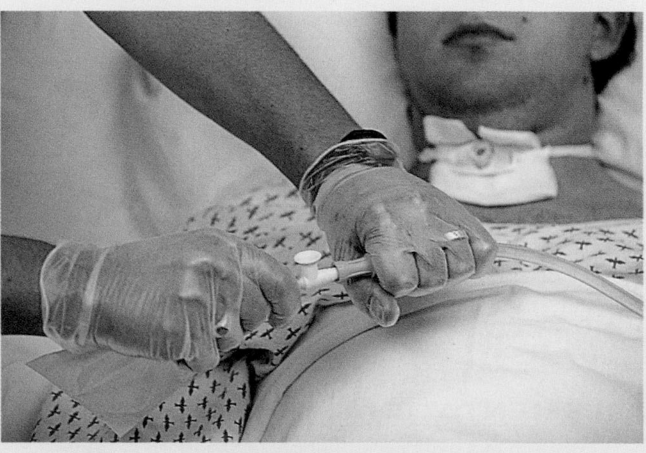

STEP 6 Attaching suction catheter to suction tubing.

STEP	RATIONALE
8. Suction airway.	
a. **Oropharyngeal suctioning:**	Clears easy-to-remove oral secretions. In patients who require sterile suctioning of airways, oropharyngeal suctioning is performed after sterile suctioning to prevent contamination of the suction catheters or tubing with bacteria present in the oral cavity (Wiegand, 2017).
(1) Remove patient's oxygen mask if present but keep it close. Nasal cannula may remain in place.	Allows access to mouth. Reduces chance of hypoxia.
(2) Insert catheter into mouth along gum line to pharynx. Move catheter around mouth until secretions have cleared. Encourage patient to cough. Replace oxygen mask.	Movement of catheter prevents suction tip from invaginating oral mucosal surfaces and causing trauma. Coughing moves secretions from lower airway into mouth and upper airway.

Safe Patient Care *If ETT is present, be careful when moving the catheter so as not to dislodge the ETT. Be careful when suctioning a patient who had recent oral or head/neck surgery. Aggressive suctioning and excessive coughing should not be used or encouraged in patients who have undergone throat surgery, such as a tonsillectomy. Aggressive suctioning in these patient populations can aggravate the operative site, increasing the risk of bleeding or infection (Hockenberry et al., 2017).*

STEP	RATIONALE
(3) Rinse catheter with water or normal saline in cup or basin until connecting tubing is cleared of secretions. Turn off suction. Place catheter in clean, dry area.	Rinses catheter and reduces probability of transmission of microorganisms. Clean suction tubing enhances delivery of set suction pressure. Medically aseptic technique saving catheter for future use is appropriate for oral catheter.
b. **Nasopharyngeal and nasotracheal suctioning:**	
(1) Have patient take deep breaths, if able, or increase oxygen flow rate with delivery device through cannula or mask (if ordered).	May help to decrease risks of hypoxemia.
(2) Be sure catheter tip is lightly coated at distal 6 to 8 cm (2–3 inches) with water-soluble lubricant.	Lubricates catheter for easier insertion.
(3) Remove oxygen-delivery device, if applicable, with nondominant hand. Advise patient that you are about to begin suctioning.	Allows access to nares and catheter.

Safe Patient Care *Be sure to insert catheter during patient inhalation, especially if inserting it into trachea, because epiglottis is open. Do not insert during swallowing or catheter will most likely enter esophagus.* ***Never apply suction during insertion.*** *Patient should cough. If patient gags or becomes nauseated, catheter is most likely in esophagus, and you need to remove it.*

STEP	RATIONALE
(4) Apply suction	
(a) *Nasopharyngeal* (without applying suction): As patient takes deep breath, insert catheter following natural course of naris; slightly slant catheter downward and advance to back of pharynx. Do not force through nares. In adults, insert catheter approximately 16 cm (6.5 inches); in older children, 8 to 12 cm (3–5 inches); in infants and young children, 4 to 7.5 cm (1.5–3 inches). Rule of thumb is to insert catheter distance from tip of nose (or mouth) to angle of mandible.	Ensure that catheter tip reaches pharynx for suctioning.

Safe Patient Care *If resistance is met during insertion, you may need to try the other naris. Do not force the catheter up the nares because this will cause mucosal damage.*

STEP	RATIONALE
i. Apply intermittent suction for no more than 10 to 15 seconds by placing and releasing nondominant thumb over catheter vent. Slowly withdraw catheter while rotating it back and forth between thumb and forefinger.	Intermittent suction up to 10 to 15 seconds safely removes pharyngeal secretions. Suction time greater than 10 to 15 seconds increases risk for suction-induced hypoxemia (AARC, 2010; Branson et al., 2014).

STEP	RATIONALE
(b) *Nasotracheal* (without applying suction): As patient takes deep breath, advance catheter following natural course of naris. Advance catheter slightly slanted and downward to just above entrance into larynx and then trachea. While patient takes deep breath, quickly insert catheter: for adults, insert approximately 16 to 20 cm (6–8 inches) into trachea (see illustration). Patient will begin to cough; then pull back catheter 1 to 2 cm (½ inch) before applying suction. **NOTE:** In older children, insert approximately 16 to 20 cm (6–8 inches) into trachea; in infants and young children, 8 to 14 cm (3–5½ inches).	Ensure that catheter tip reaches trachea for suctioning.

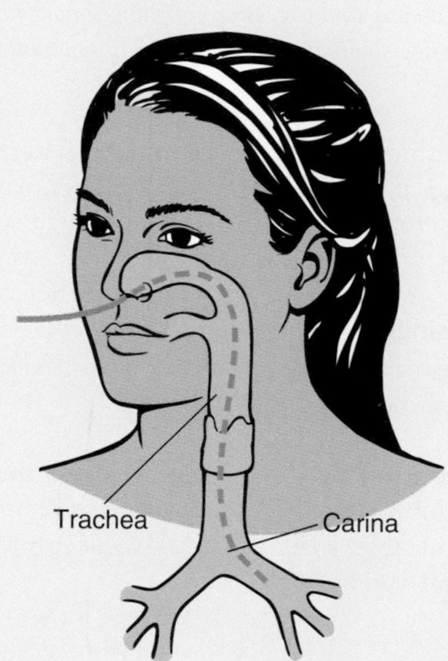

STEP 8b(4)(b) Distance of insertion of nasotracheal catheter.

Safe Patient Care *When using the nasal approach, perform tracheal suctioning before pharyngeal suctioning whenever possible. The mouth and pharynx contain more bacteria than the trachea. If copious oral secretions are present before beginning the procedure, suction mouth with oral suction device first.*

Safe Patient Care *When there is difficulty passing the catheter, ask patient to cough or say "ahh," or try to advance the catheter during inspiration. Both measures help to open the glottis to permit passage of the catheter into the trachea.*

STEP	RATIONALE
(c) *Positioning option:* In some instances, turning patient's head helps you suction more effectively. If you feel resistance after insertion of catheter, use caution; it has probably hit the carina. Pull catheter back 1 to 2 cm (0.4–0.8 inch) before applying suction (AARC, 2004).	Turning patient's head to side elevates bronchial passage on opposite side. Turning head to right helps with suctioning of left main-stem bronchus; turning head to left helps you suction right main-stem bronchus. Suctioning too deep may cause tracheal mucosa trauma.
i. Apply intermittent suction for no more than 10 to 15 seconds by placing and releasing nondominant thumb over catheter vent. Slowly withdraw catheter while rotating it back and forth between thumb and forefinger.	Suction time greater than 15 seconds increases risk for suction-induced hypoxemia (AARC, 2010; Branson et al., 2014). Intermittent suction and rotation of catheter prevents injury to tracheal mucosa. If catheter "grabs" mucosa, remove thumb to release suction.

Safe Patient Care *Monitor patient's vital signs and oxygen saturation throughout suctioning process. Stop suctioning if there is a 20-beats/min change (increase or decrease) in pulse rate or if SpO_2 falls below 90% or 5% from baseline.*

STEP	RATIONALE
(5) Reapply oxygen-delivery device and encourage patient to take some deep breaths, if able.	Helps decrease risk of hypoxia. Increases patient comfort.

STEP	RATIONALE
(6) Rinse catheter and connecting tubing with normal saline or water until cleared.	Secretions that remain in suction catheter or connecting tubing decrease suctioning efficiency.
(7) Assess for need to repeat suctioning. Do not perform more than two passes with catheter. Allow patient to rest at least 1 minute (AARC, 2010). Ask patient to deep breathe and cough.	Observe for alterations in cardiopulmonary status. Suctioning induces hypoxemia, irregular pulse, laryngospasm, and bronchospasm (AARC, 2010). Hyperoxygenation is recommended before, during, and after open suctioning to reduce suction-induced hypoxemia (Galbiati and Paola, 2015).
c. Artificial airway:	
(1) When patient has an artificial airway, hyperoxygenate with 100% oxygen for at least 30 to 60 seconds before suctioning by (1) pressing suction hyperoxygenation button on ventilator; *or* (2) increasing baseline fraction of inspired oxygen (FiO_2) level on mechanical ventilator; *or* (3) disconnecting ventilator, attaching self-inflating resuscitation bag-valve device to tube with nondominant hand (or have assistant do this), and administering 5 to 6 breaths over 30 seconds (or have assistant do this). **NOTE:** Some mechanical ventilators have a button that, when pushed, delivers 100% oxygen for a few minutes and then resets to previous setting.	Preoxygenation decreases risk of decreased arterial oxygen levels while ventilation or oxygenation is interrupted and volume is lost during suctioning (AARC, 2010). Some models of resuscitation bags do not deliver 100% oxygen; therefore this is not the best way to oxygenate patient (Wiegand, 2017).

Safe Patient Care *Suctioning can cause elevations in intracranial pressure (ICP) in patients with head injuries. Reduce this risk by presuction hyperoxygenation, which results in hypocarbia, which in turn induces vasoconstriction. Vasoconstriction reduces the potential for an increase in ICP (Urden et al., 2016).*

STEP	RATIONALE
(2) If patient is receiving mechanical ventilation, open swivel adapter or, if necessary, remove oxygen- or humidity-delivery device with nondominant hand.	Exposes artificial airway.
(3) Advise patient that you are about to begin suctioning. Without applying suction, gently but quickly insert catheter into artificial airway using dominant thumb and forefinger (it is best to try to time catheter insertion into artificial airway with inspiration; see illustration). Advance catheter until you meet resistance or patient coughs; then pull back 1 cm (0.4 inch; Wiegand, 2017).	Application of suction pressure while introducing catheter into trachea increases risk for damage to tracheal mucosa and increased hypoxia. Pulling back stimulates cough and removes catheter from mucosal wall so that catheter is not resting against tracheal mucosa during suctioning. Shallow suctioning is recommended to prevent tracheal mucosa trauma (AARC, 2010; Wiegand, 2017).

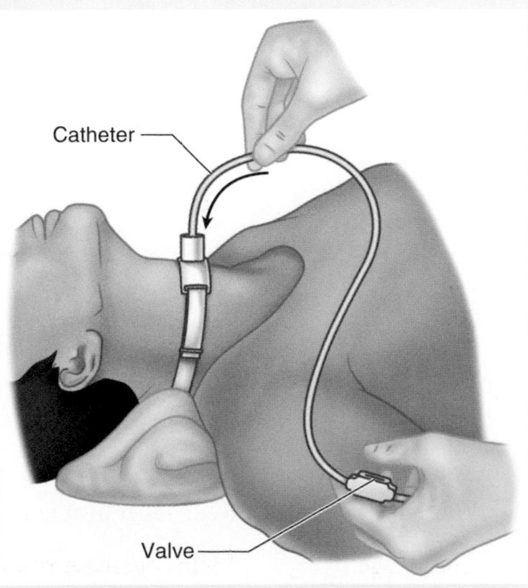

STEP 8c(3) Suctioning tracheostomy.

STEP	RATIONALE

Safe Patient Care *If unable to insert catheter past the end of an ETT, the catheter is probably caught in the Murphy eye (i.e., side hole at the distal end of the ETT that allows for collateral airflow in the event of tracheal main-stem intubation). If this happens, rotate the catheter to reposition it away from the Murphy eye or withdraw it slightly and reinsert with the next inhalation. Usually the catheter meets resistance at the carina. One indication that the catheter is at the carina is acute onset of coughing because the carina contains many cough receptors. Pull the catheter back 1 cm (½ inch).*

STEP	RATIONALE
(4) Apply intermittent suction for 10 to 15 seconds (AARC, 2010; Branson et al., 2014). Apply intermittent suction by placing and releasing nondominant thumb over vent of catheter; slowly withdraw catheter while rotating it back and forth between dominant thumb and forefinger. Do not use suction for greater than 15 seconds. Encourage patient to cough. Watch for respiratory distress.	Suction time greater than 15 seconds increases risk for suction-induced hypoxemia (AARC, 2010; Branson et al., 2014). Intermittent suction and rotation of catheter prevent injury to tracheal mucosa. If catheter "grabs" mucosa, remove thumb to release suction.

Safe Patient Care *If patient develops respiratory distress during the suction procedure, immediately withdraw catheter and supply additional oxygen and breaths as needed. In an emergency, administer oxygen directly through the catheter. Disconnect suction and attach oxygen at prescribed flow rate through the catheter. If the patient does not tolerate the suctioning procedure, you may need to consider switching to closed (in-line) suctioning or allowing longer recovery times. Notify health care provider if patient develops significant cardiopulmonary compromise during suctioning (Urden et al., 2016; Wiegand, 2017).*

STEP	RATIONALE
(5) If patient is receiving mechanical ventilation, close swivel adapter or replace oxygen-delivery device. Hyperoxygenate patient for 30 to 60 seconds.	Reestablishes artificial airway. Helps decrease risks of hypoxia.
(6) Rinse catheter and connecting tubing with normal saline until clear. Use continuous suction.	Removes catheter secretions. Secretions left in tubing decrease suctioning efficiency and provide environment for microorganism growth.
(7) Assess patient's vital signs, cardiopulmonary status, and ventilator measures for secretion clearance. Repeat Steps 8c(1) through 8c(6) once or twice more to clear secretions. Allow adequate time (at least 1 full minute) between suction passes.	Suctioning can induce dysrhythmias, hypoxia, and bronchospasm and impair cerebral circulation or adversely affect hemodynamic stability (Wiegand, 2017).

Safe Patient Care *The number of suction passes should be based on patient assessment and presence of secretions. If secretions persist after two passes, allow patient more time to rest and recover from these procedures (Wiegand, 2017).*

STEP	RATIONALE
(8) When pharynx and trachea are sufficiently cleared of secretions, perform oropharyngeal suctioning (see Step 8a) to clear mouth of secretions. Do not suction artificial airway again after suctioning mouth.	Removes upper airway secretions. More microorganisms generally are present in mouth. Upper airway is considered "clean," and lower airway is considered "sterile." You can use same catheter to suction from sterile to clean areas (e.g., tracheal suctioning to oropharyngeal suctioning) but not from clean to sterile areas.
9. When suctioning is complete, disconnect catheter from connecting tubing. Roll catheter around fingers of dominant hand. Pull glove off inside out so that catheter remains coiled in glove. Pull off other glove over first glove in same way. Discard in appropriate receptacle.	Seals contaminants in gloves. Reduces transmission of microorganisms.
10. Remove towel, place in laundry or appropriate receptacle, and reposition patient.	Reduces transmission of microorganisms. Promotes comfort.
11. If oxygen level was changed during procedure, readjust oxygen to original ordered level because patient's blood oxygen level should have returned to baseline.	Prevents absorption atelectasis (i.e., tendency for airways to collapse if proximally obstructed by secretions). Prevents oxygen toxicity while allowing patient time to reoxygenate blood.
12. Apply clean gloves to continue personal care, such as washing the face or oral hygiene.	
13. Discard remainder of normal saline into appropriate receptacle. If basin is disposable, discard into appropriate receptacle. If basin is reusable, rinse it out and place it in soiled utility room.	Reduces transmission of microorganisms.

STEP	RATIONALE
14. Remove personal protective equipment and gloves and discard into appropriate receptacle. Perform hand hygiene.	Reduces transmission of microorganisms.
15. Place unopened suction kit on suction machine table or at head of bed.	Provides immediate access to suction catheter for next procedure.
16. Help patient to comfortable position.	
17. Be sure nurse call system is in an accessible location within patient's reach.	Ensures patient can call for assistance if needed.
18. Raise side rails (as appropriate) and lower bed to lowest position.	Ensures patient safety.

EVALUATION

1. Compare patient's vital signs, cardiopulmonary assessments, $ETCO_2$ and SpO_2 values before and after suctioning. If on ventilator, compare FiO_2 and tidal volumes and peak inspiratory pressures.	Identifies physiological effects of suction procedure to restore airway patency.
2. Ask patient if breathing is easier and if congestion is decreased.	Provides subjective confirmation that suctioning procedure has relieved airway.
3. Observe character of airway secretions.	Provides data to document presence or absence of respiratory tract infection or thickened secretions.
4. **Use Teach-Back:** "I need to suction your father, and I want to be sure that I explained the suctioning procedure and when I need to do it. Please tell me in your own words why suctioning is beneficial." Revise your instruction now or develop a plan for revised patient/family caregiver teaching if patient/family caregiver is not able to teach back correctly.	Determines patient's/family caregiver's level of understanding of instructional topic.

Unexpected Outcomes	Related Interventions
1. Patient has decrease in overall cardiopulmonary status as evidenced by decreased SpO_2, increased $ETCO_2$, continued tachypnea, continued increased work of breathing, and cardiac dysrhythmias.	• Limit length of suctioning. • Determine need for more frequent suctioning, possibly of shorter duration. • Determine need for supplemental or increase in supplemental oxygen. Supply oxygen between suctioning passes. • Notify health care provider.
2. Bloody secretions are returned after suctioning.	• Determine amount of suction pressure used. May need to be decreased. • Ensure that suction is completed correctly using intermittent suction and catheter rotation. Do not apply suction until after catheter has been pulled back 1 cm (0.4 inch) to prevent applying suction while catheter is touching carina. • Evaluate suctioning frequency. • Provide more frequent oral hygiene.
3. Patient has paroxysms of coughing or bronchospasm.	• Administer supplemental oxygen. • Allow patient to rest between passes of suction catheter. • Consult with health care provider regarding need for inhaled bronchodilators or topical anesthetics.
4. Inability to obtain secretions during suction procedure.	• Evaluate patient's fluid status and adequacy of humidification on oxygen-delivery device. • Assess for signs of infection. • Determine need for chest physiotherapy.

Recording

- Document your evaluation of patient learning.
- Record quantity and quality of sputum obtained during suction procedure, including whether or not blood was present.
- Record patient's tolerance of procedure, including vital signs, oxygen saturation, and postprocedure comfort level.

Hand-Off Reporting

- Report patient tolerance of suctioning procedure, including changes in vital signs, pulse oximetry values, and $ETCO_2$ values (if applicable). Report frequency of suctioning and patient response to suctioning and oxygen requirement after procedure.

PROCEDURAL GUIDELINE 16.4 *Closed (In-Line) Suctioning*

Purpose

Closed suctioning (or in-line suctioning) involves the use of a multiuse suction catheter that is housed within a plastic sleeve and is attached to a patient's artificial airway (Fig. 16.8). This method of suctioning is recommended for patients who cannot tolerate loss of positive end-expiratory pressure (PEEP), such as those with severe respiratory disorders who require high amounts of PEEP or oxygen requirements, because in-line suctioning decreases the risk of hypoxia and cardiovascular complications compared with open suctioning (Letchford and Bench, 2018).

Delegation and Collaboration

The skill of airway suction with a closed (in-line) suction catheter cannot be delegated to nursing assistive personnel (NAP). In special situations such as suctioning a well-established permanent tracheostomy, this procedure may be delegated to the NAP. The nurse is responsible for cardiopulmonary assessment and evaluation of the patient. The nurse often collaborates with a respiratory therapist when assessing the patient and performing the suction procedure. The nurse directs the NAP about:

- Any individualized aspects of patient care that pertain to suctioning (e.g., position, duration of suction, pressure settings).
- Expected quality, quantity, and color of secretions and to inform the nurse immediately if there are changes.
- Patient's anticipated response to suction and to immediately report to the nurse changes in vital signs, complaints of pain, shortness of breath, confusion, or increased restlessness.

Equipment

Closed-system or in-line suction catheter; sterile saline vial solution containers (5–10 mL); suction machine/source with regulator; connecting tubing (6 feet); clean gloves; oral suction kit/supplies for oropharyngeal suctioning; mask, goggles, or face shield; gown if isolation precautions indicate; pulse oximeter and stethoscope.

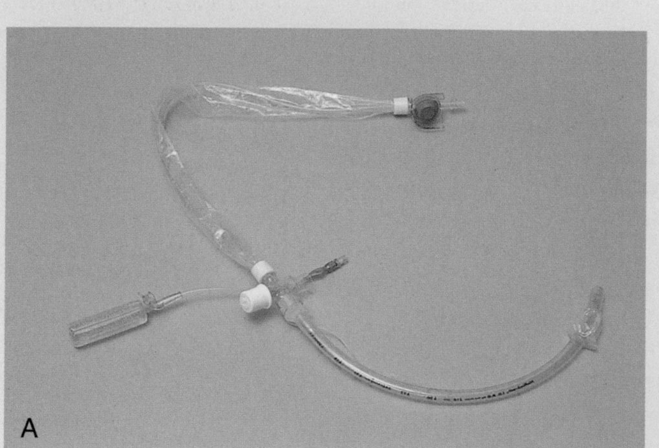

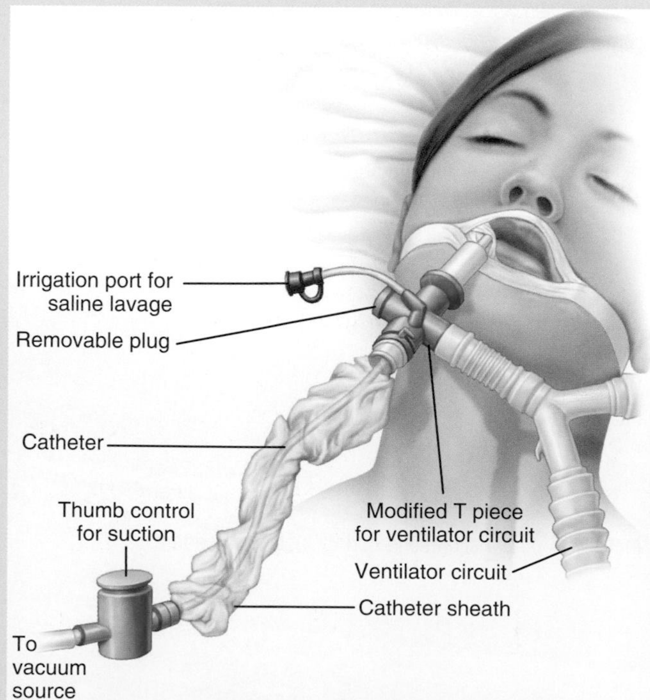

FIG 16.8 (A) Closed-system suction catheter attached to endotracheal tube. (B) Closed suction system attached to an endotracheal tube. *(B from Blanchard B: Thoracic surgery. In Rothrock JC, McEwen DR, eds.* Alexander's care of the patient in surgery, *ed 14, St. Louis, 2011, Mosby.)*

PROCEDURAL GUIDELINE 16.4 *Closed (In-Line) Suctioning—cont'd*

A manual self-inflating resuscitation bag (bag-valve-mask) with appropriate-size mask, although not necessary for the procedure, is safe to have on hand

Procedural Steps

1. Identify patient using at least two identifiers (e.g., name and birthday or name and medical record number) according to agency policy (TJC, 2019).
2. Perform assessment as in Skill 16.3
3. Perform hand hygiene. Gather equipment/supplies and close room door or curtain.
4. Explain procedure to patient and the importance of coughing during the suctioning procedure. Even if patients cannot speak, they deserve to have information regarding the procedure.
5. Adjust the bed to appropriate height and lower side rail on the side nearest you. Check locks on the bed.
6. Help patient assume a position of comfort for both patient and nurse, usually semi- or high-Fowler's position. Place towel across patient's chest.
7. Perform hand hygiene and apply clean gloves and face shield and attach suction:
   (1) Open suction catheter package using aseptic technique and attach closed suction catheter to ventilator circuit by removing swivel adapter and placing closed suction catheter apparatus on endotracheal tube (ETT) or tracheostomy tube (TT). Connect Y on mechanical ventilator circuit to closed suction catheter with flex tubing (see Fig. 16.9). **NOTE:** In many agencies a respiratory therapist attaches the catheter to the mechanical ventilator circuit.
   (2) Connect one end of connecting tubing to suction machine; connect other end to the end of a closed-system or in-line suction catheter. Turn suction device on, set vacuum regulator to appropriate negative pressure, and check pressure. Many closed-system suction catheters require slightly higher suction pressures (consult manufacturer guidelines).
8. Hyperoxygenate patient (usually 100% oxygen) by adjusting the fraction of inspired oxygen (FiO_2) setting on the ventilator or by using a temporary oxygen-enrichment program available on microprocessor ventilators according to agency policy or protocol. (Manual ventilation is not recommended.)
9. Unlock suction control mechanism if required by manufacturer. Open saline port and attach saline vial.
10. Pick up suction catheter enclosed in plastic sleeve with dominant hand.
11. Wait until patient inhales to insert catheter. Then gently insert while advancing catheter and sliding (or pulling) plastic sleeve back between thumb and forefinger until resistance is felt or patient coughs. Pull back 1 cm (0.4 inch) before applying suction to avoid tissue damage to tracheal carina.
12. Encourage patient to cough and apply suction by squeezing on suction control mechanism while withdrawing catheter. **NOTE:** It is difficult to apply intermittent pulses of suction and nearly impossible to rotate the catheter compared to standard catheter. Apply continuous suction for 10 to 15 seconds but no longer than 15 seconds as you remove the suction catheter (AARC, 2010; Branson et al., 2014). Be sure to withdraw catheter completely into plastic sheath and past the tip of the airway so that it does not obstruct airflow.
13. Reassess cardiopulmonary status, including pulse oximetry (SpO_2) and ventilator measures, to determine need for subsequent suctioning or complications. Repeat Steps 8 to 12 one more time to clear secretions if patient condition indicates. Allow adequate time (at least 1 full minute) between suction passes for ventilation and reoxygenation.
14. When airway is clear, withdraw catheter completely into sheath. Be sure that colored indicator line on catheter is visible in the sheath. Attach sterile solution lavage vial to side port of suction catheter. Squeeze vial while applying suction to rinse inner lumen of catheter. Use at least 5 to 10 mL of saline to rinse the catheter until it is clear of retained secretions, which can cause bacterial growth and increase the risk for infection (AARC, 2004). Lock suction mechanism if applicable and turn off suction.
15. Hyperoxygenate for at least 1 minute by following the same technique used to preoxygenate (Wiegand, 2017).
16. If patient requires oral or nasal suctioning, perform Skill 16.3 with separate standard suction catheter.
17. Place a Yankauer catheter on a clean, dry area for reuse with suction turned off or within patient's reach with suction on if patient can suction his or her own mouth.
18. Reposition patient. Remove gloves, face shield, and other personal protective equipment; discard into appropriate receptacle; and perform hand hygiene.
19. Be sure nurse call system is in an accessible location within patient's reach.
20. Raise side rails (as appropriate) and lower bed to lowest position.
21. Compare patient's vital signs and SpO_2 before and after suctioning.
22. Auscultate lung fields and compare with baseline.
23. Observe airway secretions.
24. Ask patient if breathing is easier and congestion is decreased.
25. Document patient's presuctioning and postsuctioning vital signs, cardiopulmonary status, character of mucus, and response to treatment.

✦ SKILL 16.4 Care of Artificial Airways

Purpose

Artificial airways relieve upper airway obstruction, protect against aspiration, or provide access to clear secretions, and are necessary for mechanical ventilation. Endotracheal tubes (ETTs) are used for short-term artificial airway support (see Fig. 16.5); following insertion, the cuff is inflated to maintain position within the trachea.

When a patient requires long-term artificial airway support, a tracheostomy tube (TT) is necessary (see Fig. 16.6). A TT offers advantages over long-term ETT placement, such as decreased laryngeal and tracheal tissue injury, ease of breathing, increased patient mobility, and access for better oral hygiene (Hyzy et al., 2018b).

Delegation and Collaboration

This skill of performing ETT care cannot be delegated to nursing assistive personnel (NAP). NAP may assist the nurse with ETT care. Often the nurse collaborates with a respiratory therapist in performing this care. In some settings, the skill of TT care for patients with a well-established TT can be delegated to NAP. The nurse directs the NAP to:

- Immediately report any signs of respiratory problems or increased airway secretions.
- Immediately report if the ETT or TT appears to have moved or become obstructed or dislodged.
- Immediately report changes in patient's mood, level of consciousness, irritability, vital signs, decreased pulse oximetry value, or changes in end-tidal CO_2 values.
- Immediately report changes in around ETT or TT and any stomal drainage.

Equipment

- Towel
- Stethoscope
- Bedside table
- Pulse oximeter and end-tidal CO_2 detector
- Personal protective equipment: Goggles/mask/face shield; clean gloves; gown
- Oral and artificial airway suction supplies and equipment (see Skill 16.3)
- Oxygen source
- Self-inflating manual resuscitation bag-valve device and appropriate-size mask
- Oral hygiene supplies (e.g., pediatric-size toothbrush, sponge toothette for edentulous patients, toothpaste, cleaning solution and non–alcohol-based mouthwash)
- Communication device—optional (letter or picture board, tablet, pen and paper)

Endotracheal Tube Care

- Additional health care team member (two people are needed to safely complete some of the ETT care steps)
- 1- to 1½-inch adhesive or waterproof tape (not paper tape) or commercial ETT stabilizer (follow manufacturer's or health care agency's instructions for securing the ETT)
- Two pairs of clean gloves
- Adhesive remover swab
- Face cleanser (e.g., wet washcloth, towel, soap, shaving supplies)
- Clean 2 × 2–inch gauze
- Tincture of benzoin or liquid adhesive
- Oral airway or bite block
- Tongue blade *(optional)*

Tracheostomy Care

- Additional health care team member (two people are needed to safely complete some of the TT care steps)
- Sterile tracheostomy care kit if available or:
  - Three sterile 4 × 4–inch gauze pads
  - Sterile cotton-tipped applicators
  - Sterile tracheostomy dressing
  - Sterile basin
  - Small sterile brush (or disposable cannula)
  - Tracheostomy ties (e.g., twill tape, manufactured tracheostomy ties, Velcro tracheostomy ties)
- Sterile normal saline or water
- Scissors
- Pair of sterile and clean gloves
- Disposable inner cannula, if patient has one
- Extra sterile tracheostomy kit
- Cuff pressure manometer
- Reintubation equipment should be available at bedside in case of accidental tube dislodgment

ASSESSMENT

1. Identify patient using at least two identifiers (e.g., name and birthday or name and medical record number) according to agency policy. *Rationale: Ensures correct patient. Complies with The Joint Commission standards and improves patient safety (TJC, 2019).*
2. Assess patient's hydration status, humidity delivered to airway/ventilator circuit, status of any existing infection, patient's nutritional status, and ability to cough. *Rationale: Determines factors that affect amount and consistency of secretions in ETT/TT and patient's ability to clear airway.*
3. Perform hand hygiene, apply clean gloves, and perform complete respiratory assessment (see Chapter 8). *Rationale: Provides baseline measure of ventilation.*
4. Assess patient's cardiopulmonary status, including pulse oximetry, end-tidal carbon dioxide ($ETCO_2$) concentration, vital signs, and level of consciousness. Keep pulse oximeter in place. *Rationale: Provides baseline to determine patient response to and tolerance of therapy.*
5. Observe condition of tissues surrounding ETT/TT for impaired skin integrity (e.g., blistering, abrasions, pressure injuries) on nares, lips, cheeks, corner of mouth, or neck; excess nasal or oral secretions; patient moving tube with tongue, biting tube or tongue; or foul-smelling mouth. *Rationale: Increased risk for developing pressure areas around ETT or TT from impaired circulation as tube is pulled or pressed against mucosal tissues (Pittman et al., 2015). Presence of ETT or TT impairs ability of patient to swallow oral secretions.*
6. Observe patency of airway: excess peristomal, intratracheal, or endotracheal secretions; diminished airflow; or signs and symptoms of airway obstruction. *Rationale: Buildup of secretions in ETT/TT impairs oxygen delivery and subsequent tissue oxygenation. Excess secretions in the artificial airways may*

indicate need for suctioning before performing any other airway cares (see Skill 16.3).

7. Observe for signs and symptoms of gurgling on expiration, decreased exhaled tidal volume (mechanically ventilated patient), signs and symptoms of inadequate ventilation (rising $ETCO_2$, patient-ventilator desynchrony, or dyspnea), spasmodic coughing, tense test balloon on tube, flaccid test balloon on tube, and ability to speak or vocalize. *Rationale: Cuff underinflation increases risk for aspiration, allows secretions to enter the trachea, and permits vocalization. Cuff overinflation may cause ischemia or necrosis of tracheal tissue from obstruction of capillary bed, resulting in tracheomalacia or tracheoesophageal fistula (Myatt, 2015; Rouzé et al., 2017). $ETCO_2$ validates the correct placement of the ETT by analyzing the exhaled gas for carbon dioxide levels (see Fig. 16.7; Wiegand, 2017).*

Safe Patient Care *For possible overinflation or underinflation of ETT/TT cuff, notify respiratory therapy and follow agency policy for correcting cuff pressures. Most sources agree that 20 cm H_2O is the lowest accepted pressure, but some sources recommend that the highest pressure to maintain the cuff is 25 cm H_2O (AACN, 2016; Myatt, 2015).*

8. Observe for factors that increase risk for complications from ETT/TT: type and size of tube, movement of tube up and down trachea (in and out), duration of tube placement, presence of facial trauma, malnutrition, and neck or thoracic radiation. *Rationale: Tube pressure can cause medical device–related pressure injuries. Tube can become dislodged from lower airway (incidental extubation), or it can enter right main-stem bronchus.*
9. **For ETT:** Determine proper ETT depth as noted by centimeters at lip or gum line. This line is marked on tube and recorded in patient's record at time of intubation and every shift. *Rationale: Ensures that tube is at proper depth to adequately ventilate both lungs and that it is not too high, which causes vocal cord damage, or too low, which results in right main-stem intubation, in which only the right lung is ventilated.*
10. Determine when oral and airway care were last performed. Know the health care agency protocols and procedures but be aware of patient-specific needs for more frequent care. Remove and dispose of gloves. Perform hand hygiene. *Rationale: Oral care is performed every 2 to 4 hours. TT care is performed every 4 to 8 hours (AACN, 2017a; Wiegand, 2017).*
11. Assess patient's or family caregiver's knowledge of procedure, experience, literacy level, and ability to provide own care, as allowed. *Rationale: Ensures patient or caregiver has the capacity to obtain, communicate, process, and understand basic health information (CDC, 2016).*

STEP	RATIONALE
PLANNING	
1. Expected outcomes following completion of procedure:	
• ETT/TT remains in correct position in patient's trachea, evidenced by depth of tube same as when started or as ordered (same centimeter marking at gums or lips for ETT); bilateral breath sounds are equal; $ETCO_2$ values remain at patient baseline	Maintaining ETT/TT position promotes adequate ventilation of lungs. Complications of lower airway and vocal cord trauma are prevented.
• Patient's skin around mouth, oral mucous membranes, and stoma remains intact without evidence of pressure or other injury from biting or from ETT/TT.	ETT/TT does not place undue pressure against corners of mouth or stoma, causing pressure area. Patient is not able to bite inner cheeks or tongue.
2. Perform hand hygiene. Gather equipment/supplies and arrange at bedside. Close room curtain or door.	Ensures an organized procedure. Ensures patient privacy.
3. Obtain assistance from available staff for this procedure. Have staff member perform hand hygiene and apply clean gloves.	Reduces risk for accidental extubation of ETT or dislodgment of the TT.
4. Assist patient in assuming comfortable position for both patient and staff. Elevate patient's head of bed at least 30 degrees, unless contraindicated.	Provides access to site and facilitates completion of procedure. Prepares patient for oropharyngeal suctioning. Position may decrease risk of aspiration (AACN, 2016, 2017b).
5. Explain procedure and patient's need to participate, including not biting or moving ETT with tongue, trying not to cough when tape or holder is off ETT/TT, keeping hands down, and not pulling on tubing.	Reduces anxiety, encourages cooperation, and reduces risk of accidental extubation or tube dislodgment.

Safe Patient Care *For patients with TT: At some agencies, it is standard practice to have an extra TT that is the same size as the patient's current TT and a TT one size smaller at the bedside at all times in case there is an emergent need to replace the TT because of obstruction or dislodgment.*

STEP	RATIONALE

IMPLEMENTATION

STEP	RATIONALE
1. Perform hand hygiene. Apply clean gloves and mask, goggles, or face shield if indicated. Have assistant do so as well.	Reduces transmission of microorganisms.
2. Place clean towel across patient's chest.	Reduces soiling of bedclothes and linen.
3. Perform airway suctioning if indicated (see Skill 16.3 and Procedural Guideline 16.4).	Removes secretions. Diminishes patient's need to cough during procedure.
4. Perform ETT care.	
a. Connect Yankauer suction catheter to suction source and have it ready to use. Ensure that suction source/machine for oral suctioning is on and functioning properly.	Need to have functioning equipment to perform oral care appropriately. Prepares suction apparatus.
b. Remove oral airway or bite block, if present, and place on towel.	Provides access to and complete observation of patient's oral cavity.

Safe Patient Care *If patient is biting the tube, do not remove bite block until necessary. This prevents obstruction of the ETT and occlusion of the artificial airway.*

STEP	RATIONALE
c. Brush teeth with soft toothbrush, using solution or toothpaste that helps break down plaque buildup on teeth. Suction oropharyngeal secretions as necessary.	There may be need for pediatric toothbrush, depending on size of patient's oral cavity. It is recommended to brush teeth at least twice a day (AACN, 2017b; Wiegand, 2017).
d. Use chlorhexidine solution and oral swabs to clean mouth. Suction oropharyngeal secretions as necessary. Apply mouth moisturizer to oral mucosa and lips after each cleaning.	This step should be completed every 2 to 4 hours (AACN, 2017a; AACN, 2017b; Wiegand, 2017). The swabs, solution, and moisturizer may come in a prepackaged kit from manufacturer. The use of chlorhexidine mouthwash or gel is effective in reducing VAP (AACN, 2017b; Munro and Ruggiero, 2014).
e. Prepare ETT securement options:	
(1) *Tape method:* Prepare tape by cutting piece of tape long enough to go completely around patient's head from naris to naris plus 15 cm (6 inches). This is typically 30 to 60 cm (12–24 inches) in total length. Lay tape adhesive-side up on bedside table. Cut and lay 8 to 15 cm (3–6 inches) of second piece of tape, adhesive sides together, in center of the long strip to prevent tape from sticking to hair. Smaller strip of tape should cover area between ears around back of head (see illustration).	Preparing tape ahead decreases amount of time one must manually hold ETT throughout procedure, therefore decreasing risk of tube dislodgement. Adhesive tape needs to encircle head below ears with sufficient tape left to wrap around tube.

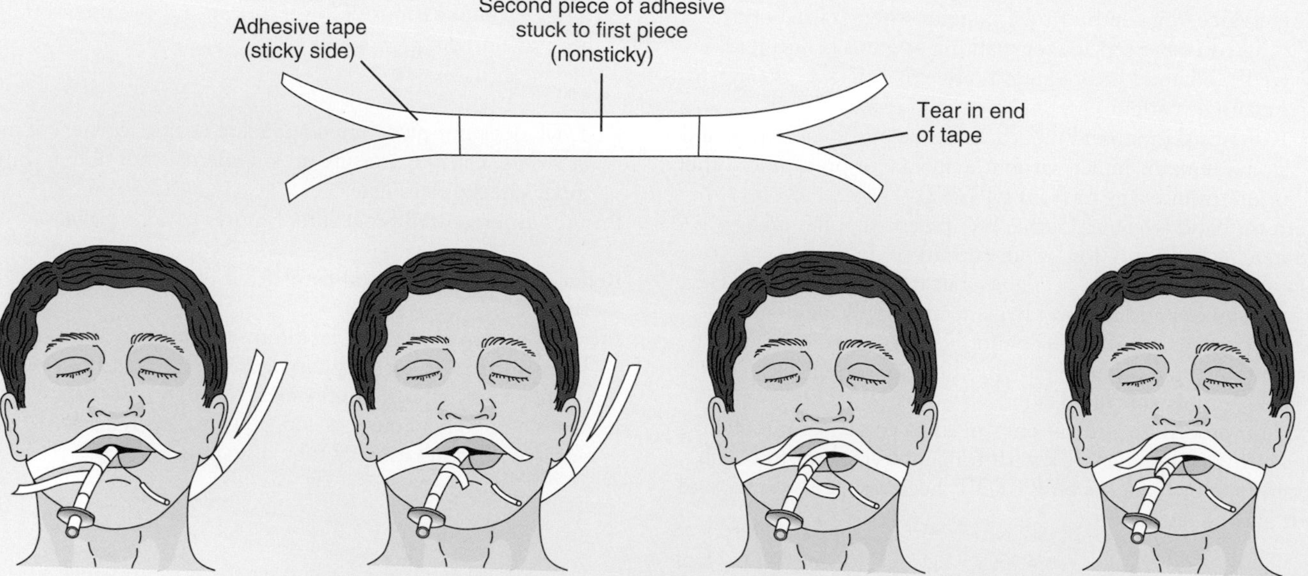

STEP 4e(1) Methods of securing adhesive tape. *(From* Wiegand's AACN procedure manual for high acuity, progressive and acuity care, *St. Louis, 2017, Elsevier.)*

STEP	RATIONALE
(2) *Commercially available ET holder:* Open package per manufacturer instructions. Set device aside with head guard in place and Velcro strips open.	Commercial devices are latex free, fast, convenient, and disposable.

Safe Patient Care *It is a nursing decision whether to use tape or a commercially available ET holder. There are advantages and disadvantages to both. The commercial tube holders allow for less slippage of the ETT and easier access for oral care but have an increased risk of the formation of pressure injuries (Branson et al., 2014; Smith and Pietrantonio, 2016).*

STEP	RATIONALE
f. Remove old tape or device.	
(1) *Tape:* While one person is holding and stabilizing ETT, the other person should remove tape from patient, using adhesive tape remover. The tape will also need to be removed from ETT itself.	Provides access to skin under tape for assessment and hygiene. Adhesive tape remover ensures easier, less traumatic removal of the tape.

Safe Patient Care *Clean ETT tube with cloth dampened in soap and water as needed. Do not apply adhesive tape remover to the ETT itself. This action will make it nearly impossible for the new tape to appropriately stick to the ETT, which increases the risk of tube dislodgement. Do not allow assistant to hold the tube away from the lips or nares. Doing so allows too much movement in the tube and increases the risk for tube movement and accidental extubation. Never let go of the ETT because it could become dislodged.*

STEP	RATIONALE
(2) *Commercially available device:* Remove Velcro strips from ETT and remove ETT holder from patient.	Velcro adhesive strips hold ETT in place and provide marker to measure distance to patient's lips or gums. These devices all permit access to patient's mouth and lips for ease in oropharyngeal suctioning and oral hygiene.

Safe Patient Care *Do not allow assistant to hold the tube away from the lips or nares. Doing so allows too much movement in the tube and increases the risk for tube movement and accidental extubation. Never let go of the ETT because it could become dislodged.*

STEP	RATIONALE
g. Remove excess secretions or adhesive from patient's face. Clean facial skin with mild soap and water and dry thoroughly. May need to apply tape-adherence product, such as tincture of benzoin, to face.	Application of tape-adherence product allows for new tape or device to stay on patient's face (Wiegand, 2017).

Safe Patient Care *Do not remove oral airway or bite block if patient is actively biting. Wait until the new tape or commercial device is partially or completely secured to ETT.*

STEP	RATIONALE
h. Note level of ETT by looking at mark or noting centimeter value on tube itself. Move oral ETT to other side of mouth and **ensure that tube marking at lip is unchanged.** Perform oral care as needed on side where tube was initially positioned. Clean oral airway or bite block with warm soapy water and rinse well. Reinsert as necessary.	Changing sides of ETT removes pressure and decreases risk of breakdown at corners of mouth and oral mucosa (Pittman et al., 2015; Wiegand, 2017).

Safe Patient Care *The patient may cough excessively when the tube is being moved. The person who is holding the tube in place should be prepared for this and take extra caution while holding. In some instances, the ETT may need to be secured with the tape before the rest of the oral care is performed. In some cases, the patient may need to be administered a dose of an antianxiety or sedating medication. The cuff of the ETT may need to be deflated before changing its position. If this step needs to be performed, deep oral suctioning should be completed before deflation of the cuff, and oral care should not be performed until the cuff is properly reinflated (Wiegand, 2017).*

STEP	RATIONALE
i. Secure tube (assistant continues to hold ET).	
(1) **Tape method:**	
(a) Slip tape under patient's head and neck, adhesive side up. Take care not to twist tape or catch hair. Do not allow tape to stick to itself. It helps to gently stick the end of tape to tongue blade, which serves as guide. Then slide tongue blade under patient's neck. Center tape so double-faced tape extends around back of neck from ear to ear.	Positions tape to secure ETT in proper position. Don't allow tape to go over earlobe.

STEP	RATIONALE
(b) On one side of face secure tape from ear to naris (nasal ETT) or over lip to ETT (oral ETT). Tear remaining tape in half lengthwise, forming two pieces that are 1 to 1.5 cm (0.4–0.6 inch) wide. Secure bottom half of tape across upper lip (oral ETT) or across top of nose (nasal ETT) to opposite ear (see illustration A). Wrap top half of tape around tube and up from bottom (see illustration B). Tape should encircle tube at least 2 times for security.	Secures tape to face. Using top tape to wrap prevents downward drag on ETT.
(c) Gently pull other side of tape firmly to pick up slack and secure to opposite side of face and ETT same as first piece. **NOTE:** ETT is secured. Assistant can release hold. Check depth mark at lips or gum line.	Secures tape to face and tube. ETT should be at same depth at lips or gum line. Check earlier assessment for verification of tube depth in centimeters.
(2) **Commercially available ETT tube securement device:**	

Safe Patient Care *Applying a new securement device will be needed only if the device is visibly soiled and cannot be cleaned or if it is no longer adhering to the face and keeping the ETT secure.*

STEP	RATIONALE
(a) Thread ETT through opening designed to secure it. Be sure that pilot balloon is accessible.	Commercially available holders have a slit in front of holder designed to secure ETT.
(b) Place strips of ETT holder under patient at occipital region of head.	
(c) Verify that ETT is at established depth using lip or gum line marker as guide.	Ensures that ETT remains at correct depth as determined during assessment.
(d) Attach Velcro strips at base of patient's head. Leave 1 cm (0.4 inch) slack in strips.	
(e) Verify that tube is secure, it does not move forward from patient's mouth or backward down into patient's throat, and there are no pressure areas on oral mucosa or occipital region of head (see illustration).	Tube must be secure so that it remains at correct depth. It can be secured without being tight and causing pressure.
j. For unconscious patient, reinsert oral airway without pushing tongue into oropharynx and secure with tape (see Chapter 30).	Prevents patient from biting ETT and allows access for oropharyngeal suctioning. An oral airway is not used in a conscious, cooperative patient because it causes excessive gagging and pressure areas to mouth and tongue.
k. Clean rest of face and neck with soapy washcloth, rinse, and dry. Shave male patient as necessary.	Moisture and beard growth prevent adhesive tape adherence.

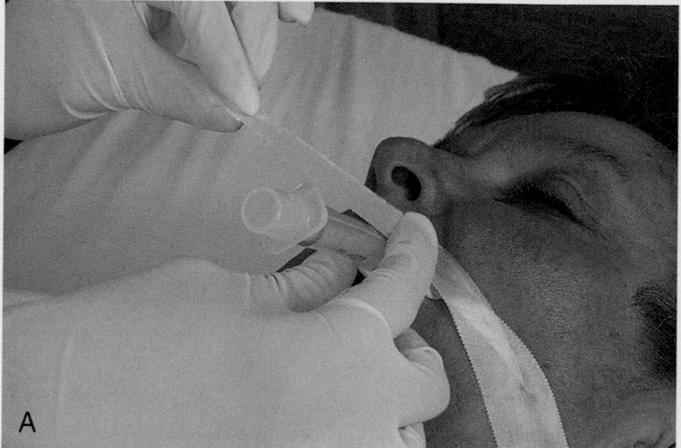

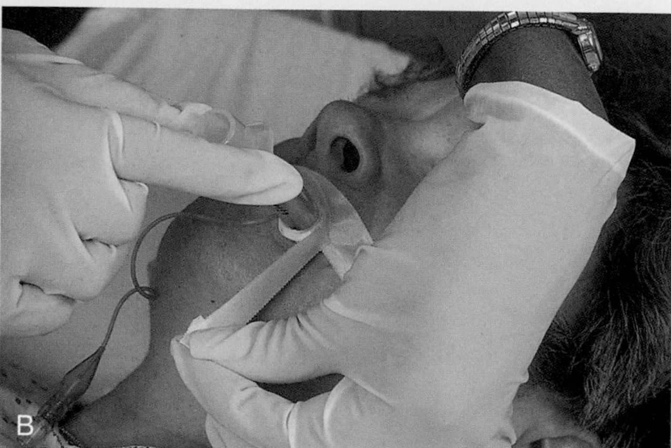

STEP 4i(1)(b) (A) Securing bottom half of tape across patient's upper lip. (B) Securing top half of tape around tube.

STEP	RATIONALE

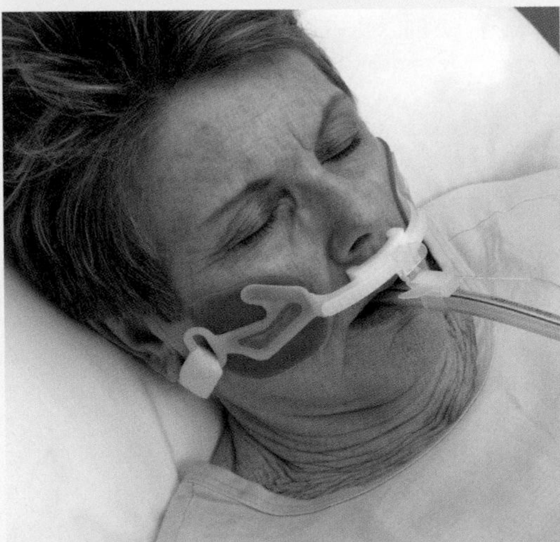

STEP 4i(2)(e) Commercial endotracheal tube holder. *(Modified from Sills JR: Entry-level respiratory therapist exam guide, St. Louis, 2000, Mosby.)*

Safe Patient Care *When shaving patients, take great care to keep the cuff inflation port away from the razor. The razor can inadvertently cut or nick the tubing, causing air loss from the cuff and the possible need for reintubation.*

Safe Patient Care *If a nasotracheal tube is in place, all the preceding steps will be completed, except that the tube will not be moved, and its position will not be changed. It is out of the scope of nurse practice to move the ETT from one naris to another and could cause great harm to the patient.*

STEP	RATIONALE
5. Perform tracheostomy tube care.	
a. Preoxygenate patient for 30 seconds or ask patient to take 5 to 6 deep breaths. Then suction tracheostomy (see Skill 16.3). Before removing gloves, remove soiled tracheostomy dressing and discard in glove with coiled catheter.	Removes secretions to avoid occluding outer cannula while inner cannula is removed. Reduces need for patient to cough.
b. Perform hand hygiene. Arrange equipment on bedside table.	Decreases risk of infection. Prepares equipment and allows for smooth, organized completion of tracheostomy care. Tracheostomy care should be performed every 4 to 8 hours or per agency protocol (Wiegand, 2017).
c. Open sterile tracheostomy kit (if available). Open two 4 × 4–inch gauze packages using aseptic technique and pour normal saline on one package. Leave second package dry. Open two cotton-tipped swab packages and pour normal saline on one package. Do not recap normal saline.	
d. Open sterile tracheostomy dressing package, keeping dressing sterile.	
e. Unwrap sterile basin and pour about 0.5 to 2 cm (0.2–1 inch) of normal saline into it.	
f. Prepare TT fixation device.	
(1) If using twill tape: Prepare length of twill tape long enough to go around patient's neck 2 times, about 60 to 75 cm (24–30 inches) for an adult. Cut ends on diagonal. Lay aside in dry area.	Cutting ends of tie on diagonal aids in inserting tie through eyelet of tracheostomy tube.
(2) If using commercially available TT holder, open package according to manufacturer directions.	
g. Open inner cannula package (if new one is to be inserted such as with disposable inner cannulas or if patient does not tolerate being disconnected from oxygen source while cleaning reusable inner cannula).	
h. Apply sterile gloves. Keep dominant hand sterile throughout procedure.	Reduces transmission of microorganisms.
i. Remove oxygen source if present.	

STEP	RATIONALE

Safe Patient Care *It is important to stabilize TT at all times during tracheostomy care to prevent injury, unnecessary discomfort, or accidental dislodgment. Have an assistant such as a NAP, nurse, or respiratory therapist help during the procedure. Instruct assistant to apply clean gloves.*

STEP	RATIONALE
j. Care of tracheostomy with reusable inner cannula:	
(1) While touching only outer aspect of tube, unlock and remove inner cannula with nondominant hand following line of tracheostomy. Drop inner cannula into normal saline basin.	Removes inner cannula for cleaning. Normal saline loosens secretions from inner cannula.

Safe Patient Care *If patient is receiving mechanical ventilation, you may want the person assisting you to hold the TT stable and remove the ventilator tube from the connection while you remove the inner cannula. This action helps ensure that the TT itself is not removed accidentally if difficulties removing the ventilator from the TT or removing the inner cannula from the TT occur.*

STEP	RATIONALE
(2) Place tracheostomy collar, T tube, or ventilator oxygen source over outer cannula. (**NOTE:** May not be able to attach T tube and ventilator oxygen devices to all outer cannulas when inner cannula is removed.)	Maintains supply of oxygen to patient as needed.

Safe Patient Care *If patient is unable to tolerate being disconnected from the ventilator, replace the inner cannula with a clean new one and reattach the ventilator to the tracheostomy. Then proceed with cleaning the original inner cannula as described in the next steps and store it in a sterile container until the next inner cannula change (Wiegand, 2017).*

STEP	RATIONALE
(3) To prevent oxygen desaturation in affected patients, quickly pick up inner cannula and use small brush to remove secretions inside and outside inner cannula (see illustration).	Tracheostomy brush provides mechanical force to remove thick or dried secretions.
(4) Hold inner cannula over basin and rinse with sterile normal saline, using nondominant (clean) hand to pour normal saline.	Removes secretions and normal saline from inner cannula.
(5) Remove oxygen source, replace inner cannula (see illustration), and secure "locking" mechanism. Reapply ventilator, tracheostomy collar, or T tube. Hyperoxygenate patient if needed.	Secures inner cannula and reestablishes oxygen supply.
k. Tracheostomy with disposable inner cannula:	
(1) Remove new cannula from manufacturer packaging.	Prepares you for change of inner cannula.
(2) While touching only outer aspect of tube, withdraw inner cannula and replace with new cannula by inserting it at a 90-degree angle then rotating downward. Lock into position.	Provides clean, sterile inner cannula for patient.

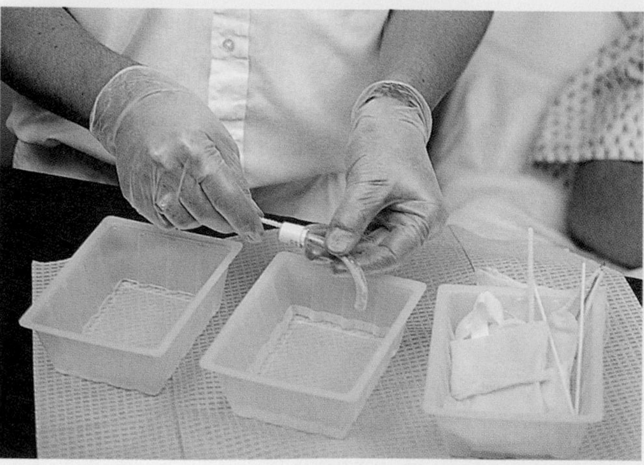

STEP 5j(3) Cleaning tracheostomy inner cannula.

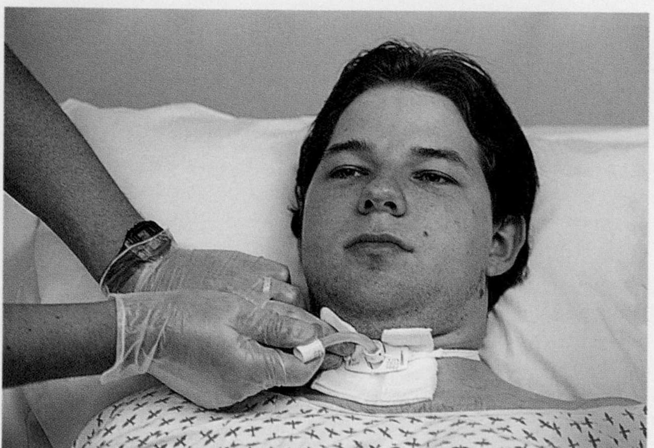

STEP 5j(5) Reinserting inner cannula.

STEP	RATIONALE

Safe Patient Care *If patient is receiving mechanical ventilation, you may want the person assisting you to hold the TT stable and remove the ventilator tube from the connection while you remove the inner cannula. This action helps ensure that the TT itself is not accidentally removed if difficulties removing the ventilator or the inner cannula from the TT occur.*

STEP	RATIONALE
(3) Dispose of contaminated cannula in appropriate receptacle and reconnect to ventilator or oxygen supply.	Prevents transmission of infection. Restores oxygen delivery.
l. Using normal saline-saturated cotton-tipped swabs and 4 × 4–inch gauze, clean exposed outer cannula surfaces and stoma under faceplate extending 5 to 10 cm (2–4 inches) in all directions from stoma (see illustration). Clean in circular motion from stoma site outward with dominant hand to handle sterile supplies. Do not go over previously cleaned area.	Aseptically removes secretions from stoma site. Moving in outward circle pulls mucus and other contaminants from stoma to periphery.
m. Using dry 4 × 4–inch gauze, pat lightly at skin and exposed outer cannula surfaces.	Dry surfaces prohibit formation of moist environment for microorganism growth and skin excoriation (Wiegand, 2017).
n. Secure tracheostomy.	

Safe Patient Care *Some agencies do not recommend changing the securement device for the first 72 hours after insertion of the TT because of risk of stoma closure if the tube were to become dislodged accidentally (Wiegand, 2017).*

STEP	RATIONALE
(1) Tracheostomy tie method:	
(a) Instruct assistant, if not already available, to apply clean gloves and securely hold TT in place. With assistant holding TT, cut old ties. Be sure to not cut pilot balloon of cuff.	Prevents transmission of infection. Secures TT to prevent incidental dislodgement. If pilot balloon is cut, there is no ability to inflate cuff (Wiegand, 2017).

Safe Patient Care *Assistant must not release hold on TT until new ties are firmly tied. If working without an assistant, do not cut old ties until new ties are in place and securely tied (Lewis et al., 2017). When ties are off, this is a good time to clean the back of the patient's neck and assess patient's skin under TT flange and under the ties or tube holder, making sure that skin is intact, free of pressure, and dry before applying securement device.*

STEP	RATIONALE
(b) Take prepared twill tape, insert one end of tie through faceplate eyelet, and pull ends even (see illustration).	Diagonal cuts ensure ease of threading end of tie through holes of eyelet (Wiegand, 2017).
(c) Slide both ends of tie behind head and around neck to other eyelet and insert one tie through second eyelet.	
(d) Pull snugly.	Secures TT.

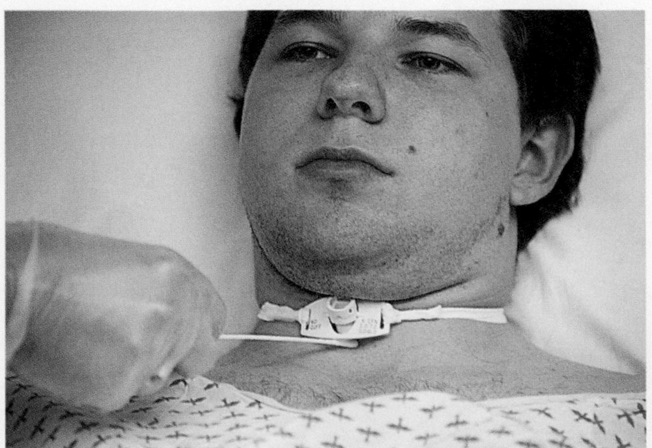

STEP 5l Cleaning around stoma.

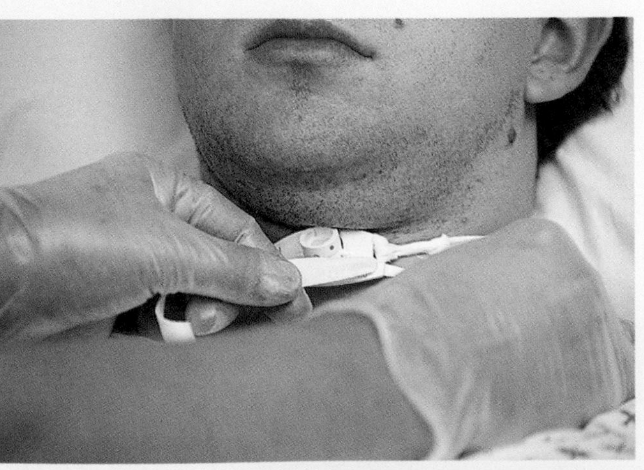

STEP 5n(1)(b) Replacing tracheostomy ties. Do not remove old tracheostomy ties until new ones are secure.

STEP	RATIONALE
(e) Tie ends securely in double square knot, allowing space for insertion of only one loose or two snug finger widths between tie and neck (see illustration).	One finger width of slack prevents ties from being too tight when tracheostomy dressing is in place and prevents movement of tracheostomy tube into lower airway (Wiegand, 2017).
(f) Insert fresh 4 × 4–inch tracheostomy dressing under clean ties and faceplate (see illustration).	Absorbs drainage. Dressing prevents pressure on clavicle heads (Wiegand, 2017).

Safe Patient Care *Never cut a 2 × 2–inch or 4 × 4–inch gauze pad because the cut edges fray and increase the risk of infection (Wiegand, 2017).*

STEP	RATIONALE
(2) Tracheostomy tube holder method:	Prevents incidental dislodgement of tube.
(a) Instruct assistant, if not already available, to apply clean gloves and securely hold TT in place. When an assistant is not available, leave old TT holder in place until new device is secure.	Ensures that tracheostomy stays in correct position.
(b) Align strap under patient's neck. Be sure that Velcro attachments are on either side of TT.	Ensures proper securement of TT.
(c) Place narrow end of ties under and through faceplate eyelets. Pull ends even and secure with Velcro closures (see illustration).	

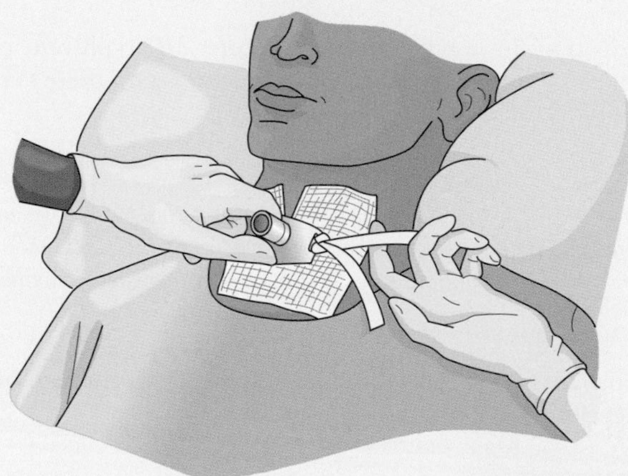

STEP 5n(1)(e) Tracheostomy ties properly placed. *(From Sorrentino SA:* Mosby's textbook for nursing assistants, *ed 8, St. Louis, 2013, Mosby.)*

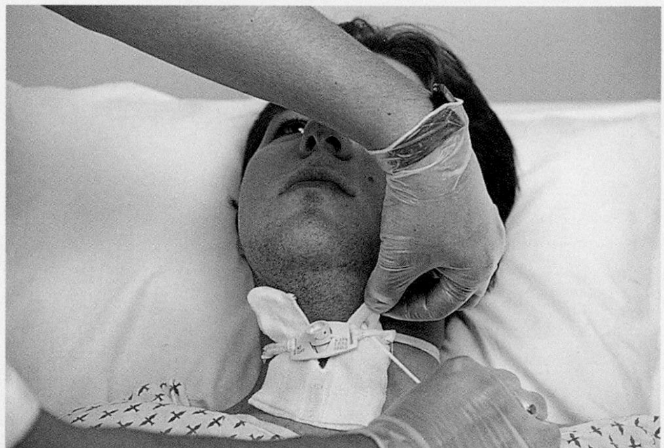

STEP 5n(1)(f) Applying tracheostomy dressing.

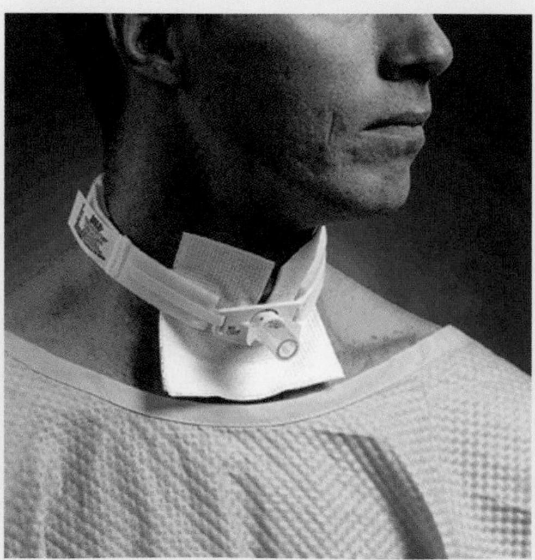

STEP 5n(2)(c) Tracheostomy tube holder in place. *(Courtesy Dale Medical Products, Plainesville, MA.)*

STEP	RATIONALE
(d) Verify that there is space for only one loose or two snug finger widths to be inserted under neck strap.	Ensures proper securement of TT without securement device being too tight.
o. Perform oral care with toothbrush or oral swabs and chlorhexidine rinse.	Use of chlorhexidine may decrease patient risk of developing a ventilator-associated event (VAE)/ventilator-associated pneumonia (VAP) and promotes patient comfort (AACN, 2017b).
p. Measure TT cuff pressure.	Cuff pressures should be measured every 8 hours and following any tracheostomy-related intervention or after the patient has been repositioned (Intensive Care Society [ICS], 2014).
(a) Attach a commercial pressure gauge/manometer to the tracheal cuff.	Allows for measurement of the pressure of TT cuff.
(b) Read the measurement. If the cuff pressure is greater than 25 cm H_2O, then release some air from the cuff (using the pressure gauge on the manometer) until the pressure reaches between 20 and 25 cm H_2O. If the pressure is less than 20 cm H_2O, add air by squeezing the bulb on the manometer until the pressure is between 20 and 25 cm H_2O.	Overinflated cuffs can lead to tracheal stenosis, necrosis, tracheomalacia, and fistula formation. Underinflated cuffs can lead to ineffective mechanical ventilation and increase risk of aspiration (Myatt, 2015; Wiegand, 2017)
6. Discard soiled items in appropriate receptacle. Remove towel and place in laundry.	Reduces transmission of microorganisms.
7. Reposition patient and ask him or her what else he or she needs.	Promotes comfort; gives patients opportunity to communicate their needs.
8. Be sure nurse call system is in an accessible location within patient's reach.	Ensures patient can call for assistance if needed.
9. Raise side rails (as appropriate) and lower bed to lowest position.	Ensures patient safety.
10. Be sure that oxygen- or humidification-delivery sources are in place and set at correct levels.	Humidification helps prevent airway obstruction and atelectasis (Hanlon, 2016).
11. Remove gloves and mask, goggles, or face shield or gown; discard in receptacle; and perform hand hygiene. (Assistant performs same steps.) Place clean items (e.g., tincture of benzoin, oral care solution, excess swabs) in place of storage.	Reduces transmission of microorganisms. Ensures that contaminated gloves and hands do not touch clean items.

EVALUATION

1. Compare respiratory assessments before and after ETT care.	Identifies any physiological changes, including presence and quality of breath sounds after procedure.
2. Observe depth and position of ETT according to health care provider recommendation.	Position of ETT should not be altered.
3. Assess security of tape by ***gently*** tugging at tube.	Tape should remain attached to face. Patient may cough during tugging.
4. Inspect skin around mouth, oral mucous membranes, and/or tracheal stoma for intactness and pressure sores.	Tape should not tear skin. Pressure areas should be absent.
5. Compare $ETCO_2$ values from before and after ETT care.	Changes in $ETCO_2$ can help identify displacement or dislodgement of ETT.
6. Observe for excessive phonation, presence of gastric secretions in airway secretions, or tracheoesophageal fistula.	Occurs with inadequate or excessive cuff inflation.

Unexpected Outcomes	Related Interventions
1. Patient is extubated accidentally.	• Remain with patient while calling for help. • Ventilate with bag-valve-mask as needed. • Assess patient for airway patency, spontaneous breathing, and vital signs. • Prepare for reintubation.

Unexpected Outcomes	Related Interventions
2. Patient has pressure injury in mouth, lips, nares, or tracheal stoma.	• Increase frequency of ETT care. • Apply antimicrobial ointment per agency protocol. • Align oxygen and humidity supply tubing so that they do not pull ETT, creating pressure sores. • Monitor for infection. If skin tear is present on cheeks or over nose or upper lip, apply protective barrier such as stoma adhesive patch or hydrocolloid dressing and apply tape to it.
3. TT only: • Excessively loose or tight tracheostomy ties/tracheostomy holder • Inflammation of tracheostomy stoma or pressure area around TT	• Adjust ties or apply new ties/tracheostomy holder. • Increase frequency of tracheostomy care. • Apply topical antibacterial solution; apply bacterial barrier if ordered. • Apply hydrocolloid or transparent dressing just under stoma to protect skin from breakdown. • Consult with skin care specialist.

Recording

- Record respiratory and skin assessments before and after tube care, size and depth of ETT or type and size of tracheostomy tube, frequency and extent of care, patient tolerance, and any complications related to presence of the tube.
- Document your evaluation of patient learning.

Hand-Off Reporting

- Report signs of infection or displacement of ETT or tracheostomy tube immediately. Report time of care and patient tolerance, including vital sign changes or any changes in pulse oximeter, $ETCO_2$, or respiratory status, and presence of any areas on impaired skin integrity on face or neck, in the mouth, or around the nares or tracheal stoma.

✦ SKILL 16.5 Managing Closed Chest Drainage Systems

Purpose

A chest tube is inserted, and a closed sterile chest drainage system is attached, to promote drainage of air and/or fluid from the pleural space so that the lung can reexpand. A closed system ensures air or fluid does not reenter to collapse a lung. This type of tube is also called a thoracostomy tube or thoracic catheter. Suction may be added to assist gravity in draining fluid (Chotai, 2016; Gross et al., 2016). In an emergent situation, a catheter is inserted through the chest wall, and a rubber flutter one-way valve (e.g., a Heimlich valve) is attached to the end (Fig. 16.9). As a patient exhales, the positive pressure generated by the air leaving the chest enters the tubing, causing the valve to open so that air is released. During inspiration, the tube collapses on itself, preventing air from reentering the chest. This device is contraindicated when the patient needs fluid drained, such as when a hemothorax or pleural effusion is present.

The placement of a chest tube depends on the type of drainage that is present. Because air rises, apical and anterior chest tube placement promotes removal of air. Chest tubes are placed low and posterior or lateral to drain fluid (Fig. 16.10). Mediastinal chest tubes are placed just below the sternum and drain blood or fluid, preventing its accumulation around the heart (e.g., after open-heart surgery) (Chotai, 2016; Gross et al., 2016).

Delegation and Collaboration

The skill of chest tube management cannot be delegated to nursing assistive personnel (NAP). The nurse directs the NAP about:

- Proper positioning of the patient to facilitate chest tube drainage and optimal functioning of the system.
- Ambulating and transferring patient with chest drainage system.
- Reporting changes in vital signs, complaints of chest pain or sudden shortness of breath, or excessive bubbling in water-seal chamber to the nurse immediately.

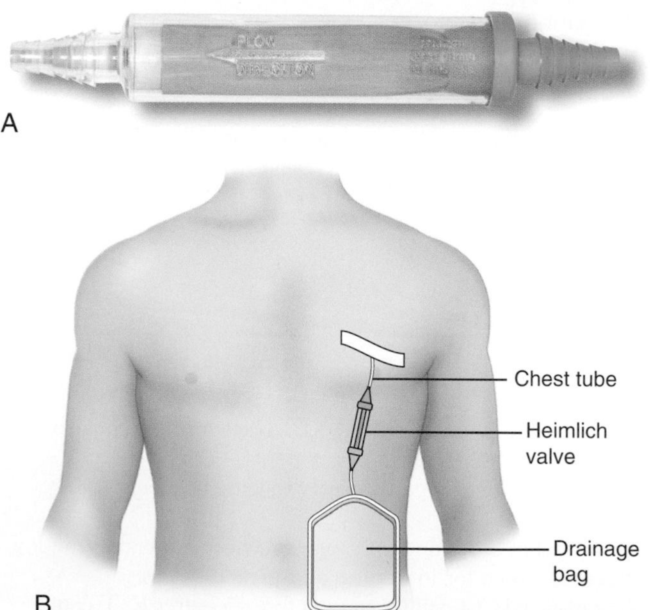

FIG 16.9 (A) Heimlich chest drain valve is a specially designed flutter valve that is used in place of a chest drainage unit for a small uncomplicated pneumothorax with little or no drainage and no need for suction. The valve allows for escape of air but prevents reentry of air into the pleural space. (B) Placement of the valve between chest tube and drainage bag, which can be worn under clothing.

- Danger of any disconnection of drainage system, change in type and amount of drainage, sudden bleeding, or sudden cessation of bubbling.

Equipment

- Local anesthetic, if not an emergent procedure
- Prescribed chest drainage system
- Water-seal system versus waterless (dry suction) system (Fig. 16.11): sterile water or normal saline per manufacturer's directions
- Clean gloves
- Suction source and setup
- Sterile skin preparation solution (povidone-iodine or chlorhexidine solutions)

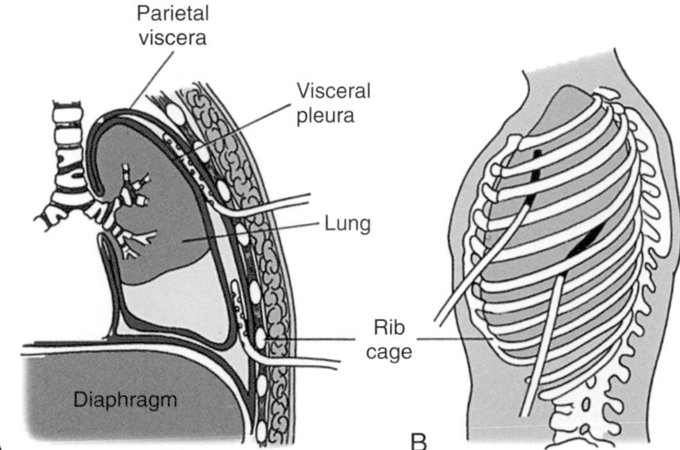

FIG 16.10 Diagram of sites for chest tube placement. (A) Anatomical drawing showing upper tube placement (for air) and lower tube placement (for blood and fluid). (B) View of tubes exiting through intracostal sites.

- Chest tube tray (all items are sterile), typically: chest tube, knife handle, clamps, small sponge forceps, needle holder, knife blade no. 10, 3-0 silk sutures, sterile drape, two clamps, 4 × 4–inch sponges, suture scissors, and sterile gloves
- Dressings: Petroleum or Xeroform gauze, large dressing of choice, split chest tube dressing, additional 4 × 4–inch dressings, 4-inch tape or elastic bandage
- Two rubber-tipped hemostats (shodded) for each chest tube
- 1-inch waterproof adhesive tape for taping connections
- Face mask, face shield, or head cover
- Sterile gloves
- 1-inch adhesive tape or zip tie for securing connections
- Stethoscope, sphygmomanometer, and pulse oximeter

ASSESSMENT

1. Identify patient using at least two identifiers (e.g., name and birthday or name and medical record number) according to agency policy. *Rationale: Ensures correct patient. Complies with The Joint Commission standards and improves patient safety (TJC, 2019).*
2. Review health care provider's order for chest tube placement. *Rationale: Insertion of chest tube requires health care provider order.*
3. Review patient's medication record for anticoagulant therapy, including aspirin, warfarin, heparin, or platelet aggregation inhibitors such as ticlopidine or dipyridamole. *Rationale: Anticoagulation therapy can increase procedure-related blood loss.*
4. Review patient's hemoglobin and hematocrit levels. *Rationale: Parameters reflect if blood loss is occurring, which may affect oxygenation.*
5. Assess patient for known allergies. Ask patient if he or she has had a problem with medications, latex, or anything applied to skin. *Rationale: Povidone-iodine and chlorhexidine are antiseptic*

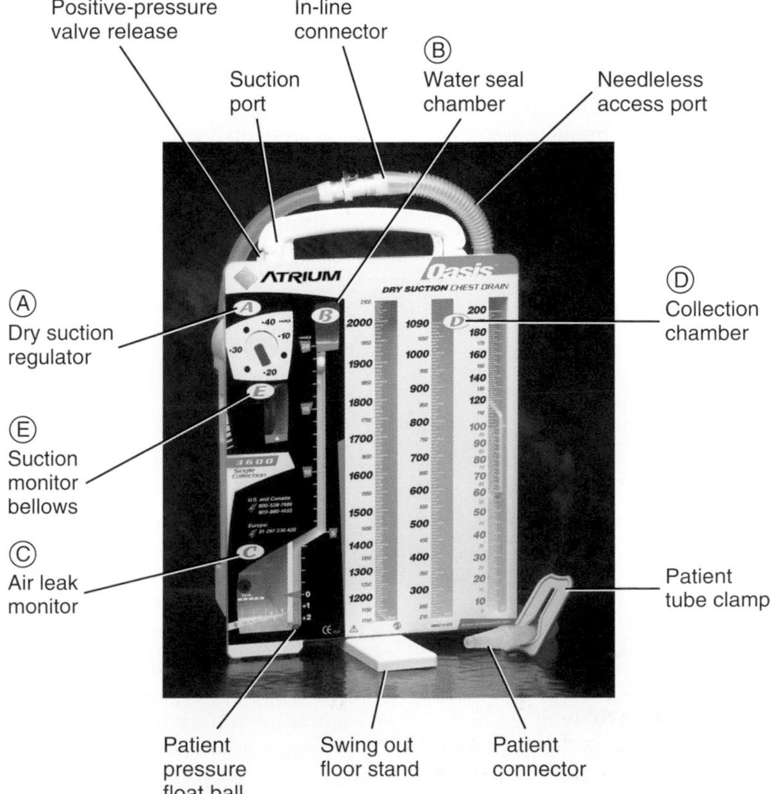

FIG 16.11 Dry suction chest drainage system. *(Courtesy Atrium Medical Corp.)*

solutions often used to clean skin before tube insertion. Lidocaine is a local anesthetic administered to reduce pain. The chest tube will be held in place with tape and sutures (Wiegand, 2017).

6. Perform hand hygiene and perform a complete respiratory assessment, baseline vital signs, and pulse oximetry (SpO_2). *Rationale: Baseline assessment and vital signs are essential for any invasive procedure. Chest tube insertion often relieves respiratory distress.*
   a. Assess for signs and symptoms of increased respiratory distress and hypoxia (e.g., decreased breath sounds over affected and unaffected lungs, marked cyanosis, asymmetrical chest movements, displaced trachea, shortness of breath, and confusion). *Rationale: Signs and symptoms associated with respiratory distress are related to type and size of pneumothorax, hemothorax, or preexisting illness. Signs of hypoxia are related to inadequate oxygen to tissues.*
   b. Assess for sharp, stabbing chest pain or chest pain on inspiration, hypotension, and tachycardia. If possible, ask patient to rate level of comfort on a scale of 0 to 10. *Rationale: Sharp stabbing chest pain with or without decreased blood pressure and increased heart rate may indicate tension pneumothorax. Presence of pneumothorax or hemothorax is painful, frequently causing sharp inspiratory pain. In addition, discomfort is associated with presence of a chest tube, not just with its insertion. As a result, patients tend to not cough or change position to minimize this pain (Chotai, 2016).*
7. For patients who have existing chest tubes, observe:
   a. Chest tube dressing and site surrounding tube insertion. *Rationale: Ensures that dr essing is intact and occlusive seal remains without air or fluid leaks and that area surrounding insertion site is free of drainage or skin irritation (Chotai, 2016).*
   b. Tubing for kinks, dependent loops, or clots. *Rationale: Maintains a patent, freely draining system, preventing fluid accumulation in chest cavity. When tubing is coiled, looped, or clotted, drainage is impeded, and there is an increased risk for tension pneumothorax or surgical emphysema (Chotai, 2016; Rajan, 2016).*
   c. Chest drainage system should remain upright and below level of tube insertion. *Rationale: An upright drainage system facilitates drainage and maintains water seal.*
8. Remove and dispose of gloves. Perform hand hygiene.
9. Assess patient's comfort level on a scale of 0 to 10. *Rationale: Provides for baseline to compare after chest tube insertion.*
10. Assess patient's or family caregiver's knowledge, experience, and health literacy. *Rationale: Ensures patient or family caregiver has the capacity to obtain, communicate, process, and understand basic health information (CDC, 2016).*
11. Determine patient's knowledge of procedure. *Rationale: Encourages cooperation, minimizes risks and anxiety. Identifies teaching needs.*

STEP	RATIONALE
PLANNING	
1. Expected outcomes following completion of procedure:	
• Patient is oriented and less anxious.	Hypoxia is relieved.
• Vital signs are stable.	Decreased hypoxia improves vital sign measures.
• Patient reports no chest pain.	Reexpansion of lung reduces chest pain.
• Breath sounds are auscultated in all lobes. Lung expansion is symmetrical, SpO_2 is stable or improved, and respirations are unlabored.	Reexpansion of lung promotes normal respirations.
• Chest tube remains in place, and chest drainage system remains airtight.	Indicates correct placement and patency of chest tube drainage system.
• Gentle tidaling (fluctuations or rocking) is evident in water-seal or diagnostic indicator.	Indicates that system is functioning normally. Reflects changes in intrapleural pressure.
2. Arrange supplies at bedside.	Ensures organized procedure.
3. Position patient to provide access to chest tubes and dressing. Usually patient is in semi-Fowler's to Fowler's position.	
4. Explain procedure to patient.	Reduces anxiety and improves patient cooperation.
IMPLEMENTATION	
1. Check agency policy and determine whether informed consent is needed. Complete "time-out" procedure.	Invasive medical procedures typically require informed consent. "Time-out" is completed to determine right patient, procedure, and location of insertion or incision site (Wiegand, 2017).
2. Perform hand hygiene.	Reduces transmission of microorganisms.
3. Set up water-seal system (or dry system with suction); see manufacturer guidelines.	The water-seal system contains two or three compartments or chambers. Fluid drains into the first chamber. The second chamber contains the water seal, which allows air to escape because of the force of expiration but not to reenter on inspiration. If suction is needed, a third chamber is used.
a. Prepare chest drainage system. Remove wrappers and prepare to set up two- or three-chamber system.	Maintains sterility of system for use under sterile operating room conditions.
b. While maintaining sterility of drainage tubing, stand system upright and add sterile water or normal saline (NS) to appropriate compartments.	Reduces possibility of contamination.

STEP	RATIONALE
(1) *Two-chamber system (without suction):* Add sterile solution to water-seal chamber (second chamber), bringing fluid to required level as indicated.	Water-seal chamber acts as one-way valve so that air cannot enter pleural space (Chotai, 2016).
(2) *Three-chamber system (with suction):* Add sterile solution to water-seal chamber (second chamber). Add amount of sterile solution prescribed by health care provider to suction-control chamber (third chamber), usually 20 cm H_2O pressure. Connect tubing from suction-control chamber to suction source. Tailor length of drainage tube to patient. **NOTE:** Suction control chamber vent must not be occluded when using suction (see illustration).	Depth of fluid level dictates highest amount of negative pressure that can be present within system. For example, 20 cm of water is approximately 20 cm of water pressure. After chest tube is inserted, turn up the wall or portable suction device until water in suction-control bottle exhibits continuous, gentle bubbling.

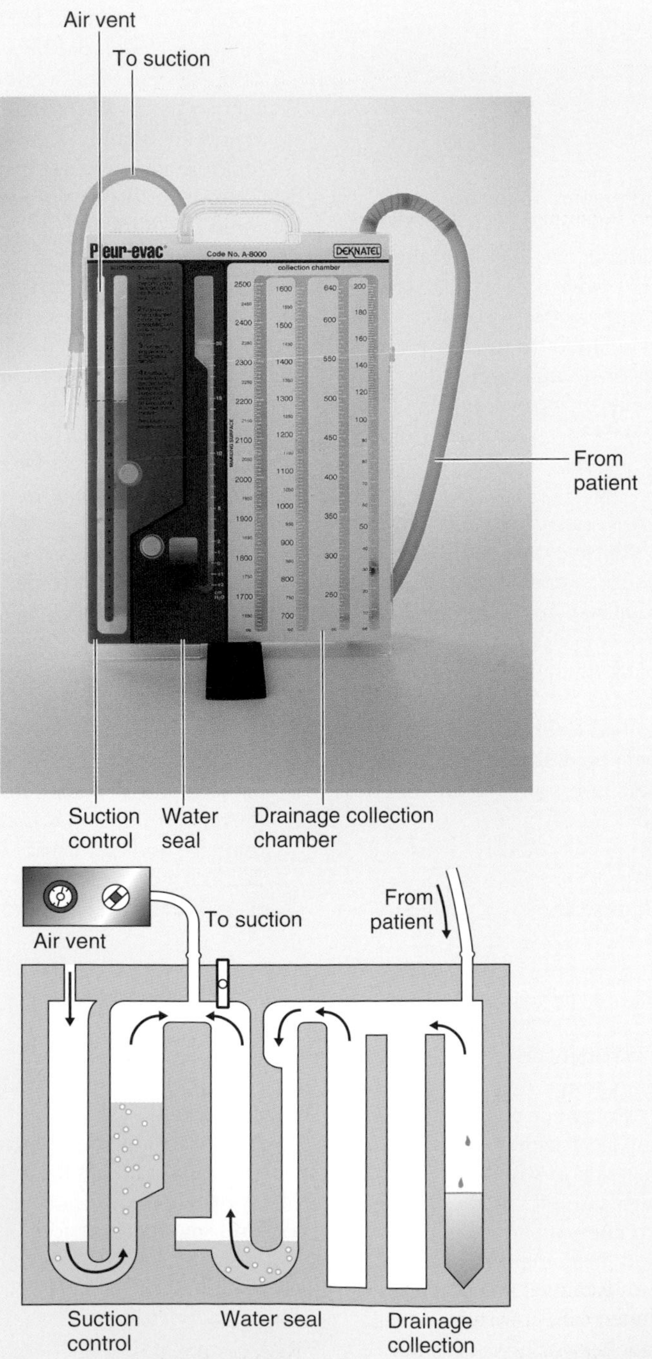

STEP 3b(2) Top, Pleur-Evac drainage system, a commercial three-chamber chest drainage device. Bottom, Schematic of drainage device.

STEP	RATIONALE

Safe Patient Care *When increasing suction, remember that increased bubbling does not result in more suction to the chest cavity but only serves to evaporate the water more quickly. The suction pressure should not exceed 20 cm H_2O because lung tissue damage may occur (Chotai, 2016).*

STEP	RATIONALE
(3) *Dry suction system* (see Fig. 16.11): Fill water-seal chamber with sterile solution. Adjust suction-control dial to prescribed level of suction; suction ranges from −10 to −40 cm of water pressure. Suction-control chamber vent is never occluded when suction is used. **NOTE:** On dry suction system, *DO NOT* obstruct positive-pressure relief valve. This allows air to escape.	Automatic control valve on dry suction-control device adjusts to changes in patient air leaks and fluctuation in suction source and vacuum to deliver prescribed amount of suction.
4. Set up waterless system (see manufacturer guidelines).	A waterless system is like a water-seal system except that sterile water is not required for suction. The suction control chamber is replaced by a one-way valve located near the top of the system. The suction control chamber contains a suction control float ball that is set by a suction control dial (between 10 and 40 cm H_2O after the suction is connected and turned on) (Zisis et al., 2015).
a. Remove sterile wrappers and prepare to set up.	Maintains sterility of system for use under sterile operating room conditions.
b. For two-chamber system (without suction), nothing is added or needs to be done to system.	Waterless two-chamber system is ready for connecting to patient's chest tube after opening wrappers.
c. For three-chamber system (with suction), connect tubing from suction-control chamber to suction source.	Suction source provides additional negative pressure to system.
d. Instill 15 mL of sterile water or normal saline (NS) into diagnostic indicator injection port located on top of system.	Allows observation of rise and fall of water in diagnostic air-leak window. Constant left-to-right bubbling or rocking is abnormal and indicates air leak. This is not necessary for mediastinal drainage because there is no tidaling. In an emergency, system *does not* require water for setup.
5. Secure all tubing connections with tape in double-spiral fashion using 2.5-cm (1-inch) adhesive tape or zip ties (nylon cable) with a clamp. Check system for patency by: a. Clamping drainage tubing that will connect to patient's chest tube. b. Connecting tubing from float ball chamber to suction source. c. Turning on suction to prescribed level.	Prevents atmospheric air from leaking into system and patient's intrapleural space. Provides chance to ensure airtight system before connection to patient.
6. Turn off suction source and unclamp drainage tubing before connecting patient to system. Suction source is turned on again after patient is connected.	Having patient connected to suction when it is initiated could damage pleural tissues from sudden increase in negative pressure. Tubing that is coiled or looped prevents adequate drainage and can cause tension pneumothorax (Wiegand, 2017).
7. Administer premedication such as sedatives or analgesics as ordered.	Reduces patient anxiety and pain during chest tube insertion.

Safe Patient Care *During procedure, carefully monitor patient for changes in level of sedation.*

STEP	RATIONALE
8. Provide psychological support to patient. a. Reinforce preprocedure explanation. b. Coach and support patient throughout procedure.	Reduces patient anxiety and helps complete procedure efficiently.
9. Perform hand hygiene and apply clean gloves. Position patient for tube insertion so that side in which tube is to be inserted is accessible to health care provider.	Reduces transmission of microorganisms. Allows ease of access for insertion of the tube.
10. Assist health care provider with chest tube insertion by providing needed equipment and local analgesic. Health care provider anesthetizes skin over insertion site, makes small skin incision, inserts clamped tube into intrapleural space, sutures it in place, and applies occlusive dressing.	Ensures smooth insertion.

STEP	RATIONALE
11. Help health care provider attach drainage tube to chest tube; remove clamp. Turn on suction to prescribed level.	Connects drainage system and suction (if ordered) to chest tube.
12. Tape or zip-tie all connections between chest tube and drainage tube. (**NOTE:** Chest tube is usually taped by health care provider at time of tube placement; check agency policy.)	Secures chest tube to drainage system and reduces risk for air leak that causes breaks in airtight system (Chotai, 2016; Wiegand, 2017).
13. Check systems for proper functioning. Health care provider orders chest x-ray film.	X-ray verifies intrapleural placement of tube.
14. After tube placement position patient:	Permits optimum drainage of fluid and/or air.
a. Semi-Fowler's or high-Fowler's position to evacuate air (pneumothorax; Chotai, 2016).	
b. High-Fowler's position to drain fluid (hemothorax; Chotai, 2016).	
15. Check patency of air vents in system.	
a. Water-seal vent must have no occlusion.	Permits displaced air to pass into atmosphere.
b. Suction-control chamber vent is not occluded when suction is used.	Provides safety factor of releasing excess negative pressure into atmosphere.
c. Waterless systems have relief valves without caps.	Provides safety factor of releasing excess negative pressure.
16. Position excess tubing horizontally on mattress next to patient. Secure on bottom sheet with clamp provided so that it does not obstruct tubing.	Prevents excess tubing from hanging over edge of mattress in dependent loop. Drainage collected in loop can occlude drainage system, which predisposes patient to tension pneumothorax (Wiegand, 2017).
17. Adjust end of tubing to hang in straight line from chest tube to drainage chamber.	Promotes drainage and prevents fluid or blood from accumulating in pleural cavity.

Safe Patient Care *Gentle lifting of the drain tubing allows gravity to help blood and other viscous material to move to the drainage bottle and avoid stasis in the tubing, which can lead to obstruction of the system and increased pressure in the thoracic cavity. Patients with recent chest surgery or trauma may need to have the chest drain tubing lifted more frequently, based on assessment of the amount of drainage (Wiegand, 2017).*

STEP	RATIONALE
18. Place two rubber-tipped hemostats (for each chest tube) in easily accessible position (e.g., taped to top of patient's headboard). These should remain with patient when ambulating.	Chest tubes are double clamped under specific circumstances: (1) to assess for air leak (Table 16.4), (2) to empty or quickly change disposable systems, or (3) to assess if patient is ready to have tube removed.

Safe Patient Care *In the event of a chest tube disconnection or if the drainage system breaks, submerge the distal part of the tube 2 to 4 cm (1 to 2 inches) below the surface of a 250-mL bottle of sterile water or NS until a new chest tube unit can be set up (Lewis et al., 2017).*

STEP	RATIONALE
19. Dispose of sharps in proper container, dispose of used supplies, remove and dispose of gloves, and perform hand hygiene.	Reduces transmission of microorganisms.
20. Care of patient after chest tube insertion/existing chest tube:	
a. Perform hand hygiene and apply clean gloves. Assess vital signs; oxygen saturation; skin color; breath sounds; rate, depth, and ease of respirations; and insertion site every 15 minutes for first 2 hours, and then at least every shift (see agency policy).	Provides immediate information about procedure-related complications such as respiratory distress and leakage. Provides information about status of patient with existing chest tube.
b. Monitor color, consistency, and amount of chest tube drainage every 15 minutes for first 2 hours after insertion. Indicate level of drainage fluid, date, and time on write-on surface of chamber.	Provides baseline for continuous assessment of type and quantity of drainage. Ensures early detection of complications.
(1) From mediastinal tube, expect less than 100 mL/hr immediately after surgery and no more than 500 mL in first 24 hours.	Sudden gush of drainage may result from coughing or changing patient's position (i.e., releasing pooled/collected blood rather than indicating active bleeding). Acute bleeding indicates hemorrhage. Health care provider should be notified if there is more than 100 to 200 mL of bloody drainage in an hour (Lewis et al., 2017; Wiegand, 2017).
(2) Expect little or no output from anterior chest tube that is inserted for a pneumothorax (Wiegand, 2017).	

TABLE 16.4
Problem Solving With Chest Tubes

Assessment	Intervention
Air leak can occur at insertion site, connection between tube and drainage device, or within drainage device itself. Continuous bubbling is noted in water-seal chamber that is attached to suction (Wiegand, 2017). If a water-seal unit is not attached to suction, a total absence of bubbling and drainage would indicate a leak.	Locate leak by quickly clamping tube at different intervals. Leaks are corrected when constant bubbling stops.
Assess for location of leak by clamping chest tube with two rubber-shod or toothless clamps close to the chest wall. If bubbling stops, air leak is inside patient's thorax or at chest insertion site.	Unclamp tube, reinforce chest dressing, and notify health care provider immediately. *Rationale:* Leaving chest tube clamped can cause collapse of lung, mediastinal shift, and eventual collapse of other lung from buildup of air pressure within the pleural cavity (Wiegand, 2017).
If bubbling continues with clamps near the chest wall, gradually move one clamp at a time down drainage tubing away from patient and toward suction-control chamber. When bubbling stops, leak is in section of tubing or connection between clamps (Wiegand, 2017).	Replace tubing, or secure connection and release clamps.
If bubbling continues, this indicates that leak is in the drainage system.	Change the drainage system.
Assess for tension pneumothorax (a medical emergency): • Severe respiratory distress • Low oxygen saturation • Chest pain • Absence of breath sounds on affected side • Tracheal shift toward unaffected side • Hypotension and signs of shock • Tachycardia	Ensure that chest tubes are patent: remove clamps, eliminate kinks, or eliminate occlusion. Notify health care provider and Rapid Response Team immediately and prepare for another chest tube insertion. You may use a flutter (Heimlich) valve or large-gauge needle for short-term emergency release of pressure in the intrapleural space. Have emergency equipment, oxygen, and code cart available because condition is life-threatening (Lewis et al., 2017).
Water-seal tube is no longer submerged in sterile fluid because of evaporation.	Add sterile water to water-seal chamber until distal tip is 2 cm (1 inch) under surface level.

STEP	RATIONALE

Safe Patient Care *Routine stripping or milking of the chest tube is not a recommended practice. Doing so can result in increased pressure in the thoracic cavity, causing damage to the lungs or the pleural tissues. If there is a visible clot in the tubing, gentle milking of the tubing (manual squeezing and releasing of parts of the tubing) may be indicated, but only if the patient is at risk of further harm from the clot, such as the development of a tension pneumothorax (Makic et al., 2015; Wiegand, 2017).*

STEP	RATIONALE
c. Observe chest dressing for drainage and to determine if it is still occlusive.	Drainage around tube may indicate blockage of the tube. Many health care agencies require the chest tube dressings to be occlusive in nature.

Safe Patient Care *If the dressing is not occlusive or is saturated with drainage, it may need to be changed. There is no standard for how chest tube dressings should be performed, such as sterile versus a nonsterile dressing change. Know the health care agency standards for this procedure. Some health care agencies require the use of Petrolatum gauze around the chest tube, whereas others do not (Gross et al., 2016).*

STEP	RATIONALE
d. Palpate around tube for swelling and crepitus (subcutaneous emphysema) as noted by crackling.	Indicates presence of air trapping in subcutaneous tissues. Small amounts are commonly absorbed. Large amounts are potentially dangerous. Most occurrences of crepitus are minor (Mao et al., 2015).

Safe Patient Care *Some patients may develop subcutaneous emphysema (i.e., a collection of air under the skin after chest tube placement), which can occur if tubing is blocked or kinked. When this occurs, a crepitus (a crackling sensation) is felt with tactile fremitus on palpation.*

STEP	RATIONALE
e. Check tubing to ensure that it is free of kinks and dependent loops.	Promotes drainage and prevents the development of a tension pneumothorax.

STEP	RATIONALE
f. Observe for fluctuation of water-seal chamber and drainage in tubing during inspiration and expiration. Observe for clots or debris in tubing.	If fluctuation or tidaling stops, it means that either the lung is fully expanded or the system is obstructed (Wiegand, 2017). In spontaneously breathing patient, fluid rises in water-seal or diagnostic indicator (waterless system) with inspiration and falls with expiration. The opposite occurs in patient who is mechanically ventilated. This indicates that system is functioning properly (Atrium, 2015).
g. Keep drainage system upright and below level of patient's chest.	Promotes gravity drainage and prevents backflow of fluid and air into pleural space.
h. Check for air leaks by monitoring bubbling in water-seal chamber: Intermittent bubbling is normal during expiration when air is being evacuated from pleural cavity, but continuous bubbling during both inspiration and expiration indicates leak in system.	Absence of bubbling may indicate that lung is fully expanded in patient with pneumothorax. Check all connections and locate sources of air leak (see Table 16.4).
21. Instruct patient on how to regularly take deep breaths and to reposition as often as possible.	Maintains lung expansion.
22. Be sure nurse call system is in an accessible location within patient's reach.	Ensures patient can call for assistance if needed.
23. Raise side rails (as appropriate) and lower bed to lowest position.	Ensures patient safety.
24. Remove gloves and dispose of used soiled equipment in appropriate biohazard container. Perform hand hygiene.	Prevents accidents involving contaminated equipment.

EVALUATION

1. Evaluate patient for decreased respiratory distress and chest pain. Auscultate patient's lungs and observe chest expansion.	Determines status of lung expansion.
2. Monitor vital signs and SpO_2.	Determines if level of oxygenation has improved.
3. Reassess patient's level of comfort on scale of 0 to 10, comparing level with comfort before chest tube insertion.	Indicates need for analgesia. Patient with chest tube discomfort hesitates to take deep breaths and as a result is at risk for pneumonia and atelectasis.
4. Evaluate patient's ability to use deep-breathing exercises and reposition self while maintaining comfort.	Indicates patient's ability to promote lung expansion and prevent complications. Patients need to be repositioned every 2 hours when a chest tube is in place (Wiegand, 2017).
5. Monitor continued functioning of system as indicated by reduction in amount of drainage, resolution of air leak, and complete reexpansion of the lung.	Detects early signs of system complications or indicates possible removal of chest tube.
6. **Use Teach-Back:** "I want to be sure I explained clearly why you have a chest tube. Tell me the reason why you have it." Revise your instruction now or develop a plan for revised patient/family caregiver teaching if patient/family caregiver is not able to teach back correctly.	Determines patient's/family caregiver's level of understanding of instructional topic.

Unexpected Outcomes	Related Interventions
1. Patient develops respiratory distress. Chest pain, decrease in breath sounds over affected and unaffected lungs, marked cyanosis, asymmetrical chest movements, presence of subcutaneous emphysema around tube insertion site or neck, hypotension, tachycardia, and/or mediastinal shift are critical and indicate severe change in patient status such as excessive blood loss or tension pneumothorax.	• Notify health care provider immediately. • Collect set of vital signs and SpO_2. • Prepare for chest x-ray film. • Provide oxygen as ordered.
2. There is no chest tube drainage.	• Observe for kink in chest drainage system. • Observe for possible clot in chest drainage system. • Observe for mediastinal shift or respiratory distress (medical emergency). • Notify health care provider.
3. Chest tube is dislodged.	• Immediately apply dressing and/or pressure over chest tube insertion site. • Notify health care provider.

Recording

- Record respiratory assessment findings; amount of suction, if used; amount of drainage since the previous assessment; type and amount of drainage in chest tubing; and presence or absence of an air leak, and patient comfort level.
- Record integrity of dressing and presence of drainage on dressing.
- Document your evaluation of patient learning.

Hand-Off Reporting

- Report patient tolerance of chest tube insertion, comfort level and any analgesia, respiratory assessment before and after chest tube insertion, and quantity and quality of chest tube drainage.

SPECIAL CONSIDERATIONS

Patient-Centered Care

- Patients with chronic conditions, such as cancer, cardiopulmonary diseases, and arthritis, often have diminished activity tolerance and cannot tolerate a complete chest physiotherapy (CPT) session. Plan CPT sessions in short intervals with rest periods between sessions.
- Patients with artificial airways (ETT/TT) have difficulties communicating their needs due to their inability to speak. Electronic tablets and pen and paper are useful items to help assist these patients communicate with families and health care team members (Rodriguez et al., 2016).
- Additional communication difficulties may occur when patients have visual or auditory deficits. Ensure that glasses and hearing aids are available and working properly.
- If patient is not English speaking, have a professional interpreter present or available.

Patient Education

- Teach patient and family caregiver about the hazards of home oxygen and how to administer oxygen safely based on which system is selected for home use (see Table 16.1). This includes eliminating mechanical or electrical toys that may be a source of a spark (Hockenberry et al., 2017).
- Teach patient and family caregiver signs and symptoms of hypoxia (see Box 16.2).
- Instruct patient and family caregiver that the best times for airway clearance therapies are before meals and not after to prevent vomiting of the meal. The optimal time to perform airway clearance therapies is within 1 hour of rising in the morning and then 1 hour before bedtime (Hockenberry et al., 2017).
- Family caregivers must know how to clean established tracheostomy tubes and stoma sites and recognize the signs and symptoms of respiratory and stoma infections.

Age-Specific

Pediatric

- Infants and children have smaller airways than adults. Even a small amount of mucus can lead to obstruction (Hockenberry et al., 2017).
- Infants and young children are not able to use the Acapella device for airway clearance. Infants who do not have adequate head control are not candidates for HFCWC therapy. Other airway clearance techniques should be utilized, such as manual chest percussion.
- When suctioning a child with an ETT or a TT, the diameter of suction catheter should be no more than one-half the internal diameter of the child's tracheostomy or other artificial airway. Unless secretions are thick, a lower range of vacuum pressure is recommended (Hockenberry et al., 2017).
- Because of infants' delicate skin, skin preparation or tape adhesive is not always used before securing ETT. ETT holders are best to use in infants.
- Normal or near-normal activities should be promoted in infants and children who receive long-term mechanical ventilation to enhance their growth and development.

Gerontological

- Older adults have stiffer chest walls and weaker respiratory muscles, which increases their risk for having a disturbance that requires oxygen therapy (Touhy and Jett, 2018).
- Because of increased tissue fragility, older adults may have bloody secretions on suctioning. Monitor the suction return for clearing and avoid unnecessary suctioning.
- Older adult skin may be more fragile and prone to breakdown from secretions or pressure or tearing when removing tape.

Home Care

- Frequent follow-up may be necessary to enhance compliance with any prescribed home treatments (oxygen, noninvasive ventilation, airway clearance therapies) and address unexpected outcomes promptly.
- Patients and family caregivers will need to be taught the rationale for any equipment that is prescribed for home use, how to troubleshoot the equipment if problems arise, whom to contact for their home medical equipment needs, and when to contact the health care provider.
- Ensure that patients on home oxygen therapy have long tubing or extension tubing that allows them more ability to ambulate through the rooms of the house or apartment. Caution patients and family caregivers that oxygen tubing can be a tripping hazard and increase the risk for falls (Walsh and Smallwood, 2017).
- Ensure patients and caregivers know and follow best practices for infection control during invasive procedures such as airway suctioning while weighing the necessity of cost-effectiveness in their chronic situation. For example, clean suctioning techniques are acceptable, with the patient or family caregiver cleaning the secretion collection container and disinfecting it every 24 hours.
- Notify power companies when patients are receiving either invasive or noninvasive mechanical ventilation. In the event of a power outage, these homes would be the priority for restoring power.

✦ PRACTICE REFLECTIONS

You are caring for a patient receiving mechanical ventilation via a tracheostomy tube (TT). You enter the room and find that the patient is anxious, tachycardic, and diaphoretic. The patient is trying to communicate with you by mouthing words to you, but you are unable to read the patient's lips. The pulse oximeter reading is 90%, the lung sounds are coarse, and there is a small amount of secretions around the stoma site.

1. What will you do? What is your priority action?
2. What other interventions will you perform for this patient?
3. What will you do if your interventions do not lead to an increase in the pulse oximeter value?

✦ CLINICAL REVIEW QUESTIONS

1. The nurse is caring for a patient receiving mechanical ventilation via an endotracheal tube. What interventions should be included in the plan of care? (Select all that apply.)
   1. Elevate the head of the bed to 90 degrees.
   2. Suction the patient every 4 hours.
   3. Perform oral care every 2 to 4 hours.
   4. Hyperoxygenate patient prior to suctioning.
   5. Ensure humidity is applied to ventilator circuit.
2. The nurse is caring for a patient receiving noninvasive ventilation via a CPAP face mask. What are the appropriate assessments for the nurse to perform? (Select all that apply.)
   1. Assess for reddened areas along bridge of nose.
   2. Auscultate lung sounds.
   3. Provide continuous monitoring of capnography waveforms.
   4. Monitor a continuous pulse oximeter.
   5. Assess for abdominal distension.
3. When caring for a patient with a chest tube, which activities can a nurse delegate to the nursing assistive personnel (NAP)? (Select all that apply.)
   1. Proper positioning of the patient to facilitate chest tube drainage.
   2. Helping with removal of the chest tube.
   3. Ambulating and transferring the patient with chest tube drainage system.
   4. Reporting any abnormal vital signs, complaints of chest pain, or shortness of breath.
   5. Reinfusion of chest tube drainage.
   6. Reporting any change in the amount of drainage or sudden bleeding.

Answers and Rationales for Clinical Review Questions can be found on the Evolve website.

REFERENCES

American Association of Critical Care Nurses (AACN): AACN practice alert: prevention of aspiration, 2016. http://www.aacn.org/wd/practice/content/practicealerts/aspiration-practice-alert.pcms?menu=practice.

American Association of Critical Care Nurses (AACN): AACN practice alert: oral care for acutely and critically ill patients, 2017a. https://www.aacn.org/~/media/aacn-website/clincial-resources/practice-alerts/oralcarepractalert2017.pdf.

American Association of Critical Care Nurses (AACN): AACN practice alert: prevention of ventilator-associated pneumonia in adults, 2017b. https://www.aacn.org/clinical-resources/practice-alerts/ventilator-associated-pneumonia-vap.

American Association of Respiratory Care (AARC): AARC clinical practice guideline: nasotracheal suctioning—2004 revision & update, 2004. http://www.rcjournal.com/cpgs/pdf/09.04.1080.pdf.

American Association for Respiratory Care (AARC): AARC clinical practice guidelines: endotracheal suctioning of mechanically ventilated patients with artificial airways: 2010, *Respir Care* 55(6):758, 2010.

American Lung Association: Using oxygen safely, 2018. http://www.lung.org/lung-health-and-diseases/lung-procedures-and-tests/oxygen-therapy/using-oxygen-safely.html.

Atrium: *Evidence-based care of patients with chest tubes*, 2015. http://www.atriummed.com/EN/chest_drainage/Documents/NTI2015Evidence-BasedCareofPatientswithChestTubes.pdf.

Branson RD, et al: Management of the artificial airway, *Respir Care* 59(6):974, 2014.

Centers for Disease Control and Prevention (CDC): What is health literacy? 2016. https://www.cdc.gov/healthliteracy/learn/index.html.

Chacko R, et al: Oral decontamination techniques and ventilator-associated pneumonia, *Br J Nurs* 26(11):594, 2017.

Chatwin M, et al: Airway clearance techniques in neuromuscular disorders: a state of the art review, *Respir Med* 136:98, 2018.

Chotai P: Tube thoracostomy management, Medscape, 2016. https://emedicine.medscape.com/article/1503275-overview.

Clinkscale D, et al: A randomized trial of conventional chest physical therapy versus high frequency chest wall compressions in intubated and non-intubated adults, *Respir Care* 57(2):221, 2012.

DeVrieze BW, Bhimji SS: Peak flow rate measurement. https://www.ncbi.nlm.nih.gov/books/NBK459325.

Drake MG: High-flow nasal cannula oxygen in adults: an evidence-based assessment, *Ann Am Thorac Soc* 15(2):145–155, 2018.

Elliott ZJ, Elliott SC: An overview of mechanical ventilation in the intensive care unit, *Nurs Stand* 32(28):41, 2018.

Galbiati G, Paola C: Effects of open and closed endotracheal suctioning on intracranial pressure and cerebral perfusion pressure in adult patients with severe brain injury: a literature review, *J Neurosci Nurs* 47(4):239, 2015.

Gale N, et al: Adapting to domiciliary non-invasive ventilation in chronic obstructive pulmonary disease: a qualitative interview study, *Palliat Med* 29(3):268, 2015.

Gerald L, et al: How to use a peak flow meter (Beyond the Basics), UpToDate, 2018. https://www.uptodate.com/contents/how-to-use-a-peak-flow-meter-beyond-the-basics#!

Gross SL, et al: Comparison of three practices for dressing chest tube insertion sites: a randomized controlled trial, *Medsurg Nurs* 25(4):229, 2016.

Hanlon P: Physiological effects of humidification, 2016. http://www.rtmagazine.com/2016/04/physiological-effects-humidification.

Hill N, Kramer N: Trouble shooting problems with noninvasive positive pressure ventilation, 2018. http://www.uptodate.com/contents/troubleshooting-problems-with-noninvasive-positive-pressure-ventilation.

Hockenberry MJ, et al: *Essentials of pediatric nursing*, ed 10, St. Louis, 2017, Mosby.

Hyzy R, et al: Noninvasive ventilation in acute respiratory failure in adults, UpToDate 2018a. https://www.uptodate.com/contents/noninvasive-ventilation-in-acute-respiratory-failure-in-adults.

Hyzy R, et al: Overview of tracheostomy, UpToDate, 2018b. https://www.uptodate.com/contents/overview-of-tracheostomy.

Institute for Healthcare Improvement (IHI): How-to guide: prevent ventilator-associated pneumonia, 2012. http://www.ihi.org/resources/Pages/Tools/HowtoGuidePreventVAP.aspx.

Institute for Healthcare Improvement (IHI): Ventilator-associated pneumonia: getting to zero…and staying there, 2016. http://www.ihi.org/resources/pages/improvementstories/vapgettingtozeroandstayingthere.aspx.

Intensive Care Society (ICS): ICS tracheostomy standards, 2014. www.ics.ac.uk.

Larrow V, Klich-Heartt EI: Prevention of ventilator-associated pneumonia in the intensive care unit: beyond the basics, *J Neurosci Nurs* 48(3):160, 2016.

Letchford E, Bench S: Ventilator-associated pneumonia and suction: a review of the literature, *Br J Nurs* 27(1):13, 2018.

Lewis SL, et al: *Medical-surgical nursing: assessment and management of clinical problems*, ed 10, St. Louis, 2017, Elsevier.

Li J, et al: Evaluation of the safety and effectiveness of the rapid flow expulsion maneuver to clear subglottic secretions in vitro and in vivo, *Respr Care* 62(8):1007, 2017.

Makic MBF, et al: Continuing to challenge practice to be evidence-based, *Crit Care Nurse* 35(2):39, 2015.

Mao M, et al: Complications of chest tubes: a focused clinical synopsis, *Curr Opin Pulm Med* 21:376, 2015.

Messika J, et al: Use of high-flow nasal cannula oxygen therapy in subjects with ARDS: a 1-year observational study, *Respir Care* 60(2):163, 2015.

Munro N, Ruggiero M: Ventilator-associated pneumonia bundle reconstruction for best care, *AACN Adv Crit Care* 25(2):163, 2014.

Myatt R: Nursing care of patients with a temporary tracheostomy, *Nurs Stand* 29(26):42, 2015.

Naswa S, et al: Comparison of acapella versus active cycle of breathing technique in post-operative pulmonary complications after valve replacement surgeries, *Indian J Physiother Occup Ther* 11(2):24, 2017.
National Heart, Lung, and Blood Institute (NHLBI): How to use a peak flow meter, 2013. http://www.nhlbi.nih.gov/files/docs/public/lung/asthma_tipsheets.pdf.
Ntoumenopoulos G: High-frequency chest wall compressions: Good for the patient? Good for the clinician? *Respir Care* 57(2):3233, 2012.
Pittman J, et al: Medical device related hospital-acquired pressure ulcers, *J Wound Ostomy Continence Nurs* 42(2):151, 2015.
Pooboni S, et al: Noninvasive ventilation procedures, 2015. http://emedicine.medscape.com/article/1417959-overview#a1.
Rajan C: Tube thoracostomy management, 2016 update. http://emedicine.medscape.com/article/1503275-overview#a5.
Restrepo RD, Walsh BK: Humidification during invasive and noninvasive mechanical ventilation, *Respir Care* 57(5):782, 2012.
Rodriguez CS, et al: Enhancing the communication of suddenly speechless critical care patients, *Am J Crit Care* 25(3):e40, 2016.
Rouzé A, et al: Tracheal tube design and ventilator-associated pneumonia, *Respir Care* 62(10):1316, 2017.
Schallom M, et al: Pressure ulcer incidence in patients wearing nasal-oral versus full-face noninvasive ventilation masks, *Am J Crit Care* 24(4):349, 2015.
Smith SG, Pietrantonio T: Best method for securing an endotracheal tube, *Crit Care Nurs* 36(2):78, 2016.
Sole ML, et al: Clinical indicators for endotracheal suctioning in adult patients receiving mechanical ventilation, *Am J Crit Care* 24(4):318, 2015.
Strickland SL, et al: AARC clinical practice guideline: effectiveness of nonpharmacologic airway clearance therapies in hospitalized patients, *Respir Care* 60(7):1071, 2015.
The Joint Commission (TJC): *2019 National Patient Safety Goals*, Oakbrook Terrace, IL, 2019, The Commission. http://www.jointcommission.org/standards_information/npsgs.aspx.
Touhy TA, Jett K: *Ebersole & Hess' gerontological nursing and healthy aging*, ed 5, St. Louis, 2018, Elsevier.
Urden L, et al: *Priorities in critical care nursing*, ed 7, St. Louis, 2016, Mosby.
Volsko TA: Airway clearance therapy: finding the evidence, *Respir Care* 58(10):1669, 2013.
Walsh BK, Smallwood CD: Pediatric oxygen therapy: a review and update, *Respir Care* 62(6):645, 2017.
Wiegand D: *AACN procedure manual for high acuity, progressive, and critical care*, ed 7, St. Louis, 2017, Elsevier.
Zisis C, et al: Chest drainage systems in use, *Ann Transl Med* 3(3):43, 2015.

17 Safe Patient Handling

SKILLS AND PROCEDURES

EVOLVE WEBSITE/RESOURCES LIST

http://evolve.elsevier.com/Perry/nursinginterventions

Audio Glossary • Checklists • Clinical Review Questions • Answers and Rationales for Clinical Review Questions • Video Clips

INTRODUCTION

Data from the Bureau of Labor Statistics (BLS) show that in 2014, the rate of overexertion injuries averaged across all industries was 33 per 10,000 full-time workers. By comparison, the overexertion injury rate for hospital workers was twice the average (68 per 10,000) (BLS, 2014). The greatest risk factor for overexertion injuries in health care workers is the manual lifting, moving, and repositioning of patients. Using principles of safe patient handling during transfer and positioning for routine activities decreases work effort and places less strain on musculoskeletal structures. It also remains important for health care providers to use good body mechanics when performing patient-handling activities (Box 17.1). Safe patient-handling laws require hospitals and nursing homes to develop programs for the use of engineering controls, lifting and transfer aids, or assistive devices by staff to perform the acts of lifting, transferring, and repositioning health care patients and residents. Safe patient-handling and mobility (SPHM) programs, if properly implemented, can drastically reduce health care worker injuries (American Nurses Association [ANA], 2013b).

PRACTICE STANDARDS

- Occupational Safety and Health Administration (OSHA), 2014: Safe patient handling: preventing musculoskeletal disorders in nursing homes—Guidelines for transfer and positioning of patients
- Occupational Safety and Health Administration (OSHA), 2015: Worker safety in hospitals—Elements of a safe patient-handling program
- Tampa Research and Education Foundation, Inc (TVAREF), 2014: VHA Safe patient handling and mobility algorithms
- The Joint Commission, 2019: National Patient Safety Goals—Patient identification

EVIDENCE-BASED PRACTICE

Efficacy of Safe Patient-Handling and Mobility Programs

Health care organizations are adopting safe patient-handling and mobility (SPHM) programs to reduce patient and health care worker injuries. Dennerlein and colleagues (2017) evaluated a hospital-wide SPHM program (Hospital A) and compared its success with that of a comparison hospital (Hospital B) over a period of 12 months. Staff self-reports of use of safe patient-handling and mobilization practices improved significantly in Hospital A compared with Hospital B. In addition, scores for ergonomic practices increased for Hospital A. In addition, Hospital A experienced a decline in the number of recordable injuries on patient care units. A smaller, unit-based study involved pre- and post-intervention measures at 12 months after implementing the use of safe patient-handling equipment on intervention and control units at two hospitals. At 12 months, the intervention groups had more positive attitudes toward patient-handling equipment and increased use of specific patient-handling equipment (Risor et al., 2017). However, no significant change was observed in musculoskeletal problems. A study involving California hospitals where SPHM programs had been implemented for 12 months showed that nurses whose agencies employed lift teams were significantly less likely to report low back pain, and nurses whose units had ceiling lifts were significantly less likely to report shoulder pain than nurses with no access to lifts (Lee, 2015).

PRACTICE ISSUES/PRINCIPLES

- A comprehensive SPHM program includes integrating the use of safe patient-handling and mobilization equipment, practices for improving patient mobility, use of patient risk assessments,

BOX 17.1

Proper Body Mechanics

- Keep the weight (patient) to be lifted as close to the body as possible; this action places the weight in the same plane as the lifter and close to the center of gravity for balance.
- Bend at the knees to help maintain your center of gravity. Let the strong muscles of the legs do the lifting.
- Avoid twisting. Twisting your spine can lead to serious injury.
- Before lifting, tighten stomach muscles and tuck the pelvis to provide balance and protect the back.
- Maintain the trunk erect and knees bent so that multiple muscle groups work together in a synchronized manner.
- The best height for lifting vertically is approximately 2 feet off the ground and close to the lifter's center of gravity.

a hospital infrastructure for maintaining and servicing equipment, patient hand-off procedures, and staff training (Dennerlein et al., 2017).

- A multi-component SPHM program has been found to be effective in reducing patient-handling injuries among nurses (Choi and Cramer, 2016).
- Use of lifting/transfer equipment and devices, ergonomic assessments and controls, no-lift policies, and training and education is recommended (Choi and Brings, 2015).

SAFETY GUIDELINES

Professional standards and guidelines, such as those from the American Nurses Association (2013a, 2013b), and the American Association for Safe Patient Handling and Movement (2012), concerning the use of assistive equipment and devices to transfer and position patients safely are invaluable for the safety of you and your patients. Follow these guidelines in the performance of skills in this chapter:

- Always promote the patient's independence (e.g., decision making for time to perform activities) while safely adhering to any prescribed rehabilitation plan.
- Communicate clearly with members of the health care team. During hand-off communication, share information about the patient's level of mobility; any restrictions; type of assist devices used; and methods being used to transfer, reposition, or ambulate.
- Clear the immediate environment where a patient will stand/walk of any obstacles or clutter.
- Monitor a patient's activity tolerance throughout any extended ambulation or period of time sitting in a chair.

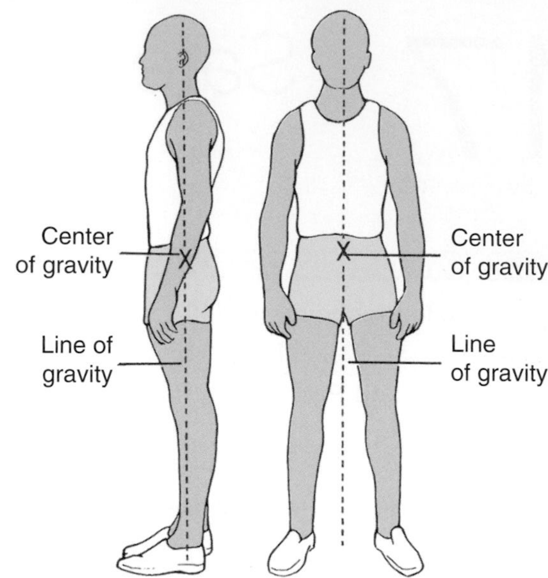

FIG 17.1 Body alignment when standing.

- Mentally review the steps of a transfer before beginning to ensure the safety of both you and the patient.
- Stand on the patient's weak side when assisting a patient able to stand (Pierson and Fairchild, 2017).
- When assisting with transfer or positioning, position the level of the bed to a comfortable and safe height.
- Determine the amount and type of assistance required for transfer, including the type of transfer equipment and the number of personnel it will take to safely transfer the patient and prevent harm to the patient and health care providers.
- Raise the side rail on the side of the bed opposite of where you are standing to prevent the patient from falling out of bed on that side.
- Make sure all personnel understand how lift and transfer equipment functions before it is used.
- Educate patients and/or family caregivers about how equipment functions to reduce their anxiety and enlist their cooperation.
- Arrange equipment (e.g., intravenous [IV] lines, feeding tube, Foley catheter) so that it will not interfere with the transfer process.
- Evaluate the patient for correct body alignment (Fig. 17.1) and pressure injury risks after a transfer.

✦ SKILL 17.1 Transfer Techniques

Purpose

Transferring patients to and from their beds or chairs includes a set of skills that protect patients and health care providers from injuries and help patients regain optimal independence as quickly as possible. When preparing to transfer patients, consider the type of problems that can develop. For example, a patient who has been immobile for several days or longer is often weak or dizzy or sometimes develops initial orthostatic hypotension; anticipate this patient being at risk for not tolerating standing or possibly falling during a transfer. If there is any doubt about safe transfer, use a transfer belt and obtain assistance when transferring patients. Follow the principles of proper body mechanics (see Box 17.1) when you are required (within safe patient-handling guidelines) to lift a patient or any patient care equipment. The guidelines will reduce lumbar injury. Remember that injuries are not only related to lifting. Activities that involve bending and twisting (e.g., carrying supplies and equipment and pushing and pulling equipment) can also cause injury (Anderson et al., 2014).

Delegation and Collaboration

The skill of effective transfer techniques can be delegated to trained nursing assistive personnel (NAP). The nurse is responsible for initially assessing the patient's readiness and ability to transfer. The nurse directs the NAP by:

- Assisting and supervising when moving patients who are transferred for the first time after prolonged bed rest, extensive surgery, critical illness, or spinal cord trauma.
- Explaining the patient's mobility restrictions, changes in blood pressure to look for, or sensory alterations that may affect safe transfer (e.g., medicated or confused).
- Explaining what to observe and report back to the nurse, such as dizziness or the patient's ability/inability to assist.

Equipment

- Gait belt, sling, or lapboard (as needed)
- Nonskid shoes, bath blankets, and pillows
- Chair with arms or wheelchair (position chair at 45- to 60-degree angle to bed, lock brakes, remove footrests, and lock bed brakes)
- Stretcher (position next to bed, lock brakes on stretcher, lock brakes on bed)
- Mechanical/hydraulic lift (use frame, canvas strips or chains, and hammock or canvas strips)
- Stand-assist lift device
- *Option:* Clean gloves (if risk of contacting soiled linen)

ASSESSMENT

1. Identify patient using at least two identifiers (e.g., name and birthday or name and medical record number) according to agency policy. *Rationale: Ensures correct patient. Complies with The Joint Commission standards and improves patient safety (TJC, 2019).*
2. Refer to medical record for most recent recorded weight and height for patient. *Rationale: Data determine if mechanical transfer device or friction-reducing device is needed for transfer.*
3. Review history for previous fall and if patient has a fear of falling. *Rationale: Previous fall history is a significant fall risk. Having a fear of falling can alter one's gait and security in walking.*
4. Assess previous mode of transferring to bed or chair (if applicable). *Rationale: Ensures some consistency in how to assist with transfer.*
5. Assess patient for presence of neuromuscular deficits, motor weakness or incoordination, calcium loss from bone, cognitive and visual dysfunction, and altered balance (see Chapter 8). *Rationale: Certain conditions increase risk of tripping, falling, or suffering potential injury during fall.*
6. Perform hand hygiene. *Rationale: Reduces transmission of microorganisms.*
7. Assess the patient's mobility, including ability to sit up on side of bed or chair and ability to stand. *Option:* Administer the Banner Mobility Assessment Tool (BMAT; Boynton et al., 2014). *Rationale: The BMAT is a tool that assesses four functional tasks to identify the level of mobility a patient can achieve (Boynton et al., 2014). The assessment aids in determining a patient's level of mobility (e.g., Mobility Level 1) and recommends equipment and tools needed to safely lift, transfer, and mobilize the patient.*
   a. **Sit and Shake**: From a semi-reclined position, ask patient to sit upright and rotate to a seated position at the side of the bed; patient may use the bedrail. Note patient's ability to maintain bedside position. Ask patient to reach out and grab your hand and shake, making sure patient reaches across his or her midline.
   b. **Stretch and Point**: With patient in seated position at the side of the bed, have patient place both feet on the floor (or stool) with knees no higher than hips. Ask patient to extend one leg and straighten the knee, then bend the ankle and point the toes. Repeat with the other leg
   c. **Stand**: Ask patient to elevate off the bed or chair (seated to standing) using an assistive device (walker, cane, bedrail). Patient should be able to raise buttocks off bed and hold for a count of five. May repeat once.
   d. **Walk** (march in place and advance step). Ask patient to march in place at bedside; then ask patient to step forward and back with each foot. Patient should display stability while performing tasks. Assess for stability and safety awareness.

If patient fails Sit and Shake: Use total lift with sling and/or positioning sheet and/or straps, and/or use lateral transfer devices such as roll board, friction-reducing device (slide sheets/tube), or air-assisted device.

If patient fails Stretch and Point: Use total lift for patient unable to bear weight on at least one leg; use sit-to-stand lift for patient who can bear weight on at least one leg.

If patient fails to Stand: Use nonpowered raising/stand aid (default to powered sit-to-stand lift if no stand aid available), total lift with ambulation accessories, or assistive device (cane, walker, crutches).

If patient cannot Walk: Use nonpowered raising/stand aid (default to powered sit-to-stand lift if no stand aid available), total lift with ambulation accessories, or assistive device (cane, walker, crutches).

Safe Patient Care *Do not rely on self-report from patient or family caregiver as to patient's ability to sit, stand, or ambulate. An objective assessment is needed to accurately determine a patient's capabilities.*

8. While assessing mobility, note any weakness, dizziness, or risk for orthostatic (postural) hypotension (e.g., previously on bed rest, first time arising from supine position after surgical procedure, history of dizziness when arising). *Rationale: Determines risk of fainting or falling during transfer. Immobilized patients have decreased ability of autonomic nervous system to equalize blood supply, resulting in initial drop of 40 mm Hg systolic or more in blood pressure when rising from sitting position (Frith et al., 2014; Mills et al., 2014).*
9. Assess activity tolerance, noting for fatigue during sitting and standing. *Rationale: Determines ability of patient to help with transfer.*
10. Assess proprioceptive function (awareness of posture and changes in equilibrium), including ability to maintain balance while sitting in bed or on side of bed and tendency to sway toward one side. *Rationale: Determines stability of patient's balance for transfer and risk for falls.*
11. Assess sensory status, including central and peripheral vision, adequacy of hearing, and presence of peripheral sensation loss. *Rationale: Visual field loss decreases patients' ability to see in direction of transfer and may impact their balance. Peripheral sensation loss decreases proprioception. Patients with visual and hearing losses need transfer techniques and communication methods adapted to their deficits.*

Safe Patient Care *Patients with hemiplegia may "neglect" one side of the body (inattention to or unawareness of one side of body or environment), which distorts perception of the visual field. If patient experiences neglect of one side, instruct him or her to scan all visual fields when transferring.*

12. Assess level of comfort (e.g., joint discomfort, muscle spasm) and measure level of pain using scale of 0 to 10. Offer prescribed analgesic 30 minutes before transfer. (**NOTE:** Patient will require assistance when analgesic has been given.) *Rationale: Pain reduces patient's motivation and ability to be mobile. Pain relief before transfer enhances patient's ability to participate (Schofield, 2014).*
13. Assess patient's cognitive status, including ability to follow verbal instructions, short-term memory, and recognition of physical deficits and limitations to movement. *Rationale: Determines patient's ability to follow directions and learn transfer techniques.*

Safe Patient Care *Patients with certain conditions that affect cognition, such as dementia, head trauma, or degenerative neurological disorders, may have perceptual cognitive defects that create safety risks. If the patient has difficulty comprehending, simplify instructions by providing one step at a time and maintain consistency.*

14. Assess patient's level of motivation, such as eagerness versus unwillingness to be mobile and perception of value of exercise. *Rationale: Will affect patient's desire to engage in activity.*
15. Assess need for special transfer equipment for home setting and previous mode of transfer (if applicable). *Rationale: Providing appropriate aids greatly enhances transfer ability at home.*
16. Assess patient's vital signs just before transfer. *Rationale: Baseline measures will determine if vital sign changes occur during activity, which will indicate activity intolerance (see Chapter 7). Patient with low blood pressure may not tolerate sudden position change and is at risk for orthostatic hypotension.*
17. Refer to mobility status and safe patient-handling algorithm (available in most agencies) to determine if a lift device or mechanical transfer device is needed and the number of people needed to help with transfer. Do not start procedure until all required caregivers are available. *Rationale: Ensures safe patient handling, reducing risk of injury to patient and caregivers.*
18. Assess patient's or family caregiver's knowledge, experience, and health literacy. *Rationale: Ensures patient or family caregiver has the capacity to obtain, communicate, process, and understand basic health information (Centers for Disease Control and Prevention [CDC], 2016).*

STEP	RATIONALE
PLANNING	
1. Expected outcomes following completion of procedure:	
• Patient sits on side of bed without dizziness, weakness, or orthostatic hypotension.	Precautions during transferring prevent vascular compromise.
• Patient tolerates increased activity.	Gradual increase in number of transfers and period of time out of bed increases tolerance and endurance.
• Patient can bear more weight on the lower extremities.	Repeated transfers usually result in improved strength/endurance and greater independence of patient.
• Patient transfers without injury.	Proper techniques avoid injury to patient and caregivers.
• Patient transfers with minimal discomfort.	Transfer procedures performed correctly.
2. Provide privacy and prepare environment.	Respects patient's dignity. Helps the student/nurse think about the need to remove clutter from the over-bed or bedside table.
3. Organize and set up any equipment/lift devices to use for transfer.	Ensures more efficiency and safe use of equipment.
4. Get additional caregivers as necessary to perform transfer.	Safe patient-handling algorithms (see agency policy) determine number of caregivers and type of devices needed to transfer a patient if lifting is required.
5. Explain to patient (in simple language) how you are going to prepare for transfer technique and safety precautions to be used. Explain benefits and reasons for getting up in a chair. Do so in a way that matches patient's beliefs and values regarding recovery or maintaining health (Shieh et al., 2015).	Provides for clearer understanding by patient. Motivates patient to be involved in transfer.
IMPLEMENTATION	
1. Perform hand hygiene.	Reduces transmission of microorganisms.
2. Assist patient from supine to sitting position on edge of bed with bed positioned so that top of mattress is even with your elbows. Refer to mobility assessment findings to confirm appropriateness to transfer patient.	Reduces strain on your back. Assessment findings offer objective measure of readiness for transfer.

STEP	RATIONALE
3. Allow patient to sit on the side of the bed for a few minutes. Have patient alternately flex and extend feet, then move lower legs up and down. Ask if patient feels dizzy; if so, check blood pressure. Have patient relax and take a few deep breaths until dizziness subsides and balance is gained. If dizziness lasts more than 60 seconds, return patient to bed (Frith et al., 2014; Mills et al., 2014). Recheck blood pressure.	Allows patient's circulation to equilibrate to reduce chance of orthostatic hypotension.

Safe Patient Care *Remain in front of patient until he or she regains balance, and continue to provide physical support to weak or cognitively impaired patient.*

STEP	RATIONALE
4. Transfer patient from bed to chair (*Option:* Apply clean gloves if bed linen soiled):	
a. Have chair in position at 45-degree angle with one side against bed, facing foot of bed.	Positions chair with easy access for transfer.
b. Place bed in low position or to point where patient's feet are comfortably flat on the floor with the hip and knees at a 90-degree angle.	Provides patient stability when transferring.
c. If patient is limited cognitively or has only partial weight bearing with upper-body strength or caregiver must lift more than 15.9 kg (35 lb), use a mechanical lift or transfer aid with minimum of two or three caregivers (see illustration). Follow manufacturer lift guidelines to apply.	The use of mechanical lift devices is strongly recommended to transfer a patient to reduce risk for musculoskeletal injury (Degelau et al., 2014; Occupational Safety and Health Administration [OSHA], 2014, 2015).

Safe Patient Care *If patient demonstrates weakness or paralysis of one side of the body, place chair on his or her strong side.*

STEP	RATIONALE
d. If patient has partial weight bearing, is cooperative and able to stand, and has upper-body strength, use stand-and-pivot technique with one caregiver.	
(1) Apply transfer belt (see illustration). Be sure that it completely circles waist. Place belt low and be sure that it is snug. Avoid placing belt over any intravenous lines, incisions, or drainage tubes.	Transfer belt allows you to maintain stability of patient during transfer and reduces risk for falling (Degelau et al., 2014; OSHA, 2014).
(2) If not already in place, help patient apply stable, nonskid shoes/socks. Place patient's weight-bearing or strong leg forward on floor, with weak foot back.	Nonskid soles decrease risk for slipping during transfer. Always have patient wear nonskid shoes during transfer; bare feet increase risk for falls. Patient will stand on stronger, or weight-bearing, leg.
(3) Spread your feet apart. Flex hips and knees, aligning knees with patient's knees.	Ensures balance with wide base of support. Flexing knees and hips lowers your center of gravity to object to be raised; aligning knees with those of patient stabilizes knees when patient stands.

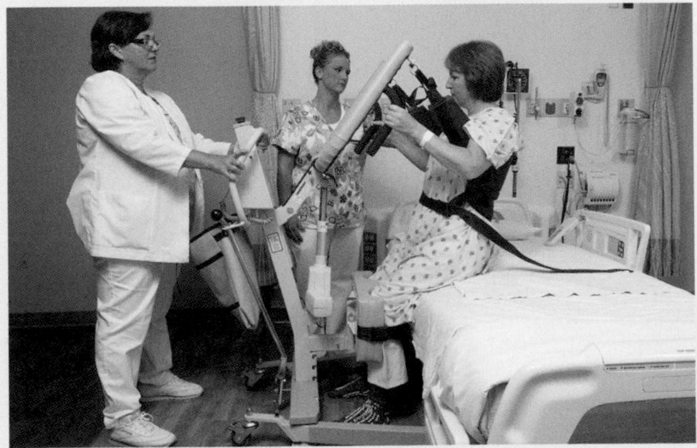

STEP 4c Patient grasps handles as nurse turns on motorized lift.

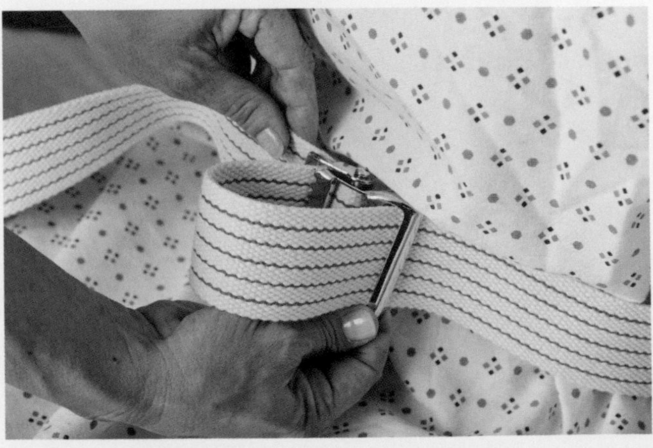

STEP 4d(1) Application of transfer belt.

STEP	RATIONALE
(4) Grasp transfer belt, keeping your palms up, along patient's sides (see illustration).	Transfer belt allows you to move patient at center of gravity. Patients should never be lifted by or under their arms.
(5) Rock patient up to standing position on count of three while straightening hips and legs and keeping knees slightly flexed (see illustration). While rocking patient in back-and-forth motion, make sure that your body weight is moving in the same direction as patient's to ensure that you and patient are moving in same direction simultaneously. Unless contraindicated, patient may be instructed to use hands to push up if applicable.	Rocking motion gives patient's body momentum and requires less muscular effort to lift him or her.
(6) Maintain stability of patient's weaker leg with your knee (if needed).	Ability to stand can often be maintained in weak limb with support of knee to stabilize.
(7) Pivot on foot farthest from chair.	Maintains support of patient while allowing adequate space for patient to move.
(8) Instruct patient to use armrests on chair for support and ease into chair (see illustration).	Increases patient stability.
(9) Flex hips and knees while lowering patient into chair.	Prevents injury from poor body mechanics.
(10) Assist patient to assume proper alignment in sitting position. Provide support for weakened extremity. You can use a sling or lap board to support an injured or flaccid arm. Stabilize leg with bath blanket or pillow.	Prevents injury to patient from poor body alignment.
i. Proper alignment for sitting position: head is erect, and vertebrae are in straight alignment. Body weight is evenly distributed on buttocks and thighs. Thighs are parallel and in horizontal plane. Both feet are supported flat on floor, and ankles are comfortably flexed. A 2.5- to 5-cm (1- to 2-inch) space is maintained between edge of seat and popliteal space on posterior surface of knee.	Prevents stress on intravertebral joints. Prevents increased pressure over bony prominences and reduces damage to underlying musculoskeletal system.

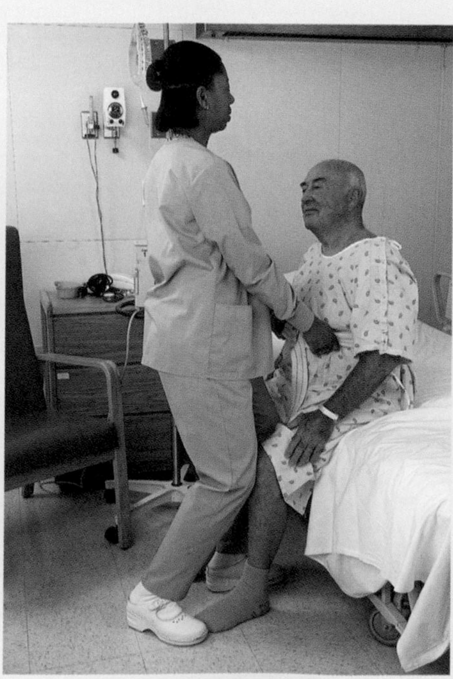

STEP 4d(4) Nurse flexes hips and knees, aligns knees with patient's knee, and grasps transfer belt palms up.

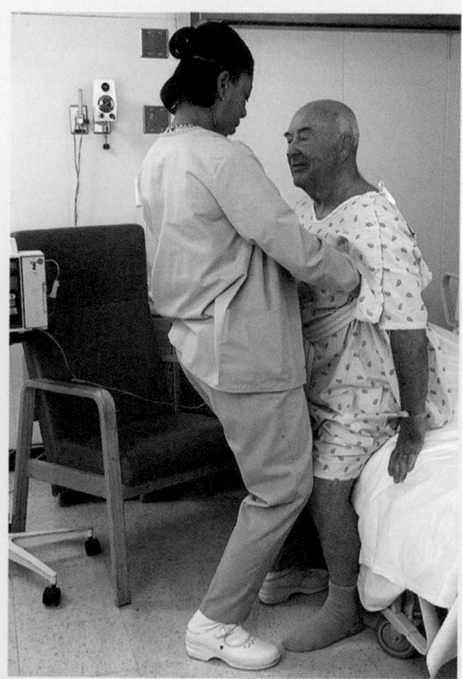

STEP 4d(5) Nurse rocks patient (who is able to help) to standing position.

STEP	RATIONALE
e. If patient is not able to cooperate (regardless of ability to bear weight) or does not have sufficient upper or lower body strength, use ceiling or floor hydraulic lift to transfer patient from bed to chair (TVAREF, 2014).	Research supports use of mechanical lifts to prevent musculoskeletal injuries (ANA, 2013a, 2013b). Use of ceiling-mounted lifts is a popular choice because of availability of lift in each patient's room (see illustration).
(1) Bring mechanical floor lift to bedside or lower ceiling lift and position properly.	Ensures safe elevation of patient off bed.
(2) Be sure chair is available along one side of bed, facing foot of bed. Allow adequate space to maneuver the lift.	Prepares environment for safe use of lift and subsequent transfer of patient into chair.
(3) Raise bed to high position with mattress flat. Lower side rail on side near chair.	Allows you to use proper body mechanics.
(4) Have second nurse positioned at opposite side of bed.	Maintains patient safety, preventing fall from bed.
(5) Roll patient on side away from you.	Positions patient for placement of lift sling.
(6) Place hammock or canvas strips under patient to form sling. With two canvas pieces, lower edge fits under patient's knees (wide piece), and upper edge fits under patient's shoulders (narrow piece).	Two types of seats are supplied with mechanical/hydraulic lift: hammock style is better for patients who are flaccid, weak, and need support; canvas strips can be used for patients with normal muscle tone. Be sure hooks face away from patient's skin. Place sling under patient's center of gravity and greatest part of body weight.
(7) Roll patient back toward you as second nurse pulls hammock (straps) through.	Ensures that sling is in proper position before lift.
(8) Return patient to supine position. Be sure that hammock or straps are smooth over bed surface. Sling should extend from shoulders to knees (hammock) to support patient's body weight equally.	Completes positioning of patient on mechanical/hydraulic sling.
(9) Remove patient's eyeglasses if appropriate.	Swivel bar is close to patient's head and could break eyeglasses.
(10) Roll the horseshoe base of floor lift under patient's bed (on side with chair).	Positions lift efficiently and promotes smooth transfer.
(11) Lower horizontal bar to sling level by following manufacturer directions. Lock valve if required.	Positions hydraulic lift close to patient. Locking valve prevents injury to patient.
(12) Attach hooks on strap (chain) to holes in sling. Short chains or straps hook to top holes of sling; longer chains hook to bottom of sling (see manufacturer directions).	Secures hydraulic lift to sling.

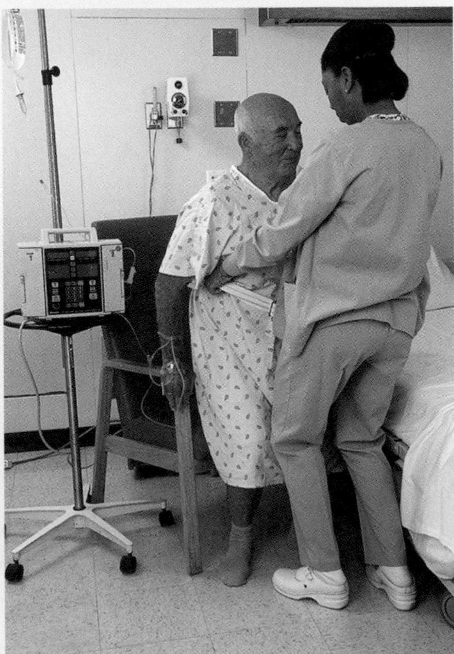

STEP 4d(8) Patient uses armrests and is guided to sit in chair.

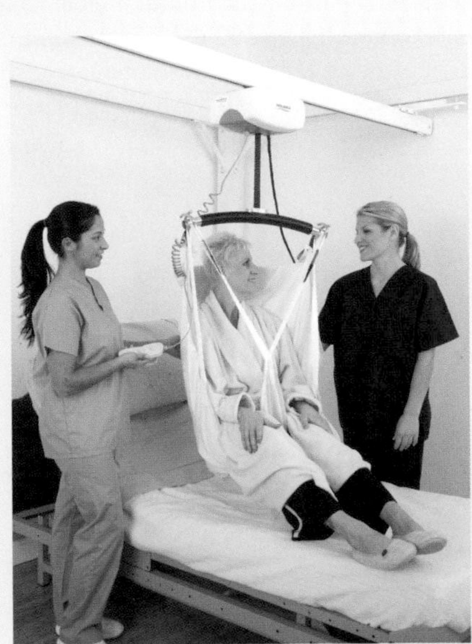

STEP 4e Ceiling lift. *(Courtesy of Handicare USA, Inc.)*

STEP	RATIONALE
(13) Elevate head of bed to Fowler's position.	Positions patient in sitting position.
(14) Have patient fold arms over chest.	Prevents injury to patient's arms during transfer.
(15) If the lift is electric, then push the button to raise the patient off the bed. If the lift is a non-electric lift, then pump the hydraulic handle using long, slow, even strokes until patient is raised off bed (see illustration). For ceiling lift, turn on control device to move lift.	Ensures safe support of patient during elevation.
(16) Use lift to raise patient off bed and use steering handle to pull lift from bed as you and another nurse maneuver patient to chair. Have second nurse alongside patient.	Lifts patient off the bed safely; nurse's position reduces any risk of patient falling from sling.
(17) Roll base of lift around chair. Release check valve slowly or push the button down and lower patient into chair (see manufacturer directions) (see illustration).	Positions lift in front of chair into which patient is to be transferred. Safely guides patient into back of chair as seat descends.
(18) Close check valve, if needed as soon as patient is down in chair and straps can be released. Newer lifts may not need this step (see manufacturer's directions).	If valve is left open, boom may continue to lower and injure patient.
(19) Remove straps and roll mechanical/hydraulic lift out of patient's path.	Prevents damage to skin and underlying tissues.
(20) Check patient's sitting alignment and correct if necessary.	Prevents injury from poor posture.
5. Perform lateral transfer from bed to stretcher:	The three-person lift (using drawsheet) for horizontal transfer from bed to stretcher is no longer recommended and is discouraged (Anderson et al., 2014; OSHA, 2014). Physical stress can be decreased significantly by using slide board or friction-reducing board positioned under drawsheet beneath patient. In addition, patient is more comfortable using this method.
a. Can patient assist? (1) If patient can assist, caregiver is only needed to stand by for safety, with stretcher and bed locked as patient moves to stretcher (TVAREF, 2014). (2) If patient is partially or not at all able to assist and is less than 91 kg (200 lb), use friction-reducing device or lateral transfer board (TVAREF, 2014). (3) If patient is partially or not at all able to assist and is greater than 91 kg (200 lb), use a ceiling lift with supine sling or a mechanical lateral-transfer device with three caregivers (TVAREF, 2014).	Patient's level of strength and weight determine level of help required for safe transfer. During any patient-transferring task, if any caregiver is required to lift more than 15.9 kg (35 lb) of patient's weight, patient is considered fully dependent, and an assist device is used (OSHA 2014, 2015).

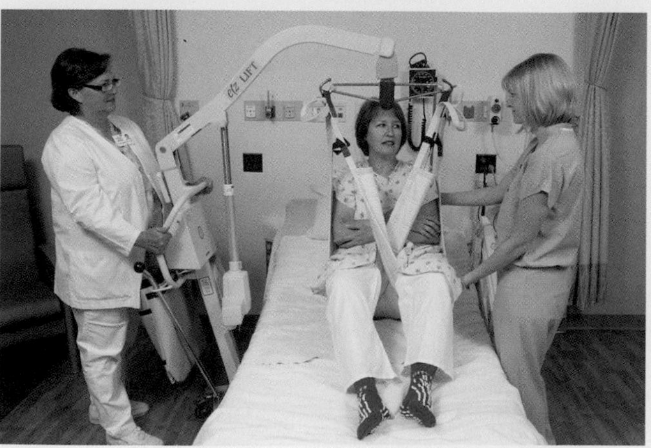

STEP 4e(15) Patient lifted in hydraulic lift above bed.

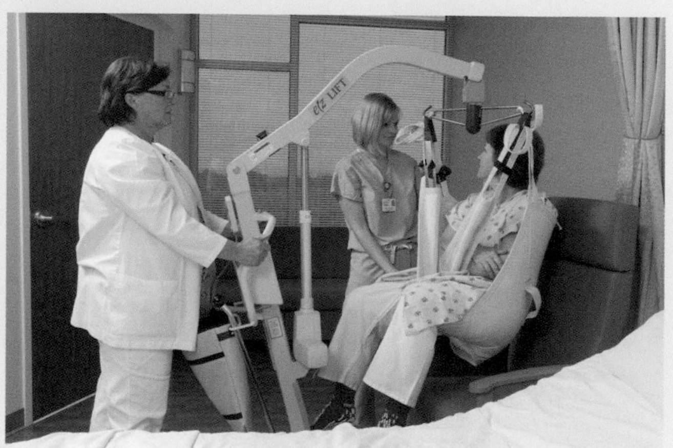

STEP 4e(17) Use of hydraulic lift lowers patient into chair.

STEP	RATIONALE
b. Lateral transfer with friction-reducing device—slide board (see illustration) or air-assisted device:	Maintains alignment of spinal column. Ensures that bed does not move inadvertently.
(1) Apply clean gloves if there is risk of soiling. Lower head of bed as much as patient can tolerate. Be sure to lock bed brakes.	Reduces transmission of microorganisms.
(2) Cross patient's arms on chest.	Prevents injury to arms during transfer.
(3) Lower side rails. To place slide board under patient, position two nurses on side of bed toward which patient will be turned. Position third nurse on other side of bed.	Distributes weight equally between nurses.
(4) Fanfold drawsheet on both sides.	Provides strong handles to grip drawsheet without slipping.
(5) On count of three, logroll patient onto side toward the two nurses. Turn patient as one unit with smooth, continuous motion.	Maintains body in alignment, preventing stress on any part.
(6) Place slide board under drawsheet (see illustration). *Option:* Apply air-assisted device.	Prevents friction from contact of skin with board.
(7) Gently roll patient back onto slide board.	
(8) Line up stretcher so that surface is ½ inch lower than bed (TVAREF, 2014). Lock brakes on stretcher. Instruct patient not to move.	Ensures that stretcher does not move inadvertently during transfer.
(9) Two nurses position themselves on side of stretcher while third nurse positions self on side of bed without stretcher. All three nurses place feet widely apart with one foot slightly in front of the other and grasp friction-reducing device.	

Safe Patient Care *A nurse may also be positioned at the head of patient's bed to protect and support his or her head and neck if patient is weak or unable to help.*

STEP	RATIONALE
(10) Holding fan-folded drawsheet and one nurse counting to three, the two nurses pull drawsheet across slide board, positioning patient onto stretcher (see illustration A). The third nurse holds slide board in place. *Option:* Inflate air-assisted device and slide patient across bed onto stretcher (see illustrations B and C).	Slide board remains stationary, provides slippery surface to reduce friction, and allows patient to transfer easily to stretcher.
(11) Position patient in center of stretcher. Raise head of stretcher if not contraindicated. Raise stretcher side rails. Cover patient with blanket.	Provides for patient comfort.
6. After transferring patient to bed or chair, be sure patient is positioned comfortably. Place nurse call system in an accessible location within patient's reach.	Ensures patient safety.

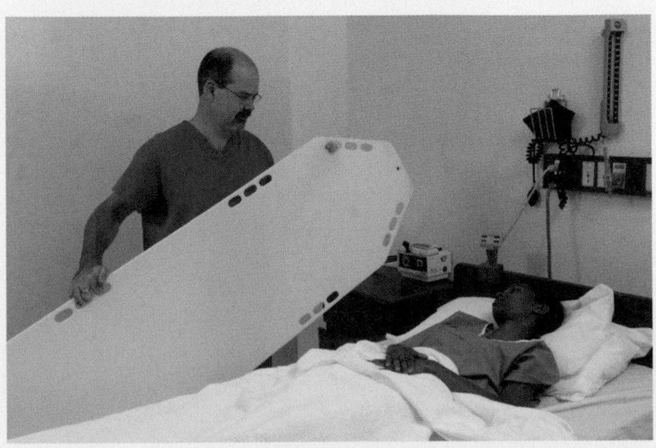

STEP 5b Slide board.

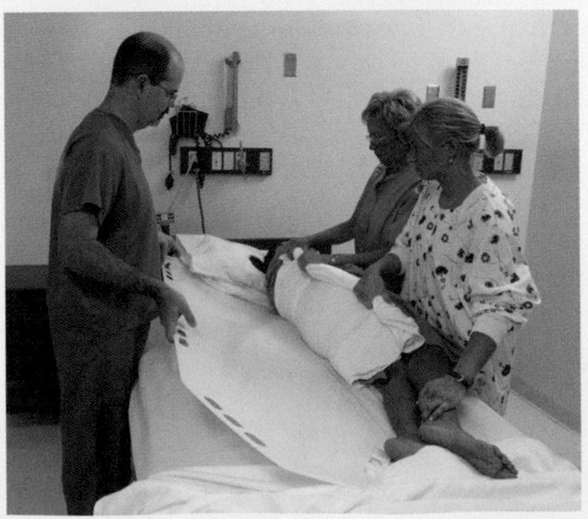

STEP 5b(6) Caregivers placing slide board under drawsheet.

STEP	RATIONALE

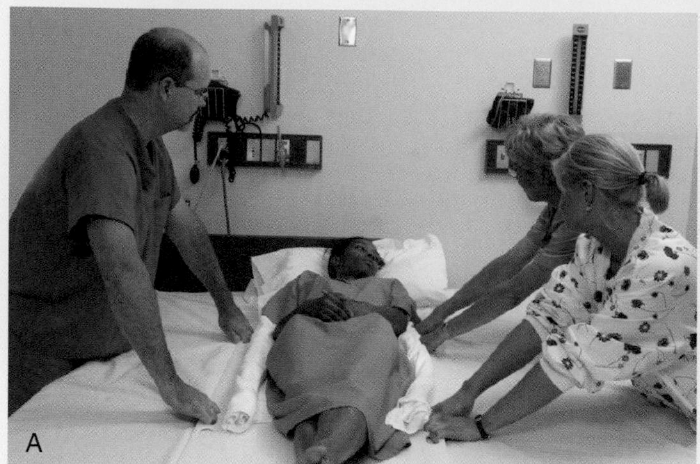

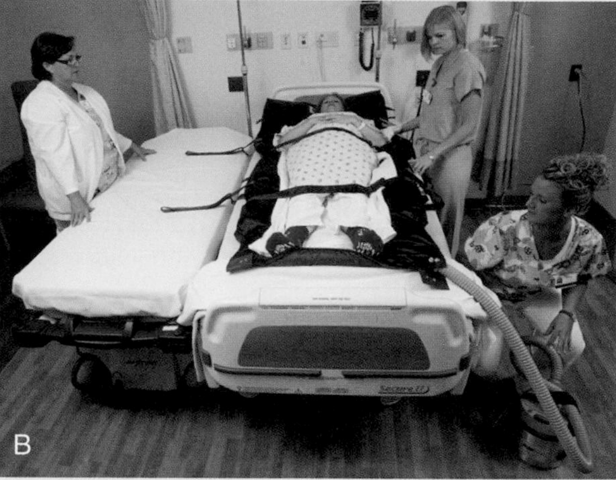

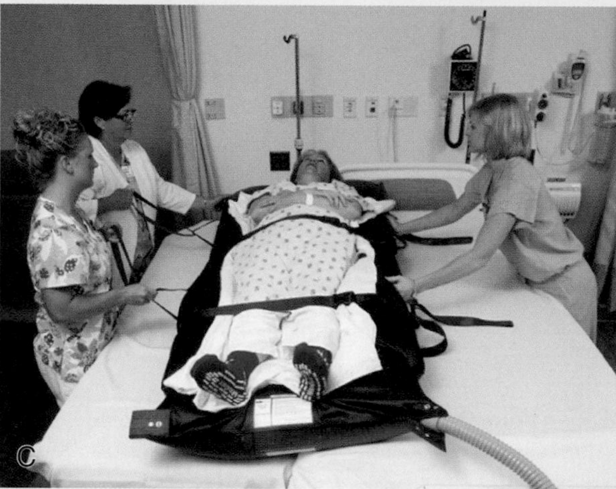

STEP 5b(10) (A) Transfer of patient to stretcher using slide board. (B) Inflating air-assisted transfer device. (C) Transfer of patient using air-assisted transfer device.

STEP	RATIONALE
7. Raise side rails (as appropriate) and lower bed to lowest position.	Ensures patient safety.
8. Remove and dispose of gloves (if used) and perform hand hygiene.	Reduces transmission of microorganisms.

EVALUATION

1. Monitor vital signs. Ask if patient feels dizzy or tired. Ask him or her to rate pain on pain scale.	Evaluates patient's response to postural changes and activity.
2. Note patient's behavioral response to transfer.	Reveals level of motivation and self-care potential.
3. **Use Teach-Back:** "I want to be sure I explained the steps we are going to use to transfer you to the chair. Tell me the steps you can take to make the transfer safe." Revise your instruction now or develop a plan for revised patient/family caregiver teaching if patient/family caregiver is not able to teach back correctly.	Determines patient's/family caregiver's level of understanding of instructional topic.

Unexpected Outcomes	Related Interventions
1. Patient is unable to comprehend or is unwilling to follow directions for transfer.	• Reassess continuity and simplicity of your instruction. • If patient is tired or in pain, allow for rest period before transferring. • Consider medicating for pain (if indicated). • Consider using hydraulic lift.
2. Patient sustains injury on transfer.	• Evaluate incident that led to injury (e.g., inadequate assessment, change in patient status, improper use of equipment). • Complete incident report according to agency policy.
3. Patient is unable to stand for time required to transfer to chair.	• Consider use of lateral transfer slide board or hydraulic lift.

Recording

- Record procedure, including pertinent observations: weakness, ability to follow directions, weight-bearing ability or restrictions, balance, ability to pivot, use of assistive devices or lifts, number of personnel needed to assist, amount of assistance (muscle strength) required, and patient's tolerance to transfer.
- Document your evaluation of patient learning.

Hand-Off Reporting

- Report transfer ability and assistance needed (including personnel and assist devices) to caregivers on next shift.
- Report progress or remission to rehabilitation staff (physical therapist, occupational therapist).

PROCEDURAL GUIDELINE 17.1 *Wheelchair Transfer Techniques*

Purpose

Wheelchair safety is very important. Patients who use wheelchairs can suffer falls, pressure injuries, and even choking if seat belts used on wheelchairs are applied too loosely (enabling a patient's torso to slide down, and the belt becomes a choking hazard). Transporting patients without proper application or engagement of safety features such as anti-tip bars, brakes, or side rails may lead to patient ejection, collisions, or entrapped limbs (Robson Forensic, 2016). Wheelchair prescription, posture, training, and maintenance are also critical components of safety for patients who use wheelchairs routinely. Transferring a patient from a bed to a wheelchair encompasses the same principles discussed in Skill 17.1. This procedural guideline focuses on the safety precautions to follow when a weight-bearing patient is being transferred to a wheelchair.

Delegation and Collaboration

The skill of transferring a patient to or from a wheelchair can be delegated to nursing assistive personnel (NAP). The nurse directs the NAP by:

- Assessing and supervising when moving patients who are transferring for the first time after prolonged bed rest, extensive surgery, critical illness, or spinal cord trauma.
- Explaining the patient's mobility restrictions, changes in blood pressure, or sensory alterations that may affect safe transfer.

Equipment

Transfer belt, nonskid shoes, wheelchair, transfer board

Procedural Steps

1. Identify patient using at least two identifiers (e.g., name and birthday or name and medical record number) according to agency policy (TJC, 2019).
2. Perform hand hygiene.
3. Review medical record to assess patient's weight, height, and strength; cognition; level of pain; and balance during previous transfer. Or complete a full assessment (see Skill 17.1) to determine patient's ability to help with transfer.
4. Check wheelchair locks, wheels, and footplates for proper functioning before use.
5. Explain to patient the steps you will be taking to help in transfer.
6. Transferring patient from a wheelchair to bed (patient is cooperative and weight bearing) using pivot technique:
   a. Adjust the height of the bed to the level of the seat of the wheelchair.
   b. Position wheelchair with one wheel against the side of the bed midway between the head and foot of the bed, with the wheelchair facing toward the foot of the bed. Remove the armrest nearest the side of the bed.
   c. Lock both wheels of the wheelchair. Locks are located above the rims of the wheels. Push handle forward to lock.
   d. Raise the footplates.
   e. Place a transfer belt on patient. Be sure that it completely circles patient's waist. Place the belt low and be sure that it is snug. Avoid placing the belt over any intravenous lines, incisions, or drainage tubes.
   f. Have patient place hands on armrests and stand by as you have him or her move to the front of the wheelchair.
   g. Stand slightly in front of patient to guard and protect him or her throughout the transfer.
   h. Instruct patient to stand at a count of three as you place both hands (palms up) under transfer belt while bending your knees.
   i. Allow patient to stand a few seconds to ensure that he or she is not dizzy and has good balance. Pivot with patient as he or she turns to face away from the side of the bed. Then have patient sit on the edge of the mattress.
   j. With patient sitting on the edge of the bed, place your arm nearest the head of the bed under his or her shoulder while supporting the head and neck. Place your other arm under patient's knees. Bend your knees and keep your back straight.
   k. Tell patient to help lift the legs when you begin to move. On a count of three, standing with a wide base of support, raise patient's legs as you pivot his or her body and lower the shoulders onto the bed. Remember to keep your back straight.
   l. Help patient return to bed and assume a comfortable position.
7. Transferring patient from a wheelchair to bed (patient is non–weight bearing and unable to stand but is cooperative and has upper-body strength) using transfer board:
   a. Follow Steps 6a–e.
   b. If not already applied, place a transfer belt on patient. Be sure that it completely circles patient's waist. Place the belt low and be that sure it is snug. Avoid placing the belt over any intravenous lines, incisions, or drainage tubes.
   c. Be sure seat of the wheelchair is level with the top of the bed mattress. Position a transfer board by placing it across the bed to the chair so patient can slide across it. Be sure the board overlaps the chair and mattress so that it will not slip out of place. Then place the other

Continued

PROCEDURAL GUIDELINE 17.1 *Wheelchair Transfer Techniques—cont'd*

part of the board under the patient's buttock that is closest to the bed.

d. Stand in front of patient and have him or her move to the front of the wheelchair.

e. Place your legs on the outside of patient's legs. Be sure that patient's feet are on the floor. Grasp the transfer belt (palms up) along both of patient's sides. Have patient place one hand on the slide board and the other on the mattress surface.

f. Bend your knees, and on a count of three, have patient use the arms to slide across the board from the chair to the bed. If the patient is struggling, the nurse can attempt to assist the patient or a lift will need to be used.

g. Have patient sit on edge of bed.

h. Follow Steps 6j–l to help patient return to bed and assume a comfortable position.

8. Place nurse call system in reach; instruct patient in use.
9. Raise side rails (as appropriate) and lower bed to lowest position.
10. Perform hand hygiene.
11. Monitor vital signs after patient has been transferred. Ask if patient feels dizzy, is fatigued, or is in pain.
12. Note patient's behavioral response to transfer.
13. **Use Teach-Back:** "I want to be sure I explained what to do as I move you from the chair to the bed. Tell me how you can help move to the bed." Revise your instruction now or develop a plan or revised patient/family caregiver teaching if patient/family caregiver is not able to teach back correctly.

✦ SKILL 17.2 Moving and Positioning Patients in Bed

Purpose

Patients with impaired nervous or musculoskeletal system functioning, patients with increased weakness, and patients restricted to bed rest benefit from therapeutic positioning. Correct positioning maintains patients' body alignment and comfort. Immobilized patients require vigilant nursing care with frequent repositioning to avoid physical complications, including pressure injuries, reduced ventilation, and muscle contractures. In general, you reposition patients as needed and at least every 2 hours if they are in bed and every 15 to 20 minutes if they are sitting in a chair or wheelchair (Agency for Healthcare Research and Quality [AHRQ], 2014; Swafford, 2016). However, research has shown that patients contribute to repositioning through their own frequent movement (Chaboyer et al., 2013). Patients often adopt positions that increase their pressure injury risk (McInnes et al., 2013). Thus the routine monitoring of patient positions is important. Caregivers are at risk for injury during positioning of patients unless safe patient-handling principles and algorithms are followed.

Delegation and Collaboration

The skills of moving and positioning patients in bed and maintaining correct body alignment can be delegated to nursing assistive personnel (NAP). The nurse instructs the NAP by:

- Explaining any moving and positioning restrictions unique to patient (e.g., avoid prone position, patient has one-sided weakness).
- Designating specific times throughout the shift that NAP must reposition patient.
- Providing information about patient's individual needs for body alignment (e.g., patient with spinal cord injury).

Equipment

- Pillows, drawsheet
- Appropriate safe patient handling assistive devices (e.g., friction-reducing device, ceiling lift, or mechanical floor lift)
- Therapeutic boots/splints *(optional)*
- Trochanter rolls *(optional)*
- Hand rolls
- Clean gloves

ASSESSMENT

1. Identify patient using at least two identifiers (e.g., name and birthday or name and medical record number) according to agency policy. *Rationale: Ensures correct patient. Complies with The Joint Commission standards and improves patient safety (TJC, 2019).*
2. Refer to medical record for most recent recorded weight and height for patient. *Rationale: Factors help to determine if mechanical lift, mechanical transfer device, or friction-reducing device is needed for moving patient up in bed.*
3. Check health care provider's orders for any restrictions in movement before positioning patient. *Rationale: Some positions may be contraindicated in situations such as spinal cord injury; hip fracture; respiratory difficulties; neurological conditions; and presence of incisions, drains, or tubing.*
4. Perform hand hygiene. *Rationale: Reduces transmission of microorganisms.*
5. Assess patient's range of motion (ROM) (see Chapter 8) and current body alignment while patient is lying down. *Rationale: Provides baseline data for later comparisons. Determines ways to improve position and alignment.*
6. Assess for risk factors that contribute to complications of immobility. *Rationale: Risk factors require patient to be repositioned more frequently.*
   a. **Reduced sensation:** Cerebrovascular accident (CVA), spinal cord injury, or neuropathy. *Rationale: With reduced sensation, a patient has difficulty moving, has poor awareness of involved body part, and is unable to position body part and protect it from pressure.*
   b. **Impaired mobility:** Traction, arthritis, CVA, spinal cord injury, hip fracture, joint surgery, or other contributing disease processes. *Rationale: Traction, bone fractures,*

surgery, or arthritic changes result in decreased ROM. Loss of function caused by CVA or spinal injury can lead to contractures.

c. **Impaired circulation:** Arterial insufficiency. *Rationale: Decreased circulation predisposes patient to pressure injury.*

d. **Age:** Very young, older adult. *Rationale: Premature and young infants require frequent turning because their skin is fragile. Normal physiological changes of aging predispose to greater risks for developing complications of immobility.*

7. Assess patient's level of consciousness. *Rationale: Determines need for special aids or devices. Patients with altered levels of consciousness may not understand instructions and may be unable to help with positioning.*
8. Assess patient for presence of pain; rate on scale of 0 to 10 (see Chapter 15). *Rationale: Pain reduces patient's motivation and ability to be mobile. Pain relief before transfer enhances patient participation.*
9. Assess condition of patient's skin, especially over bony prominences. *Rationale: Provides baseline to determine effects of positioning. Routine positioning reduces occurrence of pressure injuries.*
10. Assess patient's physical ability to help with moving and positioning, which may be affected by age, level of consciousness, disease process, strength, ROM, and coordination. *Rationale: Enables you to use patient's existing mobility, strength, and coordination during positioning. Determines need for additional help, ensuring patient and nurse safety.*
11. Assess patient's vision and hearing (see Chapter 8). *Rationale: Sensory deficits affect patient's ability to cooperate during repositioning.*
12. Apply clean gloves (as needed) to assess for presence of incisions, drainage tubes, and equipment (e.g., traction). Empty drainage bags before positioning. Remove and dispose of gloves. Perform hand hygiene. *Rationale: Alters positioning procedure and type of position in which to place patient. Eliminates barriers to moving patient.*
13. Assess motivation of patient and ability of family caregivers to participate in moving and positioning if patient to be discharged home. *Rationale: Indicates level of instruction needed before discharge.*
14. Assess patient's or family caregiver's knowledge, experience, and health literacy. *Rationale: Ensures patient or family caregiver has the capacity to obtain, communicate, process, and understand basic health information (CDC, 2016).*

STEP	RATIONALE
PLANNING	
1. Expected outcomes following completion of procedure:	
• Patient retains ROM.	Correct positioning allows patient to achieve optimal joint mobility and alignment.
• Patient's skin shows no evidence of breakdown.	Frequent position changes decrease occurrence of skin breakdown.
• Patient's comfort level increases.	Proper positioning reduces stress on joints.
• Patient's level of independence in completing activities of daily living (ADLs) increases.	Maintaining good body alignment and joint mobility increases patient's overall mobility.
2. If patient perceives level of pain to be enough to avoid movement, offer an analgesic 30 minutes (if ordered) before repositioning.	Will lessen discomfort when positioning extremities. **NOTE:** The frequency of an analgesic may not be available as frequently as a patient will require turning.
3. Remove all pillows and devices used in previous position.	Reduces interference from bedding during positioning procedure.
4. Get additional caregivers and/or necessary lift or transfer device to perform positioning.	Safe patient-handling algorithms (see agency policy) determine number of caregivers and type of devices needed to position a patient if lifting is required.
5. Explain positioning procedure to patient using plain language.	Helps decrease anxiety and increase cooperation.
6. Close door to room or bedside curtains	Provides for patient privacy
IMPLEMENTATION	
1. Perform hand hygiene.	Reduces transmission of microorganisms.
2. Raise level of bed to comfortable working height, level with your elbows.	Raises level of work toward nurse's center of gravity and reduces risk for back injuries.
3. Assist patient to move up in bed:	This is not a one-person task unless patient can help completely (OSHA, 2014). Pulling patients who have migrated in bed carries an extremely high risk of caregiver injury (Wiggermann, 2014).
a. Determine if the patient can assist.	Determines degree of risk in repositioning patient and technique required to safely help patient.
(1) **Patient is fully able to assist:**	Techniques promote patient independence.
(a) Stand at bedside to help with positioning of tubing and equipment as patient moves.	Prevents accidental tube dislodgement.

STEP	RATIONALE
(b) Have patient place feet flat on mattress, grasp either side rails or overhead trapeze and, on a count of three, lift hips up and push legs so body moves up in bed.	
(2) **Patient is partially able to assist:**	
(a) Encourage patient to help using friction-reducing device (e.g., slide board).	Repositioning device reduces friction as patient is moved up in bed.
(b) Patient weighs less than 91 kg (200 lb): use friction-reducing sheet or slide board and two or three caregivers.	
(c) Patient weighs greater than 91 kg (200 lb): use friction-reducing device and at least three caregivers.	
i. Using a friction-reducing device (three nurses). Position patient supine with head of bed flat. A nurse stands on each side of bed.	Prevents friction from contact of skin with board.
ii. Remove pillow from under head and shoulders and place it at head of bed.	
iii. Turn patient side to side to place friction-reducing device under drawsheet on bed, with device extending from shoulders to thighs/ankles.	
iv. Return patient to supine position.	
v. Have two caregivers grasp drawsheet (one on each side of bed) firmly and have third nurse hold on to end of friction-reducing device.	Slide board remains stationary, provides slippery surface to reduce friction, and allows patient to move up in bed easily.
vi. Place feet apart with forward-backward stance. Flex knees and hips. On count of three, shift weight from front to back leg and move patient and drawsheet to desired position up in bed.	Positions patient smoothly without exerting shear against skin and without risk of injury to nurses.
(3) **Patient unable to assist:**	
(a) Use appropriate number of caregivers and appropriate safe patient-handling devices (e.g., supine sling with ceiling lift or floor-based lift and two or more caregivers) to move and position patient.	Repositioning patients manually is associated with high risk of musculoskeletal injury (Wiggermann, 2014).

Safe Patient Care *Protect patient's heels from shearing force by having another caregiver lift heels while moving patient up in bed.*

STEP	RATIONALE
4. Position patient in bed in one of the following positions while ensuring correct body alignment. Protect pressure areas.	Prevents injury to patient's musculoskeletal system and integument. Even positioning patient side to side requires use of safe patient-handling techniques.
a. Determine if patient can assist.	Determines degree of risk in repositioning patient and the technique required to safely help patient.
b. Begin with patient lying supine and move up in bed following Steps 2a(1)–(3).	
c. **Position patient in supported semi-Fowler's (see illustration) or Fowler's position:**	
(1) With patient lying supine, elevate head of bed 45 to 60 degrees if not contraindicated.	Increases comfort, improves ventilation, and increases patient's opportunity to socialize or relax.
(2) Rest head against mattress or on small pillow.	Prevents flexion contractures of cervical vertebrae.

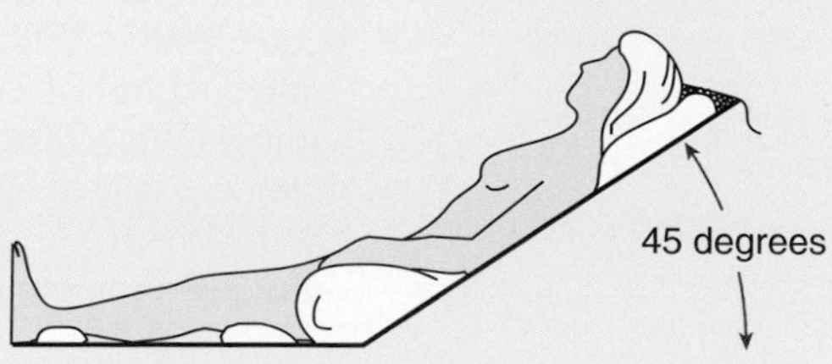

STEP 4c Supported semi-Fowler's position.

STEP	RATIONALE
(3) Use pillows to support arms and hands if patient does not have voluntary control or use of hands and arms.	Prevents shoulder dislocation from effect of downward pull of unsupported arms, promotes circulation by preventing venous pooling, and prevents flexion contractures of arms and wrists.
(4) Position small pillow at lower back.	Supports lumbar vertebrae and decreases flexion of vertebrae.
(5) Place pillows long-wise under each leg (mid-thigh to ankle) to support the knee in slight flexion (avoids hyperextension) and to allow the heels to float.	Prevents hyperextension of knee and occlusion of popliteal artery from pressure from body weight. Heels should not be in contact with bed. Floating heels prevents prolonged pressure of mattress on heels.
d. **Position hemiplegic patient in supported semi-Fowler's or Fowler's position:**	
(1) Elevate head of bed 30 to 60 degrees according to patient's condition. For example, those with increased risk for pressure injury remain at 30-degree angle (see Chapter 26).	Increases comfort, improves ventilation, and increases patient's opportunity to relax.
(2) Position patient in Fowler's position as anatomically straight as possible	Counteracts tendency to slump toward affected side. Improves ventilation and cardiac output; decreases intracranial pressure. Improves patient's ability to swallow and helps prevent aspiration of food, liquids, and gastric secretions.
(3) Position head on small pillow with chin slightly forward. If patient is totally unable to control head movement, avoid hyperextension of neck.	Prevents hyperextension of neck. Too many pillows under head may cause or worsen neck flexion contracture.
(4) Provide support for involved arm and hand by placing arm away from patient's side and supporting elbow with pillow.	Paralyzed muscles do not automatically resist pull of gravity as they do normally. As a result, shoulder subluxation, pain, and edema may occur.
(5) Place rolled blanket (trochanter roll) or pillows firmly alongside patient's legs to help prevent the patient from leaning toward the affected side.	Ensures proper alignment. Prevents external rotation of hips, which contributes to contractures.
(6) Support feet in dorsiflexion with therapeutic boots or splints.	Prevents plantar flexion contractures or footdrop by positioning patient's ankle in neutral dorsiflexion. Positions foot so heel is aligned in opening of splint to prevent pressure. Other therapeutic boots or splints are manufactured with thick padding to cushion heel and prevent pressure injury.
e. **Position patient in supported supine position:**	
(1) Place patient supine with head of bed flat.	Necessary for properly aligning patient.
(2) Place small rolled towel under lumbar area of back.	Provides support for lumbar spine.
(3) Place pillow under upper shoulders, neck, and head.	Maintains correct alignment and prevents flexion contractures of cervical vertebrae.
(4) Place trochanter rolls or sandbags parallel to lateral surface of patient's thighs.	Reduces external rotation of hip.
(5) Place patient's feet in therapeutic boots or splints.	Maintains feet in dorsiflexion. Prevents plantar flexion contractures or footdrop.
(6) Place pillows under pronated forearms, keeping upper arms parallel to patient's body (see illustration).	Reduces internal rotation of shoulder and prevents extension of elbows. Maintains correct body alignment.

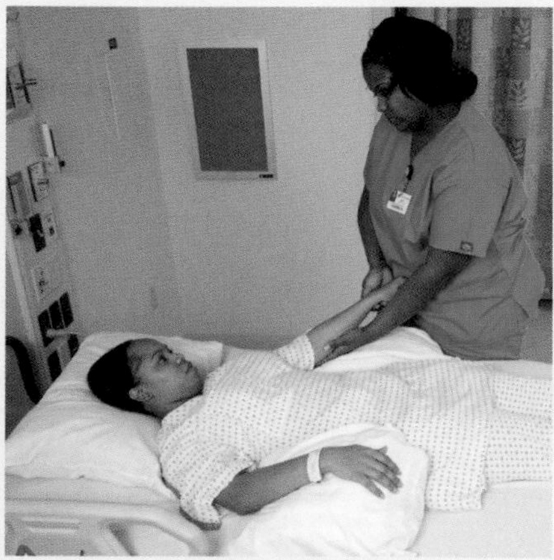

STEP 4e(6) Supported supine position with pillows in place.

STEP	RATIONALE
(7) Place hand rolls in patient's hands. Consider physical therapy referral for use of hand splints.	Reduces extension of fingers and abduction of thumb. Maintains thumb slightly adducted and in opposition to fingers.
f. Position hemiplegic patient in supine position:	
(1) Place head of bed flat.	Necessary for positioning in supine position.
(2) Place folded towel or small pillow under shoulder of affected side.	Decreases possibility of pain, joint contracture, and subluxation. Maintains mobility in muscles around shoulder to permit normal movement patterns.
(3) Keep affected arm away from body with elbow extended and palm up. Position affected hand in one of recommended positions for flaccid or spastic hand. (Alternative is to place arm out to side, with elbow bent and hand toward head of bed.)	Maintains mobility in arm, joints, and shoulder to permit normal movement patterns. (Alternative position counteracts limitation of ability of arm to rotate outward at shoulder [external rotation]. External rotation must be present to raise arm overhead without pain.)
(4) Place folded towel under hip of involved side.	Diminishes effect of spasticity in entire leg by controlling hip position.
(5) Flex affected knee 30 degrees by supporting it on pillow or folded blanket.	Slight flexion breaks up abnormal extension pattern of leg. Extensor spasticity is most severe when patient is supine.
(6) Support feet with soft pillows placed against sole of feet at right angle to leg.	Maintains foot in dorsiflexion and prevents footdrop. Pillows prevent stimulation to ball of foot by hard surface, which has tendency to increase muscle tone in patient with extensor spasticity of lower extremity.
g. Position patient in 30-degree lateral (side-lying) position (one nurse):	This position is recommended to prevent development of pressure injuries by reducing direct contact of trochanter with support surface (see Chapter 26).
(1) Lower head of bed completely or as low as patient can tolerate.	Provides position of comfort for patient and removes pressure from bony prominences on back.
(2) Lower side rail and position patient on side of bed opposite direction toward which patient is to be turned. Move upper trunk, supporting shoulders first; then move lower trunk, supporting hips.	Provides room for patient to turn to side.
(3) Raise side rail and go to opposite side of bed.	
(4) Lower side rail and flex patient's knee that will not be next to mattress. Keep foot on mattress. Place one hand on patient's upper bent leg near hip and other hand on patient's shoulder.	Use of leverage makes turning to side easy.
(5) Roll patient onto side toward you.	Rolling decreases trauma to tissues. In addition, patient is positioned so leverage on hip makes turning easy.
(6) Place pillow under patient's head and neck.	Maintains alignment. Reduces lateral neck flexion. Decreases strain on sternocleidomastoid muscle.
(7) Place hands under patient's dependent shoulder and bring shoulder blade forward.	Prevents patient's weight from resting directly on shoulder joint.
(8) Position both arms in slightly flexed position. Support upper arm with pillow level with shoulder; other arm, by mattress.	Decreases internal rotation and adduction of shoulder. Supporting both arms in slightly flexed position protects joint. Ventilation improves because chest is able to expand more easily.
(9) Place hands under dependent hip and bring hip slightly forward so angle from hip to mattress is approximately 30 degrees.	The 30-degree lateral position reduces pressure on trochanter; designed to prevent pressure injury.
(10) Place small tuck-back pillow behind patient's back. (Make by folding pillow lengthwise. Smooth area is slightly tucked under patient's back.)	Provides support to maintain patient on side.
(11) Place pillow under semiflexed upper leg level at hip from groin to foot (see illustration).	Flexion prevents hyperextension of leg. Maintains leg in correct alignment. Prevents pressure on bony prominences.
(12) *Option:* Place pillows or sandbags (if available) parallel against plantar surface of dependent foot. May also use ankle-foot orthotic on feet if available.	Maintains dorsiflexion of foot.
h. Position patient in Sims' (semi-prone) position:	
(1) Lower head of bed completely.	Provides for proper body alignment while patient is lying down flat on abdomen.

STEP	RATIONALE
(2) Place patient supine on side of bed opposite direction toward which he or she is to be turned. Move upper trunk, supporting shoulders first, followed by moving lower trunk, supporting hips.	Prepares patient for position.
(3) Move to other side of bed and turn patient on side. Position in lateral position, lying partially on abdomen, with dependent shoulder lifted out and arm placed at patient's side.	
(4) Place small pillow under patient's head.	Maintains proper alignment and prevents lateral neck flexion.
(5) Place pillow under flexed upper arm, supporting arm level with shoulder.	Prevents internal rotation of shoulder. Maintains alignment.
(6) Place pillow under flexed upper legs, supporting leg level with hip.	Prevents internal rotation of hip and adduction of leg. Flexion prevents hyperextension of leg. Reduces mattress pressure on knees and ankles.
(7) Place sandbags parallel against plantar surface of foot (see illustration).	Maintains foot in dorsiflexion. Prevents plantar flexion contractures or footdrop.
i. **Logroll patient (three nurses):**	

Safe Patient Care *A registered nurse supervises and helps the NAP when there is a health care provider's order to logroll a patient. Patients with spinal cord injuries or who are recovering from neck, back, or spinal surgery need to keep the spinal column in straight alignment to prevent further injury.*

STEP	RATIONALE
(1) Place small pillow between patient's knees.	Prevents tension on spinal column and adduction of hip.
(2) Cross patient's arms on chest.	Prevents injury to arms.
(3) Position two nurses on side toward which patient is to be turned and one nurse on side where pillows are to be placed behind patient's back (see illustration).	Distributes weight equally between nurses during turning.
(4) Fanfold drawsheet along backside of patient.	Provides strong handles for nurses to grip drawsheet without slipping.
(5) With one nurse grasping drawsheet at lower hips and thighs and the other nurse grasping drawsheet at patient's shoulders and lower back, roll patient as one unit in a smooth, continuous motion on count of three (see illustration).	Maintains proper alignment by moving all body parts at the same time, preventing tension or twisting of spinal column.
(6) Nurse on opposite side of bed places pillows along length of patient for support (see illustration).	Maintains patient in side-lying position.
(7) Gently lean patient as a unit back toward pillows for support.	Ensures continued straight alignment of spinal column, preventing injury.

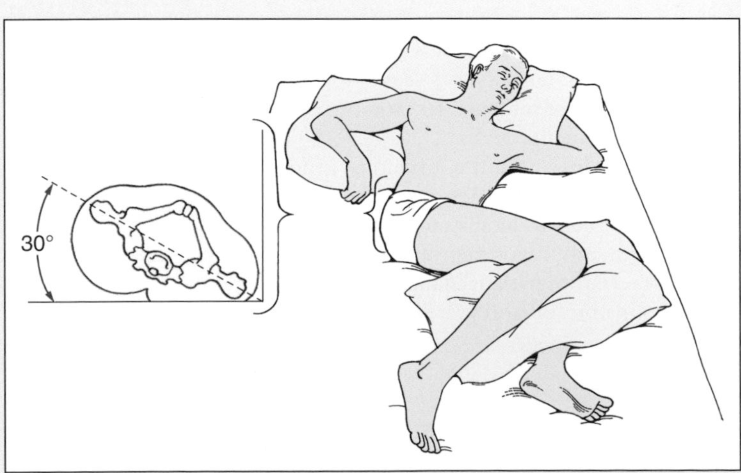

STEP 4g(11) Thirty-degree lateral position with pillows in place.

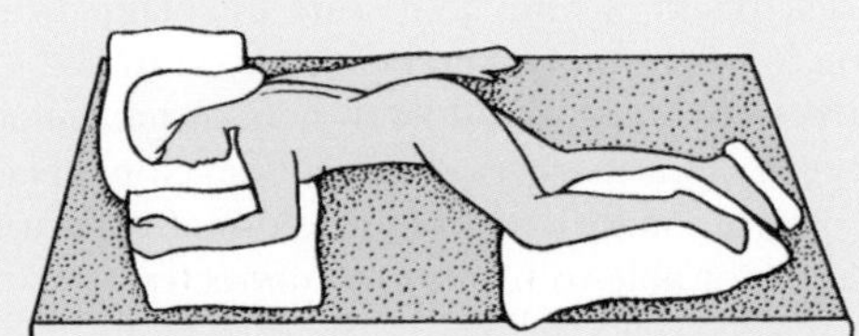

STEP 4h(7) Sandbag supporting right foot in dorsiflexion.

STEP	RATIONALE
5. Be sure patient feels comfortable in new position. Be sure nurse call system is accessible within patient's reach.	Gives patient sense of well-being. Ensures patient can call for help if needed.
6. Raise side rails (as appropriate) and lower bed to lowest position.	Ensures patient safety.
7. Perform hand hygiene.	Reduces transmission of microorganisms.

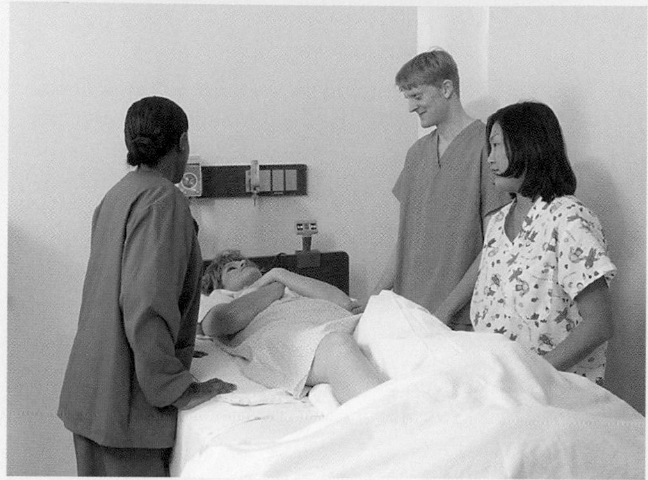
STEP 4i(3) Preparing patient for logrolling.

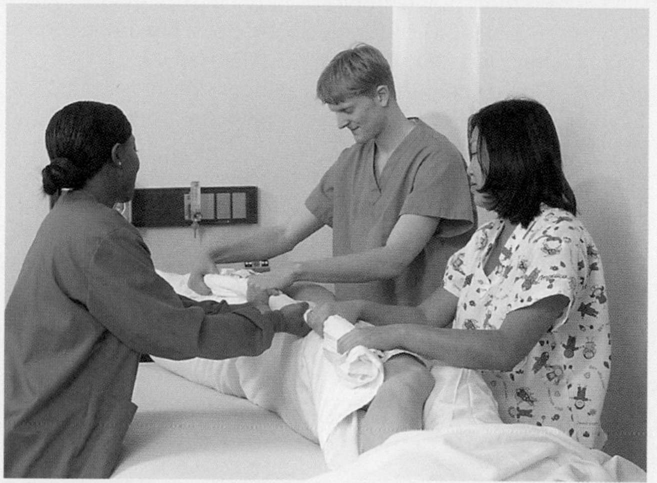
STEP 4i(5) Logrolling patient onto side.

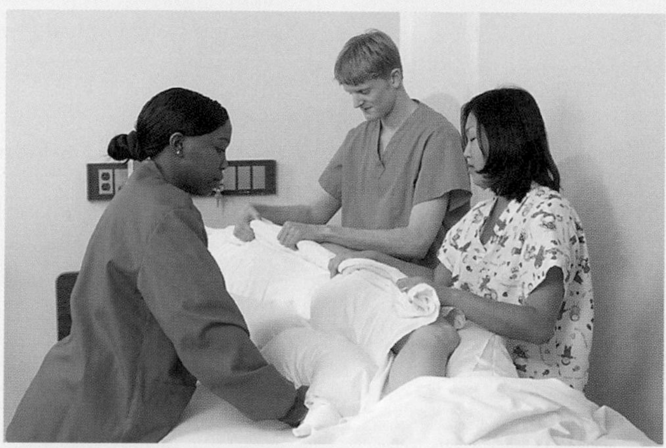
STEP 4i(6) Placing pillows along patient's back for support.

EVALUATION

1. Assess patient's respiratory status, body alignment, position, and level of comfort. Patient's body should be supported by adequate mattress, and vertebral column should be without observable curves.	Determines effectiveness of positioning and patient's tolerance. Additional supports (e.g., pillows, bath blankets) may be added or removed to promote comfort and correct body alignment.
2. Measure range of motion (ROM).	Determines if joint contracture is developing.
3. Observe for areas of erythema or breakdown involving skin (see Chapter 26).	Provides ongoing observation regarding patient's skin and musculoskeletal systems. Indicates complications of immobility or improper positioning of body part.
4. **Use Teach-Back:** "I want to be sure I explained the steps we are going to use to move and position you in bed. Can you repeat the steps you can follow to help us move you up in bed?" Revise your instruction now or develop a plan for revised patient/family caregiver teaching if patient/family caregiver is not able to teach back correctly.	Determines patient's/family caregiver's level of understanding of instructional topic.

Unexpected Outcomes	Related Interventions
1. Joint contractures develop or worsen.	• Increase frequency of ROM exercises to affected and immobilized areas (see Chapter 18). • Consider physical therapy consultation for different positioning.
2. Skin shows localized areas of erythema and breakdown.	• Increase frequency of repositioning. • Place a turning schedule above patient's bed.
3. Patient avoids moving.	• Medicate with analgesia as ordered by health care provider to ensure patient's comfort before moving. • Allow pain medication to take effect before repositioning.

Recording

- Record positioning change, time of change, and observations (e.g., condition of skin, joint movement, patient's ability to assist with positioning).
- Document your evaluation of patient learning.

Hand-Off Reporting

- Report observations of patient's tolerance of position changes to nurse at change of shift.
- Report skin or joint complications to health care provider.

SPECIAL CONSIDERATIONS

Patient-Centered Care

- It is a patient's choice to increase mobility. Hospitals have early mobility protocols to encourage early ambulation, but a patient must be willing to participate. Consider the patient's knowledge, cultural beliefs, and circumstances surrounding any loss of independence when planning mobility activities.
- A patient's values and beliefs about the nature of pain, and pain management might affect willingness to accept pain-control measures needed to promote mobility.
- For patients who are in any way sensitive to personal contact, be patient and explain in depth why it is necessary to take the steps required for proper positioning.

Patient Education

- Educate patients about the specific risk factors that predispose them to falls so that they can become partners in fall prevention (see Chapter 4).
- A family caregiver should practice patient transfer in the health care setting to achieve success before taking a patient home. Alternatively, a patient (if living alone) should practice transfer skills in bed that will be used at home. Patients should learn to transfer to chair with arms for ease of rising and sitting.
- Educate patients about the risk of pressure injuries and how they develop. This is especially important for patients with limited mobility.

Age-Specific

Pediatric

- Transporting a child by stretcher, stroller, or wheelchair outside confines of room increases environmental stimuli and provides social contact with others (Hockenberry and Wilson, 2017).
- Encourage children to be as active as their condition and restrictive devices allow. Use developmentally appropriate toys or items that stimulate activity and participation in care.
- Children who are unable to move need passive exercise and movement (see Chapter 18).

Gerontological

- As a patient's age increases, the frequency of repositioning (independently and with assistance from staff) has been shown to decrease. Targeted interventions are needed to ensure frequent repositioning of older adults (Latimer et al., 2015).
- A major health concern that threatens the function of older adults is the risk of falls. Risk increases when a patient is transferred from bed to a chair. Assess patient for the risk for falls on admission to the health care agency and implement a protocol to prevent falls (Touhy and Jett, 2018; see Chapter 4).

Home Care

- Assess the need for special transfer equipment to be used in the home setting. Assess home environment for hazards (e.g., throw rugs, electrical cords, slippery floors). If wheelchair is used, access must be possible through all doors, and space for transfer must be available in bathroom and bedroom.
- Assess home to determine compatibility of environment with assistive devices (e.g., over-bed trapeze, mechanical lift, hospital bed).
- Assess ability and motivation of patient and family caregivers to participate in moving and positioning patient in bed.
- For patients who use wheelchairs at home, recommend these safety precautions:
  - Always check wheelchair locks, wheels, and footplates for proper functioning before use.
  - Never attempt to reach an object if you must move forward in the wheelchair seat or pick them up from the floor by reaching between your knees.
  - Position wheelchair as close as possible to a desired object. Position the wheel casters so that they are extended away from the drive wheels to create the longest possible wheelbase. Reach back only as far as your arm will extend without changing your sitting position.
  - Always inspect any ramp, incline, decline, or pathway for hazards such as holes, obstacles, slippery or uneven surfaces, and so forth before proceeding. If you cannot see the entire ramp, ask someone to inspect it for you.

✦ PRACTICE REFLECTIONS

A patient who experienced a stroke that reduced movement on his right side has started his first day of rehabilitation. He can stand on his strong leg with assistance but cannot bear weight on the affected leg, and balance is very limited at this time. The patient is 185 cm (6 ft 1 inch), 109 kg (240 lb), and very cooperative.

1. What technique would you use to transfer this patient to a wheelchair? Why is this technique preferred?
2. When positioning this patient in bed, what unexpected outcomes are he particularly at risk for due to weakness in the right leg and arm?
3. What precautions should you take in transferring this patient due to the patient's weight?

✦ CLINICAL REVIEW QUESTIONS

1. A nurse is caring for a patient who requires assistance in transferring from a bed to a chair. The patient is weight bearing. The nurse should follow which of the following safe practices during the transfer process? (Select all that apply.)
   1. Clear the area around where the patient will stand/walk of over-bed table and trash can.
   2. While patient sits in chair, monitor activity tolerance.
   3. Stand on patient's strong side when assisting the patient to stand before transferring to the chair.
   4. When assisting with transfer or positioning, position the level of the bed lower than the level of the chair.
   5. Determine the amount and type of assistance required for transfer, including type of transfer equipment and the number of personnel needed.
2. When assessing a patient's ability to transfer, which of the following would suggest the patient is at risk for falling during the transfer? (Select all that apply.)
   1. Patient is able to march in place at bedside and advance a step and return each foot while remaining stable.
   2. Patient has same blood pressure reading within 10 mm Hg sitting and standing.
   3. Patient tends to sway toward weakened side while sitting on side of bed.
   4. Patient has adequate visual perception.
   5. Patient has memory and decision-making deficits.
3. Place the following steps in the correct order for positioning a patient in the 30-degree lateral side-lying position.
   a. Raise side rail and go to opposite side of bed.
   b. Lower side rail and flex patient's knee that will not be next to mattress; keep foot on mattress and place one hand on patient's upper bent leg near hip and other hand on shoulder.
   c. Lower head of bed flat if patient can tolerate.
   d. Roll patient onto side toward you.
   e. Lower side rail and position patient on side of bed opposite direction toward which patient is to be turned.
   f. Place hands under patient's dependent shoulder and bring shoulder blade forward.
   g. Place hands under dependent hip and bring hip slightly forward so that angle from hip to mattress is approximately 30 degrees.

Answers and Rationales for Clinical Review Questions can be found on the Evolve website.

REFERENCES

Agency for Healthcare Research and Quality (AHRQ): Pressure injury prevention and treatment, 2014. http://www.ahrq.gov/professionals/systems/hospital/pressureulcertoolkit/index.html.

American Association for Safe Patient Handling & Movement (AASPHM): Healthcare recipient sling and lift hanger bar compatibility guidelines, 2012. http://aasphm.org/.

American Nurses Association (ANA): Safe patient handling and mobility interprofessional national standards, Silver Spring, MD, 2013a, The American Nurses Association.

American Nurses Association (ANA): ANA leads initiative to develop national safe patient handling standards, Silver Spring, MD, 2013b, The American Nurses Association.

Anderson MP, et al: Safe moving and handling of patients: an interprofessional approach, *Nurs Stand* 28(46):37, 2014.

Boynton T, et al: Banner Mobility Assessment Tool for nurses: instrument validation, *Am J Safe Patient Handl Mov* 4(3):86, 2014.

Bureau of Labor Statistics (BLS): Table R8. Incidence rates for nonfatal occupational injuries and illnesses involving days away from work per 10,000 full-time workers by industry and selected events or exposures leading to injury or illness, private industry, 2014. https://www.bls.gov/iif/oshwc/osh/case/ostb4374.pdf.

Centers for Disease Control and Prevention (CDC): What is health literacy, 2016. https://www.cdc.gov/healthliteracy/learn/index.html.

Chaboyer W, et al: Physical activity levels and torso orientations of hospitalized patients at risk of developing a pressure injury: an observational study, *Int J Nurs Pract* 1:11–17, 2013.

Choi SD, Brings K: Work-related musculoskeletal risks associated with nurses and nursing assistants handling overweight and obese patients: a literature review, *Work* 53(2):439–448, 2015.

Choi J, Cramer E: Reports from RNs on safe patient handling and mobility programs in acute care hospital units, *J Nurs Adm* 46(11):566–573, 2016.

Degelau J, et al: Institute for Clinical Systems Improvement (ICSI): Prevention of falls (acute care): health care protocol, Bloomington, MN, 2014, Institute for Clinical Systems Improvement.

Dennerlein JT, et al: Lifting and exertion injuries decrease after implementation of an integrated hospital-wide safe patient handling and mobilisation programme, *Occup Environ Med* 74:336–343, 2017.

Frith J, et al: Measuring and defining orthostatic hypotension in the older person, *Age Ageing* 43(2):168–170, 2014.

Hockenberry MJ, Wilson D: *Wong's essentials of pediatric nursing*, ed 10, St. Louis, 2017, Elsevier.

Latimer S, et al: The repositioning of hospitalized patients with reduced mobility: a prospective study, *Nurs Open* 2(2):85–93, 2015.

Lee S: Musculoskeletal symptoms in nurses in the early implementation phase of California's safe patient handling legislation, *Res Nurs Health* 38(3):183–193, 2015.

McInnes E, et al: Acute care patient mobility patterns and documented pressure injury prevention-an observational study and survey, *Wound Pract Res* 21(3):116–125, 2013.

Mills P, et al: Five things to know about orthostatic hypotension in the older adult, *J Am Geriatr Soc* 62(9):1822, 2014.

Occupational Safety & Health Association (OSHA): Safe patient handling—preventing musculoskeletal disorders in nursing homes, *OSHA Publication* 3108, 2014. https://www.osha.gov/Publications/OSHA3708.pdf.

Occupational Safety & Health Administration (OSHA): Worker safety in hospitals, OSHA Publication, 2015. https://www.osha.gov/dsg/hospitals/patient_handling.html.

Pierson F, Fairchild S: *Principles and techniques of patient care*, ed 6, St. Louis, 2017, Saunders.

Risor BW, et al: A multi-component patient-handling intervention improves attitudes and behaviors for safe patient handling and reduces aggression experienced by nursing staff: a controlled before-after study, *Appl Ergon* 60:74, 2017.

Robson Forensic: Patient transport—expert article on injuries in healthcare facilities, 2016. http://www.robsonforensic.com/articles/patient-transport-expert-witness.

Schofield PA: The assessment and management of peri-operative pain in older adults, *Anaesthesia* 6(1):54, 2014.

Shieh C, et al: Association of self-efficacy and self-regulation with nutrition and exercise behaviors in a community sample of adults, *J Community Health Nurs* 32(4):199, 2015.

Swafford K, et al: Use of a comprehensive program to reduce the incidence of hospital-acquired pressure ulcers in an intensive care unit, *Am J Crit Care* 25:152–155, 2016.

Tampa Research and Education Foundation, Inc. (TVAREF): VHA safe patient handling and mobility algorithms (2014 revision). http://www.tampavaref.org/safe-patient-handling/Enc4-2SPHMAlgorithms.pdf.

The Joint Commission (TJC): *2019 National Patient Safety Goals*, Oakbrook Terrace, IL, 2019, The Commission. http://www.jointcommission.org/standards_information/npsgs.aspx.

Touhy T, Jett K: *Ebersole and Hess's gerontological nursing and healthy aging*, ed 5, St. Louis, 2018, Mosby.

Wiggermann N: The sliding patient: how to respond to and prevent migration in bed: migration can cause negative patient outcomes and caregiver injuries related to repositioning, *Am Nurse Today* 9(9):2014.

18 Exercise, Mobility, and Immobilization Devices

SKILLS AND PROCEDURES

EVOLVE WEBSITE/RESOURCES LIST

http://evolve.elsevier.com/Perry/nursinginterventions

Audio Glossary • Case Studies • Checklists • Clinical Review Questions • Answers and Rationales for Clinical Review Questions

INTRODUCTION

Exercise is physical activity used to condition the body, improve health, and maintain fitness. Patients benefit from regular activity and exercise that is appropriate for their current health conditions. Recently, hospitals have made efforts to increase inpatients' activity and mobility levels as soon as possible to prevent deconditioning and other complications of immobilization. The American Association of Critical Care Nurses (AACN) recommends an early progressive mobility protocol for critical care patients (refer to agency policy for protocols; Agency for Healthcare Research and Quality [AHRQ], 2013). When patients are transferred out to general nursing units, early mobility protocols should continue with routine ambulation being the end goal. Some hospitals have designated special mobility teams or mobility assistants to engage patients in early ambulation and activity. A patient's individualized exercise program depends on his or her activity tolerance, underlying medical condition, and motivation. Nurses can assist patients in maintaining or improving their level of activity and exercise by implementing a progressive mobility program that consists of ambulation, out-of-bed activities (with and without assist devices) and range-of-motion (ROM) exercises. It is useful to incorporate active exercise into activities of daily living (ADLs) whenever possible (Table 18.1). As a nurse, practicing safe patient handling (see Chapter 17) and knowing proper body mechanics will allow you to assist patients while reducing your risk of injury and their risk as well.

PRACTICE STANDARDS

- Agency for Healthcare Research and Quality (AHRQ), 2013: Implementing the ABCDE bundle at the bedside—Implementing early mobility
- National Database for Nursing Quality Indicators (NDNQI), 2017: Pressure injuries and staging—Assessing medical device–related (MDR) pressure injuries
- The Joint Commission, 2019: National Patient Safety Goals—Patient identification

EVIDENCE-BASED PRACTICE

Impact of the Use of Assist Devices

Disability and mobility problems increase with age. Assist devices such as canes, crutches, and walkers are often used to increase a patient's base of support, improve balance, and increase activity and independence, but the use of assist devices can pose significant musculoskeletal and metabolic demands. There is some evidence that the use of assist devices is a risk factor for patient falls among older adults living in residential settings (de Mettelinge et al., 2015). A study involving 10 patients who reported either gait or balance impairment from Parkinson's disease (but who usually ambulated independently) examined the effects of using a cane and a walker (Bryant et al., 2013). Both devices were properly fitted for each patient. Subjects in the study walked without any device, walked with a cane, and walked with a wheeled walker while gait parameters were measured. The patients walked with a slower gait speed when using a cane and wheeled walker compared with walking independently without a device (Bryant et al., 2013). The findings suggest that gait modification when using assist devices places patients at risk for falling. In a study involving 783 ambulatory patients with a history of spinal cord injury (1 year or longer post-injury), Saunders and colleagues (2013) found that those who used a unilateral cane or crutch had increased pain intensity and fatigue. Luz and colleagues (2017) studied a different aspect of assist devices and falls by surveying 262 people aged 60 and older who were community dwelling, cognitively intact, and current cane/walker users with a history of falls. Their study found that 75% of respondents who fell were not using their device at the time of fall despite stating that their devices help prevent falls. Reasons for nonuse included believing it was not needed, forgetfulness, the device making them feel old, and inaccessibility (Luz et al., 2017).

TABLE 18.1

Incorporating Active Range-of-Motion Exercises Into Activities of Daily Living

Joint Exercised	Activity of Daily Living	Movement
Neck	Nodding head "yes" Shaking head "no" Moving right ear to right shoulder Moving left ear to left shoulder	Flexion Rotation Lateral flexion Lateral flexion
Shoulder	Reaching to turn on overhead light Reaching to bedside stand for book Applying deodorant Combing hair Scratching back; brushing or combing hair Rotating shoulders toward chest Rotating shoulders toward back	Flexion, extension Extension Abduction Flexion Hyperextension Internal rotation External rotation
Elbow	Eating, bathing, shaving, grooming	Flexion, extension
Wrist	Eating, bathing, shaving, grooming	Flexion, extension, abduction, adduction, ulnar/radial deviation
Fingers and thumb	All activities requiring fine motor coordination (e.g., writing, eating, hobbies)	Flexion, extension, abduction, adduction, opposition
Hip	Walking Moving to side-lying position Moving from side-lying position	Flexion, extension, hyperextension Flexion, extension, abduction Extension, adduction
Knee	Walking Moving to and from side-lying position	Flexion, extension Flexion, extension
Ankle	Walking Moving toe toward head of bed Moving toe toward foot of bed	Dorsiflexion, plantar flexion Dorsiflexion Plantar flexion
Toes	Walking	Extension, hyperextension

Practice Issues/Principles

- Encourage patients to use prescribed assist devices at home and to follow instructions for safe use.
- Follow guidelines for properly fitting patients with crutches, canes, or walkers (see Skill 18.2).
- Provide patient education on the proper care of all assist devices and about risks of falling to patients and family caregivers.
- Consult with physical therapy when a patient has been ordered to have an assist device; discuss the possibility of also providing gait training.
- When patients have assist devices that they have purchased retail, be sure the devices are properly fitted.
- Inform patients that if they develop any physical problems associated with using their assist devices, they should notify their health care provider or physical therapist.

SAFETY GUIDELINES

To prevent injury to both a patient and caregiver, use of safety guidelines is essential. Follow these guidelines in the performance of the skills in this chapter:

- When ambulating patients, be sure catheters and supportive equipment are attached to patients or held in a way so that they do not become dislodged and cause injury.
- Obtain and become familiar with any type of assist device to be used. Know how to properly measure and prepare a device for a patient. Have a physical therapy consult if available.
- Prepare patients for ambulation with and without assist devices. Make sure that their vital signs are stable, they are rested and not fatigued, and their pain is under control.
- Apply safe patient-handling principles (see Chapter 17) when assisting patients out of bed or a chair for ambulation.
- Discuss with patients any risks for falling. Ask patients how they feel about walking, whether they have fallen recently, and how you intend to remove risks for falling.
- Use appropriate clinical guidelines (e.g., early mobility protocols) for advancing a patient's activity level. Follow the specific screening criteria for each protocol. Consult with physical therapy.
- Be sure the patient has a home care plan for any exercise regimen and use of an assist device.

PROCEDURAL GUIDELINE 18.1 *Promoting Early Activity and Exercise*

Purpose

A goal of the *Healthy People 2020* initiative is to improve health, fitness, and quality of life through daily physical activity (Office of Disease Prevention and Health Promotion [ODPHP], 2015). This goal is based on guidelines that suggest that regular physical activity can improve the health and quality of life of Americans of all ages and help prevent chronic diseases such as heart disease, cancer, and stroke (U.S. Department of Health and Human Services

PROCEDURAL GUIDELINE 18.1 *Promoting Early Activity and Exercise—cont'd*

[USDHHS], 2017). As a nurse, you will work in inpatient and outpatient settings with the opportunity to plan health promotion activities. It is crucial to educate patients and family caregivers about the importance of regular physical activity and exercise and how these activities can be incorporated into daily routines.

Delegation and Collaboration

The skill of promoting early activity and exercise in the outpatient setting regarding activity and exercise education cannot be delegated to nursing assistive personnel (NAP).

Equipment

Weights, resistance bands (optional based on physical therapy recommendations)

Procedural Steps

1. Identify patient using at least two identifiers (e.g., name and birthday or name and medical record number) according to agency policy (TJC, 2019).
2. Measure patient's baseline heart rate or have patient/family caregiver do measurement. *Provides baseline for activity tolerance.*
3. Identify patient's activity/exercise history:
   - Which type of regular daily exercise do you perform at home?
   - Do you exercise or play a sport at least three times a week?
   - On a scale of 0 to 5, with 0 being no daily exercise and 5 being strenuous regular daily exercise, how would you rate yourself?
   - How long have you been exercising regularly?
4. Ask patient to what extent he or she enjoys exercising and what his or her beliefs are about ability to exercise. *Rationale: Factors positively associated with adult physical activity (ODPHP, 2015).*
5. Determine if patient has social support from peers, family, or spouse.
6. Determine if patient has access to facility or area to exercise. Is neighborhood considered safe?
7. Consider these factors in your assessment: patient's age, income level, time available to exercise, rural resident, overweight, being disabled. *Rationale: Factors negatively associated with adult participation in activity (ODPHP, 2015).*
8. Have patient rate level of quality of life based on current activity level. *Rationale: Serves as baseline to measure long-term benefits of exercise.*
9. Develop an outpatient exercise program that contains any of the following components:
   - Warm-up (5–10 minutes)
   - Strengthening exercises
   - Endurance exercises
   - Balance exercises
   - Flexibility exercises

   Consult with physical therapy to help develop complete exercise program that fits the needs of your patient. A good resource is available at http://health.gov/paguidelines/guidelines. *Rationale: Warm-up directs needed blood flow to muscles and prepares body for exercise, helping to prevent injury. Flexibility exercises lessen tightness of muscles and improve joint range of motion (ROM). Cool-downs help body recover from exercises.*
10. Recommend strength training for adults in collaboration with physical therapy. *Rationale: Improves strength and bone density.*
11. Recommend aerobic exercise. The American Heart Association (AHA, 2016) recommends aerobic exercise at least 150 minutes per week of moderate exercise or 75 minutes per week of vigorous exercise (or combination of moderate and vigorous activity). This includes activities such as climbing stairs; playing sports; or aerobic activities such as walking, jogging, swimming, or biking. *Rationale: Improves overall cardiovascular health.*
12. Recommend balance exercises for older adults to decrease risk of falls. Have patient be sure to have something sturdy nearby on which to hold (wall or chair) if he or she becomes unsteady.

    Perform exercises: standing on one foot, walking heel to toe, balance walking, back leg raises, side leg raises. Have patient do strength exercises (back leg raises, side leg raises) 2 or more days per week, but not on any 2 days in a row (National Institutes of Health [NIH], n.d.).
13. Recommend that patient perform cool-down (5–10 minutes) after exercising: quadriceps stretch; hamstring/calf stretch; chest and arm stretch; neck, upper back, and shoulder stretch. *Rationale: Helps muscles relax and become more flexible.*
14. Measure heart rate during and after exercise. Compare results with baseline. Stop physical activity when (Adler and Malone, 2012):
    - >70% age predicted maximum heart rate (APMHR), or
    - Heart rate (HR) is more than a 20% decrease in resting value, or
    - HR is less than 40 beats/min, or
    - HR is greater than 130 beats/min
15. Document in outpatient record the exercises recommended. Document patient response if you witness patient exercising.

✦ SKILL 18.1 Assisting With Ambulation (Without Assist Devices)

Purpose

Early mobilization includes activities such as sitting, standing, and ambulation, as well as passive and active range-of-motion (ROM) exercises (Taito et al., 2016). Physical activity benefits a patient's overall health and reduces psychological and physical stress (Childs and deWit, 2014). Safely assisting patients with ambulation is vital to their recovery. In the normal walking posture, the head is erect; the cervical, thoracic, and lumbar vertebrae are aligned; the hips and knees have slight flexion; and the arms swing freely. Illness, surgery, injury, advanced age, and prolonged bed rest can reduce activity tolerance and affect the ability to maintain a normal postural stance and balance, so assistance is required. Patients with altered cardiovascular or respiratory function or who have been on prolonged bed rest may experience activity intolerance evidenced by chest pain, dizziness, diaphoresis, abnormal heart rate response, dyspnea, orthostatic hypotension, or fatigue. For this reason, it is important to monitor a patient carefully during ambulation.

Delegation and Collaboration

The skill of assisting patients with ambulation can be delegated to nursing assistive personnel (NAP). The nurse directs the NAP to:

- Apply safe patient-handling principles (see Chapter 17) when assisting patient out of bed or chair.
- Have a patient who has been lying in bed first sit on the side of the bed with feet touching the floor. Then have patient move legs back and forth without touching the floor (dangle) before starting ambulation. Check patient's blood pressure (BP) before ambulation.
- Immediately return a patient to the bed or chair if he or she is nauseated, dizzy, pale, or diaphoretic or if systolic BP has dropped at least 20 mm Hg within 3 minutes of sitting upright (Shibao et al., 2013). Report these signs and symptoms to the nurse immediately.
- Apply safe, nonskid shoes/socks and ensure that the environment is free of clutter and there is no moisture on the floor before ambulating the patient.

Equipment

- Nonskid footwear
- Transfer (gait) belt
- Stethoscope, sphygmomanometer, pulse oximeter (as needed)

ASSESSMENT

1. Identify patient using at least two identifiers (e.g., name and birthday or name and medical record number) according to agency policy. *Rationale: Ensures correct patient. Complies with The Joint Commission standards and improves patient safety (TJC, 2019).*
2. Review medical record for patient's most recent activity experience, including distance ambulated, use of assist device, activity tolerance, balance, and gait. Note history of orthostatic hypotension and any medications, chronic illnesses, gait alterations, or a history of falling. *Rationale: Allows you to anticipate precautions to take in ambulating patient. History may reveal factors that will influence patient's ability to ambulate and be at risk for falling*
3. Review most recently recorded weight for patient and report of patient's ability to stand and bear weight. *Rationale: Determines if assistance will be required from another health care provider.*

Safe Patient Care *Use mechanical lift or transfer aid with minimum of two or three caregivers if a patient has partial weight bearing with upper-body strength or caregiver must lift more than 15.9 kg (35 lb) (TVAREF, 2014).*

4. Review health care provider's order for activity; note any mobility, ROM, or weight-bearing restrictions. *Rationale: Order required for patient to become progressively mobile.*
5. Perform hand hygiene. Assess patient's baseline resting heart rate, blood pressure, oxygen saturation (when available), and respirations. *Rationale: Provides a baseline to compare with assessment data monitored during and after walking to evaluate patient tolerance to exercise.*
   a. If patient's strength and endurance have been affected by illness or deconditioning, assess ROM and muscle strength (see Chapter 8) of lower extremities while in bed. Assess the patient's mobility, including ability to sit up on side of bed or chair and ability to stand, by using the Banner Mobility Assessment Tool (BMAT; Boynton et al., 2014; see Chapter 17). *Rationale: Confirms patient's ability to assist with standing and walking. The BMAT is an assessment tool to guide a patient through four functional tasks in order to identify the level of mobility the patient can achieve (Boynton et al., 2014).*
   b. Ask if patient feels excessively tired or is currently experiencing any pain. Determine source and severity of pain (using a 0-to-10 pain-rating scale). Offer an analgesic 30 minutes before ambulation to improve patient's tolerance to exercise. *Rationale: Pain may delay ambulation.*
6. Assess patient's response to commands. Is he or she able to understand instructions and cooperate during ambulation? Is patient willing to ambulate? *Rationale: Determines how safe it will be to engage patient to ambulate and take precautions needed while walking.*
7. Assess patient for any hearing or visual deficits. *Rationale: May affect ability to understand instructions.*
8. Refer to patient's mobility status and safe patient-handling algorithm (available in most agencies). Do not start procedure until all required caregivers are available. *Rationale: Determines if a lift device or mechanical transfer device is needed and the number of people needed to assist patient to stand.*
9. Assess patient's or family caregiver's knowledge, experience and health literacy level. *Rationale: Ensures patient has the capacity to obtain, communicate, process, and understand basic health information (Centers for Disease Control and Prevention [CDC], 2016).*

STEP	RATIONALE
PLANNING	
1. Expected outcomes following completion of procedure:	
• Patient can ambulate without falling.	Taking safety precautions during assisted ambulation prevents falls.
• Patient can ambulate without excessive fatigue or dizziness and with return of vital signs to baseline 3 to 5 minutes after rest.	Patient ambulates without episode of orthostatic hypotension and within exercise tolerance.
2. Determine the best time to ambulate, considering other scheduled activities such as bathing or other medical procedures.	Allows you to lessen likelihood patient will be fatigued at time of ambulation.

STEP	RATIONALE
3. Provide privacy. Organize and set up any equipment/lift devices.	Ensures more efficiency, safe use of equipment, and safe ambulation.
4. Remove sequential compression device (SCD) from patient's legs if present (see Procedural Guideline 18.2). Note that if patient wears a mobile compression device, ambulation can occur safely with stockings in place.	Prevents patient from becoming tangled in cords.
5. Explain to patient in simple language how you are going to prepare for ambulation (e.g., gait belt application, distance planned to walk). Discuss benefits of walking and risks that you are adapting for to reduce chance of falling.	Allows patient to cooperate and lessens anxiety.

Safe Patient Care *If patient is on an early progressive mobility protocol, know distance walked during previous ambulation and attempt to increase distance this time.*

IMPLEMENTATION

STEP	RATIONALE
1. If hands became soiled during assessment, perform hand hygiene. Assist patient from supine position to sitting position on edge of bed with bed positioned so that top of mattress is even with your elbows.	Reduces transfer of microorganisms. Reduces strain on your back.
a. With patient in supine position in bed, raise head of bed 30 degrees and place bed in low position, level with your hips. Apply nonskid shoes or socks. If patient is fully mobile, allow to sit up on side of bed independently.	Reduces strain on back during pivot to side of bed. Nonskid soles decrease risk for slipping during transfer. Always have patient wear nonskid shoes when ambulating; bare feet increase risk for falls.
b. If patient needs assistance, turn patient onto his or her side facing you while standing on side of bed where patient will sit.	Positioning reduces strain on your back.
c. Stand opposite patient's hips. Turn diagonally to face patient and far corner of foot of bed.	
d. Place your feet apart in wide base of support with foot closer to head of bed in front of other foot.	
e. Place your arm nearer to head of bed under patient's lower shoulder, supporting his or her head and neck. Place your other arm over and around patient's thighs (see illustration).	Position provides leverage for patient to rise to sitting position.
f. Move patient's lower legs and feet over side of bed. Pivot weight onto your rear leg as you allow patient's upper legs to swing downward (see illustration). At same time, continue to shift weight to your rear leg and elevate patient's trunk to the upright position	

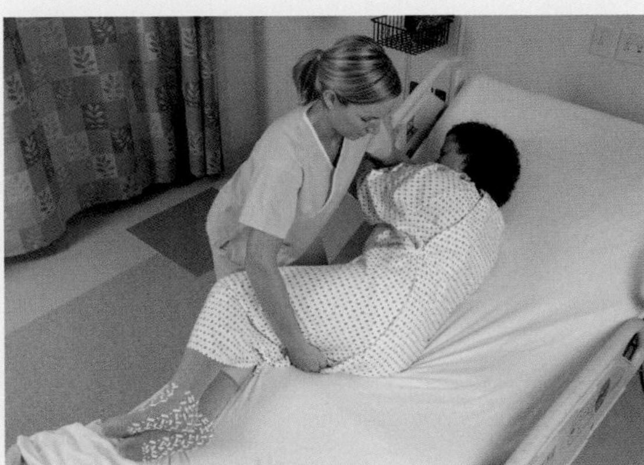

STEP 1e Nurse places arm over patient's thighs, other arm under patient's shoulder.

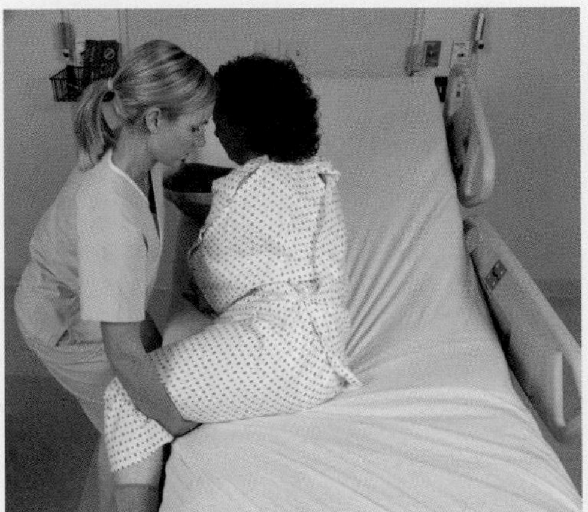

STEP 1f Nurse shifts weight to rear leg and elevates patient to sitting position.

STEP	RATIONALE
2. Allow patient to sit on the side of the bed with feet on floor for 2 to 3 minutes. Have patient alternately flex and extend feet, and move lower legs up and down without touching floor (see illustration). Ask if patient feels dizzy; if so, check blood pressure. Have patient relax and take a few deep breaths until dizziness subsides and balance is gained. If dizziness lasts more than 60 seconds or if systolic blood pressure (BP) has dropped at least 20 mm Hg within 3 minutes of sitting upright, return patient to bed (Frith et al., 2014; Mills et al., 2014; Shibao et al., 2013). Recheck blood pressure.	Allows patient's circulation to equilibrate to reduce chance of orthostatic hypotension. Patient cannot be safely ambulated if dizziness develops.

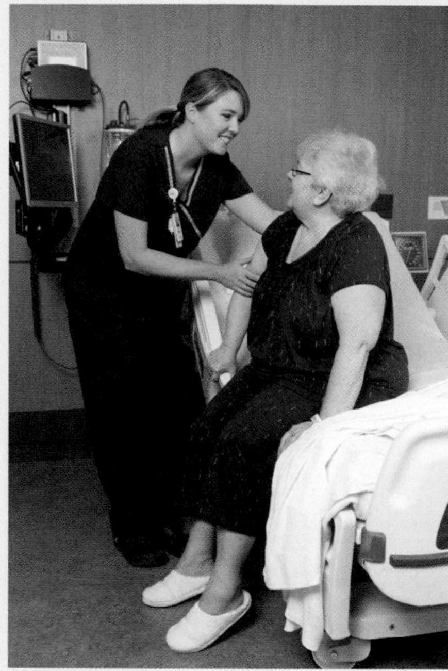

STEP 2 Patient sits on side of bed.

STEP	RATIONALE
3. Apply gait belt. Be sure that it completely circles waist. Place belt low and be sure that it is snug. Avoid placing belt over any intravenous lines, incisions, or drainage tubes.	Gait belt allows you to maintain stability of patient during transfer and reduces risk for falling (Degelau et al., 2014; Occupational Safety and Health Administration [OSHA], 2014).
4. Place patient's weight-bearing or unaffected leg forward on floor, with affected foot back.	Provides more stability as patient stands.
5. If assisting patient independently, spread your feet apart. Flex hips and knees, aligning knees with patient's knees. (If assisted by another caregiver, each of you stands toward patient on each side of patient.)	Ensures balance with wide base of support. Flexing knees and hips lowers your center of gravity to object to be raised; aligning knees with those of patient stabilizes knees when patient stands.
6. Grasp gait belt, keeping your palms up, along patient's sides.	Gait belt allows you to move patient at center of gravity. Patients should never be lifted by or under their arms.
7. Assist patient to standing position. Ask if patient feels dizzy or light-headed. If patient appears light-headed, have patient lie back down and recheck blood pressure. If patient is stable, have him or her stand fully erect with shoulders back and looking ahead (not at floor).	Allows you to detect orthostatic hypotension before ambulation begins and determine if there is a need to postpone ambulation. Stabilizes patient in normal standing position.
8. Confirm with patient distance to ambulate.	Motivates patient to reach goal.

Safe Patient Care *If any time during ambulation the patient becomes unstable or reports feeling dizzy, seat him or her in chair or return to bed immediately. May need use of mechanical lift. This prevents patient falls.*

STEP	RATIONALE
9. *Option:* If patient has an intravenous (IV) line, place the IV pole on the same side as the site of infusion and instruct patient where to hold and push the pole while ambulating. It is best if another caregiver can push IV pole.	Prevents accidental pulling on IV catheter. Assist from second caregiver allows patient to focus on walking and may lessen risk of tripping
10. If a Foley catheter is present, carry the bag below the level of the bladder and prevent tension on the tubing.	Prevents reflux of urine from the bag back into bladder.
11. For orthopedic patients stand on patient's unaffected side. For patients with neurological deficits (e.g., stroke), stand on the affected side. For all other patients requiring assistance to maintain weight bearing, stand on involved side.	This provides balance and facilitates lowering patient to the floor if he or she is unable to continue because of weakness or dizziness. Helps support the affected limb of neurological patient (i.e., prevent knee buckling).
12. Grasp belt firmly with palm facing up (see illustration A). Take a few steps, supporting patient with one hand grasping the gait belt and the other under the elbow of the patient's flexed arm (see illustration B). *Option:* Use ambulation lift or ceiling lift with gait harness for more dependent patients who are now walking for first time after being in bed.	The wall provides stable support for patients who start to fall away from nurse.

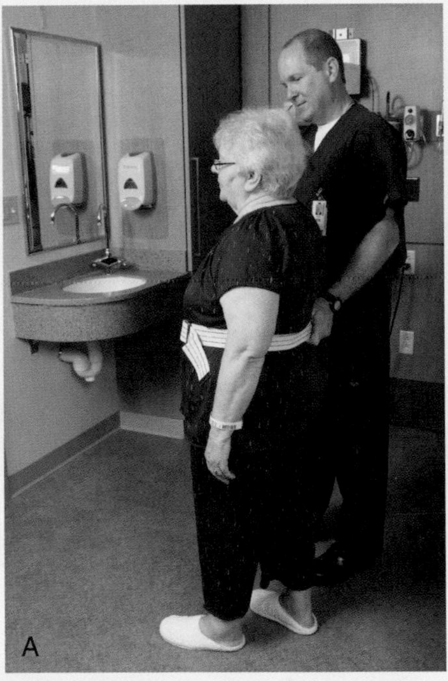

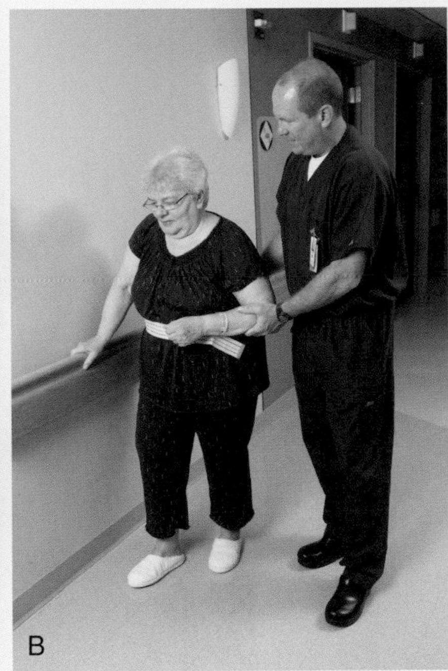

STEP 12 (A) Nurse grasps gait belt firmly. (B) Nurse helps patient by providing support under patient's flexed arm.

STEP	RATIONALE
13. When ambulating in a hallway, position patient between yourself and the wall. Encourage patient to use handrails if available.	The wall provides stable support for patients who start to fall away from nurse.
14. Observe how patient walks (posture, gait, balance) and determine distance patient can safely continue walking. Measure pulse and respirations as needed.	Monitors patient's tolerance to walking.
15. Return patient to bed or chair and assist patient to assume a comfortable position. Be sure the nurse call system is accessible within patient's reach.	Gives patient sense of well-being. Ensures patient can call for assistance if needed.
16. Raise side rails (as appropriate) and lower bed to lowest position. Perform hand hygiene.	Ensures patient safety. Reduces transmission of microorganisms.

STEP	RATIONALE

EVALUATION

1. Monitor vital signs. Ask if patient feels dizzy or tired. Ask him or her to rate pain on pain scale. — Evaluates patient's response to postural changes and activity.
2. Note patient's behavioral response to walking. — Reveals level of motivation and self-care potential.
3. **Use Teach-Back:** "I want to be sure I explained the importance of increasing your distance walking each day, and to continue once you go home. Tell me why it is important for you to be able to walk farther each day." Revise your instruction now or develop a plan for revised patient/family caregiver teaching if patient/family caregiver is not able to teach back correctly. — Determines patient's/family caregiver's level of understanding of instructional topic.

Unexpected Outcomes / Related Interventions

1. Patient starts to fall while walking.
    - Grasp patient's gait belt with both hands around his or her waist with palms up.
    - Stand with feet apart for a broad base of support (see illustration A).
    - Extend one leg slightly forward, pull patient against you, and let him or her slide down your leg as you ease him or her to the floor (see illustration B). *Caution:* If patient is obese, do not risk personal injury. If you extend leg too far, hyperextension could occur.
    - Bend your knees and lower your body as patient slides to floor (see illustration C).
    - Stay with patient until help arrives.

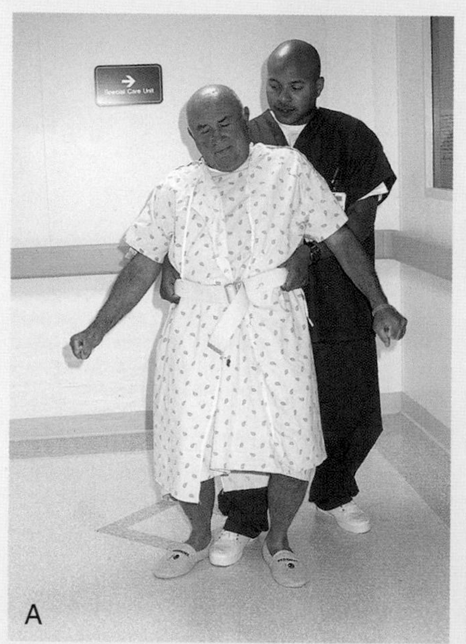

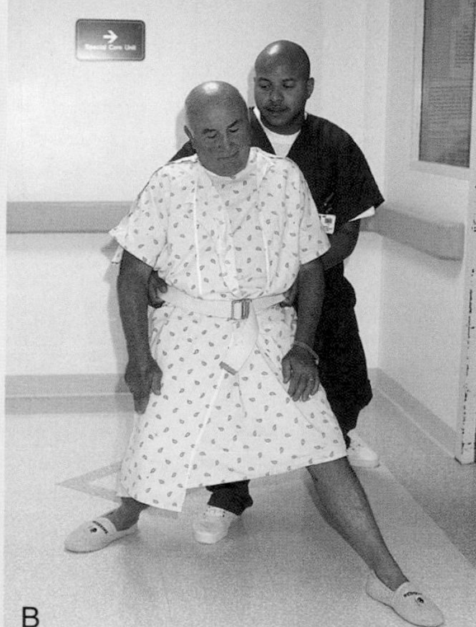

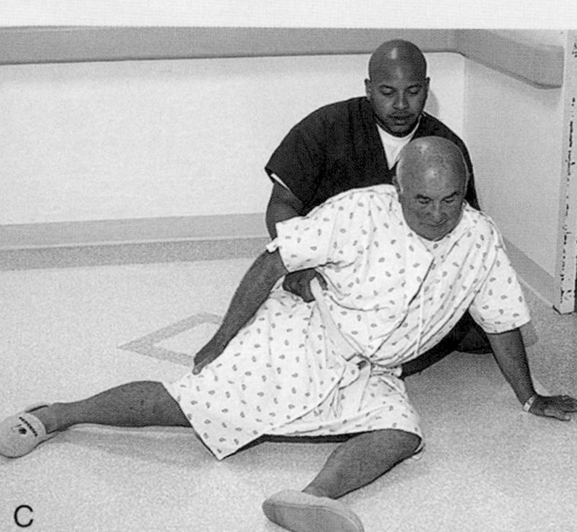

STEP 1 (A) Grasp gait belt and stand with feet apart to provide broad base of support. (B) Extend one leg and let patient slide against it to floor. (C) Bend knees to lower body as patient slides to floor.

2. Patient does not tolerate walking due to fatigue, pain, dizziness, or other symptoms.
    - Return to bed or chair immediately.
    - Measure vital signs.
    - Notify health care provider or nurse in charge.

Recording

- Record procedure and pertinent observations: distance walked, patient's tolerance, onset of weakness, fatigue, pain, poor balance or gait, changes in vital signs.
- Document evaluation of patient learning.

Hand-Off Reporting

- Report unexpected outcomes to health care provider or nurse in charge.

PROCEDURAL GUIDELINE 18.2 *Range-of-Motion Exercises*

Purpose

Range of motion (ROM) refers to the distance or amount of freedom a joint can be moved in a certain direction (e.g., rotating, bending, or twisting). A ROM exercise preserves flexibility and mobility of the involved joint. There are three types of ROM exercises: active, passive, and active assisted. An active ROM exercise allows a patient, when able, to independently move an extremity against gravity; active-assisted ROM is when a patient is able to assist in moving an extremity against gravity but requires assistance from a caregiver to complete the movement; and passive ROM exercise involves a caregiver moving the extremity because the patient is unable to due to weakness or sedation. A study involving 59 bedridden older stroke survivors who received ROM exercises 6 days a week showed benefits. Among the two intervention groups that received an exercise regimen, there was an improvement in joint angles, activity function, perception of pain, and depressive symptoms compared with the usual-care group (Tseng et al., 2007). Always encourage patients to be as active and independent as possible in every aspect of activities of daily living (ADLs; see Table 18.1). Also incorporate active-assisted and passive ROM into bathing and feeding activities.

Delegation and Collaboration

The skill of performing ROM exercises can be delegated to trained nursing assistive personnel (NAP). Patients with spinal cord injuries, burns, or orthopedic trauma usually require ROM exercises by professional nurses or physical therapists. The nurse directs the NAP to:

- Perform exercises slowly and provide adequate support to each joint being exercised.
- Not exercise joints beyond the point of resistance or to the point of fatigue or pain.
- Be aware of a patient's individual limitations or preexisting conditions, such as arthritis, that affect ROM.

Equipment

No mechanical or physical equipment needed; clean gloves *(optional)*

Procedural Steps

1. Identify patient using at least two identifiers (e.g., name and birthday or name and medical record number) according to agency policy (TJC, 2019).
2. Review patient's medical record for physical assessment findings that could affect the performance of ROM exercises (e.g., pain in joint, skin integrity or presence of wound near joint, presence of deformity; level of consciousness and ability to attend).
3. Review patient's medical record for health care provider's orders (e.g., any ROM restrictions for medical reasons), medical diagnosis, medical history, and activity progression.
4. Perform hand hygiene. Assess patient's baseline joint function. Observe for obvious limitations in joint mobility by having or assisting patient perform a ROM movement. Note any redness, or warmth over joints, joint tenderness, deformities, or edema.
5. Assess patient's or family caregiver's knowledge, experience, and health literacy.
6. Determine patient's or family caregiver's readiness and willingness to learn (e.g., desire to participate, perceived ability to perform exercise, perceived benefit of exercise). Explain in plain language reason for the ROM exercises and describe and demonstrate exercises to be performed.
7. Assess patient's level of comfort (on a scale of 0 to 10 with 10 being the worst pain) before exercises. Determine if patient would benefit from pain medication before beginning ROM exercises; then administer analgesic 30 minutes before exercise.
8. Perform hand hygiene and apply clean gloves if wound drainage or skin lesions are present.
9. Close room curtains or doors to provide privacy.
10. Help patient to a comfortable position, preferably sitting or lying down.
11. When performing passive ROM exercises (Table 18.2), support joint by holding distal part of extremity or using cupped hand to support joint (see illustration). If there is swelling or discomfort in the joint, perform the exercise slowly and steadily.
12. Complete exercises in head-to-toe sequence.
    a. Perform each exercise 10 times or move to the point of resistance and hold for 30 seconds.
    b. Begin exercises slowly, doing each exercise a few times only and gradually build up to more.
    c. Try to achieve full ROM by moving until you feel a slight stretch, but don't force a movement.
    d. Move only to the point of resistance.
    e. Inform patient how these exercises can be incorporated into ADLs (see Table 18.1).

Safe Patient Care *When resistance is noted within a joint, do not force joint motion. Consult with health care provider or physical therapist.*

13. Observe patient perform ROM activity independently (when appropriate).
14. Once completed be sure patient is in comfortable position. Place nurse call system in a location accessible within patient's reach.
15. Raise side rails (as appropriate) and lower bed to lowest position.
16. Remove and dispose of gloves, if worn. Perform hand hygiene.
17. Measure joint motion to determine level of improvement.
18. Evaluate patient during exercise by having him or her rate the severity of pain on a pain scale.
19. Record exercises performed and patient's tolerance.

Continued

PROCEDURAL GUIDELINE 18.2 *Range-of-Motion Exercises—cont'd*

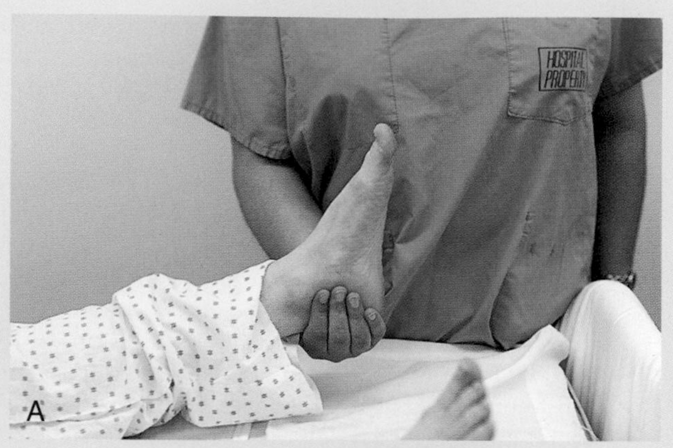

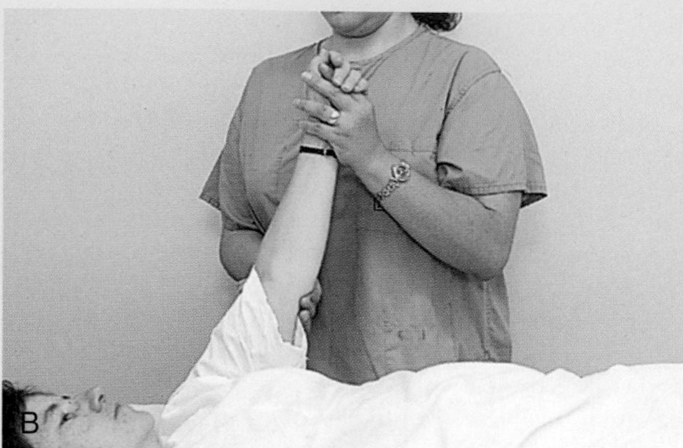

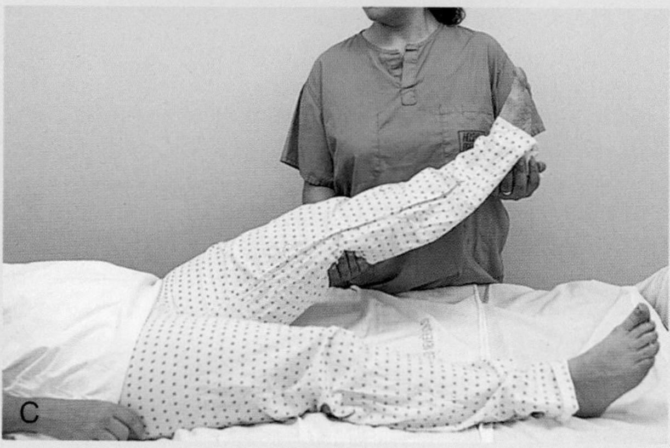

STEP 11 (A) Support joint by holding distal and proximal areas adjacent to joint. (B) Support joint by cradling distal part of extremity. (C) Use cupped hand to support joint.

TABLE 18.2

Range-of-Motion Exercises

Body Part	Type of Joint	Type of Movement	Range (Degrees)	Primary Muscles
Neck, cervical spine	Pivotal	*Flexion:* Bring chin to rest on chest.	45	Sternocleidomastoid
		Extension: Return head to erect position.	45	Trapezius
		Hyperextension: Bend head back as far as possible.	10	Trapezius
		Lateral flexion: Slowly tilt head as far as possible toward each shoulder.	40–45	Scalenes
		Rotation: Slowly turn head as far as possible in circular movement.	180	Sternocleidomastoid, upper trapezius

TABLE 18.2

Range-of-Motion Exercises—cont'd

Body Part	Type of Joint	Type of Movement	Range (Degrees)	Primary Muscles
Shoulder	Ball-and-socket	*Horizontal Flexion:* Swing arm horizontally forward.	180	Coracobrachialis, deltoid, pectoralis major
		Horizontal Extension: Swing arm horizontally backward.	45–60	Latissimus dorsi, teres major, triceps brachii
		Abduction: Raise arm from side to position above head with palm away from head.	180	Deltoid, supraspinatus, trapezius, serratus anterior
		Adduction: Lower arm sideways and across body as far as possible.	45	Pectoralis major, teres major, deltoid
		Internal rotation: With elbow flexed, rotate shoulder by moving arm until thumb is turned inward and toward back.	90	Pectoralis major, latissimus dorsi, teres major, subscapularis
		External rotation: With elbow flexed, move arm until thumb is upward and lateral to head.	90	Infraspinatus, teres major, deltoid
		Circumduction: Move arm in full circle (circumduction is combination of all movements of ball-and-socket joint).	360	Deltoid, coracobrachialis, latissimus dorsi, teres major
Elbow	Hinge	*Flexion:* Bend elbow so that lower arm moves toward its shoulder joint and hand is level with shoulder.	150	Biceps brachii, brachialis, brachioradialis
		Extension: Straighten elbow by lowering hand.	150	Triceps brachii
Forearm	Pivotal	*Supination:* Turn lower arm and hand so that palm is up.	70–90	Supinator, biceps brachii
		Pronation: Turn lower arm so that palm is down.	70–90	Pronator teres, pronator quadratus
Wrist	Condyloid	*Flexion:* Move palm toward inner aspect of forearm.	80–90	Flexor carpi ulnaris, flexor carpi radialis
		Extension: Move fingers and hand posterior to midline.	70–80	Extensor carpi radialis brevis, extensor carpi radialis longus, extensor carpi ulnaris
		Hyperextension: Bring dorsal surface of hand back as far as possible.	80–90	Extensor carpi radialis brevis, extensor carpi radialis longus, extensor carpi ulnaris
		Abduction (ulnar deviation): Bend wrist laterally toward fifth finger.	30–50	Flexor carpi ulnaris, extensor carpi ulnaris
		Adduction (radial deviation): Bend wrist medially toward thumb.	Up to 30	Flexor carpi radialis, extensor carpi radialis brevis, extensor carpi radialis longus

Continued

TABLE 18.2
Range-of-Motion Exercises—cont'd

Body Part	Type of Joint	Type of Movement	Range (Degrees)	Primary Muscles
Fingers	Condyloid hinge 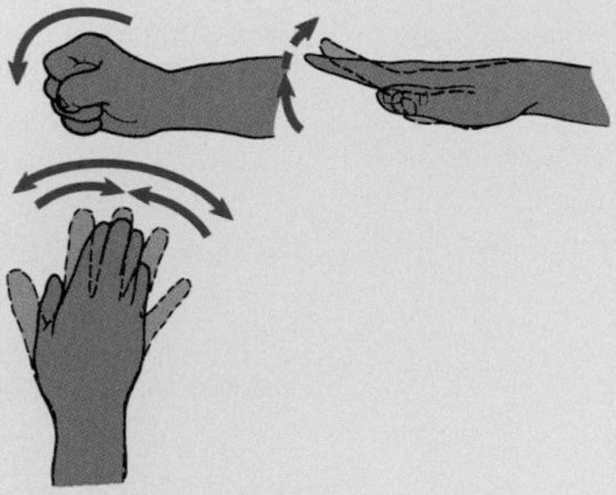	*Flexion:* Make fist.	90	Lumbricales, interosseus volaris, interosseus dorsalis
		Extension: Straighten fingers.	90	Extensor digiti quinti proprius, extensor digitorum communis, extensor indicis proprius
		Hyperextension: Bend fingers back as far as possible.	30–60	Extensor digitorum
		Abduction: Spread fingers apart.	30	Interosseus dorsalis
		Adduction: Bring fingers together.	30	Interosseus volaris
Thumb	Saddle 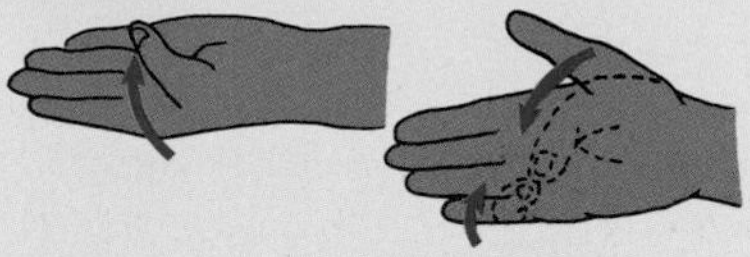	*Flexion:* Move thumb across palmar surface of hand.	90	Flexor pollicis brevis
		Extension: Move thumb straight away from hand.	90	Extensor pollicis longus, extensor pollicis brevis
		Abduction: Extend thumb laterally (usually done when placing fingers in abduction and adduction).	30	Abductor pollicis brevis and longus
		Adduction: Move thumb back toward hand.	30	Adductor pollicis obliquus, adductor pollicis transversus
		Opposition: Touch thumb to each finger of same hand.	—	Opponens pollicis, opponens digiti minimi
Hip	Ball-and-socket 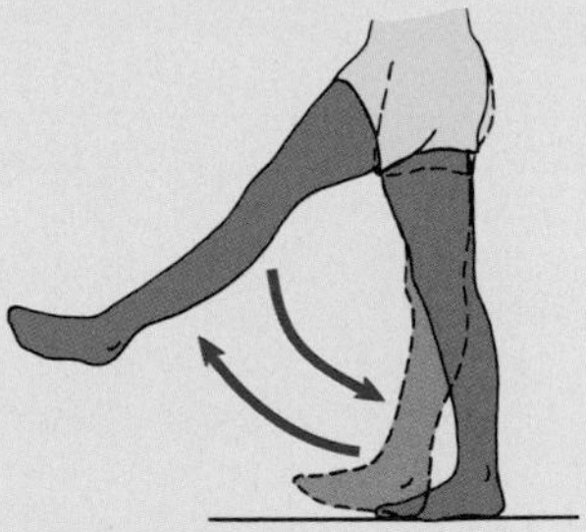	*Flexion:* Move leg forward and up.	110–120	Psoas major, iliacus, sartorius
		Extension: Move leg back, beside other leg.	90–120	Gluteus maximus, semitendinosus, semimembranosus
		Abduction: Move leg laterally away from body.	30–50	Gluteus medius, gluteus minimus
	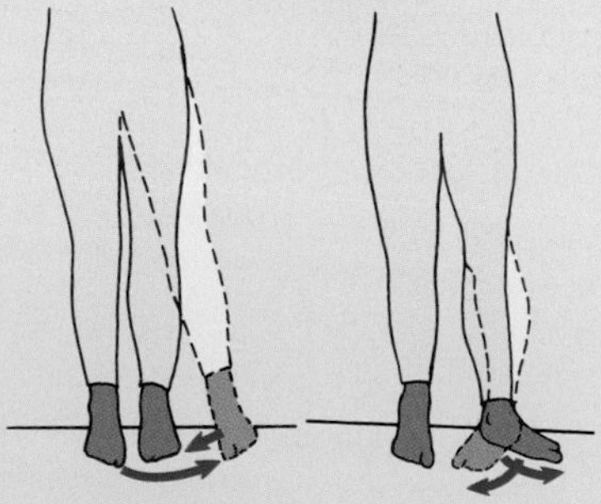	*Adduction:* Move leg back toward medial position and beyond if possible.	30–50	Adductor longus, adductor brevis, adductor magnus
		Internal rotation: Turn foot and leg toward other leg.	45	Gluteus medius, gluteus minimus, tensor fasciae latae
		External rotation: Turn foot and leg away from other leg.	45	Obturatorius internus, obturatorius externus, quadratus femoris, piriformis, gemellus superior and inferior, gluteus maximus
	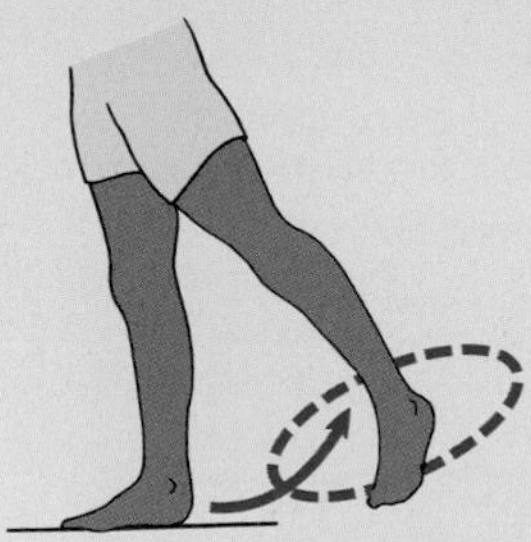	*Circumduction:* Move leg in circle.	120–130	Psoas major, gluteus maximus, gluteus medius, adductor magnus

TABLE 18.2
Range-of-Motion Exercises—cont'd

Body Part	Type of Joint	Type of Movement	Range (Degrees)	Primary Muscles
Knee	Hinge	*Flexion:* Bring heel back toward back of thigh.	120–130	Biceps femoris, semitendinosus, semimembranosus, sartorius
		Extension: Return leg to floor.	120–130	Rectus femoris, vastus lateralis, vastus medialis, vastus intermedius
Ankle	Hinge	*Dorsiflexion:* Move foot so toes are pointed upward.	20–30	Tibialis anterior
		Plantar flexion: Move foot so toes are pointed downward.	45–50	Gastrocnemius, soleus
Foot	Gliding	*Inversion:* Turn sole of foot medially.	≤35	Tibialis anterior, tibialis posterior
		Eversion: Turn sole of foot laterally.	≤10	Peroneus longus, peroneus brevis
Toes	Condyloid	*Flexion:* Curl toes downward.	30–60	Flexor digitorum, lumbricales pedis, flexor hallucis brevis
		Extension: Straighten toes.	30–60	Extensor digitorum longus, extensor digitorum brevis, extensor hallucis longus
		Abduction: Spread toes apart.	≤15	Abductor hallucis, interosseus dorsalis
		Adduction: Bring toes together.	≤15	Adductor hallucis, interosseus plantaris

PROCEDURAL GUIDELINE 18.3 *Applying Graduated Compression (Elastic) Stockings or Sequential Compression Devices*

Purpose

Prolonged recumbence (a position of lying down at rest) leads to circulatory fluid volume loss with a fluid shift to the thoracic area. A patient will diurese, excrete more urine, because of protein loss. A decrease in plasma volume causes the hematocrit to rise, but then fall as the red blood cell mass later decreases. Immobilized patients (even short term) are thus at risk for a deep vein thrombosis (DVT). A thrombus is an accumulation of platelets, fibrin, clotting factors, and cellular elements of the blood attached to the interior wall of a vein or artery, sometimes occluding the lumen of the vessel. Three factors, known as Virchow's triad, contribute to venous thrombus formation: (1) blood stasis resulting from decreased blood flow and increased viscosity, (2) hypercoagulability due to a change in clotting factors or increased platelet activity, and (3) vessel trauma (Huether and McCance, 2017). If a DVT forms, it places a patient at risk for pulmonary emboli (clot travelling to lung), a life-threatening complication. Common risk factors include conditions that affect the Virchow's triad: hypercoagulability (e.g., clotting disorders, fever, dehydration), venous wall abnormalities (e.g., orthopedic surgery, varicose veins), and blood flow stasis (e.g., immobility, obesity, pregnancy; Lewis et al., 2017). Signs of DVT include swelling in the affected leg (rarely swelling in both legs); warm, cyanotic skin; and pain in the leg that often starts in the calf and can feel like cramping or soreness. If a DVT is suspected, keep patient calm and quiet in bed and notify the health care provider. If patients are at high risk for DVT, mechanical thrombo-prophylaxis (use of compression stockings or intermittent sequential compression devices [SCDs]) along with early ambulation and use of anticoagulant therapy are recommended therapies (AHRQ, 2015; Pai and Douketis, 2016; Sachdeva et al., 2014), especially in surgical patients after surgery.

There are two types of sequential compression devices. SCDs consist of inflatable plastic sleeves wrapped around the legs and secured with Velcro. The tubing that inflates the sleeves extends

Continued

PROCEDURAL GUIDELINE 18.3 *Applying Graduated Compression (Elastic) Stockings or Sequential Compression Devices—cont'd*

from the sleeve at the patient's ankles to an air pump that alternately inflates and deflates, providing rhythmic, external extremity compression. Mobile compression devices (MCDs) act physiologically in much the same manner as SCDs. In addition, MCDs like the Active Care+SFT® have a synchronized flow technology that uses an internal sensor to apply pressure around the legs in sync with respiratory-related changes in venous phasic flow to optimize peak venous velocity at lower applied pressures (United Health Care [UHC], 2012). The disposable, inflatable compression sleeves wrap around the lower legs and fasten with Velcro (Topfer, 2016). The sleeves connect to a lightweight pump. The MCDs have an advantage over SCDs because the cords extend up from the waist and can be worn safely during ambulation.

Delegation and Collaboration

The skill of applying and maintaining graduated compression stockings and intermittent SCDs and MCDs may be delegated to nursing assist personnel (NAP). The nurse initially determines the size of elastic stockings and assesses the patient's lower extremities for any signs and symptoms of a DVT or impaired circulation. The nurse directs the NAP to:

- Remove SCD sleeves before allowing a patient to get out of bed.
- Report to the nurse if a patient's calf or thigh appears larger than the other or is red, tender, hot, or swollen or if the patient complains of calf pain.
- Report to the nurse if there is redness, itching, or irritation on the legs (signs of allergic reactions to elastic).
- Report to the nurse if the patient is routinely removing the compression device from the legs.

Equipment

Tape measure; powder or cornstarch *(optional)*; graduated compression stockings or Velcro compression device sleeves; SCD/MCD insufflator with air hoses attached; compression device pump; hygiene supplies; *Option:* cotton stockinette with MCD

Procedural Steps

1. Review medical record for order for SCDs/MCDs or graduated compression stocking.
2. Identify patient using at least two identifiers (e.g., name and birthday or name and account number) according to agency policy (TJC, 2019).
3. Review medical record to assess patient for risk factors for developing DVT (Box 18.1). *An option is to use the Wells Score, an objective and widely used measure for determining a patient's risk for a DVT (Box 18.2) (Modi et al., 2016).*
4. Assess for contraindications for use of elastic stockings or compression devices:
   a. Dermatitis or open skin lesions on area to be covered by stockings/sleeves.
   b. Recent skin graft to lower leg.
   c. Decreased arterial circulation in lower extremities as evidenced by cyanotic, cool extremities, and/or gangrenous conditions affecting the lower limb(s).

BOX 18.1

Risk Factors for Developing Deep Vein Thrombosis

- Injury to a vein, often caused by the following:
  - Fractures
  - Severe muscle injury
  - Major surgery (e g., involving the abdomen, pelvis, hip, or legs)
- Slow blood flow, often caused by the following:
  - Confinement to bed (e.g., caused by a medical condition or after surgery)
  - Limited movement (e.g., a cast on a leg to help heal an injured bone)
  - Sitting for a long time, especially with crossed legs
  - Paralysis
- Increased estrogen, often caused by the following:
  - Birth control pills
  - Hormone replacement therapy, sometimes used after menopause
  - Pregnancy, for up to 6 weeks after giving birth
- Certain chronic medical illnesses, such as the following:
  - Heart disease, lung disease, cancer and its treatment, inflammatory bowel disease (Crohn's disease or ulcerative colitis)
- Other factors include the following:
  - Previous DVT or PE
  - Family history of DVT or PE
  - Age (risk increases as age increases)
  - Obesity
  - A catheter located in a central vein

DVT, Deep vein thrombosis; *PE,* pulmonary embolism.
Data from The American College of Obstetricians and Gynecologists: Preventing deep vein thrombosis, August 2011. http://www.acog.org/Patients/FAQs/Preventing-Deep-Vein-Thrombosis; Centers for Disease Control and Prevention (CDC): Venous thromboembolism (blood clots), 2015. http://www.cdc.gov/ncbddd/dvt/facts.html.

BOX 18.2

Wells Score

Parameter	Score
Active cancer (patient receiving treatment for cancer within previous 6 months or currently receiving palliative treatment)	1
Paralysis, paresis, or recent plaster immobilization of lower extremities	1
Recently bedridden for 3 days or more, or major surgery within previous 12 weeks requiring general or regional anesthesia	1
Localized tenderness along distribution of the deep vein system	1
Entire leg swollen	1
Calf swelling at least 3 cm more when compared with asymptomatic leg	1
Pitting edema localized to symptomatic leg	1
Collateral superficial veins	1
Previously documented DVT	1
Alternative diagnosis as likely or greater than that of DVT	–2

DVT, Deep vein thrombosis.
Wells scoring system for DVT: –2 to 0: low probability, 1 to 2 points: Moderate probability, 3 to 8 points: high probability.
From Modi S, Deisler R, Gozel K, et al: Wells criteria for DVT is a reliable clinical tool to assess the risk of deep venous thrombosis in trauma patients. *World J Emerg Surg* 11:24, 2016.

PROCEDURAL GUIDELINE 18.3 *Applying Graduated Compression (Elastic) Stockings or Sequential Compression Devices—cont'd*

   d. If signs/symptoms of a DVT are present, do not manipulate the leg to apply stockings. Manipulation could cause a clot in the vein within the leg to dislodge.

5. Perform hand hygiene. Assess condition of patient's skin and circulation to the legs. Palpate pedal pulses, note any palpable veins, and inspect skin over lower extremities for edema, skin discoloration, warmth, presence of lesions. Reduces transmission of microorganisms. Determines condition of patient's skin and circulation to the legs in area that will be covered by stockings/sleeves.

6. Assess patient's or family caregiver's knowledge or experience regarding previous use of elastic compression stockings or compression devices. Assess patient's or family caregiver's health literacy.

7. Explain procedure and reason for applying elastic stockings/SCD/MCD to prevent DVT.

8. Close room curtains or door to provide privacy. Position patient in supine position.

9. Perform hand hygiene. Bathe patient's legs as needed. Dry thoroughly. Perform hand hygiene.

10. **Apply graduated compression stocking:**

   a. Use tape measure to measure patient's leg to determine proper elastic stocking size (follow package directions).

   b. *Option:* Apply a small amount of powder or cornstarch to legs provided patient does not have sensitivity.

   c. Turn elastic stocking inside out: Place one hand into stocking, holding heel of stocking. Take other hand and pull stocking inside out until reaching the heel (see illustration).

   d. Place patient's toes into foot of elastic stocking up to the heel, making sure that stocking is smooth (see illustration A). Slide remaining portion of stocking over patient's foot, making sure that toes are covered. Make sure that foot fits into toe and heel position of stocking. Stocking will now be right side out (see illustration B).

   e. Slide stocking up over patient's calf until sock is completely extended. Be sure that stocking is smooth and that no ridges or wrinkles are present (see illustration).

   f. Instruct patient not to roll stockings partially down, avoid wrinkles, avoid crossing legs, and elevate legs while sitting.

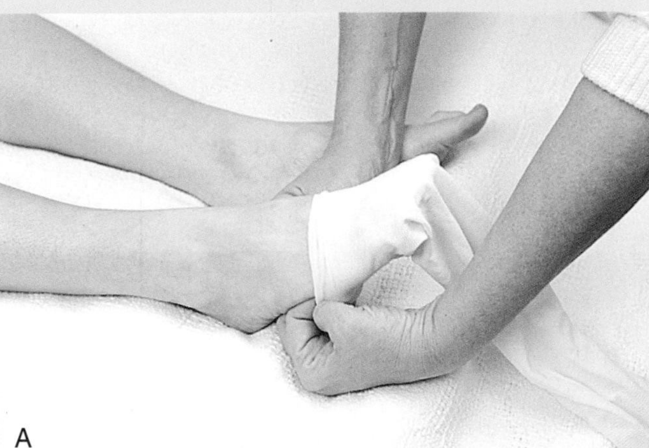

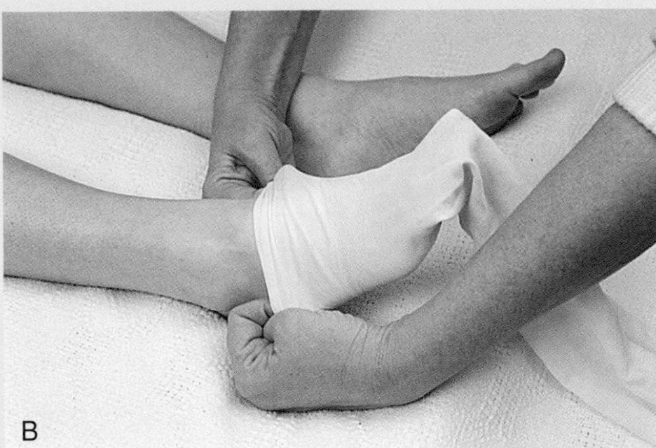

STEP 10d (A) Place toes into foot of stocking. (B) Slide remaining part of stocking over foot.

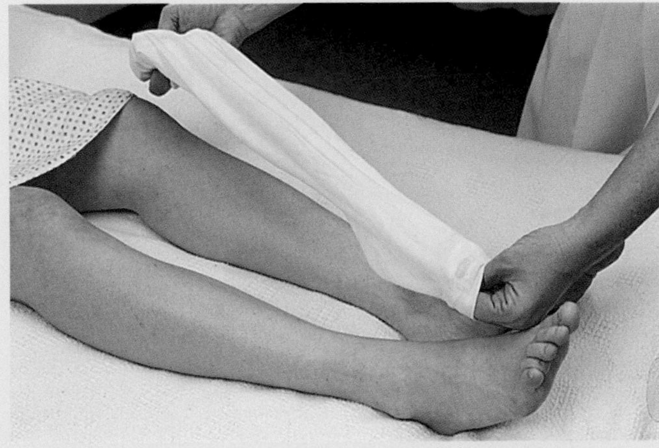

STEP 10c Turn stocking inside out; hold heel and pull through.

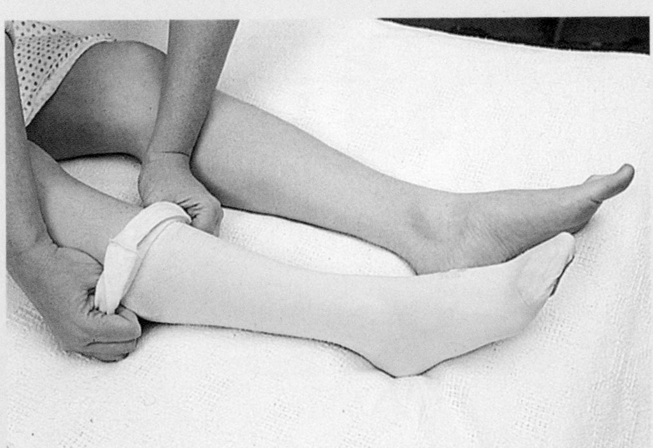

STEP 10e Slide sock up leg until completely extended.

Continued

PROCEDURAL GUIDELINE 18.3 *Applying Graduated Compression (Elastic) Stockings or Sequential Compression Devices—cont'd*

11. **Apply SCD sleeve(s):**
    a. Remove SCD sleeves from plastic cover; unfold and flatten onto bed.
    b. Arrange SCD sleeve under patient's leg according to leg position indicated on inner lining of sleeve.
    c. Place patient's leg on SCD sleeve. Back of ankle should line up with ankle marking on inner lining of sleeve.
    d. Position back of knee with popliteal opening on inner sleeve (see illustration).
    e. Wrap SCD sleeve securely around patient's leg. Check fit of SCD sleeve by placing two fingers between patient's leg and sleeve (see illustration).
    f. Attach SCD sleeve connector to plug on mechanical unit. Arrows on connector line up with arrows on plug from mechanical unit (see illustration).
    g. Turn mechanical unit on. Green light indicates that unit is functioning. Monitor functioning SCD through one full cycle of inflation and deflation.
12. **Apply MCD sleeve (example: Calf Sleeve ActiveCare+SFT® Application):**
    a. A cotton stockinette is provided along with the calf sleeves. Apply over patient's calves.

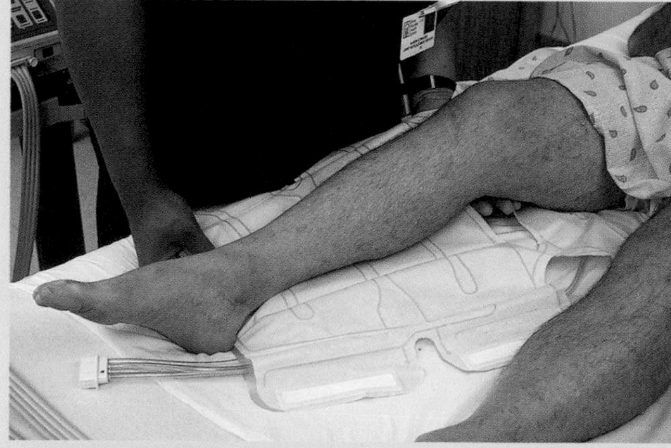

STEP 11d Position back of patient's knee with popliteal opening.

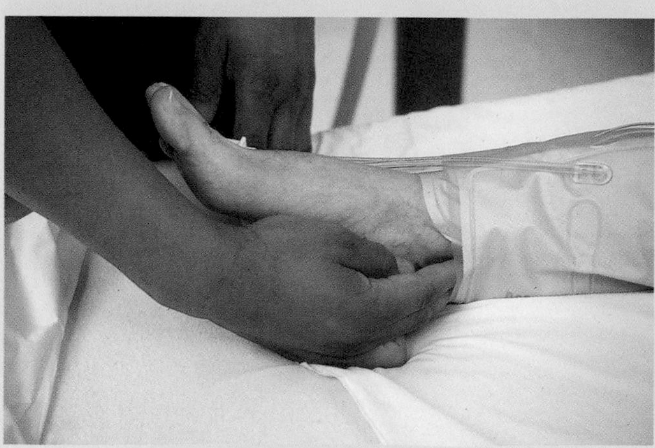

STEP 11e Check fit of SCD sleeve.

    b. Wrap the sleeve smoothly around the patient's calf and fasten it beginning at the top, moving toward the bottom.
    c. Place two fingers between patient's calf and sleeve to be sure it is snug but not too tight (see illustration).
    d. The device has two identical extension tubes (see illustration). Use either end of the extension tube to connect to the sleeve or device pump.

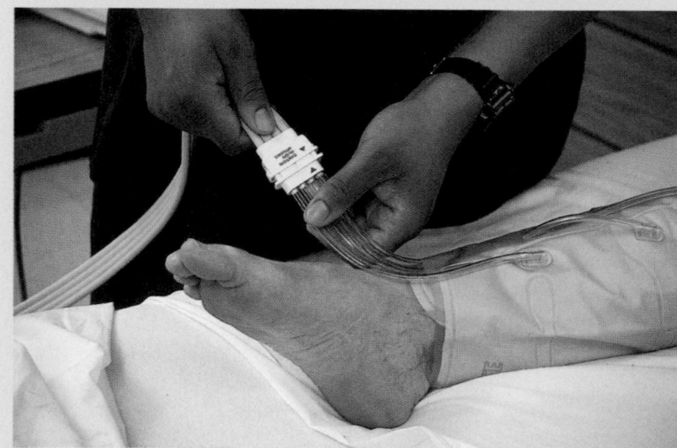

STEP 11f Align arrows when connecting plug to mechanical unit.

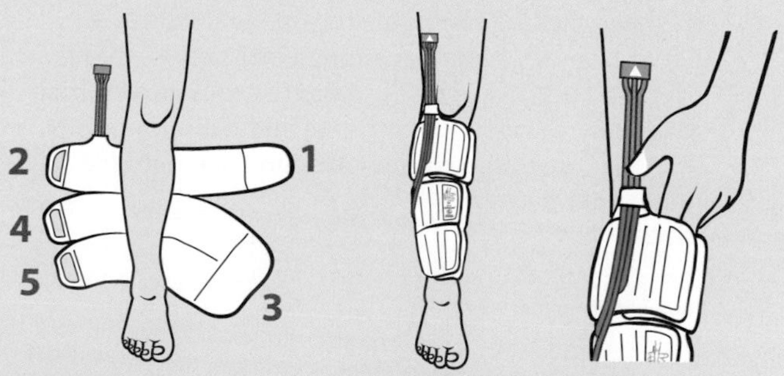

STEP 12c Application of ActiveCare+SFT® MCD to calves. *(Courtesy Zimmer Biomet.)*

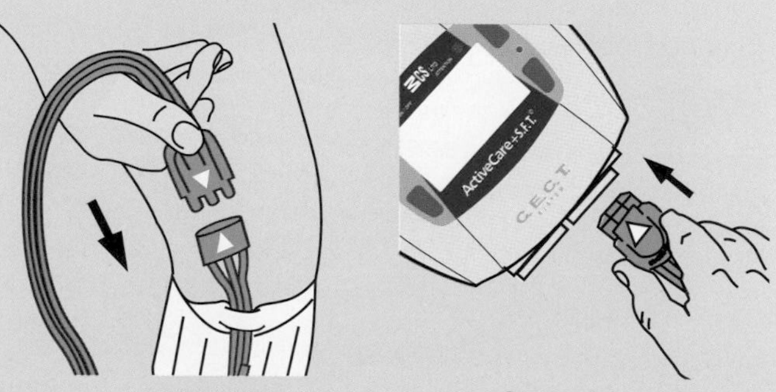

STEP 12d Application of ActiveCare+SFT® MCD connector hose to pump. *(Courtesy Zimmer Biomet.)*

PROCEDURAL GUIDELINE 18.3 *Applying Graduated Compression (Elastic) Stockings or Sequential Compression Devices—cont'd*

(1) Connect one end of the extension tube to the sleeve connector. The white arrows should be pointed toward each other.
(2) Connect the other end of the extension tube to the device pump. The white arrow should be facing upward.

e. Press the power switch located at the back of the device to ON position (see illustration). After turning the device on, the Configuration Setup Screen is shown on the liquid crystal display (LCD) screen, and the sleeves should immediately start to inflate, from the bottom to the top.

f. Wait 60 seconds for the automatic operation of the device. The device automatically identifies which sleeves are connected, selects the suitable treatment mode, and will display information on the main LCD screen.

13. Position patient comfortably, and then place the nurse call system in an accessible location within the patient's reach.

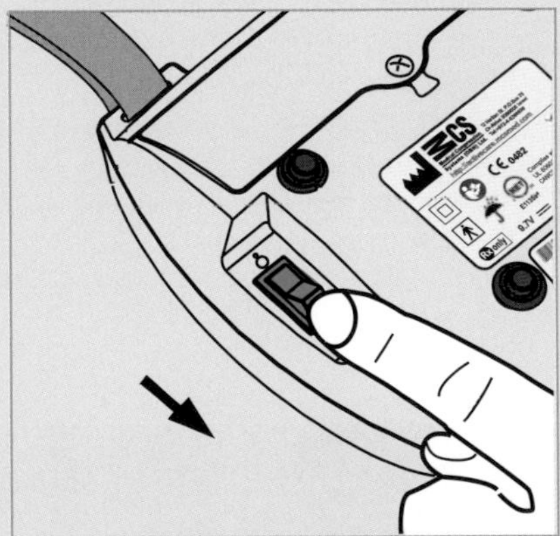

STEP 12e Powering on ActiveCare+SFT® MCD. *(Courtesy Zimmer Biomet.)*

Safe Patient Care *Caution patient to not exit bed and walk with SCDs in place. Have patient call for assistance. The patient may walk with MCD in place (see illustration).*

14. Raise side rails (as appropriate) and lower bed to lowest position. Perform hand hygiene.
15. Remove compression stockings or SCD/MCD sleeves at least once per shift (e.g., long enough to inspect skin for irritation or breakdown and to determine patient's comfort level).
16. Evaluate skin integrity and circulation to patient's lower extremities as ordered (see agency policy).
17. Record condition of lower extremities, application of stockings/SCDs/MCD, and patient response to education.

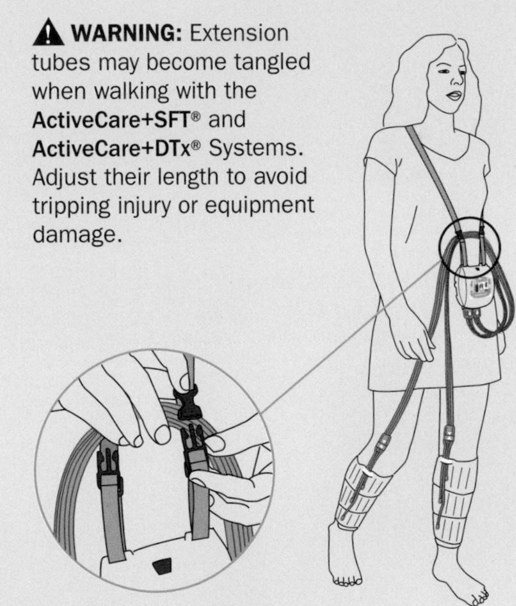

⚠ WARNING: Extension tubes may become tangled when walking with the ActiveCare+SFT® and ActiveCare+DTx® Systems. Adjust their length to avoid tripping injury or equipment damage.

STEP 13 Walking with ActiveCare+SFT® MCD. *(Courtesy Zimmer Biomet.)*

✦ SKILL 18.2 Use of Canes, Crutches, and Walkers

Purpose

Assist devices such as canes, crutches, and walkers are recommended for patients who cannot bear full weight on one or more joints of the lower extremities. Other indications for use are instability, poor balance, or pain in weight bearing. A benefit of using an assist device includes reduction in risk of falling, decreased pain with mobility, improved balance with ambulation, and increased confidence with mobility (Touhy and Jett, 2018). However, an assist device can be a risk for falling if the device is not used correctly. Know a patient's weight-bearing status, any specific movement precautions, and the type of device ordered by the health care provider. You will collaborate with a physical therapist to help a patient use the assist device correctly and safely. Table 18.3 summarizes the types of assist devices.

Delegation and Collaboration

The skill of assisting patients with ambulation using an assist device can be delegated to nursing assist personnel (NAP). The nurse should conduct the initial assessment when a patient is ambulating for the first time. The nurse directs the NAP to:

- Have a patient dangle following lying in bed before ambulation.
- Immediately return a patient to the bed or chair if he or she is nauseated, dizzy, pale, or diaphoretic or blood pressure (BP) drops, and report these signs and symptoms to the nurse immediately.
- Apply safe, nonskid shoes on the patient and ensure that the environment is free of clutter and there is no moisture on the floor before ambulating the patient.

TABLE 18.3
Types of Assist Devices

Type of Device	Features	Measurement
Canes: lightweight, easily movable devices approximately waist high, made of wood or metal. Two types: single straight-legged and quad (Fig. 18.1).	Straight canes provide support and balance for patients who have mild balance or strength impairments. Quad canes are often used for patients who have unilateral weakness from a neurological event/disease (e.g., stroke) and require more support than a straight cane. Patient keeps the cane on the stronger side of the body (Pierson et al., 2017). Nurse stands on the patient's weak side for support (Pierson et al., 2017).	Have patient stand upright with arms relaxed down with normal bend at the elbow (15–30 degrees). The handle of the cane should be close to the patient's wrist crease. Cane handle should fit comfortably in palm of hand.
Crutches: wooden or metal staff. Two types of crutches: double adjustable Lofstrand or forearm crutch (Fig. 18.2) and the axillary wooden or metal crutch.	Use of crutches is usually temporary (e.g., after ligament damage to the knee). Some patients, such as those with paralysis of the lower extremities, need crutches permanently.	Measurements include the patient's height, the angle of elbow flexion, and the distance between the crutch pad and the axilla. Standing: Position crutches with crutch tips at 15 cm (6 inches) laterally to side and 15 cm in front of patient's feet (tripod position). Crutch pads should be 3.75–5 cm (1½ to 2 inches, or 2–3 finger widths) under axilla with the elbows slightly flexed at 20–25 degrees (American College of Foot and Ankle Surgeons, 2016; Pierson et al., 2017; Fig. 18.3). Supine: Crutch pad is approximately 5 cm (2 inches, or 2–3 finger widths) under axilla with crutch tips positioned 15 cm (6 inches) lateral to patient's heel (Fig. 18.4). Height of handgrips must be adjusted so patient's elbow is flexed 15–30 degrees or it sits at approximately height of wrist crease. Both height of crutch and handgrip dimensions are adjustable on a well-made crutch.
Walkers: extremely light, movable devices, approximately waist high and made of metal tubing (Fig. 18.5). They have four widely placed, sturdy legs. They can also have 2–4 wheels.	Has a wide base of support, providing stability and security when walking.	Have patient step inside walker. When patient relaxes arms at side of body and stands up straight, top of walker should line up with crease on inside of wrist). Elbows should flex about 15–30 degrees when standing inside walker, with hands on handgrips (American Academy of Orthopaedist Surgeons, 2015; Pierson et al., 2017).

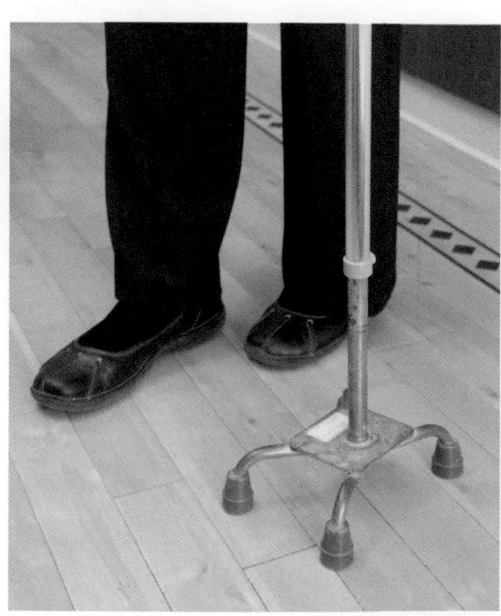

FIG 18.1 Base of quad cane.

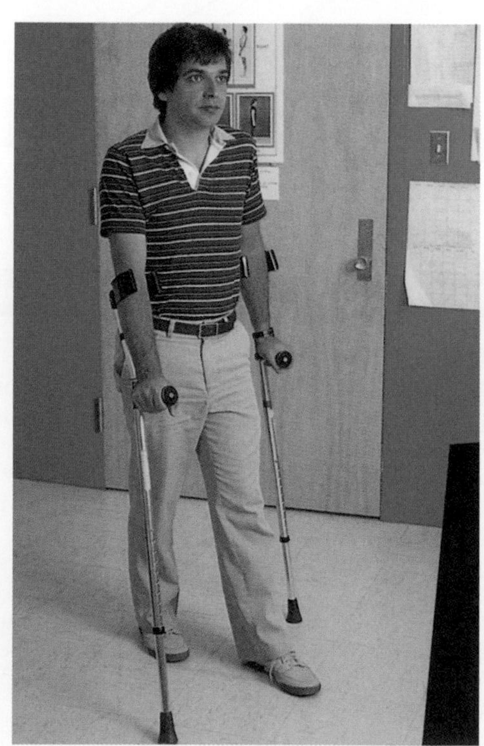

FIG 18.2 Double adjustable Lofstrand or forearm crutch.

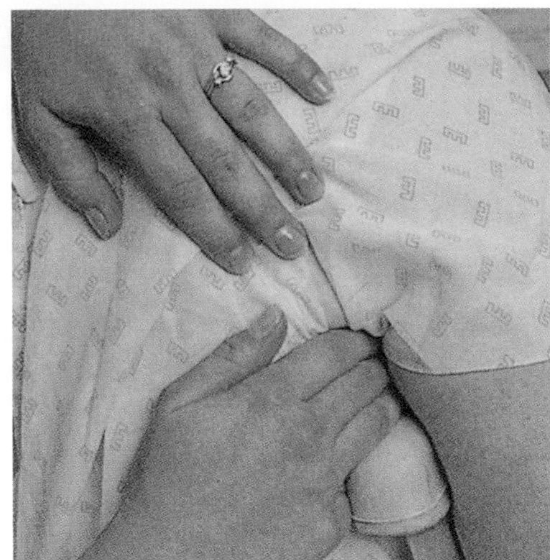
FIG 18.3 Crutch pad is 2 to 3 finger widths under axilla.

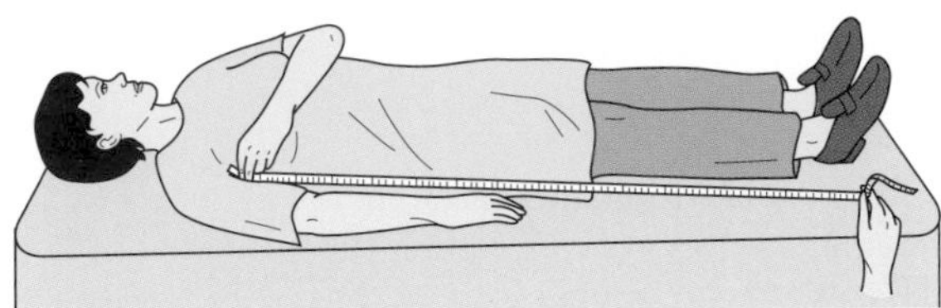
FIG 18.4 Measuring length of crutch with patient in bed.

Equipment

- Assist device (cane, crutches, walker)
- Well-fitting, nonskid flat shoes or slippers
- Robe; well-fitting pants or dress
- Transfer (gait) belt

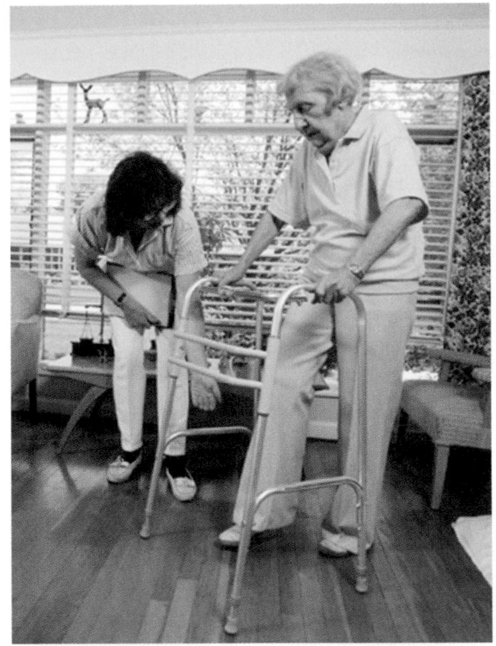
FIG 18.5 Patient using a walker.

ASSESSMENT

1. Identify patient using at least two identifiers (e.g., name and birthday or name and medical record number) according to agency policy. *Rationale: Ensures correct patient. Complies with The Joint Commission standards and improves patient safety (TJC, 2019).*
2. Complete assessment steps in Skill 18.1, Steps 2–9. *Rationale: Determines patient's ability to ambulate with a device and readiness for learning necessary gaits and precautions.*

STEP	RATIONALE
PLANNING	
1. Expected outcomes following completion of procedure:	
• Patient ambulates using assist device without injury.	Appropriate level of assistance with device ensures patient's safety.
• Patient ambulates without excessive fatigue or dizziness and with return of vital signs to baseline 3 to 5 minutes after rest.	Assist device chosen requires minimal exertion. Patient tolerates exercise.
• Patient demonstrates correct use of assist device, gait pattern, and weight-bearing status.	Demonstrates learning and physical ability to use device.
2. Explain to patient how you are going to prepare for ambulation (e.g., transfer technique out of bed and safety precautions to be used while walking). Explain benefits and reasons for activity/exercise. Do so in a way that matches patient's educational level and beliefs and values regarding recovery or maintaining health.	Exercise self-efficacy is an important predictor of the adoption and maintenance of exercise behaviors. Self-efficacy is a belief and conviction that one can successfully perform a given activity (Shieh et al., 2015).
3. Explain and demonstrate specific gait technique to patient or family caregiver.	Teaching and demonstration enhance learning, reduce anxiety, and encourage cooperation.
4. Perform hand hygiene. Check for appropriate height and fit of assist device (see Table 18.3). If physical therapist has seen patient, the device should be at appropriate height. **NOTE:** *This is usually done when patient is standing at side of bed and is stable.*	Ensures that patient is able to ambulate successfully without injury using device.
5. Make sure that ambulation device has clean, dry rubber tips.	Prevents device from slipping.
6. Provide privacy and prepare environment.	Providing privacy and preparing the environment early help you think about the need to remove clutter from the over-bed or bedside table.

STEP	RATIONALE

Safe Patient Care *Remove obstacles from pathways, including throw rugs (in the home), fall pads, and electrical cords; wipe up any spills immediately. Avoid crowds. Crowds increase the risk of the crutch, cane, or walker being kicked or jarred and patient losing balance.*

IMPLEMENTATION

STEP	RATIONALE
1. Perform hand hygiene.	
2. If using crutches, have patient report any tingling or numbness in upper torso while ambulating.	Helps indicate that crutches are being used incorrectly or that they are the wrong size.
3. Help patient from lying position to side of bed (see Skill 18.1) or up from chair.	Ensures that patient is stable and ready to ambulate.
4. Allow patient to sit on the side of the bed for 2 to 3 minutes and dangle by alternately flexing and extending feet and moving lower legs up and down. Ask if patient feels dizzy; if so, check blood pressure. Have patient relax and take a few deep breaths until dizziness subsides and balance is gained. If dizziness lasts more than 60 seconds or if systolic blood pressure has dropped at least 20 mm Hg within 3 minutes of sitting upright, return patient to bed (Frith et al., 2014; Mills et al., 2014; Shibao et al., 2013). Recheck blood pressure.	Allows patient's circulation to equilibrate to reduce chance of orthostatic hypotension. Patient cannot be safely ambulated if dizziness develops.
5. Apply gait belt around patient's waist. Be sure that it completely circles patient's waist. Place belt low and be sure that it is snug. You may need to adjust belt once patient stands. You hold belt along patient's back with your palms facing up as patient walks.	Gait belt allows you to maintain stability of patient during transfer and reduces risk for falling (Degelau et al., 2014; OSHA, 2014).
6. Help patient stand at bedside. Recheck height of device (see Table 18.3) to make sure that it is correct size. Have patient stand fully erect with shoulders back and looking ahead (not at floor). Now reassess patient's ability to bear weight and maintain balance.	Ensures that patient begins ambulation with correct posture and position. Non–weight-bearing status requires a patient to support weight on the assist device and unaffected limb. The affected leg is kept off the floor at all times. Partial or touch-down weight bearing is similar to that for non–weight-bearing status, except that less weight is placed on the affected limb. Total weight bearing allows a patient to distribute equal weight between each limb with minimal weight on the assist device.
7. If patient is unsteady, seat him or her in chair or return to bed immediately.	Patient may require strengthening exercises or evaluation of balance by physical therapist.
8. Decide with patient how far to ambulate. Attempt to walk further than previous time.	Determines mutual goal.
9. Implement ambulation around patient's other activities.	Taking scheduled rest periods between activities reduces patient fatigue.
10. Help patient walk with cane (steps are the same with standard, tripod, or quad cane):	
a. Have patient hold cane on unaffected **(strong)** side of body and stand to the side and slightly behind the patient while holding on to the gait belt. Direct patient to place cane forward 15 to 25 cm (6–10 inches) and slightly to the side of the foot, keeping body weight on both legs. Allow approximately 15- to 30-degree elbow flexion.	Offers most support when on stronger side of body. Cane and weaker leg work together with each step.
b. Instruct patient to advance affected leg forward, even with the cane.	Body weight is supported by cane and unaffected leg.
c. Have patient advance unaffected leg 15 to 25 cm (6–10 inches) even with the cane and the affected leg.	Aligns patient's center of gravity. Returns patient body weight to equal distribution.
d. Repeat sequence of three steps as patient tolerates. Once comfortable, the patient can advance the cane and affected leg together followed by the unaffected leg.	
11. Help patient crutch walk by using appropriate crutch gait:	To use crutches, patient supports self with hands and arms; therefore ability to balance body in upright position and stamina are necessary. Type of crutch gait depends on patient's weight-bearing status.

STEP	RATIONALE
a. Four-point gait:	This is most stable crutch gait. It provides at least three points of support at all times. Patient must be able to bear weight on both legs. Patient moves each leg alternately with each opposing crutch so that three points of support are on floor all the time. Often used when patient has some form of paralysis (e.g., children with spastic cerebral palsy; Hockenberry and Wilson, 2017). May also be used for arthritic patients.
(1) Begin in tripod position (see illustration). Have patient place the crutch tips about 4 to 6 inches (10–15 cm) to the side and in front of each foot (American College of Foot and Ankle Surgeons, 2016). Have patient place weight on handgrips, not under arms.	Improves balance by providing wide base of support. Patient should have posture of erect head and neck, straight vertebrae, and extended hips and knees.
(2) Move right crutch forward 10 to 15 cm (4–6 inches) (see illustration A).	Crutch and foot position is similar to arm and foot position during normal walking.
(3) Move left foot forward to level of left crutch (see illustration B).	
(4) Move left crutch forward 10 to 15 cm (4–6 inches) (see illustration C).	
(5) Move right foot forward to level of right crutch (see illustration D).	
(6) Repeat above sequence.	

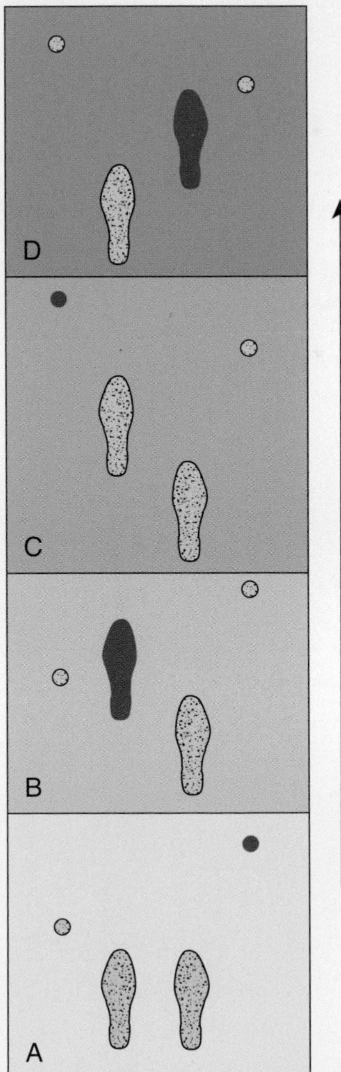

STEP 11a(2-5) Four-point gait. Solid feet and crutch tips show foot and crutch tip movement in each of four phases. (A) Right tip moves forward. (B) Left foot moves toward left crutch. (C) Left crutch tip moves forward. (D) Right foot moves toward right crutch. (Read from bottom to top.)

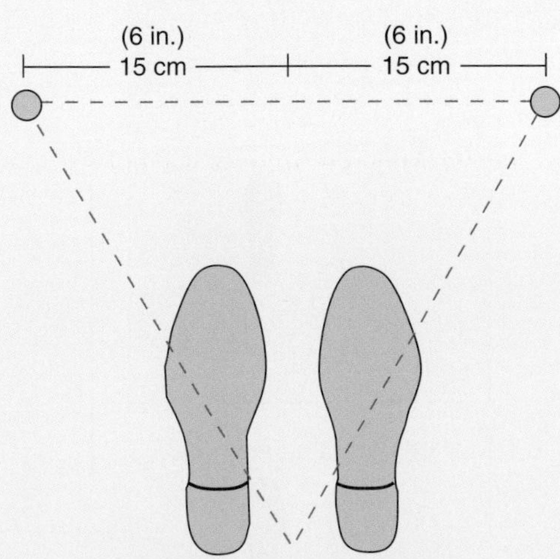

STEP 11a(1) Tripod position.

STEP	RATIONALE
b. Three-point gait (see illustrations) appropriate for patients who can toe touch, have partial weight bearing and weight bearing as tolerated:	Requires patient to bear all weight on one foot. Weight is borne on unaffected leg and then on both crutches. Affected leg does not touch ground during early phase of three-point gait. May be useful for patient with broken leg or sprained ankle.
(1) Begin in tripod position (see illustration A), with patient standing on weight-bearing foot.	Improves patient's balance by providing wide base of support.
(2) Advance both crutches and affected leg, keeping foot of involved leg off floor (see illustration B).	
(3) Move weight-bearing leg forward, stepping or hopping on floor (see illustration C).	
(4) Repeat sequence.	
c. Two-point gait (see illustrations) appropriate for weight bearing as tolerated or full weight bearing on each foot:	Is faster gait than four-point gait. Requires more balance because only two points support body at one time.
(1) Begin in tripod position (see illustration A).	Improves patient's balance by providing wide base of support.
(2) Move left crutch and right foot forward (see illustration B).	Crutch movements are similar to arm movement during normal walking; patient moves crutch at same time as opposing leg.
(3) Move right crutch and left foot forward (see illustration C).	
(4) Repeat sequence.	
d. Swing-to gait:	Used by patients whose lower extremities are paralyzed or who wear weight-supporting braces on their legs.
(1) Begin in tripod position.	This is the easier of two swinging gaits. It requires ability to partially bear body weight on both legs.
(2) Move both crutches forward.	
(3) Lift and swing legs to crutches, letting crutches support body weight.	
(4) Repeat two previous steps.	
e. Swing-through gait:	Requires that patient have ability to bear partial weight on both feet.
(1) Begin in tripod position.	Improves patient's balance by providing wide base of support.

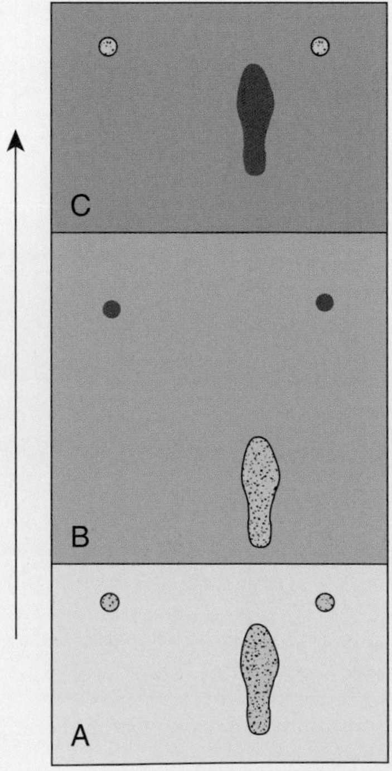

STEP 11b (A–C) Three-point gait with weight borne on unaffected right leg. Solid foot and crutch tips show weight bearing in each phase, A–C. (Read from bottom to top.)

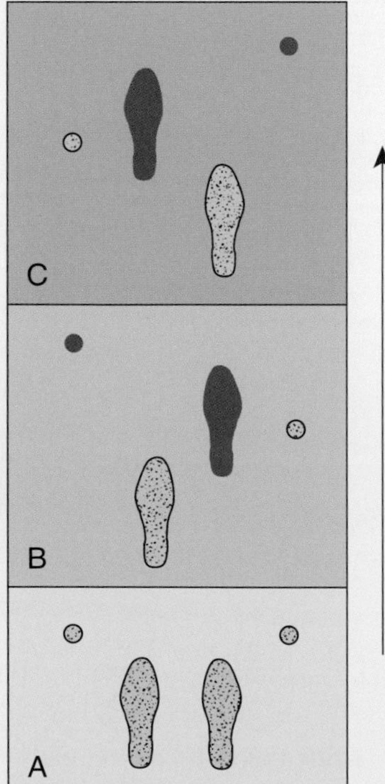

STEP 11c (A–C) Two-point gait. Solid areas indicate weight-bearing leg and crutch tips, A–C. (Read from bottom to top.)

STEP	RATIONALE
(2) Move both crutches forward.	Initial placement of crutches increases patient's base of support so that when body swings forward, patient is moving center of gravity toward additional support provided by crutches.
(3) Lift and swing legs through and beyond crutches.	
(4) Repeat previous steps.	
12. Help patient climb up stairs with a railing with crutches (partial weight bearing, one leg):	Climbing stairs with use of a railing is safest way for patient with crutches to ascend stairs.

Safe Patient Care *There is a risk for falling using this technique. Monitor patient's balance carefully. See following option (see Step 12i).*

STEP	RATIONALE
a. Be sure there are no obstacles on the stairs, such as stacks of magazines or other items. Have patient begin in tripod position and then hold the handrail with one hand (strong leg next to railing).	Improves patient's balance by providing wide base of support.
b. You carry the crutch positioned next to the handrail as the patient holds the other crutch.	
c. Patient transfers body weight to crutch.	Prepares patient to transfer weight to unaffected leg when ascending first stair.
d. Have patient hold handrail with one hand	Ensures patient safety.
e. Stay behind the patient holding the gait belt. Then have the patient support his or her weight evenly between the handrail and crutch.	Achieves better balance. Reduces risk of patient fall.
f. Patient next places some weight on crutch and then steps up with first step with weight-bearing foot (uninvolved leg). Have patient get his or her balance.	Places most weight on stronger leg. Balance reduces risk of fall.
g. Patient then straightens uninvolved knee and lifts his or her body weight, bringing crutch and affected leg up the stair.	
h. Repeat sequence of steps until patient reaches top of stairs. Observe patient's balance and level of fatigue.	Monitors patient tolerance.
i. *Option:* Have patient sit on the lower stair. If distance and reach allow, place the crutches at the top of the staircase. If this isn't possible, have patient place crutches as far up the stairs as he or she can, then patient will move them to the top as he or she progresses up the stairs (American College of Foot and Ankle Surgeons, 2018).	
(1) In the seated position, have patient reach behind with both arms.	
(2) Then have patient use arms and weight-bearing foot/leg to lift up one step.	
(3) Repeat process one step at a time.	
13. Help patient descend stairs with a railing with crutch (partial weight bearing, one leg):	

Safe Patient Care *There is a risk for falling using this technique. Monitor patient's balance carefully. See following option (see Step 13g).*

STEP	RATIONALE
a. Begin in tripod position.	Improves patient's balance by providing wide base of support.
b. Place both crutches under the patient's axilla and then have the patient hold on to the handrail.	Prepares patient to release support of body weight maintained by crutches.
c. Have patient hold handrail with one hand (affected leg next to railing). Stand below the patient while holding onto the gait belt to guard the patient on the steps.	Nurse's position reduces fall risk.
d. Have patient bend his or her unaffected knee while moving crutches followed by moving the affected leg down a step.	
e. Patient then supports his or her weight evenly between handrail and crutch. Be sure that patient has good balance.	
f. Have patient slowly bring the unaffected leg down step. Caution patient not to hop.	Hopping could injure leg and create risk for fall.

STEP	RATIONALE
g. *Option:* Have patient sit on the lower stair. If distance and reach allow, place the crutches at the top of the staircase. If this isn't possible, have patient place crutches as far up the stairs as he or she can, then patient will move them to the top as he or she progresses up the stairs (American College of Foot and Ankle Surgeons, 2018).	
(1) In the seated position, have patient reach behind with both arms.	
(2) Then have patient use arms and weight-bearing foot/leg to lift up one step.	
(3) Repeat process one step at a time.	
14. **Help patient ambulate with walker:**	Patients who are able to bear partial weight use walkers.
a. Have patient stand straight in center of walker, looking forward and grasping handgrips on upper bars.	Patient balances self before attempting to walk.
b. Have patient move walker comfortable distance forward, about 15 to 25 cm (6–10 inches). Patient then takes step forward with involved leg first and follows through with good leg. Instruct patient not to advance leg past the front bar of walker. If patient has equal strength in both legs, it makes no difference which leg advances first.	Provides broad base of support between walker and patient. Patient then moves center of gravity toward walker. Keeping all four feet of walker on floor is necessary to prevent tipping walker.
c. If patient is unable to bear weight on involved leg, have him or her slowly hop to center of walker using strong leg, supporting weight on hands.	
d. Instruct patient not to try to climb stairs with walker unless he or she has specific walker for steps.	Patient should use handrails as alternative. Using walker could cause a fall.
15. Attend to a patient when using an assist device until you are assured that the patient has sufficient strength and understands how to use device.	Promotes patient safety.
16. After patient ambulates, help him or her back to bed or chair and help assume comfortable position.	
17. Be sure nurse call system is in an accessible location within patient's reach.	Ensures patient can call for assistance if needed.
18. Raise side rails (as appropriate) and lower bed to lowest position.	Ensures patient safety.
19. Perform hand hygiene.	Reduces transmission of microorganisms.

EVALUATION

1. After ambulation, obtain patient's vital signs, observe skin color, and ask about his or her comfort and energy levels.	Evaluates how patient tolerated ambulation.
2. Evaluate patient's subjective statements regarding experience.	Evaluates activity tolerance and if any anxiety present.
3. Evaluate patient's gait pattern: observe body alignment in standing position and balance during gait.	Determines if patient is using supportive aids for ambulation correctly. Keep in mind patient's previous manner of ambulating when assessing gait.
4. **Use Teach-Back:** "You have done well walking with your walker. We reviewed with your wife how to place a gait belt. I talked about why it is important for your wife to use a gait belt to help you at first. Can both of you tell me why a gait belt is important?" Revise your instruction now or develop a plan for revised patient/family caregiver teaching if patient/family caregiver is not able to teach back correctly.	Determines patient's/family caregiver's level of understanding of instructional topic.

Unexpected Outcomes	Related Interventions
1. Patient is unable to ambulate because of fear of falling, physical discomfort, low endurance, upper-body muscles that are too weak to use ambulation device, or lower extremities that are too weak to support body weight.	• Consult with physical therapist about possible exercise program to strengthen muscles or other alternative methods that patient can use for ambulation. • Provide analgesic for discomfort. • Discuss with patient fears or concerns about walking using assist device.

Unexpected Outcomes	Related Interventions
2. Patient sustains an injury.	• Notify health care provider. • Return patient to bed if injury stable. • Document per institution/agency policy.
3. When using assist device, patient bends over and does not stand straight.	• Reinforce correct posture.

Recording

- Record type of device and gait patient used, weight-bearing status, amount of assistance required, tolerance of activity, and distance walked. Document instructions given to patient and family.
- Document your evaluation of patient learning.

Hand-Off Reporting

- Immediately report any injury sustained during attempts to ambulate, alteration in vital signs, or inability to ambulate.

✦ SKILL 18.3 Care of a Patient With an Immobilization Device

Purpose

Immobilization devices increase stability of bones and joints, support an extremity, or reduce the load on weight-bearing structures such as hips, knees, or ankles (Table 18.4). A splint immobilizes and protects a body part. Slings provide support, immobilization, and elevation of the arm or shoulder following injury or surgery. An abduction splint or pillow (Fig. 18.6) is used after hip-replacement surgery to maintain a patient's legs in an abducted position. Cloth and foam splints, known as *immobilizers*, provide long-term immobilization (Fig. 18.7). Medical device–related pressure injuries can result from the use of devices designed and applied for diagnostic or therapeutic purposes. In the case of immobilization devices, the resultant pressure injury generally conforms to the pattern or shape of the device (NDNQI, 2017). It is a nursing responsibility to carefully assess the skin prior to device placement and then evaluate on an ongoing basis. In addition, if a device is applied too tightly there can be compression, causing reduction in circulation to the extremity.

Delegation and Collaboration

The skill of caring for a patient wearing a brace/splint/sling can be delegated to nursing assistive personnel (NAP). The nurse instructs the NAP by:

- Reviewing prescribed schedule of wear and activities permitted while in the brace/splint/sling.
- Reviewing any special observations that might be required based on device.
- Instructing to inform the nurse if the patient complains of pain, rubbing, or pressure from the brace/splint/sling or if a change occurs in patient's skin condition under device develops.

TABLE 18.4
Immobilization Devices

Device	Uses and Benefits	Features
Soft splints	Temporary splints reduce pain and prevent tissue damage from further motion immediately after an injury (e.g., fracture or sprain). Air splints, Thomas splints, and improvised splints from materials on hand are examples of temporary splints applied in emergency situations.	Available commercially or can be made for almost any body part. Velcro or buckle closures permit these devices to be adjusted to fit a body part of almost any size and shape.
Molded splints	Provide support to patients with chronic injuries or diseases such as arthritis. Maintain the body part in a functional position to prevent contractures and muscle atrophy during the period of disuse.	Made of plastic, which can be cleaned with a washcloth and warm soap and water. Can be removed quickly for assessment of the skin or a wound.
Abduction pillow	Permits a patient to be turned without changing the position of the healing limb. Prevents dislocation of the hip prosthesis.	The pillow is easily removed for nursing care (e.g., skin care, dressing changes, and neurovascular assessments).
Immobilizers	Immobilizers treat sprains and dislocations that do not require complete and continuous immobilization in a cast or traction.	Common types of immobilizers include cervical collars (soft or hard), belt-type shoulder immobilizers, and knee immobilizers.
Braces	Support weakened structures during weight bearing. Chest and abdominal braces (Boston brace) immobilize the thoracic and lumbar vertebral column to treat scoliosis (curvature of the spine). Lumbar braces support lumbar and sacral tissues after spinal surgery. Leg braces hold the thigh, leg, and foot in functional positions for weight bearing and ambulation.	Made of sturdy materials such as leather, metal, and molded plastic.

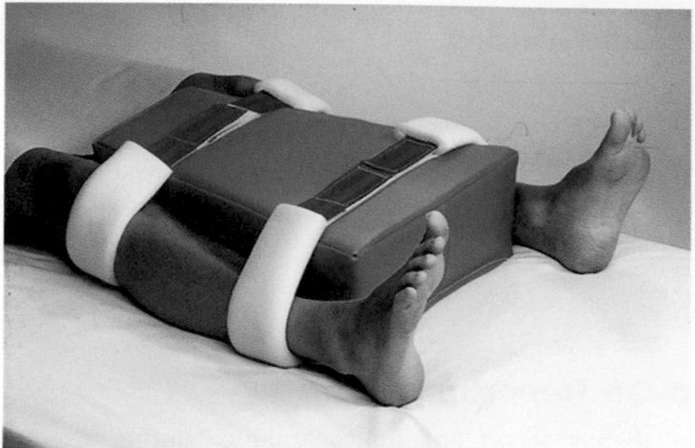

FIG 18.6 Abduction pillow.

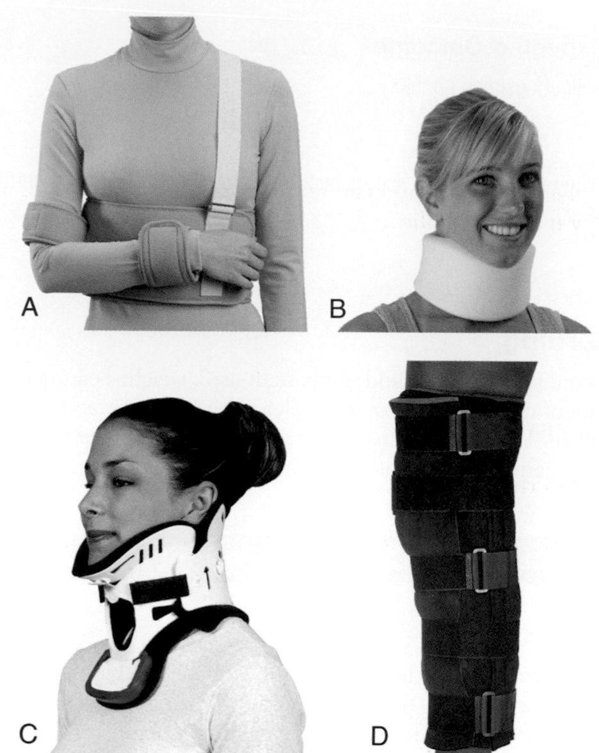

FIG 18.7 Examples of immobilizers. (A) Shoulder/arm immobilizer. (B) Soft cervical collar. (C) Hard cervical collar. (D) Knee immobilizer. *(Used with permission from [A] ProCare and [B–D] Össur Americas. All rights reserved.)*

Equipment

- Brace/splint/commercially prepared sling
- Cotton shirt or gown
- Clean gloves
- Cotton webbing or bandage *(optional)*
- Towel, washcloth, soap, basin with water

ASSESSMENT

1. Identify patient using at least two identifiers (e.g., name and birthday or name and account number) according to agency policy. *Rationale: Ensures correct patient. Complies with The Joint Commission standards and improves patient safety (TJC, 2019).*
2. Review patient's medical history, previous and current activity level, description of the condition requiring immobilization, and medical order for device. *Rationale: Reveals patient's current and previous health status and purpose for immobilization. Medical order required for use of devices.*
3. Perform hand hygiene. Inspect area of skin in contact with immobilization device or area that will be covered by a newly applied device. (Apply clean gloves if risk of contacting body fluids.) Perform hand hygiene. *Rationale: Reduces transmission of microorganisms. Provides baseline to monitor for skin breakdown. Immobile and older patients are particularly vulnerable to skin breakdown.*

Safe Patient Care *When assessing medical device–related pressure injuries, remove only those devices that can be safely removed. Nonremovable devices include those that are not normally removed during patient care (e.g., casts) or those for which a patient has a health care provider order to "not remove." Skin under the edges of nonremovable devices can be assessed if it can be done without displacing the device (NDNQI, 2017).*

4. Palpate temperature, pulse, and sensation of extremity distal to where device is to be applied. *Rationale: Provides baseline to measure circulation and neurosensory status.*
5. Assess patient's level of pain on a scale of 0 to 10. *Rationale: Provides baseline to determine if immobilization device affects comfort.*
6. Refer to occupational or physical therapy consultation to determine type of device to be used, desired position, and amount of activity and movement permitted. *Rationale: Provides direction in proper fit and use of device.*
7. Assess patient's or family caregiver's knowledge and experience with immobilization devices and their health literacy level. *Rationale: Ensures patient has the capacity to obtain, communicate, process, and understand basic health information (CDC, 2016).*

STEP	RATIONALE
PLANNING	
1. Expected outcomes following completion of procedure:	
• Patient's skin remains intact, warm, without signs of pressure, and with normal sensation.	Device applied correctly without skin irritation.
• Patient and family caregiver verbalize purpose, correct application, and care of the device.	Demonstrates learning.
• Patient reports a temporary increase in pain on a scale of 0 to 10 during device application.	Normal response to device application.
• Patient uses the device correctly, including schedule of wear, activity limitations, and positioning.	Able to perform self-care wearing device.

STEP	RATIONALE
2. Provide privacy and prepare environment.	Providing privacy and preparing the environment early help you think about the need to remove clutter from the over-bed or bedside table.
3. Explain to patient and family caregiver purpose of device and how it will be applied.	Promotes understanding needed for self-care of device.

IMPLEMENTATION

STEP	RATIONALE
1. Perform hand hygiene. Assist patient to a comfortable position: apply upper extremity brace/splint/sling with patient sitting upright; apply lower extremity brace with patient lying down.	Reduces transmission of microorganisms. Facilitates correct, aligned placement of brace/splint/sling.
2. Apply clean gloves if risk of contacting body fluids. Prepare skin that will be enclosed in brace/splint/sling by cleaning skin with soap and water; rinse, pat dry, and change any dressings (if present). If applying a back brace, put a thin cotton shirt or gown on patient. Ensure that there are no wrinkles to cause pressure.	This protects skin and keeps brace clean. Smooth cotton clothing between the brace and skin protects skin from irritation and absorbs moisture.
3. Inspect device for wear, damage, or rough edges.	Decreases potential for skin breakdown and maintains correct alignment.
4. Apply brace/splint/sling as directed by health care provider, orthotist, physical therapist, or occupational therapist.	Proper application of the brace/splint/sling is important to avoid skin breakdown, pressure injuries, neurovascular compromise, calluses, or worsening of deformity.
a. Apply even tension on any bandage or gauze padding that is ordered to be applied against skin; wrap distal to proximal.	Prevents trapping of blood and fluid distal to immobilization device.
b. Prevent padding from gathering or bunching.	Prevents irritation to underlying tissues.
c. Support joints when you position the device.	Reduces risk of musculoskeletal injury during application.
5. Apply commercial sling:	
a. Be sure correct size is chosen. Place elbow into close side of sling aligning arm into sling and slipping wrist and hand through open side of sling or through separate Velcro enclosure (see Fig. 18.7A).	Commercially available slings secure arm to chest for added support and have padding on strap for comfort.
b. Enclose Velcro strap around arm and place strap around patient's neck and tighten buckle until it fits snugly.	
c. Position arm so that the hand and forearm are higher that elbow.	
6. Remove and dispose of gloves. Perform hand hygiene.	Reduces transmission of microorganisms.
7. Teach patient/family caregiver prescribed schedule of wear and activities while in device as directed by health care provider, physical therapist, or occupational therapist.	Proper use of brace/splint/sling facilitates healing and mobility and reduces pain and stress.
8. Reinforce instruction regarding signs to report to health care provider: skin breakdown, pressure, or rubbing.	Device may need to be adjusted. Changes may also be required because of growth or atrophy, when muscles regain or lose strength, or after reconstructive surgery.
9. Teach patient/family caregiver how to care for brace/splint/sling:	Maintains integrity of device.
a. When not in use, store metal braces upright in a safe but easily accessible location.	Prevents deformity or bending of brace.
b. Store splints of molded materials away from heat.	Prevents melting and deformation of splint.
c. Treat any leather material with leather preservative.	Prevents drying or cracking.
d. Keep brace clean, dry, and in good working order. Clean plastic parts with a damp cloth and thoroughly dry. Clean metal brace joints with a pipe cleaner and oil weekly. Remove rust with steel wool and clean metal parts with a solvent.	Maintains function and integrity of devices.
10. Assist patient in ambulating with brace/splint/sling in place.	Determines if patient is able to ambulate safely.
11. Have patient or family caregiver apply and remove brace/splint/sling.	Promotes patient independence; demonstration confirms level of learning skill.
12. Help patient to comfortable position. Place nurse call system in an accessible location within patient's reach.	Gives patient sense of well-being. Ensures patient can call for assistance.
13. Raise side rails (as appropriate) and lower bed to lowest position.	Ensures patient safety.
14. Dispose of supplies or dirty linen. Perform hand hygiene.	Reduces transmission of microorganisms.

STEP	RATIONALE
EVALUATION	
1. Inspect area of skin underneath device for redness or skin breakdown. If allowed, remove device briefly to assess skin thoroughly.	Monitors for development of pressure injury.
2. Palpate temperature, pulse, and sensation of extremity distal to device. Check capillary refill by pressing on toe or finger (see illustration).	Screens for changes in circulation due to compression of device against skin.

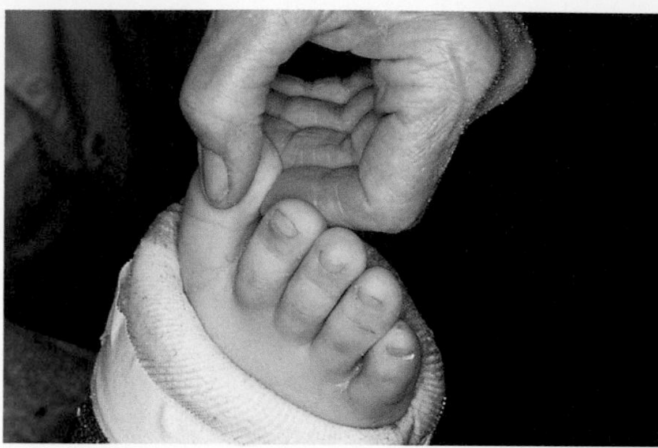

STEP 2 Inspecting toe to assess capillary refill.

STEP	RATIONALE
3. Inspect alignment of the limb after application of device.	Device is designed to support limb in a stable position.
4. Ask patient to rate level of pain on a scale of 0 to 10 after device application.	Application of device may cause temporary discomfort, but eventually the support it offers reduces pain.
5. **Use Teach-Back:** "I want to be sure I explained clearly the need for the brace/splint/sling, how to maintain the device, and the limitations related to the device. Can you tell me how you will use this brace/splint/sling safely?" Revise your instruction now or develop plan for revised patient/family caregiver teaching if patient/family caregiver is not able to teach back correctly.	Determines patient's/family caregiver's level of understanding of instructional topic.

Unexpected Outcomes	Related Interventions
1. Patient reports increased severity in pain after application of the device.	• Reposition extremity. • Administer analgesics as ordered to maintain patient's comfort level. • Increase frequency of neurovascular checks. • Inform health care provider.
2. Patient develops area of pressure, redness, or skin breakdown.	• Inspect device for proper fit and positioning and for areas of damage, wear, or rough edges. • Inform health care provider. • Inform orthoptist, physical therapist, or occupational therapist so that adjustments to device can be made.

Recording

- Record assessments of skin integrity, neurovascular status, application of and type of device, schedule of wear, activity level, movement permitted, patient's tolerance of procedure, and instructions given to patient and family caregiver.
- Record observations about patient's ability to apply device, ambulate, and remove device.
- Document your evaluation of patient learning.

Hand-Off Reporting

- Report to health care provider any unexpected outcomes.

SPECIAL CONSIDERATIONS

Patient-Centered Care

- Respect patient preferences for degree of active engagement in activity and exercise.

- Always assess a patient's level of physical and emotional comfort before implementing activity or exercise therapies (Quality and Safety Education for Nurses [QSEN], 2017). Patients with pain, nausea, or fatigue have little motivation to exercise. Patients who are anxious or afraid of injury often resist participation.
- When educating patients and family caregivers, create partnerships that promote health, safety and well-being, and self-care management (QSEN, 2017).
- During ambulation and exercise, provide a garment that protects a patient's privacy so as to prevent embarrassment.

Patient Education

- Teach patients to lift rather than slide an assist device to reduce the possibility of catching the tips, which could cause the user to lose balance, trip, or fall.
- Talk to a patient about his or her risks for falls. Let patients who have a fear of falling know that they can regain confidence with practice.
- Instruct patients that if wearing shoes with varying heel sizes, the crutches, canes, and walkers may need to be adjusted to maintain the proper height.
- All assist devices should be kept in good working condition:
  - Be sure rubber tips on canes and crutches are attached securely. Worn tips should be replaced immediately because they increase surface friction.
  - Inform patients about the importance of keeping cane and crutch tips dry. Water decreases surface friction and increases the risk of crutches slipping.
  - Inspect the structure of wooden crutches for cracks that decrease the ability of the crutch to support weight. Bends in aluminum crutches alter body alignment, increasing the risk for further damage to the musculoskeletal system.
- Give patients a list of medical suppliers in the community to obtain repairs, new rubber tips, handgrips, and pads as needed for assist devices.

Age-Specific

Pediatric

- Physical activity is essential for a child's physical growth and development (Hockenberry and Wilson, 2017).
- If a child has been immobilized for a long time, perform upper-body strengthening exercises to condition and strengthen arms and shoulders (Hockenberry and Wilson, 2017).
- For rehabilitation of a small child who has not yet learned to walk or who is unsteady, front-rolling or rear-rolling walkers are often used before progressing to special crutches (Hockenberry and Wilson, 2017).
- Monitor children closely to ensure that they do not remove an immobilization device.
- Recognize that bracing in adolescents affects body image and self-esteem.

Gerontological

- Lightweight immobilization devices are less restrictive for older adults.
- Older patients are often fearful of falling when ambulatory, especially if they have fallen previously. This fear causes a person to move less often, which causes greater problems with gait. Encouragement, reassurance, and assistance from family or caregiver decrease anxiety. Older adults may need more time in the morning to resume activity.
- Older adults may have decreased sensation, so carefully assess fit of immobilization device (Touhy and Jett, 2018).

Home Care

- Teach patient/family caregiver how to measure carotid or radial pulse before and after walking, what a normal range is for patient, how to monitor exercise tolerance, and when to notify health care provider about problems.
- Instruct patient on how to use an assist device on various terrains (e.g., carpet, stairs, rough ground, inclines) and when it is unsafe to use the device.
- Instruct patient on how to maneuver around obstacles such as doors and how to use the aid when transferring (e.g., to and from a chair, toilet, tub, and car).
- Instruct patient and family caregiver in the proper way to check that assist device is functioning.
- Have family caregiver remove scatter rugs, electrical cords, and spills.
- Have patient use a backpack, fanny pack, or apron, or attach a "saddle bag" to patient's walker to carry objects. Caution patients not to overfill bag attached to walker to prevent forward tipping of walker.
- When a patient has an immobilization device, instruct him or her to inspect skin daily for pressure or areas of breakdown. Involve family caregiver as appropriate.
- Remind patient to inspect and clean immobilization device weekly.

✦ PRACTICE REFLECTIONS

A 58-year-old man is scheduled to be transferred out of critical care to a medical-surgical unit after recovering from traumatic injuries to lower extremities following an auto accident 3 days ago. The patient has advanced from sitting on the side of the bed to sitting in a chair only two times. His transfer orders call for the man to begin ambulation. The health care provider has ordered physical therapy for gait training using crutches.

1. Consider the factors that would increase this patient's chances of developing a DVT. What would be a likely nonpharmacological intervention?
2. If the patient can bear weight only on one leg, what other information would you need to obtain in consultation with the physical therapist to determine the appropriate crutch gait? What gait do you believe would be appropriate? Provide a rationale.
3. What risks do you anticipate this patient might have that would affect his ability to ambulate?

✦ CLINICAL REVIEW QUESTIONS

1. A patient has an order for application of compression stockings. Place the following steps for application of the stockings in the correct order:
   1. Place patient's toes into foot of stocking up to the heel; keep smooth.

2. Use tape measure to measure patient's leg for proper stocking size.
3. Slide stocking up over patient's calf until sock is completely extended.
4. Turn elastic stocking inside out, keeping hand inside holding heel. Take other hand and pull stocking inside out until reaching the heel.
5. Slide remaining portion of stocking over patient's foot, covering toes. Be sure foot fits into toe and heel of stocking.

2. A family has asked for a meeting with the nursing staff of a long-term care agency to discuss care planned for their mother. In the recent week, their mother has started to use a walker. The family is worried that their mother's health is declining, and they wonder if she can use the walker safely. Which of the following instructions should the nurse give the family? (Select all that apply.)
1. A gait belt is used to prevent their mother from losing balance and falling.
2. Use of a walker is safe and reduces the chances of their mother falling.
3. If the family walks with their mother, she can go up the steps using the walker.
4. The nurses will check their mother's blood pressure before walking to be sure she is not dizzy or having blood pressure problems.
5. The patient will be less likely to fall if she assumes a bent posture over the walker.

3. Which of the following statements describes the correct technique to assist a patient in performing active assisted range of motion in the right elbow? (Select all that apply.)
1. Support elbow by holding distal part of extremity.
2. Grasp joint with fingers to provide support.
3. Have patient move joint independently.
4. Move the joint past the point of resistance.
5. Perform the exercise a few times only, and gradually build up to more.

Answers and Rationales for Clinical Review Questions can be found on the Evolve website.

REFERENCES

Adler J, Malone D: Early mobilization in the intensive care unit: a systematic review, *Cardiopulm Phys Ther J* 23(1):2012.

Agency for Healthcare Research and Quality (AHRQ): Implementing the ABCDE Bundle at the Bedside, 2013. https://innovations.ahrq.gov/qualitytools/implementing-abcde-bundle-bedside.

Agency for Healthcare Research and Quality (AHRQ): Preventing hospital-acquired venous thromboembolism prophylaxis, 2015. http://www.ahrq.gov/sites/default/files/wysiwyg/professionals/quality-patient-safety/patient-safety-resources/resources/vtguide/vteguide.pdf.

American Academy of Orthopaedist Surgeons: How to use crutches, canes, and walkers, 2015. http://orthoinfo.aaos.org/topic.cfm?topic=A00181.

American College of Foot and Ankle Surgeons: Instructions for using crutches, 2018. http://www.acfas.org/footankleinfo/crutches.htm.

American Heart Association (AHA): The American Heart Association recommendations for physical activity in adults, 2016. http://www.heart.org/HEARTORG/HealthyLiving/PhysicalActivity/FitnessBasics/American-Heart-Association-Recommendations-for-Physical-Activity-Infographic_UCM_450754_SubHomePage.jsp.

Boynton T, et al: Implementing a mobility assessment tool for nurses. A nurse-driven assessment tool reveals the patient's mobility level and guides SPHM technology choices, *American Nurse Today* 13–16, 2014. https://americannursetoday.com/wp-content/uploads/2014/09/ant9-Patient-Handling-Supplement-821a_Implementing.pdf.

Bryant MS, et al: Gait changes with walking devices in persons with Parkinson's disease, *Disabil Rehabil Assist Technol* 7(2):149–152, 2013.

Centers for Disease Control and Prevention: What is health literacy, 2016. https://www.cdc.gov/healthliteracy/learn/index.html.

Childs E, deWit H: Regular exercise is associated with emotional resilience to acute stress in healthy adults, *Front Physiol* 5:1, 2014.

de Mettelinge R, et al: Understanding the relationship between walking aids and fall in older adults: a prospective cohort study, *J Geriatr Phys Ther* 38(3):127–132, 2015.

Degelau J, et al; Institute for Clinical Systems Improvement (ICSI): *Prevention of falls (acute care): health care protocol*, Bloomington, MN, 2014, Institute for Clinical Systems Improvement.

Frith J, et al: Measuring and defining orthostatic hypotension in the older person, *Age Aging* 43(2):168, 2014.

Hockenberry MJ, Wilson D: *Wong's essentials of pediatric nursing*, ed 10, St. Louis, 2017, Mosby.

Huether S, McCance K: *Understanding pathophysiology*, ed 6, St Louis, 2017, Mosby.

Lewis L, et al: *Medical-surgical nursing: assessment and management of clinical problems*, ed 10, St. Louis, 2017, Elsevier.

Luz C, et al: Do canes or walkers make any difference? Nonuse and fall injuries, *Gerontologist* 57(2):211–218, 2017.

Mills P, et al: Five things to know about orthostatic hypotension in the older adult. *J Am Geriatr Soc* 62(9):1822, 2014.

Modi S, et al: Wells criteria for DVT is a reliable clinical tool to assess the risk of deep venous thrombosis in trauma patients, *World J Emerg Surg* 11:24, 2016. doi:10.1186/s13017-016-0078-1. Published online 2016 Jun 8.

National Database for Nursing Quality Indicators (NDNQI): Pressure injuries and staging: medical device related (MDR) pressure injuries, 2017. https://members.nursingquality.org/ndnqipressureulcertraining/Module1/MDRPressureUlcers.aspx.

National Institutes of Health (NIH): Go for life: improve your strength, n.d. https://go4life.nia.nih.gov/exercises/strength.

Occupational Safety and Health Administration (OSHA): Safe patient handling—preventing musculoskeletal disorders in nursing homes, OSHA Publication 3108, 2014. https://www.osha.gov/Publications/OSHA3708.pdf.

Office of Disease Prevention and Health Promotion (ODPHP): Healthy People 2020: Physical activity, 2015. https://www.healthypeople.gov/2020/topics-objectives/topic/physical-activity.

Pai M, Douketis J: Prevention of venous thromboembolic disease in acutely ill hospitalized medical adults, *UpToDate* 2016. http://www.uptodate.com/contents/1346.

Pierson F, et al: *Pierson's and fairchild's principles and techniques of patient care*, ed 6, St. Louis, 2017, Saunders.

Quality and Safety Education for Nurses (QSEN): Pre-licensure KSA's, 2017. http://qsen.org/competencies/pre-licensure-ksas/.

Sachdeva A, et al: Graduated compression stockings for prevention of deep vein thrombosis, *Cochrane Database Syst Rev* (12):CD001484, 2014.

Saunders LL, et al: Ambulation and complications related to assistive devices after spinal cord injury, *JSCM* 36(6):652, 2013.

Shibao C, et al: Evaluation and treatment of orthostatic hypotension, *J Am Soc Hypertens* 7:317, 2013.

Shieh C, et al: Association of self-efficacy and self-regulation with nutrition and exercise behaviors in a community sample of adults, *J Community Health Nurs* 32(4):199, 2015.

Taito S, et al: Early mobilization of mechanically ventilated patients in the intensive care unit, *J Intensive Care* 4:50, 2016.

Tampa Research and Education Foundation, Inc. (TVAREF): VHA safe patient handling and mobility algorithms (2014 revision). http://www.tampavaref.org/safe-patient-handling/Enc4-2SPHMAlgorithms.pdf.

The Joint Commission (TJC): *2019 National Patient Safety Goals*, 2019. https://www.jointcommission.org/standards_information/npsgs.aspx.

Topfer L: Portable compression to prevent venous thromboembolism after hip and knee surgery: the ActiveCare System, CADTH Issues in Emerging Health Technologies, 2016.

Touhy T, Jett K: *Ebersole and Hess's gerontological nursing and healthy aging*, ed 5, St. Louis, 2018, Mosby.

Tseng CN, et al: Effects of a range-of-motion exercise programme, *J Adv Nurs* 57(2):181–191, 2007.

United Health Care (UHC): TechFlash: ActiveCare+SFT® portable compression device for venous thromboembolism prevention after joint arthroplasty, 2012. http://www.njha.com/media/41054/vte_1_techflash.pdf.

U.S. Department of Health and Human Services (USDHHS): Importance of physical activity, 2017. https://www.hhs.gov/fitness/be-active/importance-of-physical-activity/index.html.

19 Urinary Elimination

SKILLS AND PROCEDURES

EVOLVE WEBSITE/RESOURCES LIST

http://evolve.elsevier.com/Perry/nursinginterventions
Audio Glossary • Case Studies • Checklists • Clinical Review Questions • Answers and Rationales for Clinical Review Questions

INTRODUCTION

Urinary elimination can be compromised by a wide variety of illnesses and conditions. A nurse identifies a patient's elimination problems and then implements care measures to support normal bladder emptying with privacy and dignity by assisting patients as needed in toileting. During acute illness, a patient may require urinary catheterization for close monitoring of urine output or to facilitate bladder emptying when bladder function is compromised (see Box 19.1). Some patients require long-term indwelling catheters, urethral or suprapubic, when the bladder fails to empty effectively. When invasive therapies are used to promote bladder emptying, nurses implement meticulous measures to minimize risk for infection and promote urinary emptying.

PRACTICE STANDARDS

- Gould CV et al., 2017: Guideline for prevention of catheter-associated urinary tract infections 2009, Healthcare Infection Control Practices Advisory Committee, Centers for Disease Control and Prevention, updated February 2017—Steps for preventing catheter-associated urinary tract infections (CAUTIs)
- The Joint Commission, 2019: National Patient Safety Goals—Patient identification

EVIDENCE-BASED PRACTICE

Reducing Catheter-Associated Urinary Tract Infection

A urinary tract infection related to the use of an indwelling urinary catheter is one of the most common health care–associated infections (HAIs) acquired by patients (American Association of Critical Care Nurses [AACN], 2016: Nicolle, 2014). Biofilm develops on catheter devices, and thus the major determinant for development of bacteriuria is duration of catheterization. Symptoms of a catheter-associated urinary tract infection (CAUTI) include fever, suprapubic or costovertebral angle tenderness, and otherwise unexplained systemic symptoms such as altered mental status, hypotension, or evidence of a systemic inflammatory response syndrome (Fekete, 2018). Evidence-based guidelines for reducing CAUTI include strict adherence to aseptic technique during insertion, use of proper catheter types and sizes, proper care and maintenance of any drainage systems, and reduction in the use of catheters with timely removal (Gould et al., 2017). Nurses are key members of the health care team who can reduce the incidence of CAUTI; nurse-led initiatives and peer-to-peer teaching can have a significant impact on lowering CAUTI rates and associated costs (Pashnik et al., 2017). There have been studies involving the use of nurse-directed protocols to reduce CAUTI. In health care systems where nurses are empowered to evaluate and remove indwelling catheters based on a nurse-directed protocol, there has been a decrease in rates of CAUTI (Galiczewski & Shurpin, 2017; Timmons et al., 2017). Evidenced-based interventions for the prevention of CAUTI include the following (Gould et al., 2017):

- Perform hand hygiene immediately before and after insertion or any manipulation of a catheter device or site.
- Use aseptic technique for catheter insertion, manipulation, and maintenance of indwelling catheters (AACN, 2016).
- Use aseptic technique when using all sterile equipment.
- Secure indwelling catheters to prevent movement and pulling on the catheter.
- Maintain a closed urinary drainage system.
- Maintain an unobstructed flow of urine through the catheter, drainage tubing, and drainage bag (AACN, 2016).

- Keep the urinary drainage bag below the level of the bladder at all times.
- When emptying the urinary drainage bag, use a separate measuring receptacle for each patient. Do not let the drainage spigot touch the receptacle.
- Perform routine perineal hygiene daily and after each soiling.
- Consider using a portable ultrasound device to assess urine volume in patients undergoing intermittent catheterization to reduce unnecessary catheter insertions.

SAFETY GUIDELINES

Patients requiring assistance with urinary elimination often have a limitation in mobility (due to illness or medical treatment), requiring nurses to employ safe handling and transfer techniques (see Chapter 17). The risk of exposing the sterile urinary tract requires nurses to use aseptic techniques and know a patient's risk for infection. Safety guidelines include the following:

- Assess patients' mobility and functional status to determine their ability to safely stand and/or transfer to a toilet or commode and to ambulate safely when an indwelling catheter is in place.
- Assess a patient's normal pattern of micturition. Patients taking diuretic medications should have a toilet, commode, and/or urinal close to their bed or chair. Respond to any request for toileting assistance promptly.
- Patients who need assistance with toileting should have a nurse call system within easy reach and be offered help at regular intervals, especially in the morning after awakening, after meals, and before bedtime.
- Maintain aseptic technique when catheterizing patients and performing irrigation.

PROCEDURAL GUIDELINE 19.1 *Assisting With Use of a Urinal*

Purpose

Patients who are unable to stand and ambulate (e.g., lower-extremity weakness, severe dyspnea) or who are restricted from getting out of bed because of a medical condition or treatment restriction are forced to use a urinal to urinate. A urinal is a container that collects and holds urine when access to a toilet is restricted. In some instances, a male patient may be able to stand at the bedside and use a urinal. Most urinals are used by men, but there are specially designed urinals for women (Fig. 19.1). The female urinal has a larger opening at the top with a defined rim, which helps position the urinal closely against the genitalia.

Delegation and Collaboration

The skill of assisting a patient with a urinal can be delegated to nursing assistive personnel (NAP). The nurse directs the NAP to:

- Help the patient with special needs or adaptations, such as a need to hold a urinal for a patient.
- Provide personal hygiene as necessary after urination.
- Report immediately any changes in urine color, clarity, and odor; development of incontinence (involuntary loss of urine); patient reports of dysuria, which could indicate an infection; and any changes in the frequency and amount of urine.

Equipment

Urinal; clean gloves; graduated cylinder (used for measuring volume if on intake and output [I&O]); supplies for diagnostic urine tests and specimen collection (see Chapter 9); wash basin, washcloths, towels, and soap for perineal hygiene; toilet tissue

Procedural Steps

1. Assess patient's medical history for conditions that may place him or her at risk for falling during ambulation to bathroom: arthritis, benign prostatic hyperplasia (BPH), or overactive bladder (OAB).

Safe Patient Care *These conditions do not prohibit ambulation. Your role is to promote patient independence. But if patient is not to ambulate without assistance and experiences a sudden urge to urinate without a caregiver present, a urinal can be a helpful option for toileting.*

2. Assess patient's normal urinary elimination habits, including any episodes of incontinence.
3. Determine how much help is needed to place and remove the urinal. (Ask the patient or observe previous use.)

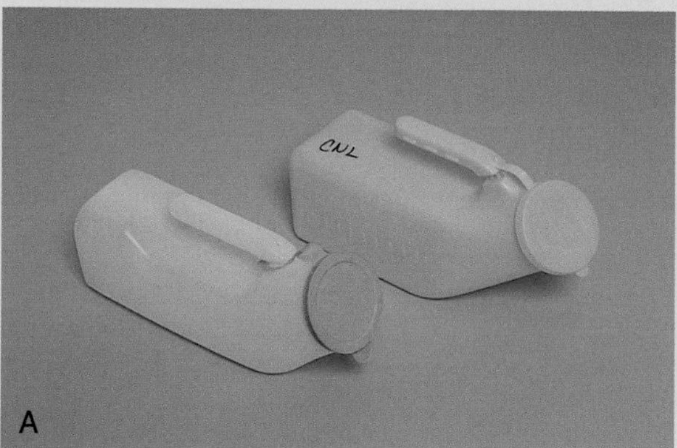

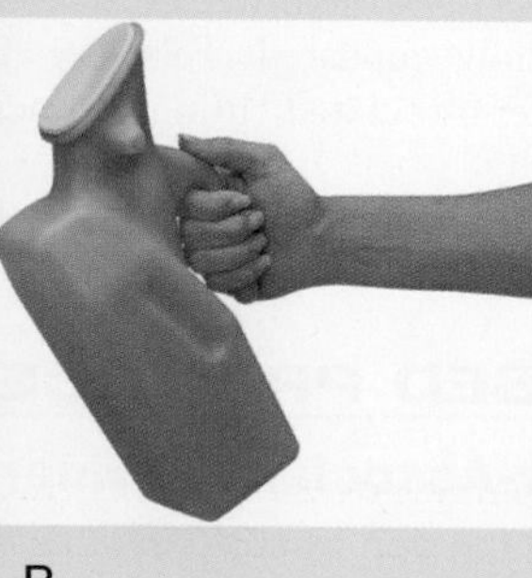

FIG 19.1 (A) Male urinal. (B) Female urinal. *(Courtesy Briggs Medical Service Company.)*

PROCEDURAL GUIDELINE 19.1 *Assisting With Use of a Urinal—cont'd*

4. Review health care provider orders to determine if a urine specimen is to be collected.
5. Perform hand hygiene.
6. Explain procedure to patient if information is required.
7. Provide privacy by closing bedside curtain and room door.
8. Apply clean gloves. Assess for a distended bladder by inspecting the lower one-third of the abdomen or palpating gently above symphysis pubis.
9. Help patient into appropriate position: for a male patient, on side, back, sitting with head of bed elevated, or in standing position; for a female patient, lying supine. If needed, place an absorbent pad under patient's buttocks to protect bed linens from accidental spills.

Safe Patient Care *Before having a patient stand to void, assess lower-extremity strength and mobility and assess blood pressure for orthostatic hypotension (see Chapter 7), especially if there has been a period of prolonged bed rest.*

10. If possible, a male patient should hold urinal and position penis in urinal. If needed, help patient by positioning penis completely in urinal and holding urinal in place or by helping him hold urinal. Ensure that the urinal is placed below the flow of urine.
11. Help a female patient by positioning the urinal against the genitalia and stabilizing it to keep it in position and below the flow of urine.
12. Cover patient with bed linens and place the nurse call system within reach. If possible, give patient further privacy by leaving the bedside after ensuring that he or she is in a safe and comfortable position. Remove gloves and perform hand hygiene.
13. After patient has finished voiding, apply gloves and remove urinal and assess characteristics of the urine for color, clarity, odor, and amount. Help him or her wash and dry penis or genitalia.
14. Empty and clean urinal. Return urinal to patient for future use.
15. Help patient perform hand hygiene as needed.
16. Remove and dispose of gloves.
17. Leave patient in comfortable position with nurse call system in place. Instruct in its use.
18. Raise side rails (as appropriate) and lower bed to lowest position.
19. Perform hand hygiene.
20. Measure urine and record output on I&O record, if needed (see Chapter 8). Note and record character of urine.

✦ SKILL 19.1 Applying a Male Incontinence Device

Purpose

An external catheter, also called a *condom catheter*, penile sheath, or Texas catheter, is a soft, pliable, condom-like sheath that fits over the penis, providing a safe and noninvasive way to contain urine for men who have complete and spontaneous bladder emptying. Most external catheters are made of soft silicone that reduces friction. They are clear to allow for easy visualization of the skin under the catheter. Latex catheters are still available, so it is important to verify that a patient does not have a latex allergy before applying this type of catheter.

Condom-type external catheters are held in place by an adhesive coating on the internal lining of the sheath, a double-sided self-adhesive strip, brush-on adhesive applied to the penile shaft, or an external strap. Never use adhesive or tape to secure a condom catheter. A catheter may be attached to a small-volume (leg) urinary drainage bag or a large-volume (bedside) drainage bag, both of which need to be kept lower than the level of the bladder. Various styles and sizes are available, so it is important to refer to the manufacturer's guidelines for fitting and correct application. For men who cannot be fitted for a condom-type external catheter, other externally applied catheters are available.

An alternative to the condom catheter is an incontinence device made of a 100% latex-free hydrocolloid material. The device fits onto the tip of the penis and not over the penile shaft. It reduces the occurrence of soiling of the skin by urine. This device is helpful for patients with retracted anatomy, large penile tip and a narrow shaft, or frequent erections, which cause the traditional condom catheter to dislodge (CliniMed, 2014).

Delegation and Collaboration

Assessment of the skin of a patient's penile shaft and determination of a latex allergy are done by a nurse before catheter application. The skill of applying a condom catheter can be delegated to nursing assistive personnel (NAP), depending on agency policy. The nurse directs the NAP to:

- Follow manufacturer directions for applying the condom catheter and securing device.
- Monitor intake and output (I&O) and record if applicable.
- Immediately report any redness, swelling, or skin irritation or breakdown of glans penis or penile shaft.

Equipment

- Condom catheter kit—condom sheath of appropriate size, securing device (internal adhesive, strap), skin preparation solution (per manufacturer's recommendations)
- *Option:* Hydrocolloid incontinence device
- Urinary collection bag with drainage tubing or leg bag and straps
- Basin with warm water and soap
- Towels, washcloth, bath blanket
- Clean gloves
- Scissors, hair guard, or paper towel

ASSESSMENT

1. Identify patient using at least two identifiers (e.g., name and birthday or name and medical record number) according to agency policy. *Rationale: Ensures correct patient. Complies with*

The Joint Commission standards and improves patient safety (TJC, 2019).

2. Review electronic health record (EHR) and assess urinary pattern, ability to empty bladder effectively, and degree of urinary continence. *Rationale: Incontinent patients are at risk for skin breakdown and thus candidates for condom catheter.*
3. Review EHR for history of allergy to rubber or latex. Confirm with patient if possible. Check patient's allergy wristband. *Rationale: Condoms are made of latex and can cause serious skin reaction. Condoms made of other material should be used if the patient has a latex allergy.*

Safe Patient Care *Apply condom catheters only when the skin on the penile surface is intact.*

4. Assess patient's or family caregiver's mental status, knowledge, prior experience with condom-type catheter, and ability to apply device. *Rationale: Ensures patient has the capacity to obtain, communicate, process, and understand basic health information (Centers for Disease Control and Prevention [CDC], 2017).*
5. Assess patient's or family caregiver's knowledge, experience, and health literacy. *Rationale: Ensures patient or family caregiver has the capacity to obtain, communicate, process, and understand basic health information (CDC, 2016).*
6. Perform hand hygiene. Verify patient's size and type of condom catheter from plan of care or use manufacturer measuring guide to measure length and diameter of penis in flaccid state (apply gloves for measurement). Perform hand hygiene. *Rationale: Identifies proper size of catheter needed. Penile shaft should be at least 2 cm (0.8 inch) in length to ensure successful application. If too small, penile strangulation and/or necrosis can occur (Özkan et al., 2015).*

STEP	RATIONALE
PLANNING	
1. Expected outcomes following completion of procedure:	
• Patient's skin is free from urine.	Catheter is applied correctly.
• Glans and penile shaft are free of skin irritation or breakdown.	Catheter is secure and not too tight.
• Patient explains procedure and what to expect.	Patient is less anxious and able to cooperate.
2. Provide privacy by closing room door or curtain. Organize and set up equipment needed.	Protects patient's privacy; reduces anxiety. Ensures more efficiency when performing skill.
3. Raise bed to appropriate working height. Lower side rail on working side.	Promotes use of good body mechanics.
4. Explain procedure to patient.	Reduces anxiety and promotes cooperation.
IMPLEMENTATION	
1. Perform hand hygiene.	Reduces transmission of microorganisms.
2. Prepare urinary drainage collection bag and tubing (large-volume drainage bag or leg bag). Clamp off drainage bag port. Place nearby ready to attach to condom after applied.	Provides easy access to drainage equipment after applying condom catheter.
3. Help patient to supine or sitting position.	Position makes it easier to apply incontinence device.
4. Place bath blanket over upper torso. Fold sheets so only penis is exposed.	Respects patient dignity; draping prevents unnecessary exposure of body parts.
5. Apply clean gloves. Provide perineal care (see Chapter 11). Dry thoroughly before applying device. In uncircumcised male, ensure that foreskin has been replaced to normal position before applying condom catheter. Do not apply barrier cream.	Prevents skin breakdown from exposure to secretions. Removes any residual adhesives. Perineal care minimizes skin irritation and promotes adhesion of new external catheter. Barrier creams prevent sheath from adhering to penile shaft.
6. Remove and dispose of gloves. Perform hand hygiene.	Reduces transmission of microorganisms.
7. Apply clean gloves. Assess skin of penis for rashes, erythema, and/or open areas.	Reduces transmission of microorganisms. Provides baseline to compare changes in condition of skin after application of condom catheter.
8. Clip hair at base of penis as necessary before application of condom sheath. Some manufacturers provide hair guard that is placed over penis before applying device. Remove hair guard after applying catheter. An alternative to hair guard is to tear a hole in a paper towel, place it over penis, and remove after application of device.	Prevents hair from adhering to condom, which can be pulled during condom application or removal.

Safe Patient Care *The pubic area should not be shaved because microabrasions in skin increase risk for skin irritation and infection.*

STEP	RATIONALE
9. Apply incontinence device:	
a. Condom catheter. With nondominant hand, grasp penis along shaft. With dominant hand, hold rolled condom sheath at tip of penis with head of penis in cone. Smoothly roll sheath onto penis. Allow 2.5 to 5 cm (1 to 2 inches) of space between tip of glans penis and end of condom catheter (see illustration).	Excessive wrinkles or creases in external catheter sheath after application may mean that patient needs smaller size.
b. Hydrocolloid device. One size fits all. Place the device onto the tip of the penis, not the shaft (see manufacturer's directions).	Hydrocolloid material makes device less irritating to the skin and is suitable for patients with latex allergy (CliniMed, 2014). Allows the skin to breath and the urine to be directed away from the body, making urination as natural as possible.
10. Apply appropriate securement device as indicated in manufacturer guidelines.	Condom must be secured firmly so that it is snug and stays on but not tight enough to cause constriction of blood flow. Application of gentle pressure ensures adherence of adhesive with penile skin.
a. Self-adhesive condom catheters: After application, apply gentle pressure on penile shaft for 10 to 15 seconds.	Secures catheter.
b. Outer securing strip-type condom catheters: Spiral wrap penile shaft with strip of supplied elastic adhesive. Strip should not overlap itself. Elastic strip should be snug, not tight (see illustration).	Using spiral wrap technique allows supplied elastic adhesive to expand so that blood flow to penis is not compromised.
c. Hydrocolloid incontinence device: Remove release papers from adhesive on faceplate of device. Center faceplate over opening of urinary meatus. Smooth hydrocolloid adhesive backing strips onto tip of penis. Then cover with hydrocolloid seal (see illustration).	Follow manufacturer's directions to ensure device covers tip of penis only.

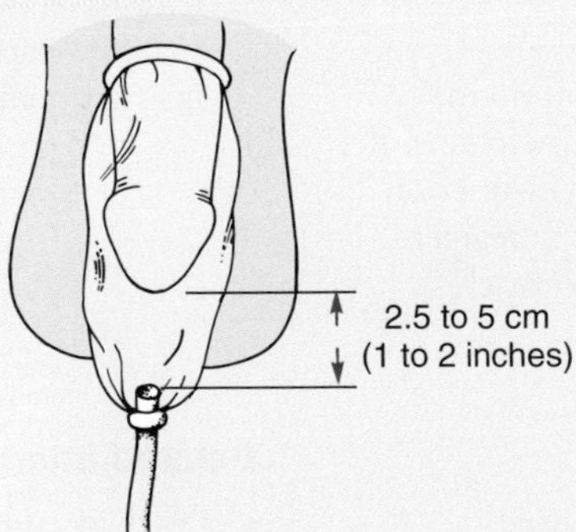

STEP 9a Condom catheter.

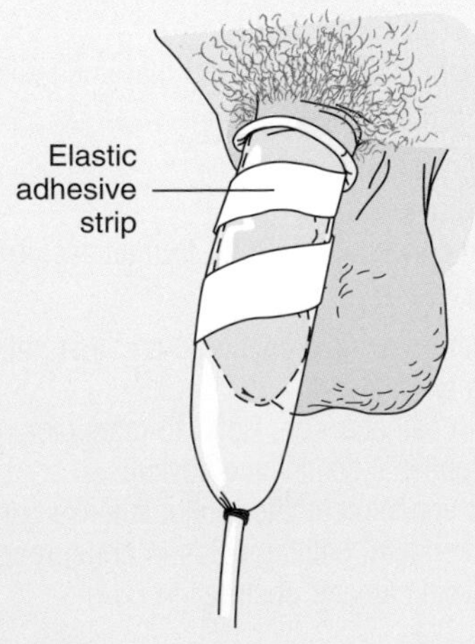

STEP 10b Spiral application of adhesive strip.

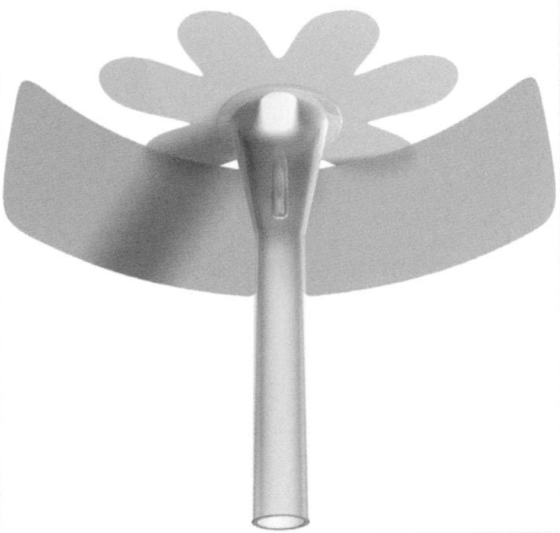

STEP 10c Men's Liberty Acute Male Incontinence Device. *(Courtesy BioDerm, Inc. Largo, Florida.)*

STEP	RATIONALE
Safe Patient Care *Never use regular adhesive tape to secure a condom catheter. Constriction from tape can reduce blood flow to tissues.*	
11. Remove hair guard or paper towel (if used). Connect drainage tubing to end of incontinence device. Be sure that a condom catheter is not twisted. If using large drainage bag, place excess tubing on bed and secure to bottom sheet.	Allows urine to be collected and measured. Keeps patient dry. Twisted condom obstructs urine flow, causing urine pooling; skin irritation; and weakening and deterioration of adhesive, causing catheter to come off.
12. Help patient to safe, comfortable position. Raise side rails (as appropriate) and lower bed to lowest position.	Promotes safety and comfort.
13. Be sure nurse call system is in an accessible location within patient's reach.	Ensures patient can call for assistance if needed.
14. Dispose of contaminated supplies, remove and dispose of gloves, and perform hand hygiene.	Reduces spread of microorganisms.
15. Remove and reapply daily following Steps 9 to 11 unless an extended-wear device is used. To remove condom, wash penis with warm, soapy water and gently roll sheath and adhesive off penile shaft.	Prevents trauma and irritation to penile sheath.

EVALUATION

STEP	RATIONALE
1. Observe urinary drainage.	Twisted condom prevents urine from draining into collection bag and could lead to urinary retention.
2. Inspect penis with condom catheter in place within 15 to 30 minutes after application. Assess for swelling and discoloration and ask patient if there is any discomfort.	Determines if condom is applied too tightly, impeding circulation to penis.
3. Inspect skin on penile shaft for signs of breakdown or irritation at least daily, when performing hygiene, and before reapplying condom or incontinence device.	Changing external catheter decreases chance of infection.
4. **Use Teach-Back:** "Let's review what I explained about your external condom catheter and the things you can do to prevent it from falling off. Tell me how you can help keep the catheter on without it slipping off." Revise your instruction now or develop a plan for revised patient/family caregiver teaching if patient/family caregiver is not able to teach back correctly.	Determines patient's/family caregiver's level of understanding of instructional topic.

Unexpected Outcomes	Related Interventions
1. Skin around penis is erythematous, ulcerated, or denuded.	• Check for latex allergy or allergy to skin preparation or adhesive device. • Remove condom and notify health care provider. • Do not reapply until penis and surrounding tissue are free from irritation. • Ensure that condom is not twisted and that urine flow is unobstructed after application.
2. Penile swelling or discoloration occurs.	• Remove external condom catheter. • Notify health care provider. • Reassess current condom size. Refer to manufacturer guidelines for sizing.
3. Condom catheter does not stay on.	• Ensure that catheter tubing is anchored and that patient understands to not pull or tug on catheter. • Reassess condom catheter size. Refer to manufacturer guidelines for sizing. Consider optional continence device. • Observe whether condom catheter outlet is kinked and urine is pooling at tip of condom, bathing penis in urine; reapply as necessary and avoid catheter obstruction.

Recording

- Record condom/device application; condition of penis, skin, and scrotum; urinary output and voiding pattern; patient response to external catheter application; and patient learning.

Hand-Off Reporting

- During hand-off report, communicate condition of skin and continence device
- Report penile erythema, rashes, or skin breakdown to health care provider.

PROCEDURAL GUIDELINE 19.2 *Bladder Scan*

Purpose

A bladder scanner (Fig. 19.2) is a noninvasive portable 3D device that creates an ultrasound image of the bladder for measuring the volume of urine in the bladder. The device makes calculations to report accurate urine volumes, especially lower volumes. Use a bladder scanner to assess bladder volume whenever inadequate bladder emptying is suspected, such as following surgery (general anesthetic and spinal) and after the removal of indwelling urinary catheters. Nurses are able to assess the presence of urinary retention, monitor the volume and excessive relaxation of the bladder, and avoid unnecessary catheterizations. The most common use for the bladder scan is to measure postvoid residual (PVR), the volume of urine in the bladder after a normal voiding. To obtain the most reliable reading, measure PVR within 5 to 15 minutes of voiding (Huether et al., 2017). A volume less than 50 mL is considered normal. Two or more PVR measurements greater than 100 mL require further investigation. If a bladder scanner is not available, obtain a PVR by measuring urine emptied from the bladder after a straight catheterization (see Skill 19.2).

Delegation and Collaboration

The skill of measuring bladder volume by bladder scan can be delegated to nursing assistive personnel (NAP). The nurse must first determine the timing and frequency of the bladder scan measurement and interpret the measurements obtained. The nurse also assesses the patient's ability to toilet before measuring PVR and the abdomen for distention if urinary retention is suspected. The nurse directs the NAP to:

- Follow manufacturer recommendations for the use of the device.
- Measure PVR volumes within 5 to 15 minutes after helping the patient to void.
- Report and record bladder scan volumes.

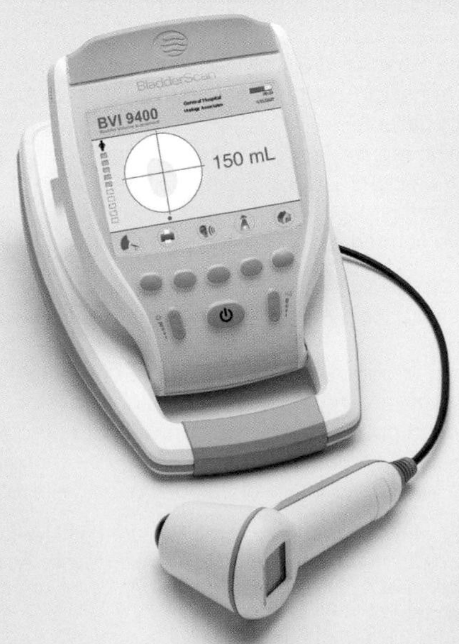

FIG 19.2 Bladder scanner. *(Courtesy Verathon, Inc.)*

Equipment

Bladder scanner, ultrasound gel, cleansing agent (e.g., alcohol pad) for scanner head, urethral catheterization tray with single-use catheter/intermittent catheter (see Skill 19.2), paper towel or washcloth

Procedural Steps

1. Identify patient using at least two identifiers (e.g., name and birthday or name and medical record number) according to agency policy (TJC, 2019).
2. Assess intake and output (I&O) record to determine urine output trends and whether patient has voided since surgery, and check the plan of care to verify correct timing of the bladder scan measurement.
3. Provide privacy by closing room door and bedside curtain.
4. Help patient to supine position with head slightly elevated. Raise bed to appropriate working height. If side rails are raised, lower side rail on working side.
5. Perform hand hygiene and apply clean gloves.
6. Discuss procedure with patient. If measurement is for PVR, ask patient to void and measure volume retained in bladder with scanner within 5 to 15 minutes of voiding:
   a. Pull back sheet to expose patient's lower abdomen.
   b. Turn on scanner per manufacturer guidelines.
   c. Set gender designation per manufacturer guidelines. Women who have had a hysterectomy should be designated as male.
   d. Wipe scanner head with alcohol pad or other cleaner and allow to air dry.
   e. Palpate patient's symphysis pubis (pubic bone). Apply generous amount of ultrasound gel (or if available a bladder scan gel pad) to midline abdomen 2.5 to 4 cm (1 to 1.5 inches) above symphysis pubis.
   f. Place scanner head on gel, ensuring that scanner head is oriented per manufacturer guidelines.
   g. Apply light pressure, keep scanner head steady, and point it slightly downward toward bladder. Press and release the scan button (see illustration).
   h. Verify accurate aim (refer to manufacturer guidelines). Complete scan and print image (if needed).
7. Remove ultrasound gel from patient's abdomen with paper towel or moist washcloth.

Continued

PROCEDURAL GUIDELINE 19.2 *Bladder Scan—cont'd*

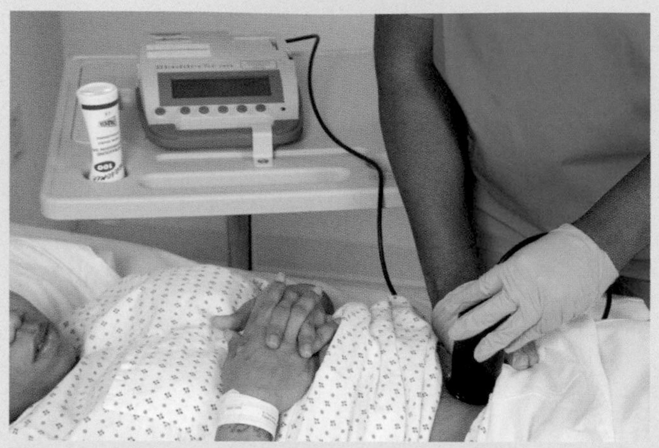

STEP 6g Placement of bladder scan head.

8. Remove ultrasound gel from scanner head and wipe with alcohol pad or other cleaner; allow to air-dry.
9. Help patient to comfortable position. Raise side rails (as appropriate) and lower bed to lowest position. Be sure nurse call system is in an accessible location within patient's reach.
10. Remove and dispose of gloves and perform hand hygiene.
11. Compare PVR results with pre-voiding scan (if available); urine volume should be less. Or if first time scan, PVR should be less than 100 mL urine.
12. Review health care provider's order to determine how often to assess residual urine or if catheterization is ordered.
13. Review I&O record to determine urine output trends.
14. Record findings of scan, PVR, and patient tolerance of procedure.

✦ SKILL 19.2 Insertion of a Straight or Indwelling Catheter

Purpose

Urinary catheterization (straight and indwelling) is the placement of a hollow tube into the bladder to remove urine. It is an invasive procedure that requires the order of a health care provider and use of strict sterile technique (Galiczewski and Shurpin, 2017). The use of an indwelling urinary catheter is associated with numerous complications, particularly catheter-associated urinary tract infection (CAUTI). This results in patient discomfort, increased hospital stay (by as much as 2 to 5 additional days), increased cost, and mortality (from sepsis). Other complications related to indwelling catheterization include prostatitis; cystitis; bladder stones; damage to the kidneys, the bladder, and the urethra; and development of antibiotic resistance (Feneley et al., 2015). Urinary tract infections (UTIs) are the fourth most common type of health care–associated infection (HAI), with an estimated 93,300 UTIs in acute care hospitals in 2011 (CDC, 2018).

Because of the risk of CAUTI, there are recommendations for the appropriate and inappropriate use of an indwelling catheter (Box 19.1). Indwelling urinary catheterization may be short term (2 weeks or less; Lam et al., 2014) or long term (more than 14 days). The steps for inserting an indwelling and a single-use straight catheter are the same. The difference lies in the inflation of a balloon to keep the indwelling catheter in place and the presence of a closed drainage system. Urinary catheters are made with one to three lumens (Fig. 19.3). Single-lumen catheters (see Fig. 19.3A) are used for intermittent catheterization (i.e., the insertion of a catheter for one-time bladder emptying). Double-lumen catheters, designed for indwelling catheters, provide one lumen for urinary drainage and a second lumen for balloon inflation to keep the catheter in place (see Fig. 19.3B). Double and triple-lumen catheters (see Fig. 19.3C) are used for continuous bladder irrigation (CBI) or to instill medications into the bladder (see Skill 19.5). One lumen drains the bladder, a second lumen is used to inflate the balloon, and a third lumen delivers fluid from an irrigation bag into the bladder. Indwelling catheters come in a variety of balloon sizes. The size of the balloon is usually printed on the catheter port

BOX 19.1

Indications for Indwelling Urethral Catheter Use

Appropriate Use

- Patients who have acute urinary retention or bladder outlet obstruction
- Need for accurate measurements of urinary output in critically ill patients
- Perioperative use for selected surgical procedures:
    - Patients undergoing urological surgery or other surgery on contiguous structures of the genitourinary tract
    - Anticipated prolonged duration of surgery (Catheters inserted for this reason should be removed in postanesthesia care unit [PACU].)
    - Anticipated need for large-volume infusions or diuretics during surgery
    - Need for intraoperative monitoring of urinary output
- To assist in healing of open sacral or perineal wounds in incontinent patients
- Patients who require prolonged immobilization (e.g., potentially unstable thoracic or lumbar spine, multiple traumatic injuries such as pelvic fractures)
- To improve comfort for end-of-life care if needed

Inappropriate Use

- As a substitute for nursing care of the patient or resident with incontinence
- As a means of obtaining urine for culture or other diagnostic tests when the patient can voluntarily void
- For prolonged postoperative duration without appropriate indications (e.g., structural repair of urethra or contiguous structures, prolonged effect of epidural anesthesia, etc.)

From Gould CV et al: Guideline for prevention of catheter-associated urinary tract infections, 2009. Healthcare Infection Control Practices Advisory Committee. Update February 2017. https://www.cdc.gov/infectioncontrol/pdf/guidelines/cauti-guidelines.pdf.

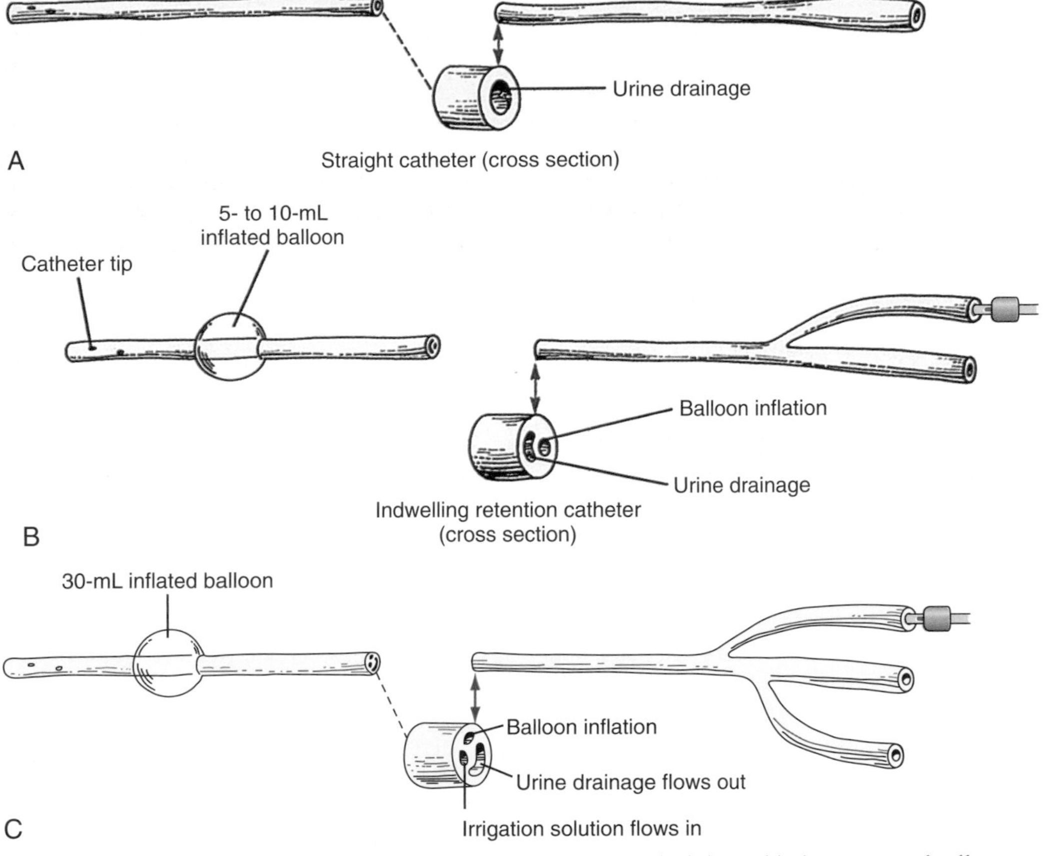

FIG 19.3 (A) Single-lumen or straight catheter (cross section). (B) Double-lumen or indwelling retention catheter (cross section). (C) Triple-lumen catheter (cross section).

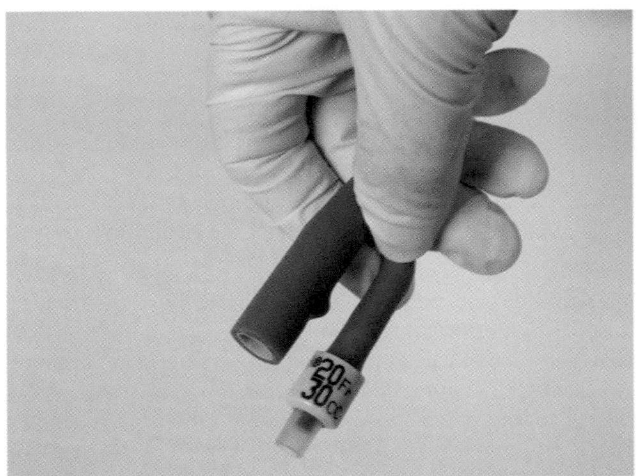

FIG 19.4 Size of catheter and balloon printed on catheter.

(Fig. 19.4). A nurse is responsible for maintaining the sterility of the urinary tract during catheter insertions and in the ongoing care and maintenance of indwelling catheters.

Delegation and Collaboration

The skill of inserting a straight or indwelling urinary catheter cannot be delegated to nursing assistive personnel (NAP). The nurse directs the NAP to:

- Assist the nurse with patient positioning, focus lighting for the procedure, maintain privacy, empty urine from collection bag, and help with perineal care.
- Report postprocedure patient discomfort or fever to the nurse.
- Report abnormal color, odor, or amount of urine in drainage bag and if the catheter is leaking or causes pain.

Equipment

- Catheter kit containing sterile items (**NOTE:** Catheter kits vary.)
  - Straight catheterization kit: Single-lumen catheter (12 to 14 Fr), drapes (one fenestrated—has an opening in the center), sterile gloves, lubricant, cleansing solution incorporated in an applicator or to be added to cotton balls, and specimen container and label.
  - Indwelling catheterization kit (Fig. 19.5): Double-lumen catheter, drapes (one fenestrated—has an opening in the center), sterile gloves, lubricant, antiseptic cleansing solution incorporated in an applicator or to be added to cotton balls, specimen container and label, and a prefilled syringe with sterile water (to inflate balloon). **NOTE:** Some kits contain a catheter with attached drainage bag; others contain only a catheter; others have no catheter.
- Sterile drainage tubing and bag (if not included in indwelling catheter insertion kit)
- Device to secure catheter (catheter strap or other device)
- Extra sterile gloves and catheter *(optional)*
- Clean gloves
- Basin with warm water, washcloth, towel, and soap for perineal care
- Flashlight or other additional light source
- Bath blanket, waterproof absorbent pad
- Measuring container for urine

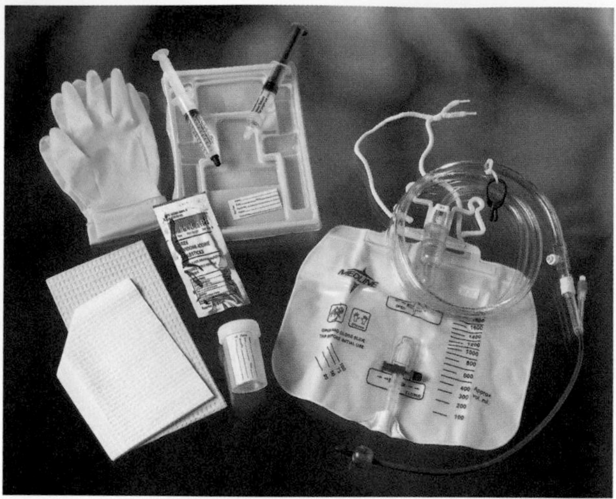

FIG 19.5 Indwelling catheterization kit. *(Image used with permission Medline Industries. All rights reserved).*

ASSESSMENT

1. Identify patient using at least two identifiers (e.g., name and birthday or name and medical record number) according to agency policy. *Rationale: Ensures correct patient. Complies with The Joint Commission standards and improves patient safety (TJC, 2019).*
2. Review patient's EHR, including health care provider's order and nurses' notes. Note previous catheterization, including catheter size, response of patient, and time of catheterization. *Rationale: Identifies purpose of inserting catheter (such as for measurement of PVR, preparation for surgery, or specimen collection) and potential difficulty with catheter insertion.*
3. Review EHR for any pathological conditions that may impair passage of catheter (e.g., enlarged prostate gland in men, urethral strictures). *Rationale: Obstruction of urethra may prevent passage of catheter into bladder.*
4. Assess patient's gender and age. *Rationale: Assists with selection of catheter size.*
5. Ask patient and check EHR for history of allergies. Check allergy bracelet. *Rationale: Catheter made of different material is needed if patient has latex allergy.*
6. Perform hand hygiene. Assess patient's weight, level of consciousness, developmental level, ability to cooperate, and mobility. *Rationale: Determines positioning to use for catheterization; indicates how much help is needed to properly position patient, ability of patient to cooperate during procedure, and level of explanation needed.*
7. Assess for pain and bladder fullness. Palpate bladder over symphysis pubis or use bladder scanner (if available; see Procedural Guideline 19.2). *Rationale: Palpation of full bladder causes pain and/or urge to void, indicating full or overfull bladder.*
8. Apply clean gloves. Inspect perineal region, observing for perineal anatomical landmarks, erythema, drainage or discharge, and odor. Remove and dispose of gloves and perform hand hygiene. *Rationale: Assessment of perineum (especially female perineal landmarks) improves accuracy and speed of catheter insertion. Reduces transmission of microorganisms.*
9. Assess patient's knowledge, prior experience with catheterization, and feelings about procedure. *Rationale: Reveals need for patient instruction and/or support.*
10. Assess patient's or family caregiver's knowledge, experience, and health literacy. *Rationale: Ensures patient or family caregiver has the capacity to obtain, communicate, process, and understand basic health information (CDC, 2016).*

STEP	RATIONALE
PLANNING	
1. Expected outcomes following completion of procedure:	
• Patient's bladder is not palpable.	Bladder successfully emptied.
• Patient verbalizes absence of abdominal discomfort or bladder pressure/fullness.	Catheterization and free flow of urine through catheter relieve bladder distention and discomfort.
• Patient has urine output of at least 30 mL/hr as measured in urinary drainage bag.	Verifies presence of catheter in bladder, catheter patency, and adequate kidney function.
• Patient verbalizes purpose and expectations about procedure.	Reflects patient understanding of procedure.
2. Explain procedure to patient.	Promotes cooperation.
3. Provide privacy. Organize and set up any equipment needed to perform procedure.	Protects patient's privacy; reduces anxiety. Ensures more efficiency when completing an assessment.
4. Arrange for extra personnel to help as necessary. Organize supplies at bedside.	Some patients are unable to assume positioning independently for procedure.
IMPLEMENTATION	
1. Check patient's plan of care for size and type of catheter (if this is a reinsertion). Use smallest-sized catheter possible. Size 14 to 16 Fr most common for adults; for older adults, 12 to 14 Fr; larger sizes (20 to 22 Fr) are needed in special circumstances, such as after urological surgery or in the presence of gross hematuria.	Ensures that patient receives correct size and type of catheter. Larger catheter diameters increase the risk for urethral trauma. Small catheter allows for adequate drainage of periurethral glands.

STEP	RATIONALE
2. Perform hand hygiene.	Reduces transmission of microorganisms.
3. Raise bed to appropriate working height. If side rails in use, raise side rail on opposite side of bed and lower side rail on working side.	Promotes good body mechanics. Use of side rails in this manner promotes patient safety.
4. Place waterproof pad under patient.	Prevents soiling bed linen.

Safe Patient Care *Obtain help to position and support patients who are weak, frail, obese, or confused.*

STEP	RATIONALE
5. Position patient:	
a. Female patient:	
(1) Help to dorsal recumbent position (on back with knees flexed). Ask patient to relax thighs so that you can rotate hips.	Exposes perineum and allows hip joints to be externally rotated.
(2) Alternate female position: Position in side-lying (Sims') position with upper leg flexed at knee and hip. Support patient with pillows if necessary to maintain position.	Alternate position is more comfortable if patient cannot abduct leg at hip joint (e.g., patient has arthritic joints or contractures).
b. Male patient:	
(1) Position supine with legs extended and thighs slightly abducted.	Comfortable position for patient aids in visualization of penis.
6. Drape patient:	Protects patient dignity and privacy by avoiding unnecessary exposure of body parts.
a. Female patient:	
(1) Drape with bath blanket. Place blanket diamond fashion over patient, with one corner at patient's midsection, side corners over each thigh and abdomen, and last corner over perineum (see illustration).	
b. Male patient:	
(1) Drape patient by covering upper part of body with small sheet or towel; drape with separate sheet or bath blanket so only perineum is exposed (see illustration).	

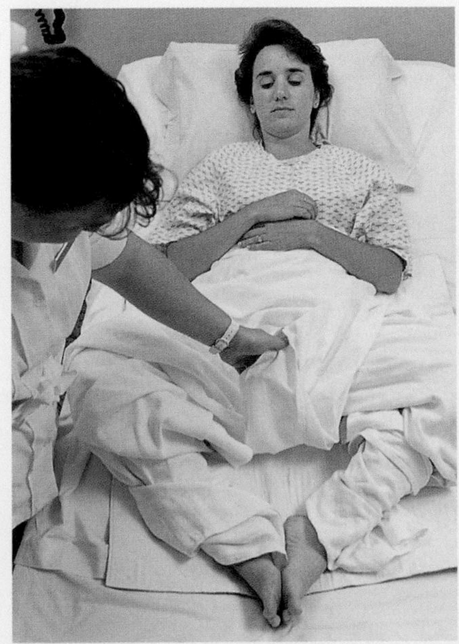

STEP 6a(1) Female patient draped and in dorsal recumbent position.

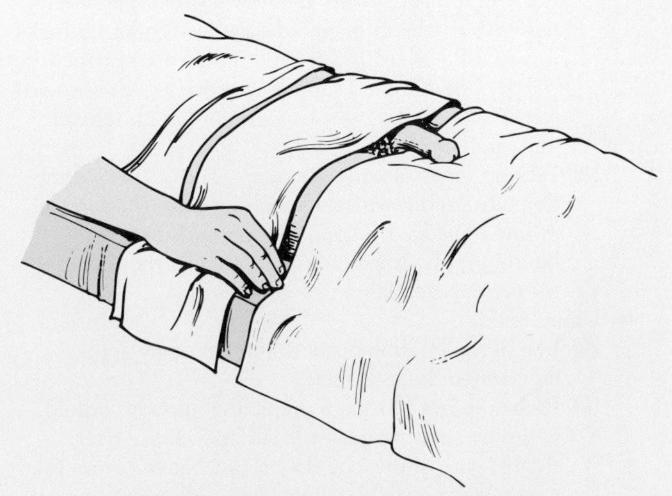

STEP 6b(1) Drape male patient with blankets.

STEP	RATIONALE
7. Apply clean gloves. Clean perineal area with soap and water, rinse, and dry (see Chapter 11). Use gloves to examine patient and identify urinary meatus. Remove and discard gloves. Perform hand hygiene.	Hygiene before initiating aseptic catheter insertion removes secretions, urine, and feces that could contaminate sterile field and increase risk for catheter-associated urinary tract infection (CAUTI). Perform hand hygiene immediately before catheter insertion (Gould et al., 2017).
8. Position portable light to illuminate genitals or have assistant available to hold light.	Adequate visualization of urinary meatus assists with accuracy of catheter insertion.
9. Open outer wrapping of catheterization kit. Place inner wrapped catheter kit tray on clean, accessible surface, such as bedside table or, if possible, between patient's open legs. Patient size and positioning dictate exact placement.	Provides easy access to supplies during catheter insertion.
10. Open inner sterile wrap covering tray containing catheterization supplies using sterile technique (see Chapter 5). Fold back each flap of sterile covering with first flap opened away from you, next two flaps open to each side one at a time, and last flap opened toward patient.	Sterile wrap serves as sterile field. Sequence prevents you from reaching over sterile field.
a. Indwelling catheterization open system: Open separate package containing drainage bag, check to make sure that clamp on drainage port is closed, and place drainage bag and tubing in easily accessible location. Open outer package of sterile catheter, maintaining sterility of inner wrapper (see Chapter 5).	Open drainage bag systems have separate sterile packaging for sterile catheter, drainage bag and tubing, and insertion kit.
b. Indwelling catheterization closed system: All supplies are in sterile tray and arranged in sequence of use.	Closed drainage bag systems have catheter preattached to drainage tubing and bag.
c. Straight catheterization: All needed supplies are in sterile tray that contains supplies and can be used for urine collection.	
11. Apply sterile gloves.	Maintains surgical asepsis.
12. *Option:* Apply sterile drape with ungloved hands when drape is packed as first item. Touch only 1-inch edges of drape. Then apply sterile gloves.	Maintains surgical asepsis.
13. Drape perineum, keeping gloves and working surface of drape sterile.	Sterile drapes provide sterile field over which you will work during catheterization.
a. Drape female:	
(1) Pick up square sterile drape touching only edges (2.5 cm [1 inch]).	
(2) Allow drape to unfold without touching unsterile surfaces. Allow top edge of drape (2.5 to 5 cm [1 to 2 inches]) to form cuff over both hands.	When creating cuff over sterile gloved hands, sterility of gloves and workspace is maintained.
(3) Place drape with shiny side down on bed between patient's thighs. Slip cuffed edge just under buttocks as you ask patient to lift hips. Take care not to touch contaminated surfaces or patient's thighs with sterile gloves. If gloves are contaminated, remove and apply new pair.	
(4) Pick up fenestrated sterile drape out of tray. Allow drape to unfold without touching unsterile surfaces. Allow top edge of drape to form cuff over both hands. Apply drape over perineum so that opening is over exposed labia (see illustration).	Opening in drape creates sterile field around labia.
b. Drape male:	
(1) Use of square drape is optional; you may apply fenestrated drape instead.	
(2) Pick up edges of square drape and allow to unfold without touching unsterile surfaces. Place over thighs, with shiny side down, just below penis. Take care not to touch contaminated surfaces with sterile gloves.	

STEP	RATIONALE
(3) Place fenestrated drape with opening centered over penis (see illustration).	
14. Move tray closer to patient. Arrange remaining supplies on sterile field, maintaining sterility of gloves. Place sterile tray with cleaning solution (premoistened swab sticks or cotton balls, forceps, and solution), lubricant, catheter, and prefilled syringe for inflating balloon (indwelling catheterization only) on sterile drape.	Provides easy access to supplies during catheter insertion and helps to maintain aseptic technique. Appropriate placement is determined by size of patient and position during catheterization.
a. If kit contains sterile cotton balls, open package of sterile antiseptic solution and pour over cotton balls. Some kits contain package of premoistened swab sticks. Open end of package for easy access (see illustration).	Use of sterile supplies and antiseptic solution reduces risk of CAUTI (Gould et al., 2017).
b. Open sterile specimen container if specimen is to be obtained (see Chapter 9).	Makes container accessible to receive urine from catheter if specimen is needed.
c. For indwelling catheterization, open sterile inner wrapper of catheter and leave catheter on sterile field. If part of closed system kit, remove tray with catheter and preattached drainage bag and place on sterile drape. Make sure that clamp on drainage port of bag is closed. If needed and if part of sterile tray, attach catheter to drainage tubing.	Indwelling catheterization trays vary. Some have preattached catheters; others need to be attached but are part of the sterile tray; others do not have catheter or drainage system as part of tray.

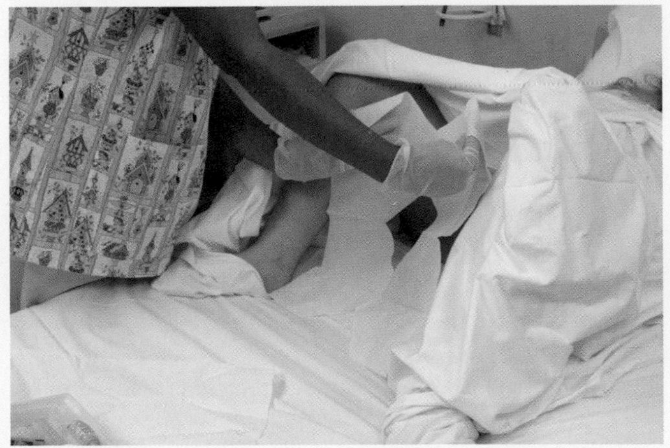

STEP 13a(4) Place sterile fenestrated drape (with opening in center) over female's perineum.

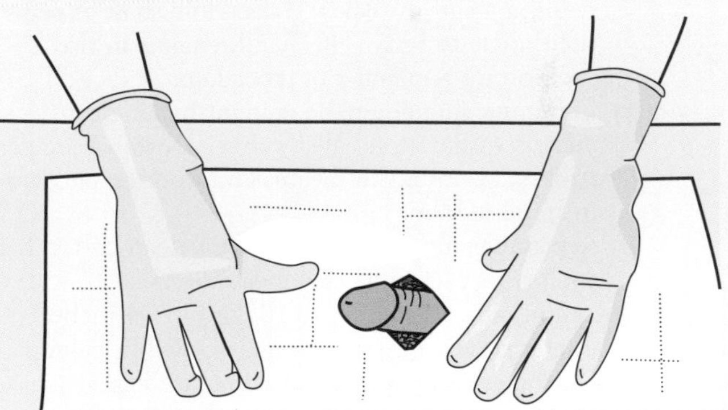

STEP 13b(3) Drape male with fenestrated drape.

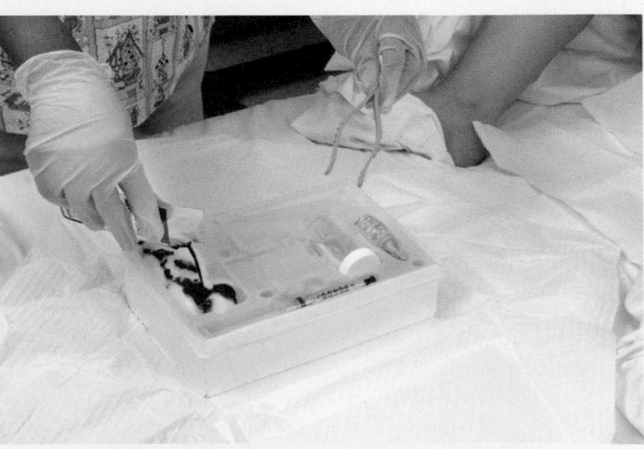

STEP 14a Sterile kit includes antiseptic swabs.

STEP	RATIONALE
d. Open packet of lubricant and squeeze out on sterile field. Lubricate catheter tip by dipping it into water-soluble gel 2.5 to 5 cm (1 to 2 inches) for women and 12.5 to 17.5 cm (5 to 7 inches) for men (see illustration).	Lubrication minimizes trauma to urethra and discomfort during catheter insertion. Male catheter needs enough lubricant to cover length of catheter inserted.

Safe Patient Care *Pretesting a balloon on an indwelling catheter by injecting fluid from the prefilled sterile normal saline syringe into the balloon port is no longer recommended. Testing the balloon may distort and stretch it and lead to damage, causing increased trauma on insertion.*

STEP	RATIONALE
15. Clean urethral meatus:	
a. Female patient:	
(1) Separate labia with fingers of nondominant hand (now contaminated) to fully expose urethral meatus.	Optimal visualization of urethral meatus is possible.
(2) Maintain position of nondominant hand throughout procedure.	Closure of labia during cleaning means that area is contaminated and requires cleaning procedure to be repeated.
(3) Holding forceps in dominant hand, pick up one moistened cotton ball or pick up one swab stick at a time. Clean labia and urinary meatus from clitoris toward anus. Use new cotton ball or swab for each area that you clean. Clean by wiping far labial fold, near labial fold, and last, directly over center of urethral meatus (see illustration).	Front-to-back cleaning moves from area of least contamination toward highly contaminated area. Follows principles of medical asepsis (see Chapter 9). Dominant gloved hand remains sterile.
b. Male patient:	
(1) With nondominant hand (now contaminated) retract foreskin (if uncircumcised) and gently grasp penis at shaft just below glans. Hold shaft of penis at right angle to body. This hand remains in this position for remainder of procedure.	When grasping shaft of penis, avoid pressure on dorsal surface to prevent compression of urethra. Losing grasp during cleaning means that area is contaminated and requires cleaning procedure to be repeated.
(2) Using uncontaminated dominant hand, clean meatus with cotton balls/swab sticks, using circular strokes, beginning at meatus and working outward in spiral motion.	Circular cleaning pattern follows principles of medical asepsis (see Chapter 5).
(3) Repeat cleaning three times using clean cotton ball/swab stick each time (see illustration).	
16. Pick up and hold catheter 7.5 to 10 cm (3 to 4 inches) from catheter tip with catheter loosely coiled in palm of hand. If catheter is not attached to drainage bag, make sure to position urine tray so that end of catheter can be placed there once insertion begins.	Holding catheter near tip allows for its easier manipulation during insertion. Coiling catheter in palm prevents distal end from striking nonsterile surface.

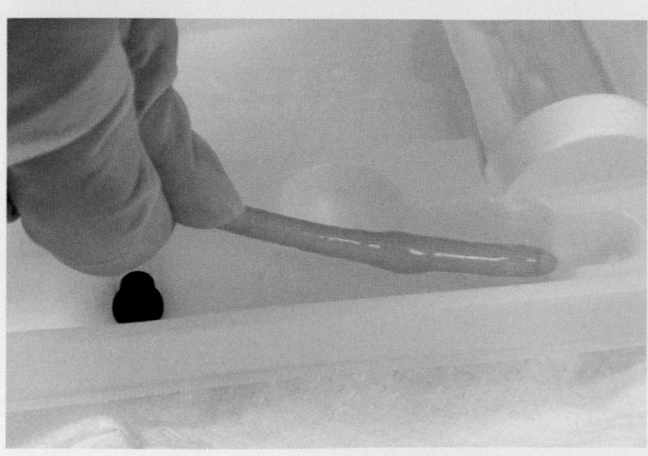

STEP 14d Lubricate catheter.

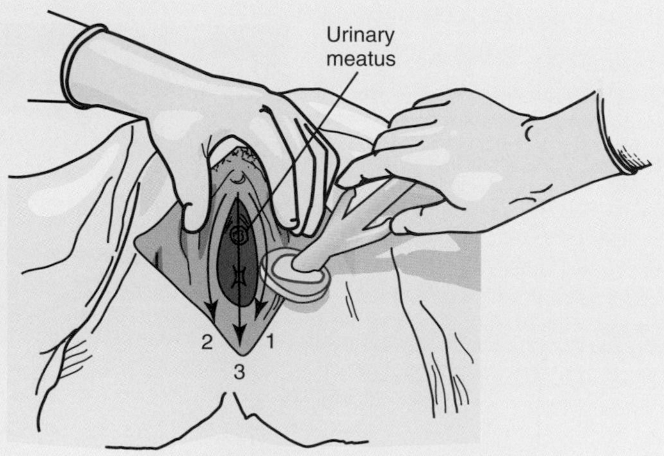

STEP 15a(3) Clean female perineum.

STEP	RATIONALE
17. Insert catheter. Explain to patient that feeling of discomfort or pressure may be experienced as catheter is inserted into urethra. This sensation is normal and will go away quickly.	Helps minimize patient anxiety.
a. Female patient:	
(1) Ask patient to bear down gently and slowly insert catheter through urethral meatus (see illustration).	Bearing down may help visualize urinary meatus and promotes relaxation of external urinary sphincter, aiding in catheter insertion.
(2) Advance catheter total of 5 to 7.5 cm (2 to 3 inches) or until urine flows out of catheter. When urine appears, advance catheter another 2.5 to 5 cm (1 to 2 inches). Do not use force to insert catheter.	Urine flow indicates that catheter tip is in bladder or lower urethra.
(3) Release labia and hold catheter securely with nondominant hand.	Prevents accidental expulsion of catheter from the patient's bladder.
b. Male patient:	
(1) Lift penis to position perpendicular (90 degrees) to patient's body and apply gentle upward traction (see illustration).	Straightens urethra to ease catheter insertion.
(2) Ask patient to bear down as if to void and slowly insert catheter through urethral meatus.	Relaxation of external sphincter aids in insertion of catheter.

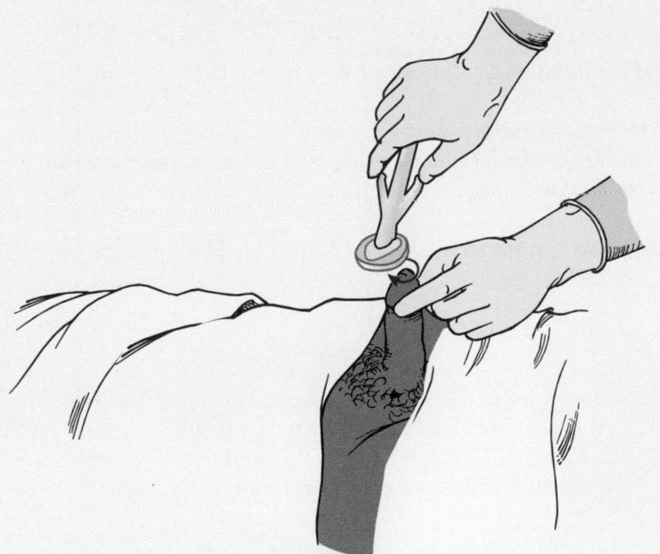

STEP 15b(3) Cleansing male urinary meatus.

STEP 17a(1) Insert catheter into female urinary meatus.

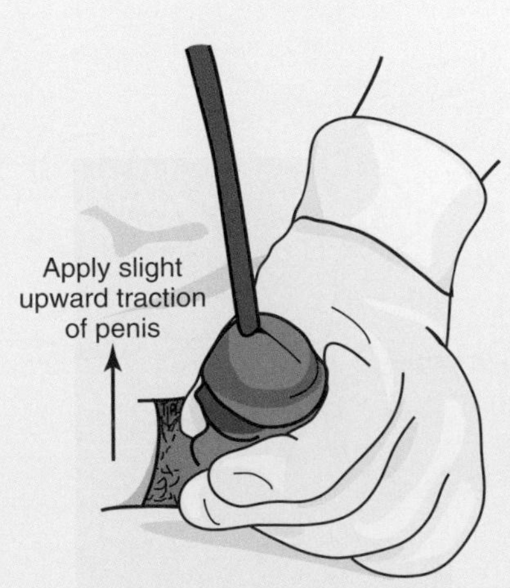

STEP 17b(1) Insert catheter into male urinary meatus.

STEP	RATIONALE
(3) Advance catheter 17 to 22.5 cm (7 to 9 inches) or until urine flows out end of catheter.	Length of male urethra varies. Flow of urine indicates that tip of catheter is in bladder or urethra but not necessarily that balloon part of indwelling catheter is in bladder.
(4) Stop advancing with straight catheter. When urine appears in indwelling catheter, advance it to bifurcation (inflation and deflation ports exposed; see illustration).	Further advancement of catheter to bifurcation of drainage and balloon inflation port ensures that balloon part of catheter is not still in prostatic urethra.
(5) Lower penis and hold catheter securely in nondominant hand.	Prevents accidental expulsion of catheter from the patient's bladder.
18. Allow bladder to empty fully unless agency policy restricts maximum volume of urine drained (see agency policy).	There is no definitive evidence regarding whether there is benefit in limiting maximal volume drained.
19. Collect urine specimen as needed (see Chapter 9). Fill specimen container to 20 to 30 mL by holding end of catheter over cup. Set aside. Keep end of catheter sterile.	Sterile specimen for culture analysis can be obtained.
20. *Option for straight catheterization:* When urine stops flowing, withdraw catheter slowly and smoothly until removed.	Minimizes trauma to urethra.
21. Inflate catheter balloon with amount of fluid designated by manufacturer.	Indwelling catheter balloon should not be underinflated. Underinflation causes balloon distortion and potential bladder damage.
a. Continue to hold catheter with nondominant hand.	Holding on to catheter before inflating balloon prevents expulsion of catheter from urethra.
b. With free dominant hand, connect prefilled syringe to injection port at end of catheter.	
c. Slowly inject total amount of solution (see illustration).	Full amount of solution needed to inflate balloon properly.

Safe Patient Care *If patient reports sudden pain during inflation of a catheter balloon or when resistance is felt when inflating the balloon, stop inflation, allow the fluid from the balloon to flow back into the syringe, advance catheter farther, and reinflate balloon. The balloon may have been inflating in the urethra. If pain continues, remove catheter and notify the health care provider.*

STEP	RATIONALE
d. After inflating catheter balloon, release catheter from nondominant hand. *Gently* pull catheter until resistance is felt. Then advance catheter slightly.	By moving catheter slightly back into bladder, pressure on bladder neck is avoided.
e. Connect drainage tubing to catheter if it is not already preconnected.	
22. Secure indwelling catheter with catheter strap or other securement device. Leave enough slack to allow leg movement. Attach securement device at tubing just above catheter bifurcation.	Securing catheter reduces risk of movement, urethral erosion, CAUTI, or accidental catheter removal (Gould et al., 2017; McNeill, 2017). Attachment of securement device at catheter bifurcation prevents occlusion of catheter.

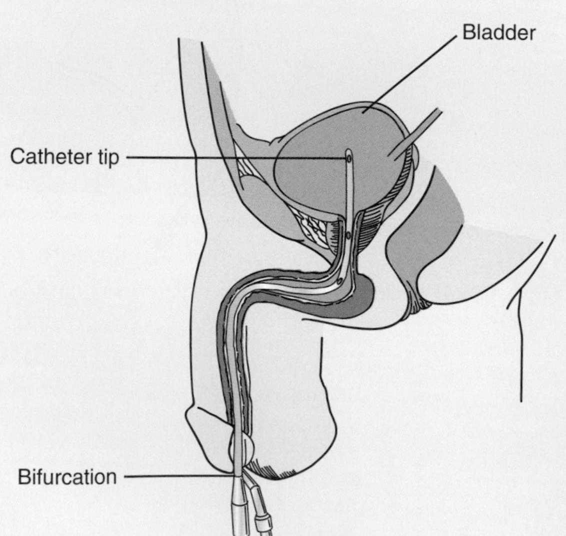

STEP 17b(4) Male anatomy with correct catheter insertion to bifurcation.

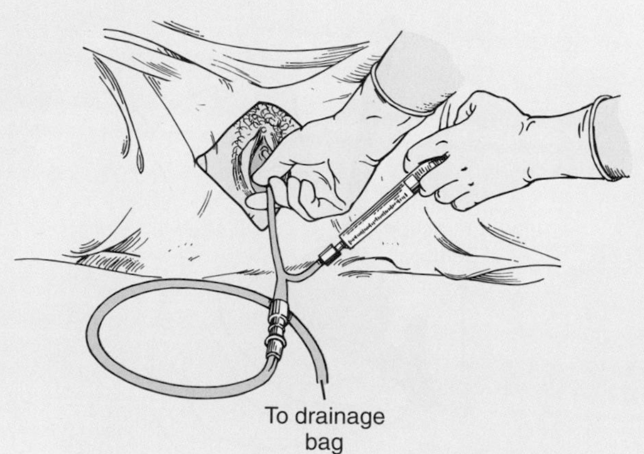

STEP 21c Inflate balloon (indwelling catheter).

STEP	RATIONALE
a. Female patient:	
(1) Secure catheter tubing to inner thigh, allowing enough slack to prevent tension (see illustration).	
b. Male patient:	
(1) Secure catheter tubing to upper thigh (see illustration) or lower abdomen (with penis directed toward chest). Allow slack in catheter so that movement does not create tension on catheter.	Anchoring catheter reduces traction on urethra and minimizes urethral injury (Gould et al., 2017; McNeill, 2017).
(2) If retracted, replace foreskin over glans penis.	Leaving foreskin retracted can cause discomfort and dangerous edema.
23. Clip drainage tubing to edge of mattress. Position drainage bag below level of bladder by attaching to bedframe (Gould et al., 2017). Do not attach to side rails of bed and do not rest on floor (see illustration).	Keeping the collection bag below the level of the bladder at all times prevents backflow into bladder which can cause risk for CAUTI (Gould et al., 2017). Bags attached to movable objects such as side rail increase risk for urethral trauma because of pulling or accidental dislodgement.
24. Check to ensure that there is no obstruction to urine flow. Coil excess tubing on bed and fasten to bottom sheet with clip or other securement device.	Keeping the catheter and collecting tube free from kinking may reduce risk of CAUTI (Gould et al., 2017).

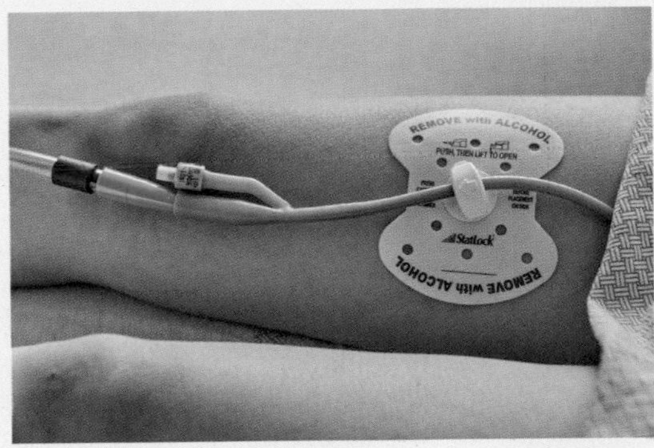

STEP 22a(1) Secure indwelling catheter on female with adhesive securement device.

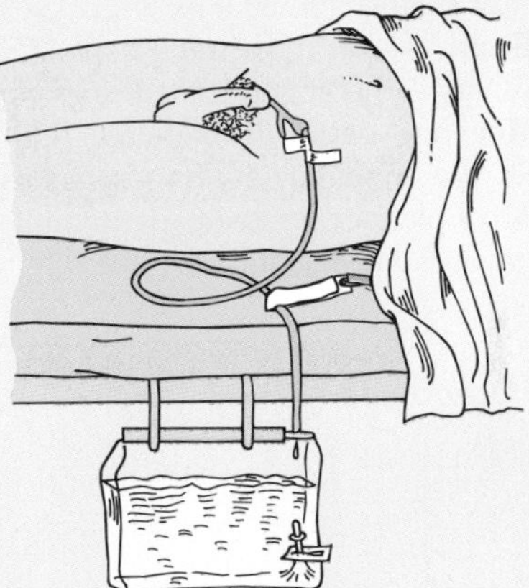

STEP 22b(1) Secure indwelling catheter on male with tape.

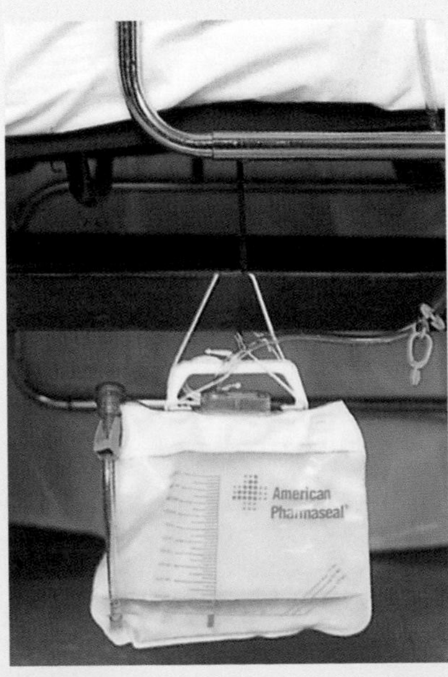

STEP 23 Drainage bag below level of bladder.

STEP	RATIONALE
25. Provide perineal hygiene as needed. Help patient to comfortable position.	Promotes patient comfort.
26. Dispose of supplies in appropriate receptacles.	Reduces transmission of microorganisms.
27. Label and bag specimen according to agency policy. Label specimen in front of patient. Send to laboratory as soon as possible.	Fresh urine specimen ensures more accurate findings. Labeling ensures that diagnostic results will be connected to correct patient.
28. Measure urine and record.	Provides baseline for urine output.
29. Remove gloves and perform hand hygiene.	Reduces transmission of infection.
30. Raise side rails (as appropriate) and lower bed to lowest position. Be sure nurse call system is in an accessible location within patient's reach.	Promotes patient comfort and safety. Ensures patient can call for assistance if needed.

EVALUATION

1. Palpate bladder for distention or use bladder scan (see Procedural Guideline 19.2) as per agency protocol.	Determines if distention is relieved.
2. Ask patient to describe level of comfort.	Determines if patient's sensation of discomfort or fullness has been relieved.
3. Indwelling catheter: Observe character and amount of urine in drainage system.	Determines if urine is flowing adequately.
4. Indwelling catheter: Determine that there is no urine leaking from catheter or tubing connections.	Prevents injury to patient's skin and ensures closed sterile system.
5. Use Teach-Back: "I want to be sure I explained clearly about your urinary catheter and some things you can do to ensure the urine flows out of the catheter. Tell me what you can do to keep the urine flowing." Revise your instruction now or develop a plan for revised patient/family caregiver teaching if patient/family caregiver is not able to teach back correctly.	Determines patient's/family caregiver's level of understanding of instructional topic.

Unexpected Outcomes	Related Interventions
1. Catheter goes into vagina.	• Leave first catheter in vagina so that you can correctly identify the urinary meatus. • Clean urinary meatus again. Using another catheter kit, reinsert sterile catheter into meatus (check agency policy). **NOTE:** If gloves become contaminated, start procedure again. • Remove first catheter that was left in vagina after successful insertion of second catheter.
2. Sterility is broken during catheterization by nurse or patient.	• Replace gloves if contaminated and start over. • If patient touches sterile field but equipment and supplies remain sterile, avoid touching that part of sterile field. • If equipment and/or supplies become contaminated, replace with sterile items or start over with new sterile kit.
3. Patient reports bladder discomfort, and catheter is patent as evidenced by adequate urine flow.	• Check catheter to ensure that there is no traction on it. • Notify health care provider. Patient may be experiencing bladder spasms or symptoms of UTI. • Monitor catheter output for color, clarity, odor, and amount.

Recording

- Record reason for catheterization, type and size of catheter inserted, amount of fluid used to inflate balloon, specimen collection (if applicable), characteristics and amount of urine, patient's response to procedure, and evaluation of patient learning.
- Record I&O on flow sheet record.

Hand-Off Reporting

- Report reason for catheterization, type and size of catheter inserted, amount of fluid used to inflate balloon, specimen collection (if applicable), characteristics and amount of urine, patient's response to procedure, and any education.
- Report to health care provider persistent catheter-related pain and discomfort.

✦ SKILL 19.3 Care and Removal of an Indwelling Catheter

Purpose

If an indwelling catheter is in place, ongoing monitoring for signs of a urinary tract infection (UTI) and proper cleansing of the external portion of the catheter and the patient's perineum are necessary to reduce risk of infection. The maintenance of a closed drainage system is also essential to reduce entrance of microorganisms into the urinary tract. Timely removal of indwelling catheters has been shown to reduce the risk of catheter-associated urinary tract infection (CAUTI; Gould et al., 2017). When removing a catheter, always be sure that the catheter balloon is fully deflated to minimize trauma to the urethra. Evidence is unclear that the practice of clamping a catheter to achieve bladder fullness for several minutes before removal improves bladder function after removal (Gould et al., 2017).

All patients should have their voiding monitored after catheter removal for at least 24 to 48 hours by using a voiding record or bladder diary to record the time and amount of each voiding, including any incontinence. A bladder scanner can be used to monitor bladder functioning by measuring postvoid residual (PVR; see Procedural Guideline 19.2). Abdominal pain and distention, a sensation of incomplete emptying, incontinence, constant dribbling of urine, and voiding in very small amounts can indicate inadequate bladder emptying that requires intervention. Symptoms of infection can develop 2 or more days after catheter removal. Always inform patients about the risk for infection, prevention measures, and signs and symptoms that need to be reported right away to the health care provider.

Delegation and Collaboration

The skill of performing routine catheter care can be delegated to nursing assistive personnel (NAP). Depending on agency policy, the skill of removing an indwelling catheter may be delegated to NAP; however, a nurse must first assess a patient's status and verify the order. The nurse directs the NAP to:

- Report characteristics of the urine (color, clarity, odor, and amount) before and after removal.
- Report the condition of the patient's genital area (e.g., color, rashes, open areas, odor, soiling from fecal incontinence, trauma to tissues around urinary meatus).
- If allowed to remove catheter per agency policy, check size of balloon and syringe needed to deflate balloon; report if balloon does not deflate and if there is bleeding after removal.
- Report time and amount of first voiding after catheter is removed.
- Report if patient experiences fever, chills, change in mental status, burning, flank or back pain, and/or hematuria (signs of UTI); dysuria after catheter removal.

Equipment

Catheter Care

- Clean gloves
- Waterproof pad
- Bath blanket
- Basin with warm water, washcloth, towel, and soap for perineal care

Removing a Catheter

- Clean gloves
- 10-mL syringe or larger without a needle (size depends on volume of solution used to inflate the balloon)
- Graduated cylinder to measure urine
- Waterproof pad
- Toilet, bedside commode, urine "hat," urinal, or bedpan
- Bladder scanner (if indicated)

ASSESSMENT

1. Identify patient using at least two identifiers (e.g., name and birthday or name and medical record number) according to agency policy. *Rationale: Ensures correct patient. Complies with The Joint Commission standards and improves patient safety (TJC, 2019).*
2. Perform hand hygiene. Apply clean gloves. *Rationale: Reduces transmission of microorganisms.*
3. Assess need for catheter care:
   a. Observe urinary output and urine characteristics. *Rationale: Sudden decrease in urine output may indicate occlusion of catheter. Cloudy, foul-smelling urine associated with other systemic symptoms may indicate CAUTI.*
   b. Assess for history or presence of bowel incontinence. *Rationale: Most common bacteria to cause CAUTI are* Escherichia coli, *a major colonizer of the bowel; thus fecal incontinence increases risk for CAUTI (Fekete, 2018).*
   c. Position patient and retract labia or foreskin to observe for any discharge, redness, bleeding, or presence of tissue trauma around urethral meatus (this may be deferred until catheter care). *Rationale: Indicates inflammatory process, possible infection, or erosion of catheter through urethra.*
   d. Remove and dispose of gloves; perform hand hygiene. *Rationale: Reduces transmission of microorganisms.*
4. Assess need for catheter removal:
   a. Review patient's electronic health record (EHR), including health care provider's order and nurses' notes. Note length of time catheter has been in place. *Rationale: Catheters in place for more than a few days cause higher risk for catheter encrustation and UTI.*
   b. Perform hand hygiene. Assess urine color, clarity, odor, and amount. Note any urethral discharge, irritation of genital region, or trauma to urinary meatus (this requires clean gloves or may be deferred until just before removal). Remove and dispose of gloves if worn. *Rationale: May be indicator of inflammation or UTI and source of discomfort during catheter removal. Reduces transmission of microorganisms.*
   c. Determine size of catheter inflation balloon by looking at balloon inflation valve. *Rationale: Determines size of syringe needed to deflate balloon and amount of fluid expected in syringe after deflation.*
5. Assess patient's or family caregiver's knowledge and prior experience with catheter care and/or catheter removal. *Rationale: Ensures patient has the capacity to obtain, communicate, process, and understand basic health information (CDC, 2016).*

STEP	RATIONALE
PLANNING	
1. Expected outcomes following catheter care:	
• Genital area is free of secretions, fecal matter, and irritation.	Basic hygiene, especially perineal care, reduces risk for CAUTI (McNeill, 2017).
• Patient verbalizes feeling of comfort around catheter exit site.	Cleaning relieves local discomfort from irritation of catheter.
2. Expected outcomes after catheter removal:	
• Patient voids at least 150 mL with each voiding no more than 6 to 8 hours after removal.	Indicates return of voluntary bladder function without urinary retention.
• Patient verbalizes feeling of complete bladder emptying and absence of discomfort.	Urinary retention does not develop after catheter removal.
• Patient identifies signs and symptoms of UTI.	Indicates patient learning.
3. Close room door and bedside curtain.	Provides patient privacy.
4. Obtain and organize equipment for perineal care/catheter removal at bedside.	Ensures more efficient procedure.
5. Explain procedure to patient. Discuss signs and symptoms of UTI. If applicable, teach patient or family caregiver how to perform catheter hygiene.	Reduces anxiety and promotes cooperation. Self-care supports patient's sense of autonomy.
IMPLEMENTATION	
1. Perform hand hygiene.	Reduces transmission of microorganisms.
2. Raise bed to appropriate working height. If side rails are raised, lower side rail on working side.	Promotes use of proper body mechanics.
3. Position patient with waterproof pad under buttocks and cover with bath blanket, exposing only genital area and catheter (see Skill 19.2).	Shows respect for patient dignity by only exposing genital area and catheter.
a. Female in dorsal recumbent position.	
b. Male in supine position.	
4. Apply clean gloves.	Reduces transmission of microorganisms.
5. Remove catheter securement device while maintaining connection with drainage tubing.	Provides ability to easily clean around catheter and to remove it.
6. Catheter care:	
a. *Female:* Use nondominant hand to gently separate labia to fully expose urethral meatus and catheter. Maintain position of hand throughout procedure.	Provides full visualization of urethral meatus. Full separation of labia prevents contamination of meatus during cleaning.
b. *Male:* Use nondominant hand to retract foreskin if not circumcised and hold penis at shaft just below glans. Maintain hand position throughout procedure.	Retraction of foreskin provides full visualization of urethral meatus.
c. Grasp catheter with two fingers of nondominant hand to stabilize it.	Prevents unnecessary traction on catheter. Pulling on catheter is cause of discomfort for patient and can damage urethra and bladder neck.
d. If not performed earlier, assess urethral meatus and surrounding tissues for inflammation, swelling, discharge, or tissue trauma and ask patient if burning or discomfort is present.	Determines frequency and type of ongoing care required. Indicates possibility of CAUTI or catheter erosion through urethra.
e. Provide perineal hygiene using mild soap and warm water (see Chapter 11). *Option:* Use chlorhexidine gluconate (CHG) 2% cloth.	Antiseptic cleaners have not been shown to definitively decrease CAUTI; mild soap and water is appropriate (McNeill, 2017). Although CHG cloth can be used, there is no clear scientific evidence for use of antiseptics versus nonantiseptics to reduce rates of CAUTI (Fasugba et al., 2017).
f. Using clean washcloth or CHG cloth, clean catheter.	
(1) Starting close to urinary meatus, clean catheter in circular motion along its length for about 10 cm (4 inches), moving away from body (see illustration). Remove all traces of soap. *For male patients:* Reduce or reposition foreskin after care.	Reduces presence of secretions or drainage on outside catheter surface.

STEP	RATIONALE

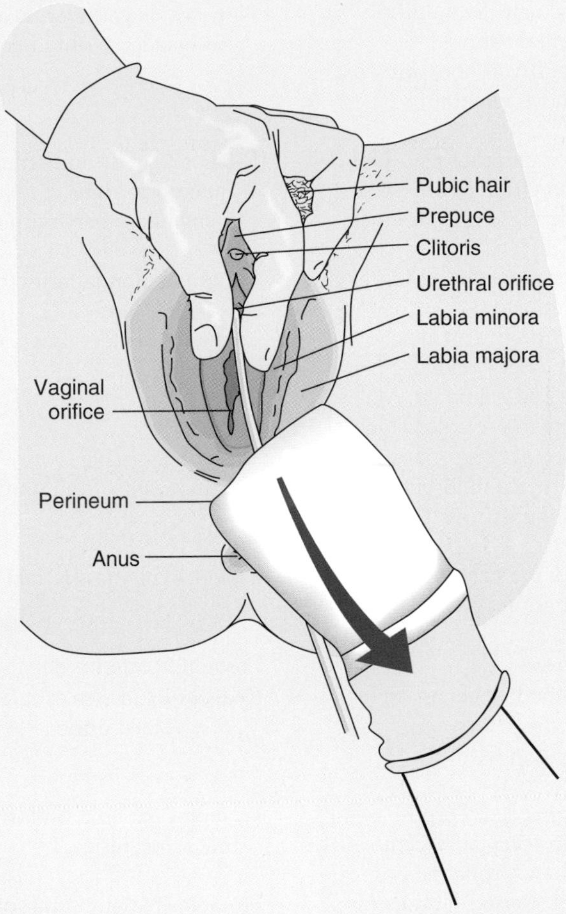

STEP 6f(1) Clean catheter starting at meatus and moving downward while holding it securely.

STEP	RATIONALE
g. Reapply catheter securement device. Allow slack in catheter so that movement does not create tension on it.	Securing indwelling catheter reduces risk of urethral trauma, urethral erosion, CAUTI, or accidental removal (Gould et al., 2017; McNeill, 2017).
7. Routinely check drainage tubing and bag.	
a. Catheter is secured to upper thigh.	Maintains unobstructed flow of urine out of bladder (Gould et al., 2017; McNeill, 2017).
b. Tubing is coiled and secured onto bed linen.	
c. Tubing is not looped or positioned above level of bladder.	
d. Tubing is not kinked or clamped.	
e. Drainage bag is positioned below level of bladder with urine flowing freely into bag.	
f. Drainage bag is not overfull. Empty drainage bag when ½ full.	Overfull drainage bag creates tension and pulls on catheter, resulting in trauma to urethra and/or urinary meatus. Facilitates unobstructed flow of urine (Gould et al., 2017).
8. Catheter removal: (Follow Step 6 before catheter removal.)	
a. With clean gloves still on, move syringe plunger up and down to loosen, and then pull it back to 0.5 mL. Insert hub of syringe into inflation valve (balloon port). Allow balloon fluid to drain into syringe automatically by itself. Syringe should fill. Make sure that entire amount of fluid is removed by comparing removed amount to volume needed for inflation.	Partially inflated balloon can traumatize urethral wall during removal. Passive drainage of catheter balloon prevents formation of ridges in balloon. These ridges can cause discomfort or trauma during removal.

STEP	RATIONALE
b. Pull catheter out smoothly and slowly. Examine it to ensure that it is whole. Catheter should slide out easily. Do not use force. If you note any resistance, repeat Step 8a to remove remaining inflation fluid.	Non–whole catheter means that pieces of catheter may still be in bladder. Notify health care provider immediately.
c. Wrap contaminated catheter in waterproof pad. Unhook collection bag and drainage tubing from bed.	Promotes safety and reduces the risk for transmission of microorganisms.
d. Empty, measure, and record urine present in drainage bag (see Chapter 9).	Documents urinary output.
e. Encourage patient to maintain or increase fluid intake (unless contraindicated by restrictions).	Maintains normal urine output.
f. Initiate voiding record or bladder diary. Instruct patient to tell you when need to empty bladder occurs and that all urine needs to be measured. Make sure that patient understands how to use collection container.	Evaluates bladder function.
g. Explain that many patients experience mild burning, discomfort, or small-volume voiding with first voiding, which soon subsides.	Burning results from urethral irritation.
h. Measure PVR volume (if ordered; see Procedural Guideline 19.2) within 5 to 15 minutes after helping the patient to void.	Provides the most reliable PVR reading (Huether et al., 2017).
i. Inform patient to report any signs of UTI.	Promotes patient safety.
j. Ensure easy access to toilet, commode, bedpan, or urinal. Place urine "hat" on toilet seat if patient is using toilet. Place nurse call system within easy reach.	Reduces incidence of falls during toileting. Urine hat collects first voided urine.
9. Provide patient personal hygiene as needed. Dispose of all contaminated supplies in appropriate receptacle, remove and dispose of gloves, and perform hand hygiene.	Promotes patient comfort and safety. Reduces transmission of microorganisms.
10. Help patient to comfortable position. Raise side rails (as appropriate) and lower bed to lowest position. Be sure nurse call system is in an accessible location within patient's reach.	Promotes patient comfort and safety. Ensures patient can call for assistance if needed.

EVALUATION

1. Inspect catheter and genital area for soiling, irritation, and skin breakdown. Ask patient about discomfort.	Determines if area is cleaned properly and/or if patient has any irritation.
2. Observe time and measure amount of first voiding after catheter removal.	Indicates return of bladder function after catheter removal.
3. Evaluate patient for signs and symptoms of UTI.	Any patient who has a catheter or has had a catheter removed recently is at risk for UTI.
4. **Use Teach-Back:** "I want to be sure I clearly explained the signs of a urinary tract infection and some things you should do to prevent infection. Tell me some ways in which you can prevent a urinary tract infection." Revise your instruction now or develop plan for revised patient/family caregiver teaching if patient/family caregiver is not able to teach back correctly.	Determines patient's/family caregiver's level of understanding of instructional topic.

Unexpected Outcomes	Related Interventions
1. Normal saline from inflation balloon does not return into syringe.	• Reposition patient; ensure that catheter is not pinched or kinked. • Remove syringe. Attach new syringe and allow enough time for passive emptying. • Attempt to empty balloon by gently pulling back on syringe plunger. • If catheter balloon does not deflate, *do not* cut balloon inflation valve to drain fluid. Notify health care provider.

2. Patient has cloudy foul-smelling urine, fever, chills, dysuria, flank pain, back pain, hematuria, urgency, frequency, lower abdominal pain, change in mental status, and lethargy (U.S. National Library of Medicine, 2016).	• Assess for bladder distention and tenderness. • Monitor vital signs and urine output. • Report findings to health care provider; signs and symptoms may indicate UTI. • Consult with health care provider for order to remove catheter.
3. Patient is unable to void within 6 to 8 hours after catheter removal, has sensation of not emptying, strains to void, or experiences small voiding amounts with increasing frequency.	• Assess for bladder distention. Perform bladder scan (see Procedural Guideline 19.2). • Help to normal position for voiding and provide privacy. • If patient is unable to void within 6 to 8 hours of catheter removal and/or experiences abdominal pain, notify health care provider.

Recording

- Record time catheter was removed; teaching related to increasing fluid intake and signs and symptoms of UTI; and time, amount, and characteristics of first voiding.
- Record intake and voiding times and amounts on voiding record or bladder diary as indicated.
- Record patient symptoms experienced upon and after catheter removal.
- Document your evaluation of patient learning.

Hand-Off Reporting

- Report time catheter was removed; teaching related to increasing fluid intake and signs and symptoms of UTI; and time, amount, and characteristics of first voiding.
- Report hematuria, dysuria, inability or difficulty voiding, and any new incontinence after a catheter is removed to health care provider.

✦ SKILL 19.4 Suprapubic Catheter Care

Purpose

A suprapubic catheter is a urinary drainage tube inserted surgically through a small cut in the abdominal wall above the symphysis pubis into the bladder (Fig. 19.6). The catheter may be sutured to the skin, secured with an adhesive material, or retained in the bladder with a fluid-filled balloon like an indwelling catheter. Suprapubic catheters are placed when there is blockage of the urethra (e.g., enlarged prostate, urethral stricture, after urological surgery) and in situations when a long-term urethral catheter causes irritation or discomfort or interferes with sexual functioning. A review of scientific studies comparing suprapubic with indwelling urethral catheters showed that suprapubic catheters reduced the number of study participants with asymptomatic bacteriuria, recatheterization, and pain (Kidd et al., 2015). Evidence from the same review showed reduction in urinary tract infections (UTIs) to be inconclusive.

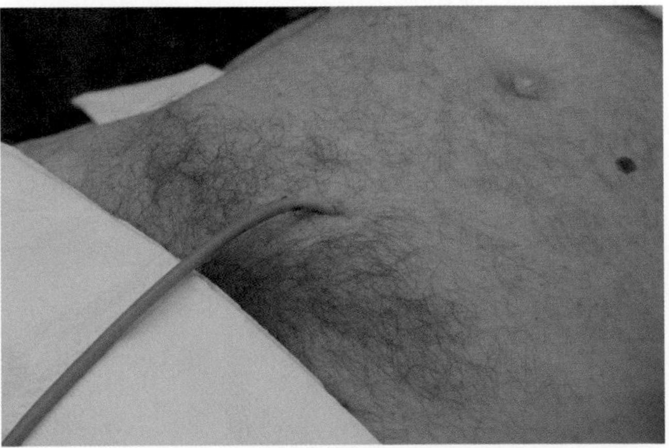

FIG 19.6 Suprapubic catheter without dressing.

Delegation and Collaboration

The skill of caring for a newly established suprapubic catheter cannot be delegated to nursing assistive personnel (NAP); however, care of an established suprapubic catheter may be delegated (if permitted per agency policy). The nurse directs the NAP to:

- Report patient's discomfort (bladder fullness, abdominal pain, skin irritation) related to the suprapubic catheter.
- Empty drainage bag and document urinary output on intake and output (I&O) record.
- Report any change in the amount and character of the urine and signs of redness, foul odor, or drainage around catheter insertion site to the nurse.

Equipment

- Clean gloves (sterile gloves may be needed in some cases; refer to agency policy)
- Cleansing agent (sterile normal saline solution)
- Sterile cotton-tipped applicators
- Sterile surgical drainage sponge (split gauze)
- Sterile gauze dressing
- Washcloth, towel, soap, and water
- Tape
- Velcro tube holder or tube stabilizer *(optional)*

ASSESSMENT

1. Identify patient using at least two identifiers (e.g., name and birthday or name and medical record number) according to agency policy. *Rationale: Ensures correct patient. Complies with*

The Joint Commission standards and improves patient safety (TJC, 2019).

2. Review electronic health record (EHR) and ask patient about any history of allergies. Check allergy armband. *Rationale: Determines supplies used for catheter care. Identifies known patient allergies.*
3. Inspect urine in drainage bag for amount, clarity, color, odor, and sediment. *Rationale: Abnormal findings indicate potential complications, such as UTI, decreased urinary output, and catheter occlusion.*
4. Perform hand hygiene and apply clean gloves. Observe dressing for drainage and intactness. *Rationale: Reduces transmission of microorganisms. Drainage indicates potential complication, such as infection. Dressing may become nonocclusive because of tape choice or drainage.*
5. Assess catheter insertion site (may be deferred until you clean site) for signs of inflammation (i.e., pain, erythema, edema, and drainage) and for growth of overgranulation tissue. Ask patient if there is any pain at site; if so, have him or her rate on scale of 0 to 10. Remove gloves and perform hand hygiene. *Rationale: If insertion is new, slight inflammation may be expected as part of normal wound healing but can also indicate infection. Overgranulation tissue can develop at insertion site as reaction to catheter. In some instances, intervention may be needed. Reduces transmission of microorganisms.*
6. Assess for elevated temperature and chills. *Rationale: Increased temperature may indicate UTI or skin site infection.*
7. Assess patient's or family caregiver's knowledge, experience, and health literacy. *Rationale: Ensures patient has the capacity to obtain, communicate, process, and understand basic health information (CDC, 2016).*

STEP	RATIONALE
PLANNING	
1. Expected outcomes following completion of procedure:	
• Patient verbalizes no pain or discomfort at insertion site and over bladder.	Patent catheter system keeps bladder empty and patient comfortable.
• Urine output is 30 mL or greater per hour.	Indicates that catheter is patent.
• Urine remains clear without foul odor, and patient is afebrile.	Indicates that patient is free of catheter-associated urinary tract infection (CAUTI).
• Catheter exit site is free of infection (i.e., erythema, edema, drainage, tenderness).	Indicates absence of infection and irritation of skin.
• Patient and/or family caregiver can explain purpose of and methods for catheter care.	Evaluates learning.
2. Provide privacy by closing room door and beside curtain.	Promotes patient's comfort.
3. Prepare and organize equipment at bedside.	Ensures efficient procedure.
4. Raise bed to appropriate working height. If side rails are raised, lower side rail on working side.	Promotes use of good body mechanics.
5. Explain procedure to patient and/or family caregiver.	Reduces anxiety and promotes cooperation. Patients with a suprapubic catheter frequently rely on family caregivers for support.
IMPLEMENTATION	
1. Perform hand hygiene.	Reduces transmission of microorganisms.
2. Prepare supplies by opening gauze packets in same manner as for applying dry dressing (see Chapter 27).	Keeps dressing sterile until application.
3. Apply clean gloves. Loosen tape and remove existing dressing. Note type and presence of drainage. Remove gloves and perform hand hygiene.	Provides baseline for condition of suprapubic wound. Reduces transmission of infection from dressing.
4. **Clean insertion site using sterile aseptic technique for newly established catheter:** Option is used less frequently; review agency policy or consider individual patient need (such as reduced immunity). In some agencies, clean gloves are appropriate.	Catheter site is made surgically and therefore is treated similarly to other incisions. Confirm if using either medical aseptic or sterile technique based on agency policy.
a. Apply sterile gloves (see previous note about agency policy).	
b. Without creating tension, hold catheter up with nondominant hand while cleaning. Use sterile gauze moistened in saline and clean skin around insertion site in circular motion, starting near insertion site and continuing in outward widening circles for approximately 5 cm (2 inches; see illustration).	Moves from area of least contamination to area of most contamination. Tension on catheter may cause discomfort or damage to wall of bladder or catheter to slip out of place.

STEP	RATIONALE
c. With fresh, moistened gauze, gently clean body of catheter, starting at base of catheter, moving up and away from site of insertion (proximal to distal).	Removes microorganisms that reside on any drainage that adheres to tubing.
d. Once insertion site is dry, use sterile gloved hand to apply drain dressing (split gauze) around catheter (see illustration). Tape in place.	Moist skin can cause maceration and breakdown. Dressing collects drainage that develops around catheter insertion site.
5. **Clean long-term/established catheter:**	
a. Apply clean gloves.	Reduces transmission of microorganisms.
b. Without creating tension, hold catheter erect with nondominant hand while cleaning. Clean skin with soap and water in circular motion, starting near catheter insertion site and continuing in outward widening circles for approximately 5 cm (2 inches).	Cleaning and drying suprapubic insertion site requires general hygienic measures; dressing is optional if drainage is not present.
c. With a fresh washcloth or gauze, gently clean body of catheter, staring at base of catheter, moving up and away from site of insertion (proximal to distal).	Removes microorganisms that reside in any drainage that adheres to tubing. Soap can cause drying of skin.
d. Rinse skin well removing soap residue. Pat completely dry.	Moisture can macerate skin, causing breakdown.
e. *Option:* Apply drain dressing (split gauze) around catheter and tape in place.	
6. Secure catheter to lateral abdomen with tape or Velcro multipurpose tube holder.	Secures catheter and reduces risk of excessive tension on suture and/or catheter.
7. Coil excess tubing on bed. Keep drainage bag below level of bladder at all times.	Maintains free flow of urine, thus decreasing risk for CAUTI (Gould et al., 2009; McNeill, 2017).
8. Assist patient to comfortable position. Be sure nurse call system is in an accessible location within patient's reach.	Promotes patient comfort and safety. Ensures patient can call for assistance if needed.
9. Raise side rails (as appropriate) and lower bed to lowest position.	Promotes patient safety.
10. Dispose of all contaminated supplies in appropriate receptacle, remove gloves, and perform hand hygiene.	Reduces transmission of microorganisms.

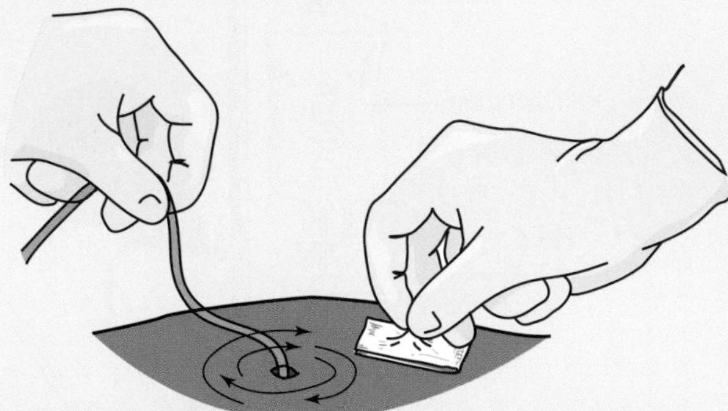

STEP 4b Clean around suprapubic catheter in circular pattern.

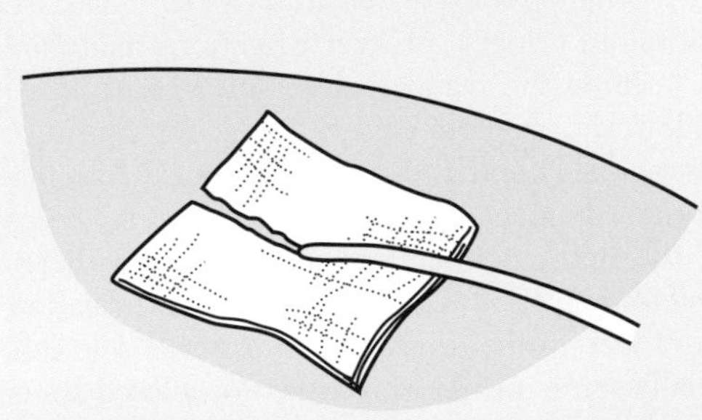

STEP 4d Split drain dressing for suprapubic catheter.

EVALUATION

1. Ask patient to rate pain or discomfort from suprapubic catheter on scale of 0 to 10.	Determines if bladder is draining and patient is free of skin irritation or infection.
2. Monitor for signs of infection (e.g., fever, elevated white blood count) and observe urine for clarity, sediment, unusual color, or odor.	Suprapubic catheters increase risk for UTI.
3. Observe catheter insertion site for erythema, edema, discharge, tenderness. Check dressing at minimum of every 8 hours.	Indicators of an insertion site infection.
4. **Use Teach-Back:** "I want to be sure I explained clearly about the care of your suprapubic catheter. Tell me about some of the things you need to do to care for it at home." Revise your instruction now or develop plan for revised patient/family caregiver teaching if patient/family caregiver is not able to teach back correctly.	Determines patient's/family caregiver's level of understanding of instructional topic.

Unexpected Outcomes	Related Interventions
1. Patient develops symptoms of UTI or catheter site infection.	• Increase fluid intake to at least 2200 mL in 24 hours (unless contraindicated). • Monitor vital signs, I&O; observe amount, color, consistency of urine; assess site. • Notify health care provider.
2. Suprapubic catheter becomes dislodged.	• Cover site with sterile dressing. • Notify health care provider. If newly established catheter, it will need to be reinserted immediately.
3. Skin surrounding catheter exit site becomes red or irritated and/or develops open areas.	• Notify health care provider. • Change dressing (if used) more frequently to keep site dry. • Consult with wound care nurse.

Recording

- Record condition of insertion site, character of urine, type of dressing change, and patient's comfort level with the catheter and dressing change.
- Record urine output on I&O flow sheet. In a situation in which there is both a suprapubic and a urethral catheter, record outputs from each catheter separately.
- Document your evaluation of patient learning.

Hand-Off Reporting

- Report condition of insertion site, character of urine, type of dressing change, and patient's comfort level with the catheter and dressing change.
- Report any complications with catheter to health care provider.

✦ SKILL 19.5 Performing Catheter Irrigation

Purpose

Following surgery on the bladder and other genitourinary (GU) structures, it is common to have hematuria for several days. Intermittent or continuous urinary catheter irrigations maintain catheter patency by keeping the bladder clear and free of blood clots or sediment. However, irrigation poses a risk for causing a urinary tract infection (UTI) and thus must be done while maintaining a closed urinary drainage system. Closed catheter irrigations do not disrupt the sterile connection between the catheter and the drainage system (Fig. 19.7). Continuous bladder irrigation (CBI) is an example of a continuous infusion of a sterile solution into the bladder, usually using a three-way irrigation closed system with a triple-lumen catheter.

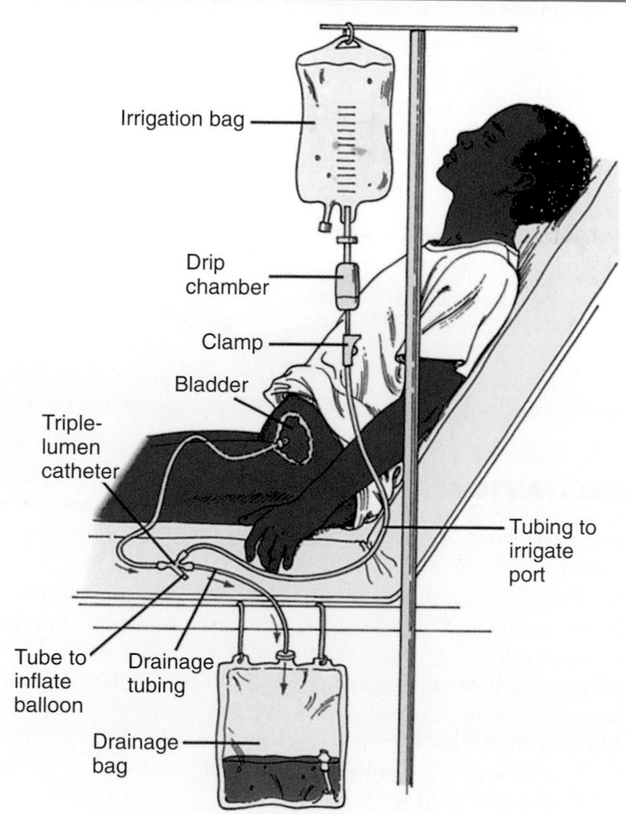

FIG 19.7 Continuous bladder irrigation setup.

Delegation and Collaboration

The skill of catheter irrigation cannot be delegated to nursing assistive personnel (NAP). The nurse directs the NAP to:

- Report if the patient has concerns of pain, discomfort, or leakage of fluid around the catheter.
- Monitor and record intake and output (I&O); report immediately any decrease in urine output to the nurse.
- Report any change in the color of the urine, especially if blood clots are noted.

Equipment

- Clean gloves
- Antiseptic swabs
- Container of sterile irrigation solution at room temperature as prescribed
- Intravenous (IV) pole (closed continuous or intermittent)

Closed Intermittent Irrigation

- Sterile 50-mL syringe to access system: Luer-Lok syringe for needleless access port (per manufacturer's instructions)
- Screw clamp or rubber band (used to occlude catheter temporarily as irrigant is instilled)

Closed Continuous Irrigation

- Sterile irrigation tubing with clamp to regulate irrigation flow rate
- Y connector *(optional)* to connect irrigation tubing to triple-lumen catheter

ASSESSMENT

1. Identify patient using at least two identifiers (e.g., name and birthday or name and medical record number) according to agency policy. *Rationale: Ensures correct patient. Complies with The Joint Commission standards and improves patient safety (TJC, 2019).*
2. Verify in electronic health record (EHR):
   a. Order for irrigation method (continuous or intermittent), solution type (sterile saline or medicated solution), and amount of irrigant. *Rationale: Health care provider's order is required to initiate therapy. Frequency and volume of solution used for irrigation may be in the order or standardized as part of agency policy.*
   b. Type of catheter in place (see Fig. 19.3). *Rationale: Triple-lumen catheters are used for intermittent and continuous closed irrigation.*
3. Perform hand hygiene. Palpate bladder for distention and tenderness or use bladder scan (see Procedural Guidelines 19.2). *Rationale: Reduces transmission of microorganisms. Bladder distention indicates that flow of urine may be blocked from draining.*
4. Assess patient for abdominal pain or spasms, sensation of bladder fullness, or catheter bypassing (leaking). (Wear clean gloves if risk of contacting urine.) *Rationale: May indicate overdistention of bladder caused by catheter blockage. Offers baseline to determine if therapy is successful.*
5. Observe urine for color; amount; clarity; and presence of mucus, clots, or sediment. *Rationale: Indicates if patient is bleeding or sloughing tissue, which would require increased irrigation rate or frequency of catheter irrigation.*
6. Monitor I&O. If CBI is being used, amount of fluid draining from bladder should exceed amount of fluid infused into bladder. *Rationale: If output does not exceed irrigant infused, catheter obstruction (i.e., blood clots, kinked tubing) should be suspected, irrigation stopped, and prescriber notified (Ignatavicius et al., 2018).*
7. Assess patient's or family caregiver's knowledge, experience, and health literacy. *Rationale: Ensures patient has the capacity to obtain, communicate, process, and understand basic health information (CDC, 2016).*

STEP	RATIONALE
PLANNING	
1. Expected outcomes following completion of this procedure:	
• With CBI: Urine output is greater than volume of irrigating solution instilled.	Indicates patency of drainage system, allowing for drainage of urine and irrigating solution.
• Patient reports relief of bladder pain or spasms.	Indicates bladder emptying.
• Urine output has decreased, with an absence of blood clots and sediment. (NOTE: Urine will be bloody following bladder/urethral surgery, gradually becoming lighter and blood tinged in 2 to 3 days.)	Indicates that catheter is at decreased risk for occlusion with blood clots.
• Absence of fever, lower abdominal pain, cloudy and/or foul-smelling urine.	Signs of UTI are not present.
• Patient or family caregiver can explain purpose of procedure and what to expect.	Demonstrates learning.
2. Provide privacy by closing room door and bedside curtain.	Protects patient comfort and privacy.
3. Obtain supplies and set up at bedside.	Ensures more efficient procedure.
4. Raise bed to appropriate working height. If side rails are raised, lower side rail on working side.	Promotes use of good body mechanics. Position provides access to catheter and promotes patient dignity as much as possible.
5. Explain procedure to patient.	Reduces anxiety and promotes cooperation.
IMPLEMENTATION	
1. Perform hand hygiene.	Reduces transmission of microorganisms.
2. Position patient supine and expose catheter junctions (catheter and drainage tubing).	Position provides access to catheter and promotes patient dignity as much as possible.
3. Remove catheter securement device.	Eases access to catheter parts.
4. Organize supplies according to type of irrigation prescribed. Apply clean gloves.	Ensures an efficient procedure.

STEP	RATIONALE
5. Closed continuous irrigation:	
a. Close clamp on new irrigation tubing and hang bag of irrigating solution on IV pole. Insert (spike) tip of sterile irrigation tubing into designated port of irrigation solution bag using aseptic technique (see illustration).	Prevents air from entering tubing. Air can cause bladder spasms. Technique prevents transmission of microorganisms.

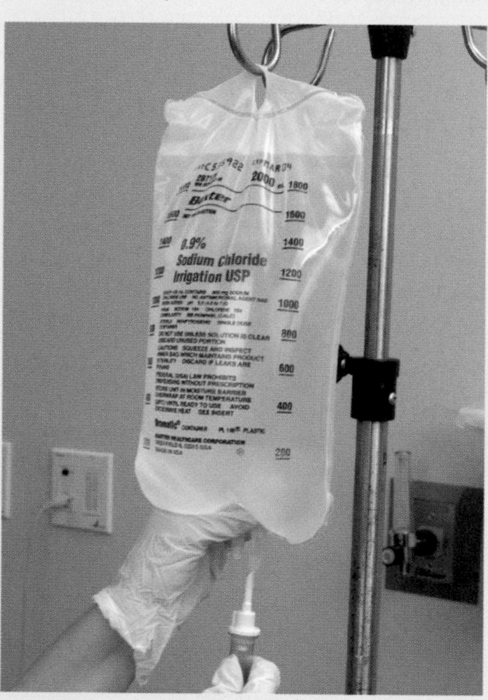

STEP 5a Spiking bag of sterile irrigation solution for continuous bladder irrigation.

STEP	RATIONALE
b. Fill drip chamber half full by squeezing chamber. Remove cap at end of tubing, and then open clamp and allow solution to flow (prime) through tubing, keeping end of tubing sterile. Once fluid has completely filled tubing, close clamp and recap end of tubing.	Priming tubing with fluid prevents introduction of air into bladder.
c. Using aseptic technique, remove cap and connect end of tubing securely to port for infusing irrigation fluid into double- or triple-lumen catheter.	Reduces transmission of microorganisms.
d. Adjust clamp on irrigation tubing to begin flow of solution into bladder. If set volume rate is ordered, calculate drip rate and adjust rate at roller clamp (see Chapter 28). If urine is bright red or has clots, increase irrigation rate until drainage appears pink (according to ordered rate or agency protocol).	Continuous drainage is expected. It helps to prevent clotting in presence of active bleeding in bladder and flushes clots out of bladder.
e. Observe for outflow of fluid into drainage bag. Empty catheter drainage bag as needed.	Discomfort, bladder distention, and possible injury can occur from overdistention of bladder when bladder irrigant cannot adequately flow from bladder. Bag will fill rapidly and may need to be emptied every 1 to 2 hours.
6. Closed intermittent irrigation:	Fluid is instilled through catheter in a bolus, flushing system. Fluid drains out after irrigation is complete.
a. Pour prescribed sterile irrigation solution into sterile container.	
b. Draw prescribed volume of irrigant (usually 30 to 50 mL) into sterile syringe using aseptic technique. Place sterile cap on tip of needleless syringe.	Ensures sterility of irrigating fluid.
c. Clamp catheter tubing below soft injection port with screw clamp (or fold catheter tubing onto itself and secure with rubber band).	Occluding catheter tubing below point of injection allows irrigating solution to enter catheter and flow into bladder.

STEP	RATIONALE
d. Using circular motion, clean catheter port (specimen port) with antiseptic swab.	Reduces transmission of microorganisms.
e. Insert tip of needleless syringe using twisting motion into port.	Ensures that catheter tip enters lumen of catheter.
f. Inject solution using slow, even pressure.	Gentle instillation of solution minimizes trauma to bladder mucosa.
g. Remove syringe and clamp (or rubber band), allowing solution to drain into urinary drainage bag. (**NOTE:** Some medicated irrigants may need to dwell in bladder for prescribed period, requiring catheter to be clamped temporarily before being allowed to drain.)	Allows drainage to flow out by gravity. Medications must be instilled long enough to be absorbed by lining of bladder. Clamped drainage tubing and bag should not be left unattended.
7. Anchor catheter with catheter securement device (see Skill 19.1).	Prevents trauma to urethral tissue caused by pulling catheter.
8. Help patient to safe and comfortable position. Lower bed and place side rails accordingly. Place nurse call system in reach and instruct patient in use.	Promotes patient comfort and safety.
9. Dispose of all contaminated supplies in appropriate receptacle, remove and dispose of gloves, and perform hand hygiene.	Reduces transmission of microorganisms.

EVALUATION

1. Measure actual urine output by subtracting total amount of irrigation fluid infused from total volume drained into collection bag or basin.	Determines accurate urinary output.
2. Review I&O flow sheet to verify that hourly output into drainage bag is in appropriate proportion to irrigating solution entering bladder. Expect more output than fluid instilled because of urine production.	Determines urinary output in relation to irrigation.
3. Inspect urine for blood clots and sediment and be sure that tubing is not kinked or occluded.	Decrease in blood clots means that therapy is successful in maintaining catheter patency. System is patent.
4. Evaluate patient's comfort level.	Indicates catheter patency by absence of symptoms of bladder distention.
5. Monitor for signs and symptoms of infection.	Patients with indwelling catheters remain at risk for infection.
6. **Use Teach-Back:** "I want to be sure I explained clearly about why we are irrigating your catheter. Tell me in your own words the reason we are doing the irrigation." Revise your instruction now or develop plan for revised patient/family caregiver teaching if patient/family caregiver is not able to teach back correctly.	Determines patient's/family caregiver's level of understanding of instructional topic.

Unexpected Outcomes	Related Interventions
1. Irrigating solution does not return (closed intermittent irrigation) or is not flowing at prescribed rate (CBI).	• Examine tubing for clots, sediment, and kinks. • Notify health care provider if irrigant does not flow freely from bladder, patient complains of pain, or bladder distention occurs.
2. Drainage output is less than amount of irrigation solution infused.	• Examine drainage tubing for clots, sediment, or kinks. • Inspect urine for presence of or increase in blood clots and sediment. • Evaluate patient for pain and distended bladder. • Notify health care provider.
3. Bright-red bleeding with the irrigation (CBI) infusion wide open.	• Assess for hypovolemic shock (vital signs, skin color and moisture, anxiety level). • Leave irrigation infusion wide open and notify health care provider.
4. Patient experiences pain with irrigation.	• Examine drainage tubing for clots, sediment, or kinks. • Evaluate urine for presence of or increase in blood clots and sediment. • Evaluate for distended bladder. • Notify health care provider.

Recording

- Record irrigation method, amount of and type of irrigation solution, amount returned as drainage, characteristics of output, and urine output.
- Record I&O.
- Document your evaluation of patient learning.

Hand-Off Reporting

- Report catheter occlusion, sudden bleeding, infection, or increased pain.

SPECIAL CONSIDERATIONS

Patient-Centered Care

- The personal level of touch required when performing urinary elimination procedures requires you to understand patients' values and preferences.
- Determine a patient's feelings about having to undergo procedures such as catheterization or application of a continence device. Adapt your approach to minimize the invasive nature of a procedure and maintain a patient's dignity.
- Variations within a cultural group are common. Assess each patient to provide care that incorporates the patient's specific beliefs and practices related to elimination, privacy, and gender-specific care:
  - Patients who emphasize female/male modesty and prohibit nonrelated males and females from touching require a same-gender caregiver.
  - Some cultures emphasize interdependence over independence; thus family presence at the bedside for important decision making is common.

Patient Education

- Teach patients and family caregivers appropriate assessments, such as signs and symptoms of UTI and how to prevent UTI, signs of skin irritation, and signs of poor-fitting catheter sheath.
- Patients who have suprapubic catheters may shower. Caution against use of creams, powders, or sprays near the catheter entrance site.
- If a patient or family caregiver must handle or empty a urine drainage bag, instruct on proper way to empty and importance of hand hygiene.

Age-Specific

Pediatric

- Condom catheters are not commonly used for children. When used in adolescents, take precautions to minimize embarrassment of application and use.
- When caring for an infant or young child, explain procedures to parents. Describe procedure to child at level the child can understand (Hockenberry et al., 2017).
- Catheterization in infants and children may be more comfortable with the use of an adequate amount of lubricant containing 2% lidocaine (Xylocaine; Hockenberry et al., 2017).

Gerontological

- Evaluate older adults with neuropathy carefully before application of an external catheter, and assess penile skin at more frequent intervals, at least twice daily.
- Condom catheters are not recommended for patients with prostatic obstruction.
- The urethral meatus of an older woman may be difficult to identify because of urogenital atrophy.
- Older adults may exhibit atypical signs and symptoms of UTI, such as a change in mental status, which may be wrongly attributed to delirium (Ignatavicius et al., 2018). A change in mental status may include confusion, agitation, or lethargy.
- Older adults have an increased risk for UTI related to increased prevalence of chronic disease such as diabetes, prostatic hypertrophy in men, and a higher prevalence of incontinence (Ignatavicius et al., 2018).

Home Care

- Collaborate with patients to adapt the home so that those with urinary frequency, urgency, nocturia, and urinary incontinence can reach toileting facilities quickly and safely. Conduct a safety review of the bedroom and bath (see Chapter 32; Soliman et al., 2016).
- In the non–acute care setting, clean (i.e., nonsterile) technique for intermittent catheterization is an acceptable and more practical alternative to sterile technique for patients requiring chronic intermittent catheterization (Gould et al., 2017).
- Loose-fitting clothing may be needed to accommodate an indwelling and drainage system.
- Patients who are at home with an indwelling catheter may use a leg bag during the day and switch to a larger-volume bag at night. If a patient changes from a large-volume bag to a leg bag, instruct in the importance of handwashing and cleansing of the connection ports with alcohol before changing bags.
- Ensure that patient and caregiver understand the correct steps in applying an external continence device and how to empty the drainage bag. Manufacturers often supply educational materials for patients.
- Patient or family caregiver will learn how to change a suprapubic catheter every 4 to 6 weeks using sterile technique. Patients with suprapubic catheters should drink 8 to 12 glasses of water every day for a few days after changing a catheter and avoid physical activity for a week or two (National Institutes of Health, 2017).
- Teach patients and family caregivers how to position a urinary drainage bag properly; how to empty the bag; signs of catheter obstruction and wound infection; and to observe urine color, clarity, odor, and amount.

✦ PRACTICE REFLECTIONS

A 78-year-old female patient returns to a medical-surgical unit following abdominal surgery for a colon tumor. The patient has an indwelling urinary catheter, an intravenous line, and a surgical dressing. As the nurse assigned to the patient, you begin your care after the patient has been on the unit for 2 hours. The nurse leaving for the end of shift reports to you the following: IV line in right forearm is patent and infusing at 80 mL/hr on intravenous pump. The indwelling catheter is draining clear, yellow urine. The surgical dressing is dry and intact. The patient is awake, oriented, and asking questions.

1. What is your first priority in regard to promoting this patient's normal urinary elimination?
2. The patient's sister will be staying with her for a few weeks once the patient is discharged home. The sister asks if the patient will still have the urinary catheter and what the risks are. What would you explain to the patient and sister?
3. What clinical signs of a UTI might you expect in this patient? Give a rationale.

✦ CLINICAL REVIEW QUESTIONS

1. Which of the following nursing interventions decrease the risk for CAUTI? (Select all that apply.)
   1. Cleansing the urinary meatus with antiseptic cleansing solution
   2. Hanging the urinary drainage bag below the level of the bladder
   3. Changing the urinary drainage bag daily
   4. Performing daily urinary catheter irrigations with normal saline
   5. Performing hand hygiene before manipulation of urinary drainage system
   6. Eliminating any kinking in urinary drainage tubing
2. Place the following steps for application of a condom catheter in the correct order:
   1. Smoothly roll sheath onto penis.
   2. Assess skin of penis for rashes, erythema, and/or open areas.
   3. Apply appropriate securement device.
   4. Prepare urinary drainage collection bag and tubing (large-volume drainage bag or leg bag). Clamp off drainage bag port.
   5. Verify patient's size and type of condom catheter.
   6. Apply clean gloves. Provide perineal care.
   7. With nondominant hand, grasp penis along shaft.
   8. Review EHR for history of allergy to rubber or latex.
3. A male patient returned to a nursing unit after a surgical procedure involving administration of spinal anesthesia. While in recovery, the patient had an indwelling urinary catheter removed. Eight hours later, the patient has not yet voided. He is drinking water and has no episodes of nausea. Which of the following actions should the nurse expect to perform? (Select all that apply.)
   1. Insert an intermittent urinary catheter to determine bladder volume.
   2. This is a normal response following spinal anesthesia, and ongoing monitoring is all that is needed.
   3. Encourage the patient to continue drinking clear liquids, and then offer a urinal and encourage an attempt to void.
   4. After the first time the patient voids, perform a bladder scan in 10 minutes.
   5. Prepare to reinsert an indwelling urinary catheter.

Answers and Rationales for Clinical Review Questions can be found on the Evolve website.

REFERENCES

American Association of Critical Care Nurses: Practice Alert. Prevention of catheter-associated urinary tract infections in adults, 2016. http://ccn.aacnjournals.org/content/36/4/e9.full.pdf.

Centers for Disease Control and Prevention (CDC): What is health literacy? 2016. https://www.cdc.gov/healthliteracy/learn/index.html.

Centers for Disease Control and Prevention: Urinary tract infection (catheter-associated urinary tract infection [CAUTI] and non-catheter-associated urinary tract infection [UTI]) and other urinary system infection [USI]) events, 2018. https://www.cdc.gov/nhsn/pdfs/pscmanual/7psccauticurrent.pdf.

CliniMed: Bioderm male continence device, 2014. http://www.clinimed.co.uk/Urology-Continence-Care/Incontinence-Products/BioDerm/Detail.aspx.

Fasugba O, et al: Systematic review and meta-analysis of the effectiveness of antiseptic agents for meatal cleaning in the prevention of catheter-associated urinary tract infections, *J Hosp Infect* 95(3):233, 2017.

Fekete T: Catheter-associated urinary tract infection in adults, 2018. https://www.uptodate.com/contents/catheter-associated-urinary-tract-infection-in-adults.

Feneley RCL, et al: Urinary catheters: history, current status, adverse events and research agenda, *J Med Eng Technol* 39(8):459, 2015.

Galiczewski JM, Shurpin KM: An intervention to improve the catheter associated urinary tract infection rate in a medical intensive care unit: direct observation of catheter insertion procedure, *Intensive Crit Care Nurs* 40:26, 2017.

Gould CV, et al: Guideline for prevention of catheter-associated urinary tract infections 2009, Healthcare Infection Control Practices Advisory Committee, Centers for Disease Control and Prevention, updated February 2017. https://www.cdc.gov/infectioncontrol/pdf/guidelines/cauti-guidelines.pdf.

Hockenberry MJ, et al: *Wong's essentials of pediatric nursing e-book*, St. Louis, 2017, Elsevier.

Huether SE, et al: *Understanding pathophysiology*, ed 6, St. Louis, 2017, Elsevier.

Ignatavicius D, et al: *Medical-surgical nursing: concepts for interprofessional collaborative care*, ed 9, St. Louis, 2018, Elsevier.

Kidd EA, et al: Urethral (indwelling or intermittent) or suprapubic routes for short-term catheterisation in hospitalised adults, *Cochrane Database Syst Rev* (12):CD004203, 2015.

Lam T, et al: Types of indwelling urinary catheters for short-term catheterization in hospitalized adults, Cochrane Incontinence Group/Cochrane Database of Systematic Reviews, 2014. https://www.ncbi.nlm.nih.gov/pubmed/25248140.

McNeill L: Back to basics: how evidence-based nursing practice can prevent catheter-associated urinary tract infections, *Urol Nurs* 37:204, 2017.

National Institutes of Health: Medline Plus: Suprapubic catheter care, 2017. https://medlineplus.gov/ency/patientinstructions/000145.htm.

Nicolle LE: Catheter associated urinary tract infections, *Antimicrob Resist Infect Control* 3:23, 2014.

Özkan HS, et al: Penile strangulation and necrosis due to condom catheter, *Int Wound J* 12(3):248, 2015.

Pashnik B, et al: Effectiveness of a nurse-led initiative, peer-to-peer teaching, on organizational CAUTI rates and related costs, *J Nurs Care Qual* 32(4):324, 2017.

Soliman Y, et al: Falls in the elderly secondary to urinary symptoms, *Rev Urol* 18(1):26, 2016.

The Joint Commission (TJC): *2019 National Patient Safety Goals*, Oakbrook Terrace, IL, 2019, The Commission. http://www.jointcommission.org/standards_information/npsgs.aspx.

Timmons B, et al: Nurse-driven protocol to reduce indwelling catheter dwell time: a health care improvement initiative, *J Nurs Care Qual* 32(2):104, 2017.

U.S. National Library of Medicine: MedlinePlus: catheter-related UTI, 2016. https://medlineplus.gov/ency/article/000483.htm.

20 Bowel Elimination and Gastric Decompression

SKILLS AND PROCEDURES

EVOLVE WEBSITE/RESOURCES LIST

http://evolve.elsevier.com/Perry/nursinginterventions

Audio Glossary • Animations • Case Studies • Checklists • Nursing Skills Online • Clinical Review Questions • Answers and Rationales for Clinical Review Questions • Video Clips

INTRODUCTION

Regular elimination of bowel waste products is essential for normal body functioning. Alterations in bowel elimination, such as diarrhea or constipation, are often early signs or symptoms of problems within either the gastrointestinal (GI) system or other body systems. When patients undergo surgery or experience an alteration in GI peristalsis, the insertion of a nasogastric (NG) tube is needed for gastric decompression. Gastric decompression keeps the stomach empty and reduces nausea and vomiting.

PRACTICE STANDARDS

- American Association of Critical-Care Nurses (AACN), 2017: AACN practice alert: Prevention of aspiration in adults—Patient positioning
- Emergency Nurses Association, 2015: Clinical practice guideline—Gastric tube placement—X-ray confirmation
- The Joint Commission (TJC), 2019: National Patient Safety Goals—Patient identification
- Wound Ostomy and Continence Nurses (WOCN) Society, 2016: Guideline for prevention and management of pressure ulcers

EVIDENCE-BASED PRACTICE

Medical Device–Related Pressure Injuries

All patients with a medical device, such as a nasogastric tube, are at risk for medical device–related pressure injuries (Delmore and Ayello, 2017). When pressure from a nasogastric (NG) decompression tube is applied to the mucous membranes lining the nasal passages, tissue ischemia and pressure injury result. Nasal mucosal tissues are especially vulnerable to pressure from medical devices such as NG and feeding tubes, especially in patients who are dehydrated, immunocompromised, or septic (Padula et al., 2017; Pittman et al., 2015). These devices and their securement products cause pressure on the skin. Patients who cannot convey discomfort may have a higher risk for the development of pressure injuries than an alert patient. The National Pressure Ulcer Advisory Panel (NPUAP, 2014) recommends these best practices for prevention of medical device–related pressure injury (MDPI):

- Perform routine and ongoing assessment of nares and the skin under and around the device at least twice per day for signs of pressure-related injury. If necessary, reposition the tube in the nose when the patient is in the side-lying position (Padula et al., 2017; Pittman et al., 2015).
- Implement skin-care practices, such a pressure-relief taping method or commercial fixation device, to reduce risk for MDPI (NPUAP, 2014; Pittman, 2015; Wound Ostomy and Continence Nurses [WOCN], 2016).
- Frequently remove tape or fixation device to inspect underlying skin and tissue and provide skin care (Pittman, 2015).
- Be aware of other devices, such as oxygen tubing and other respiratory equipment, that can place secondary pressure on the NG tube and drainage tubing (Padula et al., 2017).
- Position NG drainage tubing in such a manner as not to cause secondary pressure on the nares from the weight of the drainage tubing itself (Pittman, 2015).

SAFETY GUIDELINES

When assisting patients with bowel elimination or inserting an NG tube for gastric decompression, safe nursing practices are essential. Use safe patient-handling techniques when positioning patients to promote bowel elimination. Safety guidelines include the following:

- Patients with neurological sensory and/or motor deficits are prone to constipation as a result of immobility. Place patients on an individualized bowel training schedule and offer assistance with toileting at these intervals.

- If a patient has cardiac disease or is taking cardiac or hypertensive medication, obtain a pulse rate before an enema because manipulation of rectal tissue stimulates the vagus nerve and can cause a sudden decline in pulse rate, which can increase the patient's risk for fainting while on the bedpan, commode, or toilet (Ball et al., 2019).
- Instruct patients who self-administer enemas to use the side-lying position. Administering an enema with the patient sitting on the toilet is unsafe because it is impossible to safely guide the tubing into the rectum.
- Keep patient in sitting high-Fowler's position during NG intubation to prevent aspiration (AACN, 2017; Metheny, 2016).
- Always follow agency policy and best practices to verify NG tube placement (McFarland, 2017).

PROCEDURAL GUIDELINE 20.1 *Providing and Positioning a Bedpan*

Purpose

A patient restricted to bed must use a bedpan for bowel elimination. Two types of bedpans are available (Fig. 20.1). The regular and most commonly used bedpan has a curved, smooth upper end and a tapered lower end. The upper end (wide end) of the regular pan fits under a patient's buttocks toward the sacrum, with the lower end (tapered end) fitting just under the upper thighs toward the foot of the bed. A fracture pan, designed for patients with body or leg casts or those who are restricted from raising their hips (e.g., following total hip joint replacement), slips easily under a patient. The shallow upper end of the pan with a flat, wide rim fits under a patient's buttocks toward the sacrum, with the deep lower open end toward the foot of the bed.

Delegation and Collaboration

The skill of providing a bedpan can be delegated to nursing assistive personnel (NAP). The nurse instructs the NAP to:

- Correctly position patients with mobility restrictions or those who have therapeutic equipment such as wound drains, intravenous (IV) catheters, or traction.
- Provide perineal and hand hygiene for patient as necessary after using a bedpan.

Equipment

Clean gloves; bedpan (regular or fracture; see Fig. 20.1); bedpan cover; toilet tissue or premoisturized perineal wipes; specimen container with label (if necessary); plastic bag clearly labeled with date, patient's name, and identification number; washbasin; washcloths; towels; soap; waterproof, absorbent pads (if necessary); clean drawsheet (if necessary); stethoscope

Procedural Steps

1. Assess patient's normal bowel elimination habits: routine pattern, character of stool, effect of certain foods/fluids and eating habits on bowel elimination, effect of stress and level of activity on normal bowel elimination patterns, current medications, and normal fluid intake.
2. Determine need for stool specimen before bedpan use.
3. Perform hand hygiene. Auscultate abdomen for bowel sounds and palpate lower abdomen for distention.
4. Assess patient to determine level of mobility, including ability to sit upright and lift hips or turn.
5. Assess patient's level of comfort. Ask about presence of rectal or abdominal pain, presence of hemorrhoids, or irritation of skin surrounding anus.
6. Apply clean gloves. Inspect condition of perianal and perineal skin (Whiteley and Sinclair, 2014). Remove and dispose of gloves and perform hand hygiene.
7. For patient comfort, prepare metal bedpan by running warm water over it for a few minutes.

Safe Patient Care *Use a fracture pan if the patient had a total hip replacement. An abduction pillow must be placed between the legs when turning patient to prevent dislocation of new joint.*

8. Provide privacy by closing curtains around bed or door of room.
9. Raise side rail on opposite side of bed.
10. Raise bed horizontally according to your height.
11. Assist patient to the supine position.
12. Place patient who can assist on bedpan.
    a. Perform hand hygiene and apply clean gloves. Raise head of patient's bed 30 to 60 degrees.
    b. Remove upper bed linens so that they are out of the way but do not expose patient.
    c. Have patient flex knees and lift hips upward.
    d. Place hand closest to patient's head palm up under patient's sacrum to help lift. Ask patient to bend knees

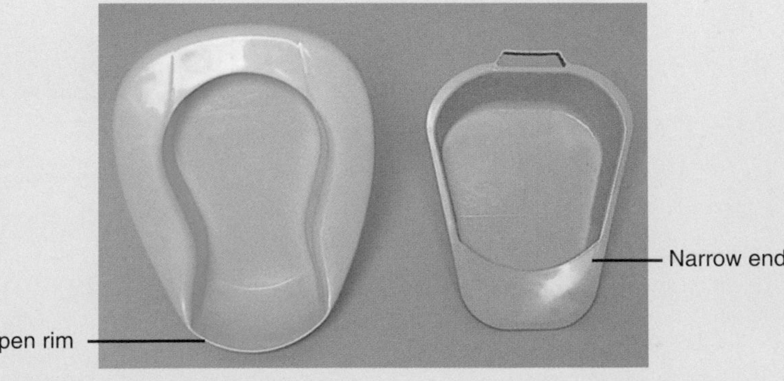

FIG 20.1 Types of bedpans. *Left,* Regular bedpan. *Right,* Fracture bedpan.

Continued

PROCEDURAL GUIDELINE 20.1 ***Providing and Positioning a Bedpan—cont'd***

and raise hips. As patient raises hips, use other hand to slip bedpan under him or her (see illustrations). Be sure that open rim of bedpan is facing toward foot of bed. Do not force pan under patient's hips. (*Optional:* Have patient use overhead trapeze frame to raise hips.)

 e. *Optional:* If using fracture pan, slip it under patient as hips are raised (see illustration). Be sure that deep, open, lower end of bedpan is facing toward foot of bed.

13. Place patient who is immobile or has mobility restrictions on bedpan.

 a. Perform hand hygiene and apply clean gloves. Lower head of bed flat or raise head slightly (if tolerated by medical condition).

 b. Remove top linens as necessary to turn patient while minimizing exposure.

 c. Assist patient to roll onto side with back toward you. Place bedpan firmly against patient's buttocks and down into mattress. Be sure that open rim of bedpan is facing toward foot of bed (see illustrations).

 d. Keep one hand against bedpan; place other around far hip of patient. Assist patient to roll back onto bedpan, flat in bed. Do not force pan under patient.

 e. Raise patient's head 30 degrees or to a comfortable level (unless contraindicated).

 f. Have patient bend knees (unless contraindicated).

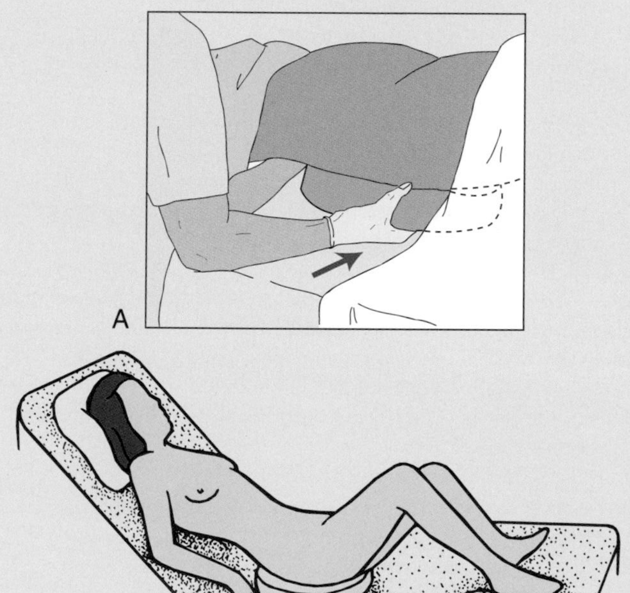

STEP 12d (A) Placing bedpan under patient's hips. (B) Correct positioning for placing mobile patient on bedpan.

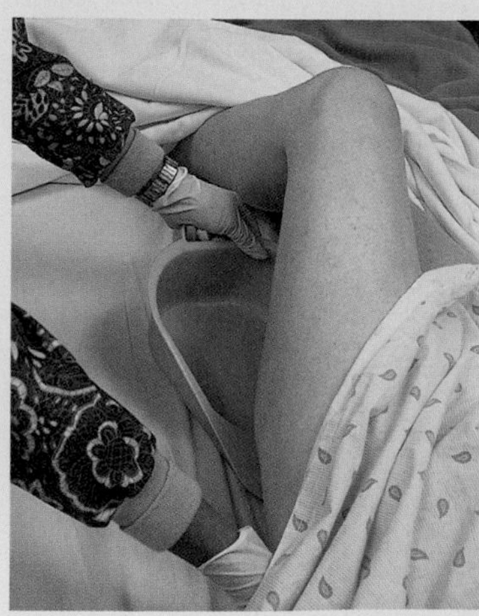

STEP 12e Patient lifts hips as fracture pan is positioned.

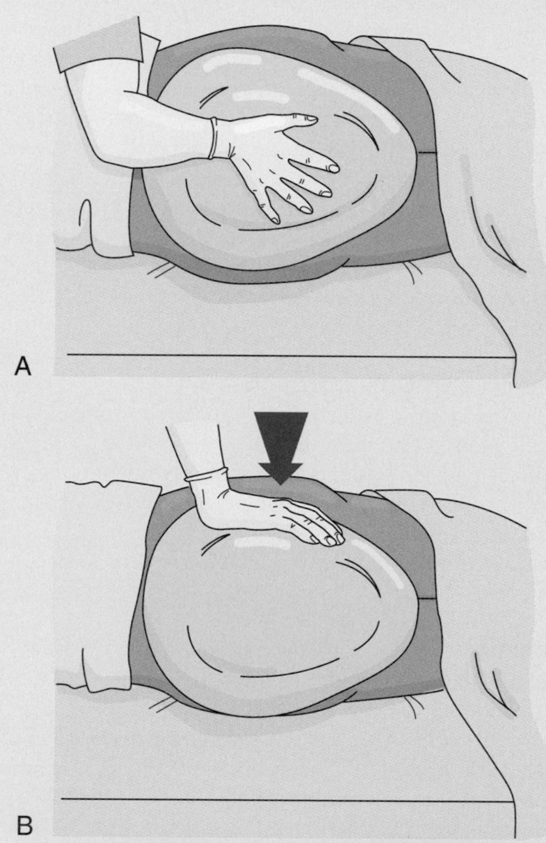

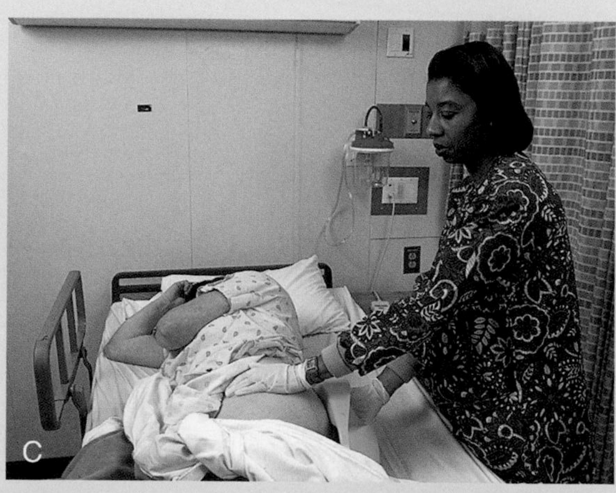

STEP 13c (A) Position patient on one side and place bedpan firmly against buttocks. (B) Push down on bedpan and toward patient. (C) Nurse places bedpan in position. (**A** *and* **B** *from Sorrentino SA: Mosby's textbook for nursing assistants, ed 7, St. Louis, 2009, Mosby.)*

PROCEDURAL GUIDELINE 20.1 ***Providing and Positioning a Bedpan—cont'd***

14. Maintain patient's comfort, privacy, and safety. Cover patient for warmth. Place small pillow or rolled towel under lumbar curve of back. Leave room but stay close by.
15. Place nurse call system and toilet tissue within reach for patient.
16. Ensure that bed is in lowest position and raise upper side rails.
17. Remove and discard gloves and perform hand hygiene.
18. Allow patient to be alone but monitor status and respond promptly.
19. Perform hand hygiene and apply clean gloves.
20. Remove bedpan:
    a. Place patient's bedside chair close to working side of bed.
    b. Maintain privacy; determine if patient is able to wipe own perineal area. If you clean perineal area, use several layers of toilet tissue or disposable washcloths. For female patients, clean from mons pubis toward rectal area.
    c. Deposit contaminated tissue in bedpan if no specimen or intake and output (I&O) is needed.
    d. **For mobile patient:** Ask patient to flex knees, placing body weight on lower legs, feet, and upper torso; lift buttocks up from bedpan. At same time, place hand farthest from patient on side of bedpan to support it (prevent spillage) and place other hand (closest to patient) under sacrum to help lift. Have patient lift and remove bedpan. Place bedpan on draped bedside chair and cover.
    e. **For immobile patient:** Lower head of bed. Help patient roll onto side away from you and off bedpan. Hold bedpan flat and steady while patient is rolling off; otherwise spillage will occur. Place bedpan on draped bedside chair and cover.
    f. Remove and dispose of gloves. Perform hand hygiene. Assist patient with hand and perineal hygiene as needed.
21. Change soiled linens (apply clean gloves if risk of contacting fecal fluids). Remove and dispose of gloves, perform hand hygiene, and return patient to comfortable position.
22. Place bed in its lowest position. Ensure that nurse call system, drinking water, and desired personal items (e.g., books) are within easy access.
    Option: Obtain stool specimen as ordered (see Skill 9.2), wearing clean gloves. Use spray faucet attached to most institution toilets to rinse bedpan thoroughly. Use disinfectant if required by agency; store pan. Remove gloves.
23. Perform hand hygiene and apply clean gloves to assess characteristics of stool. Note color, odor, consistency, frequency, amount, shape, and constituents. Assess characteristics of urine if patient voided in bedpan. Remove and dispose of gloves. Perform hand hygiene.
24. Evaluate patient's ability to use bedpan.
25. Inspect patient's perianal area and surrounding skin while removing bedpan.
26. Document character of stool.

✦ SKILL 20.1 Administering an Enema

Purpose

An enema is the instillation of a solution into the rectum and sigmoid colon to promote defecation by stimulating peristalsis. Enemas are prescribed to treat constipation, to empty the bowel before diagnostic procedures or abdominal surgeries, and to begin a program of bowel training (Table 20.1). Cleansing enemas help to evacuate feces from the colon.

Delegation and Collaboration

The skill of administering an enema can be delegated to nursing assistive personnel (NAP). **NOTE:** If a medicated enema is ordered, then it must be administered by a nurse. The nurse instructs the NAP about:

- How to properly position patients who have mobility restrictions or therapeutic equipment such as drains, intravenous (IV) catheters, or traction.
- Informing the nurse immediately about patient's report of new abdominal pain (exception: a patient reports cramping) or rectal bleeding.
- Informing the nurse immediately about the presence of blood in the stool or around the rectal area or any change in vital signs.

Equipment

- Clean gloves
- Water-soluble local anesthetic lubricant (**NOTE:** Some agencies require use of water-soluble lubricant without anesthetic when nurse performs procedure.)
- Waterproof, absorbent pads
- Bedpan
- Bedpan cover *(optional if available)*
- Bath blanket
- Washbasin, washcloths, towels, and soap
- Stethoscope

Enema Bag Administration

- Enema container (Fig. 20.2)
- IV pole
- Tubing and clamp (if not already attached to container)
- Appropriate-size rectal tube (adult, 22 to 30 Fr; child, 12 to 18 Fr)
- Correct volume of warmed (tepid) solution (adult, 750 to 1000 mL; adolescent, 500 to 700 mL; school-age child, 300 to 500 mL; toddler, 250 to 350 mL; infant, 150 to 250 mL)

TABLE 20.1
Types of Enemas

Type of Enema	Description and Implications
Tap water (hypotonic) enema	Do not repeat after first installation because water toxicity or circulatory overload can develop.
Physiological normal saline	Safest enema to administer. Infants and children can tolerate only this type because of their predisposition to fluid imbalance.
Hypertonic solution (e.g., Fleet enema)	Useful for patients who cannot tolerate large fluid volumes.
Harris flush enema	A return-flow enema that helps to expel intestinal gas. Administer a small amount (100 to 200 mL) of enema solution into patient's rectum and colon. Then lower the enema container to allow the total volume of solution to flow back. The repeated back-and-forth administration and return of the fluid reduces flatus and promotes return of peristalsis.
Sodium polystyrene sulfonate (Kayexalate) enema	Prescribed to reduce severely high serum potassium levels.
Soapsuds enema	Used to relieve constipation or bowel cleansing. Pure castile soap added to bag filled with tap water or normal saline. Use only pure castile soap. Recommended ratio of pure soap to solution is 5 mL (1 tsp) soap to 1000 mL (1 quart) warm water or saline.
Oil retention	Oil-based solution, slow acting. The colon absorbs a small volume, which softens stool for easier evacuation.
Carminative solution	Relieves gaseous distention. Example: MGW enema (30 mL magnesium, 60 mL glycerin, 90 mL water)

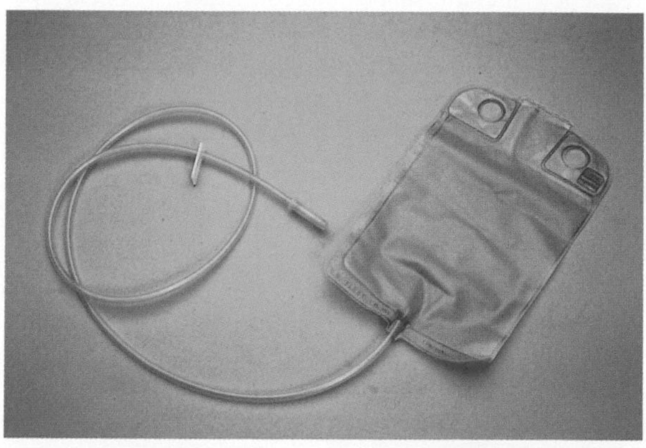

FIG 20.2 Enema bag with tubing.

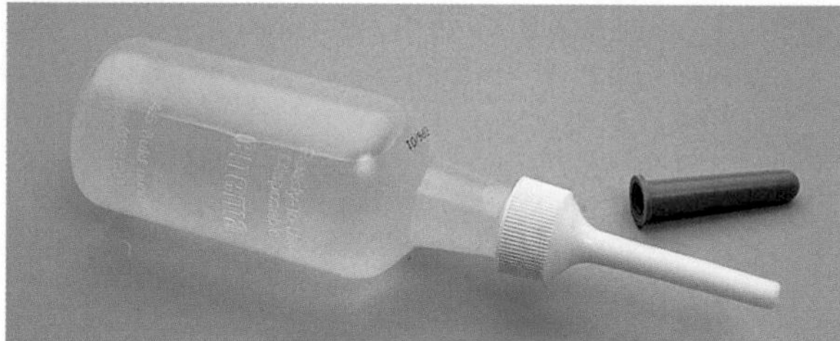

FIG 20.3 Prepackaged enema container with rectal tip.

Prepackaged Enema

- Prepackaged enema container with lubricated rectal tip (Fig. 20.3)

ASSESSMENT

1. Identify patient using at least two identifiers (e.g., name and birthday or name and medical record number) according to agency policy). *Rationale: Ensures correct patient. Complies with The Joint Commission standards and improves patient safety (TJC, 2019).*
2. Review health care provider's order for enema and clarify reason for administration. *Rationale: Order by health care provider is usually required for hospitalized patient. Order states which type of enema patient will receive.*
3. Review medical record and assess last bowel movement, normal versus most recent bowel pattern, presence of hemorrhoids, and presence of abdominal pain or cramping. *Rationale: Determines need for enema and type of enema used. Also establishes baseline for bowel function. Hemorrhoids may obscure rectal opening and cause discomfort or bleeding during evacuation.*
4. Assess patient's mobility and ability to turn and position on side. *Rationale: Determines if assistance is needed for positioning patient.*
5. Assess patient for allergy to any active ingredients of Fleet enema. *Rationale: Reduces risk for allergic reaction.*
6. Perform hand hygiene and inspect and palpate abdomen for presence of distention and auscultate for bowel sounds. *Rationale: Reduces transmission of microorganisms. Establishes baseline for determining effectiveness of enema.*
7. Assess patient's/family caregiver's knowledge, experience, and health literacy. *Rationale: Ensures patient/family caregiver has the capacity to obtain, communicate, process, and understand basic health information (Centers for Disease Control and Prevention [CDC], 2016).*

Safe Patient Care *When "enemas until clear" is ordered, the water expelled may be tinted but should not contain solid fecal material. It is essential to observe contents of solution passed. Check agency policy, but a patient should receive only three consecutive enemas to prevent fluid and electrolyte imbalance.*

STEP	RATIONALE

PLANNING

STEP	RATIONALE
1. Expected outcomes following completion of procedure:	
• Stool is evacuated.	Solution clears rectum and lower colon of stool.
• Enema return is clear.	Indicates that all solid fecal material in colon has passed.
• Abdomen is flat, nontender, with no distention.	Gas and feces are expelled.
2. Perform hand hygiene. Arrange supplies at bedside.	Ensures access to supplies during procedure.
3. Provide privacy by closing curtains around bed or closing door.	Reduces embarrassment for patient.
4. Place bedpan or bedside commode in easily accessible position. If patient will be expelling contents in toilet, ensure that toilet is available and place patient's nonskid slippers and bathrobe in easily accessible position.	Bedpan is used if patient is unable to get out of bed. Nonskid slippers help prevent patient who may be rushing to bathroom from falling. Extra gown provides modesty for patient.

IMPLEMENTATION

STEP	RATIONALE
1. Check accuracy and completeness of each medication administration record (MAR) with health care provider's written order. Check patient's name, type of enema, and time for administration. Compare MAR with label of enema solution. **NOTE:** If enema is medicated, the skill may not be delegated to a NAP (see agency policy).	The health care provider's order is the most reliable source and only legal record of drugs or procedure that patient is to receive. Ensures that patient receives correct enema.
2. Perform hand hygiene.	Reduces transmission of microorganisms.
3. With side rail raised on patient's right side and bed raised to appropriate working height, help patient turn onto left side-lying (Sims') position with right knee flexed. Determine that patient is comfortable and encourage patient to remain in position until procedure is complete. **NOTE:** Place a child in the dorsal recumbent position.	Allows enema solution to flow downward by gravity along natural curve of sigmoid colon and rectum, thus improving retention of solution.

Safe Patient Care *Patients with poor sphincter control require placement of a bedpan under the buttocks. Administering enema with patient sitting on toilet is unsafe because curved rectal tubing can abrade rectal wall.*

STEP	RATIONALE
4. Apply clean gloves and place waterproof pad, absorbent side up, under hips and buttocks. Cover patient with bath blanket, exposing only rectal area, clearly visualizing anus.	Pad prevents soiling of linen. Blanket provides warmth, reduces exposure of body parts, and allows patient to feel more relaxed and comfortable.
5. Separate buttocks and examine perianal region for abnormalities, including hemorrhoids, anal fissure, and rectal prolapse.	Findings influence approach for inserting enema tip. Prolapse contraindicates enema.
6. Administer enema.	
a. **Administer prepackaged disposable enema:**	
(1) Remove plastic cap from tip of container. Tip may already be lubricated. Apply more water-soluble lubricant as needed.	Lubrication provides for smooth insertion of rectal tube without causing rectal irritation or trauma. With presence of hemorrhoids, extra lubricant provides added comfort.
(2) Gently separate buttocks and locate anus. Instruct patient to relax by breathing out slowly through mouth.	Breathing out promotes relaxation of external rectal sphincter.
(3) Hold container upright and expel any air from enema container.	Introducing air into colon causes further distention and discomfort.
(4) Insert lubricated tip of container gently into anal canal toward umbilicus (see illustration). ***Adult:*** 7.5 to 10 cm (3 to 4 inches) ***Adolescent:*** 7.5 cm to 10 cm (3 to 4 inches) ***Child:*** 5 to 7.5 cm (2 to 3 inches) ***Infant:*** 2.5 to 3.75 cm (1 to 1½ inches)	Gentle insertion prevents trauma to rectal mucosa.

Safe Patient Care *If pain occurs or you feel resistance at any time during procedure, stop and discuss with health care provider. Do not force insertion.*

STEP	RATIONALE

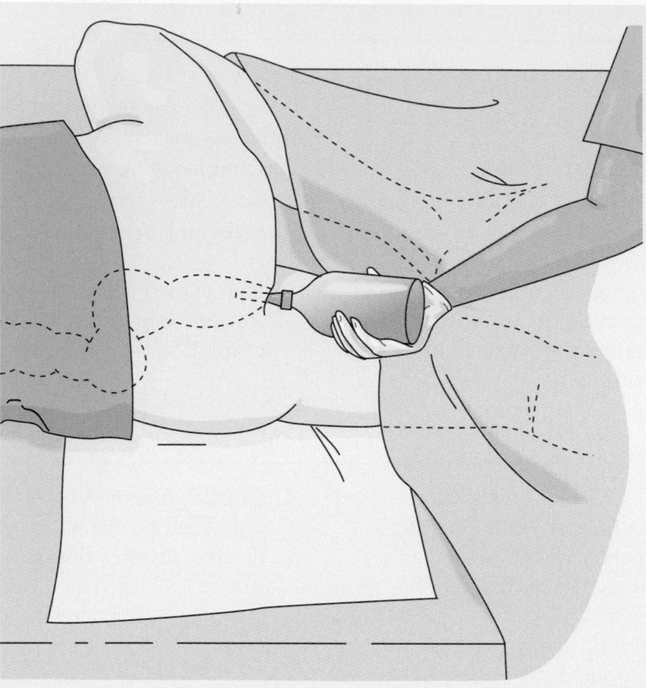

STEP 6a(4) With patient in left lateral Sims' position, insert tip of commercial enema into rectum. *(From Sorrentino SA: Mosby's textbook for nursing assistants, ed 9, St. Louis, 2017, Elsevier.)*

STEP	RATIONALE
(5) Squeeze and roll plastic bottle from bottom to tip until all of solution has entered rectum and colon. Tell patient procedure is completed and that you will remove tip.	Prevents instillation of air into colon and ensures that all content enters rectum. Hypertonic solutions require only small volumes to stimulate defecation.
b. **Administer enema in standard enema bag:**	
(1) Add warmed prescribed type of solution and amount to enema bag. Warm tap water as it flows from faucet. Place saline container in basin of warm water before adding saline to enema bag. Check temperature of solution by pouring small amount of solution over inner wrist.	Hot water burns intestinal mucosa. Cold water causes abdominal cramping and is difficult to retain.
(2) If soapsuds enema (SSE) is ordered, add castile soap after water.	Reduces suds in enema bag.
(3) Raise container, release clamp, and allow solution to flow long enough to fill tubing.	Removes air from tubing.
(4) Reclamp tubing.	Prevents further loss of solution.
(5) Lubricate 6 to 8 cm (2½ to 3 inches) of tip of rectal tube with lubricant.	Allows smooth insertion of rectal tube without risk for irritation or trauma to mucosa.
(6) Gently separate buttocks and locate anus. Instruct patient to relax by breathing out slowly through mouth. Touch patient's skin next to anus with tip of rectal tube.	Breathing out and touching skin with tube promotes relaxation of external anal sphincter.
(7) Insert tip of rectal tube slowly by pointing it in direction of patient's umbilicus. Length of insertion varies (see Step 6a[4]).	Careful insertion prevents trauma to rectal mucosa from accidental lodging of tube against rectal wall. Insertion beyond proper limit can cause bowel perforation.

Safe Patient Care *If tube does not pass easily, do not force. Consider allowing a small amount of fluid to infuse and then trying to reinsert the tube slowly. The instillation of fluid relaxes the sphincter and provides additional lubrication. If fecal impaction is present, remove it before administering the enema.*

STEP	RATIONALE
(8) Hold tubing in rectum constantly until end of fluid instillation.	Prevents expulsion of rectal tube during bowel contractions.

STEP	RATIONALE
(9) Open regulating clamp and allow solution to enter slowly with container at patient's hip level.	Rapid infusion stimulates evacuation of tubing and can cause cramping.
(10) Raise height of enema container slowly to appropriate level above anus: 30 to 45 cm (12 to 18 inches) for high enema (see illustration); 30 cm (12 inches) for regular enema; 7.5 cm (3 inches) for low enema. Instillation time varies with volume of solution administered (e.g., 1 L may take 10 minutes). You may use an intravenous (IV) pole to hold an enema bag once you establish a slow flow of fluid.	Allows for continuous, slow instillation of solution. Raising container too high causes rapid instillation and possible painful distention of colon. High pressure can result in bowel rupture.

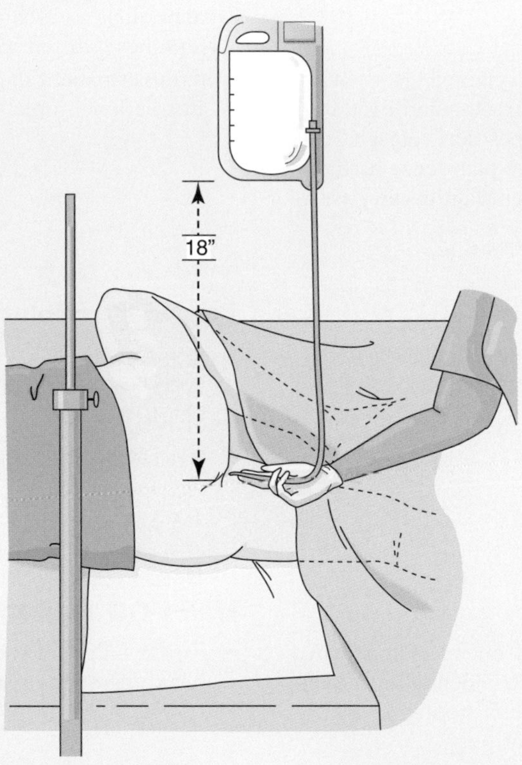

STEP 6b(10) Intravenous (IV) pole is positioned so bottom of enema bag is 45 cm (18 inches) above anus. *(From Sorrentino SA: Mosby's textbook for nursing assistants, ed 9, St. Louis, 2017, Elsevier.)*

Safe Patient Care *Temporary cessation of infusion minimizes cramping and promotes ability to retain solution. Lower container or clamp tubing if patient complains of cramping or if fluid escapes around rectal tube.*

STEP	RATIONALE
(11) Instill all solution and clamp tubing. Tell patient that procedure is completed and that you will remove tubing.	Prevents entrance of air into rectum. Patients may misinterpret sensation of removing tube as loss of control.
7. Place layers of toilet tissue around tube or container tip at anus and gently withdraw rectal tube or container tip.	Provides for patient's comfort and cleanliness.
8. Instruct patient to retain solution until urge to defecate, usually 2 to 5 minutes.	Length of retention varies with type of enema and patient's ability to contract rectal sphincter.
9. Explain to patient that some distention and abdominal cramping are normal. Stay at bedside. Have patient lie quietly in bed if possible. (For infant or young child, gently hold buttocks together for few minutes.)	Solution distends bowel. Longer retention promotes stimulation of peristalsis and defecation.
10. Discard enema container or disposable bag and tubing in proper receptacle.	Reduces transmission and growth of microorganisms.

STEP	RATIONALE
11. Help patient to bathroom or commode if possible. If using bedpan, help patient to as near a normal position for evacuation as possible (see Skill 20.1).	Normal squatting position promotes defecation.
12. Observe character of stool and solution (instruct patient not to flush toilet before inspection). Remove and discard gloves and perform hand hygiene.	Determines if enema was effective. Reduces transmission of microorganisms.
13. Help patient as needed to wash anal area with warm soap and water (use gloves for perineal care).	Fecal contents irritate skin. Hygiene promotes patient's comfort.

EVALUATION

1. Inspect color, consistency, and amount of stool; odor; and fluid passed.	Determines if stool is evacuated or fluid is retained. Note abnormalities such as presence of blood or mucus.
2. Palpate for abdominal distention.	Determines if distention is relieved.
3. Use Teach-Back: "I want to be sure I explained clearly how to position yourself in bed if you need to self-administer a Fleet enema. Show me how you would position yourself." Revise your instruction now or develop a plan for revised patient/family caregiver teaching if patient/family caregiver is not able to teach back correctly.	Determines patient's/family caregiver's level of understanding of instructional topic.

Unexpected Outcomes	Related Interventions
1. Severe abdominal cramping, bleeding, or sudden abdominal pain develops and is unrelieved by temporarily stopping or slowing flow of solution.	• Stop enema. • Notify health care provider. • Obtain vital signs.
2. Patient is unable to hold enema solution.	• If this occurs during installation, slow rate of infusion.

Recording

- Record the time, type, and volume of enema administered; patient's signs and symptoms; response to enema; and results, including color, amount, and appearance of stool.
- Document your evaluation of patient learning.

Hand-Off Reporting

- Report failure of patient to defecate or any adverse reactions to health care provider.

✦ SKILL 20.2 Insertion, Maintenance, and Removal of a Nasogastric Tube for Gastric Decompression

Purpose

Normal peristalsis is sometimes temporarily altered, either following major surgery or from conditions affecting the gastrointestinal (GI) tract. When peristalsis is slowed or absent, a patient cannot eat or drink fluids without causing abdominal distention. The temporary insertion of a nasogastric (NG) tube into the stomach serves to decompress the stomach, keeping it empty until normal peristalsis returns.

An NG tube is a hollow, pliable tube inserted through a patient's nasopharynx into the stomach. The Levin and Salem sump tubes are the most common for stomach decompression. The Levin tube is a single-lumen tube with holes near the tip (Fig. 20.4); the Salem sump tube (Fig. 20.5) is preferable for stomach decompression, this tube has two lumina: one for removal of gastric contents and one

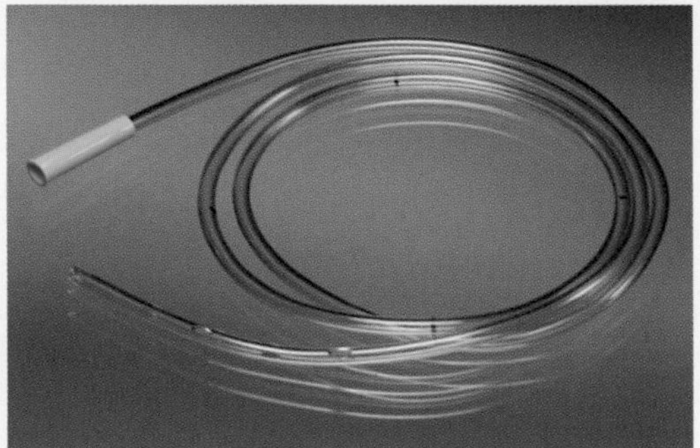

FIG 20.4 Levin tube. *(Copyright © 2018 C.R. Bard, Inc. Used with permission.)*

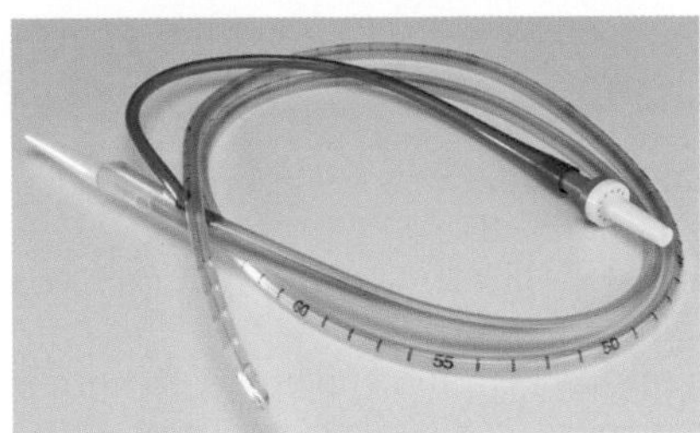

FIG 20.5 Salem sump tube. *(Copyright © 2010 Covidien. All rights reserved. Used with permission of Covidien.)*

to provide an air vent, which prevents suctioning of gastric mucosa into eyelets at the distal tip of the tube.

Delegation and Collaboration

The skill of inserting and maintaining an NG tube cannot be delegated to nursing assistive personnel (NAP). The nurse instructs the NAP to:

- Measure and record the drainage from an NG tube.
- Provide oral and nasal hygiene measures.
- Perform selected comfort measures such as positioning or offering ice chips if allowed.
- Anchor the tube to patient's gown during routine care to prevent accidental displacement.
- Immediately report to the nurse any patient complaints of burning or signs of redness or irritation to nares.

Equipment

- 14 Fr or 16 Fr NG tube (smaller lumen catheters are not used for decompression in adults because they must be able to remove thick secretions)
- Water-soluble lubricating jelly
- pH test strips 1.0 to 11.0 or higher (measure gastric aspirate acidity)
- Tongue blade
- Clean gloves
- Flashlight
- Emesis basin
- Asepto bulb or catheter-tipped syringe
- Commercial fixation device or 2.5-cm-wide (1-inch-wide) hypoallergenic tape (*option:* Bridle nasal tube system)
- Rubber band and plastic clip to attach tube to gown
- Clamp, drainage bag, or suction machine or pressure gauge if wall suction is to be used
- Towel
- Glass of water with straw
- Facial tissues
- Normal saline
- Tincture of benzoin *(optional)*
- Gastric suction equipment
- Stethoscope
- Pulse oximeter

ASSESSMENT

1. Identify patient using at least two identifiers (e.g., name and birthday or name and medical record number) according to agency policy. *Rationale: Ensures correct patient. Complies with The Joint Commission standards and improves patient safety (TJC, 2019).*
2. Verify health care provider order for type of NG tube to be placed and whether tube is to be attached to suction or drainage bag. *Rationale: Requires order from health care provider. Adequate decompression depends on NG suction.*
3. Perform hand hygiene (apply clean gloves if risk of body fluid exposure). Inspect condition of skin integrity around patient's nares and nasal and oral cavity. *Rationale: Provides baseline data on the condition of the patient's skin prior to NG tube insertion. All patients with any medical device are at risk for pressure injury (Delmore and Ayello, 2017).*
4. Ask if patient has history of nasal surgery or congestion and allergies and note if deviated nasal septum is present. *Rationale: Alerts nurse to potential obstruction. Insert tube into uninvolved nasal passage. Procedure may be contraindicated if surgery is recent.*
5. Auscultate for bowel sounds. Palpate patient's abdomen for distention, pain, and rigidity. Remove and discard gloves if applied and perform hand hygiene. In presence of diminished or absent bowel sounds, auscultate abdomen at least 1 minute in each quadrant (Ball et al., 2019). *Rationale: Documents baseline for any abdominal distention, GI ileus, and general GI function, which later serves as comparison once tube is inserted.*
6. Assess patient's level of consciousness and ability to follow instructions. *Rationale: Determines patient's ability to help in procedure.*

Safe Patient Care *If patient is confused, disoriented, or unable to follow commands, get help from another staff member to insert the tube.*

7. Determine if patient had previous NG tube and, if so, which naris was used. *Rationale: Patient's previous experience complements any explanations and prepares patient for NG tube placement.*
8. Assess patient's caregiver's knowledge, experience, and health literacy. *Rationale: Ensures patient or family caregiver has the capacity to obtain, communicate, process, and understand basic health information (CDC, 2016).*

STEP	RATIONALE
PLANNING	
1. Expected outcomes following completion of procedure:	
• Abdomen is soft, nontender, and without distention.	Correctly positioned NG tube remains patent, drains gastric secretions, and relieves gastric distention.
• Nares and nasal mucosa remain intact, clear, without abrasions or excoriation.	Ensures absence of irritation or pressure injury formation from NG tube.
• Patient's level of comfort improves or remains the same.	Correctly inserted NG tube prevents abdominal discomfort from progressing.

STEP	RATIONALE
2. Pull curtain around bed or close room and prepare environment.	Provides privacy. A clutter-free environment assists in smooth implementation of skill.
3. Perform hand hygiene and arrange supplies at bedside.	Reduces transmission of microorganisms. Ensures access to supplies during procedure.
4. Inform patient that procedure may cause gagging and there may be a burning sensation in nasopharynx as tube is passed. Develop hand signal with patient.	Increases patient's cooperation and ability to anticipate nurse's action. If patient is unable to tolerate procedure, use of hand signal will alert nurse.

IMPLEMENTATION

STEP	RATIONALE
1. Raise bed to working height. Position patient upright in high-Fowler's position unless contraindicated. If patient is comatose, raise head of bed as tolerated in semi-Fowler's position with head tipped forward, chin to chest.	Promotes patient's ability to swallow during procedure. Good body mechanics prevent injury to you or patient.
2. Place bath towel over patient's chest; give facial tissues to patient. Allow to blow nose if necessary. Place emesis basin within reach.	Prevents soiling of patient's gown. Tube insertion through nasal passages may cause tearing and coughing with increased salivation.
3. Wash bridge of nose with soap and water or alcohol swab. Dry thoroughly.	Removes oils from nose to allow fixation devices to adhere completely.
4. Stand on patient's right side if right-handed, left side if left-handed. Lower side rail.	Allows easiest manipulation of tubing.
5. Instruct patient to relax and breathe normally while occluding one naris. Then repeat this action for other naris. Select nostril with greater airflow.	Tube passes more easily through naris that is more patent.

Safe Patient Care *Insertion of an NG tube is a painful procedure. Research provides evidence that in some instances, topical lidocaine, either as a gel or spray, significantly reduces pain (Solomon and Jurica, 2017).*

STEP	RATIONALE
6. Determine length of tube to be inserted and mark location with tape or indelible ink.	Ensures organized procedure and estimation of the proper length of tube to insert into patient.
a. *Option for adult:* Measure distance from tip of nose to earlobe to xyphoid process (NEX) of sternum (see illustration). Mark this distance on tube with tape.	Most traditional method. Length approximates distance from nose to stomach. Research has shown this method may be least effective compared with others, although more research is needed (Santos et al., 2016).

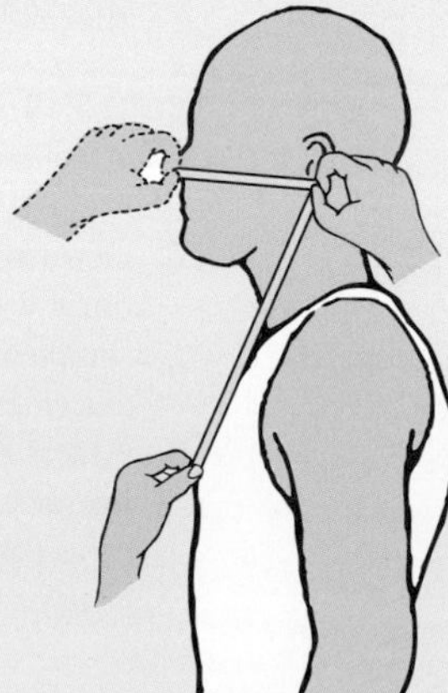

STEP 6a Determine length of tube to be inserted.

STEP	RATIONALE
b. *Option for adult:* Measure distance from tip of nose to earlobe to mid-umbilicus (NEMU).	Promotes placement of the tube end holes in or closer to the gastric fluid pool (Bolutta et al., 2017).
c. *Option for adult:* Measure distance from xyphoid process to earlobe to nose (XEN) + 10 cm (Taylor et al., 2014).	Shown to be more accurate than NEX (Taylor et al., 2014).
d. *Option for children:* Use the NEMU method.	Estimates proper length of tube insertion for the pediatric patient.

Safe Patient Care *Tip of NG tube must reach stomach to avoid the risk for pulmonary aspiration, which occurs when tubes terminate in the esophagus. Research has mixed findings in regard to the best technique for estimating tube length (Santos et al., 2016). Confirmation of placement via x-ray immediately after completed insertion is still needed.*

STEP	RATIONALE
7. With small piece of tape placed around tube, mark length that will be inserted.	Indicates length of tube you will insert.
8. Prepare materials for tube fixation. Tear off a 10-cm (4-inch) length of hypoallergenic tape or open membrane dressing or other fixation device (see Step 22a[2]).	Tape is traditionally used to anchor tubing. Fixation devices allow tube to float free of nares, thus reducing pressure on nares and preventing medical device–related pressure injuries (MDRPIs; Pittman et al., 2015).
9. Perform hand hygiene and apply clean gloves.	Reduces transmission of infection.
10. Apply pulse oximetry/capnography device and measure vital signs. Monitor oximetry/capnography during insertion.	Provides objective assessment of respiratory status before and during tube insertion.
11. Lubricate 7.5 to 10 cm (3 to 4 inches) of end of tube with water-soluble lubricant (see manufacturer directions).	Water-soluble lubricant is less toxic than oil-based lubricant if aspirated.
12. Hand an alert patient a cup of water if able to hold cup and swallow. Explain that you are about to insert tube.	Swallowing water facilitates tube passage. Explanation decreases patient anxiety and increases patient cooperation.
13. Explain next steps. Insert tube gently and slowly through naris to back of throat (posterior nasopharynx). Aim back and down toward patient's ear.	Natural contour facilitates passage of tube into GI tract and reduces gagging.
14. Have patient relax and flex head toward chest after tube is passed through nasopharynx.	Closes off glottis and reduces risk of tube entering trachea.
15. Encourage patient to swallow by taking small sips of water when possible. Advance tube as patient swallows. Rotate tube gently 180 degrees while inserting.	Swallowing facilitates passage of tube past oropharynx. A tug may be felt as patient swallows, indicating that tube is following desired path.
16. Emphasize need to mouth breathe during procedure.	Helps facilitate passage of tube and alleviates patient's anxiety and fear during procedure.
17. Do not advance tube during inspiration or coughing because it will likely enter respiratory tract. Monitor oximetry/capnography.	When tube inadvertently enters airway, changes in oxygen saturation or end-tidal CO_2 (capnography) occur.
18. Advance tube each time patient swallows until you reach desired length.	Reduces discomfort and trauma to patient.

Safe Patient Care *Do not force NG tube. If patient starts to cough or has a drop in O_2 saturation or an increased CO_2, withdraw tube into the posterior nasopharynx until normal breathing resumes.*

STEP	RATIONALE
19. Using penlight and tongue blade, check to be sure that tube is not positioned in back of throat.	Tube could become coiled, become kinked, or enter trachea.
20. Temporarily anchor tube to patient's cheek with small piece of tape.	Temporarily securing tube prevents movement of tube and subsequent gagging. Allows for verification of tube placement.
21. Verify tube placement. Check agency policy for recommended methods of checking tube placement.	
a. Follow order for bedside x-ray film and notify radiology for examination of chest and abdomen.	Radiography remains the gold standard for verification of initial placement of tube (McFarland, 2017; Mordiffi et al., 2016).
b. While waiting for x-ray film to be performed, follow these procedures: Attach Asepto or catheter-tipped syringe to end of tube. Aspirate gently back on syringe to obtain gastric contents, observing amount, color, and quality of return (see illustration).	Observation of gastric contents is useful to determine initial tube placement. Gastric contents are usually green but are sometimes off-white, tan, bloody, or brown in color. Other common aspirate colors include yellow or bile-stained (duodenal placement) or possibly saliva-appearing (esophagus) (Mordiffi et al., 2016).
c. Use pH test paper to measure aspirate for pH with color-coded pH paper. Be sure that paper range of pH is at least from 1.0 to 11.0 (see illustration).	Evidence supports pH test to be used as indicator for placement (McFarland, 2017; Tho et al., 2011). A pH of 1.0 to 4.0 is a good indicator of gastric placement.
22. After tube is properly inserted and positioned, either clamp end or connect it to drainage bag or suction source. Anchor tube with a fixation device, avoiding pressure on the nares. Select one of the following fixation methods:	Drainage bag is used for gravity drainage. Intermittent low suction is most effective for decompression. Proper anchoring and marking of tube help prevent migration of tube and pressure injury formation.
a. Apply tape.	
(1) Apply small amount of tincture of benzoin or other skin adhesive on bridge of patient's nose and allow it to become "tacky."	Helps tape adhere better. Protects underlying skin.

STEP	RATIONALE
(2) Tear small horizontal slits at ⅓ and ⅔ length of tape without splitting entire tape (see illustration). Fold middle sections toward one another to form a closed strip.	The strip holds tubing to lessen rubbing against soft palate and naris.
(3) Print date and time on top end of tape and place it over bridge of patient's nose.	
(4) Wrap bottom end of tape around tube as it exits nose (see illustration).	
b. Apply tube fixation device using shaped adhesive patch (see manufacturer directions).	Secures tube and reduces friction on nares; decreases risk for MDRPI (Delmore and Ayello, 2017).
(1) Apply wide end of patch to bridge of nose (see illustration).	
(2) Slip connector around tube as it exits nose (see illustration).	

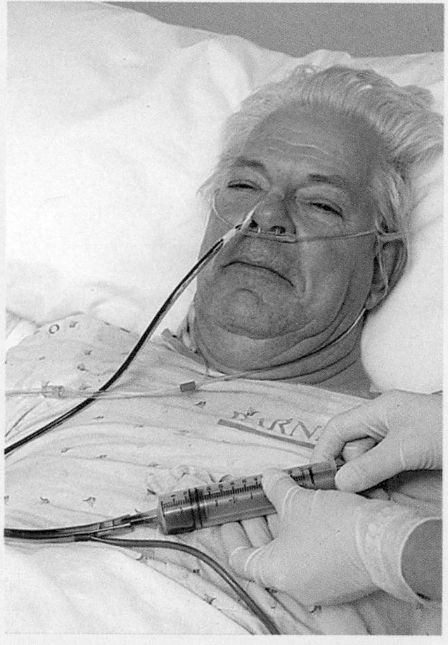

STEP 21b Aspiration of gastric contents.

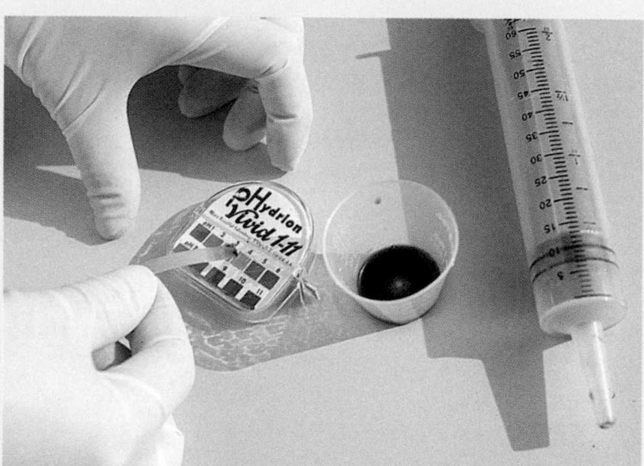

STEP 21c Checking pH of gastric aspirate.

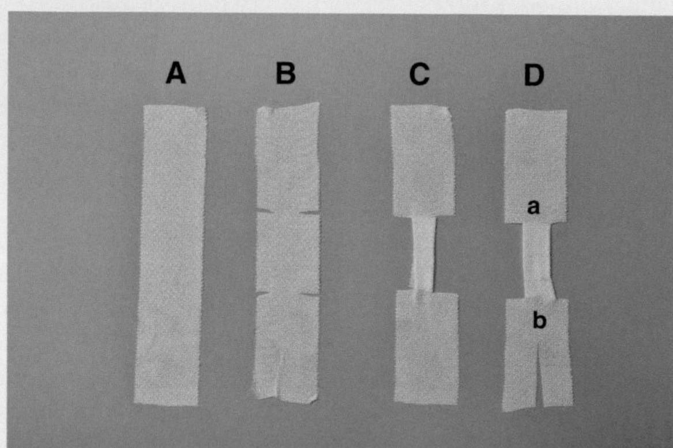

STEP 22a(2) Taping method. (A) Start with piece of tape. (B) Make two slits on both sides of tape. (C) Fold middle section inward. (D) Tear a new slit in bottom of tape. Top part (a) should attach to patient's nose; bottom part (b) should be wrapped around tube.

STEP	RATIONALE

Safe Patient Care *Assess at least twice daily the condition of the naris and mucosa for inflammation, blistering, excoriation, or any type of skin or tissue injury (Karadag, 2017). Injury can develop for many reasons: rigidity of device rubbing against mucosa, difficulty in securing or adjusting the device to the body, increased moisture surrounding the tubing, tight securement of the device, and poor positioning or fixation of the device (Delmore and Ayello, 2017).*

STEP	RATIONALE
23. Fasten end of NG tube to patient's gown with piece of tape (see illustration). Do not use safety pins to fasten tube to gown.	Anchors tubing to prevent pulling on nose.
24. Keep head of bed elevated 30 to 45 degrees (preferably 45 degrees) unless contraindicated (AACN, 2017; Metheny and Franz, 2013).	Head-of-bed elevation reduces risk for aspiration of stomach contents if tube becomes clogged and patient regurgitates (Metheny, 2016; AACN, 2017).

Safe Patient Care *If inserting a Salem sump tube, keep the blue "pigtail" of the tube above level of the stomach. This prevents a siphoning action that clogs the tube. The blue "pigtail" is the air vent that connects with the second lumen. When the main lumen of the sump tube is connected to suction, the air vent permits free, continuous drainage of secretions.* ***Never clamp off the air vent, connect to suction, or use for irrigation.***

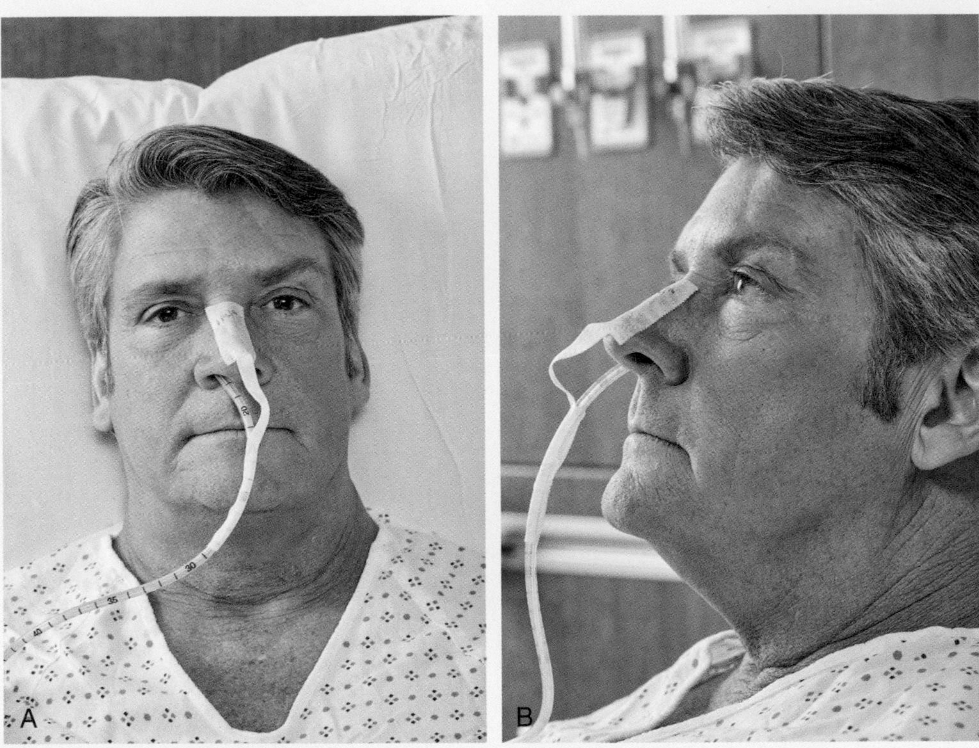

STEP 22a(4) (A) Tape applied to anchor nasogastric tube. (B) Nares are free of pressure from tape and tube.

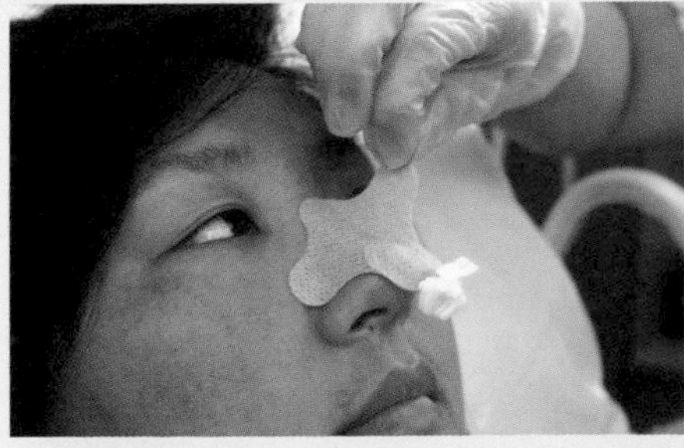

STEP 22b(1) Apply patch to bridge of nose.

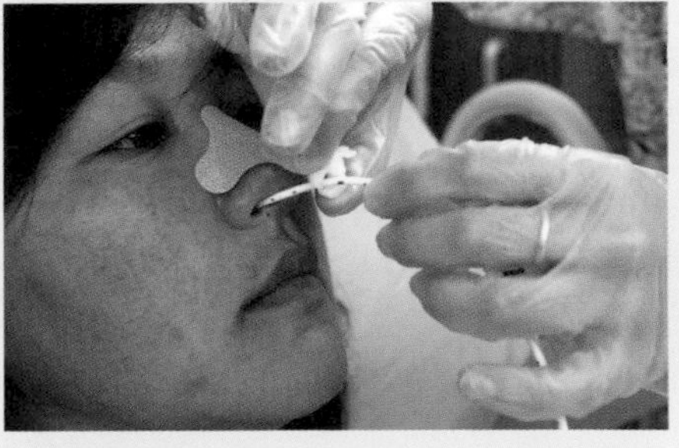

STEP 22b(2) Slip connector around NG tube.

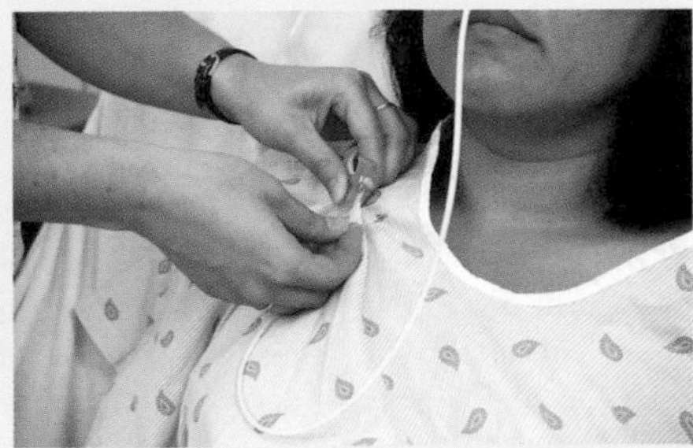

STEP 23 Fasten NG tube to patient gown.

STEP	RATIONALE
25. Remove gloves, perform hand hygiene, and help patient to comfortable position.	Reduces transmission of microorganisms.
26. Once placement is confirmed by x-ray, measure amount of tube that is external and mark exit of tube at nares with indelible marker as guide for any tube displacement. Record this information in nurses' notes in electronic health record (EHR) or chart.	The mark alerts nurses and other health care providers to possible tube displacement, which will require confirmation of tube placement.

Safe Patient Care *Never reposition an NG tube of a gastric surgical patient because positioning can rupture the suture line.*

STEP	RATIONALE
27. Attach NG tube to suction as ordered.	Suction setting is usually ordered low intermittent, which decreases gastric irritation from NG tube.

Safe Patient Care *If lumen of tube is narrow and secretions are thick, NG will not drain as desired. Irrigate tube (see Step 29). Consult with health care provider for higher suction setting if unable to irrigate tube because of thick secretions.*

STEP	RATIONALE
28. NG tube irrigation:	
a. Perform hand hygiene and apply clean gloves.	Reduces transmission of microorganisms.
b. Verify tube placement in stomach by disconnecting NG tube, connecting irrigating syringe, and aspirating contents (see Step 21b). Temporarily clamp NG tube or reconnect to connecting tube after removing syringe.	pH of gastric aspirate must measure between 1.0 and 4.0 to ensure that NG tube is in the stomach (McFarland, 2017). Prevents accidental entrance of irrigating solution into lungs.
c. Empty syringe of aspirate and use it to draw up 30 mL of normal saline.	Use of saline minimizes loss of electrolytes from stomach fluids.
d. Disconnect NG from connecting tubing and lay end of connection tubing on towel.	Reduces soiling of patient's gown and bed linen.
e. Insert tip of irrigating syringe into end of NG tube. Remove clamp (if present). Hold syringe with tip pointed at floor and inject saline slowly and evenly. Do not force solution.	Position of syringe prevents introduction of air into vent tubing, which causes gastric distention. Solution introduced under pressure causes gastric trauma.

Safe Patient Care *Do not introduce saline through blue "pigtail" air vent of Salem sump tube.*

STEP	RATIONALE
f. If resistance occurs, check for kinks in tubing. Turn patient onto left side. Repeated resistance should be reported to health care provider.	Tip of tube may lie against stomach lining. Repositioning on left side may dislodge tube away from stomach lining. Buildup of secretions causes distention.
g. After instilling saline, immediately aspirate or pull back slowly on syringe to withdraw fluid. If amount aspirated is greater than amount instilled, record difference as output. If amount aspirated is less than amount instilled, record difference as intake.	Irrigation clears tubing, so stomach should remain empty. Measure and document amount of irrigant fluid inserted in tube as intake.
h. Use an Asepto syringe to place 10 mL of air into blue pigtail.	Ensures patency of air vent.
i. Reconnect NG tube to drainage or suction. (Repeat irrigation if solution does not return.)	Reestablishes drainage collection; may repeat irrigation or repositioning of tube until NG tube drains properly.
j. Remove and dispose of gloves. Perform hand hygiene.	Reduces transmission of microorganisms.
29. Removal of NG tube:	
a. Verify order to remove NG tube.	A health care provider order is required for procedure.
b. Auscultate abdomen for presence of bowel sounds.	Verifies return of peristalsis.
c. Explain procedure to patient and reassure that removal is less distressing than insertion.	Minimizes anxiety and increases cooperation. Tube passes out smoothly.
d. Perform hand hygiene and apply clean gloves.	Reduces transmission of microorganisms.
e. Turn off suction and disconnect NG tube from drainage bag or suction. With irrigating syringe, insert 20 mL of air into lumen of NG tube. Remove tape or fixation device from bridge of nose and patient's gown.	Have tube free of connections before removal. Clears gastric fluids from tube to prevent aspiration of contents or soiling of clothing and bedding.

STEP	RATIONALE
f. Hand patient facial tissue; place clean towel across chest. Instruct patient to take and hold breath as tube is removed.	Some patients wish to blow nose after tube is removed. Towel keeps gown from soiling. Temporary airway obstruction occurs during tube removal.
g. Clamp or kink tubing securely and pull tube out steadily and smoothly into towel held in other hand while patient holds breath.	Clamping prevents tube contents from draining into oropharynx. Reduces trauma to mucosa and minimizes patient's discomfort. Towel covers tube, which is an unpleasant sight. Holding breath helps to prevent aspiration.
h. Inspect intactness of tube.	
i. Measure amount of drainage and note character of content. Dispose of tube and drainage equipment into proper container.	Provides accurate measure of fluid output. Reduces transfer of microorganisms.
j. Clean nares and provide mouth care.	Promotes comfort.
k. Position patient comfortably and explain procedure for drinking fluids if not contraindicated. Instruct patient to notify you if nausea occurs.	Sometimes patients are not allowed anything by mouth (NPO) for up to 24 hours. When fluids are allowed, orders usually begin with small amount of ice chips each hour and increase as patient is able to tolerate more.
l. Remove and dispose of gloves. Perform hand hygiene.	Reduces transmission of microorganisms.
30. For all procedures, clean equipment and return to proper place. Place soiled linen in utility room or proper receptacle. Perform hand hygiene.	Proper disposal of equipment prevents spread of microorganisms and ensures proper exchange procedures.

EVALUATION

1. Observe amount and character of contents draining from NG tube. Ask if patient feels nauseated.	Determines if tube is decompressing stomach of contents.
2. Auscultate for presence of bowel sounds. Turn off suction while auscultating.	Sound of suction apparatus is sometimes misinterpreted as bowel sounds.
3. Palpate patient's abdomen periodically. Note any distention, pain, and rigidity.	Determines success of abdominal decompression and return of peristalsis.
4. Inspect condition of nares, nose, and all skin and tissue around NG tubing.	Evaluates onset of skin and tissue irritation.
5. Observe position of tubing.	Prevents tension applied to nasal structures.
6. Explain that it is normal if patient feels sore throat or irritation in pharynx.	Result of tube irritation.
7. **Use Teach-Back:** "I need to be sure I explained the importance of letting me know if you are nauseated. Tell me why it is important for me to know if you feel nauseated." Revise your instruction now or develop a plan for revised patient/family caregiver teaching if patient/family caregiver is not able to teach back correctly.	Determines patient's/family caregiver's level of understanding of instructional topic.

Unexpected Outcomes	Related Interventions
1. Patient complains of nausea, or patient's abdomen is distended and painful.	• Assess patency of tube. NG tube may be occluded or no longer in stomach. • Irrigate tube. • Verify that suction is on as ordered. • Notify health care provider if distention is unrelieved.
2. Patient develops irritation or erosion of skin around naris.	• Provide frequent skin care to area. • Use taping method designed to reduce MDRPI (see taping methods in Steps 22a and 22b). • Consider switching tube to other naris.
3. Patient develops signs and symptoms of pulmonary aspiration: fever, shortness of breath, or pulmonary congestion.	• Perform complete respiratory assessment. • Notify health care provider. • Obtain chest x-ray film examination as ordered.

Recording

- Record length, size, and type of gastric tube inserted and naris in which tube was introduced. Also record patient's tolerance of procedure, confirmation of tube placement, character and pH of gastric contents, results of x-ray film, whether the tube is clamped or connected to drainage bag or to suction, and amount of suction supplied.
- Document your evaluation of patient learning.
- When irrigating NG tube, record difference between amount of normal saline instilled and amount of gastric aspirate removed on intake and output (I&O) sheet. Record amount and character of contents draining from NG tube every shift in nurses' notes or flow sheet.
- Record removal of tube "intact," patient's tolerance to procedure, and final amount and character of drainage.

Hand-Off Reporting

- Report occurrence of abdominal distention, unexpected increase or sudden stoppage in gastric drainage, and patient complaining of gastric distress to health care provider.

PROCEDURAL GUIDELINE 20.2 *Applying a Fecal Management System*

Purpose

A fecal management system (FMS) protects the perineum from fecal enzymes and prevents feces from spreading to wounds (Whiteley and Sinclair, 2014). An FMS is useful for patients with severe fecal incontinence such as those with *Clostridium difficile*–associated diarrhea (Tiwari et al., 20017). FMS systems are latex-free, indwelling rectal catheters with a low-pressure balloon to hold the catheter in place in the rectum and a soft, flexible drainage tubing attached to a containment device. These systems have an irrigation port to maintain the patency of the catheter and promote fecal drainage. Risks associated with use of this indwelling device include rectal bleeding, rectal necrosis, loss of rectal tone, pressure injury, or fistula formation (Lachenbrunch et al., 2016; Sammon et al., 2015; Tiwari et al., 2017).

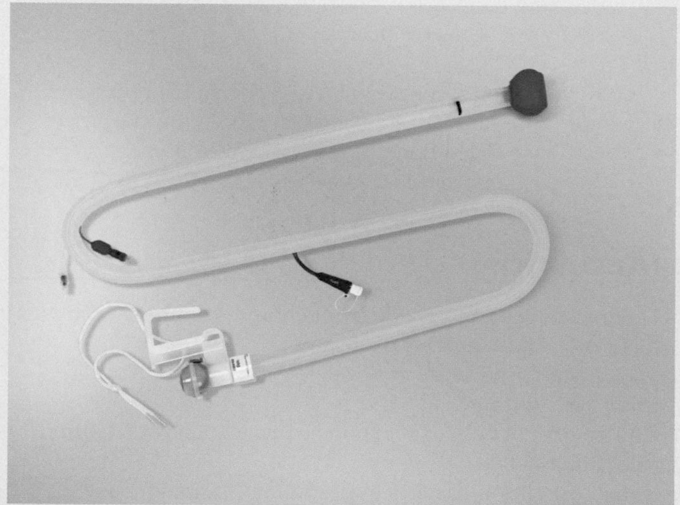

FIG 20.6 DIGNICARE® Stool Management System. *(Copyright © 2018 C.R. Bard, Inc. Used with permission.)*

Delegation and Collaboration

The skill of applying a topical (external) fecal containment device cannot be delegated to nursing assistive personnel (NAP). The NAP can assist the nurse by helping to position a patient during device application. The nurse instructs the NAP to:

- Report to the nurse any instances of leakage or change in appearance of skin around device noted during routine care.
- Report to the nurse immediately any increase in patient's rectal pain or sensation of pressure or rectal bleeding.

Equipment

FMS, also called fecal containment device (FCD), kit (Fig. 20.6); clean gloves; protective bed pad; bath basin

BOX 20.1

Contraindications for Use of Fecal Management Systems

- Pediatric population
- Suspected or confirmed anal pathology (e.g., anorectal stricture or stenosis; severe hemorrhoids)
- Surgeries: anorectal surgery; colorectal surgery in the preceding 12 months
- Existing poor anal sphincter
- Severe hemorrhoids
- Rectal tumor
- Fecal impaction
- Inflammatory processes of the rectum: Crohn's disease, radiation proctitis
- Anticoagulated patients

From Whiteley I, Sinclair G: Faecal management systems for disabling incontinence or wounds: literature review, *Br J Nurs* 23(16):881, 2014.

Procedural Steps

1. Identify patient using at least two identifiers (e.g., name and birthday or name and medical record number) according to agency policy (TJC, 2019).
2. Review medical record for contraindications for use of an FMS (Box 20.1).
3. Review medical record for frequency and amount of diarrhea over the past 24 to 48 hours.
4. Assess patient for allergy to silicone. Note that these devices are latex-free.
5. Perform hand hygiene and apply clean gloves. Perform perineal hygiene; observe patient's anal region for swelling, hemorrhoids, redness, irritation, or drainage. Presence of these findings may contraindicate placement of the device or may indicate need for other interventions to the perianal skin.
6. Change gloves and perform digital rectal examination to ensure that there is no rectal impaction. Remove and discard gloves. Perform hand hygiene.

PROCEDURAL GUIDELINE 20.2 *Applying a Fecal Management System—cont'd*

7. Pull curtain around bed or close room and prepare environment. Raise bed to working height.
8. Inform patient that you will insert device through the anus and that inflation of balloon will cause sense of fullness but should not cause discomfort.
9. Apply new clean gloves.
10. Apply the FMS.
    a. Prepare system by connecting collection bag to catheter tube assembly.
    b. Deflate cuff, usually done with 60-mL syringe supplied in the kit.
    c. Fill 60-mL syringe with 45 mL of tap water and attach syringe to inflation port. *DO NOT* inflate at this time. Inflation port is color coded.
    d. Position patient in left knee-chest position to help maximize sphincter relaxation.
    e. Place protective pad under patient's dependent hip.
    f. Fold cuff according to manufacturer directions and lubricate cuff. Note that folded cuff should be the size of your index finger.
    g. Generously lubricate anal sphincter.
    h. Gently separate patient's buttocks (NAP can assist), exposing perianal area for entire procedure. Make sure that perianal area is clean and dry. It may be necessary to perform perineal hygiene again, being sure to completely dry area.
    i. Insert cuff using index finger as a guide. Once the cuff is in the rectal vault, it will open to its original shape.
        (1) Inflate cuff with 45 mL water by slowly depressing syringe plunger; the cuff will inflate. ***Use the pilot balloon as a guide: If the balloon indicates overinflation or underinflation, withdraw all fluid from the cuff, reposition it in the rectal vault, and reinflate.***
        (2) Remove syringe from injection port and gently pull on the catheter to ensure that cuff seats against rectal floor.
    j. Note position of indicator line in relation to patient's anus. Changes in indicator line position may indicate need for cuff to be repositioned. Remove gloves and perform hand hygiene.
11. Irrigate cuff as needed: Fill syringe with 45 mL of tap water and attach to clear irrigation port. Observe flow; if leakage occurs, cuff may need repositioning (see manufacturer instructions).

Safe Patient Care *If the catheter tubing is obstructed with fecal contents, irrigate the catheter. Attach a filled syringe to the flush port and irrigate. Ensure that the flush port remains parallel to the catheter to prevent kinking.*

12. If stool sampling is needed, use sample port (see Fig. 20.6). Apply clean gloves, open sample port, and either tilt or milk catheter tubing to collect sample or insert a slip-tip catheter to withdraw fecal material. Close sample port when finished. Remove gloves and perform hand hygiene.
13. Replace collection bag as needed. Perform hand hygiene and apply clean gloves.
    a. Disconnect drainage tubing from collection bag.
    b. If necessary, attach bag plug into collection bag hub.
    c. Connect new bag to tubing.
    d. Dispose of fecal contents per agency policy. Remove gloves and perform hand hygiene.
14. Remove FMS. Perform hand hygiene and apply clean gloves.
    a. Attached depressed syringe 60 mL to cuff infusion port and slowly withdraw all water.
    b. Once cuff is deflated, grasp catheter as close to patient as possible and slowly slide out of anus.
    c. Dispose of FMS according to agency policy, remove gloves, and perform hand hygiene.
15. Position patient in comfortable position and perform any hygiene as needed. To avoid injury, do not insert anything into the anal canal while the device is in place (e.g., thermometer probe, suppositories).
16. Monitor patient for diarrhea and record amounts on intake and output (I&O) record every shift.
17. Record application of device and appearance of skin in nurses' notes in electronic health record (EHR) or chart.

SPECIAL CONSIDERATIONS

Patient-Centered Care

- Show respect for a patient's privacy, provide necessary comfort and hygiene measures, and attend to his or her emotional needs when performing required skills.
- Determine patient's normal pattern of bowel elimination and accommodate that pattern while the patient is in a health care setting. Determine the time the patient normally has a bowel movement.

Age-Specific

Pediatric

- Constipation in early childhood results from environmental changes such as being hospitalized and reluctance to use a toilet. Toilet-trained children often regress during hospitalization (Hockenberry and Wilson, 2017).
- Repeated withholding of stool leads to stretching or dilating of the rectum and decreases the sensation or "urge" to defecate (Hockenberry and Wilson, 2017).

Gerontological

- Older adults have some loss of sphincter control and often require a quick response when requesting a bedpan (Ball et al., 2019).
- The incidence of constipation is greater because there is impaired rectal sensation to defecate. As a result, the older adult does not perceive the need to defecate (Touhy and Jett, 2018).

✦ PRACTICE REFLECTIONS

One of your classmates is caring for a patient with severe vomiting and abdominal pain. He has a preliminary diagnosis of pancreatitis. The health care provider ordered a series of laboratory tests and abdominal scans. However, before the scan, the health care provider wants a nasogastric (NG) tube inserted for gastric decompression and placed on low intermittent suction.

1. The patient has never had an NG tube inserted; however, he did break his nose. In addition to assessing what the patient knows about NG tubes, identify additional pertinent assessment data needed before insertion of the NG tube.
2. Following completion, NG tube verification was confirmed by fluoroscopy. Before each NG tube irrigation, the nurse aspirates gastric contents and observes it for color and measures pH. The patient wants to know why this is important. Think about what you would tell the patient and his family.
3. You know that patients with medical devices are at risk for medical device–related pressure injuries (MDRPIs). Think about important assessments and related interventions to reduce this risk.

✦ CLINICAL REVIEW QUESTIONS

1. Match each of the following enemas with the appropriate description for use.

1. Sodium polystyrene sulfonate (Kayexalate) enema	a. Return flow enema that helps reduce intestinal gas and restore peristalsis
2. Oil retention	b. Used to promote easy evacuation after softening hard stool
3. Soapsuds	c. Prescribed to reduce severely elevated serum potassium
4. Harris flush	d. Used to relieve constipation or bowel cleansing

2. A patient just had three episodes of emesis consisting of bile and partially digested food. The last bowel movement was 4 to 5 days ago, the patient remains nauseated, the abdomen is slightly distended, and no active bowel sounds are auscultated. Place the steps of the procedure to place a Salem sump NG tube in proper order.
   1. Place patient in high-Fowler's position.
   2. Verify tube placement (check hospital policy).
   3. Measure distance to insert tube (tip of nose to earlobe to xiphoid process).
   4. Assess patient's nares and history of nasal and facial injury.
   5. Check for health care provider's order for the procedure.
   6. Properly identify the patient.
3. What are appropriate interventions to reduce the risk for medical device–related pressure injuries for an underweight older adult who had a nasogastric tube placed 1 day ago? (Select all that apply.)
   1. Obtain baseline skin assessment around nares and adjacent tissues.
   2. Assess nares and adjacent tissues once a day for pressure injuries.
   3. Use smallest NG tube possible for insertion.
   4. Avoid placement of respiratory equipment over NG tubing.
   5. Secure NG tube firmly against mucosal surface of naris.
   6. Maintain clean, dry skin under NG tube, tape or fixation device, and drainage tubing.

Answers and Rationales for Clinical Review Questions can be found on the Evolve website.

REFERENCES

American Association of Critical-Care Nurses: AACN practice alert: prevention of aspiration in adults, *Crit Care Nurse* 37(3):88, 2017.

Ball J, et al: *Seidel's guide to physical examination*, ed 9, St. Louis, 2019, Mosby.

Bolutta J, et al: ASPEN safe practices for enteral nutrition therapy, *JPEN J Parenter Enteral Nutr* 41910:15, 2017.

Centers for Disease Control and Prevention: What is health literacy?, 2016. https://www.cdc.gov/healthliteracy/learn/index.html.

Delmore BA, Ayello EA: Pressure injuries caused by medical devices and other objects: a clinical update, *Am J Nurs* 117(12):36, 2017.

Emergency Nurses Association: Clinical practice guideline, gastric tube placement, 2015. https://www.ena.org/docs/default-source/resource-library/practice-resources/cpg/gastrictubecpg7b5530b71c1e49e8b155b6cca1870adc.pdf?sfvrsn=a8e9dd7a_8.

Hockenberry MJ, Wilson D: *Essentials of pediatric nursing*, ed 10, St. Louis, 2017, Mosby.

Karadag A: A prospective, descriptive study to assess nursing staff perceptions of and interventions to prevent medical device-related pressure injury, *Ostomy Wound Manage* 63(1):34, 2017.

Lachenbruch C, et al: Pressure ulcer risk in the incontinent patient, *J Wound Ostomy Continence Nurs* 43(3):235, 2016.

McFarland A: A cost utility analysis of the clinical algorithm for nasogastric tube placement confirmation in adult hospital patients, *J Adv Nurs* 73(1):201, 2017.

Metheny NA: AACN practice alert: prevention of aspiration in adults, *Crit Care Nurse* 36(1):e20, 2016.

Metheny NA, Franz RA: Head-of-bed elevation in critically ill patients: a review, *Crit Care Nurse* 33(3):53, 2013.

Mordiffi SZ, et al: Confirming nasogastric tube placement: is the colorimeter as sensitive and specific as x-ray? Diagnostic accuracy study, *Int J Nurs Stud* 61:248, 2016.

National Pressure Ulcer Advisory Panel (NPUAP): Prevention and treatment of pressure ulcers: Clinical Practice Guideline, 2014. http://www.npuap.org/wp-content/uploads/2014/08/Quick-Reference-Guide-DIGITAL-NPUAP-EPUAP-PPPIA-Jan2016.pdf.

Padula CA, et al: Prevention of medical device-related pressure injuries associated with respiratory equipment use in a critical care unit, *J Wound Ostomy Continence Nurs* 44(2):138, 2017.

Pittman J, et al: Medical device related hospital-acquired pressure ulcers, *J Wound Ostomy Continence Nurs* 42(2):151, 2015.

Sammon MA, et al: Randomized controlled study of the effects of 2 fecal management systems on incidence of anal erosion, *J Wound Ostomy Continence Nurs* 42(3):279, 2015.

Santos SCV, et al: Methods to determine internal length of nasogastric feeding tubes: an integrative review, *Int J Nurs Stud* 61:95, 2016.

Solomon R, Jurica K: Closing the research-practice gap: increasing evidence-based practice for nasogastric tube insertion using education and an electronic order set, *J Emerg Nurs* 43(2):133, 2017.

Taylor SJ, et al: Nasogastric tube depth: the NEX guideline is incorrect, *Br J Nurs* 23(912):641, 2014.

The Joint Commission (TJC): *2019 National Patient Safety Goals*, Oakbrook Terrace, IL, 2019, The Commission. http://www.jointcommission.org/standards_information/npsgs.aspx.

Tho PC, et al: Implementation of the evidence-review on best practice for confirming the correct placement of nasogastric tube in patients in an acute care hospital, *Int J Evid Based Healthc* 9(1):51, 2011.

Tiwari T, et al: The traumatic tube: bleeding rectal ulcer caused by Flexi-seal device, *Case Rep Gastrointest Med* 2017:5278971, 2017.

Touhy T, Jett K: *Ebsersole and Hess' gerontological nursing and healthy aging*, ed 5, St. Louis, 2018, Elsevier.

Whiteley I, Sinclair G: Faecal management systems for disabling incontinence or wounds: literature review, *Br J Nurs* 23(16):881, 2014.

Wound Ostomy and Continence Nurses (WOCN) Society: *Guideline for prevention and management of pressure ulcers*, *WOCN clinical practice guidelines series*, ed 2, Mount Laurel, NJ, 2016, WOCN Society.

21 Ostomy Care

SKILLS AND PROCEDURES

EVOLVE WEBSITE/RESOURCES LIST

http://evolve.elsevier.com/Perry/nursinginterventions

Audio Glossary • Checklists • Clinical Review Questions • Answers and Rationales for Clinical Review Questions • Video Clips

INTRODUCTION

An ostomy is created surgically when a segment of intestine is brought to the surface of the abdominal wall. The opening is called a stoma, and it allows for the excretion of urine or feces into a pouch placed over the stoma. If the opening is in the colon, it is called a colostomy (Fig. 21.1), and in the small intestine, an ileostomy (Fig. 21.2). When it is necessary to remove the bladder or divert urine from the bladder, a segment of the ileum is used to form a conduit for urinary excretion called an ileal conduit or urostomy (Fig. 21.3).

Although the optimal type of stoma is one that is budded (Fig. 21.4), there are situations that make this difficult or impossible from a surgical standpoint. The stoma may be flush with the skin (Fig. 21.5) or retracted below skin level (Fig. 21.6).

PRACTICE STANDARDS

- The Joint Commission (TJC), 2019: National Patient Safety Goals—Patient identification
- Wound, Ostomy, Continence Nurses (WOCN) Society, Guideline Development Task Force, 2018: Clinical guideline: Management of the adult patient with a fecal or urinary ostomy—An executive summary

EVIDENCE-BASED PRACTICE

Health-Related Quality of Life in Patients With Ostomies

The presence of an ostomy has a negative impact on health-related quality of life (HRQOL), but evidence shows that this impact decreases over time from surgery (Nichols, 2015b). Many factors influence this impact on HRQOL, such as overall health, disease- and treatment-related symptoms, coping ability, resilience, and social support (Nichols, 2015a). The Wound, Ostomy, Continence Nurses panel of experts made four evidenced-based recommendations to promote HRQOL (WOCN Society, 2018):

- Include information about the HRQOL in preoperative education.
- Provide 12 months of follow-up after surgery to promote effective coping.
- Refer individuals with new ostomies who have severe or prolonged decrease in HRQOL to appropriate health care providers.
- Provide information about community-based support services (e.g., social worker, counselor).

SAFETY GUIDELINES

- Preoperative stoma site marking improves the chances that the patient will have a stoma that is in an optimal location and enhances the patient's ability to provide self-care. Proper stoma placement reduces the risk of pouch leakage and impaired skin integrity related to drainage on the skin (Salvadalena et al., 2015a, 2015b).
- Postoperative edema in the stoma and abdominal distention may require pouch changes and adjustments to the pouch opening for an appropriate fit during the postoperative period. Use of a transparent pouch helps to monitor these changes.
- Assessment of the abdominal contours and the type of stoma is essential to choosing a pouch that will provide a reliable and predictable wear time. Whenever possible, have an ostomy nurse evaluate the patient for the most appropriate pouching system (Carmel et al., 2016).
- The presence of blisters, rash, or excoriated peristomal skin is abnormal. Normally the peristomal skin is intact with some erythema after removal of wafer on drainage bag.
- It is important to observe the same hand hygiene measures that you would use for any patient using the bathroom. A patient should be allowed to wash his or her hands before and after participating in ostomy care.

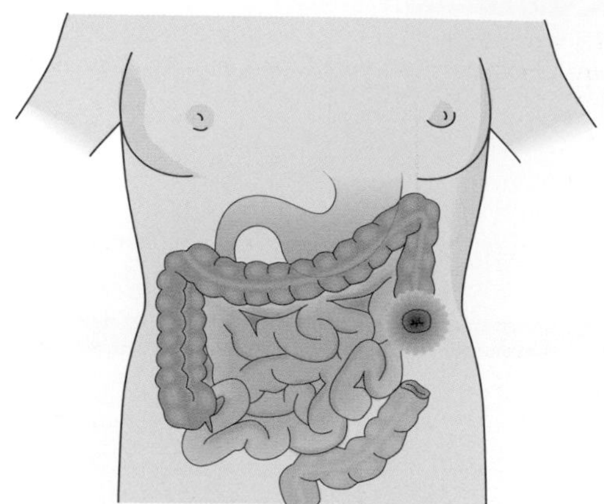
FIG 21.1 Sigmoid colostomy.

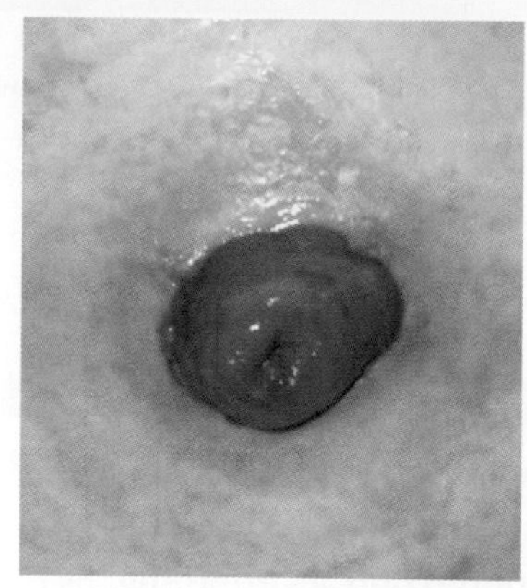
FIG 21.4 Budded stoma. *(Courtesy Jane Fellows.)*

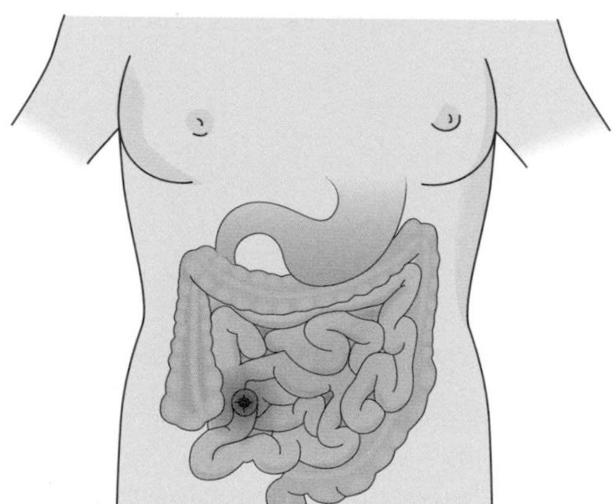
FIG 21.2 Ileostomy.

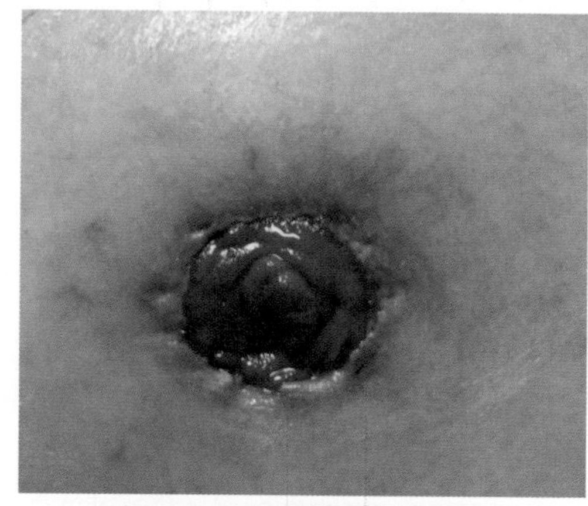
FIG 21.5 Flush stoma. *(Courtesy Jane Fellows.)*

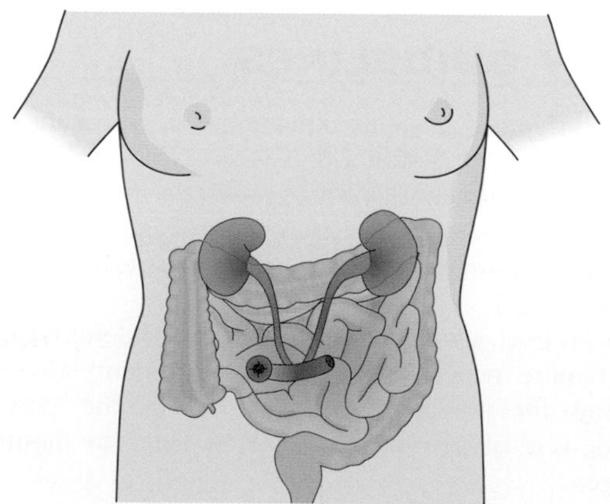
FIG 21.3 Urostomy (ileal conduit).

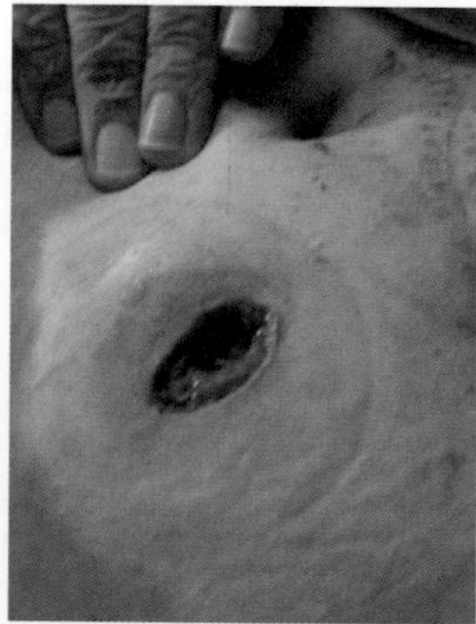
FIG 21.6 Retracted stoma. *(Courtesy Jane Fellows.)*

✦ SKILL 21.1 Pouching a Bowel Diversion

Purpose

Immediately after surgery it is necessary to place a pouch over the newly created fecal stoma to contain effluent (fecal contents) when the ostomy begins to function. The pouch keeps the patient clean and dry, protects the skin from drainage, and provides a barrier against odor. All pouches have a protective layer that adheres to the skin, called a skin barrier or wafer, and a pouch. A one-piece pouching system has the two parts integrated together (Fig. 21.7A). A two-piece system has a separate skin barrier and pouch that snaps in place on to the barrier (Fig. 21.7B).

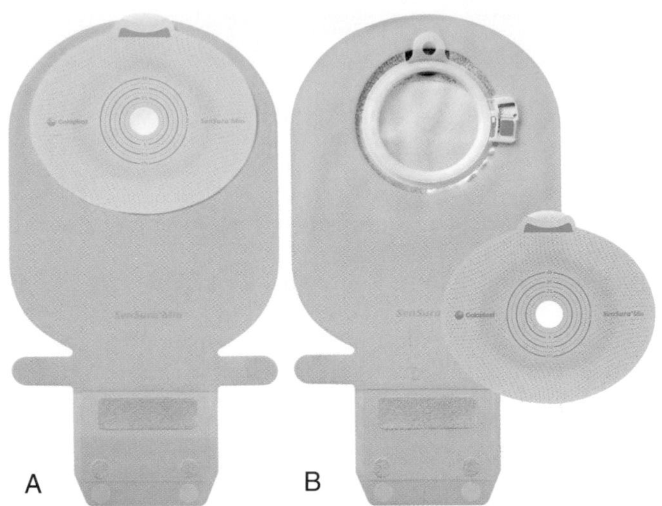

FIG 21.7 (A) One-piece pouch with Velcro closure. (B) Two-piece pouching system with separate skin barrier and attachable pouch. *(Courtesy Coloplast, Minneapolis, MN.)*

Delegation and Collaboration

The skill of pouching a new ostomy should not be delegated to nursing assistive personnel (NAP). In some agencies, care of an established ostomy (4–6 weeks or more after surgery) can be delegated to NAP. The nurse directs the NAP about:

- The expected amount, color, and consistency of effluent from an ostomy.
- The expected appearance of the stoma.
- Special equipment needed to complete a patient's pouching.
- The changes in a patient's stoma and surrounding skin integrity that should be reported.

Equipment

- Pouch: drainable one-piece or two-piece; skin barrier: cut-to-fit, precut size, or moldable
- Pouch closure device such as a clip if needed
- Measuring guide
- Adhesive releaser *(optional)*
- Clean gloves
- Washcloth
- Towel or disposable waterproof barrier
- Basin with warm tap water
- Scissors
- Waterproof bag for disposal of pouch
- Gown and goggles (if there is a risk of splashing when emptying the pouch)

ASSESSMENT

1. Identify patient using at least two identifiers (e.g., name and birthday or name and medical record number) according to agency policy. *Rationale: Ensures correct patient. Complies with The Joint Commission standards and improves patient safety (TJC, 2019).*
2. Perform hand hygiene and apply clean gloves. *Rationale: Reduces transmission of microorganisms.*
3. Observe existing skin barrier and pouch for leakage and length of time in place. Pouch should be changed every 3 to 7 days, not daily (Carmel et al., 2016). If an opaque pouch is being used, remove it to fully observe stoma. Dispose of such a pouch in proper receptacle. *Rationale: Assesses effectiveness of pouching system and detects potential for problems. To minimize skin irritation, avoid unnecessary changing of entire pouching system. When pouch leaks, skin damage from effluent causes more skin trauma than early removal of wafer.*

Safe Patient Care *Repeated leaking may indicate need for different type of pouch or addition of accessory products such as rings, seals, or paste. If the pouch is leaking, change it. Taping or patching it to contain effluent leaves the skin exposed to chemical or enzymatic irritation.*

4. Remove used pouch and skin barrier gently and observe amount of effluent. Empty it into a container for measurement of output. Note consistency of effluent and record intake and output. **NOTE:** Ileostomy may ooze effluent, so it is advised to delay pouch removal until implementation when pouch is changed. *Rationale: Monitors fluid balance and bowel function after surgery. Normal colostomy effluent is soft or formed stool, whereas normal ileostomy effluent is liquid.*
5. Observe stoma for type, location, color, swelling, presence of sutures, trauma, and healing or irritation of peristomal skin. *Rationale: Stoma characteristics influence selection of an appropriate pouching system. Convexity in skin barrier is often necessary with a flush or retracted stoma.*
6. Observe placement of stoma in relation to abdominal contours and presence of scars or incisions. Remove and dispose of gloves; perform hand hygiene. *Rationale: Determines if current pouching system is effective or if new selection is needed. Abdominal contours, scars, or incisions affect type of system and adhesion to skin surface. Reduces transmission of microorganisms.*
7. Assess patient's or family caregiver's knowledge, experience, and health literacy. *Rationale: Ensures patient or family caregiver has the capacity to obtain, communicate, process, and understand basic health information (Centers for Disease Control and Prevention [CDC], 2016).*
8. Explore patient's attitudes, perceptions, knowledge, and acceptance of stoma; discuss interest in learning self-care. Identify others who will be helping patient after leaving hospital. *Rationale: Determines patient's willingness to learn. Facilitates teaching plan and timing of care to coincide with availability of family caregivers.*

STEP	RATIONALE
PLANNING	
1. Expected outcomes following completion of procedure:	
• Stoma is red and moist; peristomal skin is intact and free of irritation; sutures are intact.	Normal findings in patient with postoperative ostomy that is healing.

STEP	RATIONALE
• Stoma drains moderate amount of liquid or soft stool, and flatus is in pouch, which can be seen with bulging of pouch. (Flatus may not be observable if pouch has gas filter.)	Stoma is functioning normally. Snug seal around stoma has been attained. Flatus indicates return of peristalsis after surgery.
• Patient and/or family caregiver observe stoma and steps of procedure.	Reveals acceptance of alteration in body image and interest in self-care.
• Patient asks questions about procedure and attempts to help with pouch change.	Indicates readiness to learn and begin self-care.
2. Assemble and prepare equipment and provide privacy.	Providing privacy and preparing the environment promotes patient comfort and ensures an organized procedure.
3. Explain procedure to patient; encourage patient's interaction and questions.	Lessens patient's anxiety and promotes patient's participation.

IMPLEMENTATION

STEP	RATIONALE
1. Have patient assume semi-reclining or supine position (same position assumed during assessment and pouching). (**NOTE:** Some patients with established ostomies prefer to stand.) If possible, provide patient with mirror for observation.	When patient is semi-reclining, there are fewer skinfolds, which allows for ease of application of pouching system.
2. Perform hand hygiene and apply clean gloves.	Reduces transmission of microorganisms.
3. Place towel or disposable waterproof barrier under patient and across patient's lower abdomen.	Protects bed linen; maintains patient's dignity.
4. If not done during assessment, remove used pouch and skin barrier gently by pushing skin away from barrier. Use adhesive releaser to facilitate removal of skin barrier. Empty pouch and dispose of it in an appropriate receptacle. Measure output, if needed. **NOTE:** There may be no output at time of first pouch change.	Reduces skin trauma. Improper removal of pouch and barrier can cause peristomal skin irritation or breakdown.
5. Clean peristomal skin gently with warm tap water using washcloth; do not scrub skin. **NOTE:** If you touch stoma, minor bleeding is normal. Pat skin dry. Have washcloth handy for additional cleaning if there is output from the stoma while preparing pouch.	Soap leaves residue on skin, which may irritate skin. Pouch does not adhere to wet skin. Ileostomies have frequent output, especially after eating.
6. Measure stoma (see illustration). Expect size of stoma to change for first 4 to 6 weeks after surgery.	Allows for proper fit of pouch that will protect peristomal skin.
7. Trace pattern of stoma measurement on pouch backing or skin barrier (see illustration).	Prepares for cutting opening in pouch.

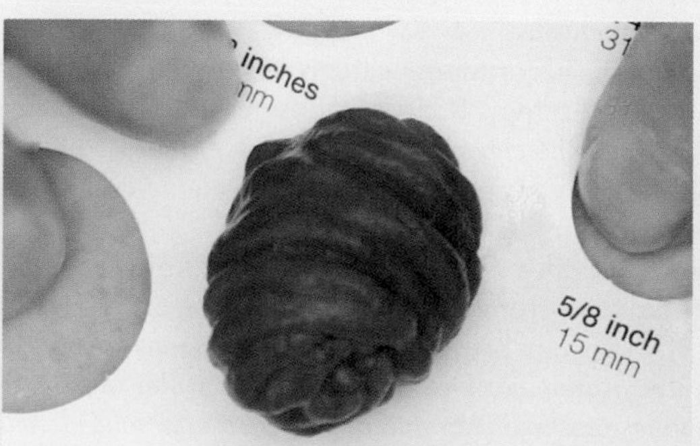

STEP 6 Measure stoma. *(Courtesy Coloplast, Minneapolis, MN.)*

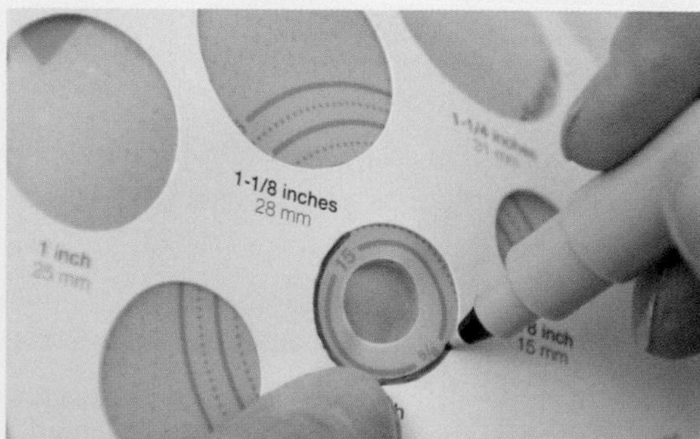

STEP 7 Trace measurement on skin barrier. *(Courtesy Coloplast, Minneapolis, MN.)*

STEP	RATIONALE
8. Cut opening on backing or skin barrier wafer (see illustration). If using moldable or shape-to-fit barrier, use fingers to mold shape to fit stoma.	Customizes pouch to provide appropriate fit over stoma.
9. Remove protective backing from adhesive backing or wafer (see illustration).	Prepares skin barrier for placement.
10. Apply pouch over stoma (see illustration). Press firmly into place around stoma and outside edges. Have patient hold hand over pouch to apply heat to secure seal.	Pouch adhesives are heat and pressure sensitive and hold more securely at body temperature.
11. Close end of pouch with clip or integrated closure. Remove drape from patient. Help patient to assume comfortable position.	Ensures that pouch is secure and will contain effluent. Gives patient sense of well-being.
12. Be sure nurse call system is in an accessible location within patient's reach.	Ensures patient can call for assistance if needed.
13. Raise side rails (as appropriate) and lower bed to lowest position.	Ensures patient safety.
14. Remove and dispose of gloves and other disposables. Perform hand hygiene.	Reduces transmission of microorganisms.

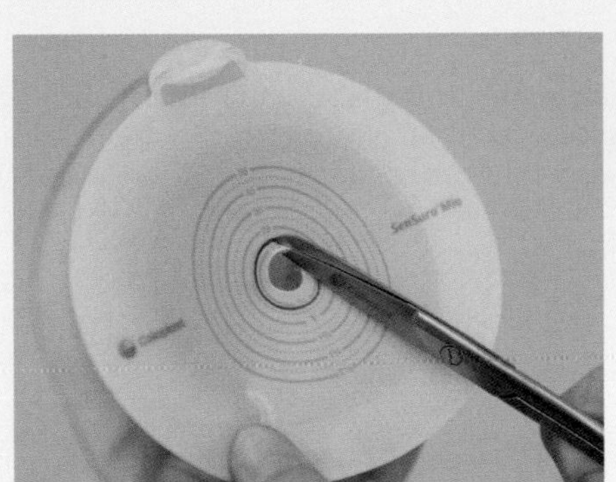

STEP 8 Cut opening in wafer. *(Courtesy Coloplast, Minneapolis, MN.)*

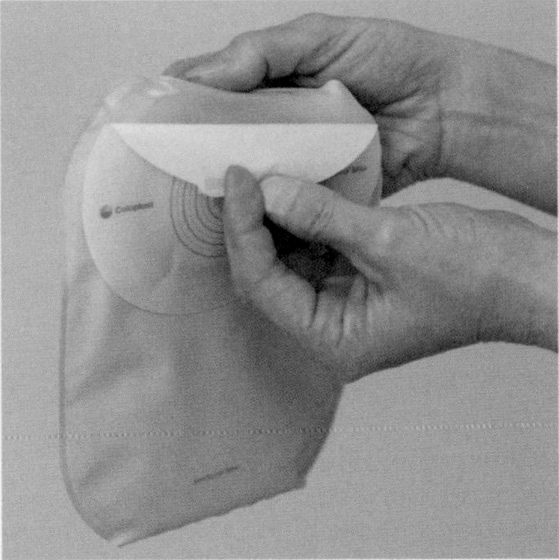

STEP 9 Remove protective backing. *(Courtesy Coloplast, Minneapolis, MN.)*

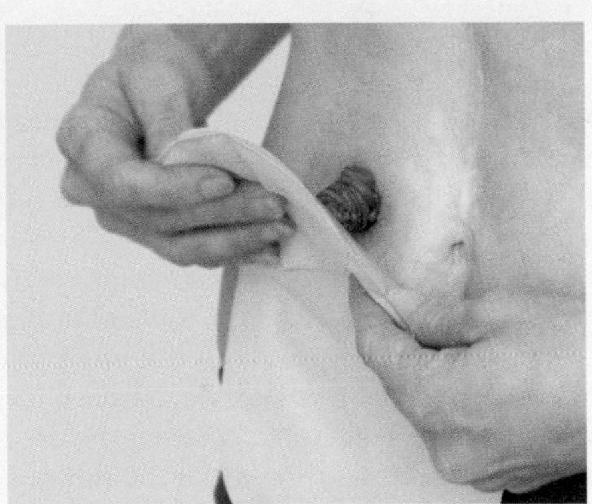

STEP 10 Apply pouch over stoma. *(Courtesy Coloplast, Minneapolis, MN.)*

EVALUATION

STEP	RATIONALE
1. Observe condition of skin barrier and adherence of pouch to abdominal surface.	Determines presence of leaks.
2. Compare appearance of stoma, peristomal skin, abdominal contours, and suture line with appearance and findings during previous pouch change.	Determines condition of stoma and peristomal skin and progress of wound healing.
3. Note if there is presence of any flatus during pouch change	Determines if peristalsis is returning.
4. Observe patient's and family caregiver's willingness to view stoma and ask questions about procedure.	Determines level of adjustment and understanding of stoma care and pouch application. Allows planning for future education needs and progress toward acceptance of altered body image.
5. **Use Teach-Back:** "I want to be sure you understand why it is important to change your ostomy pouch regularly. Tell me what you should do to prevent your skin from becoming irritated and the frequency with which you should empty your pouch." Revise your instruction now or develop a plan for revised patient/family caregiver teaching if patient/family caregiver is not able to teach back correctly.	Determines patient's/family caregiver's level of understanding of instructional topic.

Unexpected Outcomes	Related Interventions
1. Skin around stoma is irritated, blistered, or bleeding, or a rash is noted. May be caused by undermining of pouch seal by fecal contents, causing irritant dermatitis, or by adhesive removal, causing skin stripping or fungal or other skin eruption.	• Remove pouch more carefully. • Change pouch more frequently or use different type of pouching system. • Consult ostomy care nurse.
2. Necrotic stoma is manifested by purple or black color, dry instead of moist texture, failure to bleed when washed gently, or tissue sloughing.	• Report to nurse in charge or health care provider. • Document appearance.
3. Patient refuses to view stoma or participate in care.	• Obtain referral for ostomy care nurse. • Allow patient to express feelings. • Encourage family support.

Recording

- Record type of pouch and skin barrier applied, amount and appearance of effluent in pouch, size and appearance of stoma, and condition of peristomal skin. Record what patient and family caregivers are able to demonstrate and level of participation.
- Document your evaluation of patient learning.

Hand-Off Reporting

- Abnormal appearance of stoma, suture line, or peristomal skin or change in volume, consistency or color of output.
- If pouch change was done, patient's response to pouch change and participation in process.

✦ SKILL 21.2 Pouching a Urostomy

Purpose

When creating an ileal conduit or urostomy, the surgeon places stents into the ureters to keep them from becoming stenosed at the site where the ureters are attached to the conduit, and these extend out from the stoma (Fig. 21.8) The stents are removed during the hospital stay or at the first postoperative visit with the surgeon. A urinary pouch is placed over the stoma immediately after surgery to contain urine (Fig. 21.9). While the patient is in bed, the pouch may be connected to a bedside drainage bag using an adaptor that comes with the pouches to decrease the need for frequent emptying. A patient must understand the importance of draining the pouch when it is ⅓ to ½ full.

Delegation and Collaboration

The skill of pouching a new urostomy cannot be delegated to nursing assistive personnel (NAP). In some agencies, care of an established urostomy (4–6 weeks or more after surgery) can be delegated to NAP. The nurse directs the NAP about:

- Expected appearance of the stoma.
- Expected amount and character of the output and when to report changes.
- Change in patient's stoma and surrounding skin integrity that should be reported.
- Special equipment for a particular patient needed to complete procedure.

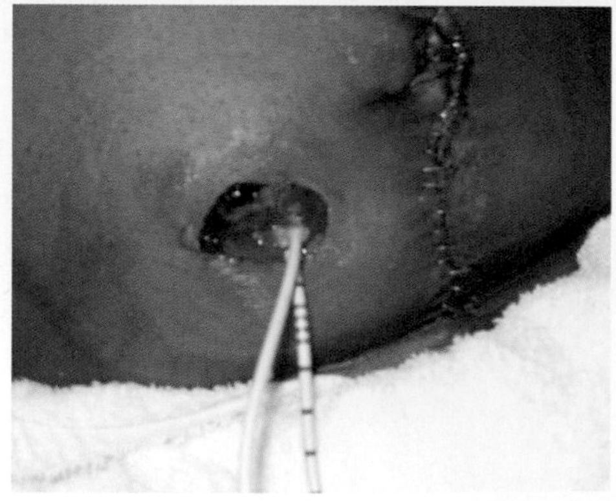

FIG 21.8 Urostomy stoma with stents in place. *(Courtesy Jane Fellows.)*

Equipment

- Urinary pouch (with antireflux flap) and skin barrier; drainable one-piece or two-piece, cut-to-fit, precut size, or moldable barrier with appropriate adapter for connection to bedside drainage bag
- Measuring guide
- Bedside urinary drainage bag
- Clean gloves
- Washcloth
- Towel or disposable waterproof barrier
- Mirror
- Basin with warm tap water
- Scissors
- Adhesive releaser *(optional)*
- Absorbent wick made from gauze rolled tightly in the shape of a tampon
- Waterproof bag for disposal of pouch
- Gown and goggles (if there is a risk of splashing when emptying the pouch)

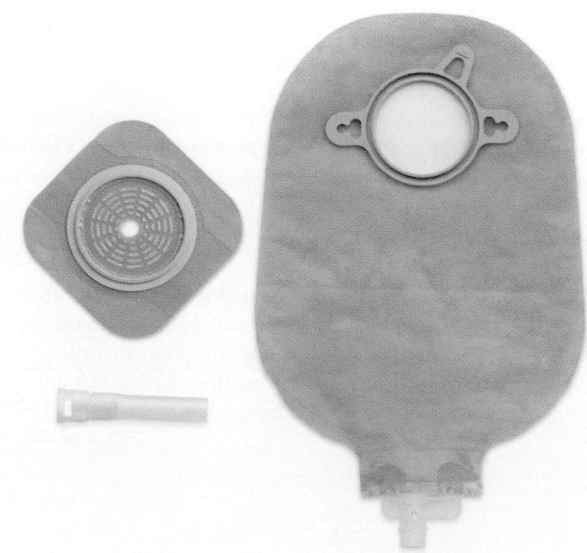

FIG 21.9 Urostomy pouching system with adapter to connect pouch to bedside drainage bag. *(Courtesy Hollister, Inc., Libertyville, IL.)*

ASSESSMENT

1. Identify patient using at least two identifiers (e.g., name and birthday or name and medical record number) according to agency policy. *Rationale: Ensures correct patient. Complies with The Joint Commission standards and improves patient safety (TJC, 2019).*
2. Perform hand hygiene and apply clean gloves. *Rationale: Reduces transmission of microorganisms.*
3. Observe existing skin barrier and pouch for leakage and length of time in place. Pouch should be changed every 3 to 7 days, not daily (Carmel et al., 2016). If urine is leaking under wafer, change pouch. *Rationale: Assesses effectiveness of pouching system and allows for early detection of potential problems. To minimize skin irritation, avoid changing entire pouching system unnecessarily. Repeated leakage may indicate need for different type of pouch to provide reliable seal.*
4. Observe characteristics of urine in pouch or bedside drainage bag. Empty pouch by opening valve and draining it into container for measurement. *Rationale: There may be blood or large amounts of mucus in urine after surgery, but this should resolve in the first 1 to 2 weeks after surgery. Urine from ileal conduit will contain mucus because of flow through intestinal segment.*
5. If visible through pouch, observe stoma for color, swelling, presence of sutures, trauma, and healing of peristomal skin. Assess type of stoma. If stoma not visible, observe just before pouch change. Remove and dispose of gloves. Perform hand hygiene. *Rationale: Consider stoma characteristics in selecting appropriate pouching system. Convexity in skin barrier is often necessary with flush or retracted stoma.*
6. Assess patient's or family caregiver's knowledge, experience, and health literacy. *Rationale: Ensures patient or family caregiver has the capacity to obtain, communicate, process, and understand basic health information (CDC, 2016).*
7. Explore patient's perceptions, acceptance and knowledge of stoma, and interest in learning self-care. Identify others who will be helping patient after leaving hospital. *Rationale: Facilitates teaching plan and timing of care to coincide with availability of family caregivers.*

STEP	RATIONALE
PLANNING	
1. Expected outcomes following completion of procedure:	
• Stoma is red and moist, with stents protruding from it. Peristomal skin is free of irritation and intact. Sutures are intact.	Normal findings for postoperative urostomy.
• Urine drains freely from stents or stoma.	These are normal findings after surgery.
• Urine is yellow with mucus shreds and is without foul odor. **NOTE:** Following surgery, urine may be pink or contain small blood clots.	Mucus shreds are normal when urine flows through intestinal segment.
• Volume of output is within acceptable limits (≥30 mL/hr).	Normal output reveals urine draining without obstruction.
• Patient and family caregiver observe stoma and procedural steps.	Shows adjustment to body-image change and willingness to learn self-care.
• Patient asks questions about procedure and may help with pouch change.	Indicates readiness to learn and begin self-care.
2. Assemble and prepare equipment and provide privacy.	Providing privacy and preparing the environment promotes patient comfort and ensures an organized procedure.
3. Explain procedure to patient; encourage his or her interaction and questions.	Lessens patient's anxiety and promotes participation.
IMPLEMENTATION	
1. Position patient in semi-reclining or supine position. If possible, provide patient with mirror for observation.	When patient is semi-reclining, there are fewer skin wrinkles, which allows for ease of pouch application. Direct view of stoma aids instruction.
2. Perform hand hygiene and apply clean gloves.	Reduces transmission of microorganisms.
3. Place towel or disposable waterproof barrier under patient and across patient's lower abdomen.	Protects bed linen; maintains patient's dignity.
4. If not done during assessment, remove used pouch and skin barrier gently by pushing skin away from barrier. If stents are present, pull pouch gently around them and lay towel underneath. Empty pouch and measure output. Dispose of pouch in appropriate receptacle.	Reduces risk for trauma to skin and for dislodging stents. Keeps urine from leaking onto skin. Urine output provides information about renal status and whether volume is within acceptable limits (≥30 mL/hr).
5. Place rolled gauze at stoma opening. Maintain gauze at stoma opening continuously during pouch measurement and change.	Using wick at stoma opening prevents peristomal skin from becoming wet with urine during pouch change.

STEP	RATIONALE
6. While keeping rolled gauze in contact with stoma, clean peristomal skin gently with warm tap water and washcloth; do not scrub skin. If you touch stoma, minor bleeding is normal. Pat skin dry.	Avoid soap. It leaves residue on skin, which can irritate it. Pouch does not adhere to wet skin.
7. Measure stoma (see illustration, Skill 21.1, Step 6). Expect size of stoma to change for first 4 to 6 weeks after surgery.	Allows for proper fit of pouch that will protect peristomal skin.
8. Trace pattern on pouch backing or skin barrier (see illustration, Skill 21.1, Step 7).	Prepares for cutting opening in pouch.
9. Cut opening in pouch (see illustration, Skill 21.1, Step 8). If using moldable or shape-to-fit barrier, use fingers to mold shape to fit stoma.	Customizes pouch to provide appropriate fit over stoma.
10. Remove protective backing from wafer surface and adhesive border (see illustration, Skill 21.1, Step 9). Remove rolled gauze from stoma.	Prepares pouch for application to skin.
11. Apply pouch (see illustration Skill 21.1, Step 10) over stents. Press wafer firmly into place around stoma and outside edges. Have patient hold hand over pouch 1 to 2 minutes to secure seal.	Pouch adhesives are heat and pressure sensitive and will hold more securely at body temperature.
12. Use adapter provided with pouches to connect pouch to bedside urinary bag. Keep tubing below level of bag.	Allows patient to rest without frequent emptying of pouch. Tubing position allows for collection and measurement of urine and prevents backflow of urine into stoma.
13. Remove drape from patient. Help patient to assume comfortable position.	Promotes comfort and ensures patient safety.
14. Remove and dispose of gloves and other disposables; perform hand hygiene.	Reduces transmission of microorganisms.
15. Be sure nurse call system is in accessible reach of patient. Instruct patient in use.	Promotes patient safety. Ensures patient can call for assistance if needed.

EVALUATION

1. Compare appearance of stoma, peristomal skin, and suture line during pouch change with appearance and findings from previous pouch change.	Determines condition of stoma and peristomal skin and progress of wound healing.
2. Evaluate character and volume of urinary drainage.	Determines if stoma and/or stents are patent. Character of urine reveals degree of concentration and whether there is possible urinary tract infection.
3. Observe patient's and family caregiver's willingness to view stoma and ask questions about procedure.	Determines level of adjustment and understanding of stoma care and pouch application.
4. **Use Teach-Back:** "I want to be sure you understand what is involved in changing your ostomy pouch. Let's review what we discussed. First, tell me how often you should empty your pouch and how often you should change it." Revise your instruction now or develop a plan for revised patient/family caregiver teaching if patient/family caregiver is not able to teach back correctly.	Determines patient's/family caregiver's level of understanding of instructional topic.

Unexpected Outcomes	Related Interventions
1. Skin around stoma is irritated, blistered, or bleeding, or maceration is noted as result of chronic exposure to urine.	• Check stoma size and opening in skin barrier. • Resize skin barrier opening if necessary. • Remove pouch more carefully. • Consult ostomy care nurse.
2. No urine output for several hours, or output is less than 30 mL/h. Urine has foul odor.	• Increase fluid intake (if allowed). • Notify health care provider. • Obtain urine specimen for culture and sensitivity if ordered.
3. Patient and family caregiver are unable to observe stoma, ask questions, or participate in care.	• Consult ostomy care nurse. • Allow patient to express feelings. • Encourage family support.

Recording

- Record type of pouch and skin barrier applied, amount and appearance of urine emptied from pouch, size and appearance of stoma, and condition of peristomal skin.
- Record what patient and family caregivers are able to demonstrate and level of participation.
- Document your evaluation of patient learning.

Hand-Off Reporting

- Abnormal appearance of stoma, suture line, or peristomal skin or change in volume, color, or odor of urine output.
- If pouch change was done and patient's response.

✦ SKILL 21.3 Catheterizing a Urostomy

Purpose

Catheterization of a urostomy is the only way to obtain an accurate culture and sensitivity specimen when screening for infection. When it is necessary to obtain a urine specimen from a urostomy, the best method is to insert a sterile catheter into the stoma (Mahoney et al., 2013). When a urine specimen is taken from the urostomy pouch or bedside drainage bag, the specimen will likely be contaminated, and the accuracy of results is questionable.

Delegation and Collaboration

The skill of catheterizing a urostomy cannot be delegated to nursing assistive personnel (NAP). The nurse directs the NAP to:

- Inform nurse if patient complains of flank pain or has a fever or new onset of altered mental status (signs of kidney infection).
- Inform nurse if there is a change in the color, odor, or amount of urine or if there is blood in the urine.

Equipment

- Urinary catheterization supplies (may be contained in prepackaged sterile catheter kit or may need to be gathered separately):
  - 14 to 16 Fr sterile catheter
  - Water-soluble lubricant
  - Antiseptic swabs (e.g., chlorhexidine)
- Sterile gloves
- Sterile specimen container
- Absorbent gauze wick
- Gauze pad
- Towels or disposable waterproof barrier
- Urostomy pouch if patient is using one-piece system (if using two-piece system, same pouch can be removed and replaced after procedure if skin barrier adhesive remains intact)
- Clean gloves
- Specimen label and labelled biohazard bag for specimen delivery

ASSESSMENT

1. Identify patient using at least two identifiers (e.g., name and birthday or name and medical record number) according to agency policy. *Rationale: Ensures patient safety. Complies with The Joint Commission standards and improves patient safety (TJC, 2019).*
2. Review accuracy of care provider's order for catheterization. *Rationale: Invasive procedure requires health care provider's order.*
3. Observe for signs and symptoms of urinary tract infection (UTI): elevated temperature, chills, foul-smelling urine, flank pain, and elevated white blood cell (WBC) count. *Rationale: Determines need to perform catheterization to obtain sterile specimen from a urostomy. Having a urostomy poses risk for reflux of urine back to kidneys, resulting in infection.*
4. Assess patient's or family caregiver's knowledge, experience, and health literacy. *Rationale: Ensures patient or family caregiver has the capacity to obtain, communicate, process, and understand basic health information (CDC, 2016).*
5. Assess patient's understanding of need for procedure and how it is done. *Rationale: Determines willingness to cooperate and reduces patient's anxiety.*

STEP	RATIONALE
PLANNING	
1. Expected outcomes following completion of procedure:	
• Urine specimen is not contaminated with bacteria during procedure.	Urine obtained correctly. Laboratory results are accurate.
• Patient describes risks for infection and techniques to prevent infection.	Demonstrates patient's learning.
2. Assemble and prepare equipment and provide privacy.	Providing privacy and preparing the environment promotes patient comfort and ensures an organized procedure.
3. Explain procedure to patient, including sensations that will be felt. If possible, obtain specimen when patient is due to change pouch if using one-piece system.	Lessens anxiety and promotes patient's cooperation. Cleaning stoma and surrounding skin may cause cool sensation. Insertion of catheter may cause sensation of mild pressure, or it may not be felt at all. Changing pouch too frequently could result in skin trauma.

STEP	RATIONALE

IMPLEMENTATION

STEP	RATIONALE
1. If possible, position patient sitting and drape towel across lower abdomen.	Gravity facilitates flow of urine. Maintains patient's dignity. Towel absorbs urine.
2. Perform hand hygiene and apply clean gloves.	Reduces transmission of microorganisms.
3. Remove pouch. (See Skill 21.1, Step 4.)	Allows access to stoma.

Safe Patient Care *If patient uses two-piece system, remove pouch but leave barrier attached to skin.*

STEP	RATIONALE
4. Remove gloves and perform hand hygiene.	Avoids contamination.
5. Open sterile catheterization set according to instructions or open needed equipment and place on sterile barrier using aseptic technique (see Chapter 5). If not using catheterization kit, place gauze pad on sterile field and squeeze small amount of lubricant onto gauze. Apply sterile gloves.	Prepares sterile work field.
6. If needed, have patient hold absorbent gauze wick on stoma while you prepare catheterization supplies.	Prevents leakage of urine on peristomal skin, linens, and clothing.
7. Clean surface of stoma with antiseptic swabs using circular motion from center outward. Use new swab each time; repeat twice. Allow antiseptic to dry or wipe off excess antiseptic with dry sterile gauze or cotton ball (check agency policy).	Removes surface bacteria. Antiseptic solution must dry to achieve antibacterial effect. More research is needed on use of antiseptic solutions versus sterile water or saline for cleansing (WOCN Society, 2016).

Safe Patient Care *If patient has stents in place, use antiseptic swab to clean the ends of the stents, and place the stents in the sterile cup. Allow urine to drip into the cup until you obtain an adequate amount for a specimen. Then go directly to Step 13.*

STEP	RATIONALE
8. Remove lid from sterile specimen container.	Sterile container collects small volume of urine.
9. Lubricate tip of catheter with water-soluble lubricant, keeping catheter sterile.	Facilitates passage of catheter through stoma.
10. With dominant hand, gently insert catheter tip into stoma. Do not force catheter; redirect course as needed until urine appears. Place distal end of catheter into specimen container. Have patient cough; massage abdomen near stoma or turn on his or her side.	Use care to avoid trauma to conduit. Movement and coughing may facilitate flow of urine from conduit.
11. Hold container below level of stoma. If needed, wait several minutes to get adequate amount of urine.	Culture and sensitivity studies only require 3 to 5 mL of urine (check agency policy).
12. Withdraw catheter slowly; place absorbent pad over stoma.	Keeps skin dry.
13. Apply lid to specimen container.	Prevents accidental spillage.
14. Reapply new pouch or reattach pouch if patient uses two-piece system (see Skill 21.2).	Pouch is necessary to contain urine.
15. Dispose of used pouch and equipment properly.	Avoids unpleasant odor in room.
16. Help patient to comfortable position.	Gives patient sense of well-being.
17. Raise side rails (as appropriate) and lower bed to lowest position.	Ensures patient safety.
18. Remove gloves; perform hand hygiene. Label specimen in presence of patient, place in labeled biohazard bag, and send to laboratory at once.	Ensures that laboratory results are assigned to correct patient. Labeling ensures acceptance and processing of specimen by laboratory. Urine that sits for long periods at room temperature will adversely affect laboratory results.
19. Be sure nurse call system is in accessible reach of patient. Instruct patient in use.	Promotes patient safety. Ensures patient can call for assistance if needed.

STEP	RATIONALE
EVALUATION	
1. Compare results of culture and sensitivity with expected findings. Mucus is a normal finding if patient has ileal conduit.	Determines presence of infection. If contamination appears likely, second specimen will be needed.
2. Use Teach-Back: "I want to be sure you understand the reason we needed to collect the urine. Tell me in your own words why we did this procedure to get urine from your stoma. What are the signs of a urinary tract infection when you have a urostomy?" Revise your instruction now or develop a plan for revised patient/family caregiver teaching if patient/family caregiver is not able to teach back correctly.	Determines patient's/family caregiver's level of understanding of instructional topic.

Unexpected Outcomes	Related Interventions
1. Unable to obtain urine specimen.	• Reposition patient. • If there is still no urine, push fluids and try again later. • Inform health care provider if unable to obtain specimen on second attempt.
2. Skin or stoma reveals complications.	• Notify nurse and/or health care provider. • Consult with ostomy care nurse about pouching system or skin barrier to use.

Recording

- Record type of specimen, time collected, patient's tolerance of procedure, and appearance of urine, skin, and stoma.

Hand-Off Reporting

- Report signs patient is exhibiting that suggests patient may have a urinary tract infection.
- Report time specimen obtained and sent to laboratory.
- Report results of laboratory test to nurse in charge or health care provider.

FIG 21.10 Convex skin barrier wafer. *(Courtesy Jane Fellows.)*

SPECIAL CONSIDERATIONS

Patient-Centered Care

- If patient does not speak English, have interpreter present or available for care and teaching.
- Financial concerns about cost of ostomy supplies and reimbursement are an important issue for patients on fixed income or for those without health insurance.
- There are many types of pouching systems available. Familiarize yourself with the pouches available to you in your agency. If a patient has a flush or retracted stoma (see Fig. 21.5) or a large, soft abdomen, a convex wafer (Fig. 21.10) may be needed because this will press against the abdomen and push the stoma through the opening in the wafer.
- An ostomy creates a major change in body image. Be aware of the need to help the patient normalize this change for him- or herself, and do not convey an attitude of discomfort or disgust when emptying or changing the pouch.
- For patients admitted to the hospital with an ostomy, respect their routine of care and assist them as needed.

Patient Education

- Whenever possible, patient should have preoperative and postoperative education and preoperative stoma site marking by a qualified medical professional (e.g., ostomy nurse) (Salvadalena et al., 2015a, 2015b).
- Have patient and/or family caregiver demonstrate ability to empty and change pouch before discharge from the hospital.
- Explain common symptoms of urinary tract infection: flank pain, dark or bloody urine, foul-smelling urine, fever (≥38.3° C [101° F]), confusion.
- Encourage patient to notify health care provider if symptoms of infection develop.
- Reinforce importance of fluid intake (2 L/day).

Age-Specific

Pediatric

- Ostomy pouches designed especially for neonates, infants, and children are smaller and have a more skin-sensitive adhesive on the barrier.
- The peristomal skin of a preterm infant is not fully developed; as a result, you should not use skin sealants and adhesive removers because they may damage the epithelium.

Gerontological

- Evaluate an older adult's cognitive status for understanding of ostomy self-care instructions.
- Some older patients have impaired manual dexterity or limited vision; make adaptations for this while teaching.

Home Care

- Evaluate patient's home toileting facilities and ability to position self to empty pouch directly into the toilet.
- Patient may shower without covering pouch.
- At home, a patient with a urostomy can open pouch spout and connect it to straight drainage at night. Make sure that patient understands that an adapter will be needed to connect the pouch to the bedside drainage bag.
- Be sure the patient has a way to obtain supplies after being discharged from home care agency.

✦ PRACTICE REFLECTIONS

Consider the importance of assisting patients who have had ostomy surgery to accept the change in how they perform a basic bodily function in a new way.

1. How can you help them to become comfortable with this change in body image?
2. You will likely be the first person to care for a patient's ostomy. How will your response to emptying and changing the pouch affect their ability to do this for themselves?
3. Can you relate how your feelings toward an ostomy will affect your ability to help patients accept their ostomies?

✦ CLINICAL REVIEW QUESTIONS

1. A patient with a urostomy has symptoms of a urinary tract infection. Which of the following should the nurse consider when obtaining a specimen from a urostomy? (Select all that apply.)
   1. It is acceptable to take the specimen from the pouch that the patient is wearing.
   2. A sterile catheter should be used to obtain the specimen.
   3. It should be an early morning specimen taken from the night drainage bag.
   4. The patient should be instructed to restrict fluids for several hours before the specimen is obtained.
   5. The stoma should be cleansed with an antiseptic solution prior to inserting the catheter.
2. Arrange the following steps for changing an ileostomy pouch in the correct order.
   1. Wash the skin around the stoma with warm water.
   2. Remove the old pouch.
   3. Press the new pouch into place.
   4. Measure the stoma.
   5. Make sure the skin is clean and dry.
   6. Have the patient place his or her hand over the pouch for 1 to 2 minutes.
   7. Cut an opening of the correct size in the pouch.
3. Which of the following statements is true about ostomy care? (Select all that apply.)
   1. The patient will always need a caregiver to change the pouch.
   2. If the patient experiences frequent episodes of leakage from under the wafer, another type of pouching system may need to be used.
   3. Stents in a urostomy stoma are temporary and will be removed after surgery.
   4. Liquid output from an ileostomy indicates the patient is having diarrhea.
   5. Regardless of stoma type, the pouch should be emptied when it is ⅓ to ½ full.
   6. Whenever possible, the patient with a new ostomy should see an ostomy nurse.

Answers and Rationales for Clinical Review Questions can be found on the Evolve website.

REFERENCES

Carmel JE, et al, editors: *Wound, Ostomy, and Continence Nurses Society: core curriculum: ostomy management*, Philadelphia, 2016, Wolters Kluwer.

Centers for Disease Control and Prevention (CDC): What is health literacy? 2016. https://www.cdc.gov/healthliteracy/learn/index.html.

Mahoney M, et al: Procedure for obtaining a urine sample from urostomy, ileal conduit, and colon conduit: best practice guideline for clinician, *J Wound Ostomy Continence Nurs* 40(3):277, 2013.

Nichols TR: Health-related quality of life in community-dwelling persons with ostomies, *J Wound Ostomy Continence Nurs* 42(4):374–377, 2015a.

Nichols TR: Quality of life of US residents with ostomies as assessed using the SF36v2, *J Wound Ostomy Continence Nurs* 42(1):71–78, 2015b.

Salvadalena G, et al: Wound, Ostomy and Continence Nurses (WOCN) Society: WOCN Society and ASCRS position statement on preoperative stoma site marking for patients undergoing colostomy or ileostomy surgery, *J Wound Ostomy Continence Nurs* 42(3):249–252, 2015a.

Salvadalena G, et al: Wound, Ostomy and Continence Nurses (WOCN) Society: WOCN Society and AUA position statement on preoperative stoma site marking for patients undergoing urostomy surgery, *J Wound Ostomy Continence Nurs* 42(3):253–256, 2015b.

The Joint Commission (TJC): *2019 National Patient Safety Goals*, 2019. Oakbrook Terrace, IL, The Commission. http://www.jointcommission.org/standards_information/npsgs.aspx.

Wound, Ostomy and Continence Nurses (WOCN) Society: *Core curriculum: ostomy management*, Philadelphia, 2016, Walters Kluwer.

Wound, Ostomy and Continence Nurses (WOCN) Society, Guideline Development Task Force: Clinical guideline: management of the adult patient with a fecal or urinary ostomy—an executive summary, *J Wound Ostomy Continence Nurs* 45(1):50–58, 2018.

22 Preparation for Safe Medication Administration

CHAPTER OUTLINE

EVOLVE WEBSITE/RESOURCES LIST

http://evolve.elsevier.com/Perry/nursinginterventions
Audio Glossary • Case Studies • Clinical Review Questions • Answers and Rationales for Clinical Review Questions

INTRODUCTION

Safe and accurate medication administration is a challenging and important nursing responsibility. As a nurse, you are responsible for having a full understanding of medication therapy and the related nursing implications. Nurses play an essential role in assessing for factors that place patients at risk when receiving medications and in preparing, administering, and evaluating the effects of medications. Nurses are also responsible for teaching a patient and family caregiver about medications and their side effects and evaluating a patient's and family caregiver's ability to administer medications safely at home.

PRACTICE STANDARDS

- Institute for Safe Medication Practices (ISMP), 2011: Acute care guidelines for timely administration of scheduled medications
- Institute for Safe Medication Practices (ISMP), 2016c: Oral dosage forms that should not be crushed—Reference to Do Not Crush list
- The Joint Commission (TJC), 2019: National Patient Safety Goals—Patient identification

EVIDENCE-BASED PRACTICE

Preventing Medication Errors

Adverse drug effects account for the largest number of adverse events patients experience in health care agencies. They can occur prior to admission, during the stay, or after discharge. A multi-system approach including the provider, nurse, and health care system should be used to prevent medication errors (Zhu and Weingart, 2017). Guidelines include the following:

- Everyone administering medications should review the medication list at each patient encounter.
- Be vigilant when handling and administering high-risk medications.
- Consider medications as the cause of any new symptoms.
- Use computerized physician order entry (CPOE) when possible to:
  - Standardize practice.
  - Improve the legibility of orders.
  - Alert and update health care providers on side effects, drug–drug interactions, and new orders.
- Use an electronic health record (EHR) when possible and interface this with CPOE if available to improve communication and alert all providers to administration times.
- Bar-coding of medications linked to patient identification bracelets improves safety and provides one last opportunity to identify a medication error (Hutton et al., 2017).
- Medication reconciliation identifies medication discrepancies and prevents errors.
- Patient, family caregiver, and provider education can be used to prevent medication errors.

SAFETY GUIDELINES

Medication administration safety is a priority goal for safe nursing practice. It begins by having a thorough understanding of the medications you administer and whether patients have any drug allergies. It is then important for you to follow safe preparation and administration standards, which are part of the seven rights of medication administration. The Institute for Safe Medication Practices (ISMP, 2016a) is recommending a seventh right of administration to include the right indication as a method to improve safety. Box 22.1 summarizes common causes of medication errors. Medication safety also requires you to understand the principles of pharmacokinetics, growth and development, nutrition, and mathematics.

The Joint Commission (2019) has specific National Patient Safety Goals for using medications safely. The 2019 goals include the following:

- Before a procedure, label medications that are not labeled, such as medications in syringes, cups, and basins. Do this in the area where medications and supplies are set up.
- Take extra care with patients who take anticoagulants (e.g., aspirin-containing drugs, warfarin [Coumadin], heparin) because of the risk of bleeding.
- Record and pass along correct information about a patient's medications to all health care providers. Find out what medications the patient is taking. Compare those medications with new medications given to the patient. Make sure the patient knows which medications to take when the patient is at home. Tell the patient it is important to bring an up-to-date list of medications to every visit with a health care provider.

PHARMACOKINETICS

When administering medications, know the mechanism of action, the therapeutic and desired effects of the drugs, and the purpose of the medications for each specific patient. It is equally important to be knowledgeable of possible side effects and adverse reactions. Pharmacokinetics is the study of how drugs enter the body (absorption), reach the site of action (distribution), are metabolized, and are excreted from the body. Absorption describes how a drug enters the body and passes into body fluids and tissues. Absorption influences the route of drug administration. Distribution is the way drugs move to the sites of action in the body. Metabolism refers to the chemical reactions by which a medication is broken down (e.g., in the liver) until it becomes chemically inactive. Excretion is the process of drug elimination from the body through the gastrointestinal tract, kidneys, or lungs (Burchum and Rosenthal, 2016).

BOX 22.1

Common Causes of Medication Errors

- Distraction (e.g., talking on phone, texting, talking with colleague) while preparing medications
- Ambiguous strength designation on labels or in packaging
- Drug product nomenclature (look-alike or sound-alike names, use of lettered or numbered prefixes and suffixes in drug names)
- Equipment failure or malfunction (e.g., infusion pumps)
- Illegible handwriting
- Improper transcription
- Inaccurate dosage calculation
- Inadequately trained personnel
- Inappropriate abbreviations used in prescribing
- Labeling errors
- Excessive workload
- Lapses in individual performance
- Medication unavailable

DRUG ACTIONS

Mechanism of Action

When giving a drug to a patient, you can expect a predictable chemical reaction that changes the physiological activity of the body. This reaction occurs as the medication bonds chemically at a specific site in the body called a *receptor site*. The reactions are possible only when the receptor site and the chemical fit together like a key in a lock. When the chemical fits well, the chemical response is initiated. These drugs are called *agonists* (Burchum and Rosenthal, 2016). Some drugs attach at the receptor site but do not produce a new chemical reaction. These drugs are called *antagonists*. Other drugs attach and produce only a small response or prevent other reactions from occurring. These drugs are called *partial agonists*.

Understanding pharmacokinetics enables you to make the decisions necessary to ensure that drugs are given by the appropriate route and to recognize and act based on the nature and extent of drug actions, interactions, and adverse actions. In addition, this knowledge helps in planning drug administration schedules. For example, knowing when the peak action of an analgesic occurs allows you to administer the drug at a time when you anticipate that the patient's pain will increase (e.g., before ambulation or a painful dressing change). Most health care agencies have standard administration schedules.

Medication Dose Responses

Pharmacokinetics affects how much of a drug dose reaches the site of action. Except when administered intravenously, medications take time to enter the bloodstream. The goal in administering a medication is to achieve a constant blood level within a safe therapeutic range. The minimum effective concentration (MEC) is the plasma level of the medication below which the effect of the medication does not occur. The toxic concentration is the level at which toxic effects occur. The safe therapeutic range is between the MEC and the toxic concentration (Fig. 22.1). When a medication

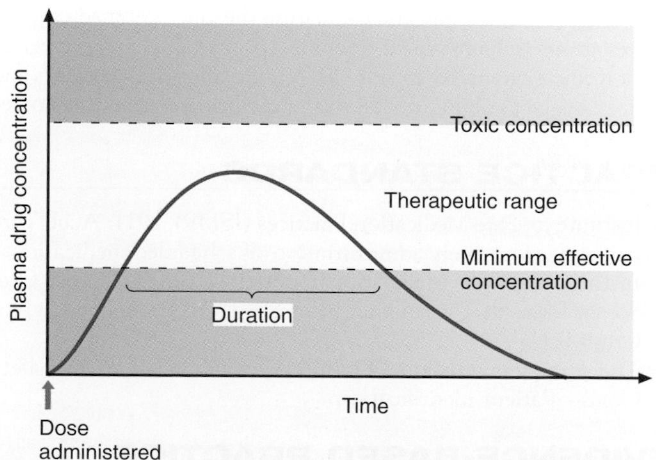

FIG 22.1 The therapeutic range of medication occurs between the minimum effective concentration and the toxic concentration. *(From Burchum J, Rosenthal L:* Lehne's pharmacology for nursing care, *ed 9, St. Louis, 2016, Elsevier.)*

is administered repeatedly, its serum level fluctuates between doses. The highest level is called the *peak concentration,* and the lowest level is the *trough concentration*. After peaking, the serum concentration falls progressively. With intravenous (IV) infusions, the peak concentration occurs quickly, but the serum level also begins to decrease immediately. Some medications (e.g., vancomycin or gentamicin) are based on peak and trough serum levels. You obtain a patient's trough level in a blood sample drawn 30 minutes before administering the drug. You draw a peak level whenever the drug is expected to reach its peak concentration. In the example of vancomycin, a peak is 1.5 to 2.0 hours after completing an IV infusion (Burchum and Rosenthal, 2016). Results of peak and trough tests reveal if a drug is reaching its therapeutic level.

All medications have a biological half-life, which is the time it takes for excretion processes to decrease the serum medication concentration by half. To maintain a therapeutic plateau, a patient needs regular fixed doses. The patient and nurse must follow regular dosage schedules and administer prescribed doses at correct intervals. Knowledge of the following time intervals of drug action helps you to anticipate the effect of a drug:

1. *Onset of action:* The time interval between when a drug is given and the first sign of its effect
2. *Peak action:* The time it takes for a drug to reach its highest effective concentration
3. *Duration of action:* The time period from onset of drug action to the time when a response is no longer seen
4. *Plateau:* Blood serum concentration reached and maintained after repeated, fixed doses
5. *Therapeutic range:* The range of plasma concentration that produces the desired drug effect without toxicity (see Fig. 22.1)

TYPES OF MEDICATION ACTION

Therapeutic Effects

A therapeutic effect is the intended or desired physiological response of a medication. A single medication may have many therapeutic effects. For example, aspirin creates analgesia, reduces inflammation and fever, and slows blood clotting. Other drugs have more limited therapeutic effects. For example, an antihypertensive medication lowers blood pressure.

Adverse Effects

Adverse drug events or effects (ADEs) are unintended, undesirable, and often unpredictable and include allergic reactions, side effects, overmedication, and medication errors (Centers for Disease Control and Prevention [CDC], 2016a). Some adverse reactions occur immediately, whereas others take weeks or months to develop. Early clinical recognition of ADEs is the important first step in identification. ADEs range from mild (e.g., rashes or photosensitivity to light) to severe (fatal anaphylaxis). Prompt recognition and reporting of ADEs prevent serious injury to patients. Always assess patients who may be at high risk for an ADE, such as pregnant women and patients with chronic disorders (e.g., hypertension, epilepsy, heart disease, psychoses) (Burchum and Rosenthal, 2016; Zhu and Weingart, 2017). When adverse responses to medications occur, the health care provider discontinues the medication immediately. Health care providers report ADEs to the U.S. Food and Drug Administration (FDA) using the MedWatch program (FDA, 2017b).

Side Effects

Every medication has the potential for harming a patient. Side effects are predictable and often unavoidable secondary effects produced at a usual therapeutic dose. They are not the same as adverse effects. Some side effects may be harmless, whereas others cause injury. For example, a common side effect of codeine phosphate is constipation, which can be managed with a change in diet and fluid intake. If side effects are serious enough to outweigh the beneficial effects of the therapeutic action of a drug, the health care provider may discontinue the drug. Patients often stop taking medications because of side effects such as fatigue, anorexia, drowsiness, or dry mouth. Report any side effects to a health care provider or pharmacist so that they can determine if the symptoms indicate a serious adverse reaction.

Toxic Effects

Toxic medication effects develop after prolonged intake of high doses of medication, after ingestion of drugs intended for external application, or when a drug builds up in the blood because of impaired metabolism or excretion. Toxic effects may be lethal, depending on the action of a drug. For example, morphine, an opioid analgesic, relieves pain by depressing the central nervous system. However, toxic levels of morphine cause severe respiratory depression and death.

Idiosyncratic Reactions

An idiosyncratic reaction is an unpredictable overreaction or underreaction to a drug. Predicting which patients will have an idiosyncratic response is impossible. For example, lorazepam, an antianxiety medication, when given to an older adult may worsen anxiety and cause agitation and delirium.

Allergic Reactions

Allergic reactions are also unpredictable responses to medications. Taking a medication for the first time may cause an immunological response. When this response occurs, the drug acts as an antigen, causing the production of antibodies. With repeated administration of the medication, the patient develops an allergic response to the drug, its chemical preservatives, or a metabolite of it.

The antibodies create a mild or severe reaction, depending on the patient and the drug. Among the different classes of drugs, antibiotics cause a high incidence of allergic reactions. Table 22.1 summarizes common allergy symptoms. Severe, or

TABLE 22.1

Common Allergic Reactions

Symptom	Description
Angioedema	Acute, painless, dermal, subcutaneous, or submucosal swelling involving the face, neck, lips, larynx, hands, feet, or genitalia
Eczema (rash)	Small, raised vesicles that are usually reddened; often distributed over the entire body
Pruritus	Itching of the skin; accompanies most rashes
Rhinitis	Inflammation of mucous membranes lining the nose, causing swelling and clear, watery discharge
Urticaria (hives)	Raised, irregularly shaped skin eruptions with varying sizes and shapes; eruptions have reddened margins and pale centers
Wheezing	Constriction of smooth muscles surrounding bronchioles that decreases diameter of airways; occurs primarily on expiration because of severely narrowed airways; development of edema in pharynx and larynx further obstructs airflow

anaphylactic, reactions are characterized by sudden constriction of bronchiolar muscles, edema of the pharynx and larynx, and severe wheezing and shortness of breath. The patient may become severely hypotensive, necessitating emergency resuscitation measures.

It is common practice for hospitalized patients with known drug allergies to have their allergy information recorded in a clearly identifiable place; this allows all caregivers to be aware of the patient's allergies. In many agencies, this information is recorded on the front of the patient's medical record on a brightly colored sticker. The patient also wears a wristband that contains the name of the medications to which he or she is allergic. Patient allergies must be recorded on the patient's medication administration record (MAR). Patients cared for in other settings (e.g., home) and who have a known history of an allergy to a medication should wear an identification bracelet or medal that alerts all health care providers to the allergy in case the patient is unconscious when receiving medical care.

Medication Interactions

When one medication modifies the action of another, a medication interaction occurs. A medication can enhance or reduce the action of other medications and alter the way in which the body absorbs, metabolizes, or eliminates the drug. When two drugs have a synergistic effect, the effect of the two medications combined is greater than the effect of one drug given separately. For example, alcohol is a central nervous system depressant that has a synergistic effect with antihistamines, antidepressants, and opioid analgesics.

A drug interaction may be desirable. Often a health care provider orders combination drug therapy to create a drug interaction for therapeutic benefit. For example, a patient with moderate hypertension may receive several drugs, such as diuretics and vasodilators, which act together to keep blood pressure at a desirable level.

Medication Tolerance and Dependence

Medication tolerance is the diminished response to a medication with repeated use and occurs over time. It is usually noted clinically when patients receive increasing amounts of medication (higher doses) to achieve the same therapeutic effect (Bartlett et al., 2013). Medications that produce tolerance include opium alkaloids, nitrates, and ethyl alcohol. Patients hospitalized for acute illnesses usually do not develop tolerance. It may take a month or longer for tolerance to occur.

Medication tolerance is not the same as medication dependence. Two types of medication dependence exist: psychological (or addiction) and physical. In psychological dependence, the patient desires the medication for a benefit other than the intended effect. Physical dependence implies that a patient will suffer withdrawal effects if the medication is stopped abruptly. When patients receive medications for a short time, such as for postoperative pain, dependence is rare. The CDC (2016b) has developed evidence-based guidelines for health care providers who prescribe opioids.

Medication Misuse

Misuse of medication includes overuse, underuse, and nonadherence. Patients of all ages misuse medications. Older adults are at greatest risk because of polypharmacy, the concurrent use of five or more medications (including both prescription and nonprescription products) by a single individual (ISMP Canada, 2018). The incidence of prescription and over-the-counter (OTC) drug misuse and abuse is also increasing. The most commonly abused prescription medications are opioids, stimulants, tranquilizers, and sedatives. Common over-the-counter (OTC) medications that patients misuse or abuse include cough syrup and cold medication containing dextromethorphan (National Institutes of Health and National Institute on Drug Abuse [NIH NIDA], 2015). You are ethically and legally responsible to understand the problems of persons using medications improperly. When caring for patients with suspected medication abuse or dependence, be aware of your values and attitudes about the willful use of harmful substances. Do not let your personal values interfere with understanding a patient's needs and concerns.

ADMINISTERING MEDICATIONS

You are not solely responsible for medication administration. The health care provider and pharmacist also help to ensure that the right medication gets to the right patient. You are accountable for knowing which medications are ordered, understanding their therapeutic effects, recognizing undesired effects, and administering medications correctly.

Medication Orders

A health care provider's order is required for all medications to be administered by a nurse (except in states where Nurse Practice Acts allows advanced practice nurses and nurse practitioners to prescribe). A health care provider's order sheet is in written or electronic form. The health care provider writes the date, time, and medication order, including the following:

1. The name of the medication, which may be either the trade name (e.g., Percocet) or the generic name (e.g., oxycodone)
2. The dose (e.g., 5 mg)
3. The route (e.g., by mouth [PO])
4. The frequency (e.g., every 4 hours [q4h])
5. Orders for medications to be given prn (as needed) also include the reason they are to be given (e.g., for pain)
6. The signature of the health care provider

Verbal and telephone orders are optional forms of orders when written or electronic communication between a health care provider and nurse is not possible. Student nurses cannot accept verbal or telephone orders. When a nurse receives a verbal or telephone order, he or she enters the order on the health care provider's order sheet. The name of the health care provider and the nurse's signature are included. The health care provider countersigns the order later, usually within 24 hours after making the order (see agency policy). Box 22.2 provides guidelines for safely taking verbal or telephone orders for medications.

BOX 22.2

Guidelines for Telephone Orders and Verbal Orders

- Only authorized staff members receive and record telephone or verbal orders. Agency identifies in writing the staff members who are authorized.
- Clearly identify patient's name, room number, and diagnosis.
- Read back all orders to health care provider (TJC, 2019).
- Use clarification questions to avoid misunderstandings.
- Write "TO" (telephone order) or "VO" (verbal order), including date and time, name of patient, and complete order; sign the name of the health care provider and nurse.
- Follow agency policies; some agencies require documentation of the "read-back" or require two nurses to review and sign telephone or verbal orders.
- Health care provider co-signs the order within the time frame required by the agency (usually 24 hours; verify agency policy).

There are five common types of medication orders. The type of order is based on the frequency or urgency of medication administration.

You carry out a *standing order* until the health care provider cancels it by another order or until a prescribed number of days have elapsed. A standing order sometimes indicates a final date or number of doses. Many agencies have a policy for automatically discontinuing standard orders.

A health care provider may order a medication to be given only when a patient requires or requests it. This is a *prn* order. As a nurse, you assess a patient thoroughly to determine whether the patient needs the medication, based on the indication for the drug (e.g., pain or nausea). Sometimes a different type of therapy is more appropriate. A prn order usually has minimum intervals set for the time of administration. This means that you cannot give the drug any more frequently than what is prescribed.

Single (one-time) orders are common for preoperative medications or medications given before diagnostic examinations. The medication is ordered to be given only once at a specified time. A *stat* order means that you give a single dose of a medication immediately and only once. Stat orders are used for emergencies when a patient's condition changes suddenly. A *now order* is more specific than a one-time order. It is used when a patient needs a medication quickly but not as soon as a stat order. When you receive a now order, you have up to 90 minutes to give the drug (see agency policy).

Although The Joint Commission allows the use of range orders (range allowed for a medication dosage), there continues to be concerns about providing enough guidance to nurses while still allowing them to address the individual needs of patients. An example of a poorly written range order is "give morphine sulfate 2 to 6 mg IV push every 4h prn for pain." This order is not specific with regard to guidelines needed to give a correct dose. A range order must provide objective measures for nurses to use to determine the correct dose. An example of a good order is "give Lortab 1 to 2 q 4 hours prn pain. For pain 1 to 5, 1 tab; for pain 5 to 10, 2 tabs." A range order should include specific indications such as a pain rating score or temperature level, especially for use of a medication indicated for more than one reason (e.g., ibuprofen, which could be indicated for pain or fever).

Communication and Transcription of Orders

After new medication orders are entered into a computer or written, the drugs must be obtained from the pharmacy. A health care provider's order is transmitted to the pharmacy automatically through the use of the EHR, but in the case of a written system, copies of orders are sent. Before updating medication orders, pharmacists assess the medication plan and ensure that orders are valid. The pharmacist is responsible for preparing the correct medications and delivering them to the nursing unit, where they are stocked in a medication administration station.

Medication Errors

The National Coordinating Council for Medication Error Reporting and Prevention (2017) defines a medication error as any preventable event that may cause inappropriate medication use or jeopardize patient safety. Medication errors include:

- Inaccurate prescribing
- Administration of the wrong medication, by the wrong route, or at the wrong time interval
- Administration of extra doses or failure to administer a medication

Hospital medication delivery systems have a system of checks, such as warning notifications, that help prevent medication errors.

BOX 22.3

Steps to Prevent Medication Errors

- Follow the seven rights of medication administration.
- Only prepare medications for one patient at a time.
- Be sure to read labels at least three times (comparing MAR with label): when removing medication from storage, before taking to patient's room, before giving medication.
- Use at least two patient identifiers every time you administer medications (e.g., patient's name, birthday, hospital number).
- Double-check all calculations and other high-risk medication administration processes (e.g., patient-controlled analgesia) and verify with another nurse.
- Do not attempt to interpret illegible handwriting; clarify with the health care provider.
- Question unusually large or small doses.
- Document all medications as soon as they are given.
- When you have made or discovered an error, reflect on what went wrong, and ask how you could have prevented it. Complete an occurrence report per agency policy.
- Evaluate the context or situation in which a medication error occurred. This helps to determine if nurses have the necessary resources for safe medication administration.
- When repeated medication errors occur within a work area, identify and analyze the factors that may have caused the errors, and take corrective action.
- Attend in-service programs on the medications you commonly administer.
- Ensure that you are well rested when caring for patients. Nurses make more errors when they are tired.
- Involve and educate patient when administering medications. Address patient's concerns about medications before administering them (e.g., concerns about their appearance or side effects).
- Follow established agency policies and procedures when using technology to administer medications (e.g., automated medication dispensing system [AMDS] and bar-code scanning). Medication errors occur when nurses "work around" the technology (e.g., override alerts without thinking about them) (Voshall et al., 2013).

MAR, Medication administration record.

Conscientious adherence to the seven rights of medication administration is your best way to prevent errors (Box 22.3).

Many medication errors occur when nurses become distracted or lose focus during preparation and administration of medications. Errors also occur when nurses do not follow best-practice protocols and procedures related to medication administration. Research reveals that nurses are frequently distracted during three phases of medication administration: the acquisition of the medication, transportation to the bedside, and during actual administration (Bravo and Cochran, 2016). Areas where nurses prepare medications are highly visible locations with high levels of staff traffic. Nurses become interrupted while accessing dispensing systems, depositing medications into delivery containers, and confirming orders on computer screens. Work-related interruptions and distractions have been identified as questions from staff or family, equipment alarms, and personal conversations (Bravo and Cochran, 2016; Yoder et al., 2015). Follow these tips:

- Reduce distractions (e.g., turn off pager) and interruptions around automated medication dispensing machines (Bravo and Cochran, 2016).
- In areas where medications are being prepared, use a brightly colored sign or tape to alert staff to avoid interruptions (e.g., discussions) (Connor et al., 2016).

When an error occurs, acknowledge it immediately, and then assess the patient. You have an ethical and professional obligation to report an error to the patient's health care provider, the nurse manager, and any other persons indicated by the agency policy regarding errors. Appropriate follow-up may include administering an antidote, withholding a subsequent dose, and monitoring the effects of the medication. A patient's medical record should include a notation that indicates what was given, who was notified, the observed effects of the medication, and follow-up measures taken.

You are also responsible for completing a report describing the incident. Most agencies have a policy or protocol for reporting adverse events. This report provides an objective analysis of what went wrong. It provides information for the risk management team to identify factors contributing to errors and develop ways to avoid similar errors in the future.

DISTRIBUTION SYSTEMS

Systems for storing and distributing medications vary. Agencies providing nursing care have special areas for stocking and dispensing medications such as special medication rooms, portable locked carts, computerized medication cabinets, and individual storage units in patients' rooms. Medication storage areas must be locked when unattended.

Unit-Dose System

The standard for medication distribution is the unit-dose system. The system uses an automated medication dispensing system (AMDS) or a cart containing a drawer with a 24-hour supply of medications for each patient (Fig. 22.2). Each drawer has a label with the name of the patient in each designated room. The unit dose is the ordered dose of medication that the patient receives at one time. Each medication form is wrapped separately. At a designated time, each day, the drawers in the cart are refilled by a pharmacy technician. A cart also contains limited amounts of prn and stock medications for special situations. The unit-dose system is designed to reduce the number of medication errors and saves steps in dispensing medications.

Automated Medication Dispensing Systems

Automated medication dispensing systems (AMDSs) within a health care agency are networked with one another and with other computer systems in the agency (e.g., the computerized medical record). AMDSs control the dispensing of all medications, including narcotics. Each nurse has a personal security code, allowing access to the system. If your agency uses a system that requires bioidentification, you must place your finger on a screen to access the computer. Once logged onto an AMDS, you select a patient's name and medication profile. Then you select the medication, dosage, and route from a list on the computer screen. The system opens the medication drawer or dispenses the medication to the nurse, records the event, and charges it to the patient. If the system is connected to the patient's medical record, information about the medication (e.g., name, dose, time) and the name of the nurse who retrieved the medication from the AMDS is recorded in the patient's medical record. Some systems require nurses to scan bar codes before recording this information in the patient's computerized medical record. AMDS and bar-code scanning are designed to improve the accuracy of patient identification and to ensure correct medication administration and medical record keeping, reducing the chance of medication errors (Chapuis et al., 2015; Fanning et al., 2016; Zhu and Weingart, 2017).

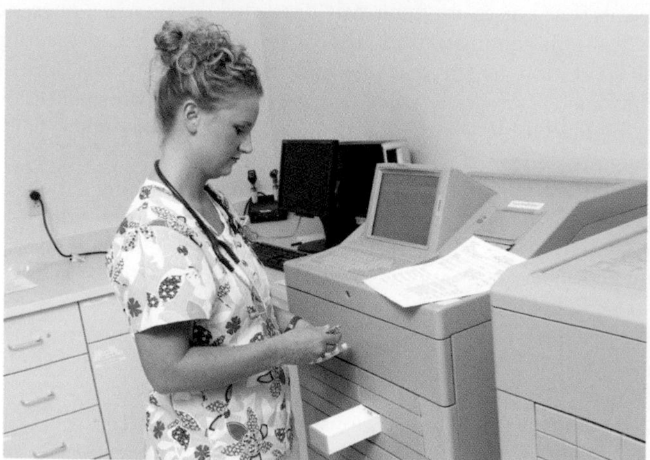

FIG 22.2 Automated medication dispensing system.

MEDICATION ADMINISTRATION RECORD

The medication administration record (MAR) is a form used to verify that the right medications are being administered at the correct times. The process of verification of medications varies among health care agencies. During the order transcription process, a nurse and pharmacist check all medication orders for accuracy and thoroughness several times, and the health care provider's complete order is placed on the appropriate MAR. The MAR includes the patient's name, room, and bed number and the names, doses, frequencies, and routes of administration for each medication. Most health care agencies have computers to generate and display electronic MARs. If the MAR is handwritten, a registered nurse (RN) completes or updates the MAR routinely. Nurses record medications administered on the MAR. In many agencies, computer stations in patient rooms allow for easy accessible entry.

Regardless of the type of MAR your agency uses, be sure that you refer to the MAR each time you prepare a medication and have the MAR available at the patient's bedside when administering medications. It is essential that you verify the accuracy of every medication you give to the patient with the patient's orders. If the medication order is incomplete, incorrect, or inappropriate or if there is a discrepancy between the written order and what is on the MAR, consult with the health care provider. Do not give a medication until you are certain that you are able to follow the seven rights of medication administration. When you give the wrong medication or an incorrect dose, *you* are legally responsible for the error.

SEVEN RIGHTS OF MEDICATION ADMINISTRATION

Preparing and administering medications require accuracy and your full attention. To ensure safe medication administration, be aware of the seven rights of medication administration.

Right Medication

The Joint Commission includes medication reconciliation as a National Patient Safety Goal for 2019 (TJC, 2019). When a patient enters a hospital setting, a complete list of the patient's current medications must be reviewed and documented with the patient involved. You will compare the medications health care providers order with medications on a patient's list. When the patient is transferred to another service or health care setting, you again must reconcile the patient's current list of medications. The goal of medication reconciliation is to ensure one list of medications and to address or correct any discrepancies before discharge from the health care setting (TJC, 2019).

In 2004, The Joint Commission created its "do not use" list of abbreviations (Table 22.2) as part of the requirements for meeting a national safety goal set in 2001. The list of unacceptable abbreviations contains abbreviations that have been found to increase the incidence of errors in medication administration. You are responsible for using correct abbreviations and verifying that an order was accurately transcribed. Electronic health records using CPOE are now incorporating the "do not use" abbreviations. Many agencies have a policy that requires nurses on a specific shift to verify the accuracy of MAR forms printed for each patient each day. Whenever new orders are handwritten on the MAR, the nurse adding the orders must verify that they are added accurately. When verification is complete, you initial and sign the order.

During medication administration, you compare a health care provider's order with the MAR when a medication is ordered initially. Nurses verify information whenever new MARs are written or distributed or when patients transfer from one nursing unit to another or a different health care setting. At the time of medication administration, you compare the label of a medication (Fig. 22.3) with the MAR three times: (1) when removing the medication from the storage bin, (2) before placing the medication in the medications cup or before taking the medication to the patient's room, and (3) again at the bedside before giving the medication to the patient. If the medication is ordered by trade name and dispensed from the pharmacy by generic name, verify that there is no discrepancy.

If a patient questions a medication, stop and recheck to be certain that there is no mistake. In most cases, the medication order has been changed. Never give a medication until you investigate the patient's concerns and recheck it against the health care provider's

TABLE 22.2

Prohibited and Error-Prone Abbreviations[a]

Do Not Use	Problem	Use Instead
U (unit) or u	Mistaken for 0 (zero), the number 4 (four), or cc	Write "unit."
IU (international unit)	Mistaken for IV (intravenous), the number 10 (ten), or unit	Write "international unit."
q.d. or QD (daily)	Mistaken for qid	Write "daily."
Q.O.D., QOD, q.o.d., qod (every other day)	Mistaken for qd (daily) or qid (4 times daily) if "o" is poorly written	Write "every other day."
Trailing zero (e.g., 1.0 mg)[b]	Decimal point is missed	Write X mg (e.g., 1 mg).
Lack of leading zero (e.g., .1 mg)	Decimal point is missed	Write 0.X mg (e.g., 0.1 mg).
MS	Can mean morphine sulfate or magnesium sulfate	Write "morphine sulfate" or write "magnesium sulfate."
MSO_4 and $MgSO_4$	Confused for one another	Write "morphine sulfate" or write "magnesium sulfate."

[a]Applies to all orders and medication-related documentation that is handwritten (including free-text computer entry or on preprinted forms).
[b]Exception: A "trailing zero" may be used only where required to show precision of a reported value (e.g., laboratory test results), studies that report the size of lesions, or catheter and tube sizes. A "trailing zero" cannot be used in medication orders or medication-related documentation.
From The Joint Commission (TJC): *Facts about the Official "Do Not Use" List of Abbreviations,* 2017, https://www.jointcommission.org/facts_about_do_not_use_list/ Reprinted with permission.

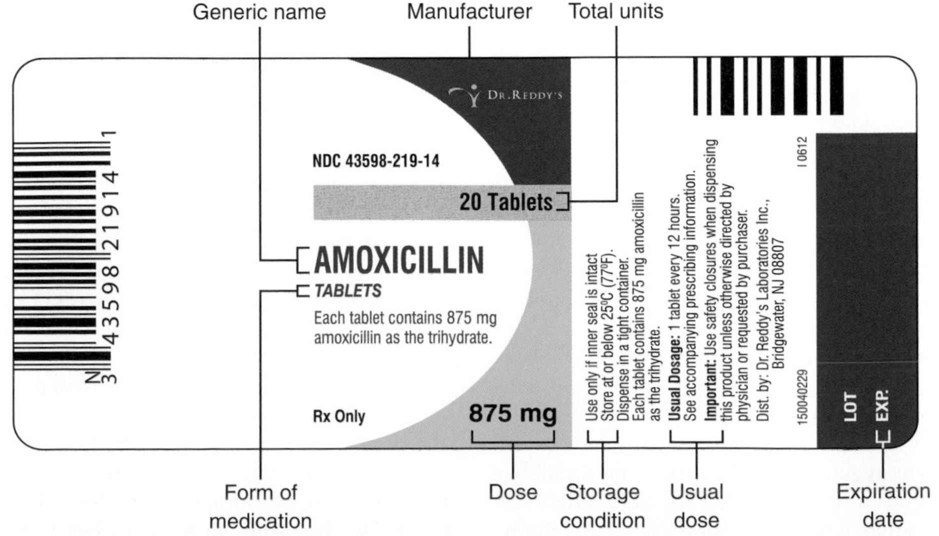

FIG 22.3 Interpreting a medication label. *(Courtesy Dr. Reddy's Laboratories, Inc.)*

order. Attention to a patient's question is one way in which errors are identified and prevented.

Right Dose

The unit-dose system is designed to minimize errors. When a medication is prepared from a larger volume or strength than needed or when the health care provider orders a system of measurement different from that which the pharmacist supplies, the chance of error increases. After calculating a dose of a high-risk medication such as insulin or warfarin, compare the calculation with one done independently by a second nurse (see agency policy). This verification is especially important if it is an unusual calculation or involves a potentially toxic drug.

Prepare medications accurately by using standard measurement devices such as graduated cups, syringes, and scaled droppers. Educate patients to use similar measurement devices at home, such as measuring spoons with metric calibrations rather than household teaspoons and tablespoons, which are inaccurate. Medication errors occur when pills need to be split. Studies show that the accuracy of split tablets is questionable, even if a tablet is scored (ISMP, 2015). In addition, in the home setting, patients may assume that tablets in containers have already been split when they have not or split them again when they have been split already (ISMP, 2015).

To promote patient safety in some inpatient settings, pharmacists split medications, label and package them, and return them to the nurse for administration. Because pill splitting can be problematic in the home, determine if a patient has the manual dexterity or visual acuity to split tablets. If possible, determine if his or her pharmacy can split the pill, or encourage the health care provider to order medications that do not require splitting.

Tablets are sometimes crushed and mixed with food. Be sure to clean a crushing device completely before crushing a tablet. Remnants of previously crushed medications increase the concentration of the medication or result in a patient receiving part of an unprescribed medication. Mix crushed medications with very small amounts of food or liquid. Do not use a patient's favorite foods or liquids because medications alter their taste and decrease the patient's desire for them. This is especially a concern for pediatric patients. *Always check to determine whether a medication can be crushed.* Some medications (e.g., enteric-coated or slow-release) have special coatings to prevent them from being absorbed too quickly. These medications should not be crushed. Refer to the "Do Not Crush List" (ISMP, 2016c) to ensure that a medication is safe to crush.

Right Patient

Before administering a medication, identify the patient using at least two patient identifiers, such as the patient's name, birthday, or hospital account number. The patient's room number or his or her physical complaint cannot be used as identifiers (TJC, 2019). Check the MAR against the patient's identification bracelet, and ask the patient to state his or her full name. In some agencies, a nurse also compares the medical record number on the MAR with the identification bracelet. If an identification bracelet becomes smudged or illegible or is missing, a new one should be obtained for the patient. In health care settings that are not acute care, The Joint Commission does not require the use of armbands for identification. However, there must be a system in place to verify a patient's identification with at least two identifiers.

Some agencies use a wireless bar-code scanner to identify the right patient. This system requires you to scan a personal bar code that is commonly placed on your name tag first. Then you scan a bar code on the single-dose medication package. Finally, you scan the patient's armband. This information is stored in a computer for documentation purposes. This system helps eliminate medication errors because it provides another step to ensure that the right patient receives the right medication (Hutton et al., 2017).

Right Route

The health care provider's order must designate a route of administration (Table 22.3). If the route of administration is missing or if the specified route is not the recommended route, you must consult the health care provider immediately. When oral medications are prepared in syringes, there is a risk of giving the medication through the parenteral route. When injections are administered, use only preparations intended for parenteral use. Injection of a liquid intended for oral use can produce local skin complications such as a sterile abscess or fatal systemic effects. Medication companies label parenteral medications "for injectable use only." The ISMP (2016b) recommends that pharmacists, *not nurses*, prepare all oral medications as a unit product to ensure patient safety. Medications prepared commercially are an exception.

The accidental IV injection of a liquid designed for oral use produces local complications, such as sterile skin abscess, or systemic effects, such as a fatality. If you work in a setting that requires you to prepare oral medications, use only enteral syringes (e.g., ENFit) when you prepare oral medications. Enteral syringes often use a color different from the parenteral syringes and are clearly labeled for oral or enteral use. The syringe tips of enteral syringes will not connect with parenteral medication administration systems. Needles do not attach to enteral syringes, and the syringes cannot be inserted into any type of IV line. Label the syringe after preparing the medication, and be sure to remove any caps from the tip of an oral syringe before administering the medication.

Right Time

Safe medication administration involves adherence to prescribed doses and dosage schedules. Some agencies set schedules for medication administration. For example, medications to be given three times a day (tid) may be routinely scheduled for 0800, 1400, and 2000 or for 0900, 1300, and 1900, depending on agency policy. Nurses can alter this schedule based on knowledge about a medication. For example, a medication ordered for once a day might typically be given at 9 AM, but if the medication works best for a patient at bedtime, the nurse can administer it before the patient goes to sleep. Acute care settings use guidelines from the ISMP and Centers for Medicaid and Medicare Services (CMS, 2011; ISMP, 2011) to determine safe, effective, and timely administration of scheduled medications.

According to ISMP (2011) and CMS (2011) guidelines, hospitals need to determine which medications are not eligible for scheduled dosing times and must be given at precise times (e.g., stat doses or first-time loading doses). In addition, hospitals must determine which medications are time-critical scheduled and which are non–time-critical scheduled. With time-critical medications (e.g., antibiotics, insulin, anticoagulants), early or delayed administration of maintenance doses of more than 20 minutes before or after the scheduled dose will most likely cause harm or result in subtherapeutic responses in a patient. Non–time-critical medications (e.g., stool softeners, vitamins) include medications in which the timing of administration most likely will not affect the desired effect of the medication if the drug is given 1 to 2 hours before or after its scheduled time. You administer time-critical scheduled medications at a precise time or within 30 minutes before or after the scheduled time. You administer non–time-critical medications within 1 to 2 hours of their scheduled time.

TABLE 22.3

Forms of Medication by Route of Administration

Form	Description
Medication Forms Commonly Prepared for Administration by Oral Route	
Solid Forms	
Caplet	Shaped like a capsule and coated for ease of swallowing
Capsule	Medication encased in a gelatin shell
Tablet	Powdered medication compressed into a hard disk or cylinder; in addition to primary medication, contains binders (adhesive to allow powder to stick together), disintegrators (to promote table dissolution), lubricants (for ease of manufacturing), and fillers (for convenient tablet size)
Enteric coated	Coated tablet that does not dissolve in stomach; coating dissolves in intestine, where medication is absorbed
Liquid Forms	
Elixir	Clear fluid containing water and alcohol; often sweetened
Extract	Syrup or dried form of pharmacologically active medication, usually made by evaporating solution
Aqueous solution	Substance dissolved in water and syrups
Aqueous suspension	Finely dissolved drug particles in liquid medium; must be shaken; when left standing, particles settle to bottom of container
Syrup	Medication dissolved in concentrated sugar solution
Tincture	Alcohol extract from plant or vegetable
Other Oral Forms and Terms Associated With Oral Preparations	
Troche (lozenge)	Flat, round tablet that dissolves in mouth to release medication; not meant for ingestion
Aerosol	Aqueous medication sprayed and absorbed in mouth and upper airway; not meant for ingestion
Sustained release	Tablet or capsule that contains small particles of a medication coated with material that requires a varying amount of time to dissolve
Medication Forms Commonly Prepared for Administration by Topical Route	
Ointment (salve or cream)	Semisolid, externally applied preparation, usually containing one or more medications
Liniment	Usually contains alcohol, oil, or soapy emollient applied to skin
Lotion	Liquid suspension that usually protects, cools, or cleans skin
Paste	Medication preparation that is thicker than ointment; absorbed through skin more slowly than ointment; often used for skin protection
Transdermal patch or disk	Disk or patch embedded with medication that is applied to skin Drug absorbed through the skin over a designated period of time (e.g., 24 hours)
Medication Forms Commonly Prepared for Administration by Parenteral Route	
Solution	Sterile preparation that contains water/normal saline with one or more dissolved compounds
Powder	Sterile particles of medication that are dissolved in a sterile liquid (e.g., water, normal saline) before administration
Medication Forms Commonly Prepared for Instillation Into Body Cavities	
Suppository	Solid dosage form mixed with gelatin and shaped in form of a pellet for insertion into body cavity (rectum or vagina) (Suppository melts when it reaches body temperature and is then absorbed.)
Intraocular disk	Small, flexible oval (similar to a contact lens) consisting of two soft outer layers and a middle layer containing medication; slowly releases medication when moistened by ocular fluid

A medication may be ordered for special circumstances. A preoperative medication may be ordered stat, to be given immediately; now, which means as soon as available, usually within an hour; or on call, which means that the operating or procedure room personnel will notify the nurse when it is the appropriate time. A drug may be ordered before meals (ac) or after meals (pc).

Give priority to medications that must act at certain times. For example, give insulin at a precise interval before a meal. Give antibiotics on time around the clock to maintain therapeutic blood levels.

To combat the prescription drug overdose epidemic, many states have enacted laws that set time limits on the prescribing or dispensing of controlled substances (CDC, 2015). For example, there are laws that set forth time limits (hours' or days' supply) on the supply of prescription drugs. These time limit laws can be further classified by their applicability to certain drugs, certain patient populations, or certain situations (CDC, 2015).

Right Documentation

Nurses and other health care providers use documentation to communicate with one another. Many medication errors result from inaccurate documentation. Therefore always document medications accurately at the time of administration and identify any inaccurate documentation before you give medications.

Before you administer a medication, ensure that the MAR clearly shows the following:

- The patient's full name
- The full name of the ordered medication (without abbreviations of medication names)
- The time the medication is to be administered
- The dosage, route, and frequency of administration

Do not give medications that have incomplete or illegible orders. Verify inaccurate orders before giving medications. It is better to give the correct medication later than to give your patient the wrong medication. Record the administration of each medication on the MAR as soon as you give it. Never document that you have given a medication until you have given it. Document the name of the medication, the dose, the time of administration, and the route. Also document the site of any injections you give. Document the patient's response to the medication in the nurses' notes.

Right Indication

ISMP (2016a) is considering a seventh right of medication administration that would enhance the safety of every medication order, the *right indication*. Indication-based prescribing would narrow medication choices, dosage forms, and dosing regimens, which would reduce the risk of a wrong medication being chosen (Schiff et al., 2016). In addition, indication-based prescribing would empower and educate patients, which can improve medication adherence. Communication would be improved between the interprofessional team and the patients and family caregivers. Medication reconciliation would improve because indication-based prescribing would aid in preventing re-prescribing.

MEDICATION PREPARATION

It is legally advisable to administer only the medications that you prepare. Administering a medication prepared by another nurse increases the opportunity for error. The nurse who gives the wrong medication or an incorrect dose is legally responsible for the error. The importance of checking similar patient names and verifying for the correct drug cannot be overemphasized.

Interpreting Medication Labels

Medication labels include several basic pieces of information: the trade name of the drug in large letters, the generic name in smaller letters, the form of the drug, the dosage, the expiration date, the lot number, and the name of the manufacturer. The trade name given by the manufacturer often suggests the action of the drug, and the generic name is the chemical name (see Fig. 22.3).

Dosage Calculations

To administer medications safely, use your mathematics skills to calculate medication dosages and mix solutions. The ability to calculate doses safely is important because you will not always dispense medications in the unit of measure in which they are ordered. Medication companies package and bottle certain standard equivalents. For example, a patient's health care provider orders 250 mg of a medication that is available only in grams. You are responsible for converting available units of volume and weight to the desired doses. Be aware of approximate equivalents in all major measurement systems, and use conversion tables. An example follows:

The order reads: vancomycin 1 g IV.

The pharmacy supplies vancomycin in 500-mg vials.

Because the dose on the medication label is in milligrams, conversion should be from grams to milligrams; 1 g = 1000 mg.

Systems of Measurement

The proper administration of medication depends on your ability to compute drug dosages accurately and measure medications correctly. A careless mistake in placing a decimal point or adding a zero to a dosage can lead to a fatal error. The health care provider and patient depend on you to check the dosage before giving a drug. The metric system is the most common system used in the measurement of medications.

Metric System

As a decimal system, the metric system is the most logically organized of the measurement systems. Each basic unit of measure is organized into units of 10. Multiplying or dividing by 10 forms secondary units. In multiplication, the decimal point moves to the right; in division, the decimal moves to the left. To convert grams to milligrams, you multiply by 1000 or move the decimal point three places to the right (0.5 g = 500 mg). Conversely, to convert milligrams to grams, you divide by 1000 or move the decimal point three places to the left (500 mg = 0.5 g).

The basic units of measure in the metric system are the meter (length), liter (volume), and gram (weight). For drug calculations, you will use primarily volume and weight units. In the metric system, small or large letters designate the basic units:

Gram: g or gm

Liter: l or L

Small letters are abbreviations for subdivisions of major units:

Milligram: mg

Milliliter: mL

Household Measurements

Most people are familiar with household measures, which include liquid measures such as drops, teaspoons, tablespoons, cups, pints, and quarts. Even though household measurements are convenient and familiar, they are inaccurate. Dose errors have occurred when household measures are used (Consumer Med Safety, 2017; ISMP, 2016b). As a result, the ISMP recommends a best practice for all oral liquids that are not commercially available as unit-dose products. The liquids should be dispensed by the pharmacy in an oral syringe using metric measurement (ISMP, 2016b). The ISMP also recommends that patients or family caregivers purchase oral liquid dosing devices (oral syringes/cups/droppers) that only display the metric scale. Encourage patients to never use household measuring devices with liquid medications (Table 22.4). Today's over-the-counter

TABLE 22.4

Equivalents of Measurement

Metric	Household
1 mL	15 drops (gtt)
5 mL	1 teaspoon (tsp)
15 mL	1 tablespoon (tbsp)
30 mL	2 tablespoons (tbsp)
240 mL	1 cup (c)
480 mL (approximately 500 mL)	1 pint (pt)
960 mL (approximately 1 L)	1 quart (qt)
3785 mL (approximately 4 L)	1 gallon (gal)

BOX 22.4

Formula Method

$$\frac{D}{H} \times V = \text{Amount to give}$$

D is the desired dose or the dose ordered by the health care provider for the patient (e.g., 250 mg of penicillin PO 4 times daily).
H is the drug dose on hand or available for use. The dose is on the drug label (e.g., penicillin tablets of 250 mg each).
V is the volume (liquid) or vehicle (number of tablets, capsules) that delivers the available dose (e.g., 1 tablet).
NOTE: The desired dose **(D)** and the on-hand dose **(H)** must be in the same unit of measurement. If they are in different units, you must perform conversions before completing the formula.

BOX 22.5

Dimensional Analysis

Follow these steps to solve medication problems using dimensional analysis:

1. Identify the unit of measure that you need to administer. For example, if you are giving a pill, you will usually be giving a tablet or a capsule; for parenteral or oral medications, the unit is milliliters.
2. Estimate the answer in your mind.
3. Place the name or appropriate abbreviation for *x* on the left side of the equation (e.g., *x* tab, *x* mL).
4. Place available information from the problem in a fraction format on the right side of the equation. Place the abbreviation or unit that matches what you are going to administer (determined in Step 1) in the numerator.
5. Look at the medication order and add other factors into the problem. Set up the numerator so that it matches the unit in the previous denominator.
6. Cancel out like units of measurement on the right side of the equation. You should end up with only one unit left in the equation, and it should match the unit on the left side of the equation.
7. Reduce to the lowest terms if possible and solve the problem or solve for *x*. Label your answer.
8. Compare your estimate from Step 2 with your answer in Step 7.

(OTC) liquid medications almost always have their own measuring devices (Consumer Med Safety, 2017).

Solutions

Nurses administer solutions of various concentrations for injections, irrigations, and infusions. A solution is a given mass of solid substance dissolved in a known volume of fluid or a given volume of fluid dissolved in a known volume of another fluid. Solutions are available in units of mass per units of volume (e.g., g/mL, g/L). You can also express a concentration of a solution as a percentage. A 10% solution is 10 g of solid dissolved in 100 mL of solution.

Dosage Calculations

Dosage calculations are necessary when the dose on the medication label differs from the dose ordered. There are several dose-calculation methods, including formula (Box 22.4), dimensional analysis (Box 22.5), and ratio and proportion (Box 22.6). The most common methods are ratio-proportion and the formula methods.

BOX 22.6

The Ratio-and-Proportion Method

1. The numbers in a ratio are separated by a colon (:).
2. A proportion is an equation that has two ratios of equal value.
3. The first and last numbers are called the *extremes*. The second and third numbers are called the *means*.
4. Write a proportion in one of three ways:
   a. 1 : 2 = 5 : 10
   b. 1 : 2 :: 5 : 10
   c. $\frac{1}{2} = \frac{5}{10}$
5. Make sure that all the terms are in the same unit or system of measurement.
6. Label all the terms in the proportion.
7. Place the ratio you know (e.g., information on the drug label) first.
8. Put the terms of the ratio in the same sequence (e.g., mg: mL = mg: mL).
9. Cross-multiply the means and the extremes, and then divide both sides by the number for the *x* to obtain the dosage.
10. Always label the answer.

Formula Method

Dose ordered: Demerol 50 mg IM
Medication available: 100 mg in 1 mL
Step 1.

$$\frac{\text{Dose ordered}}{\text{Dose on hand}} \times \text{Amount on hand} = \text{Amount to administer}$$

Step 2. Calculate your answer:

$$\frac{50 \text{ mg}}{100 \text{ mg}} \times 1 \text{ mL} = 0.5 \text{ mL}$$

Dimensional Analysis Method

Dose ordered: 0.5 g tablet
Tablets available: 0.25 g per tablet
Step 1. The starting factor is 0.5 g.

The answer label is tablets (i.e., how many tablets should be given?)

Step 2. Formulate the conversion equation:
The equivalent needed is 1 tablet = 0.25 g.

$$\frac{0.5 \text{ g}}{1} \times \frac{1 \text{ tab}}{0.25 \text{ g}} = \text{tabs}$$

Cancel labels (g). **NOTE:** If properly written, all labels except the answer label will cancel.

Step 3. Solve the equation. Reduce the numerical values and multiply the numerators and denominators.

$$\frac{{}^{2}\cancel{0.5 \text{ g}}}{1} \times \frac{1 \text{ tab}}{\cancel{0.25 \text{ g}}} = 2 \text{ tabs}$$

Ratio-and-Proportion Method

A ratio indicates the relationship between two numbers.

Dose ordered: Phenytoin solution 100 mg by mouth
Available: 125 mg/5 mL
Step 1. Set up the proportion:

$$\frac{125\ \text{mg}}{5} \times \frac{100\ \text{mg}}{x\ \text{mL}}$$

Step 2. Cross-multiply the equation:

$$125x = 100 \times 5$$

$$125x = 500$$

Step 3. Divide both sides by the number before x:

$$\frac{125x}{125} = \frac{500}{125}$$

$$x = \frac{500}{125}$$

$$x = 4\ \text{mL}$$

NURSING PROCESS

Applying the nursing process to medication administration ensures that you use critical thinking and clinical judgment. As a nurse, your role extends beyond simply giving drugs to a patient. You are responsible for monitoring patients' responses to medications; providing education to the patient and family caregivers about the medication regimen; and informing the health care provider when medications are effective, ineffective, or no longer necessary.

Assessment

History

Begin your assessment by reviewing a patient's medical history. This will yield information about any indications or contraindications for medication therapy. Certain diseases or illnesses place patients at risk for adverse medication effects. For example, if a patient has a gastric ulcer, forms of aspirin increase the chance of bleeding. Long-term health problems require specific medications. This knowledge helps you anticipate the medications that your patient requires.

Allergies

Include an assessment of patient allergies. Determine if a patient has actual allergic reactions or drug intolerances, which are uncomfortable side effects. *Never give a patient a medication when there is a known allergy*. Many medications have ingredients found in food sources. For example, propofol, which is used for anesthesia and sedation, contains inactive ingredients of egg lecithin and soybean oil. Therefore patients who have an egg or soy allergy should not receive propofol (Skidmore-Roth, 2019). If a patient has a latex allergy, latex-free gloves are worn when administering parenteral or topical medications. In an acute care setting, patients with allergies wear identification bands that list each medication allergy. All allergies and the types of reactions are noted on the patient's admission notes, medication records, and history and physical examination.

Medication History

Your assessment also involves identifying all medications that the patient takes every day at home, including prescriptions, over-the-counter (OTC) preparations, and herbal supplements. Determine how long the patient has taken each medication, the current dosage schedule, and whether the patient has had any adverse effects from any of the medications. The patient should know the name, purpose, dosage, route, and side effects of medications and supplements that are being taken. Often patients take many medications and carry a list that includes this information. Patients have different levels of understanding. One patient may describe a diuretic as a "water pill," whereas another may describe it as a drug to minimize swelling and lower blood pressure. Still another may describe it as "the little white pill I take in the morning." If possible, assess if the patient takes medications correctly (e.g., count doses or have patient keep diary). By assessing the patient's level of knowledge and practices, you determine the need for teaching. If a patient is unable to understand or remember pertinent information, it may be necessary to involve a family caregiver.

Diet History

Collect a diet history of a patient's normal eating patterns and food preferences so that you can plan an effective dosage schedule. This is important when patients take medicines around meal times. Some medications interact with food (e.g., green leafy vegetables and warfarin, grapefruit juice and statins). In these cases, assess whether patients avoid the foods that interact with their medications.

Physical Examination and Other Data

Complete appropriate physical assessments of the body systems likely to reveal physical findings that will indicate or contraindicate the medications you are administering. For example, observe the integrity of the skin before applying a topical medication. A physical examination should focus on a patient's sensory, motor, and cognitive functions (e.g., ability to open medication bottles) if the patient is self-administering medications. You will also assess vital signs, laboratory data, and the nature and severity of symptoms. It is important to have a baseline assessment to be able to determine adverse effects from medication versus an existing condition (e.g., a skin rash can be a first indicator of a serious reaction or could be an existing skin condition unrelated to medication). If data contraindicate medication administration, hold the drug and notify the health care provider.

Patient Attitude About Medication Use

Patients' attitudes about medications affect their willingness to take medication therapy. Sometimes their attitudes reveal medication dependence or avoidance. Include a family caregiver in your assessment if appropriate. In the home setting, observe a patient's behavior for evidence of dependence or avoidance.

Patient's Health Literacy Level

Health literacy involves the ability to obtain, communicate, process, and understand basic health information and services to make appropriate health decisions (CDC, 2016c). Your assessment should determine whether a patient is likely to be at risk for low health literacy and his or her understanding of medication use. A common measure for defining drug adherence is taking at least 90% of one's prescribed doses correctly (Sawkin et al., 2015). A patient with low health literacy will have difficulty reading prescriptions, preparing doses that require simple calculation, and reading drug information. Use literacy assessment tools made available by the institution where you work. Ask patients to read prescription labels and explain the implications. Have patients perform simple calculations if that is part of their ordered routine. Do the same with family caregivers if they are administering medications to patients.

Planning

During planning, organize nursing activities to ensure the safe administration of medications. Current evidence shows that distractions (e.g., discussion with staff, phone call, use of pager) or hurrying during medication preparation administration increases the risk of medication errors (Westbrook et al., 2017). Minimize distractions by closing the door of the medication room as you prepare medications. Do not stop and perform other tasks while preparing medications.

Other suggestions to reduce distraction include signage identifying the medication administration area, development of a checklist that includes all the components of medication administration, and wearing some identifying clothing (e.g., vest) when preparing medications (Westbrook et al., 2017). The following are general goals of medication administration:

1. Patient achieves therapeutic effect of the prescribed medication.
2. Patient complications related to the prescribed medication are absent.
3. Patient and family caregivers understand medication therapy.
4. Patient and family caregivers administer medication safely (when appropriate).

Implementation

Nursing interventions for safe and effective drug administration include careful medication preparation, accurate and timely administration, and relevant patient education.

Preadministration Activities

1. Identify the medication action, purpose, side effects, and nursing implications for administering and monitoring. Ensure that the medication order has not expired.
2. Make sure the information on the electronic MAR or printed MAR corresponds exactly with the health care provider's order and with the medication container label. Clarify orders that are unclear or illegible.
3. Calculate medication doses accurately and use appropriate measuring devices. Verify that the dose prescribed is within a safe dosage range and is appropriate for the patient situation.
4. Take medications to the patient at the correct time (see the section Seven Rights of Medication Administration), especially time-critical and non–time-critical medications (see agency policy).
5. Review any preadministration assessments (e.g., vital signs, laboratory test results).
6. Use thorough hand-hygiene technique. Avoid touching tablets and capsules. Wear clean gloves if you are administering topical medications, parenteral medications, or oral chemotherapy agents.
7. Use sterile technique for parenteral medications.
8. Keep medications secure. Administer only medications that you personally prepare. Never ask another nurse to administer medications that you prepare.
9. When preparing medications, be sure that the label is clear and legible and that the drug is properly mixed; has not changed in color, clarity, or consistency; and has not expired.
10. Keep tablets and capsules in their wrappers and open them at the patient's bedside. This allows you to review each medication with the patient. If a patient refuses medication, there is no question about which one is withheld.
11. TJC (2019) has a standard for labeling syringes, including before a procedure labeling all medications that are not labeled (e.g., medications in syringes, cups, and basins). This should be done in the area where medications and supplies are set up.

Drug Administration

1. Follow the *seven rights* for medication administration.
2. Inform the patient of the name, purpose, action, and common side effects of each medication. Evaluate the patient's knowledge of the medication, and provide appropriate teaching using teach-back technique.
3. Stay with the patient until the medication is taken. Provide assistance as necessary. Do not leave medication without a health care provider's order at the bedside. For example, some patients may take their own vitamins or birth control pills while in the hospital.
4. Respect the patient's right to refuse medication. If the medication wrapper is intact, the medication may be returned to the patient's storage bin. When medication is refused, determine the reason for this and take action accordingly. For example, if the patient has unpleasant side effects, it may be possible to eliminate them by giving the pills with food or using a different time schedule.

Postadministration Activities

1. Properly document medications administered (see the section Seven Rights of Medication Administration).
2. Document data pertinent to a patient's response; this is especially important when giving drugs ordered prn. Include the ability of patient and family caregiver to teach back the education provided.
3. If a medication is refused, document that it was not given, the reason for the refusal, and when the health care provider was notified.

Evaluation

1. Monitor for evidence of therapeutic effects, side effects, and adverse reactions. Monitor physical responses (e.g., heart rhythm, blood pressure, urine output, skin integrity).
2. When a medication is given for relief of symptoms, ask the patient within 30 to 60 minutes of drug administration to report if symptoms have diminished or been relieved. In the case of pain, has severity lessened?
3. Observe injection sites for bruises, inflammation, localized pain, numbness, or bleeding.
4. Evaluate patient's understanding of medication therapy and ability to self-administer medication.

REPORTING MEDICATION ERRORS

Medication errors often harm patients because of inappropriate medication use. Errors include inaccurate prescribing; administering the wrong medication, by the wrong route, and in the wrong time interval; and administering extra doses or failing to administer a medication. Medication errors are related to professional practice, health care product design, or procedures and systems such as product labeling and distribution. When an error occurs, the patient's safety and well-being become the top priority. A nurse assesses and examines the patient's condition and notifies the health care provider of the incident as soon as possible. Once the patient is stable, the nurse reports the incident to the appropriate person in the agency (e.g., manager or supervisor).

As a nurse, you are responsible for preparing a written incident or occurrence report that must usually be filed within 24 hours of an incident (see agency policy). The incident report is an internal audit tool and not a permanent part of the medical record. To legally protect the health care professional and agency, do not refer to an incident report in the nurses' notes in the EHR or chart.

Agencies use incident reports to track incident patterns and initiate performance improvement programs as needed. Depending on the circumstances and the severity of the outcome, the nurse or agency may be responsible for reporting the incident to TJC, MedWatch (FDA Medical Products Reporting Program), or the USP Medication Errors Reporting Program.

It is good risk management to report all medication errors, including mistakes that do not cause obvious or immediate harm or near misses. You should feel comfortable in reporting an error and not fear repercussions from managerial staff. Even when a patient suffers no harm from a medication error, the agency can still learn why the mistake occurred and what to do in the future to avoid similar errors. There are strategies that you can implement to prevent medication errors.

PATIENT AND FAMILY CAREGIVER TEACHING

A well-informed patient is more likely to take medications correctly and maintain adherence. However, many patients have limited health literacy, meaning that they do not understand how to read medication labels and calculate doses. You will also care for patients who do not speak English. Thus any education requires a thorough assessment of a patient's learning needs and abilities. It is legally mandated by the National Standards for Culturally and Linguistically Appropriate Services (CLAS) in health care to provide easy-to-understand print and multimedia materials in the languages commonly used by the populations in a service area (U.S. Department of Health and Human Services, Office of Minority Health, n.d.).

Provide an individualized approach to teaching, using visual aids, instructional booklets written in simple language or the patient's language, or even videotapes or DVDs. When teaching patients about their medications, include people identified as being significant to the patient's recovery (e.g., family caregivers or home care providers).

Begin instruction as soon as possible so that you can have several teaching sessions. It is ideal to use instructional materials written no higher than a sixth-grade reading level. Provide instructions written in the patient's language if available. When providing instruction, have the patient or family caregiver repeat the name and use for each medication plus the dosing instructions. Current recommendations suggest the use of teach-back as a method to confirm patient learning and improve health care provider education (Centrella-Nigro et al., 2017). Have the patient explain for you the topic you taught him or her so that you can confirm understanding. Have the patient demonstrate the preparation of each medication. Provide time to discuss problem scenarios (e.g., when side effects develop or a syringe becomes contaminated) to test the patient's knowledge of what to do should something go wrong. Determine if the patient requires a compliance aid or memory cue. This is especially important for older adults. If the patient speaks another language, have a professional interpreter available during instruction. Do not use a family member as an interpreter. Medication dose containers organized by the hours and days of the week are very useful. If patients miss a dose of medication, they need to know how to adjust their medication schedule safely.

Evaluating the effectiveness of teaching ensures that a patient can administer medications in a safe manner. One method of evaluating patient understanding is to create medication cards with the generic and trade names of the medication on the front of the card and all pertinent medication information on the back of the card. Another method is to have patients read labels on prepared medications. Remember that medication bottles often have fine print and are difficult to read for the patient with impaired vision. For these patients, have the pharmacy prepare medications with large-print labels. If the patient correctly identifies the name of the medication, ask him or her the following questions:

- Why are you taking this medication?
- How often do you take this medication and at what time of day?
- What side effects can occur with this medication?
- If this side effect occurs, what are you going to do about it?

Be sure to review your assessment of the patient's sensory, motor, and cognitive functions (e.g., ability to open medication bottles). Impairments may affect the patient's ability to safely self-administer medications, and family caregivers or home health aides may need to help with medication administration. Many self-help devices are also available for purchase (e.g., pill boxes with times displayed and electronic dispensers). Specific nursing interventions for educating about self-administration within the home setting are summarized in Box 22.7.

Teaching Patients About Side Effects

You are responsible for teaching a patient and family caregiver about possible side effects associated with each prescribed medication. Remember to ask the patient about the use of herbal remedies and OTC medications. If you do not inform the patient properly about medications or if your patients have problems with health literacy, it is possible that they will take their medications incorrectly or they will not take their medications at all. Because medications can have many side effects, teaching a patient about all of them can be overwhelming. Remember that patient learning is a continual process. When beginning to teach a patient about a new medication, evaluate each of the side effects. Then teach the patient about the ones that are most likely to occur and occur early after administration. For example, some antibiotics cause hypersensitivity reactions, hepatotoxicity, nephrotoxicity, and platelet dysfunction. Hypersensitivity reactions are likely to occur shortly after taking a few doses of an antibiotic. The other side effects tend to occur after long-term antibiotic administration. Teach patients about side effects in terms of things that they can see, feel, touch, or hear. For example, thrombocytopenia, a reduction in the number of platelets in the blood, can be a medication side effect. The patient cannot see, feel, touch, or hear thrombocytopenia. However, thrombocytopenia can cause bleeding with petechiae visible on the skin. Teach the patient how to look for petechiae. Be sure to teach the patient what to do about side effects when they are discovered.

Patient's Activities of Daily Living

Design interventions that enable patients to self-administer medications and maintain a patient's activities of daily living. When medications are initiated in the acute care setting, they are often given around the clock. In the home, it may be unreasonable for patients to administer medications according to this schedule. Thus it can be difficult for them to adhere to medication schedules. In collaboration with the health care provider or the pharmacist, teach the patient and family caregiver how to adjust medication schedules to be compatible with the patient's lifestyle. Include what to do for missed doses.

HANDLING OF SPECIAL MEDICATIONS

Controlled Substances

As a nurse, you are responsible for following legal regulations when administering controlled substances (medications with potential

BOX 22.7

Medication Administration in Home Care

1. Assess all of the patient's prescription and nonprescription medications at each visit, including herbal medications. Review information about medications, including desired effect, dose, frequency, adverse effects, and what to do if adverse effects develop.
2. Teach the complications and interactions of all food, over-the-counter (OTC) medications, and herbal medications to patients and family caregivers.
3. Collaborate with social workers to identify community resources for financial assistance with pharmaceutical needs.
4. Monitor and evaluate the effectiveness of the prescribed medications:
   a. Note changes in physical and functional status (e.g., vital signs, sleeping, elimination).
   b. Note changes in mental status (e.g., level of alertness, memory).
   c. Monitor blood levels as needed.
   d. Communicate potential problems to health care provider.
5. Monitor urinary output status of patients because changes in renal excretion may require a decrease or increase in medication dosage.
6. For patients who cannot remember when to take medications, make a chart that lists the times to take each medication, or prepare a special container that organizes and stores medications according to days and times when the patient needs to take them. Collaborate with family caregivers to assist in organization and administration of medications.
7. Reduce the chance of medication error by labeling or color-coding medication bottles.
8. Keep an accurate record of a homebound patient's weight, especially an older-adult patient, because many medication dosages are calculated by body weight.
9. Teach medication safety in the home environment:
   a. Keep medications in original, labeled containers. Read labels carefully and follow all instructions.
   b. Follow specific disposal instructions on the prescription drug label or patient information that comes with the medication. *Do not flush* medications down the sink or toilet unless this information specifically instructs you to do so. Have patients use community drug take-back programs that allow the public to bring unused drugs to a central location for proper disposal. If there are no disposal instructions on a prescription drug label and no take-back program is available, have patient throw the drugs in the household trash following these steps: (1) Remove drugs from their original containers and mix them with an undesirable substance, such as used coffee grounds or kitty litter. (2) Place the mixture in a sealable bag, empty can, or other container to prevent the drug from leaking or breaking out of a garbage bag (FDA, 2017a).
10. Never "share" medications with friends or family members.
11. Always finish a prescribed medication; do not save it for a future illness.
12. Instruct patients with arthritis or debilitating illness who have difficulty opening child-proof containers to request non-childproof containers from their health care providers.

Data from Touhy T, Jett K: *Ebersole and Hess's gerontological nursing and healthy aging,* ed 5, St. Louis, 2017, Mosby.

BOX 22.8

Storage and Accountability for Controlled Substances

- All controlled substances are stored in a securely locked, substantially constructed cabinet (i.e., automated medication dispensing system [AMDS] or safe) or a locked room.
- Authorized nurses carry a computer entry code for an AMDS or a set of keys.
- An inventory record is kept to record all controlled substances used, including patient's name, date, name of medication, and time of medication administration.
- Before any medication is removed from the cabinet, the number available is compared with the number indicated on the controlled substance record. If a discrepancy exists, it must be rectified before proceeding.
- If any part of a dose of a controlled substance is discarded, a second nurse witnesses disposal of the unused portion, and the record is signed by both nurses.
- At change of shift, one nurse going off duty counts all controlled substances with a nurse coming on duty. Both nurses sign the record to indicate that the count is correct. (Computerized storage has eliminated this process.)
- Discrepancies in controlled substance counts are reported immediately.

for abuse). Controlled substances must be properly stored to prevent diversion. Violations of the Controlled Substances Act may result in fines, imprisonment, and loss of license. Health care agencies have policies for the proper storage and distribution of controlled substances, including opioids (Box 22.8). Most agencies use computerized systems for medication access and distribution.

Chemotherapy Medications

A common treatment for cancer is chemotherapy, antineoplastic drugs that act by killing cells that divide rapidly, one of the main properties of most cancer cells. Chemotherapy is administered in both intravenous (IV) and oral forms. In 2016 the American Oncology Association in conjunction with the Oncology Nursing Society updated the chemotherapy administration standards to improve both patient and nurse safety related to administration of these medications (Neuss et al., 2017). Nurses must undergo certification to administer IV chemotherapy. However, oral chemotherapy is becoming more common and can be administered by an RN.

Oral chemotherapy has the same exposure risks to health care providers, patients, and their family caregivers as IV forms (Neuss et al., 2017). Physically touching a chemotherapy tablet is dangerous. Chemotherapy is highly toxic not only to cancer cells but also to normal cells. Chemotherapy drugs cause DNA damage leading to cell death or cell-growth arrest. The damage to others may not be known for months or years because the injuries could include cancer, birth defects, or immune dysfunction. It is critical for health care providers, patients, and family caregivers to use proper protective techniques to avoid exposure to oral chemotherapy tablets.

A patient excretes chemotherapy chemicals through urine, stool, vomit, sweat, and saliva. When patients self-administer chemotherapy at home, families should be warned of the dangers of exposure. For example, patients' toilets should be double-flushed after use, during and 48 hours after discontinuing chemotherapy. Toilets are a hazard for children and pets.

Accidental exposure to oral chemotherapeutic agents can occur during handling (i.e., unpacking, storage, handling, administration, and disposal) (Neuss et al., 2017). Guidelines for health care providers, patients, and family caregivers to handle these drugs safely and appropriately are essential:

- In health care agencies, cytotoxic agents should be stored in a designated area per the manufacturer's instructions and separate from noncytotoxic agents.
- Use disposable gloves when preparing and handling chemotherapy medications and after handling any body secretions.
- Perform thorough hand hygiene before and after glove application.
- Do not crush, cut, or split chemotherapy drugs.
- Use separate equipment to prepare chemotherapy and regular medications.
- All disposable protective clothing as well as any disposable materials used while handling oral chemotherapeutic agents should be disposed of as cytotoxic waste according to the local waste disposal regulatory guidelines.
- Patients and their family members should avoid deep kissing and sharing food or drinks because chemotherapy can be in saliva. Clean flatware and dishes thoroughly with soap and warm water and rinse well before washing a second time with other dishes.
- Any clothes or sheets that have body fluids on them should be washed in a washing machine—not by hand. Wash them twice in hot water with regular laundry detergent. Do not wash them with other clothes. If they cannot be washed right away, seal them in a plastic bag. (Guidelines are adapted from American Cancer Society [ACS], 2013.)

SPECIAL CONSIDERATIONS

Patient-Centered Care

- Culturally, a patient's values and beliefs affect medication response and adherence.
- Ethnicity, financial resources, education, and previous experiences are additional factors to consider when assisting patients with medication management. A family's influence on a patient's behaviors, such as their attitudes about health care or demands on a patient's daily schedule, can influence medication adherence.
- Regarding ethnicity, there are cultures in which it is unacceptable to verbalize complaints about stomach problems; it is common for these patients not to report nausea, vomiting, and bowel changes related to medication side effects.
- For patients whose cultures support the use of herbal and homeopathic remedies, it is important for them to know how these agents alter their responses to medications.

Age-Specific

Pediatric

- Children vary in age; weight; and ability to absorb, metabolize, and excrete medications. Children's doses are lower than doses for adults, and caution is needed in preparing medications. Medication may or may not be prepared and packaged in doses appropriate for children. Preparing appropriate doses often requires calculation based on body weight (Hockenberry and Wilson, 2016). A child's parents may be helpful in determining the best way to give a child medication.

Gerontological

- Individuals older than age 65 are the largest users of prescription and OTC medication (Touhy and Jett, 2017). Because of the physiological changes associated with aging, nursing interventions are needed to promote safe and effective medication administration, including spacing medication times to not interfere with meals, substituting liquid preparation for solid form if the older adult has difficulty swallowing, or providing memory aids in large print. Always observe an older adult opening and preparing his or her medication safely. Be aware of the following patterns related to medication use:
    - *Polypharmacy*. Polypharmacy is the concurrent use of five or more medications (including both prescription and nonprescription products) by a single individual (ISMP Canada, 2018). Polypharmacy also occurs when a patient mixes nutritional supplements or herbal products with medications. To decrease the risks associated with polypharmacy, work with your patient's health care providers to ensure that the patient's medication regimen is as simple as possible.
    - *Self-prescribing*. Older adults often attempt to seek relief from a variety of problems with OTC preparations, folk medications, and herbs.
    - *Misuse of drugs*. Misuse by older adults includes overuse, underuse, erratic use, and contraindicated use.
    - *Nonadherence*. Deliberate misuse of medication is considered nonadherence. Older adults alter doses because of ineffectiveness, unpleasant side effects, and lack of financial resources.

✦ PRACTICE REFLECTIONS

Consider that you are a new nurse and have started a staff nurse position on a busy medical-surgical unit. You must administer many medications to four different patients throughout the shift and feel overwhelmed.

1. How would you organize safe medication administration for these patients?
2. How might you ensure you are correctly identifying each patient every time you administer medications?
3. What would you do if you administered the wrong medication to a patient?

✦ CLINICAL REVIEW QUESTIONS

1. The health care provider has written the following orders. Which orders do you need to clarify before administering the medication? Provide rationales for your answers, and rewrite each unclear order so that it follows the ISMP current medication order safety guidelines.
    1. Timoptic .25% solution 1 drop OD BID
    2. Metoprolol 12.50 mg QD
    3. Insulin Glargine 6 u SC twice a day
    4. Enalapril 2.5 mg. PO three times a day, hold for systolic blood pressure <100

2. An older adult states that she cannot see her medication bottles clearly to determine when to take her prescription. What should the nurse do? (Select all that apply.)
   1. Provide a dispensing bottle for each day of the week.
   2. Provide larger, easier-to-read labels.
   3. Tell the patient what is in each container.
   4. Have a family caregiver administer the medication.
   5. Use teach-back to ensure the patient knows what medication to take and when.

3. The nurse must take a verbal order during an emergency on the unit. Which of the following guidelines can be used for taking verbal or telephone orders? (Select all that apply.)
   1. Only authorized staff members receive and record verbal or telephone orders. Agency identifies in writing the staff members who are authorized.
   2. Clearly identify patient's name, room number, and diagnosis.
   3. Read back all orders to health care provider.
   4. Use clarification questions to avoid misunderstandings.
   5. Write "VO" (verbal order) or "TO" (telephone order), including date and time, name of patient, and complete order; sign the name of the health care provider and nurse.

Answers and Rationales for Clinical Review Questions can be found on the Evolve website.

REFERENCES

American Cancer Society (ACS): Chemotherapy principles: an in-depth discussion of the techniques and its role in cancer treatment, 2013. https://www.academia.edu/8460728/Chemotherapy_Principles_An_In-depth_Discussion_of_the_Techniques_and_Its_Role_in_Cancer_Treatment.

Bartlett R, et al: Harm reduction: compassionate care of persons with addictions, *Medsurg Nurs* 22(6):349, 2013.

Bravo K, Cochran G: Nursing strategies to increase medication safety in inpatient settings, *J Nurs Care Qual* 31(4):335, 2016.

Burchum J, Rosenthal L: *Lehne's pharmacology for nursing care*, ed 9, St. Louis, 2016, Elsevier.

Centers for Disease Control and Prevention (CDC): Public Health Law: Prescription Drug Time and Dosage Limit Laws, 2015. https://www.cdc.gov/phlp/docs/menu_prescriptionlimits.pdf.

Centers for Disease Control and Prevention (CDC): Medication safety basics, 2016a. https://www.cdc.gov/medicationsafety/basics.html.

Centers for Disease Control and Prevention (CDC): CDC guideline for prescribing opioids for chronic pain, *Recomm Rep* 65(1):1, 2016b.

Centers for Disease Control and Prevention (CDC): Health literacy? 2016c. https://www.cdc.gov/healthliteracy/index.html.

Centers for Medicare and Medicaid Services (CMS): Update guidance on medication administration, Hospital Appendix A of the State Operations Manual, 2011. https://www.cms.gov/Medicare/Provider-Enrollment-and-Certification/SurveyCertificationGenInfo/downloads/SCLetter12_05.pdf.

Centrella-Nigro A, et al: Using the teach-back method in patient education to improve patient satisfaction, *J Contin Educ Nurs* 48(1):47, 2017.

Chapuis C, et al: Automated drug dispensing systems in the intensive care unit: a financial analysis, *Crit Care* 19:318, 2015.

Connor J, et al: Implementing a distraction free practice with the red zone medication safety initiative, *Dimens Crit Care Nurs* 35(3):116, 2016.

Consumer Med Safety: Tips for measuring liquid medicines safely, 2017. http://www.consumermedsafety.org/tools-and-resources/medication-safety-tools-and-resources/taking-your-medicine-safely/measure-liquid-medications.

Fanning L, et al: Impact of automated dispensing cabinets on medication selection and preparation error rates in an emergency department: a prospective and direct observational before-and-after study, *J Eval Clin Pract* 22(2):156, 2016.

Hockenberry MJ, Wilson D: *Wong's essentials of pediatric nursing*, ed 10, St. Louis, 2016, Mosby.

Hutton K, et al: The effects of bar-coding technology on medication errors: a systematic literature review, *J Patient Saf* 24, 2017.

Institute for Safe Medication Practices (ISMP): Acute care guidelines for timely administration of scheduled medications, 2011. http://www.ismp.org/tools/guidelines/acutecare/tasm.pdf.

Institute for Safe Medication Practices (ISMP): Tablet splitting: do it only if you "half" to, and then do it safely, 2015. https://www.ismp.org/newsletters/acutecare/articles/20060518.asp.

Institute for Safe Medication Practices (ISMP): Is an indication-based prescribing system in our future?, 2016a. https://www.ismp.org/Newsletters/acutecare/showarticle.aspx?id=1153.

Institute for Safe Medication Practices (ISMP): 2016-2017 targeted medication safety best practices for hospitals, 2016b. www.ismp.org/tools/bestpractices/TMSBP-for-Hospitals.pdf.

Institute for Safe Medication Practices (ISMP): Oral dosage forms that should not be crushed, 2016c. http://www.ismp.org/tools/donotcrush.pdf.

Institute for Safe Medication Practices Canada: Deprescribing: managing medications to reduce polypharmacy, vol 18, Issue 3, 2018. https://www.ismp-canada.org/download/safetyBulletins/2018/ISMPCSB2018-03-Deprescribing.pdf.

National Coordinating Council for Medication Error Reporting and Prevention (NCCMERP): What is a medication error, 2017. http://www.nccmerp.org/about-medication-errors.

National Institutes of Health, National Institute on Drug Abuse (NIH NIDA): Drug facts: prescription and over-the-counter medications, 2015. https://www.drugabuse.gov/publications/drugfacts/prescription-over-counter-medications.

Neuss M, et al: 2016 Updated American Society of Clinical Oncology/ Oncology Nursing Society Chemotherapy Administration safety standards, including standards for pediatric oncology, *Oncol Nurs Forum* 44(1):3, 2017.

Sawkin MT, et al: Health literacy and medication adherence among patients treated in a free health clinic: a pilot study, *Health Serv Res Manag Epidemiol* 2, 2015. https://www.ncbi.nlm.nih.gov/pmc/articles/PMC5266426/.

Schiff G, et al: Incorporating indications into medication ordering-time to enter the age of reason, *N Engl J Med* 375(4):306, 2016.

Skidmore-Roth L: *Mosby's 2019 nursing drug reference*, ed 32, St. Louis, 2019, Mosby.

The Joint Commission (TJC): *2019 National Patient Safety Goals*, Oakbrook Terrace, IL, 2019, The Commission. http://www.jointcommission.org/standards_information/npsgs.aspx.

Touhy T, Jett K: *Ebersole and Hess's gerontological nursing and healthy aging*, ed 5, St. Louis, 2017, Mosby.

U.S. Department of Health and Human Services Office of Minority Health (USDHHSOMH): National standards for culturally and linguistically appropriate services (CLAS) in health and health care, n.d. https://www.thinkculturalhealth.hhs.gov/pdfs/EnhancedNationalCLASStandards.pdf.

U.S. Food and Drug Administration (FDA): How to dispose of unused medicines, 2017a. https://www.fda.gov/Drugs/ResourcesForYou/Consumers/BuyingUsingMedicineSafely/EnsuringSafeUseofMedicine/SafeDisposalofMedicines/ucm186187.htm.

U.S. Food and Drug Administration (FDA): Med Watch, the FDA safety information and adverse event reporting program, 2017b. https://www.fda.gov/Safety/MedWatch/default.htm.

Voshall B, et al: Barcode medication administration work-arounds, *J Nurs Adm* 43(10):530, 2013.

Westbrook J, et al: Effectiveness of a 'do not interrupt' bundled intervention to reduce interruptions during medication administration: a cluster randomized controlled feasibility study, *BJM Qual Saf* 0:1, 2017.

Yoder M, et al: The effect of a safe zone on nurse interruptions, distractions, and medication administration errors, *J Infus Nurs* 38(2):140, 2015.

Zhu J, Weingart S: Prevention of adverse drug events in hospitals, UpToDate, 2017. https://www.uptodate.com/contents/prevention-of-adverse-drug-events-in-hospitals/contributor-disclosure.

23 Nonparenteral Medications

SKILLS AND PROCEDURES

EVOLVE WEBSITE/RESOURCES LIST

http://evolve.elsevier.com/Perry/nursinginterventions
Audio Glossary • Checklists • Clinical Review Questions • Answers and Rationales for Clinical Review Questions • Video Clips

INTRODUCTION

Nonparenteral medications include medications that are not given by injection, such as oral medications, topical skin preparations, eyedrops, and eardrops. The route chosen depends on the properties and desired effects of the medication and the physical and mental condition of the patient. The oral route (by mouth) is the easiest and most efficient way to administer medications. Each route has advantages and disadvantages (Table 23.1). There are many reasons why you may find it necessary to recommend a change from one route to another. When a recommended change occurs, you are responsible for consulting with the health care provider for an order or conferring with a pharmacist to meet the patient's needs safely.

PRACTICE STANDARDS

- Institute for Safe Medication Practices (ISMP), 2011: ISMP acute care guidelines for timely administration of scheduled medications
- Institute for Safe Medication Practices (ISMP), 2016a: Oral dosage forms that should not be crushed 2016—Reference to Do Not Crush list
- The Joint Commission (TJC), 2019: National Patient Safety Goals—Patient identification
- U.S. Department of Health and Human Services (USDHHS), 2015: Tablet splitting a risky practice—Pharmacy role in pill splitting

EVIDENCE-BASED PRACTICE

Preventing Adverse Drug Events

Medication administration is an essential role of the nurse. Nurses must be competent in all aspects of administering medications, assessing medication dosage and desired effects, evaluating the effectiveness of medications, and observing for adverse effects. Medication administration technologies are designed to assist nurses in administering medications safely. Knowledge of the technology and nurse competencies is essential in increasing patient safety and promoting best practices for medication administration (Zhu and Weingart, 2017). Guidelines include the following:

- Be vigilant when administering high-risk medications (e.g., heparin).
- Consider medications and their effects and side effects as the cause of any new symptom.
- Use computerized physician order entry (CPOE) whenever possible to avoid errors.
- Electronic medication administration records are designed to address errors related to the transcription of orders.
- Correct use of bar coding ensures a match between a patient and his or her medication during medication administration.
- Ensure that all three steps of medication reconciliation (verification, clarification, reconciliation) are done at all transitions of care.
- Education programs can provide another step in the prevention of errors in medication administration.

SAFETY GUIDELINES

Be aware of the conditions in the area where you prepare medications. Because nurses rely on visual stimulation to make critical decisions, both artificial light and natural light are important to patient safety (Ball et al., 2019). Always have sufficient lighting when locating equipment, reading labels, calculating doses, and preparing medications. Construction noise, foot traffic, and interruptions from colleagues, monitoring machines, telephones, and hallway conversations are some of the factors that decrease your ability

TABLE 23.1
Nonparenteral Routes of Administration

Route	Advantages	Disadvantages
Inhalation	Directly acts on lung tissues and provides rapid relief of respiratory distress	It is difficult for some patients to hold or manipulate inhaler canisters correctly. Patients must be taught how to use equipment.
Mucous membranes: eyes, ears, nose; vaginal, rectal	Local application to involved site; limited side effects; rectal route is an alternative when oral route unavailable	Insertion of vaginal or rectal products may cause embarrassment. Rectal suppositories are contraindicated in patients with rectal surgery or active rectal bleeding.
Oral (swallowed)	Easy, comfortable, economical; may produce local or systemic effects	Some drugs are destroyed by gastric secretions. Cannot be given if patient is on "nothing by mouth" (NPO) status, is unable to swallow, is nauseated, has gastric suction, or is unconscious or confused and unwilling to cooperate. Drugs may irritate lining of GI tract, discolor teeth, or have unpleasant taste.
Skin: topical application or transdermal patches	Provides primarily local effect; painless; limited side effects; transdermal application provides systemic effects and bypasses the liver and its first-pass effects	Extensive topical applications may be bulky or cause difficulty in maneuvering. They may leave oily or pasty substance on skin and may soil clothing. Systemic absorption can be unreliable. Allergies to adhesive in transdermal patches may develop.

GI, Gastrointestinal.

Modified from Burchum JR, Rosenthal LD: *Lehne's pharmacology for nursing care*, ed 8, Philadelphia, 2016, Saunders.

to concentrate and attend properly to medication administration. Other safety guidelines include the following:

- Assess the patient's sensory function, including sight, hearing, touch, and physical coordination and dexterity. Sensory function and coordination deficits impair the patient's ability to see medications, read labels at home, and discriminate one medication from another. Coordination and dexterity impairments hinder the patient's ability to open prescription bottles and dispense the correct dosage.
- Patients often receive more than one oral medication at a time. Evaluate each medication for potential drug–drug or drug–food interactions. When unsure, consult with a pharmacist to clarify the risk, and determine measures to reduce the risk of an interaction.
- Always assess for drug allergies. If a patient reports having an allergy, ask about the type of reaction that occurred.
- Evaluate whether the patient can take medication with food. In most cases the presence of food in the stomach delays drug absorption. However, some medications must be taken prior to meals, whereas other drugs irritate the stomach lining and need to be taken with food.
- For all medications administered, review the order for the patient's name, drug, dosage, route, and time of administration.
- For all medications, use the correct equipment for administering the medication. For example, use metric system medication cups that use the milliliter (mL) as the standard of measure. The dosing cup should not include fluid dram measures (NAN, 2015).
- For all medications administered, gather information pertinent to the drug(s) ordered: purpose, normal dosage and route, common side effects, time of onset and peak, contraindications, and nursing implications.
- Determine if medications require any specific nursing actions (e.g., obtaining vital signs, drug levels, or electrolytes) before administration.
- If patients are mentally and physically able, prepare them for discharge by instructing them in self-administration techniques. Include family caregivers if possible.

✦ SKILL 23.1 Administering Oral Medications

Purpose

Patients usually can ingest or self-administer oral medications with few problems. However, situations may arise that contraindicate patients receiving medications by mouth, including the presence of gastrointestinal (GI) alterations, the inability of a patient to swallow food or fluids, and the use of gastric suction. An important precaution to take when administering any oral preparation is to protect patients from aspiration (see Chapter 13, Skill 13.2).

Absorption of an oral medication after it is ingested depends largely on its form or preparation. Solutions and suspensions that are already in a liquid state (Fig. 23.1) are absorbed more readily than tablets or capsules.

Delegation and Collaboration

The skill of administering oral medications cannot be delegated to nursing assistive personnel (NAP). The nurse instructs the NAP about:

- Potential side effects of medications and to report their occurrence.
- Informing the nurse if patient condition changes or worsens (e.g., pain, itching, or rash) after medication administration.

Equipment

- Automated, computer-controlled drug-dispensing system or medication cart
- Disposable medication cups (mL-only cup)
- Glass of water, juice, or preferred liquid and drinking straw

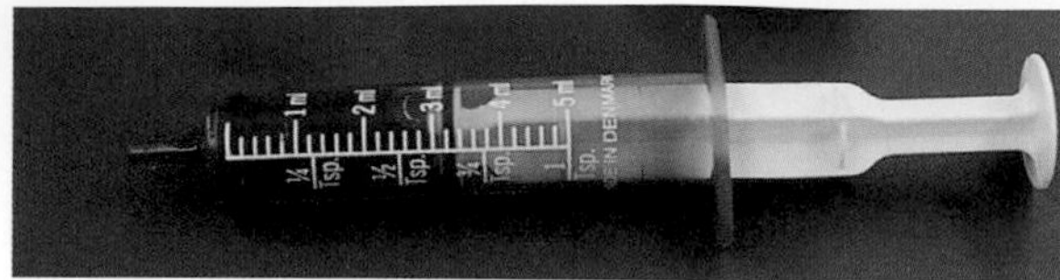

FIG 23.1 Oral medicine in syringe.

- Pill-crushing device *(optional)*
- Paper towels
- Medication administration record (MAR; electronic or printed)
- Clean gloves (if handling an oral medication)

ASSESSMENT

1. Check accuracy and completeness of each MAR or computer printout with health care provider's written medication order. Check patient's name, medication name and dosage, route of administration, and time of administration. Recopy or reprint any portion of MAR that is difficult to read. *Rationale: The order sheet is the most reliable source and only legal record of medications that patient is to receive. Ensures that patient receives the correct medications (Westbrook et al., 2017). Transcription errors are a source of medication errors (Truitt et al., 2016).*
2. Review pertinent information related to medication, including action, purpose, normal dose and route, side effects, time of onset and peak action, indications, and nursing implications. *Rationale: Allows you to anticipate effects of drug and observe patient's response.*
3. Assess for any contraindications to patient receiving oral medication, including being on "nothing by mouth" (NPO) status, inability to swallow, nausea/vomiting, bowel inflammation, reduced peristalsis, recent GI surgery, gastric suction, and decreased level of consciousness (LOC). Notify health care provider if any contraindications are present. *Rationale: Alterations in GI function can interfere with drug absorption, distribution, and excretion. Patients with GI suction do not receive actions of oral medications because the medications are suctioned from the GI tract before they are absorbed.*
4. Assess risk for aspiration using a dysphagia screening tool if available (see Skill 13.2). Protect patient from aspiration by assessing swallowing ability (Box 23.1). *Rationale: Aspiration occurs when food, fluid, or medication given orally inadvertently enters the respiratory tract. Patients with altered ability to swallow are at higher risk for aspiration (Forough et al., 2017).*
5. Assess patient's medical, medication, and diet history and history of allergies. List any drug allergies on each page of MAR and prominently display on patient's medical record. When allergies are present, patient should wear an allergy bracelet. *Rationale: Information reflects patient's need for and potential responses to medication. Information reveals potential food and drug interactions. Communication of allergies is essential for safe, effective care.*
6. Gather and review physical assessment findings and laboratory data that influence drug administration, such as vital signs and results of renal and liver function studies. *Rationale: Data may reveal need to contraindicate drug administration. Renal and liver function status affects metabolism and excretion of medications (Burchum and Rosenthal, 2016).*
7. Assess patient's or family caregiver's knowledge, experience, and health literacy. *Rationale: Ensures patient or family caregiver has the capacity to obtain, communicate, process, and understand basic health information (Centers for Disease Control and Prevention [CDC], 2016).*
8. Assess patient's knowledge regarding health and medication use, medication schedule, and ability to prepare medications. *Rationale: Determines patient's need for medication education and guidance needed to achieve drug adherence (e.g., involvement of family caregiver).*
9. Assess patient's preference for fluids and determine if medications can be given with these fluids. Maintain fluid restrictions as prescribed. *Rationale: Some fluids interfere with medication absorption (e.g., dairy products affect tetracycline). Offering fluids during drug administration is an excellent way to increase patient's fluid intake. Fluids ease swallowing and facilitate absorption from the GI tract.*

BOX 23.1

Protecting a Patient From Aspiration

- Assess patient's ability to swallow and cough, and check for presence of gag reflex.
- Prepare oral medication in form that is easiest to swallow.
- Allow patient to self-administer medications if possible.
- If patient has unilateral (one-sided) weakness, place medication in stronger side of mouth.
- Administer pills one at a time, ensuring that each medication is properly swallowed before the next one is introduced.
- Thicken regular liquids or offer fruit nectars if patient cannot tolerate thin liquids.
- Avoid straws because they decrease control patient has over volume intake, which increases risk of aspiration.
- Have patient hold and drink from a cup if possible.
- Time medications to coincide with mealtimes or when patient is well rested and awake if possible.
- Administer medications using another route if risk of aspiration is severe.

STEP	RATIONALE
PLANNING	
1. Expected outcomes following completion of procedure:	
• Patient responds appropriately to desired medication effect.	Drug has exerted its therapeutic action.
• Patient denies any GI discomfort or symptoms of alterations.	Oral medications can irritate GI mucosa.

STEP	RATIONALE
• Patient explains purpose of medication and drug dosage schedule.	Demonstrates understanding of drug therapy.
2. Provide privacy and prepare environment.	Providing privacy and preparing the environment promotes patient comfort and ensures safe, efficient procedure.
3. Discuss purpose of each medication, action, indication, and possible adverse effects. Allow patient to ask any questions.	Patient has right to be informed, and patient's understanding of each medication improves adherence to drug therapy. Helps minimize patient's anxiety.

IMPLEMENTATION

STEP	RATIONALE
1. Prepare medications.	
a. Perform hand hygiene. Arrange medication tray and cups in medication preparation area or move medication cart to position outside patient's room.	Reduces transmission of microorganisms. Organization of equipment saves time and reduces error.
b. Log on to automated dispensing system (ADS) or unlock medicine drawer or cart.	Medications are safeguarded when locked in cabinet, cart, or ADS.
c. Prepare medication using aseptic technique for one patient at a time. Follow the seven rights of medication administration. Keep all pages of MARs or computer printouts for one patient together or look at only one patient's electronic MAR at a time.	Ensures that medication is sterile. Preventing distractions reduces medication preparation errors. Use a no-interruption zone (NIZ) when possible (Prakash et al., 2014; Yoder et al., 2015).
d. Select correct medication from unit dose drawer, ADS, or stock supply. Compare name of medication on label with MAR (see illustration). Exit ADS after removing drugs.	*This is the first check for accuracy* and ensures that correct medication is administered.

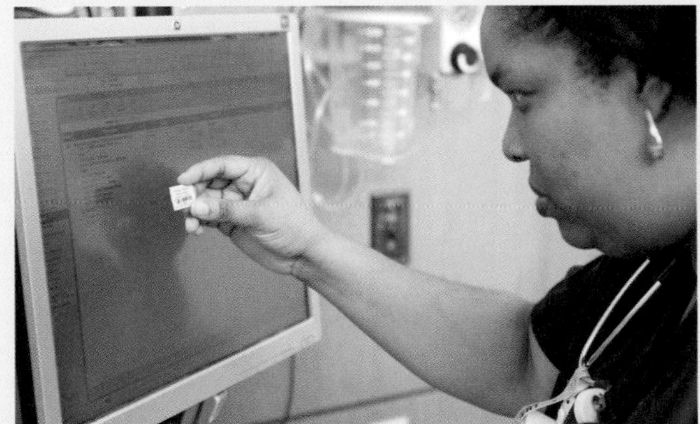

STEP 1d Nurse compares label of medication with transcribed medication order on computerized medication administration record (MAR).

STEP	RATIONALE
e. Check or calculate medication dose as necessary. Double-check any calculation. Check expiration date on all medications and return outdated medication to pharmacy.	Double-checking pharmacy calculations reduces risk for error. Agency policy may require you to check calculations of certain medications, such as insulin, with another nurse. Expired medications may be inactive or harmful to patient.
f. If preparing a controlled substance, check record for previous medication count and compare current count with available supply. Controlled drugs may be stored in computerized locked cart (see Chapter 22).	Controlled substance laws require nurses to carefully monitor and count dispensed narcotics.
g. Prepare solid forms of oral medications.	
(1) To prepare unit-dose tablets or capsules, place packaged tablet or capsule directly into medication cup without removing wrapper. Administer medications only from containers with labels that are clearly marked.	Wrappers maintain cleanliness and identify drug name and dose, which can facilitate teaching.
(2) When using a blister pack, "pop" medications through foil or paper backing into a medication cup.	Packs provide a 1-month supply, with each "blister" usually containing a single dose.

STEP	RATIONALE
(3) When preparing tablet or capsule from a floor stock bottle, pour required number into bottle cap and transfer to medication cup. Do not touch medication with fingers. Return unused medications to container.	Avoids contamination and waste of medications.
(4) If it is necessary to give half the dose of medication, pharmacy should split, label, package, and send medication to unit.	In health care agencies, only pharmacy should split tablets to ensure patient safety (U.S. Department of Health and Human Services [USDHHS], 2015). Reduces contamination of tablet.
(5) Place all tablets or capsules that patient will receive in one medicine cup, except for those requiring pre-administration assessments (e.g., pulse rate or blood pressure). Place those medications in separate additional cup with wrapper intact.	Keeping medications that require pre-administration assessments separate from others serves as reminder and makes it easier to withhold drugs as necessary.
(6) If patient has difficulty swallowing and liquid medications are not an option, use a pill-crushing device. Clean device before using. Place medicine between two cups, and grind and crush (see illustration). Mix ground tablet in small amount (teaspoon) of soft food (custard or applesauce).	Large tablets are often difficult to swallow. Ground tablet mixed with palatable soft food is usually easier to swallow.

Safe Patient Care *Not all medications can be crushed safely. Consult with a pharmacist or the ISMP Do Not Crush List (ISMP, 2016a).*

STEP	RATIONALE
h. Prepare liquids.	
(1) Use unit-dose container with correct amount of medication. Gently shake container. Administer medication directly from the single-dose cup. Do not pour medicine into another cup.	Using unit-dose container with correct dosage of medication provides most accurate dose of medication (ISMP, 2016b). Shaking container ensures that medication is mixed before administration.

Safe Patient Care *Based on current best practice (ISMP, 2016b; Paparella, 2014), liquid medications that are not available or are not in correct dose in a unit-dose container should be dispensed by the pharmacy in special oral syringes marked "Oral Use Only." These syringes do not connect to any type of parenteral (e.g., intravenous [IV]) tubing. In addition, current evidence shows that liquid measuring devices on patient care units result in inaccurate dosing. Having oral medications prepared in the pharmacy ensures that you give the most accurate dose of a medication possible and prevents parenteral administration of oral medications.*

STEP	RATIONALE
(2) Administer medications only in oral use syringes prepared by pharmacy (see illustration). *Do not* use hypodermic syringe or syringe with needle or syringe cap (see Chapter 22).	Only use syringes specifically designed for oral use when administering liquid medications. These syringes provide more accurate measurement of small amounts. A medication may be administered parenterally accidentally if hypodermic syringe used; or the syringe cap or needle, if not removed from the syringe before administration, may become dislodged and accidentally aspirated (ISMP, 2016b).

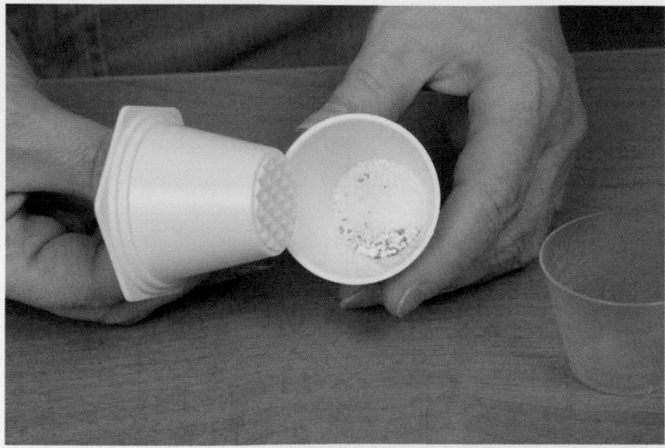

STEP 1g(6) Crushing tablet with pill-crushing device.

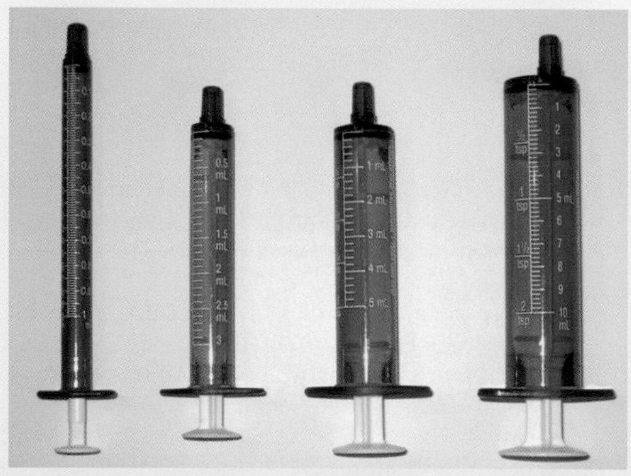

STEP 1h(2) Use special oral medication syringes to prepare small amounts of liquid medications.

STEP	RATIONALE
i. Return stock containers or unused unit-dose medications to shelf or drawer. Label medication cups with patient's name before leaving medication preparation area. Do not leave drugs unattended.	Ensures that correct medications are prepared for correct patient.
j. Before going to patient's room, compare patient's name and name of medication on label of prepared drugs with the MAR.	*This is the second check for accuracy.* Reading labels second time reduces error.
2. Administer medications.	
a. Take medication(s) to patient at correct time (see agency policy). Medications that require exact timing include STAT, first-time or loading doses, and one-time doses. Give time-critical scheduled medications (e.g., antibiotics, anticoagulants, insulin, anticonvulsants, immunosuppressive agents) at exact time ordered (no later than 30 minutes before or after scheduled dose). Give non–time-critical scheduled medications within a range of 1 or 2 hours of scheduled dose (ISMP, 2011). During administration, apply seven rights of medication administration (see Chapter 22).	Hospitals must adopt medication administration policy and procedure for timing of medication administration that considers nature of the prescribed medication, specific clinical application, and patient needs (Department of Health and Human Services, Centers for Medicare and Medicaid [DHHS], 2011; ISMP, 2011). Time-critical scheduled medications are those for which early or delayed administration of maintenance doses of greater than 30 minutes before or after the scheduled dose may cause harm or result in substantial suboptimal therapy or pharmacological effect. Non–time-critical medications are those for which early or delayed administration within a specified range of either 1 or 2 hours should not cause harm or result in substantial suboptimal therapy or pharmacological effect (DHHS, 2011; ISMP, 2011).
b. Identify patient using at least two identifiers (e.g., name and birthday or name and medical record number) according to agency policy. Compare identifiers with information on patient's MAR or medical record.	Ensures correct patient. Complies with The Joint Commission standards and improves patient safety (TJC, 2019).
c. At patient's bedside, again compare MAR or computer printout with names of medications on medication labels and patient name.	*This is the third check for accuracy* and ensures that patient receives correct medication.
d. Perform necessary pre-administration assessment (e.g., blood pressure, pulse) for specific medications. Ask patient if he or she has allergies.	Determines whether specific medications should be withheld at that time. Confirms patient's allergy history.

Safe Patient Care *If patient expresses concern regarding accuracy of a medication, do not give the medication. Explore patient's concern and verify prescriber's order before administering. Listening to patient's concerns may prevent a medication error.*

STEP	RATIONALE
e. Help patient to sitting or Fowler's position. Use side-lying position if he or she is unable to sit. Have patient stay in this position for 30 minutes after administration.	Decreases risk for aspiration during swallowing.
f. **For tablets:** Patient may wish to hold solid medications in hand or cup before placing in mouth. Offer water or preferred liquid to help patient swallow medications.	Patient can become familiar with medications by seeing each drug. Choice of fluid can improve fluid intake.

Safe Patient Care *When administering an oral chemotherapy medication, never use bare hands to touch a chemotherapy medication because residue can be absorbed through your skin (Occupational Safety and Health Administration [OSHA], 2016).*

STEP	RATIONALE
g. **For orally disintegrating formulations (tablets or strips):** Remove medication from packet just before use. Do not push tablet through foil. Place medication on top of patient's tongue. Caution against chewing it.	Orally disintegrating formulations begin to dissolve when placed on tongue. Water is not needed. Careful removal from packaging is necessary because tablets and strips are thin and fragile.
h. **For sublingually administered medications:** Have patient place medication under tongue and allow it to dissolve completely (see illustration). Caution patient against swallowing tablet.	Drug is absorbed through blood vessels of undersurface of tongue. If swallowed, it is destroyed by gastric juices or rapidly detoxified by liver, preventing therapeutic blood level.
i. **For buccally administered medications:** Have patient place medication in mouth against mucous membranes of cheek and gums until it dissolves (see illustration).	Buccal medications act locally or systemically as they are swallowed in saliva.

Safe Patient Care *Avoid administering anything by mouth until orally disintegrating buccal or sublingual medication is completely dissolved.*

STEP	RATIONALE

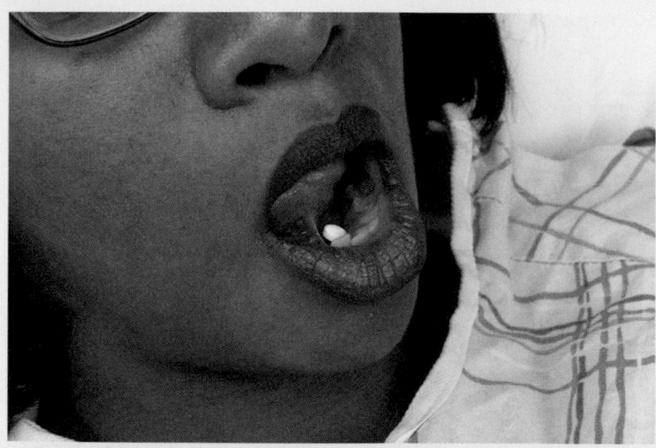

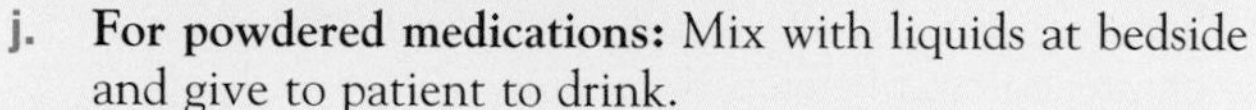

STEP 2h Proper placement of sublingual tablet in sublingual pocket.

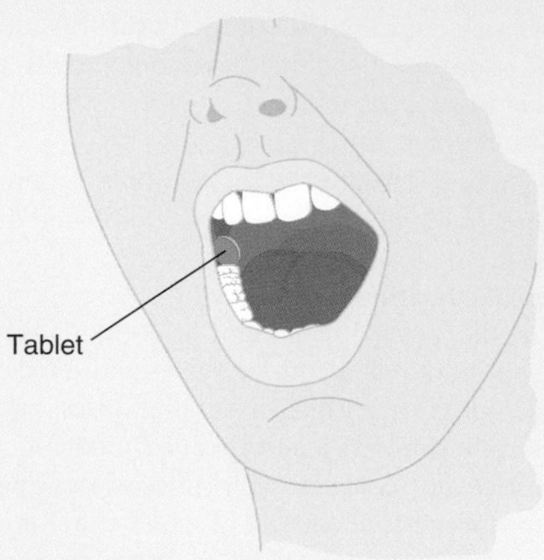

STEP 2i Buccal administration of tablet.

STEP	RATIONALE
j. **For powdered medications:** Mix with liquids at bedside and give to patient to drink.	When prepared in advance, powdered drugs thicken; some even harden, making swallowing difficult.
k. **For crushed medications mixed with food:** Give each medication separately in teaspoon of food.	Ensures that patient swallows all of medicine.
l. **For lozenge:** Have patient allow lozenge to dissolve in mouth. Caution against chewing or swallowing lozenge.	Lozenges act through slow absorption through oral mucosa, not gastric mucosa.
m. **For effervescent medication:** Add tablet or powder to glass of water. Administer immediately after dissolving.	Effervescence improves unpleasant taste and often relieves GI problems.
n. If patient is unable to hold medications, place medication cup to lips and gently introduce each drug into mouth one at a time. A spoon can also be used to place pill in patient's mouth. Do not rush or force medications.	Administering a single tablet or capsule eases swallowing and decreases risk for aspiration.
o. Stay until patient swallows each medication completely or takes it by the prescribed route. Ask patient to open mouth if uncertain whether medication has been swallowed.	Ensures that patient receives ordered dose. If left unattended, patient may not take dose or may save drugs, causing health risks.
p. For highly acidic medications (e.g., aspirin), offer patient a nonfat snack (e.g., crackers) if not contraindicated by his or her condition.	Reduces gastric irritation. Fat content of foods may delay drug absorption.
3. Help patient to comfortable position.	Gives patient sense of well-being.
4. Be sure nurse call system is in an accessible location within patient's reach.	Ensures patient can call for assistance if needed.
5. Raise side rails (as appropriate) and lower bed to lowest position.	Ensures patient safety.
6. Dispose of soiled supplies, remove and dispose of gloves if worn, and perform hand hygiene.	Reduces tranmission of microorganisms.
7. Stay with patient for several minutes and observe for any allergic reactions.	Dyspnea, wheezing, and circulatory collapse are signs of severe anaphylactic reaction.

EVALUATION

STEP	RATIONALE
1. Return to bedside to evaluate patient's response to medications at times that correlate with onset, peak, and duration of the medication.	Evaluates therapeutic benefit of medication and helps detect onset of side effects or allergic reactions. Sublingual medications act in 15 minutes; most oral medications act in 30 to 60 minutes.
2. Ask patient or family caregiver to identify medication name and explain purpose, indication, action, dose schedule, and potential side effects.	Determines level of knowledge gained by patient and family caregiver.
3. **Use Teach-Back:** "I want to be sure I showed you how to use your sublingual nitroglycerin. Show me where you will place the tablet in your mouth." Revise your instruction now or develop a plan for revised patient/family caregiver teaching if patient/family caregiver is not able to teach back correctly.	Determines patient's/family caregiver's level of understanding of instructional topic.

Unexpected Outcomes	Related Interventions
1. Patient exhibits adverse effects (e.g., side effect, toxic effect, allergic reaction).	• Notify health care provider and pharmacy. • Withhold further doses. • Assess vital signs. • Symptoms such as urticaria, rash, pruritus, rhinitis, and wheezing may indicate an allergic reaction and need for emergency medications. • Add allergy information to patient's medical record.
2. Patient refuses medication.	• Assess why patient is refusing medication. • Provide further instruction. • Do not force patient to take medications. • Notify health care provider.
3. Patient is unable to explain drug information.	• Further assess patient's or family caregiver's knowledge of medications and guidelines for drug safety. • Further instruction or different approach to instruction is necessary.

Recording

- Record drug, dose, route, and time administered immediately *after* administration, not before.
- Document your evaluation of patient learning.
- If drug is withheld, record reason and follow agency policy for marking held medications. Most agencies require that you circle the time the drug normally would have been given.

Hand-Off Reporting

- Report adverse effects or patient response and withheld drugs to nurse in charge or health care provider.

✦ SKILL 23.2 Administering Medications Through a Feeding Tube

Purpose

Patients who have enteral feeding tubes are unable to receive food or medication by mouth. Chapter 13 describes the clinical indications and nursing care implications for enteral feeding tubes. Medications administered by enteral tubes preferably should be in liquid form. If a medication is unavailable in a liquid, you need to prepare an oral medication tablet or capsule by crushing or dissolving it. However, you cannot crush sublingual, slow-release, chewable, long-acting, or enteric-coated medications. Check with a pharmacist about whether you can crush or dissolve a medication. Pierce gel caps with a sterile needle and empty contents into 30 mL of warm water to dissolve. Use oral syringes when preparing medications for this route to prevent accidental parenteral administration. Always verify the position of an enteral tube before administering any medication (see agency policy; see Skill 13.4).

Delegation and Collaboration

The skill of administering medications by enteral feeding tubes cannot be delegated to nursing assistive personnel (NAP). The nurse instructs the NAP to:

- Keep the head of the bed elevated a minimum of 30 degrees (preferably 45 degrees) for 1 hour after medication administration; follow agency policy.
- Report immediately to the nurse coughing, choking, gagging, or drooling of liquid or dissolved pills.
- Report to the nurse occurrence of possible medication side effects (specific to medication).

Equipment

- Medication administration record (MAR; electronic or printed)
- Appropriate medication syringe (see Skill 23.1, Step 1h(2) and Fig. 23.1) with appropriate tip for small-bore tube, or 60 mL Asepto syringe for large-bore tubes only
- 50-mL oral, enteral, or catheter-tipped syringe for irrigation
- Enteral-only connector (ENFit) designed to fit syringes to the enteral tube (TJC, 2014; Fig. 23.2)
- Gastric pH test strip (scale of 1 to 11.0)
- Graduated container
- Medication to be administered (usually prepared in the medication syringe)
- Pill crusher if medication in tablet form
- Water or sterile water for immunocompromised patients
- Tongue blade or straw to stir dissolved medication
- Clean gloves
- Stethoscope (for evaluation)

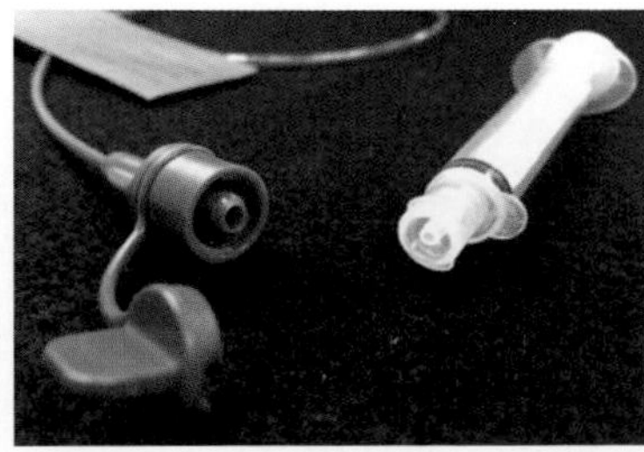

FIG 23.2 Enteral connector.

ASSESSMENT

1. Check accuracy and completeness of each MAR or computer printout with health care provider's written medication order. Check patient's name, medication name and dosage, route of administration, and time of administration. Recopy or reprint any portion of MAR that is difficult to read. *Rationale: The order sheet is the most reliable source and only legal record of medications that patient is to receive. Ensures that patient receives the correct medications (Westbrook et al., 2017). Transcription errors are a source of medication errors (Truitt et al., 2016).*
2. Review pertinent information related to medication, including action, purpose, normal dose and route, side effects, time of onset and peak action, indication, and nursing implications. *Rationale: Allows you to anticipate effects of drug and observe patient's response.*
3. Assess for any contraindications to receiving enteral medications, including presence of bowel inflammation, reduced peristalsis, recent gastrointestinal (GI) surgery, and gastric suction that cannot be turned off. *Rationale: Alterations in GI function can interfere with drug absorption, distribution, and excretion. Patients with GI suction do not benefit from medication because it may be suctioned from the GI track before it is absorbed.*
4. Assess patient's medical, medication, and diet history and history of allergies. List patient's food and drug allergies on each page of the MAR and prominently display it on the patient's medical record per agency policy. When patient has an allergy, provide allergy bracelet. If you identify contraindications, withhold medication and inform health care provider. *Rationale: Information reflects patient's need for and potential responses to medications. Information also indicates potential food and drug interactions. Some drugs may require tube feeding to be stopped for an hour before and 2 hours after dose (Burchum and Rosenthal, 2016). Communication of allergies is essential for safe, effective care.*
5. For postoperative patient, review postoperative orders for type of enteral tube care. *Rationale: Manipulation and irrigation of tube or instillation of medications may be contraindicated.*
6. Gather and review physical assessment data (e.g., bowel sounds, abdominal distention) and laboratory data (e.g., renal and liver function) that may influence drug administration. *Rationale: Physical examination findings or laboratory data may contraindicate drug administration.*
7. Check with pharmacy for availability of liquid preparation for patient's medications. The health care provider may need to change dosage form. *Rationale: When possible, liquid formulation of the medication is the best option. The agency pharmacy may have the ability to provide a liquid preparation that is compatible with the enteral nutrition formula (Boullata et al., 2017).*
8. Avoid complicated medication schedule that interrupts enteral feedings. Check with health care provider and use alternative medication route when possible.
   a. Assess where medication is absorbed and ensure that point of absorption is not by-passed by feeding tube. For example, some antacids are absorbed in stomach. If feeding tube is placed in intestines, medications are not absorbed.
   b. Determine if medication interacts with enteral feeding. If risk of interaction, stop feeding for at least 20 minutes before giving medication (see agency policy).

   Rationale: Ensures proper medication administration route. Avoids medication interactions.
9. Assess patient's or family caregiver's knowledge, experience, and health literacy. *Rationale: Ensures patient or family caregiver has the capacity to obtain, communicate, process, and understand basic health information (CDC, 2016).*

STEP	RATIONALE
PLANNING	
1. Expected outcomes following completion of procedure:	
• Patient experiences desired medication effect within period of onset of medication.	Drug has exerted its therapeutic action.
• Patient's feeding tube remains patent after administration of medication.	Patent enteral tube indicates passage of medication into stomach, ensuring proper absorption. If tube becomes blocked, administration of other medications and feedings is not possible.
• Patient does not aspirate during or after medication administration.	Patient safety in medication administration is maintained.
2. Provide privacy and prepare environment.	Providing privacy and preparing the environment promotes patient comfort and ensures efficient, safe procedure.
3. Discuss purpose of each medication, indication, action, and possible adverse effects. Allow patient to ask any questions.	Patient has right to be informed, and patient's understanding of each medication improves adherence to drug therapy. Helps minimize patient's anxiety.
IMPLEMENTATION	
1. Perform hand hygiene. Prepare medications for instillation into feeding tube (see Skill 23.1). When selecting medication, check medication label against MAR. Fill graduated container with 50 to 100 mL of tepid water. Use sterile water for immunocompromised or critically ill patients (Boullata et al., 2017).	*This is the first check for accuracy*. Preparation process ensures that right patient receives right medication. Tepid water prevents abdominal cramping, which can occur with cold water.

STEP	RATIONALE

Safe Patient Care *Whenever possible, use liquid medications instead of crushed tablets. If you must crush tablets, flush the tubing before and after the medication administration to prevent the drug from adhering to the inside of the tube. In addition, make sure that concentrated medications are thoroughly diluted. Never add crushed medications directly to a tube feeding (Boullata et al., 2017).*

STEP	RATIONALE
a. *Tablets:* Crush each tablet into a fine powder, using pill-crushing device or two medication cups (see Skill 23.1). Dissolve each tablet in separate cup of 30 mL of warm water.	Fine powder dissolves more easily, reducing chance of occluding feeding tube.
b. *Capsules:* Ensure that contents of capsule (granules or gelatin) can be expressed from covering (consult with pharmacist). Apply gloves and open capsule or pierce gel cap with sterile needle and empty contents into 30 mL of warm water (or solution designated by drug company). Gel caps dissolve in warm water, but this may take 15 to 20 minutes.	Ensures that contents of capsules are in solution to prevent occlusion of tube.
c. Prepare liquid medication according to Skill 23.1.	
2. Never add medications directly to a container or bag of tube feeding. Sometimes tube feeding needs to be held. Verify this and the amount of time that you hold a feeding with agency policy (Guenter and Boullata, 2013).	Prevents feeding tube occlusion and ensures timely administration of full dose.
3. Before going to patient's room, compare patient's name and name of medication on label of prepared drugs with MAR a second time.	Reduces medication error. *This is the second check for accuracy.*
4. Take medication(s) to patient at correct time (see agency policy). Medications that require exact timing include STAT, first-time or loading doses, and one-time doses. Give time-critical scheduled medications (e.g., antibiotics, anticoagulants, insulin, anticonvulsants, immunosuppressive agents) at exact time ordered (no later than 30 minutes before or after scheduled dose). Give non–time-critical scheduled medications within a range of 1 or 2 hours of scheduled dose (ISMP, 2011). During administration, apply seven rights of medication administration.	Hospitals must adopt medication administration policy and procedure for timing of medication administration that considers nature of the prescribed medication, specific clinical application, and patient needs (DHHS, 2011; ISMP, 2011). Time-critical scheduled medications are those for which early or delayed administration of maintenance doses of greater than 30 minutes before or after the scheduled dose may cause harm or result in substantial suboptimal therapy or pharmacological effect. Non–time-critical medications are those for which early or delayed administration within a specified range of either 1 or 2 hours should not cause harm or result in substantial suboptimal therapy or pharmacological effect (DHHS, 2011; ISMP, 2011).
5. Identify patient using at least two identifiers (e.g., name and birthday or name and medical record number) according to agency policy. Compare identifiers with information on patient's MAR or medical record.	Ensures correct patient. Complies with The Joint Commission standards and improves patient safety (TJC, 2019).
6. At patient's bedside, again compare MAR or computer printout with names of medications on medication labels and patient name. Ask patient if he or she has allergies.	*This is the third check for accuracy* and ensures that patient receives correct medication. Confirms patient's allergy history.
7. Assist patient to sitting position. Elevate head of bed to minimum of 30 degrees and preferably 45 degrees (unless contraindicated) or sit patient up in a chair (Boullata et al., 2017).	Reduces risk for aspiration, keeping head above stomach.
8. If continuous enteral tube feeding is infusing, adjust infusion pump setting to hold tube feeding.	Feeding solution should not infuse while residuals are checked or medications are administered. The presence of a feeding solution may impede drug absorption (Boullata et al., 2017).
9. Perform hand hygiene and apply clean gloves. Check placement of feeding tube (see Skill 13.4) by observing gastric contents and checking pH of aspirate contents. The position of a PEG or surgical/radiological jejunostomy can be assessed by checking that the length of tube outside the body remains constant and the suture remains intact. *Gastric pH less than 5.0 is a good indicator that tip of tube is correctly placed in stomach* (Boullata et al., 2017; Clifford et al., 2015).	Ensures proper tube placement and reduces risk of introducing fluids into respiratory tract.

STEP	RATIONALE
10. Check for gastric residual volume (GRV). Draw up 10 to 30 mL of air into a 60-mL irrigation syringe and connect syringe to feeding tube connector. Flush tube with air and pull back slowly to aspirate gastric contents. Determine GRV using either scale on syringe or a graduated container. If GRV is is 250 mL or less, return aspirated contents to stomach (see agency policy). If GRV exceeds 250 to 500 mL (see agency policy), hold medication and contact health care provider (Boullata et al., 2017).	GRV categories have been identified in studies as significant when patients have two or more GRVs exceeding 500 mL (Boullata et al., 2017). Large residuals indicate delayed gastric emptying and put patient at increased risk for aspiration (Boullata et al., 2017; Burcham and Rosenthal, 2016).
11. Irrigate the feeding tube.	
a. Be sure the appropriate enteral connector (see Fig. 23.2) is attached to end of enteral tube.	Standardization of connector tubing improves patient safety. Tubing standards are designed to reduce tubing misconnections that result in patient injury (Boullata et al., 2017; TJC, 2014).
b. Pinch or clamp enteral tube and remove syringe used to obtain GRV. Draw up 30 mL of water into syringe. Reinsert tip of syringe into tube, release clamp, and flush tubing. Clamp tube again and remove syringe.	Pinching or clamping tubing prevents leakage or spillage of stomach contents. Flushing ensures that tube is patent.

Safe Patient Care *Verify that the connector meets the ISO tubing connector standards (Boullata et al., 2017; TJC, 2014). Do not attach the enteral tubing to a standardized Luer-Lok syringe or needleless device (Guenther, 2015; TJC, 2014).*

STEP	RATIONALE
12. Attach the medication syringe to connector port on the enteral feeding tube. Ensure there is an airtight connection between the syringe and enteral tube, and administer the medication slowly.	Delivers medication.
13. *Option:* For a large-bore feeding tube, attach Aspeto syringe to ENFit connector. Administer dose of liquid or dissolved medication by pouring into syringe (see illustration). Allow to flow by gravity.	

Safe Patient Care *Sometimes it is necessary to transfer oral medications into a medication cup for enteral administration. If medication does not flow freely, raise the height of the syringe to increase the rate of flow, or try having the patient change position slightly because the end of the feeding tube may be against the gastric mucosa. If these measures do not improve the flow, a gentle push with bulb of Asepto syringe or plunger of the syringe may facilitate flow of fluid.*

STEP	RATIONALE
a. After giving only one dose of medication, flush tubing with 30 to 60 mL of water after administration.	Maintains patency of enteral tube and ensures that medication passes through tube to stomach (Boullata et al., 2017).
b. To administer more than one medication, give each separately and flush between medications with 15 to 30 mL of water.	Allows for accurate identification of medication if dose is spilled. In addition, some medications may be incompatible, and giving medication separately followed by a flush solution decreases the risk for medication incompatibilities (Boullata et al., 2017).
c. Follow last dose of medication with 30 to 60 mL of water.	Maintains patency of enteral tube and ensures passage of medication into stomach (Boullata et al., 2017).

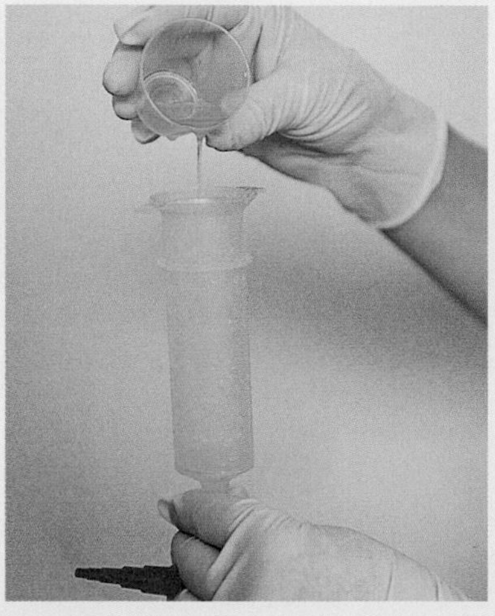

STEP 13 Pour liquid medication into syringe.

STEP	RATIONALE
14. Clamp proximal end of feeding tube if tube feeding is not being administered, and cap end of tube.	Prevents air from entering stomach between medication doses.
15. When continuous tube feeding is being administered by infusion pump, follow medication administration. If medications are not compatible with feeding solution, hold feeding for additional 30 to 60 minutes (Boullata et al., 2017).	Allows for adequate absorption of medication and avoids potential drug–food interaction between medication and enteral feeding (Boullata et al., 2017).
16. Help patient to comfortable position and keep head of bed elevated for 1 hour (see agency policy).	Gives patient sense of well-being. Reduces risk of aspiration.
17. Dispose of soiled supplies, rinse graduated container and syringe with tap water, remove and dispose of gloves, and perform hand hygiene.	Reduces spread of microorganisms.
18. Be sure nurse call system is in an accessible location within patient's reach.	Ensures patient can call for assistance if needed.
19. Raise side rails (as appropriate) and lower bed to lowest position.	Ensures patient safety.

EVALUATION

1. Observe patient for signs of aspiration such as choking, gurgling, gurgling speech, breath sounds, and difficulty breathing.	Provides for prompt intervention if aspiration has occurred.
2. Return within 30 minutes to evaluate patient's response to medications.	Monitoring patient's response evaluates therapeutic benefit of drug and helps detect onset of side effects or allergic reactions.
3. **Use Teach-Back:** "I want to be sure I explained clearly why your father must take his medications through his feeding tube. Tell me why he is receiving his medications through his feeding tube." Revise your instruction now or develop a plan for revised patient/family caregiver teaching if patient/family caregiver is not able to teach back correctly.	Determines patient's/family caregiver's level of understanding of instructional topic.

Unexpected Outcomes	Related Interventions
1. Patient exhibits signs of aspiration, including respiratory distress, changes in vital signs, or changes in oxygen saturation.	• Stop all medications/fluids through feeding tube. • Elevate head of bed and stay with patient. Be prepared to provide airway suctioning. • Assess vital signs and breath sounds while another staff member notifies health care provider.
2. Patient does not receive medication because of blocked enteral tube.	• For newly inserted tube, notify health care provider and obtain x-ray film for confirmation of placement. • Requires interventions to unclog tube to ensure drug delivery (Box 23.2).
3. Patient exhibits adverse effects (side effect, toxic effect, allergic reaction).	• Withhold further doses. • Always notify health care provider and pharmacy when patient exhibits adverse effects. • Symptoms such as urticaria, rash, pruritus, rhinitis, and wheezing indicate allergic reaction. • Enter patient allergy in medical record.

BOX 23.2

Unclogging a Blocked Feeding Tube

- Prevent tube from becoming blocked by flushing it with at least 15 to 30 mL of tepid water before and after administering each dose of medication, 30 to 60 mL after last dose of medication, before and after checking gastric residual volumes, and every 4 to 12 hours around the clock (refer to agency policies).
- Gently flush tube with large-bore syringe and warm water. Do not use small-bore syringe because this exerts too much pressure and may rupture tube.
- If irrigation with water is not effective, obtain an order for a pancrelipase tablet and follow manufacturer guidelines for tube irrigation. In addition, a declogging stylus may be used (see agency policy).
- The tube may need to be removed, and a new one inserted, if the medication is urgent.

Modified from Boullata J et al: ASPEN safe practices for enteral nutrition therapy, *J Parenter Enteral Nutr* 41(1):15, 2017.

Recording

- Record in nurses' notes method used to check for tube placement, GRV, and pH of aspirate. Record drug, dose, route, and time administered immediately after administration, not before.
- Record patient teaching and validation of understanding.
- Record total amount of water used for medication administration.

Hand-Off Reporting

- Report adverse effects or patient response and withheld drugs to nurse in charge or health care provider.

✦ SKILL 23.3 Applying Topical Medications to the Skin

Purpose

Topical administration of medications involves applying drugs directly to skin, mucous membranes, or tissues. Topical drugs such as lotions, patches, pastes, and ointments primarily produce local effects, but they can also create systemic effects if absorbed through the skin. Systemic effects are more likely to occur if the skin is thin, drug concentration is high, contact with the skin is prolonged, or the drug is applied to broken skin. To protect from accidental exposure, apply topical drugs using gloves and applicators. Always cleanse the skin or a wound thoroughly before applying a dose of a topical drug. Apply each type of medication in the proper way to ensure penetration and absorption.

Delegation and Collaboration

The skill of administering most topical medications, including skin patches, cannot be delegated to nursing assistive personnel (NAP). However, some agencies (e.g., long-term care) may allow NAP to apply some forms of topical agents (e.g., skin barriers) to irritated skin or for the protection of the perineum during morning or perineal care. Check agency policies. The nurse instructs the NAP to:

- Report immediately to the nurse any skin irritation, burning, blistering, or increased itching.
- Not apply any dressing over the topical medication unless instructed to do so.

Equipment

- Clean gloves (for intact skin) or sterile gloves (for nonintact skin)
- *Option:* Cotton-tipped applicators or tongue blades
- Ordered medication (powder, cream, lotion, ointment, spray, patch)
- Basin of warm water, washcloth, towel, nondrying soap
- *Option:* Sterile dressing, tape
- Felt-tip pen
- Medication administration record (MAR; electronic or printed)
- *Option:* Plastic wrap, transparent dressing (if ordered)

ASSESSMENT

1. Check accuracy and completeness of each MAR or computer printout with health care provider's written medication order. Check patient's name, medication name and dosage, route of administration, and time of administration. Recopy or reprint any portion of MAR that is difficult to read. *Rationale: The order sheet is the most reliable source and only legal record of medications that patient is to receive. Ensures that patient receives the correct medications (Westbrook et al., 2017). Transcription errors are a source of medication errors (Truitt et al., 2016).*
2. Review pertinent information related to medication, including action, purpose, normal dose and route, side effects, time of onset and peak action, indication, and nursing implications. *Rationale: Allows you to anticipate effects of drug and observe patient's response.*
3. Perform hand hygiene. Assess condition of skin or membrane where medication is to be applied (see Chapter 8). If there is an open wound, perform hand hygiene and apply clean gloves. First wash site thoroughly with mild, nondrying soap and warm water, rinse, and dry. Be sure to remove any previously applied medication or debris. Also remove any blood, body fluids, secretions, or excretions. Assess for symptoms of skin irritation such as pruritus or burning. Remove gloves when finished. Perform hand hygiene. *Rationale: Cleaning site thoroughly promotes proper assessment of skin surface. Assessment provides baseline to determine change in condition of skin after therapy. Application of certain topical agents can lessen or aggravate these symptoms. Cleaning removes any residual medication from the previous dose, which reduces potential adverse medication reactions or skin irritation (Lilley et al., 2015).*
4. Assess patient's medical and medication history and history of allergies (including latex and topical agent). Ask if patient has had reaction to a cream or lotion applied to skin. List drug allergies on each page of the MAR and prominently display it on the patient's medical record per agency policy. When patient has allergy, provide allergy bracelet. *Rationale: Information reflects patient's need for and potential responses to medications. Allergic contact dermatitis is relatively common and can worsen dermatological (skin) conditions. In addition, some patients may be allergic to preservatives or fragrances in topical medications. Latex allergy requires use of nonlatex gloves. Communication of allergies is essential for safe and effective care.*
5. Determine amount of topical agent required for application by assessing skin site, reviewing health care provider's order, and reading application directions carefully (a thin, even layer is usually adequate). *Rationale: An excessive amount of topical agent can irritate skin chemically, negate effectiveness of drug, and/or cause adverse systemic effects such as decreased white blood cell (WBC) counts.*
6. Assess patient's or family caregiver's knowledge, experience, and health literacy. *Rationale: Ensures patient or family caregiver has the capacity to obtain, communicate, process, and understand basic health information (CDC, 2016).*
7. Assess patient's knowledge of purpose of medication being given, application schedule, and willingness to adhere to drug regimen. *Rationale: Reveals patient's level of understanding and whether instruction is necessary.*
8. Determine if patient or family caregiver is physically able to apply medication by assessing grasp, hand strength, reach, and coordination. *Rationale: Necessary if patient is to self-administer drug at home.*

STEP	RATIONALE
PLANNING	
1. Expected outcomes following completion of procedure:	
• Patient can identify drug and describe action, purpose, dose, side effects, indication and schedule of medication.	Demonstrates learning.
• Patient can apply medication without help on prescribed schedule.	Demonstrates learning and compliance.
• With repeated applications, skin becomes clear, without inflammation or drainage from lesions.	Existing lesions heal and/or disappear as result of therapeutic action of medication.
2. Provide privacy and prepare environment.	Providing privacy and preparing the environment promotes patient comfort and safe and efficient care.
3. Discuss purpose of each medication, action, and possible adverse effects. Allow patient to ask any questions.	Patient has right to be informed, and patient's understanding of each medication improves adherence to drug therapy. Helps minimize patient's anxiety.
IMPLEMENTATION	
1. Perform hand hygiene and prepare medication using aseptic technique (see Skill 23.1). Prepare medications for one patient at a time. Keep all pages of MARs or computer printouts for one patient together or look at only one patient's electronic MAR at a time. Select medication and check label of medication carefully with MAR or computer printout.	Ensures that medication is sterile. Preventing distractions reduces medication preparation errors. Use a no-interruption zone (NIZ) when possible (Prakash et al., 2014; Yoder et al., 2015). *This is the first check for accuracy* and ensures that correct medication is administered.
2. Before going to patient's room, compare patient's name and name of medication on label of prepared drugs with MAR a second time.	Reduces medication error. *This is the second check for accuracy*.
3. Take medication(s) to patient at correct time (see agency policy). Medications that require exact timing include STAT, first-time or loading doses, and one-time doses. Give time-critical scheduled medications (e.g., antibiotics, anticoagulants, insulin, anticonvulsants, immunosuppressive agents) at exact time ordered (no later than 30 minutes before or after scheduled dose). Give non–time-critical scheduled medications within a range of 1 or 2 hours of scheduled dose (ISMP, 2011). During administration, apply seven rights of medication administration.	Hospitals must adopt medication administration policy and procedure for timing of medication administration that considers nature of the prescribed medication, specific clinical application, and patient needs (DHHS, 2011; ISMP, 2011). Time-critical scheduled medications are those for which early or delayed administration of maintenance doses of greater than 30 minutes before or after the scheduled dose may cause harm or result in substantial suboptimal therapy or pharmacological effect. Non–time-critical medications are those for which early or delayed administration within a specified range of either 1 or 2 hours should not cause harm or result in substantial suboptimal therapy or pharmacological effect (DHHS, 2011; ISMP, 2011).
4. Help patient to comfortable position. Arrange supplies at bedside.	Allows easy access to application site.
5. Identify patient using at least two identifiers (e.g., name and birthday or name and medical record number) according to agency policy. Compare identifiers with information on patient's MAR or medical record.	Ensures correct patient. Complies with The Joint Commission standards and improves patient safety (TJC, 2019).
6. At patient's bedside, again compare MAR or computer printout with names of medications on medication labels and patient name. Ask patient if he or she has allergies.	*This is the third check for accuracy* and ensures that patient receives correct medication. Confirms patient's allergy history.
7. Perform hand hygiene. If skin is broken apply sterile gloves. Otherwise apply clean gloves.	Reduces spread of microorganisms.
8. Apply topical creams, ointments, and oil-based lotions.	
a. Expose affected area while keeping unaffected areas covered.	Provides visualization for application and protects privacy.
b. Wash, rinse, and dry affected area before applying medication if not done earlier (see Assessment, Step 3).	Cleaning removes microorganisms from remaining debris and any surface medication (Burcham and Rosenthal, 2016).
c. If skin is excessively dry and flaking, apply topical agent while skin is still damp.	Increased skin hydration and surface humidity enhance absorption of topical medication (Goldstein et al., 2017).

STEP	RATIONALE
d. After washing, remove gloves, perform hand hygiene, and apply new clean or sterile gloves.	Sterile gloves are used when applying agents to open, noninfectious skin lesions. Changing gloves prevents cross-contamination of infected or contagious lesions. Gloves also protect you from topical absorption of the medication and subsequent drug effects (Lilley et al., 2015).
e. Place required amount of medication in palm of gloved hand and soften by rubbing briskly between hands.	Softening topical agent makes it easier to spread on skin.
f. Tell patient that initial application of agent may feel cold. Once medication is softened, spread it evenly over skin surface, using long, even strokes that follow direction of hair growth. Do not vigorously rub skin. Apply to thickness specified by manufacturer instructions.	Ensures even distribution and sufficient dosage of medication. Technique prevents irritation of hair follicles.
g. Explain to patient that skin may feel greasy after application.	Ointments often contain oils.
9. Apply antianginal (nitroglycerin) ointment.	
a. Remove previous dose paper. Fold used paper containing any residual medication with used sides together and dispose of it in biohazard trash container. Wipe off residual medication with tissue.	Prevents overdose that can occur with multiple-dose papers left in place. Proper disposal protects you and others from accidental exposure to medication.
b. Write date, time, and your initials on new application paper.	Label provides reference to prevent missing doses.
c. Antianginal (nitroglycerin) ointments are usually ordered in inches and can be measured on small sheets of paper marked off in 1.25-cm (½-inch) markings. Unit-dose packages are available. Apply desired number of inches of ointment to paper-measuring guide (see illustration).	Ensures correct dose of medication.

Safe Patient Care *Unit-dose packages are available.* **NOTE:** *One package equals 2.5 cm (1 inch); smaller amounts should not be measured from this package.*

STEP	RATIONALE
d. Select new application site: Apply nitroglycerin to chest area, back, abdomen, or anterior thigh (Burchum and Rosenthal, 2016). Do not apply on nonintact skin or hairy surfaces or over scar tissue.	Application sites are rotated to reduce skin irritation. Application on nonintact skin may result in increased absorption of medication. Application on hairy surfaces or scar tissue may decrease absorption (Burchum and Rosenthal, 2016).
e. Apply ointment to skin surface by holding edge or back of paper-measuring guide and placing ointment and wrapper directly on skin (see illustration). Do not rub or massage ointment into skin.	Minimizes chance of ointment covering gloves and later touching nurse's hands. Medication is designed to absorb slowly over several hours; massaging increases absorption rate.

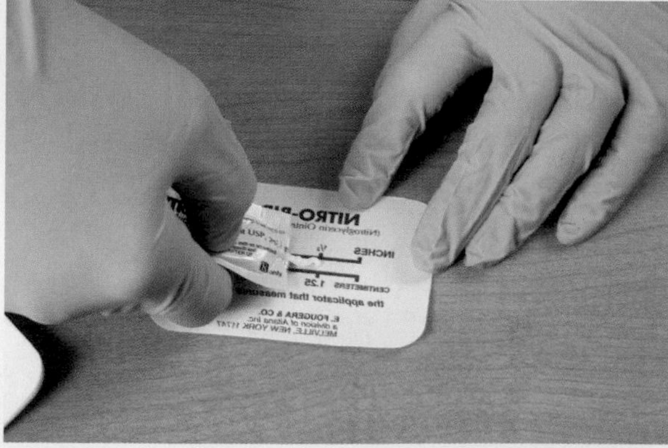

STEP 9c Ointment spread in inches over measuring guide.

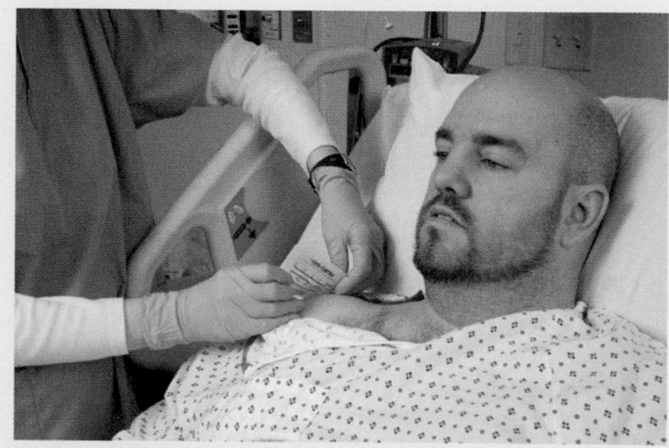

STEP 9e Nurse applies wrapper with medication to patient's skin.

STEP	RATIONALE
f. Secure ointment and paper with transparent dressing or strip of tape. Apply dressing or plastic wrap only when instructed by pharmacy (Lilley et al., 2015).	Prevents staining of clothing or inadvertent removal of medication. Covering topical medications with dressing or plastic wrap increases heat and skin humidity and rate of absorption of medication (Goldstein et al., 2017).
g. Explain to patient not to remove wrapper or dressing.	Ensures drug delivery.
10. Apply transdermal patches (e.g., analgesic, nicotine, nitroglycerin, estrogen).	
a. If old patch is present, remove it and clean area. Be sure to check between skinfolds for patch.	Failure to remove old patch can result in overdose. Many patches are small, clear, or flesh colored and can be easily hidden between skinfolds. Cleaning removes residual medication traces of previous patch.
b. Dispose of old patch by folding in half with sticky sides together. Some agencies require patch to be cut before disposal (see agency policy). Dispose of it in biohazard trash bag.	Proper disposal prevents accidental exposure to medication.
c. Date and initial outer side of new patch before applying it and note time of administration. Use soft-tip or felt-tip pen.	Visual reminder prevents missing or extra doses. Ballpoint pen damages patch and alters medication delivery.
d. Choose a new site that is clean, intact, dry, and free of hair. Some patches have specific instructions for placement locations (e.g., Testoderm patches are placed on scrotum; a scopolamine patch is placed behind the ear; *never apply* an estrogen patch to breast tissue or waistline). Do not apply patch on skin that is oily, burned, cut, or irritated in any way.	Ensures complete medication absorption. Estrogen patches should never be placed on the breast, genitals, or other reproductive organs. There is a risk for systemic absorption of the hormone, which can increase patient's risk for breast, testicular, or ovarian cancers (Lilley et al., 2015).
e. Carefully remove patch from its protective covering by pulling off liner. Hold patch by edge without touching adhesive edges.	Touching only edges ensures that patch will adhere and that medication dose has not changed. Removing protective covering allows medication to be absorbed through skin.
f. Apply patch. Hold palm of one hand firmly over patch for 10 seconds. Make sure that it sticks well, especially around edges. Apply overlay if provided with patch.	Adequate adhesion prevents loss of patch, which results in decreased dose and effectiveness.

Safe Patient Care *Never apply heat, such as with a heating pad, over a transdermal patch because this results in an increased rate of absorption, with potentially serious adverse effects (Lawton, 2013).*

STEP	RATIONALE
g. Do not apply patch to previously used sites for at least 1 week.	Rotation of site reduces skin irritation from medication and adhesive (Lilley et al., 2015).
h. Instruct patient that transdermal patches are never to be cut in half; a change in dose would require prescription for new strength of transdermal medication.	Cutting transdermal patch in half would alter intended medication delivery of transdermal system, resulting in inadequate or altered drug levels.

Safe Patient Care *It is recommended to have a daily "patch-free" interval of 10 to 12 hours because tolerance develops if patches are used every day for 24 hours a day (Burchum and Rosenthal, 2016). Apply a new patch each morning, leave in place for 12 to 14 hours, and remove in the evening.*

STEP	RATIONALE
i. Instruct patient to always remove old patch and clean skin before applying new one. Patients should not use alternative forms of medication when using patches. For example, patients should not apply nitroglycerin ointment in addition to patch unless specifically ordered to do so by their health care provider.	Use of patch with additional or alternative drug preparation can result in toxicity or other side effects.
11. Administer aerosol sprays (e.g., local anesthetic sprays).	
a. Shake container vigorously. Read container label for distance recommended to hold spray away from area, usually 15 to 30 cm (6 to 12 inches).	Mixing ensures delivery of fine, even spray. Proper distance ensures that fine spray hits skin surface. Holding container too close results in thin, watery distribution.
b. Ask patient to turn face away from spray or briefly cover face with towel while spraying neck or chest.	Prevents inhalation of spray.
c. Spray medication evenly over affected site (in some cases, time spray for a period of seconds).	Ensures that affected area of skin is covered with thin spray.

STEP	RATIONALE
12. Apply suspension-based lotion.	
a. Shake container vigorously.	Mixes powder throughout liquid to form well-mixed suspension.
b. Apply small amount of lotion to small gauze dressing or pad and apply to skin by stroking evenly in direction of hair growth.	Method of application leaves protective film of powder on skin after water base of suspension dries. Technique prevents irritation to hair follicles.
c. Explain to patient that area will feel cool and dry.	Water evaporates to leave thin layer of powder.
13. Apply powder.	
a. Be sure that skin surface is thoroughly dry. With your nondominant hand, fully spread apart any skinfolds, such as between toes or under axilla, and dry with towel.	Minimizes caking and crusting of powder. Fully exposes skin surface for application.
b. If area of application is near face, ask patient to turn face away from powder or briefly cover face with towel.	Prevents inhalation of powder.
c. Dust skin site lightly with dispenser so that area is covered with fine, thin layer of powder. *Option:* Cover skin area with dressing if ordered by health care provider.	Thin layer of powder has slight lubricating properties, which reduces friction and promotes drying (Burchum and Rosenthal, 2016).
14. Help patient to comfortable position, reapply gown, and cover with bed linen as desired.	Provides for patient's sense of well-being.
15. Raise side rails (as appropriate) and lower bed to lowest position.	Ensures patient safety.
16. Be sure nurse call system is in an accessible location within patient's reach.	Ensures patient can call for assistance if needed.
17. Dispose of soiled supplies in receptacle especially designated for such articles, remove and dispose of gloves, and perform hand hygiene.	Keeps patient's environment neat and reduces spread of infection and residual medication to others.

EVALUATION

STEP	RATIONALE
1. Inspect condition of skin between applications.	Determines if skin condition is improving or verifies that skin is intact and not irritated.
2. Have patient keep diary of doses taken.	Confirms adherence to prescribed therapy.
3. Observe patient or family caregiver apply topical medication.	Return demonstration measures learning.
4. **Use Teach-Back:** "I want to be sure I explained the action of the cortisone cream you are taking and its side effects. In your own words, tell me how the medication works, your correct dose, and any side effects." Revise your instruction now or develop a plan for revised patient/family caregiver teaching if patient/family caregiver is not able to teach back correctly.	Determines patient's/family caregiver's level of understanding of instructional topic.

Unexpected Outcomes	Related Interventions
1. Skin site appears inflamed and edematous with blistering and oozing of fluid from lesions. These signs indicate subacute inflammation or eczema that can develop if skin lesions are getting worse.	• Hold medication. • Notify health care provider; alternative therapies may be needed.
2. Patient is unable to explain information about drug or does not administer as prescribed.	• Identify possible reasons for noncompliance and explore alternative approaches or options.

Recording

- Record drug, dose or strength, site of application, and time administered immediately after administration, not before.
- Document your evaluation of patient learning.
- Describe condition of skin before each application.

Hand-Off Reporting

- Report adverse effects or changes in appearance and condition of skin lesions to health care provider.

✦ SKILL 23.4 Instilling Eye and Ear Medications

Purpose

Common eye (ophthalmic) medications are in the form of drops and ointments, including over-the-counter (OTC) preparations such as artificial tears and vasoconstrictors (e.g., Visine, Murine). Care must be taken to prevent instilling medication directly onto the cornea. The conjunctival sac is much less sensitive and a more appropriate site for medication instillation.

Many patients receive prescribed ophthalmic drugs for eye conditions such as glaucoma and eye infections and after cataract extraction. In addition, a third type of delivery system is the intraocular disk.

When administering ear medications, be aware of certain safety precautions. Internal ear structures are sensitive to temperature extremes; administer eardrops at room temperature. Administering cold eardrops can cause severe dizziness (vertigo) or nausea; either of these conditions can debilitate a patient for several minutes. Although the structures of the outer ear are not sterile, use sterile drops and solutions in case the eardrum is ruptured. A final safety precaution is to avoid forcing any solution into the ear.

Delegation and Collaboration

The skill of administering eye and ear medications cannot be delegated to nursing assistive personnel (NAP). The nurse instructs the NAP about:

- The specific potential side effects of medications and to report their occurrence.
- The potential for temporary burning or blurring of vision after administration of eye medications.
- The potential for dizziness or irritation after administration of ear medications.

Equipment

- Appropriate medication (eyedrops with sterile dropper, ointment tube, medicated intraocular disk, or eardrops)
- Clean gloves (for eyedrops and if ear has drainage)
- Medication administration record (MAR; electronic or printed)
- Eyedrops or ointment
- Cotton balls or facial tissue
- Warm water and washcloth
- Eye patch and tape *(optional)*
- Eardrops
- Cotton-tipped applicator, cotton balls

ASSESSMENT

1. Check accuracy and completeness of each MAR or computer printout with health care provider's written medication order. Check patient's name, medication name and dosage, route of administration, and time of administration. Recopy or reprint any portion of MAR that is difficult to read. *Rationale: The order sheet is the most reliable source and only legal record of medications that patient is to receive. Ensures that patient receives the correct medications (Westbrook et al., 2017). Transcription errors are a source of medication errors (Truitt et al., 2016).*
2. Review pertinent information related to medication, including action, purpose, normal dose and route, side effects, time of onset and peak action, indication, and nursing implications. *Rationale: Allows you to anticipate effects of drug and observe patient's response.*
3. Determine whether patient has any symptoms of discomfort of eye or ear or visual or hearing impairment. *Rationale: Certain medications act to either lessen or increase these symptoms.*
4. Assess patient's medical and medication history and history of allergies (including latex). List drug allergies on each page of the MAR and prominently display it on the patient's medical record per agency policy. When patient has allergy, provide allergy bracelet. *Rationale: Factors influence how certain drugs act. Reveals patient's need for and likely response to medication. Communication of allergies is essential for safe and effective care.*
5. Perform hand hygiene. Assess condition of external eye and ear structures (see Chapter 8). This may be done just before drug instillation (if drainage is present, apply clean gloves). *Rationale: Provides baseline to determine if local response to medications occurs. Also indicates need to clean eye or ear before drug application.*
6. Assess patient's level of consciousness (LOC) and ability to follow directions. *Rationale: If patient becomes restless or combative during procedure, greater risk for accidental eye injury exists.*
7. Assess patient's or family caregiver's knowledge, experience, and health literacy. *Rationale: Ensures patient or family caregiver has the capacity to obtain, communicate, process, and understand basic health information (CDC, 2016).*
8. Assess patient's knowledge regarding drug therapy and desire to self-administer medication. *Rationale: Indicates need for health teaching. Motivation influences teaching approach.*
9. Assess patient's ability to manipulate and hold dropper or ocular disk. *Rationale: Reflects patient's ability to learn to self-administer drug.*

STEP	RATIONALE
PLANNING	
1. Expected outcomes following completion of procedure:	
• Patient experiences desired effect of medication.	Drug is administered correctly without injury to patient.
• Patient denies discomfort.	Drug is administered correctly without injury to patient.
• Patient experiences no side effects, and symptoms (e.g., irritation) are relieved.	Drug is distributed and absorbed properly.

STEP	RATIONALE
• Patient can discuss information about medication and technique correctly.	Demonstrates learning.
• Patient demonstrates self-instillation of eyedrops or eardrops.	Demonstrates learning.
2. Provide privacy and prepare environment.	Providing privacy and preparing the environment promotes comfort and a safe and efficient procedure.
3. Discuss purpose of each medication, action, indication, and possible adverse effects. Allow patient to ask any questions. Tell patients receiving eyedrops (mydriatics) that vision will be blurred temporarily and that sensitivity to light may occur.	Patient has right to be informed, and patient's understanding of each medication improves adherence to drug therapy. Helps minimize patient's anxiety.

IMPLEMENTATION

STEP	RATIONALE
1. Perform hand hygiene and prepare medication using aseptic technique (see Skill 23.1). Prepare medications for one patient at a time. Keep all pages of MARs or computer printouts for one patient together or look at only one patient's electronic MAR at a time. Check label of medication carefully with MAR or computer printout when preparing medication. Preparation usually involves taking eyedrops or eardrops out of refrigerator and rewarming to room temperature before administering to patient. Check expiration date on container.	Ensures that medication is sterile. Preventing distractions reduces medication preparation errors. Use a no-interruption zone (NIZ) when possible (Prakash et al., 2014; Yoder et al., 2015). *This is the first check for accuracy* and ensures that correct medication is administered. Warming eyedrops reduces eye irritation. Ear structures are very sensitive to temperature extremes. Cold may cause vertigo and nausea.
2. Before going to patient's room, compare patient's name and name of medication on label of prepared drugs with MAR a second time.	Reduces medication error. *This is the second check for accuracy.*
3. Take medication(s) to patient at correct time (see agency policy). Medications that require exact timing include STAT, first-time or loading doses, and one-time doses. Give time-critical scheduled medications (e.g., antibiotics, anticoagulants, insulin, anticonvulsants, immunosuppressive agents) at exact time ordered (no later than 30 minutes before or after scheduled dose). Give non–time-critical scheduled medications within a range of 1 or 2 hours of scheduled dose (ISMP, 2011). During administration, apply seven rights of medication administration.	Hospitals must adopt medication administration policy and procedure for timing of medication administration that considers nature of the prescribed medication, specific clinical application, and patient needs (DHHS, 2011; ISMP, 2011). Time-critical scheduled medications are those for which early or delayed administration of maintenance doses of greater than 30 minutes before or after the scheduled dose may cause harm or result in substantial suboptimal therapy or pharmacological effect. Non–time-critical medications are those for which early or delayed administration within a specified range of either 1 or 2 hours should not cause harm or result in substantial suboptimal therapy or pharmacological effect (DHHS, 2011; ISMP, 2011).
4. Help patient to comfortable sitting position. Arrange supplies at bedside.	Ensures an organized procedure.
5. Identify patient using at least two identifiers (e.g., name and birthday or name and medical record number) according to agency policy. Compare identifiers with information on patient's MAR or medical record.	Ensures correct patient. Complies with The Joint Commission standards and improves patient safety (TJC, 2019).
6. At patient's bedside, again compare MAR or computer printout with names of medications on medication labels and patient name. Ask patient if he or she has allergies.	*This is the third check for accuracy* and ensures that patient receives correct medication. Confirms patient's allergy history.

Safe Patient Care *Instruct and reinforce that patient should not drive or operate machinery or perform any activity that requires clear vision until vision and sensitivity to light return to normal.*

STEP	RATIONALE
7. Administer eye medications.	
a. Perform hand hygiene and apply clean gloves. Ask patient to lie supine or sit back in chair with head slightly hyperextended, looking up.	Position provides easy access to eye for medication instillation and minimizes drainage of medication into tear duct.

Safe Patient Care *Do not hyperextend the neck of a patient with cervical spine injury.*

STEP	RATIONALE
b. If drainage or crusting is present along eyelid margins or inner canthus, gently wash away. Soak any dried crusts with warm, damp washcloth or cotton ball over eye for several minutes. Always wipe clean from inner to outer canthus (see illustration). Remove gloves and perform hand hygiene.	Soaking allows easy removal of crusts without applying pressure to eye. Cleaning from inner to outer canthus avoids entrance of microorganisms into lacrimal duct (Burchum and Rosenthal, 2016).
c. Explain that there might be temporary burning sensation from drops.	Corneas are highly sensitive.
d. Instill eyedrops.	
(1) Hold clean cotton ball or tissue in nondominant hand on patient's cheekbone just below lower eyelid.	Cotton or tissue absorbs medication that escapes eye.
(2) With tissue or cotton ball resting below lower lid, gently press downward with thumb or forefinger against bony orbit, exposing conjunctival sac. Never press directly against patient's eyeball.	Prevents pressure and trauma to eyeball and prevents fingers from touching eye.
(3) Ask patient to look at ceiling. Rest dominant hand on patient's forehead; hold filled medication eyedropper approximately 1 to 2 cm (¼ to ½ inch) above conjunctival sac.	Action moves cornea up and away from conjunctival sac and reduces blink reflex. Prevents accidental contact of eyedropper with eye and reduces risk of injury and transfer of microorganisms to dropper (ophthalmic medications are sterile).
(4) Drop prescribed number of drops into conjunctival sac (see illustration).	Conjunctival sac normally holds 1 or 2 drops. Provides even distribution of medication across eye.
(5) If patient blinks or closes eye, causing drops to land on outer lid margins, repeat procedure.	Therapeutic effect of drug is obtained only when drops enter conjunctival sac.
(6) When administering drops that may cause systemic effects, apply gentle pressure to patient's nasolacrimal duct with clean tissue for 30 to 60 seconds over each eye, one at a time (see illustration). Avoid pressure directly against patient's eyeball.	Prevents overflow of medication into nasal and pharyngeal passages. Prevents absorption into systemic circulation (Lilley et al., 2015).
(7) After instilling drops, ask patient to close eyes gently.	Helps distribute medication. Squinting or squeezing eyelids forces medication from conjunctival sac (Lilley et al., 2015).
e. Instill ophthalmic ointment.	
(1) Holding applicator above lower lid margin, apply thin ribbon of ointment evenly along inner edge of lower eyelid on conjunctiva (see illustration) from inner to outer canthus.	Distributes medication evenly across eye and lid margin.

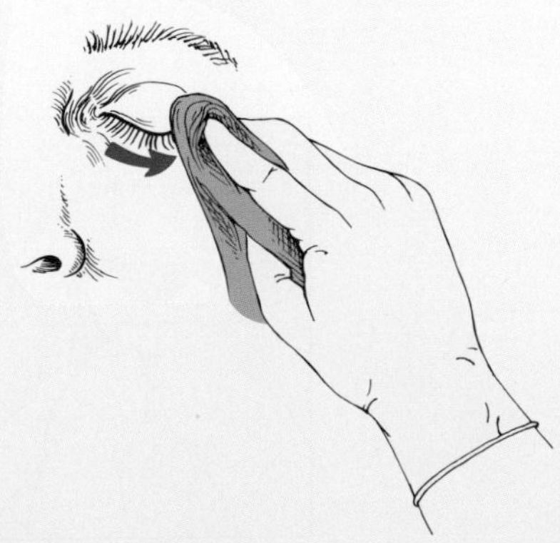

STEP 7b Clean eye, washing from inner to outer canthus, before administering drops or ointment.

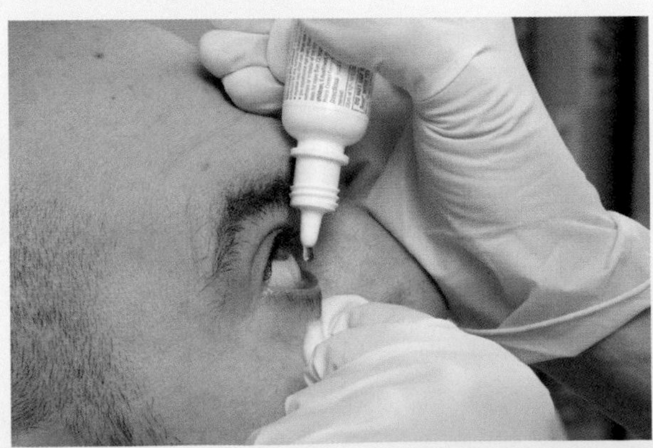

STEP 7d(4) Hold eyedropper over lower conjunctival sac.

STEP	RATIONALE
(2) Have patient close eye and rub lid lightly in circular motion with cotton ball if not contraindicated. Avoid placing pressure directly against patient's eyeball.	Further distributes medication without traumatizing eye.
(3) If excess medication is on eyelid, gently wipe it from inner to outer canthus.	Promotes comfort and prevents trauma to eye.
(4) If patient needs an eye patch, apply clean one by placing it over affected eye so that entire eye is covered. Tape securely without applying pressure to eye.	Clean eye patch reduces risk of infection.
f. Insert intraocular disk.	
(1) Open package containing disk. Gently press your fingertip against disk so that it adheres to your finger. It may be necessary to moisten gloved finger with sterile saline. Position convex side of disk on your fingertip.	Allows you to inspect disk for damage or deformity.
(2) With your other hand, gently pull patient's lower eyelid away from eye. Ask patient to look up.	Prepares conjunctival sac for receiving medicated disk and moves sensitive cornea away.
(3) Place disk in conjunctival sac so that it floats on sclera between iris and lower eyelid (see illustration).	Ensures delivery of medication.
(4) Pull patient's lower eyelid out and over disk (see illustration). You should not be able to see disk at this time. Repeat if you can see disk.	Ensures accurate medication delivery.
g. After administering eye medications, remove and dispose of gloves and soiled supplies; perform hand hygiene.	Reduces spread of microorganisms1

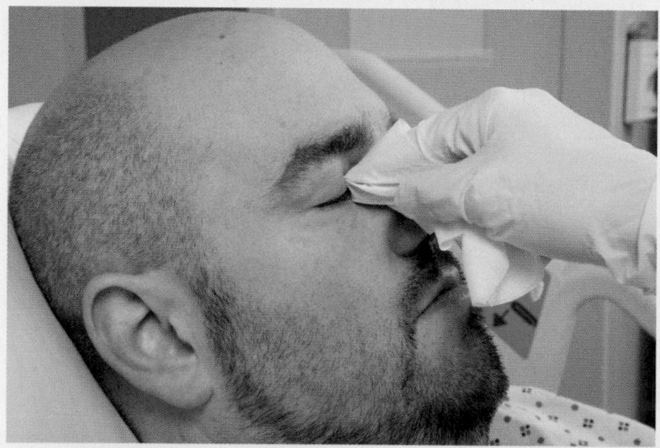

STEP 7d(6) Apply gentle pressure against nasolacrimal duct after giving eye medications.

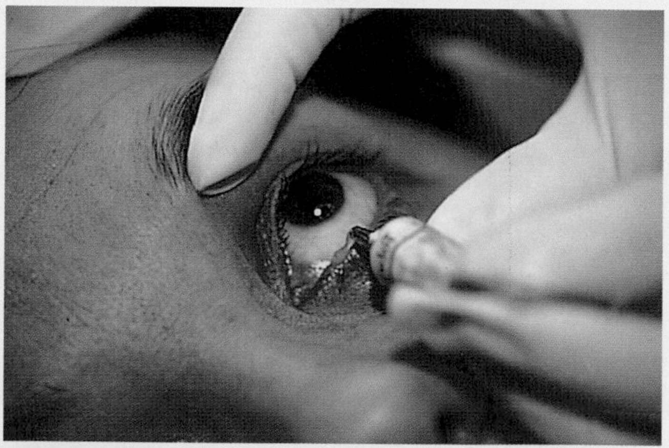

STEP 7e(1) Nurse applies ointment along inner edge of lower eyelid from inner to outer canthus.

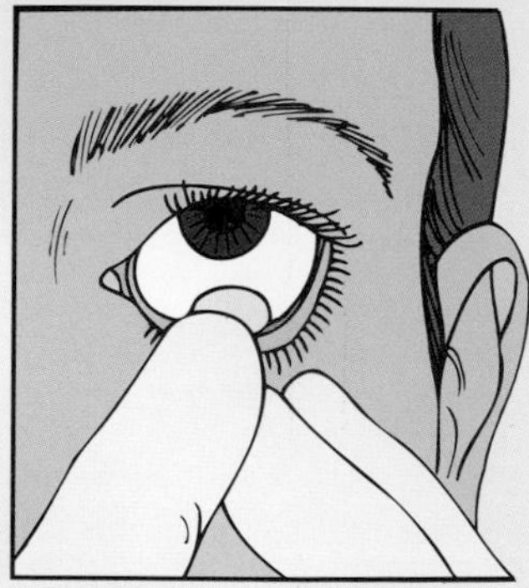

STEP 7f(3) Place intraocular disk in conjunctival sac between iris and lower eyelid.

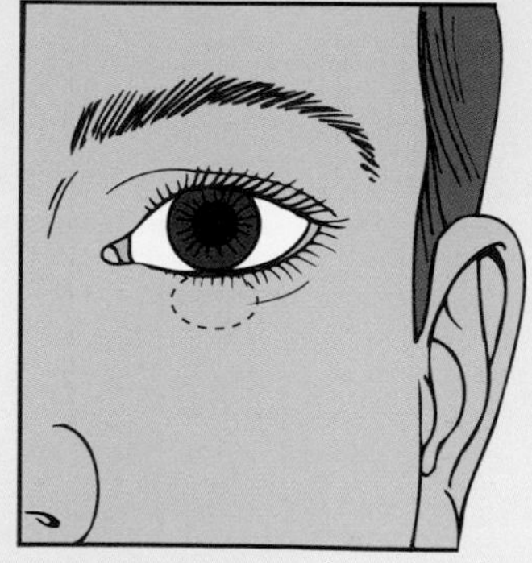

STEP 7f(4) Gently pull patient's lower eyelid over disk.

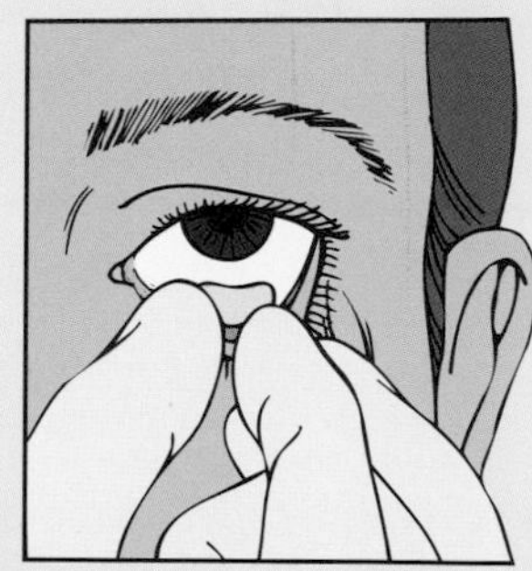

STEP 8b Carefully pinch disk to remove it from patient's eye.

STEP	RATIONALE
8. Remove intraocular disk.	
a. Perform hand hygiene and apply clean gloves. Gently pull downward on lower eyelid using your nondominant hand.	Exposes disk.
b. Using forefinger and thumb of your dominant hand, pinch disk and lift it out of patient's eye (see illustration). Remove and dispose of gloves and perform hand hygiene.	Technique avoids traumatizing eye tissue. Reduces transmission of infection.
9. Instill ear medications.	
a. Perform hand hygiene. Position patient on side (if not contraindicated) with ear to be treated facing up, or patient may sit in chair or at bedside. Stabilize patient's head with his or her own hand. *Option:* Apply clean gloves if ear drainage present.	Facilitates distribution of medication into ear.
b. Straighten ear canal by pulling pinna up and back to 10 o'clock position (adult or child older than age 3; see illustration) or down and back to 6 to 9 o'clock position (child under age 3).	Straightening ear canal provides direct access to deeper ear structures. Anatomical differences in younger children and infants necessitate different methods of positioning canal (Hockenberry and Wilson, 2017).
c. If cerumen or drainage occludes outermost part of ear canal, wipe out gently with cotton-tipped applicator (see illustration). Take care not to force cerumen into canal.	Cerumen and drainage harbor microorganisms and can block distribution of medication into canal. Occlusion blocks sound transmission.
d. Instill prescribed drops holding dropper 1 cm (½ inch) above ear canal.	Avoiding contact with external ear canal prevents contamination of dropper, which could contaminate medication in container.
e. Ask patient to remain in side-lying position for a few minutes. Apply gentle massage or pressure to tragus of ear with finger (see illustration).	Allows complete distribution of medication. Pressure and massage move medication inward.
f. If ordered, gently insert part of cotton ball into outermost part of canal. Do not press cotton into canal.	Prevents escape of medication when patient sits or stands.
g. Remove cotton after 15 minutes. Help patient to comfortable position after drops are absorbed.	Allows time for drug distribution and absorption.
h. After administering ear drops, dispose of soiled supplies, remove and dispose of gloves, and perform hand hygiene.	Reduces transmission of infection.
10. Help patient to comfortable position.	Gives patient sense of well-being.
11. Be sure nurse call system is in an accessible location within patient's reach.	Ensures patient can call for assistance if needed.
12. Raise side rails (as appropriate) and lower bed to lowest position.	Ensures patient safety.

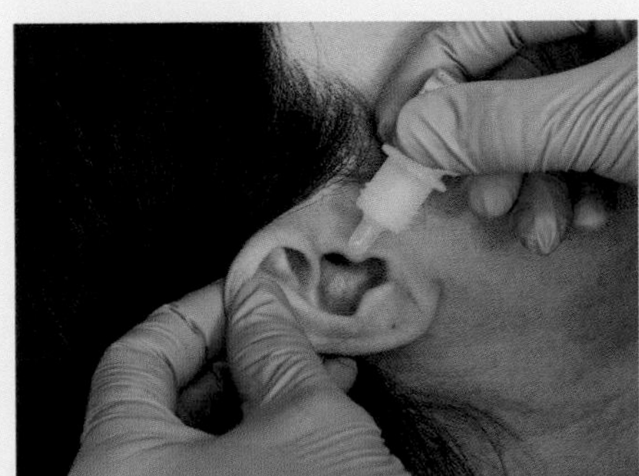

STEP 9b Pull pinna up and back for adults and children older than 3 years.

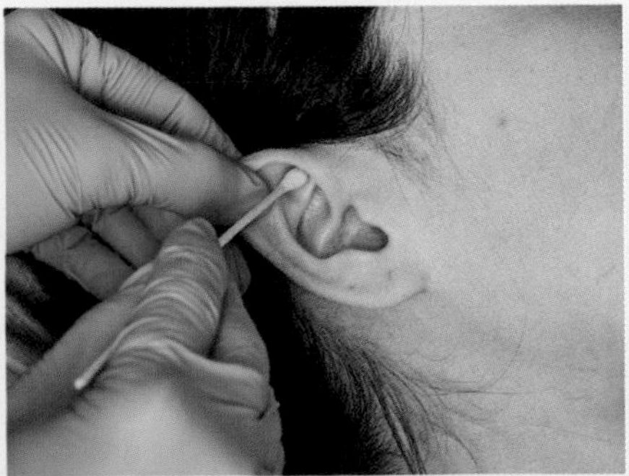

STEP 9c Always clean only outer canal. Do not push cerumen or secretions into ear.

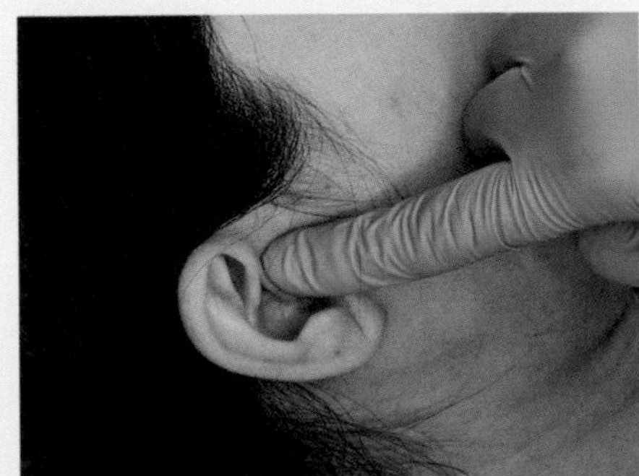

STEP 9e Nurse applies gentle pressure to tragus of ear after instilling drops.

STEP	RATIONALE
EVALUATION	
1. Observe response to medication by assessing visual or hearing changes, asking if symptoms are relieved, and noting any side effects or discomfort felt.	Evaluates effects of medication.
2. Ask patient to discuss purpose of drug, indication, action, side effects, and technique of administration.	Determines patient's level of understanding.
3. **Use Teach-Back:** "I want to be sure I showed you how to insert the intraocular disk. Show me how to insert it into your left eye." Revise your instruction now or develop a plan for revised patient/family caregiver teaching if patient/family caregiver is not able to teach back correctly.	Determines patient's/family caregiver's level of understanding of instructional topic.

Unexpected Outcomes	Related Interventions
1. Patient complains of burning or pain in eye or experiences local side effects (e.g., headache, bloodshot eyes, local eye irritation). Drug concentration and patient's sensitivity both influence chances of side effects developing.	• Eyedrops may have been instilled onto cornea, or dropper touched surface of eye. • Notify health care provider for possible adjustment in medication type and dosage.
2. Patient experiences systemic effects from eyedrops (e.g., increased heart rate and blood pressure from epinephrine, decreased heart rate and blood pressure from timolol).	• Notify health care provider immediately. • Remain with patient. Assess vital signs. • Withhold further doses.
3. Ear canal remains inflamed, swollen, or tender to palpation. Drainage is present.	• Hold next dose. • Notify health care provider for possible adjustment in medication type and dosage.

Recording

- Record drug, dose or strength, site of application (e.g., right eye or ear, left eye or ear, both), and time administered immediately after administration, not before.
- Document your evaluation of patient learning.
- Record objective data related to condition of tissues involved (e.g., redness, drainage, irritation), any subjective data (e.g., pain, itching, altered vision or hearing), and patient's response to medications. Note evidence of any side effects.

Hand-Off Reporting

- Report any side effects or continued complaints of visual or hearing deficits to nurse in charge or health care provider.

✦ SKILL 23.5 Using Metered-Dose Inhalers

Purpose

Medications administered with handheld inhalers are dispersed through an aerosol spray, mist, or powder that penetrates the airways. Pressurized metered-dose inhalers (pMDIs; Fig. 23.3), breath-actuated metered-dose inhalers (BAIs) such as Respiclick®, and dry powder inhalers (DPIs) deliver medications that produce local effects, such as bronchodilation. Some of these medications are absorbed rapidly through the pulmonary circulation and create systemic side effects; for example, albuterol may cause palpitations, tremors, or tachycardia. Patients who receive drugs by inhalation frequently have chronic respiratory disease. Because they depend on these medications for disease control, they must learn about them and how to administer them safely. Small-volume nebulizers (see Skill 23.6) are devices that also deliver inhaled medications. Box 23.3 summarizes common problems that occur when using an inhaler.

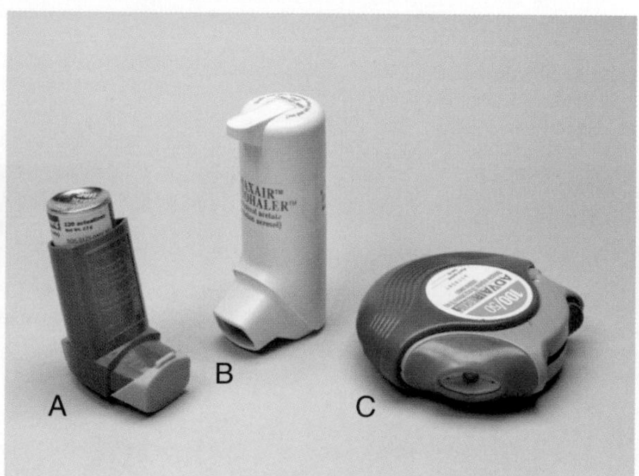

FIG 23.3 Types of inhalers. (A) Metered-dose inhaler (MDI). (B) Breath-actuated metered-dose inhaler (BAI). (C) Dry powder inhaler (DPI). *(From Lilley LL et al: Pharmacology and the nursing process, ed 8, St. Louis, 2015, Mosby.)*

Delegation and Collaboration

The skill of administering MDIs cannot be delegated to nursing assistive personnel (NAP). The nurse instructs the NAP about:

BOX 23.3

Common Problems When Using an Inhaler

- *Not taking medication as prescribed:* Either too much or too little is taken.
- *Incorrect activation:* This usually occurs through pressing the canister before taking a breath. Both actions should be done simultaneously so that the drug can be carried down to the lungs with the breath.
- *Forgetting to shake the inhaler:* The drug is in a suspension, and particles may settle. If the inhaler is not shaken, it may not deliver the correct dose of the drug.
- *Not waiting long enough between puffs:* The process of inhalation should be repeated when taking the second puff; otherwise, an incorrect dose may be delivered, or the drug may not penetrate into the lungs.
- *Failure to clean the valve:* Particles may jam the valve in the mouthpiece unless it is cleaned occasionally. This is a frequent cause of failure to get 200 puffs from one inhaler.
- *Failure to observe whether the inhaler is actually releasing a spray:* If it is not, this should be checked with the pharmacist.
- *Failure to recognize when the canister is empty.* This occurs when a metered-dose inhaler (MDI) has no built-in dose counter or instructions for dose counting.

- Potential side effects of medications and to report their occurrence to the nurse.
- Reporting breathing difficulty (e.g., paroxysmal or sustained coughing, audible wheezing) to the nurse.

Equipment

- Inhaler device with medication canister (MDI or DPI; see Fig. 23.3)
- Spacer device such as AeroChamber or Inspirease *(optional)*
- Facial tissues *(optional)*
- Medication administration record (MAR; electronic or printed)
- Stethoscope and peak flow device
- Pulse oximeter *(optional)*

ASSESSMENT

1. Check accuracy and completeness of each MAR or computer printout with health care provider's written medication order. Check patient's name, medication name and dosage, route of administration, and time of administration. Recopy or reprint any portion of MAR that is difficult to read. *Rationale: The order sheet is the most reliable source and only legal record of medications that patient is to receive. Ensures that patient receives the correct medications (Westbrook et al., 2017). Transcription errors are a source of medication errors (Truitt et al., 2016).*
2. Review pertinent information related to medication, including action, purpose, normal dose and route, side effects, time of onset and peak action, indication, and nursing implications. *Rationale: Allows you to anticipate effects of drug and observe patient's response.*
3. Assess patient's medical and medication history and history of allergies. List drug allergies on each page of the MAR and prominently display it on the patient's medical record per agency policy. When patient has an allergy, provide allergy bracelet. *Rationale: Factors influence how certain drugs act. Reveals patient's need for medication. Communication of allergies is essential for safe and effective care.*
4. Perform hand hygiene. Assess respiratory pattern and auscultate breath sounds (see Chapter 8). Also assess exercise tolerance and peak flow rate (see Chapter 16); does patient develop shortness of breath easily? *Rationale: Establishes baseline of airway status for comparison during and after treatment.*
5. Assess patient's ability to hold, manipulate, and depress canister and inhaler. *Rationale: Any impairment of grasp or presence of hand tremors interferes with patient's ability to depress canister within inhaler. Spacer device is often necessary.*
6. Assess patient's or family caregiver's knowledge, experience, and health literacy. *Rationale: Ensures patient or family caregiver has the capacity to obtain, communicate, process, and understand basic health information (CDC, 2016).*
7. If patient was previously instructed in self-administration, have him or her demonstrate how to use the device. *Rationale: Often patients who have adequate understanding of how to use an inhaler forget the procedure. Ongoing assessment of inhaler technique identifies areas for further education and reinforcement (Ari, 2015).*

STEP	RATIONALE
PLANNING	
1. Expected outcomes following completion of procedure:	
• Patient correctly self-administers a metered dose.	Demonstrates learning.
• Patient describes proper time during respiratory cycle to inhale and spray and number of inhalations for each administration.	Demonstrates learning and ensures correct administration of medication.
• Patient's breathing pattern improves, and lung sounds indicate that airways are less restrictive.	Demonstrates therapeutic effect of medication in improving gas exchange.
2. Provide privacy and prepare environment.	Providing privacy and preparing the environment promotes patient comfort and a safe and efficient procedure.
3. Discuss purpose of each medication, indication, action, and possible adverse effects. Allow patient to ask any questions.	Patient has right to be informed, and patient's understanding of each medication improves adherence to drug therapy. Helps minimize patient's anxiety.

STEP	RATIONALE

IMPLEMENTATION

STEP	RATIONALE
1. Perform hand hygiene and prepare medication using aseptic technique (see Skill 23.1). Prepare medications for one patient at a time. Keep all pages of MARs or computer printouts for one patient together or look at only one patient's electronic MAR at a time. Check label of medication carefully with MAR or computer printout when preparing medication.	Ensures that medication is sterile. Preventing distractions reduces medication preparation errors. Use a no-interruption zone (NIZ) when possible (Prakash et al., 2014; Yoder et al., 2015). *This is the first check for accuracy* and ensures that correct medication is administered.
2. Before going to patient's room, compare patient's name and name of medication on label of prepared drugs with MAR a second time.	Reduces medication error. *This is the second check for accuracy.*
3. Take medication(s) to patient at correct time (see agency policy). Medications that require exact timing include STAT, first-time or loading doses, and one-time doses. Give time-critical scheduled medications (e.g., antibiotics, anticoagulants, insulin, anticonvulsants, immunosuppressive agents) at exact time ordered (no later than 30 minutes before or after scheduled dose). Give non–time-critical scheduled medications within a range of 1 or 2 hours of scheduled dose (ISMP, 2011). During administration, apply seven rights of medication administration.	Hospitals must adopt medication administration policy and procedure for timing of medication administration that considers nature of the prescribed medication, specific clinical application, and patient needs (DHHS, 2011; ISMP, 2011). Time-critical scheduled medications are those for which early or delayed administration of maintenance doses of greater than 30 minutes before or after the scheduled dose may cause harm or result in substantial suboptimal therapy or pharmacological effect. Non–time-critical medications are those for which early or delayed administration within a specified range of either 1 or 2 hours should not cause harm or result in substantial suboptimal therapy or pharmacological effect (DHHS, 2011; ISMP, 2011).
4. Identify patient using at least two identifiers (e.g., name and birthday or name and medical record number) according to agency policy. Compare identifiers with information on patient's MAR or medical record.	Ensures correct patient. Complies with The Joint Commission standards and improves patient safety (TJC, 2019).
5. At patient's bedside, again compare MAR or computer printout with names of medications on medication labels and patient name. Ask patient if he or she has allergies.	*This is the third check for accuracy* and ensures that patient receives correct medication. Confirms patient's allergy history.
6. Allow adequate time for patient to manipulate inhaler, canister, and spacer device (if provided). Explain and demonstrate how canister fits into inhaler.	Patient must be familiar with how to use equipment.

Safe Patient Care *If using an MDI that is new or has not been used for several days, push a "test spray" into the air to prime the device before using. This ensures that the MDI is patent and the metal canister is positioned properly.*

STEP	RATIONALE
7. Explain and demonstrate steps for administering MDI without spacer.	Simple one-on-one instruction and demonstration of step-by-step administration allows patient to ask questions at any point during procedure and increases patient adherence to inhaler use (Ari, 2015).
a. Remove mouthpiece cover from inhaler after inserting MDI canister into holder.	
b. Shake inhaler well for 2 to 5 seconds (five or six shakes).	Ensures mixing of medication in canister.
c. Hold inhaler in dominant hand.	
d. Have patient stand or sit and instruct him or her to position inhaler in one of two ways:	
(1) Have patient place the mouthpiece in the mouth between the teeth and over the tongue, aimed toward back of throat, with lips closed tightly around it. Do not block the mouthpiece with the teeth or tongue (see illustration).	Ensures proper fit to inhale medication.
(2) Position mouthpiece 2 to 4 cm (1 to 2 inches) in front of widely opened mouth (see illustration), with opening of inhaler toward back of throat. Lips should not touch inhaler.	Directs aerosol spray toward airway. This is best way to deliver medication without a spacer.

STEP	RATIONALE
e. While holding the mouthpiece either in or away from the mouth, have patient take deep breath and exhale completely.	Empties lung volume and prepares airway to receive medication.
f. With inhaler positioned, have patient hold it with thumb at mouthpiece and index and middle fingers at top. This is a three-point or bilateral hand position.	Hand position ensures proper activation of MDI and distribution of dosage (Burchum and Rosenthal, 2016).
g. Instruct patient to tilt head back slightly and inhale slowly and deeply through mouth for 3 to 5 seconds while depressing canister fully.	Medication is distributed to airways during inhalation.
h. Have patient hold breath for about 10 seconds.	Allows tiny drops of aerosol spray to reach deeper branches of airways.
i. Remove MDI from mouth before exhaling and exhale slowly through nose or pursed lips.	Keeps small airways open during exhalation.
8. Explain and demonstrate steps to administer MDI using spacer device.	Simple one-on-one instruction and demonstration of step-by-step administration allows patient to ask questions at any point during procedure and increases patient adherence to inhaler use (Ari, 2015).
a. Remove mouthpiece cover from MDI and mouthpiece of spacer device.	Inhaler fits into end of spacer device.
b. Shake inhaler well for 2 to 5 seconds (five or six shakes).	Ensures mixing of medication in canister.
c. Insert MDI into end of spacer device.	Spacer device traps medication released from MDI; patient then inhales drug from device. These devices improve delivery of correct dose of inhaled medication.
d. Instruct patient to place spacer device mouthpiece in mouth and close lips. Do not insert beyond raised lip on mouthpiece. Avoid covering small exhalation slots with lips.	Medication should not escape through mouth.
e. Have patient breathe normally through spacer device mouthpiece (see illustration).	Allows patient to relax before delivering medication.
f. Instruct patient to depress medication canister, spraying one puff into spacer device.	Device contains fine spray and allows patient to inhale more medication. The spacer increases drug delivery and deposition of the medication on the oropharyngeal mucosa (Burchum and Rosenthal, 2016).
g. Patient breathes in slowly and fully (for 5 seconds).	Ensures that particles of medication are distributed to deeper airways.
h. Instruct patient to hold full breath for 10 seconds.	Ensures full drug distribution.

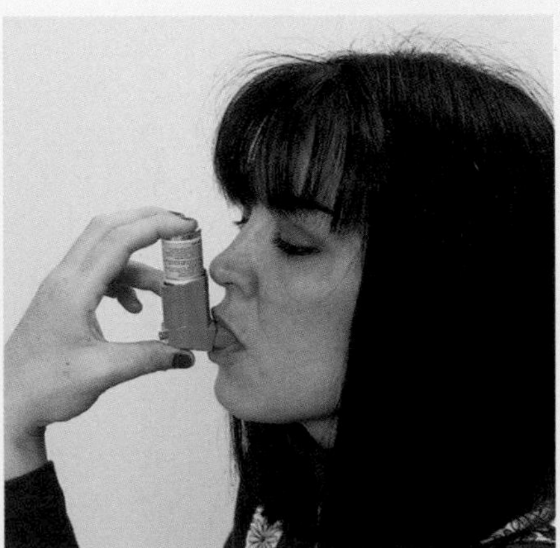

STEP 7d(1) Patient opens lips and places inhaler mouthpiece in mouth with opening toward back of throat.

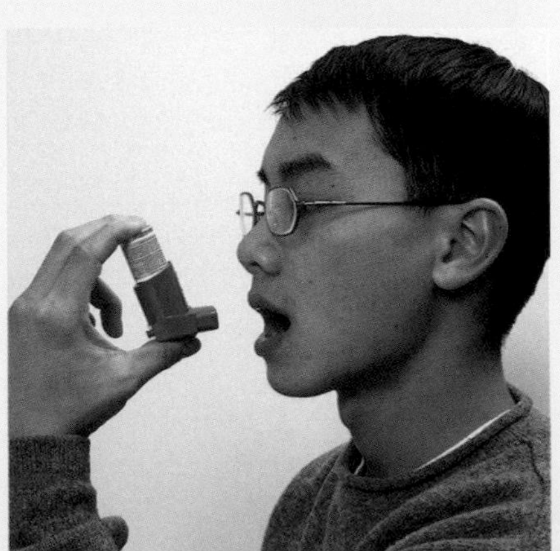

STEP 7d(2) Patient positions inhaler mouthpiece 2 to 4 cm (1 to 2 inches) from widely open mouth. This is considered the best way to deliver medication without a spacer.

STEP	RATIONALE

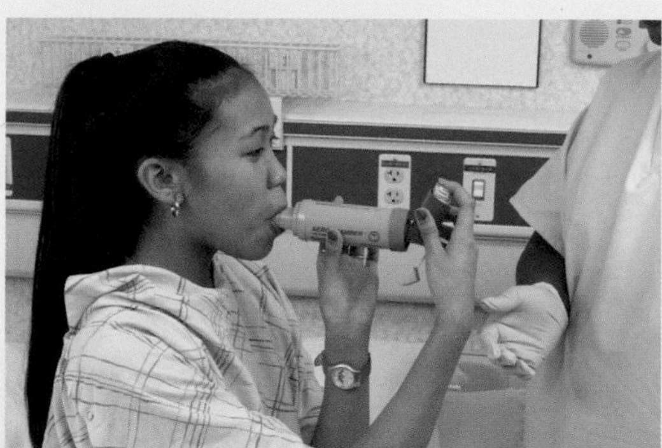

STEP 8e Using spacer device with a metered-dose inhaler (MDI).

STEP	RATIONALE
9. Explain steps to administer DPI or BAI (demonstrate when possible).	
a. Remove mouthpiece cover. Do not shake inhaler.	
b. Prepare medication as directed by manufacturer (e.g., hold inhaler upright and turn wheel to the right and then to the left until a click is heard; load medication pellet).	Primes inhaler, ensuring medication is delivered correctly.
c. Exhale away from inhaler.	Prevents loss of powder.
d. Position mouthpiece between lips.	Keeps medication from escaping through mouth.
e. Inhale deeply and forcefully through mouth.	Creates an aerosol.
f. Hold full breath for 5 to 10 seconds.	Allows medication distribution.
10. Instruct patient to wait 20 to 30 seconds between inhalations (if same medication) or 2 to 5 minutes between inhalations (if different medications).	Drugs must be inhaled sequentially. Always administer bronchodilators before steroids so that dilators can open airway passages (Burchum and Rosenthal, 2016).
11. Instruct patient to not repeat inhalations before next scheduled dose.	Drugs are prescribed at intervals during day to provide constant drug levels and minimize side effects. Beta-adrenergic MDIs are used either on an "as needed" basis or regularly every 4 to 6 hours.
12. Warn patients that they may feel gagging sensation in throat caused by droplets of medication on pharynx or tongue.	This occurs when medication is sprayed and inhaled incorrectly.
13. About 2 minutes after last dose, instruct patient to rinse mouth with warm water and spit water out.	Steroids may alter normal flora of oral mucosa and lead to development of fungal infection. Rinsing out patient's mouth reduces risk of fungal infection (Ari, 2015).
14. Clean the MDI.	Removes residual medication and reduces spread of microorganisms.
a. For daily cleaning, instruct patient to remove medication canister, rinse inhaler and cap with warm running water, and be sure that inhaler is completely dry before reuse. Do not get valve mechanism of canister wet.	Water damages valve mechanism of canister.
b. Instruct patient to clean mouthpiece twice a week with a mild dishwashing soap, rinse thoroughly, and dry completely before storage.	
15. Help patient to comfortable position.	Gives patient sense of well-being.
16. Be sure nurse call system is in an accessible location within patient's reach.	Ensures patient can call for assistance if needed.
17. Raise side rails (as appropriate) and lower bed to lowest position.	Ensures patient safety.
18. Remove and dispose of gloves and perform hand hygiene.	Reduces transmission of microorganisms.

EVALUATION

STEP	RATIONALE
1. Auscultate patient lungs, listen for abnormal breath sounds, and obtain peak flow measures if ordered.	Determines patient response to medication.
2. Have patient explain and demonstrate steps in use and cleaning of inhaler.	Return demonstration provides feedback for measuring patient's learning.

STEP	RATIONALE
3. Ask patient to explain drug schedule and dose of medication.	Improves likelihood of adherence to therapy.
4. Ask patient to describe side effects of medication and criteria for calling health care provider.	Allows patient to recognize signs of overuse and need to seek medical support when drugs are ineffective.
5. **Use Teach-Back:** "I want to be sure I clearly showed you how to use your inhaler. Let's take this time; show me how you will use the inhaler to take your medicine." Revise your instruction now or develop a plan for revised patient/family caregiver teaching if patient/family caregiver is not able to teach back correctly.	Determines patient's/family caregiver's level of understanding of instructional topic.

Unexpected Outcomes	Related Interventions
1. Patient's respirations are rapid and shallow; breath sounds indicate wheezing; patient reports no relief from shortness of breath.	• Evaluate vital signs and respiratory status. • Notify health care provider. • Reassess type of medication and/or delivery method.
2. Patient experiences cardiac dysrhythmias (light-headedness, syncope), especially if receiving beta-adrenergic medications.	• Withhold all further doses of medication. • Evaluate cardiac and pulmonary status (see Chapter 8). • Notify health care provider for reassessment of type of medication and delivery method.

Recording

- Record drug, dose or strength, number of inhalations, and time administered immediately after administration, not before. Include initials or signature.
- Document your evaluation of patient learning.
- Record patient's response to MDI (e.g., respiratory rate and pattern, breath sounds), evidence of side effects (e.g., arrhythmia, patient's feelings of anxiety), and patient's ability to use MDI.

Hand-Off Reporting

- Report any side effects of medication to health care provider.

✦ SKILL 23.6 Using Small-Volume Nebulizers

Purpose

Nebulization is a process of adding medications or moisture to inspired air by mixing particles of various sizes with air. Adding moisture to the respiratory system through nebulization improves clearance of pulmonary secretions. Medications such as bronchodilators, mucolytics, and corticosteroids are often administered by nebulization. Small-volume nebulizers are machines that convert a drug solution into a mist that a patient then inhales into the tracheobronchial tree. The droplets in the mist are much finer than the droplets created by inhalers. Inhalation of the nebulized mist is delivered via face mask or a mouthpiece held between the teeth. A nebulized medication is designed to create a local effect, but it can be absorbed into the bloodstream through the alveoli. As a result, systemic effects from the medications may occur.

Delegation and Collaboration

In many health care agencies, a respiratory therapist performs the skill of administering medications by nebulizer. The nurse must be aware of the type and actions of the inhaled medication that the patient is receiving. The skill of administering medications by nebulizer cannot be delegated to nursing assistive personnel (NAP). The nurse instructs the NAP about:

- Potential side effects of medications and to report their occurrence to the nurse.
- Reporting paroxysmal coughing, ineffective breathing patterns, and other respiratory difficulties to the nurse.

Equipment

- Medication ordered and diluent (if needed)
- Medicine dropper or syringe
- Nebulizer bottle and tubing assembly
- Small-volume nebulizer machine (often called handheld nebulizer or simply nebulizer)
- Pulse oximeter and peak flow device
- Stethoscope
- Medication administration record (MAR; electronic or printed)
- Clean gloves

ASSESSMENT

1. Check accuracy and completeness of each MAR or computer printout with health care provider's written medication order. Check patient's name, medication name and dosage, route of administration, and time of administration. Recopy or reprint any portion of MAR that is difficult to read. *Rationale: The order sheet is the most reliable source and only legal record of medications that patient is to receive. Ensures that patient receives the correct medications (Westbrook et al., 2017). Transcription errors are a source of medication errors (Truitt et al., 2016).*
2. Review pertinent information related to medication, including action, purpose, normal dose and route, side effects, time of onset and peak action, indication and nursing

implications. *Rationale: Allows you to anticipate effects of drug and observe patient's response.*

3. Assess patient's medical and medication history and history of allergies. List drug allergies on each page of the MAR and prominently display it on the patient's medical record per agency policy. When patient has allergy, provide allergy bracelet. *Rationale: These factors influence how certain drugs act. Information also reflects patient's need for medications and risk for side effects. Communication of allergies is essential for safe and effective care.*
4. Assess patient's grasp and ability to assemble, hold, and manipulate nebulizer mouthpiece and tubing. *Rationale: Any impairment of cognition or grasp or the presence of hand tremors affects patient's ability to use equipment.*
5. Perform hand hygiene. Assess pulse, respirations, breath sounds, pulse oximetry, and peak flow measurement (if ordered) before beginning treatment. *Rationale: Establishes baseline for comparison during and after treatment.*
6. Assess patient's or family caregiver's knowledge, experience, and health literacy. *Rationale: Ensures patient or family caregiver has the capacity to obtain, communicate, process, and understand basic health information (CDC, 2016).*
7. If patient was previously instructed in self-administration, have him or her demonstrate how to use device. *Rationale: Determines level of understanding and whether additional instruction is needed.*

STEP	RATIONALE
PLANNING	
1. Expected outcomes following completion of procedure:	
• Patient's breathing pattern and peak flow rate are effective.	Demonstrates therapeutic effect of medication.
• Patient's oxygen saturation level is adequate.	Demonstrates therapeutic effect of medication.
• Patient describes side effects of medication and criteria for calling health care provider (e.g., low peak flow rate).	Increases likelihood of adherence to therapeutic regimen.
• Patient demonstrates self-administration of nebulized dose of medication correctly.	Demonstrates proper administration of medication and documents learning.
2. Provide privacy and prepare environment.	Providing privacy and preparing the environment promotes patient comfort and ensures a safe and efficient procedure.
3. Discuss purpose of each medication, indication, action, and possible adverse effects. Allow patient to ask any questions.	Patient has right to be informed, and patient's understanding of each medication improves adherence to drug therapy. Helps minimize patient's anxiety.
IMPLEMENTATION	
1. Perform hand hygiene and prepare medication using aseptic technique (see Skill 23.1). Prepare medications for one patient at a time. Keep all pages of MARs or computer printouts for one patient together or look at only one patient's electronic MAR at a time. Check label of medication carefully with MAR or computer printout when preparing medication.	Ensures that medication is sterile. Preventing distractions reduces medication preparation errors. Use a no-interruption zone (NIZ) when possible (Prakash et al., 2014; Yoder et al., 2015). *This is the first check for accuracy* and ensures that correct medication is administered.
2. Before going to patient's room, compare patient's name and name of medication on label of prepared drugs with MAR a second time.	Reduces medication error. *This is the second check for accuracy.*
3. Take medication(s) to patient at correct time (see agency policy). Medications that require exact timing include STAT, first-time or loading doses, and one-time doses. Give time-critical scheduled medications (e.g., antibiotics, anticoagulants, insulin, anticonvulsants, immunosuppressive agents) at exact time ordered (no later than 30 minutes before or after scheduled dose). Give non–time-critical scheduled medications within a range of 1 or 2 hours of scheduled dose (ISMP, 2011). During administration, apply seven rights of medication administration.	Hospitals must adopt medication administration policy and procedure for timing of medication administration that considers nature of the prescribed medication, specific clinical application, and patient needs (DHHS, 2011; ISMP, 2011). Time-critical scheduled medications are those for which early or delayed administration of maintenance doses of greater than 30 minutes before or after the scheduled dose may cause harm or result in substantial suboptimal therapy or pharmacological effect. Non–time-critical medications are those for which early or delayed administration within a specified range of either 1 or 2 hours should not cause harm or result in substantial suboptimal therapy or pharmacological effect (DHHS, 2011; ISMP, 2011).
4. Identify patient using at least two identifiers (e.g., name and birthday or name and medical record number) according to agency policy. Compare identifiers with information on patient's MAR or medical record.	Ensures correct patient. Complies with The Joint Commission standards and improves patient safety (TJC, 2019).

STEP	RATIONALE
5. At patient's bedside, again compare MAR or computer printout with names of medications on medication labels and patient name. Ask patient if he or she has allergies.	*This is the third check for accuracy* and ensures that patient receives correct medication. Confirms patient's allergy history.
6. Perform hand hygiene and apply clean gloves (if risk of contacting secretions). Assemble nebulizer equipment per manufacturer directions.	Reduces transmission of infection. Assembly may vary slightly with different manufacturers. Proper assembly ensures safe delivery of medication.
7. Add prescribed medication by pouring medicine into nebulizer cup. (*Option:* You may use a medicine dropper or syringe to instill medication.)	Ensures proper dose and delivery of ordered medication.
8. Attach top to nebulizer cup and be sure that it is secure. Then connect cup to mouthpiece or face mask.	Prevents loss of medication.
9. Connect tubing to both aerosol compressor and nebulizer cup.	Ensures aerosol delivery to mouthpiece.
10. Have patient hold mouthpiece between lips with gentle pressure, but be sure lips are sealed (see illustration).	Prevents escape of nebulized medication.

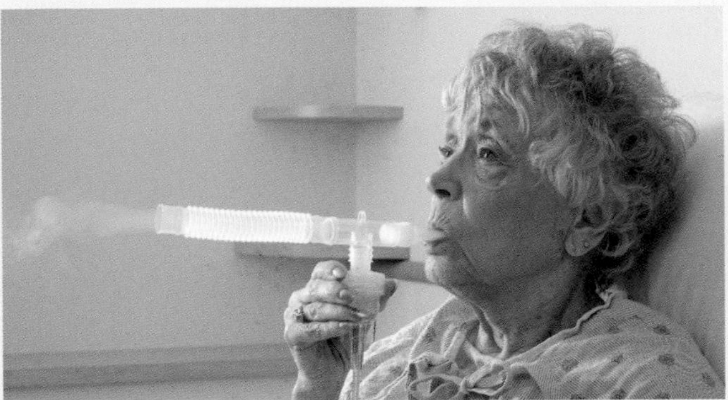

STEP 10 Nebulizer mouthpiece placed between patient's lips.

STEP	RATIONALE
a. If patient is an infant, child, or tired adult or unable to follow instructions, use face mask.	Use of face mask does not require patient to remember to hold mouthpiece correctly. Correct delivery ensures sufficient deposition of medication.
b. Use special adapters for patients with tracheostomy.	Promotes greater deposition of medication in airways.
11. Turn on small-volume nebulizer machine and ensure that a sufficient mist begins to flow.	Verifies that equipment is working properly during delivery of medication.
12. Instruct patient take deep breath, slowly, to a volume slightly greater than normal. Encourage brief, end-inspiratory pause for about 2 to 3 seconds; then have patient exhale passively. *Option:* If needed, use a nose clip so that patient breathes only through the mouth.	Improves effectiveness of medication.
a. If patient is dyspneic, encourage him or her to hold every fourth or fifth breath for 5 to 10 seconds.	Maximizes effectiveness of medication.
b. Remind patient to repeat breathing pattern until drug is completely nebulized. This usually takes about 10 to 15 minutes. Some health care providers set time limit as length of treatment rather than waiting for medication to completely nebulize.	Maximizes effectiveness of medication.
c. Tap nebulizer cup occasionally during and toward end of treatment.	Releases droplets that are clinging to side of cup, thus allowing for renebulization of solution.
d. Monitor patient's pulse during procedure, especially if beta-adrenergic bronchodilators are used.	Enables you to observe for potential side effects of medications.
13. When medication is completely nebulized, turn off machine. Rinse nebulizer cup per agency policy. Dry completely and store tubing assembly per agency policy.	Proper storage reduces transfer of microorganisms.
14. If steroids are nebulized, instruct patient to rinse mouth and gargle with warm water 2 minutes after nebulizer treatment. Have patient spit out solution.	Removes medication residue from oral cavity and helps prevent oral candidiasis, a possible adverse effect of inhaled steroid therapy.

STEP	RATIONALE
15. After nebulizer treatment is complete, have patient take several deep breaths and cough to expectorate mucus.	Nebulized medication is often ordered to open airways and promote expectoration of mucus.
16. Help patient to comfortable position.	Gives patient sense of well-being.
17. Be sure nurse call system is in an accessible location within patient's reach.	Ensures patient can call for assistance if needed.
18. Raise side rails (as appropriate) and lower bed to lowest position.	Ensures patient safety.
19. Remove and dispose of gloves and perform hand hygiene.	Reduces transmission of microorganisms.

EVALUATION

STEP	RATIONALE
1. Assess patient's respirations, breath sounds, cough effort, sputum production, pulse oximetry, and peak flow measure (if ordered).	Determines status of breathing pattern and adequacy of ventilation/gas exchange. Allows comparison with baseline data and evaluation of effectiveness of procedure.
2. Ask patient to explain drug schedule.	Improves likelihood of adherence to therapy.
3. Ask patient to describe side effects of medication and criteria for calling health care provider.	Allows patient to recognize signs of overuse and need to seek medical support when drugs are ineffective.
4. **Use Teach-Back:** "I want to be sure I was clear about how to put together the nebulizer and add medications. Show me the steps for assembling the nebulizer and adding medications." Revise your instruction now or develop a plan for revised patient/family caregiver teaching if patient/family caregiver is not able to teach back correctly.	Determines patient's/family caregiver's level of understanding of instructional topic.

Unexpected Outcomes	Related Interventions
1. Patient's breathing pattern is ineffective; respirations are rapid and shallow; breath sounds indicate wheezing.	• Reassess type of medication and/or delivery method. • Notify health care provider.
2. Patient experiences paroxysms of coughing. Aerosolized particles can irritate posterior pharynx.	• Reassess type of medication and/or delivery method. • Notify health care provider.
3. Patient experiences cardiac dysrhythmias (light-headedness, syncope), especially if receiving beta-adrenergics.	• Withhold all further doses of medication. Assess vital signs. • Notify health care provider for reassessment of type of medication and delivery method.

Recording

- Record drug, dose or strength, length of treatment, route, and time administered immediately after administration, not before.
- Document your evaluation of patient learning.
- Document patient's assessment findings and response to treatment.

Hand-Off Reporting

- Report adverse effects or patient response and withheld drugs to nurse in charge or health care provider.

PROCEDURAL GUIDELINE 23.1 *Administering Vaginal Medications*

Purpose

Female patients who develop vaginal infections often require topical application of antiinfective agents. Vaginal medications are available in foam, jelly, cream, or suppository form (Fig. 23.4). Medicated irrigations or douches can also be given. However, their excessive use can lead to vaginal irritation. You insert a suppository into the vagina with an applicator or a gloved hand. After insertion, body temperature causes the suppository to melt for effective medication distribution. You can insert foam, jellies, and creams with an inserter or applicator.

Delegation and Collaboration

The skill of administering vaginal medications cannot be delegated to nursing assistive personnel (NAP). The nurse instructs the NAP about:

- Potential side effects of medications and to report their occurrence to the nurse.

PROCEDURAL GUIDELINE 23.1 *Administering Vaginal Medications—cont'd*

- Reporting any change in comfort level or new or increased vaginal discharge or bleeding to the nurse.

Equipment

Vaginal cream, foam, jelly, tablet, suppository, or irrigating solution; applicators (see Fig. 23.4) (if needed); clean gloves; tissues; towels and/or washcloths; perineal pad; drape or sheet; water-soluble lubricants; bedpan; irrigation or douche container (if needed); medication administration record (MAR; electronic or printed); *Option:* Gooseneck lamp

Procedural Steps

1. Check accuracy and completeness of each MAR or computer printout with health care provider's written medication order. Check patient's name, medication name and dosage, route of administration, and time of administration. Recopy or reprint any portion of MAR that is difficult to read.
2. Review pertinent information related to medication, including action, indication, purpose, normal dose and route, side effects, time of onset and peak action, and nursing implications.
3. Assess patient's medical and medication history and history of allergies. List drug allergies on each page of the MAR and prominently display it on the patient's medical record per agency policy. When patient has an allergy, provide allergy bracelet.
4. Perform hand hygiene and apply clean gloves. During perineal care, inspect condition of vaginal tissues; note if drainage is present. Remove gloves and perform hand hygiene.
5. Ask if patient is experiencing any symptoms of pruritus, burning, or discomfort.
6. Assess patient's ability to manipulate applicator, suppository, or irrigation equipment and to properly position self to insert medication (may be done just before insertion).
7. Assess patient's or family caregiver's knowledge, experience, and health literacy.
8. Provide privacy and prepare environment.
9. Discuss purpose of each medication, action, and possible adverse effects. Allow patient to ask any questions.

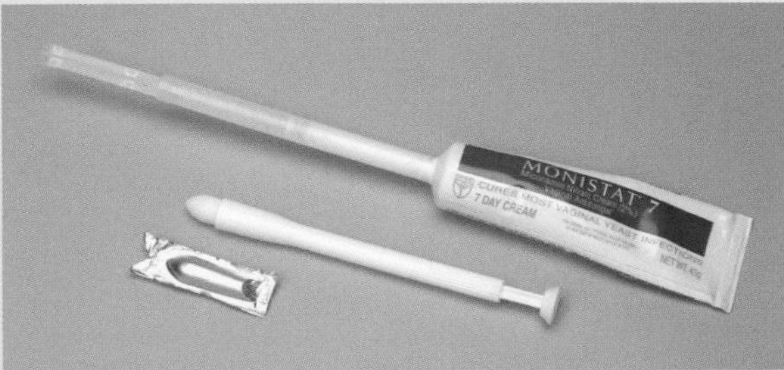

FIG 23.4 From top: Vaginal cream with applicator, applicator, and vaginal suppository. *(From Lilley LL et al:* Pharmacology and the nursing process, *ed 8, St. Louis, 2015, Mosby.)*

10. Perform hand hygiene and prepare medication using aseptic technique (see Skill 23.1). Prepare medications for one patient at a time. Keep all pages of MARs or computer printouts for one patient together or look at only one patient's electronic MAR at a time. Check label of medication carefully with MAR or computer printout when preparing medication.
11. Before going to patient's room, compare patient's name and name of medication on label of prepared drugs with MAR a second time.
12. Take medication(s) to patient at correct time (see agency policy). Medications that require exact timing include STAT, first-time or loading doses, and one-time doses.
13. Identify patient using at least two identifiers (e.g., name and birthday or name and medical record number) according to agency policy. Compare identifiers with information on patient's MAR or medical record (TJC, 2019).
14. At patient's bedside, compare MAR or computer printout a third time with names of medications on medication labels and patient name. Ask patient if he or she has allergies.
15. Have patient void (using bathroom or bedpan). Help her lie in bed in dorsal recumbent position. Patients with restricted mobility in knees or hips may lie supine with legs abducted.
16. Keep abdomen and lower extremities draped.
17. Be sure that vaginal orifice is well illuminated by room light. Otherwise position portable gooseneck lamp.
18. Perform hand hygiene and apply gloves.
19. Insert vaginal suppository.
    a. Remove suppository from wrapper and apply liberal amount of water-soluble lubricant to smooth or rounded end (see illustration). Be sure that suppository is at room temperature. Lubricate gloved index finger of dominant hand.
    b. With nondominant gloved hand, gently separate labial folds in front-to-back direction.
    c. With dominant gloved hand, insert rounded end of suppository along posterior wall of vaginal canal the

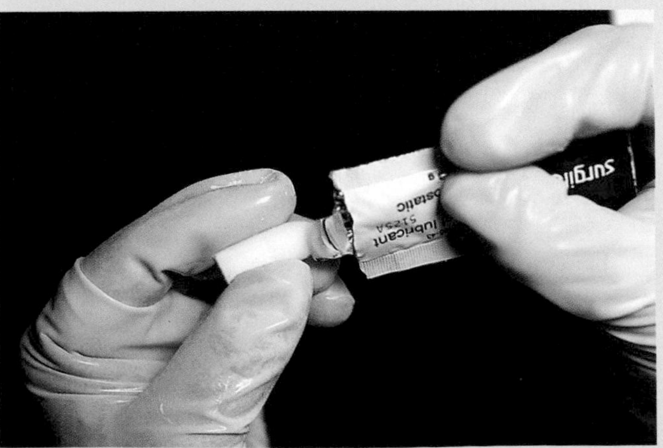

STEP 19a Lubricate tip of suppository.

Continued

PROCEDURAL GUIDELINE 23.1 *Administering Vaginal Medications—cont'd*

entire length of finger (7.5 to 10 cm [3 to 4 inches]; see illustration).

- **d.** Withdraw finger and wipe away remaining lubricant from around orifice and labia with tissue or cloth.

20. Apply cream or foam.

- **a.** Fill cream or foam applicator following package directions.
- **b.** With nondominant gloved hand, gently separate labial folds.
- **c.** With dominant gloved hand, gently insert applicator approximately 5 to 7.5 cm (2 to 3 inches). Push applicator plunger to deposit medication into vagina (see illustration).
- **d.** Withdraw applicator and place on paper towel. Wipe off residual cream from labia or vaginal orifice with tissue or cloth.

21. Administer irrigation or douche.

- **a.** Place patient on bedpan with absorbent pad underneath.
- **b.** Be sure that irrigation or douche fluid is at body temperature. Run fluid through container nozzle (priming the tubing).
- **c.** Gently separate labial folds and direct nozzle toward sacrum, following floor of vagina.
- **d.** Raise container approximately 30 to 50 cm (12 to 20 inches) above level of vagina. Insert nozzle 7 to 10 cm (3 to 4 inches). Allow solution to flow while rotating nozzle. Administer all irrigating solution.
- **e.** Withdraw nozzle and help patient to comfortable sitting position.
- **f.** Allow patient to remain on bedpan for a few minutes. Clean perineum with soap and water.
- **g.** Help patient off bedpan. Dry perineal area.

22. Instruct patient who received suppository, cream, or foam to remain on her back for at least 10 minutes.

23. If using an applicator, wash with soap and warm water, rinse, air dry, and then store for future use.

24. Offer perineal pad when patient resumes ambulation.

25. Remove and dispose of gloves. Perform hand hygiene. Help patient to comfortable position.

26. Be sure nurse call system is in an accessible location within patient's reach.

27. Raise side rails (as appropriate) and lower bed to lowest position.

28. Perform hand hygiene and apply clean gloves. Thirty minutes after administration, inspect condition of vaginal canal and external genitalia between applications. Assess vaginal discharge if present. Remove gloves and perform hand hygiene.

29. Record drug (or solution if vaginal installation), dose, type of installation, and time administered immediately after administration, not before.

30. Report to health care provider if patient states that symptoms do not disappear or symptoms get worse.

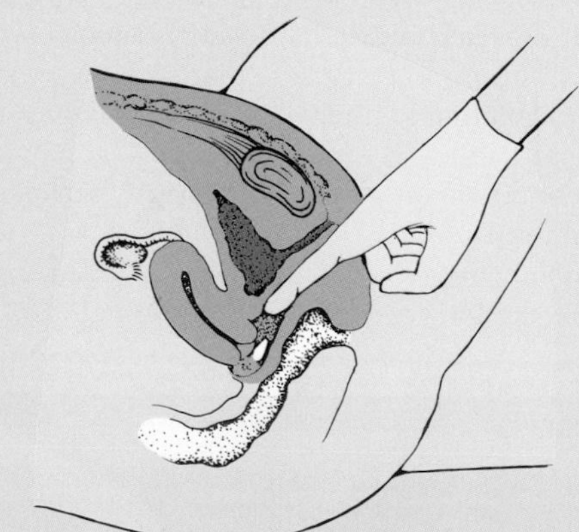

STEP 19c Angle of vaginal suppository insertion.

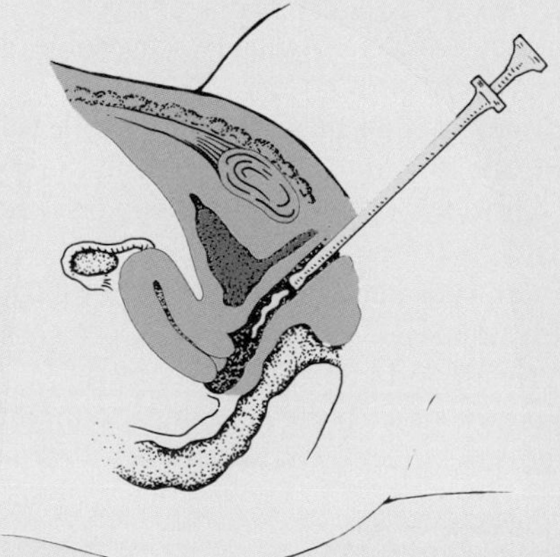

STEP 20c Applicator inserted into vaginal canal. Plunger pushed to instill medication.

PROCEDURAL GUIDELINE 23.2 *Administering Rectal Suppositories*

Purpose

A rectal suppository (Fig. 23.5) is a form of medication that acts when it melts and is absorbed into the rectal mucosa. Rectal medications exert either local effects on gastrointestinal (GI) mucosa (e.g., promoting defecation) or systemic effects (e.g., relieving nausea or providing analgesia). The rectal route is not as reliable as oral or parenteral routes in terms of drug absorption and distribution. However, the medications are relatively safe because they rarely cause local irritation or side effects. Rectal medications are contraindicated in patients with recent surgery

PROCEDURAL GUIDELINE 23.2 *Administering Rectal Suppositories—cont'd*

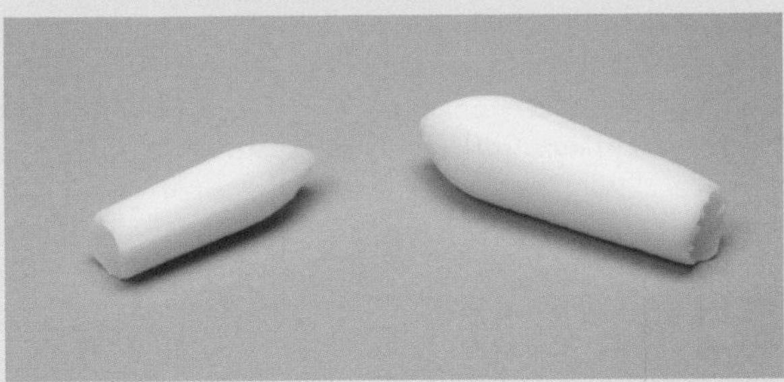

FIG 23.5 Vaginal suppositories (right) are larger and more oval than rectal suppositories (left). *(From Lilley LL et al:* Pharmacology and the nursing process, *ed 8, St. Louis, 2015, Mosby.)*

on the rectum, bowel, or prostate gland; rectal bleeding or prolapse; and very low platelet counts (Burchum and Rosenthal, 2016).

Delegation and Collaboration

The skill of rectal medication administration cannot be delegated to nursing assistive personnel (NAP). The nurse instructs the NAP about:

- Reporting expected fecal discharge or bowel movement to the nurse.
- Potential side effects of medications and to report their occurrence to the nurse.
- Informing nurse of any rectal pain or bleeding.

Equipment

Rectal suppository; water-soluble lubricating jelly; clean gloves; tissue; drape; medication administration record (MAR; electronic or printed)

Procedural Steps

1. Check accuracy and completeness of each MAR or computer printout with health care provider's written medication order. Check patient's name, medication name and dosage, route of administration, and time of administration. Recopy or reprint any portion of MAR that is difficult to read.
2. Review pertinent information related to medication, including action, purpose, normal dose and route, side effects, time of onset and peak action, indication, and nursing implications.
3. Assess patient's medical and medication history and history of allergies. List drug allergies on each page of the MAR and prominently display it on the patient's medical record per agency policy. When patient has allergy, provide allergy bracelet.
4. Review any presenting signs and symptoms of gastrointestinal (GI) alterations (e.g., constipation or diarrhea).
5. Assess patient's ability to hold suppository and position self to insert medication.
6. Assess patient's or family caregiver's knowledge, experience, and health literacy.
7. Provide privacy and prepare environment.
8. Discuss purpose of each medication, action, indication, and possible adverse effects. Allow patient to ask any questions.
9. Perform hand hygiene and prepare medication using aseptic technique (see Skill 23.1). Prepare medications for one patient at a time. Keep all pages of MARs or computer printouts for one patient together or look at only one patient's electronic MAR at a time. Check label of medication carefully with MAR or computer printout when preparing medication.
10. Before going to patient's room, compare patient's name and name of medication on label of prepared drugs with MAR a second time.
11. Take medication(s) to patient at correct time (see agency policy). Medications that require exact timing include STAT, first-time or loading doses, and one-time doses.
12. Identify patient using at least two identifiers (e.g., name and birthday or name and medical record number) according to agency policy. Compare identifiers with information on patient's MAR or medical record (TJC, 2019).
13. At patient's bedside, again compare MAR or computer printout a third time with names of medications on medication labels and patient name. Ask patient if he or she has allergies.
14. Perform hand hygiene and apply clean gloves.
15. Help patient assume left side-lying Sims' position with upper leg flexed upward.
16. If patient has mobility impairment, help into lateral position. Obtain help to turn patient, and use pillows under upper arm and leg.
17. Keep patient draped with only anal area exposed.
18. Examine condition of anus externally. *Option:* Palpate rectal walls as needed (e.g., if impaction is suspected; see Chapter 8). If you palpate rectal walls, dispose of gloves by turning them inside out and placing them in proper receptacle if they become soiled. Otherwise keep gloves on your hands and proceed to Step 19.

Safe Patient Care *Do not palpate patient's rectum if there is a recent history of rectal surgery. A suppository is contraindicated in the presence of active bleeding and diarrhea (Burchum and Rosenthal, 2016).*

19. If you disposed of gloves, perform hand hygiene and apply new pair of clean gloves.
20. Remove suppository from foil wrapper and lubricate rounded end with water-soluble lubricant. Lubricate gloved index finger of dominant hand. If patient has hemorrhoids, use liberal amount of lubricant and touch area gently.
21. Ask patient to take slow, deep breaths through mouth and relax anal sphincter.
22. Retract patient's buttocks with nondominant hand. With gloved index finger of dominant hand, insert suppository gently through anus, past internal sphincter, and against rectal wall, 10 cm (4 inches) in adults (see illustration) or 5 cm (2 inches) in infants and children. You should feel rectal sphincter close around your finger.

Safe Patient Care *Do not insert suppository into a mass of fecal material; this will reduce effectiveness of medication.*

Continued

PROCEDURAL GUIDELINE 23.2 ***Administering Rectal Suppositories—cont'd***

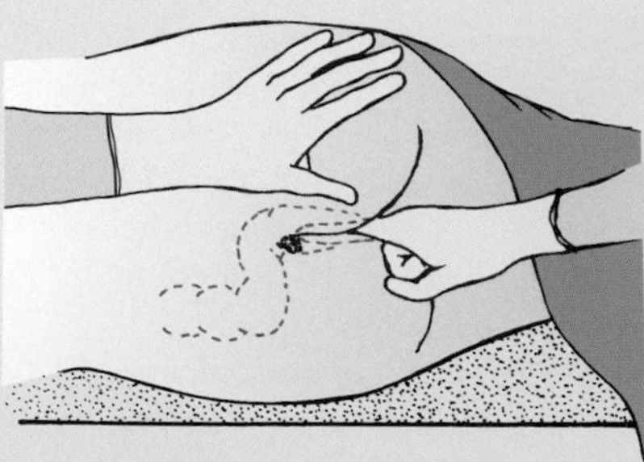

STEP 22 Insert rectal suppository past sphincter and against rectal wall.

23. *Option:* A suppository may be given through a colostomy (not ileostomy) if ordered. Patient should lie supine. Use small amount of water-soluble lubricant for insertion.
24. Withdraw finger and wipe patient's anal area.
25. Ask patient to remain flat or on side for 5 minutes.
26. Remove and discard gloves by turning them inside out and dispose of them and used supplies in appropriate receptacle. Perform hand hygiene.
27. If suppository contains laxative or fecal softener, place nurse call system within reach so that patient can obtain help to reach bedpan or toilet.
28. If suppository was given for constipation, remind patient not to flush commode after bowel movement.
29. Return to bedside within 5 minutes to determine if suppository was expelled.
30. Help patient to comfortable position.
31. Be sure nurse call system is in an accessible location within patient's reach.
32. Raise side rails (as appropriate) and lower bed to lowest position.
33. Record drug, dose or strength, length of treatment, route, and time administered immediately after administration, not before.
34. Report adverse effects or patient response and withheld drugs to health care provider.

SPECIAL CONSIDERATIONS

Patient-Centered Care

- Health beliefs vary by culture and influence how patients manage and respond to medication therapy. Differences in values, attitudes, and beliefs affect a patient's adherence to medication therapy. Herbal remedies and alternative therapies may be common practice in some cultures and can interfere with prescribed medications. It is also important to consider cultural influences on drug response, metabolism, and side effects if a patient is not responding to drug therapy as expected.
- Certain food preferences may have food–drug interactions. Vegetarian diets can affect warfarin or medications for glycemic control. A change in the medication may be necessary by the prescriber, or the patient may need counseling on how to change dietary patterns.

Patient Education

- Health care provider issues include inappropriate prescriptions, poor instruction, and lack of health care provider knowledge about adherence.
- Simply explaining medications and offering printed information are not enough.
- Adapt your instructional approach to the patient's values, beliefs, readiness and willingness to learn, and resources available. For example, repetition of information is important, especially when caring for older adults and patients with cognition problems (e.g., changes in consciousness, inability to attend because of symptoms).

Age-Specific

Pediatric

- Pediatric doses are usually calculated based on body weight.
- Infants often clench the eyes tightly to avoid eyedrops. Place the drops in the nasal corner where the lids meet as the infant lies supine. When the infant opens the eye, the medication will flow into the eye.
- Insert cotton pledgets loosely into ear canal to prevent medication from flowing out of the external ear canal. To prevent cotton from absorbing medication in ear, premoisten cotton with a few drops of medication (Hockenberry and Wilson, 2017).
- Ensure that parents and other caregivers are aware of the proper method of administration (e.g., for children <3 years old, gently pull the pinna of the ear downward and straight back).

Gerontological

- Physiological changes of aging influence distribution, absorption, and excretion. Common changes include dry mouth; delayed esophageal clearance and impaired swallowing; reduction in gastric acidity and stomach peristalsis; reduced liver function, resulting in altered drug metabolism; and reduced renal function and colon motility, slowing drug excretion (Lilley et al., 2015).
- If possible, provide a written medication schedule for the patient to follow at home. Use large print in written materials if vision is impaired.
- An older adult may be unable to depress the medication canister because of weakened grasp. If there is difficulty with coordinating activation of the inhaler and inhalation, the use of a spacer device may be helpful.

Home Care

- Help patients/family caregivers to set up medication reminders at home (e.g., pillboxes arranged by day of week).
- When measuring liquid medications at home, provide patients and family members with calibrated spoons and oral syringes.
- Provide patient or primary caregiver with resources to determine which medications can be crushed, which medications should

not be crushed, and how to obtain liquid formulations of medications.

- Instruct patient on safe disposal techniques at home. Fold used patches with medication sides together and wrapped in newspaper before discarding. Used applicators or patches are placed into cardboard or plastic disposable containers. Children and pets may become ill if they ingest or handle used patches; careful disposal is necessary to ensure safety in the home.
- Teach patients how to count doses in MDI and how to plan for renewal of medication. Failure to do so might result in a patient using an empty inhaler during an acute episode of a respiratory problem. To track doses:
  - Note first day of use on a calendar.
  - Note number of inhalations in the canister (e.g., 200 inhalations per MDI).
  - Note number of inhalations used per day (e.g., 2 inhalations a day, 3 times a day, equals 6 inhalations a day).
  - Divide the total number of inhalations in canister by the number of inhalations needed per day to determine number of days inhaler should last (e.g., 200/6 = 33 days of 3-times-a-day dosing).
  - Mark on calendar the date inhaler will be empty; obtain a refill a few days before.

✦ PRACTICE REFLECTIONS

Consider all the nonparenteral routes of medication your patients may be receiving during their admission to a health care agency. Consider the need for different approaches to administering these medications.

1. How would you determine how to administer topical medications to patients with wounds?
2. When might it be acceptable to allow patients to administer some of these routes of medications themselves?
3. In the clinical setting, what has helped you organize yourself to administer multiple nonparental medications to a patient safely?

✦ CLINICAL REVIEW QUESTIONS

1. A nurse is administering ophthalmic ointment to a patient. Place the following steps in correct order for the administration of the ointment.
   1. Clean eye, washing from inner to outer canthus.
   2. Assess patient's level of consciousness and ability to follow instructions.
   3. Apply thin ribbon of ointment evenly along inner edge of lower eyelid on conjunctiva.
   4. Have patient close eye and rub lightly in a circular motion with a cotton ball.
   5. Ask patient to look at ceiling and explain the steps to patient.
2. A nurse is administering a metered-dose inhaler (MDI) with a spacer to a patient with chronic obstructive pulmonary disease. Place the steps of the procedure in the correct order.
   1. Insert MDI into end of spacer.
   2. Perform a respiratory assessment.
   3. Remove mouthpiece from MDI and spacer device.
   4. Place the spacer mouthpiece into patient's mouth and instruct patient to close lips around the mouthpiece.
   5. Depress medication canister, spraying 1 puff into spacer device.
   6. Shake inhaler for 2 to 5 seconds.
   7. Instruct patient to hold breath for 10 seconds.
   8. Instruct patient to breathe in slowly through mouth for 3 to 5 seconds.
3. A patient is to receive medications through a small-bore nasogastric feeding tube. Which nursing actions are appropriate? (Select all that apply.)
   1. Verifying tube placement after medications are given
   2. Mixing all medications together and give all at once
   3. Using an enteral tube syringe to administer medications
   4. Flushing tube with 30 to 60 mL of water after the last dose of medication
   5. Checking for gastric residual before giving the medications
   6. Keeping the head of the bed elevated 30 to 60 minutes after the medications are given

Answers and Rationales for Clinical Review Questions can be found on the Evolve website.

REFERENCES

Ari A: Patient education and adherence to aerosol therapy, *Respir Care* 60(6):941, 2015.

Ball JW, et al: *Seidel's guide to physical examination*, ed 9, St Louis, 2019, Mosby.

Boullata J, et al: ASPEN safe practices for enteral nutrition therapy, *JPEN J Parenter Enteral Nutr* 41(1):15, 2017.

Burchum JR, Rosenthal LD: *Lehne's pharmacology for nursing care*, ed 8, Philadelphia, 2016, Saunders.

Centers for Disease Control and Prevention (CDC): What is health literacy, 2016. https://www.cdc.gov/healthliteracy/learn/index.html.

Clifford P, et al: Following the evidence: enteral tube placement and verification in neonates and young children, *J Perinat Neonatal Nurs* 29(2):149, 2015.

Department of Health and Human Services, Centers for Medicare & Medicaid (DHHS): *Updated guidance on medication administration, Hospital Appendix A of State Operations Manual*, Baltimore, 2011, Department of Health and Human Services.

Forough A, et al: Nurses' experiences of medication administration to people with swallowing difficulties in aged care agencies: a systematic review protocol, *JBI Database System Rev Implement Rep* 15(4):932, 2017.

Goldstein B, et al: General principles of dermatologic therapy and topical corticosteroid use, UpToDate 2017. https://www.uptodate.com/contents/general-principles-of-dermatologic-therapy-and-topical-corticosteroid-use.

Guenther P: New enteral connectors: raising awareness, *Nut Clin Pract* 29:612, 2015.

Guenter P, Boullata J: Drug administration by enteral feeding tube, *Nursing* 43(12):26, 2013.

Hockenberry M, Wilson D: *Wong's essentials of pediatric nursing*, ed 10, St. Louis, 2017, Mosby.

Institute for Safe Medication Practices (ISMP): ISMP acute care guidelines for timely administration of scheduled medications, 2011. http://www.ismp.org/Tools/guidelines/acutecare/tasm.pdf.

Institute for Safe Medication Practices (ISMP): Oral dosage forms that should not be crushed, 2016a, http://www.ismp.org/tools/donotcrush.pdf.

Institute for Safe Medication Practices (ISMP): 2016-2017 targeted medication safety best practices for hospitals, 2016b. www.ismp.org/tools/bestpractices/TMSBP-for-Hospitals.pdf.

Lawton S: Safe and effective application of topical treatments to the skin, *Nurs Stand* 27(42):49, 2013.

Lilley LL, et al: *Pharmacology and the nursing process*, ed 8, St. Louis, 2015, Mosby.

National Alert Network (NAN): Move toward full use of metric dosing: Eliminate dosage cups that measure liquids in fluid drams, 2015. https://www.nccmerp.org/sites/default/files/nan-alert-june-2015.pdf.

Occupational Safety and Health Administration (OSHA): Safety and health topics: hazardous drugs, 2016. http://www.osha.gov/?SLTC/?hazardousdrugs/?controlling_occex_hazardousdrugs.html.

Paparella S: Adopt the 2014-2015 Targeted best practices for medication safety, *J Emerg Nurs* 40(3):263, 2014.

Prakash V, et al: Mitigating errors caused by interruptions during medication verification and administration: interventions in a simulated ambulatory chemotherapy setting, *BMJ Qual Saf* 23(11):884, 2014.

The Joint Commission (TJC): Sentinel event alert: Managing risk during transition to new ISO tubing connector standards, 2014. https://www.jointcommission.org/assets/1/6/SEA_53_Connectors_8_19_14_final.pdf.

The Joint Commission (TJC): *2019 National Patient Safety Goals*, Oakbrook Terrace, IL, 2019, The Commission. http://www.jointcommission.org/standards_information/npsgs.aspx.

Truitt E, et al: Effect of the implementation of barcode technology and an electronic medication administration record on adverse drug events, *Hosp Pharm* 51(6):474–483, 2016.

U.S. Department of Health and Human Services (USDHHS): Tablet splitting a risky practice, 2015. https://www.fda.gov/ForConsumers/ConsumerUpdates/ucm171492.htm.

Westbrook J, et al: Effectiveness of a 'do not interrupt' bundled intervention to reduce interruptions during medication administration: a cluster randomized controlled feasibility study, *BJM Qual Saf* 0:1, 2017.

Yoder M, et al: The effect of a safe zone on nurse interruptions, distractions, and medication administration errors, *J Infus Nurs* 38(2):140, 2015.

Zhu J, Weingart S: Prevention of adverse drug events in hospitals, UpToDate 2017. https://www.uptodate.com/contents/prevention-of-adverse-drug-events-in-hospitals/contributor-disclosure.

24 Parenteral Medications

SKILLS AND PROCEDURES

EVOLVE WEBSITE/RESOURCES LIST

http://evolve.elsevier.com/Perry/nursinginterventions
Audio Glossary • Checklists • Clinical Review Questions • Answers and Rationales for Clinical Review Questions • Video Clips

INTRODUCTION

The route of medication administration is the path by which a drug comes in contact with the body. Medications administered by the parenteral route enter body tissues and the circulatory system by injection. Injected medications are more quickly absorbed than oral medications; parenteral routes are used when patients are vomiting, cannot swallow, or are restricted from taking oral fluids. There are four routes for parenteral administration:

1. Subcutaneous injection: Injection into tissues just under the dermis of the skin
2. Intramuscular (IM) injection: Injection into the body of a muscle
3. Intradermal (ID) injection: Injection into the dermis just under the epidermis
4. Intravenous (IV) injection or infusion: Injection into a vein

PRACTICE STANDARDS

- Infusion Nurses Society, 2016: Infusion nursing standards of practice
- Institute for Safe Medication Practices (ISMP), 2011: Acute care guidelines for timely administration of scheduled medications—Medication safety
- Institute for Safe Medication Practices (ISMP), 2015: List of error-prone abbreviations, symbols, and dose designations—Medication safety
- The Joint Commission (TJC), 2019: National Patient Safety Goals—Patient identification

EVIDENCE-BASED PRACTICE

Guidelines for Administering Subcutaneous Insulin

There is increasing evidence that addresses practice guidelines for the administration of subcutaneous insulin injections. Insulin injection technique has been modified over the past several years in response to evidence and research about best practices for patient assessment and site selection (McCulloch et al., 2017). There is now enough consensual evidence to develop guidelines for the administration of insulin injections. Based on this evidence (McCulloch et al., 2017):

- Use the same technique for both insulin syringes and insulin pens.
- Use a body area where 2.5 cm (1 inch) of subcutaneous fat can be pinched.
- Use a 27-gauge needle, perpendicular to the pinched skin.
- Do not aspirate the injection, and hold the needle in place for several seconds. This is especially important with insulin pens to prevent leakage of medication.
- Insulin is absorbed rapidly through the abdominal wall, so this should be the first choice for sites when using rapid-acting insulin.

SAFETY GUIDELINES

Patient safety in administering medication involves following the seven rights of medication administration (see Chapter 22). When managing a patient's medications, communicate clearly with members of the interprofessional team, assess and incorporate the patient's priorities of care and preferences, and use the best evidence when making decisions about drug administration. Follow these guidelines to ensure safe medication administration:

- Be vigilant during medication administration. Avoid distractions while preparing a parenteral medication. No-interruption zones (NIZs) have been recommended to reduce distractions during medication preparation and administration (Bravo and Cochran, 2016; Yoder et al., 2015). NIZs are created by placing signs, red tape, or tile borders on the floor around medication carts or areas. Nurses standing in these zones are not to be interrupted. Be sure that your patients receive the appropriate medications. Know why your patient is receiving each medication; know what you need to do before, during, and after medication administration; and evaluate the effectiveness of medications and any adverse effects.
- Verify that medications have not expired by checking labels.
- Avoid use of error-prone abbreviations, symbols, and dose designations (ISMP, 2015).
- Use at least two identifiers before administering medications, and check against the medication administration record (MAR). Follow agency policy for patient identification.
- Before administering medication, it is critical to ensure that all information is correct; you should check for accuracy three times:
  1. The first check is when the medications are pulled or retrieved from the automated dispensing machine, the medication drawer, or whatever system is in place at the agency.
  2. The second check is when preparation of the medications for administration takes place.
  3. The final check occurs at the patient's bedside just before medications are given.
- Clarify unclear medication orders and ask for help whenever you are uncertain about an order or calculation. Consult with your peers, pharmacists, and other health care providers, and be sure that you have resolved all concerns related to medication administration before preparing and giving medications.
- Use the technology (e.g., bar scanning, electronic MARs) available in your agency when preparing and giving medications. Follow all policies related to use of the technology, and do not use "workarounds." A workaround bypasses a procedure, policy, or problem in a system. Nurses who use workarounds fail to follow agency protocols, policies, or procedures during medication administration in an attempt to get medications administered to patients in a timelier fashion.
- Use strict aseptic technique during parenteral medication preparation and administration.
- Educate patients about each medication they take while you are administering medications. It is important for a patient to know each medication with respect to its purpose, the daily dose and when to take the medication, the most common side effects, and the problems to report to the health care provider. Make sure that you answer all the patient questions before administering medications. Educate family caregivers if appropriate.
- Most of the time you cannot delegate medication administration. Ensure that you follow standards set by the Nurse Practice Act in your state and guidelines established by your health care agency. Licensed practical nurses or licensed vocational nurses usually can administer medications via the oral (PO), subcutaneous, intramuscular (IM), and intradermal (ID) routes. Sometimes they can give medications intravenously if they have had special training and if the medications are not high-alert medications. Some states also allow certified medical assistants to administer some types of medications (e.g., oral medications) in long-term care facilities.

NEEDLESTICK PREVENTION

The most frequent route of exposure to bloodborne disease for health care workers is from needlestick injuries (Occupational Safety and Health Administration [OSHA], 2012). These injuries occur when health care workers recap needles, mishandle intravenous (IV) lines and needles, or leave needles at a patient's bedside. However, the implementation of safe needle devices can prevent needlestick injuries (OSHA, 2012). The Needlestick Safety and Prevention Act is a federal law that mandates health care agencies to use safe needle devices to reduce the frequency of needlestick injury. Employers are required to maintain a current exposure control plan and seek employee input when considering changing medical devices (OSHA, 2012).

A sharp with engineered sharps injury protection (SESIP) is a device effective in preventing needlesticks. One type of SESIP is a blunt-end cannula; another is a safety syringe equipped with a plastic guard or sheath that slips over the needle as it is withdrawn from the skin (Fig. 24.1). The guard immediately covers the needle, eliminating the chance for a needlestick injury. A variety of other SESIP devices are found in needleless IV-line connection systems (see Chapter 28). Box 24.1 lists recommendations for health care workers to reduce their risk of needlestick injuries.

Special puncture-proof and leak-proof containers are available in health care agencies for the disposal of sharps. Containers are made so that only one hand needs to be used when disposing of uncapped needles. In addition, containers must stand upright, not be allowed to overfill, and be colored red or labeled with a biohazard symbol (Fig. 24.2).

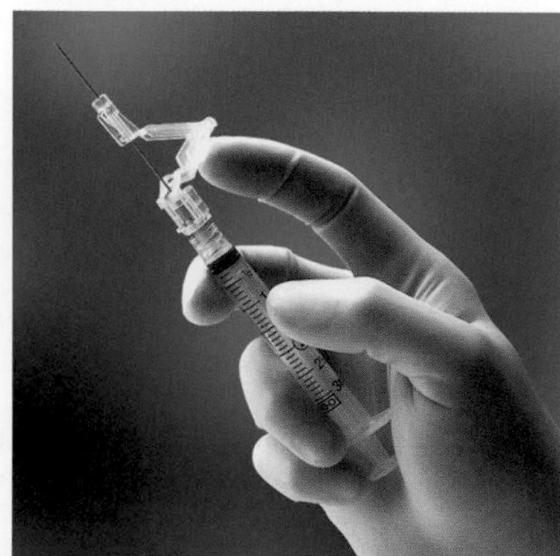

FIG 24.1 Needleless system. Safety syringe with guard.

BOX 24.1

Recommendations for Prevention of Needlestick Injuries

- Avoid using needles when effective needleless systems or sharp with engineered sharps injury protection (SESIP) devices are available.
- Do not recap needles after medication administration.
- Plan safe handling and disposal of needles before beginning a procedure that requires the use of a needle.
- Immediately dispose of used needles, needleless systems, and SESIP into puncture- and leak-proof sharps disposal containers.
- Maintain a sharps injury log that reports the following: type and brand of device involved in the incident; location of the incident (e.g., department or work area); description of the incident; privacy of the employees who have had sharps injuries (see agency policy).
- Attend educational offerings regarding bloodborne pathogens, and follow recommendations for infection prevention, including receiving the hepatitis B vaccine.
- Report all needlestick and sharps-related injuries immediately, according to agency policies.
- Participate in the selection and evaluation of SESIP devices with safety features within your agency whenever possible.

Data from Occupational Safety and Health Administration (OSHA): Bloodborne pathogens and needlestick injuries, 77 FR 19934, 2012. https://www.osha.gov/FedReg_osha_pdf/FED20120403.pdf.

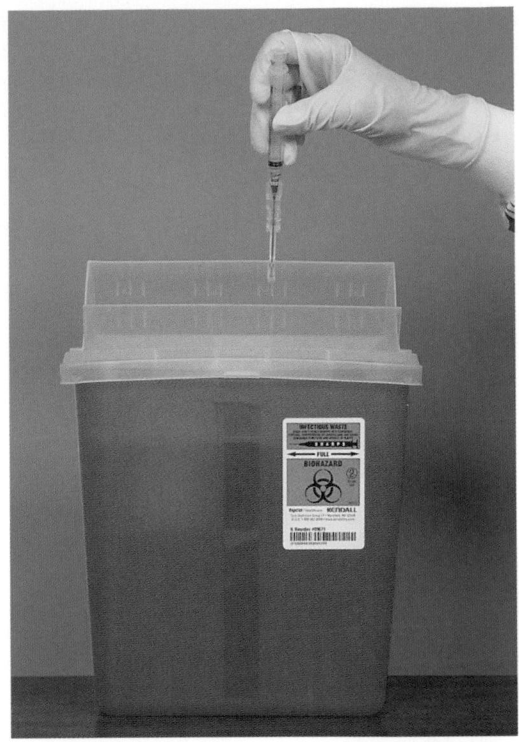

FIG 24.2 Sharps disposal using only one hand.

✦ SKILL 24.1 Preparing Injections: Vials and Ampules

Purpose

Medications may be dispensed from a pharmacy or from a manufacturer in a vial or ampule. There will be the need for nurses administering this type of parenteral medication to have the knowledge base to prepare injections from ampules and vials.

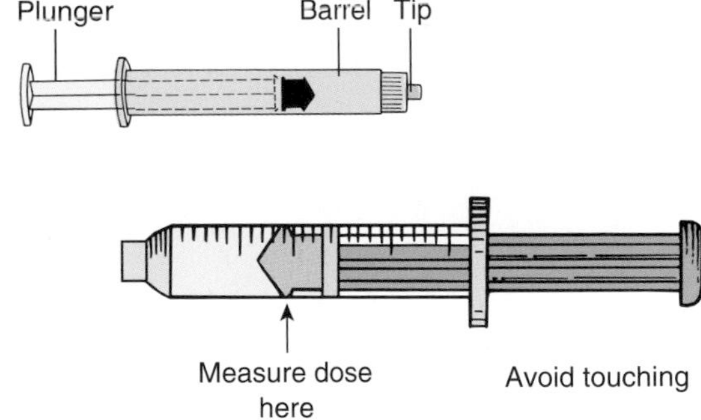

FIG 24.3 Parts of a syringe.

Preparation

Administer parenteral medication by using a needle and a syringe, available in a variety of sizes. Determine the appropriate size of syringe, length and gauge of needle, volume of solution, and medication route. These decisions are based on the quantity and type of medication prescribed and the body size of a patient. Most syringes come with needleless systems or safety needles that help prevent needlestick injuries. A variety of electronic infusion pumps deliver intravenous (IV) or continuous subcutaneous infusions. Infusion pumps ensure a constant and accurate delivery of medication.

Syringes

Syringes are single use, are disposable, and have tips that are either Luer-Lok or non–Luer-Lok. They are packaged separately, in paper wrappers or rigid plastic containers. Syringes come with or without a sterile needle or with a needleless SESIP device. The parts of a syringe are shown in (Fig. 24.3). Non–Luer-Lok syringes use needles or needleless devices that slip onto the tip. Luer-Lok syringes (Fig. 24.4A) use standard needles or needleless devices that twist onto the syringe tip and lock in place to prevent the accidental removal of the needle from the syringe.

Syringes come in various sizes, ranging in capacity from 0.5 to 60 mL (see Fig. 24.4). When you select a syringe, choose the smallest syringe size possible to improve the accuracy of medication preparation. In addition, avoid injecting a large volume of fluid into tissues. A 1- to 3-mL syringe is usually adequate for a subcutaneous or intramuscular (IM) injection. Larger volumes create pain and discomfort for a patient. Syringes are most commonly marked in a scale by tenths of a milliliter (see Fig. 24.4A–B). You use tuberculin syringes to prepare small amounts of medications for intradermal (ID) and subcutaneous injections (see Fig. 24.4C). Insulin syringes (see Fig. 24.4D) hold 0.3 to 1 mL, come with preattached needles, and are calibrated in units. Most insulin syringes are U-100s, designed for use with U-100–strength insulin. Each milliliter of solution contains 100 units of insulin.

Use a larger syringe to administer some IV medications and irrigate drainage tubes. Some syringes are packaged with their needle attached, and some syringes require you to change the needle based on the viscosity of the medication, route of administration, and gender and size of the patient. Before use, carefully examine a syringe to determine the measurement scale and ensure that you use the correct syringe for preparing the ordered medication.

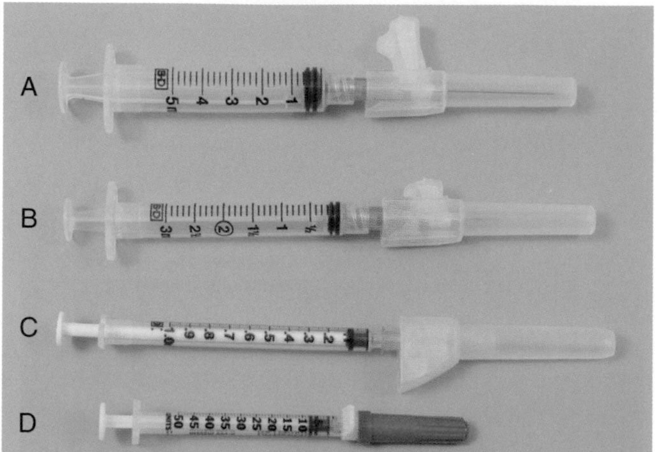

FIG 24.4 Types of syringes. (A) 5-mL syringe. (B) 3-mL syringe. (C) Tuberculin syringe marked in 0.01 (hundredths) for doses less than 1 mL. (D) Insulin syringe marked in units (50).

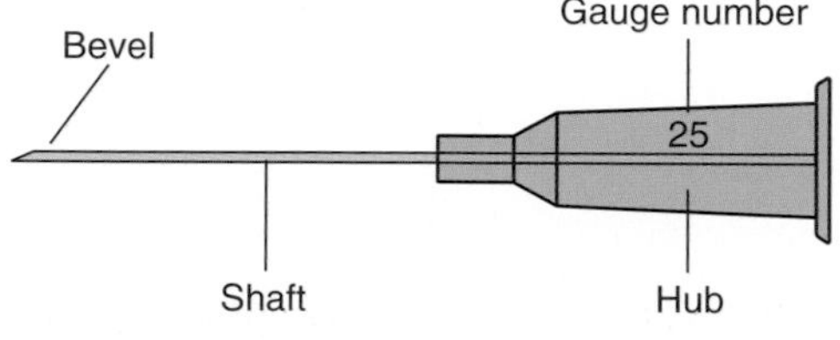

FIG 24.5 Parts of a needle.

Needles

Some needles come attached to syringes. Others come packaged individually to allow flexibility in selecting the right needle for a patient. Needles are disposable, and most are made of stainless steel. A needle has three parts: the hub, which fits onto the tip of the syringe; the shaft, which connects to the hub; and the bevel, or slanted tip (Fig. 24.5). The needle hub, shaft, and bevel must remain sterile at all times. To prevent contamination, use gentle force to place the needle onto a syringe with the cap intact.

The tip of a needle, or the bevel, is always slanted. The bevel creates a narrow slit when injected into tissue, which quickly closes as the needle is removed to prevent leakage of medication, blood, or serum. Longer beveled tips are sharper and narrower, which minimizes discomfort from a subcutaneous or IM injection.

Most needles vary in length from ¼ to 3 inches. Choose the needle length according to a patient's size and weight and the type of tissue into which the medication is to be injected. Current evidence suggests that needle length should be based on a patient's weight (Holliday et al., 2016). There should be a 5-mm depth of muscle penetration for an IM injection (Hibbard et al., 2017). A child or slender adult generally requires a shorter needle. Use longer needles (1 to 1½ inches) for IM injections and a shorter needle (⅜ to ⅝ inch) for subcutaneous injections. Needles come in different gauges or outer diameters. As a needle gauge becomes smaller, the needle diameter is larger. The selection of a gauge depends on the viscosity of the fluid to be injected or infused.

Disposable Injection Units

Single-dose, prefilled, disposable syringes are available for some medications. You do not need to prepare medication doses except perhaps to expel unneeded portions of medication or air. However, it is important to check the medication and concentration carefully because prefilled syringes appear very similar. Prefilled unit-dose systems, such as Tubex and Carpuject, include reusable plastic syringe holders and disposable, prefilled, sterile, glass cartridge units (Fig. 24.6). To assemble a prefilled system, place the cartridge, barrel

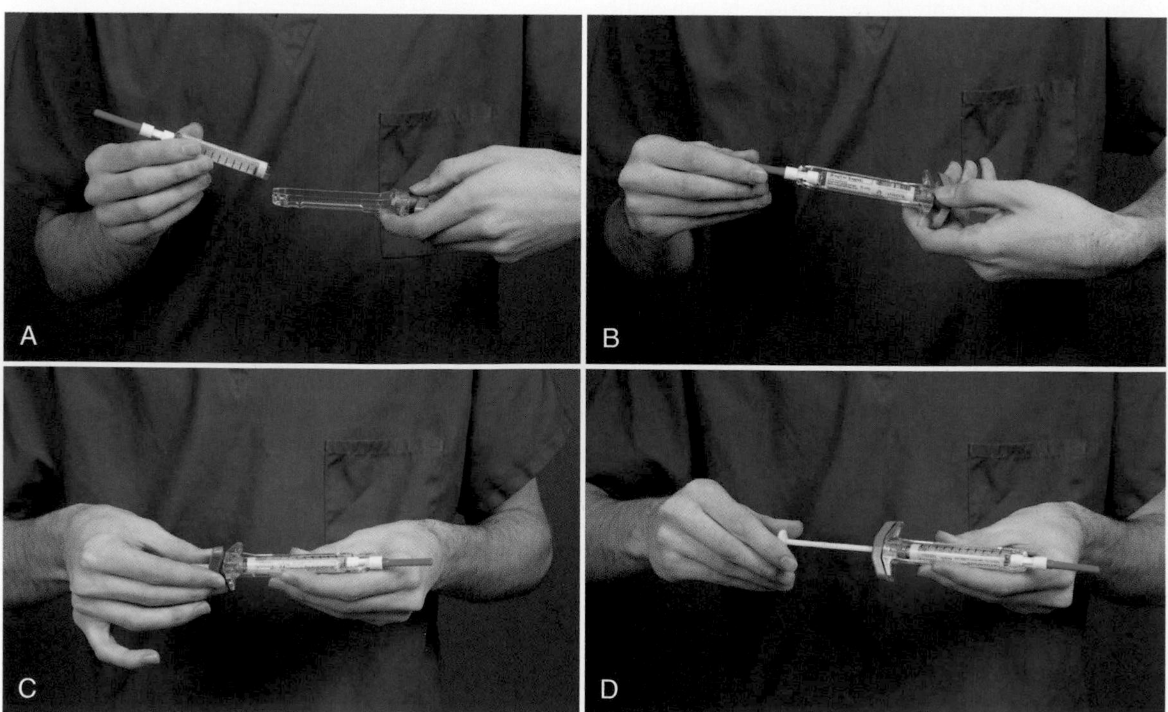

FIG 24.6 (A–D) Carpuject syringe holder and needleless, prefilled, sterile cartridge.

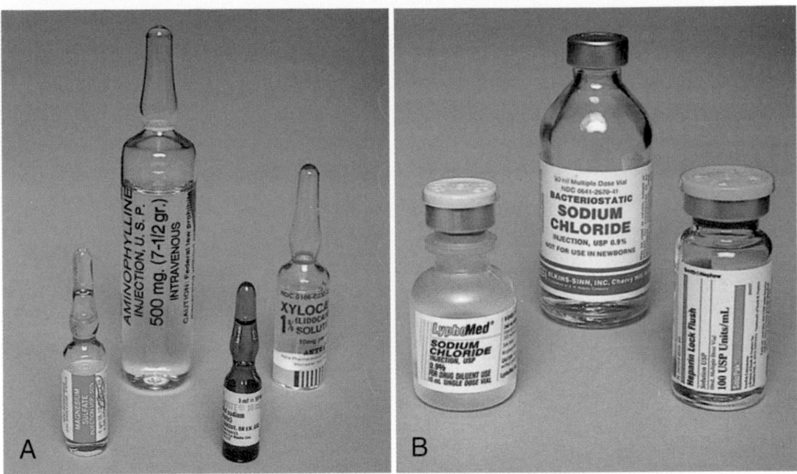

FIG 24.7 (A) Medication in ampules. (B) Medication in vials.

first, into the plastic syringe holder. Following manufacturer's instructions, turn the plunger rod to the left (counterclockwise) and the lock to the right (clockwise) until it "clicks." Finally, remove the needle guard and advance the plunger to expel air and excess medication, as with a regular syringe. The cartridge may be used with SESIP needles. After administering a medication, dispose of the glass cartridge safely in a puncture-proof and leak-proof container. This design reduces the risk for needlestick injury.

Ampules and Vials

Ampules contain single doses of injectable medication in a liquid form and are available in sizes ranging from 1 to 10 mL or more. An ampule is made of glass with a constricted, prescored neck that is snapped off to allow access to the medication (Fig. 24.7A). A colored ring around the neck indicates where the ampule is prescored to be broken easily. Medication is easily withdrawn from an ampule by aspirating the fluid with a filter needle and syringe. Filter needles must be used when preparing medication from a glass ampule to prevent glass particles from being drawn into the syringe (Joo et al., 2016). Do not use a filter needle to administer a medication. Place an appropriate-sized needle on the syringe after withdrawing the medication.

A vial is a single-dose or multi-dose plastic or glass container with a rubber seal at the top (see Fig. 24.7B). After you open a single-dose vial, discard it, regardless of the amount of medication used (Alexander et al., 2014). A multi-dose vial contains several doses of medication and can be entered several times, although only for a single patient (Alexander et al., 2014). When using a multi-dose vial, write the date and time that the vial is opened on the vial label. Verify with the agency how long an opened multi-dose vial may be used. Vials that exceed the time allowed by agency policy must be properly discarded.

A metal or plastic cap protects the rubber seal of a vial. Remove the cap when you first prepare a vial for use. Vials may contain liquid or dry forms of medications; medications that are unstable in solution are packaged in dry form. A vial label specifies the solvent or diluents used to dissolve the dry medication and the amount needed to prepare a desired medication concentration. Normal saline and distilled water are the most common diluents.

Some vials have two chambers separated by a rubber stopper. One chamber contains a liquid diluent, and the other chamber contains a dry medication. Before preparing a medication, push on the upper chamber to dislodge the rubber stopper and allow the powder and the diluent to mix. In contrast to an ampule, a vial is a closed system. You must inject air into the vial to permit easy withdrawal of the solution. Some medications, even when in a vial, may need to be drawn up with a filter needle because of the nature of the medication. Agency policies and package inserts from the manufacturer indicate drugs that should be prepared with a filter needle.

A health care provider may order an injectable medication that requires reconstitution because it comes in a powdered form. This frequently occurs with time-sensitive injectable medications, which must be administered within a specific time period to guarantee full drug effectiveness.

Delegation and Collaboration

The skill of preparing injections from ampules and vials cannot be delegated to nursing assistive personnel (NAP).

Equipment

Medication in an Ampule

- Syringe, needle, and filter needle
- Small sterile gauze pad or alcohol swab

Medication in a Vial

- Syringe and two needles
- Needles:
  - Needleless blunt-tip vial-access cannula or needle (with safety sheath) for drawing up medication (if needed)
  - Filter needle if indicated
- Small sterile gauze pad or alcohol swab
- Diluent (e.g., 0.9% sodium chloride or sterile water if indicated)

Both

- Sharps with engineered sharps injury protection (SESIP) safety needle for injection
- Medication administration record (MAR) or computer printout
- Medication in vial or ampule
- Puncture-proof container for disposal of syringes, needles, and glass

ASSESSMENT

1. Check accuracy and completeness of each MAR or computer printout with health care provider's written medication order. Check patient's name, medication name and dosage, route of administration, and time of administration. Recopy or reprint any portion of MAR that is difficult to read. *Rationale: The order sheet is the most reliable source and only legal record of medications that patient is to receive. Ensures that patient receives the correct medications (Westbrook et al., 2017). Transcription errors are a source of medication errors (Truitt et al., 2016).*
2. Assess patient's medical and medication history. *Rationale: Determines need for medication or possible contraindications for medication administration.*
3. Assess patient's history of allergies. Know type of allergies and normal allergic response. *Rationale: Do not prepare medication if there is a known patient allergy.*
4. Review medication reference information for action, purpose, side effects, and nursing implications. *Rationale: Allows you to administer drug properly and monitor patient's response.*
5. Assess patient's body build, muscle size, and weight if giving subcutaneous or IM medication. *Rationale: Determines type and size of syringe and needle for injection.*

STEP	RATIONALE
PLANNING	
1. Expected outcomes following completion of procedure:	
• Proper dose is prepared. No air bubbles are in syringe barrel.	Ensures right dose. Air bubbles displace medication. Elimination of air ensures accuracy of medication dose.
IMPLEMENTATION	
1. Perform hand hygiene and prepare supplies.	Reduces transmission of microorganisms.
2. Prepare medications.	
a. If using a medication cart, move it outside patient's room.	Organization of equipment saves time and reduces error.
b. Unlock medication drawer or cart or log onto computerized medication dispensing system.	Medications are safeguarded when locked in cabinet, cart, or computerized medication dispensing system.
c. Follow the agency's no-interruption zone (NIZ) policy. Prepare medications for one patient at a time. Keep all pages of MARs or computer printouts for one patient together or look at only one patient's electronic MAR at a time.	Preventing distractions reduces medication preparation errors. Use NIZ when possible (Prakash et al., 2014; Yoder et al., 2015).
d. Select correct drug from stock supply or unit-dose drawer. Compare label of medication with MAR computer printout or computer screen.	Reading label and comparing it with transcribed order reduce errors. *This is the first check for accuracy.*
e. Check expiration date on each medication, one at a time.	Medications used past their expiration date are sometimes inactive, less effective, or harmful to patients.
f. Calculate drug dose as necessary. Double-check your calculation. In the case of high-risk medications, ask another nurse to perform an independent double check of dosage (see agency policy).	Double-checking reduces error. Research has shown the ability of independent double checks to detect up to 95% of errors (Institute for Safe Medication Practices [ISMP], 2013). Independent double checks should only be used for very selective high-alert medications (not all) that most warrant their use (ISMP, 2013).
g. If preparing a controlled substance, check record for previous drug count and compare with supply available.	Controlled substance laws require careful monitoring of dispensed narcotics.
h. Do not leave drugs unattended.	Nurse is responsible for safekeeping of drugs.
3. Prepare ampule.	
a. Tap top of ampule lightly and quickly with finger until fluid moves from its neck (see illustration).	Dislodges any fluid that collects above neck of ampule. All solution moves into lower chamber.
b. Place small gauze pad around neck of ampule (see illustration).	Protects fingers from trauma as glass tip is broken off. Do not use opened alcohol swab to wrap around top of ampule because alcohol may leak into ampule.
c. Snap neck of ampule quickly and firmly away from hands (see illustration).	Protects your fingers and face from shattering glass.
d. Draw up medication quickly, using filter needle long enough to reach bottom of ampule to access medication.	System is open to airborne contaminants. Filter needles filter out any fragments of glass (Joo et al., 2016).
e. Hold ampule upside down or set it on flat surface. Insert filter needle into center of ampule opening. Do not allow needle tip or shaft to touch rim of ampule.	Broken rim of ampule is considered contaminated. When ampule is inverted, solution dribbles out if needle tip or shaft touches rim of ampule.

STEP	RATIONALE
f. Aspirate medication into syringe by gently pulling back on plunger (see illustration).	Withdrawal of plunger creates negative pressure within syringe barrel, which pulls fluid into syringe.
g. Keep needle tip under surface of liquid. Tip ampule to bring all fluid within reach of needle.	Prevents aspiration of air bubbles.
h. If you aspirate air bubbles, do not expel air into ampule.	Air pressure forces fluid out of ampule, and medication will be lost.
i. To expel excess air bubbles, remove needle from ampule. Hold syringe vertically with needle pointing up. Tap side of syringe to cause bubbles to rise toward needle. Draw back slightly on plunger and push plunger upward to eject air. Do not eject fluid.	Withdrawing plunger too far removes it from barrel. Holding syringe vertically allows fluid to settle in bottom of barrel. Pulling back on plunger allows fluid within needle to enter barrel so fluid is not expelled. You then expel air at top of barrel and within needle.

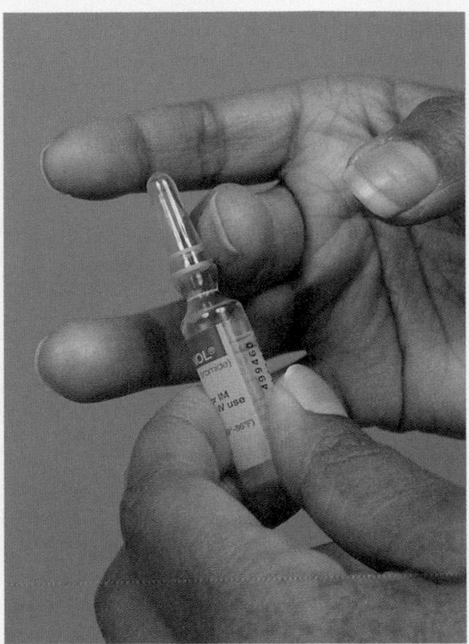

STEP 3a Tapping ampule moves fluid down neck.

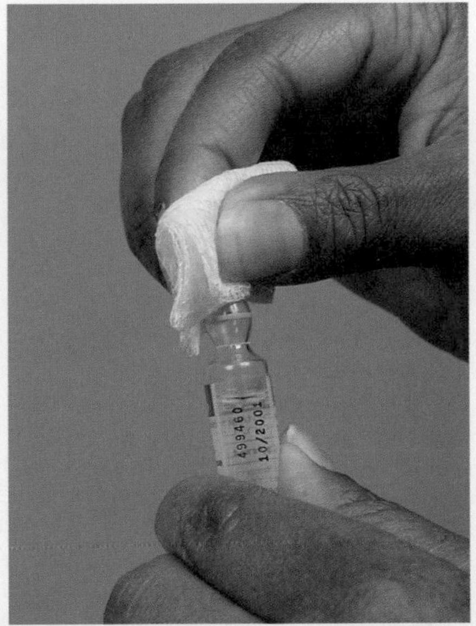

STEP 3b Gauze pad placed around neck of ampule.

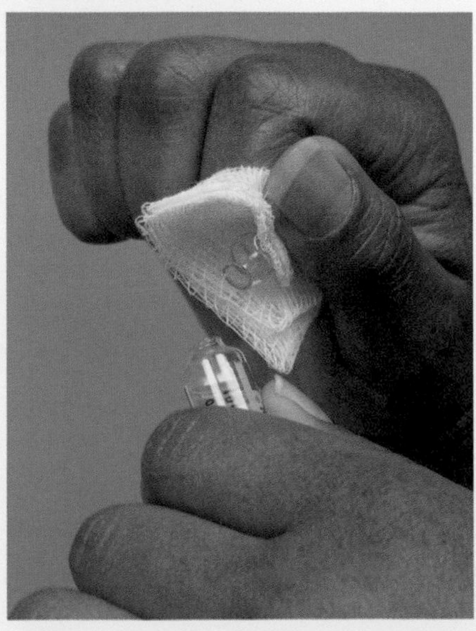

STEP 3c Neck snapped away from hands.

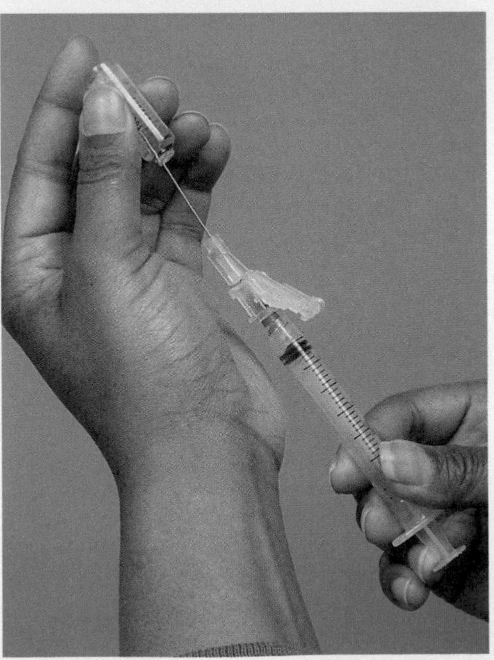

STEP 3f Medication aspirated with ampule inverted.

STEP	RATIONALE
j. If syringe contains excess fluid, use sink for disposal. Hold syringe vertically with needle tip up and slanted slightly toward sink. Slowly eject excess fluid into sink. Recheck fluid level in syringe by holding it vertically.	Safely disperses excess medication into sink. Position of needle allows you to expel medication without having it flow down needle shaft. Rechecking fluid level ensures proper dose.
k. Cover needle with its safety sheath or cap. Replace filter needle with regular SESIP needle.	Minimizes needlesticks. Filter needles cannot be used for injection.
4. Prepare vial containing a solution.	
a. Remove cap covering top of unused vial to expose sterile rubber seal. If a multi-dose vial has been used before, cap is already removed. Firmly and briskly wipe surface of rubber seal with alcohol swab and allow it to dry.	Vial comes packaged with cap that cannot be replaced after seal removal. Not all drug manufacturers guarantee that rubber seals of unused vials are sterile. Swabbing with alcohol reduces transmission of microorganisms. Allowing alcohol to dry prevents alcohol from coating needle and mixing with medication.
b. Pick up syringe and remove needle cap or cap covering needleless access device. Pull back on plunger to draw amount of air into syringe equivalent to volume of medication to be aspirated from vial.	Injecting air into vial prevents buildup of negative pressure in vial when aspirating medication.

Safe Patient Care *Some medications and agencies require use of a filter needle when preparing medications from vials. Check agency policy or medication reference. If you use a filter needle to aspirate medication, you need to change it to a regular SESIP needle of the appropriate size to administer medication (Alexander et al., 2014).*

STEP	RATIONALE
c. With vial on flat surface, insert tip of needle or needleless device through center of rubber seal (see illustration). Apply pressure to tip of needle during insertion.	Center of seal is thinner and easier to penetrate. Using firm pressure prevents dislodging rubber particles that could enter vial or needle.
d. Inject air into air space of vial, holding on to plunger. Hold plunger firmly; plunger is sometimes forced backward by air pressure within vial.	Injection of air creates vacuum needed to get medication to flow into syringe. Injecting into air space of vial prevents formation of bubbles and an inaccurate dose.
e. Invert vial while keeping firm hold on syringe and plunger. Hold vial between thumb and middle fingers of nondominant hand (see illustration). Grasp end of syringe barrel and plunger with thumb and forefinger of dominant hand to counteract pressure in vial.	Inverting vial allows fluid to settle in lower half of container. Position of hands prevents forceful movement of plunger and permits easy manipulation of syringe.
f. Keep tip of needle or needleless device below fluid level.	Prevents aspiration of air.
g. Allow air pressure from vial to fill syringe gradually with medication. If necessary, pull back slightly on plunger to obtain correct amount of medication.	Positive pressure within vial forces fluid into syringe.

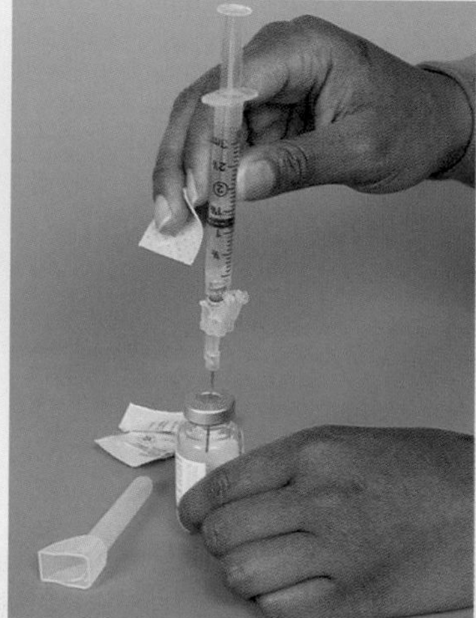

STEP 4c Insert safety needle through center of vial diaphragm (with vial flat on table).

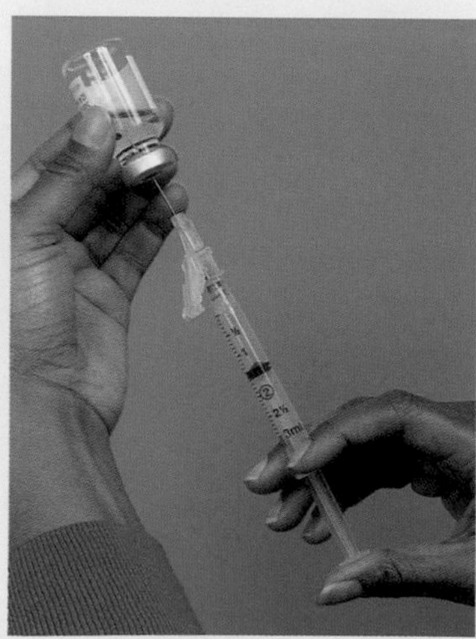

STEP 4e Withdraw fluid with vial inverted.

STEP	RATIONALE
h. When you obtain desired volume, position needle or needleless device into air space of vial; tap side of syringe barrel gently to dislodge any air bubbles (see illustration). Eject any air remaining at top of syringe into vial.	Forcefully striking barrel while needle is inserted in vial may bend needle. Accumulation of air displaces medication and causes dose errors.

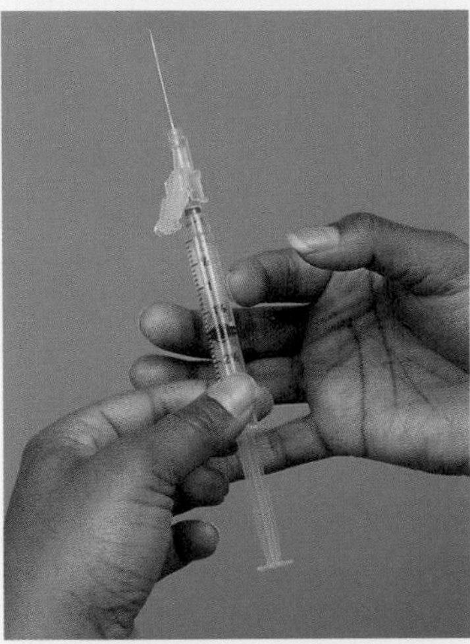

STEP 4h Hold syringe upright; tap barrel to dislodge air bubbles.

STEP	RATIONALE
i. Remove needle or needleless access device from vial by pulling back on barrel of syringe.	Pulling plunger rather than barrel causes plunger to separate from barrel, resulting in loss of medication.
j. Hold syringe at eye level at 90-degree angle to ensure correct volume and absence of air bubbles. Remove any remaining air by tapping barrel to dislodge any air bubbles. Draw back slightly on plunger; then push it upward to eject air. Do not eject fluid. Recheck volume of medication.	Holding syringe vertically allows fluid to settle in bottom of barrel. Tapping dislodges air to top of barrel. Pulling back on plunger allows fluid within needle to enter barrel so that you do not expel fluid. You then expel air at top of barrel and within needle.

Safe Patient Care *When preparing medication from single-dose vial, do not assume that volume listed on label is total volume in vial. Some manufacturers provide a small amount of extra liquid, expecting loss during preparation. Be sure to draw up and verify the correct volume.*

STEP	RATIONALE
k. Before you inject medication into patient's tissue, change needle with regular SESIP to appropriate gauge and length according to route of medication administration.	Inserting needle through rubber stopper dulls beveled tip. New needle is sharper and, because no fluid is along shaft, does not track medication through tissues. Filter needles cannot be used for injection.
l. Cover needle with its safety sheath or cap.	Minimizes needlesticks.
m. For multi-dose vial, make label that includes date of opening, concentration of drug per milliliter, and your initials.	Ensures that nurses will prepare future doses correctly. You discard some drugs within a certain time frame after mixing.
5. Prepare vial containing powder (reconstituting medications).	
a. Remove cap covering vial of powdered medication and cap covering vial of proper diluent. Firmly swab both rubber seals with alcohol swab and allow alcohol to dry.	Allowing alcohol to dry prevents it from coating needle and mixing with medication.
b. Draw up manufacturer suggestion for volume and type of diluent into syringe following Steps 4b through 4j.	Prepares diluent for injection into vial containing powdered medication.
c. Insert tip of needle or needleless device through center of rubber seal of vial of powdered medication. Inject diluent into vial. Remove needle.	Diluent begins to dissolve and reconstitute medication.
d. Mix medication thoroughly. Roll in palms. Do not shake.	Ensures proper dispersal of medication throughout solution and prevents formation of air bubbles.
e. Reconstituted medication in vial is ready to be drawn into new syringe. Read label carefully to determine dose after reconstitution.	Once you add diluent, concentration of medication (mg/mL) determines dose you give. Reading medication label carefully decreases medication errors.
f. Draw up reconstituted medication into syringe. Insert needleless device/needle into vial. Do not add air. Then follow Steps 4e through 4l.	Prepares medication for administration.

STEP	RATIONALE

Safe Patient Care *Some agencies require that doses of certain medications (e.g., insulin and heparin) be checked using an independent double check by another nurse (ISMP, 2013). Check policies and procedures before administering medication.*

STEP	RATIONALE
6. Compare label of medication with MAR, computer screen, or computer printout.	*This is the second check for accuracy.*
7. Dispose of soiled supplies. Place broken ampule and/or used vials and used needle or needleless device in puncture- and leak-proof container. Clean work area and perform hand hygiene.	Proper disposal of glass and needle prevents accidental injury to staff. Controls transmission of infection.

EVALUATION

STEP	RATIONALE
1. Just before administering drug to patient, compare MAR with label of prepared drug and compare dose in syringe with desired dose.	Ensures that dose is accurate. *This is the third check for accuracy.*

Unexpected Outcomes	Related Interventions
1. Air bubbles remain in syringe.	• Expel air from syringe and add medication to it until you prepare correct dose.
2. Incorrect dose of medication is prepared.	• Discard prepared dose. • Prepare correct new dose.

PROCEDURAL GUIDELINE 24.1 *Mixing Parenteral Medications in One Syringe*

Purpose

Some medications need to be mixed from two vials or from a vial and an ampule. Mixing compatible medications avoids the need to give a patient more than one injection. Most patient care units have medication compatibility charts that are in drug reference guides, posted within patient care unit rooms, or available electronically. If you are uncertain about medication compatibilities, consult a pharmacist. When mixing medications, you must correctly aspirate fluid from each type of container. When using multi-dose vials, do not contaminate the contents of the vial with medication from another vial or ampule.

Delegation and Collaboration

The skill of mixing medications in one syringe cannot be delegated to nursing assistive personnel (NAP). The nurse directs the NAP about:

- Potential side effects of medications and the need to immediately report their occurrence to the nurse.

Equipment

- Single- or multi-dose vials and ampules containing medication; syringe and two needles; alcohol swab; puncture-proof container for disposing of syringes, needles, and glass; medication administration record (MAR) or computer printout; medication in vial or ampule
- Needles: Needleless blunt-tip vial access cannula or needle for drawing up medication; filter needle if indicated; sharps with engineered sharps injury protection (SESIP) needle for injection

Procedural Steps

1. Check accuracy and completeness of MAR or computer printout with health care provider's written medication order. Check patient's name, medication name and dosage, route of administration, and time of administration. Recopy or reprint any part of MAR that is difficult to read.
2. Review pertinent information related to medication, including action, purpose, side effects, and nursing implications.
3. Perform hand hygiene. Assess patient body build, muscle size, and weight if giving subcutaneous or intramuscular (IM) medication.
4. Consider compatibility of medications to be mixed and type of injection.
5. Check expiration date of medication printed on vial or ampule.
6. Perform hand hygiene.
7. Prepare medication for one patient at a time following the seven rights of medication administration (see Chapter 22). Select an ampule or vial from the unit-dose drawer or automated dispensing system. Compare the label of each medication with the MAR or computer printout. In the case of insulin, ensure that correct type or types of insulin are prepared. *This is the first check for accuracy.*
8. Mixing medications from two vials (see illustration):
   a. Take syringe with needleless device or filter needle and aspirate volume of air equivalent to first medication dose (vial A).

PROCEDURAL GUIDELINE 24.1 *Mixing Parenteral Medications in One Syringe—cont'd*

- **b.** Inject air into vial A, making sure that needle or needleless device does not touch solution (see illustration A).
- **c.** Holding on to plunger, withdraw syringe from vial A. Aspirate air equivalent to second medication dose (vial B) into syringe.
- **d.** Insert needle or needleless device into vial B, inject volume of air into vial B, and withdraw medication from vial B into syringe (see illustration B).
- **e.** Withdraw needle or needleless device and syringe from vial B. Ensure that proper volume has been obtained.
- **f.** Determine on syringe scale what the combined volume of medications should measure.
- **g.** Insert needle or needleless device into vial A, being careful not to push plunger and expel medication within syringe into vial. Invert vial and carefully withdraw the desired amount of medication from vial A into syringe (see illustration C).
- **h.** Withdraw needle or needleless device and expel any excess air from syringe. Check fluid level in syringe for proper dose. Medications are now mixed.

Safe Patient Care *If too much medication is withdrawn from second vial, discard syringe and start over. Do not push medication back into either vial.*

- **i.** Change needle or needleless device for appropriate-sized needle if medication is being injected. Keep needle or needleless device capped until administration time.

9. Mixing insulin:

- **a.** If patient takes insulin that is cloudy, roll bottle of insulin between hands to resuspend insulin preparation.
- **b.** Wipe off tops of both insulin vials with alcohol swab.
- **c.** Verify insulin dose against MAR.

Safe Patient Care *If long-acting insulin glargine (Lantus) is ordered, note that this is a clear insulin, and it should not be mixed with other insulin preparations.*

- **d.** If mixing rapid- or short-acting insulin with intermediate-acting insulin, take insulin syringe and aspirate volume of air equivalent to dose to be withdrawn from intermediate-acting insulin first (see illustration). If two intermediate-acting insulins are mixed, it makes no difference which vial is prepared first.
- **e.** Insert needle and inject air into vial of intermediate-acting insulin. Do not let tip of needle touch solution.
- **f.** Remove syringe from vial of insulin without aspirating medication.
- **g.** With the same syringe, inject air equal to the dose of rapid- or short-acting insulin into vial and withdraw correct dose into syringe (see illustration).
- **h.** Remove syringe from rapid- or short-acting insulin and remove any air bubbles to ensure accurate dose.
- **i.** Verify short-acting insulin dosage with MAR. Have another nurse perform an independent double check of dosage to verify that correct dosage of insulin was prepared. Determine which point on syringe scale the combined units of insulin should measure by adding the number of units of both insulins together (e.g., 4 units Regular + 10 units NPH = 14 units total). Verify combined dosage.
- **j.** Place needle of syringe back into vial of intermediate-acting insulin. Be careful not to push plunger and inject insulin in syringe into vial.
- **k.** Invert vial and carefully withdraw desired amount of insulin into syringe (see illustration).
- **l.** Withdraw needle and check fluid level in syringe. Verify with another nurse that correct total dose was prepared. Keep needle of prepared syringe sheathed or capped until ready to administer medication.

10. Mixing medications from a vial and an ampule:

- **a.** Prepare medication from vial first, following Skill 24.1, Step 4.
- **b.** Determine on syringe scale what combined volume of medications should measure.

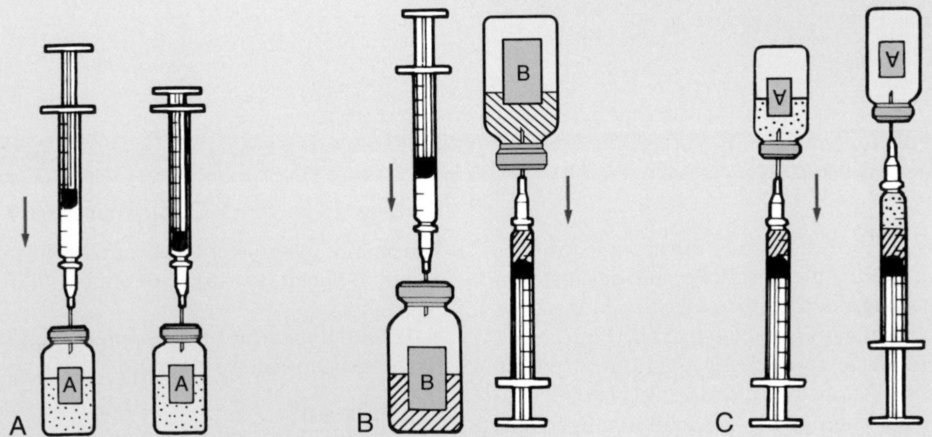

STEP 8 (A) Inject air into vial A. (B) Inject air into vial B and withdraw dose. (C) Withdraw medication from vial A; medications are now mixed.

Continued

PROCEDURAL GUIDELINE 24.1 *Mixing Parenteral Medications in One Syringe—cont'd*

Safe Patient Care *If needleless access device was used in preparing medication from vial, change needleless system to a filter needle to remove medication from ampule.*

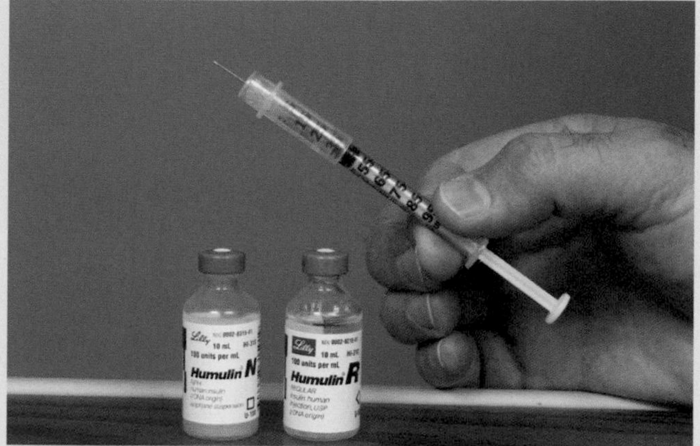

STEP 9d Aspirate air equivalent to dose to be withdrawn from intermediate insulin.

c. Next, using the same syringe, prepare second medication from ampule, following Step 3 in Skill 24.1.
d. Withdraw filter needle from ampule and verify fluid level in syringe. Change filter needle to appropriate SESIP needle. Keep device or needle sheathed or capped until administering medication.
e. Check syringe carefully for total combined dose of medications. If a high-risk medication is being administered, have a second nurse perform an independent check of dosage.

11. Compare MAR, computer screen, or computer printout with prepared medication and labels on vials/ampules. *This is the second check for accuracy.*
12. Dispose of soiled supplies. Place used ampules and/or vials and needle or needleless device in puncture- and leak-proof container.
13. Clean work area and perform hand hygiene.
14. Check syringe again carefully for total combined dose of medications.
15. Compare MAR, computer screen, or computer printout with prepared medication. *The third check for accuracy occurs at patient's bedside.*

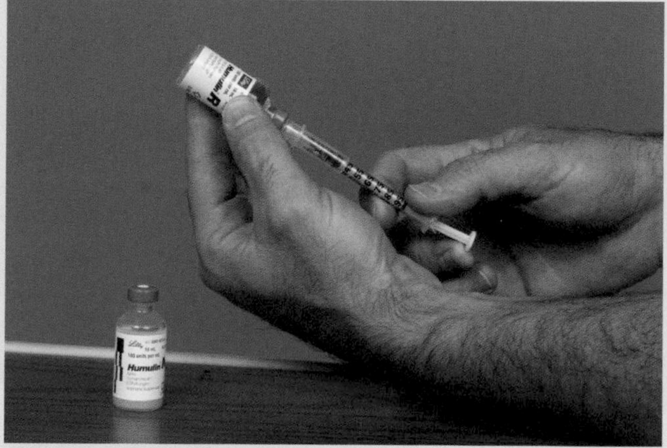

STEP 9g Withdraw short-acting insulin.

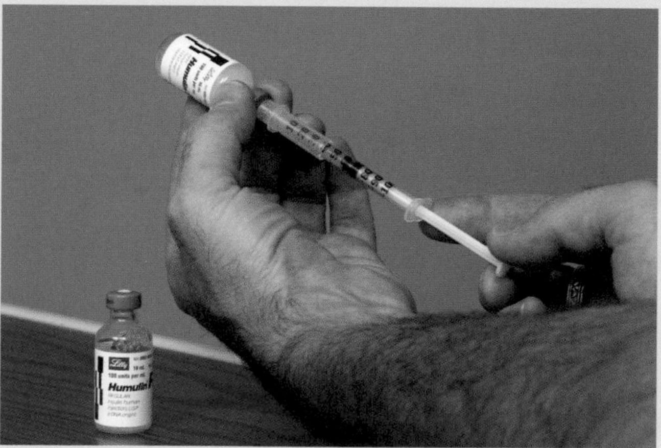

STEP 9k Withdraw intermediate insulin.

✦ SKILL 24.2 Administering Subcutaneous Injections

Purpose

Subcutaneous injections involve depositing medication into the loose connective tissue underlying the dermis. Because subcutaneous tissue does not contain as many blood vessels as muscles, medications are absorbed more slowly than with intramuscular (IM) injections. Subcutaneous tissue is sensitive to irritating solutions and large volumes of medications. Injection into blood vessels is rare; thus you do not need to aspirate when giving subcutaneous injections (Lilley et al., 2016). Thus you only administer small volumes (0.5 to 1.5 mL) of water-soluble medications subcutaneously to adults. Examples of subcutaneous medications include epinephrine, insulin (Box 24.2), allergy medications, opioids, and heparin (Box 24.3).

Delegation and Collaboration

The skill of administering subcutaneous injections cannot be delegated to nursing assistive personnel (NAP). The nurse directs the NAP about:

- Potential medication sides effects and to immediately report their occurrence to the nurse.

Equipment

- Proper size syringe and sharp with engineered sharps injury protection (SESIP) needle:
  - Subcutaneous: syringe (1 to 3 mL) and needle (25 to 27 gauge, ⅜ to ⅝ inch)

BOX 24.2

General Guidelines for Insulin Administration

- Store vials of insulin in the refrigerator, not the freezer. Keep vials currently being used at room temperature. Do not inject cold insulin.
- Inspect vials before each use for changes in appearance (e.g., clumping, frosting, precipitation, change in clarity or color) indicating lack of potency.
- Do not interchange insulin types unless approved by the patient's health care provider.
- Preferred injection site includes the abdomen, avoiding a 5-cm (2-inch) radius around the umbilicus and the outer aspect of the thighs.
- Research in insulin administration now shows that insulin needles that are 5/16 inch (8 mm) or longer often enter the muscles of men and people with a body mass index (BMI) of 25 or less. Shorter (3/16-inch or 4- to 5-mm) needles were associated with less pain, adequate control of blood sugars, and minimal leakage of medication (Diggle, 2014; Hirsch et al., 2012).
- Thus, when administering insulin, you should use needles of 3/16 inch (4 to 5 mm) administered at a 90-degree angle to reduce pain and achieve adequate control of blood sugars with minimal adverse effects for people of all BMIs, including children (Levitsky et al., 2017).
- Have patient self-administer insulin whenever possible.
- Patients who take insulin need to self-monitor their blood glucose.
- Teach patients appropriate use, storage, and maintenance of syringes or insulin pens (Fig. 24.8).
- All patients who take insulin should carry at least 15 g carbohydrate (e.g., 4 ounces of fruit juice, 4 ounces of regular soft drink, 8 ounces of skim milk, 6 to 10 hard candies) in the event of a hypoglycemic reaction.

Adapted from American Diabetes Association (ADA): Diabetes care in the hospital, nursing home, and skilled nursing agency, *Diabetes Care* 38(S1): S80, 2015. http://care.diabetesjournals.org/content/38/Supplement_1/S80.full.

BOX 24.3

General Guidelines for Heparin Administration

- Before administering heparin, assess for preexisting conditions that contraindicate its use, including cerebral or aortic aneurysm, cerebrovascular hemorrhage, severe hypertension, and blood dyscrasias.
- Assess the patient's current medication regimen, including use of over-the-counter (OTC) and herbal medications, for possible interaction with heparin. Other medications that interact with heparin include aspirin and nonsteroidal antiinflammatory drugs.
- Choose an injection site that is free of skin lesions, bony prominences, and large underlying muscles or nerves.
- A patient's body weight and amount of adipose tissue indicate the depth of the subcutaneous layer.
- Base the needle length and angle of needle insertion on the patient's weight and an estimate of subcutaneous tissue. Generally, a 25-gauge, 5/8-inch needle inserted at a 45-degree angle or a 1/2-inch needle inserted at a 90-degree angle deposits medication into the subcutaneous tissue of a normal-sized patient (Fig. 24.9).
- To minimize the pain and bruising associated with low-molecular-weight heparin (LMWH), it is given subcutaneously on the right or left side of the abdomen, at least 5 cm (2 inches) away from the umbilicus (the patient's "love handles").
- A child usually requires a 26- to 30-gauge needle inserted at a 90-degree angle (Hockenberry and Wilson, 2017).
- There is some new evidence to support a slower injection rate of 30 seconds to reduce bruising and pain (Akbari Sari et al., 2014; RCN, 2016).

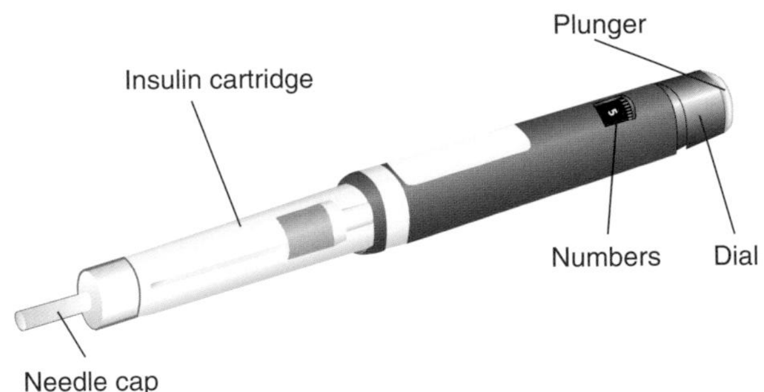

FIG 24.8 Insulin injection pen.

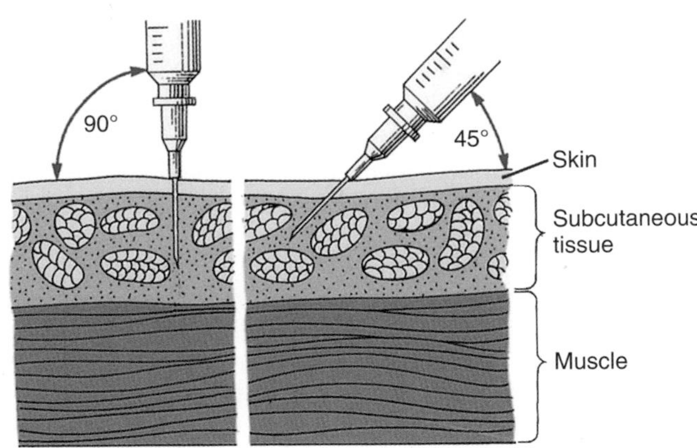

FIG 24.9 Subcutaneous injection. Angle and needle length depend on thickness of skinfold.

  - Immunizations: 5/8-inch, 23- to 25-gauge needle (Centers for Disease Control and Prevention [CDC], 2015)
  - Subcutaneous U-100 insulin: insulin syringe (1 mL) with preattached needle (28 to 31 gauge, 3/8 to 5/8 inch)
  - Subcutaneous U-500 insulin: 1-mL tuberculin (TB) syringe with needle (25 to 27 gauge, 1/2 to 5/8 inch)
- Small gauze pad *(optional)*
- Alcohol swab
- Medication vial or ampule
- Clean gloves
- Medication administration record (MAR) or computer printout
- Puncture-proof container

ASSESSMENT

1. Check accuracy and completeness of each MAR or computer printout with health care provider's written medication order. Check patient's name, medication name and dosage, route of administration, and time of administration. Recopy or reprint any portion of MAR that is difficult to read. *Rationale: The order sheet is the most reliable source and only legal record of medications that patient is to receive. Ensures that patient receives the correct medications (Westbrook et al., 2017). Transcription errors are a source of medication errors (Truitt et al., 2016).*
2. Assess patient's medical and medication history. *Rationale: Determines need for medication or possible contraindications for medication administration.*

3. Assess patient's history of allergies: known type of allergies and normal allergic reaction. *Rationale: Do not prepare medication if there is known patient allergy.*
4. Review medication reference information for medication action, purpose, normal dose, side effects, time and peak of onset, and nursing implications. *Rationale: Allows you to administer medication safely and monitor patient's response to therapy.*
5. Check date of expiration for medication. *Rationale: Dose potency increases or decreases when outdated.*
6. Observe patient's previous verbal and nonverbal responses toward injection. *Rationale: Anticipating patient's anxiety allows you to use distraction to reduce pain awareness.*
7. Assess patient's symptoms before initiating medication therapy. *Rationale: Provides information to evaluate desired effect of medication.*
8. Perform hand hygiene. Assess for contraindication to subcutaneous injections, such as circulatory shock or reduced local tissue perfusion. *Rationale: Reduced tissue perfusion interferes with drug absorption and distribution.*
9. Assess adequacy of patient's adipose tissue. *Rationale: Adipose tissue influences methods for administering injections.*
10. Assess relevant laboratory results (e.g., blood glucose, partial thromboplastin). *Rationale: Provides baseline for measuring drug response.*
11. Assess patient's or family caregiver's knowledge, experience, and health literacy. *Rationale: Ensures patient or family caregiver has the capacity to obtain, communicate, process, and understand basic health information (CDC, 2016).*

STEP	RATIONALE
PLANNING	
1. Expected outcomes following completion of procedure:	
• Patient experiences no pain or mild burning at injection site.	Medications may cause minor tissue irritation.
• Patient achieves desired effect of medication with no signs of allergies or undesired effects.	Medication administered without patient injury.
• Patient explains purpose, dosage, effects of medication, and side effects to be aware of.	Demonstrates learning.
2. Provide privacy and prepare environment.	Providing privacy and preparing the environment early help the student/nurse think about the need to remove clutter from the over-bed or bedside table.
3. Discuss purpose of each medication, action, and possible adverse effects. Allow patient to ask any questions. Tell patient that injection will cause slight burning or sting.	Patient has right to be informed, and patient's understanding of each medication improves adherence to drug therapy. Helps minimize patient's anxiety.
IMPLEMENTATION	
1. Perform hand hygiene and prepare medication using aseptic technique. Prepare medications for one patient at a time. Keep all pages of MARs or computer printouts for one patient together or look at only one patient's electronic MAR at a time. Check label of medication carefully with MAR or computer printout two times (see Skill 24.1 or Procedural Guideline 24.1) when preparing medication.	Ensures that medication is sterile. Preventing distractions reduces medication preparation errors. Use no-interruption zone (NIZ) when possible (Prakash et al., 2014; Yoder et al., 2015). *These are the first and second checks for accuracy* and ensure that correct medication is administered.
2. Take medication(s) to patient at correct time (see agency policy). Medications that require exact timing include STAT, first-time or loading doses, and one-time doses. Give time-critical scheduled medications (e.g., antibiotics, anticoagulants, insulin, anticonvulsants, immunosuppressive agents) at exact time ordered (no later than 30 minutes before or after scheduled dose). Give non–time-critical scheduled medications within a range of 1 or 2 hours of scheduled dose (ISMP, 2011). During administration, apply seven rights of medication administration.	Hospitals must adopt medication administration policy and procedure for timing of medication administration that considers nature of the prescribed medication, specific clinical application, and patient needs (Department of Health and Human Services, Centers for Medicare and Medicaid [DHHS], 2011; ISMP, 2011). Time-critical scheduled medications are those for which early or delayed administration of maintenance doses of greater than 30 minutes before or after the scheduled dose may cause harm or result in substantial suboptimal therapy or pharmacological effect. Non–time-critical medications are those for which early or delayed administration within a specified range of either 1 or 2 hours should not cause harm or result in substantial suboptimal therapy or pharmacological effect (DHHS, 2011; ISMP, 2011).

STEP	RATIONALE
3. Identify patient using at least two identifiers (e.g., name and birthday or name and medical record number) according to agency policy. Compare identifiers with information on patient's MAR or medical record.	Ensures correct patient. Complies with The Joint Commission standards and improves patient safety (TJC, 2019). Some agencies are now using a bar-code system to help with patient identification.
4. At patient's bedside, again compare MAR or computer printout with names of medications on medication labels and patient name. Ask patient again if he or she has allergies.	*This is the third check for accuracy* and ensures that patient receives correct medication. Confirms patient's allergy history.
5. Perform hand hygiene and apply clean gloves. Keep sheet or gown draped over body parts not requiring exposure.	Reduces transmission of infection. Respects dignity of patient while exposing injection area.
6. Select appropriate injection site (Fig. 24.10). Inspect skin surface over sites for bruises, inflammation, or edema. Do not use an area that is bruised or has signs associated with infection.	Injection sites are free of abnormalities that interfere with drug absorption. Sites used repeatedly become hardened from lipohypertrophy (increased growth in fatty tissue).

Safe Patient Care *Applying ice to the injection site for 1 minute before the injection may decrease the patient's perception of pain (Hockenberry and Wilson, 2017).*

STEP	RATIONALE
7. Palpate sites and avoid those with masses or tenderness. Be sure that needle is correct size by grasping skinfold at site with thumb and forefinger. Measure fold from top to bottom. Make sure that needle is one-half length of fold.	You can mistakenly give subcutaneous injections in muscle, especially in abdomen and thigh sites. Appropriate size of needle ensures that you inject medication into subcutaneous tissue (Hirsch et al., 2012; Ogston-Tuck, 2014a).
a. When administering insulin or heparin, use abdominal injection sites first, followed by thigh injection site.	Risk for bruising is not affected by site.
b. When administering low-molecular-weight heparin (LMWH) subcutaneously, choose site on right or left side of abdomen, at least 5 cm (2 inches) away from umbilicus.	Injecting LMWH on side of abdomen helps decrease pain and bruising at injection site (Royal College of Nursing [RCN], 2016).
c. Rotate insulin site within an anatomical area (e.g., abdomen) and systematically rotate sites within that area.	Rotating injection sites within same anatomical site maintains consistency in day-to-day insulin absorption.
8. Help patient into comfortable position. Have him or her relax arm, leg, or abdomen, depending on site selection.	Relaxation of site minimizes discomfort.
9. Relocate site using anatomical landmarks.	Injection into correct anatomical site prevents injury to nerves, bone, and blood vessels.
10. Clean site with antiseptic swab. Apply swab at center of site and rotate outward in circular direction for about 5 cm (2 inches; see illustration).	Mechanical action of swab removes secretions containing microorganisms.

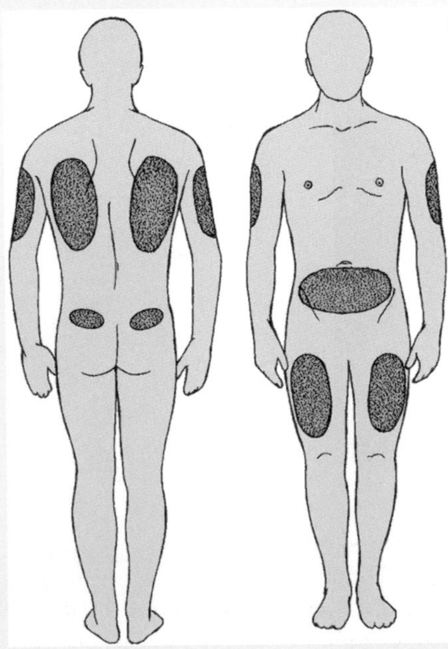

FIG 24.10 Common sites for subcutaneous injections.

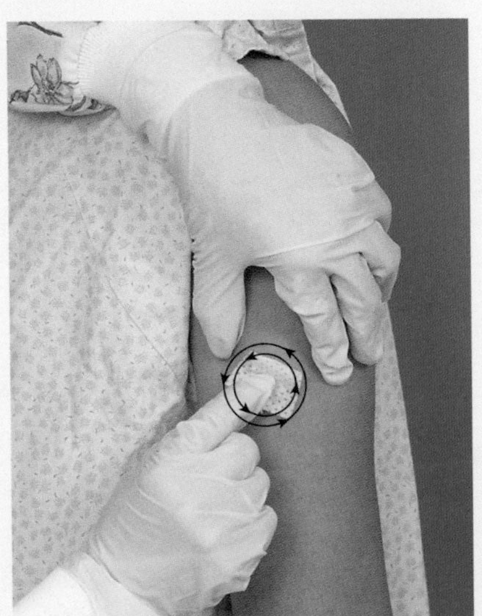

STEP 10 Clean site with circular motion.

STEP	RATIONALE
11. Hold swab or gauze between third and fourth fingers of nondominant hand.	Swab or gauze remains readily accessible for use when withdrawing needle after the injection.
12. Remove needle cap or protective sheath by pulling it straight off.	Preventing needle from touching sides of cap prevents contamination.
13. Hold syringe between thumb and forefinger of dominant hand; hold as dart (see illustration).	Quick, smooth injection requires proper manipulation of syringe parts.
14. Administer injection:	
a. For average-size patient, hold skin across injection site or pinch skin with nondominant hand.	Needle penetrates tight skin more easily than loose skin. Pinching elevates subcutaneous tissue and desensitizes area.
b. Inject needle quickly and firmly at 45- to 90-degree angle (see illustration). Release skin if pinched. *Option:* When using injection pen or giving heparin, continue to pinch skin while injecting medicine.	Quick, firm insertion minimizes discomfort. (Injecting medication into compressed tissue irritates nerve fibers.) Correct angle prevents accidental injection into muscle.
c. For obese patient, pinch skin at site and inject needle at 90-degree angle below tissue fold.	Obese patients have fatty layer of tissue above subcutaneous layer.
d. After needle enters site, grasp lower end of syringe barrel with nondominant hand to stabilize it. Move dominant hand to end of plunger and slowly inject medication over several seconds (see illustration). When giving heparin, inject over 30 seconds (Akbari Sari et al., 2014; RCN, 2016). Avoid moving syringe.	Movement of syringe may displace needle and cause discomfort. Slow injection of medication minimizes discomfort.

Safe Patient Care *Aspiration after injecting a subcutaneous medication is not necessary. Piercing a blood vessel in a subcutaneous injection is very rare. Aspiration after injecting heparin and insulin is not recommended (CDC, 2015; Sepah, 2017).*

STEP	RATIONALE
e. Withdraw needle quickly while placing antiseptic swab or gauze gently over site.	Supporting tissues around injection site minimizes discomfort during needle withdrawal. Dry gauze may minimize patient discomfort associated with alcohol on nonintact skin.
15. Apply gentle pressure to site. Do not massage site. (If heparin is given, hold alcohol swab or gauze to site for 30 to 60 seconds.)	Aids absorption. Massage can damage underlying tissue. Time interval prevents bleeding at site.
16. Help patient to comfortable position.	Gives patient sense of well-being.
17. Discard uncapped needle or needle enclosed in safety shield (see illustrations) and attached syringe into puncture- and leak-proof receptacle.	Prevents injury to patients and health care personnel. Recapping needles increases risk for needlestick injury (OSHA, 2012).

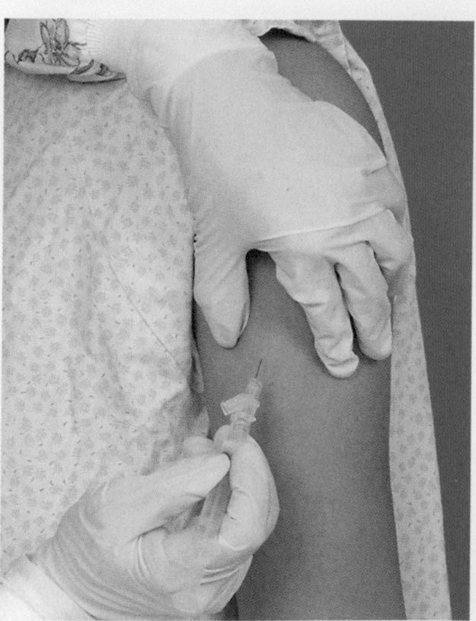

STEP 13 Hold syringe as if grasping a dart.

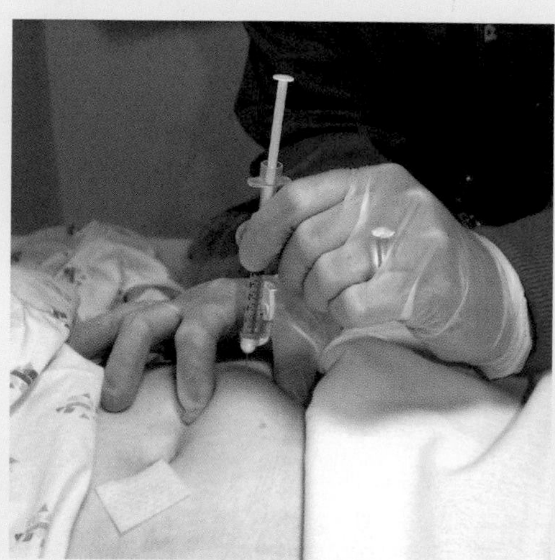

STEP 14b Subcutaneous injection. Angle and needle length depend on thickness of skinfold.

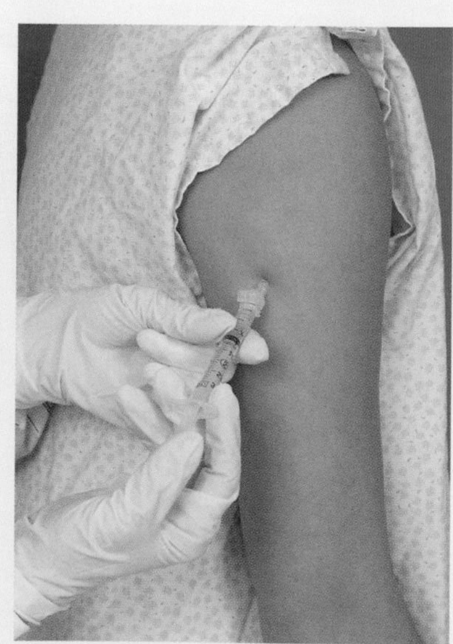

STEP 14d Inject medication slowly.

STEP	RATIONALE

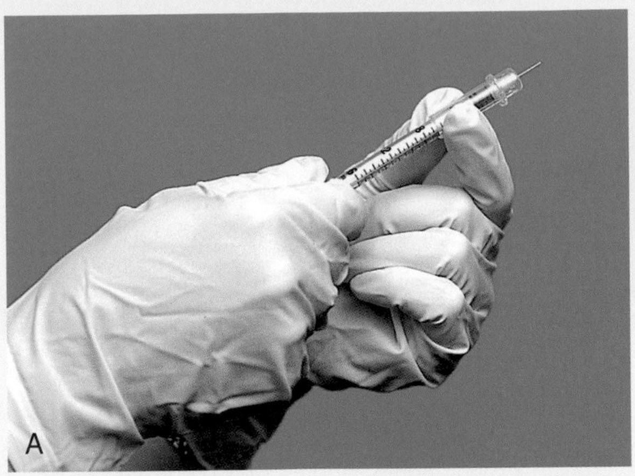
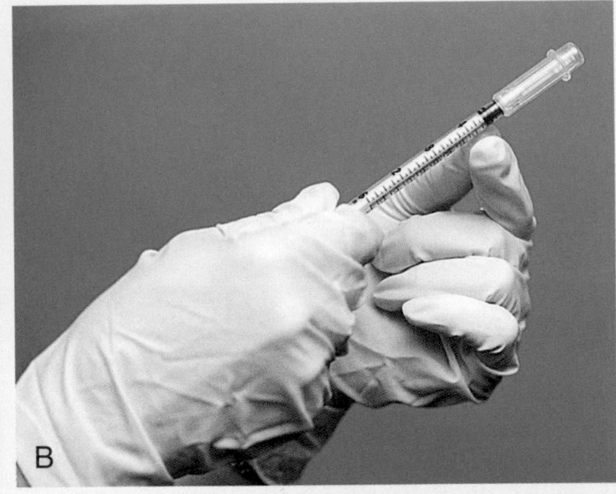

STEP 17 Needle with plastic guard to prevent needlesticks. (A) Position of guard before injection. (B) After injection guard locks in place, covering needle.

STEP	RATIONALE
18. Be sure nurse call system is in an accessible location within patient's reach.	Ensures patient can call for assistance if needed.
19. Raise side rails (as appropriate) and lower bed to lowest position.	Ensures patient safety.
20. Remove and dispose of gloves and perform hand hygiene.	Reduces transmission of microorganisms.
21. Stay with patient for several minutes and observe for any allergic reactions.	Dyspnea, wheezing, and circulatory collapse are signs of severe anaphylactic reaction.

EVALUATION

STEP	RATIONALE
1. Return to room in 15 to 30 minutes and ask if patient feels any acute pain, burning, numbness, or tingling at injection site.	Continued discomfort may indicate injury to underlying bones or nerves.
2. Inspect site, noting bruising or induration. Provide warm compress to site.	Bruising or induration indicates complication associated with injection.
3. Observe patient's response to medication at times that correlate with onset, peak, and duration of medication. Review laboratory results as appropriate (e.g., blood glucose, partial thromboplastin).	Adverse effects of parenteral medications develop rapidly. Evaluates effect of medication at key therapeutic times.
4. Use Teach-Back: "I want to be sure I explained to you the reason for this subcutaneous injection. Tell me why you are receiving this injection." Revise your instruction now or develop a plan for revised patient/family caregiver teaching if patient/family caregiver is not able to teach back correctly.	Determines patient's/family caregiver's level of understanding of instructional topic.

Unexpected Outcomes	Related Interventions
1. Patient complains of localized pain, numbness, tingling, or burning at injection site.	• Assess injection site; may indicate potential injury to nerve or tissues. • Notify patient's health care provider and do not reuse site.
2. Patient displays adverse reaction, with signs of urticaria, eczema, pruritus, wheezing, and dyspnea.	• Monitor patient's heart rate, respirations, blood pressure, and temperature. • Follow agency policy or guidelines for appropriate response to allergic reactions (e.g., administration of antihistamine such as diphenhydramine or epinephrine) and notify patient's health care provider immediately. • Add allergy information to patient's record.
3. Hypertrophy of skin develops from repeated subcutaneous injection.	• Do not use site for future injections. • Instruct patient not to use site for 6 months.

Recording

- Immediately after administration, record medication, dose, route, site, time, and date given.
- Record patient's response to medication, including any adverse effects.
- Document your evaluation of patient learning.

Hand-Off Reporting

- Report any undesirable effects from medication to patient's health care provider.

✦ SKILL 24.3 Administering Intramuscular Injections

Purpose

The intramuscular (IM) injection route deposits medication into deep muscle tissue, which has a rich blood supply, allowing medication to absorb more quickly than the subcutaneous route. However, there is an increased risk of injecting drugs directly into blood vessels. Any factor that interferes with local tissue blood flow affects the rate and extent of drug absorption. In addition, if a medication is not injected correctly into a muscle, complications can arise, such as abscess, hematoma, ecchymosis, pain, and vascular and nerve injury (Gülnar and Çalışkan, 2014; Kaya et al., 2015; Nicoll and Hesby, 2002). Therefore, whenever administering a medication by the IM route, first verify that the injection is justified (Nicoll and Hesby, 2002; World Health Organization [WHO], 2016). Some medications, such as hepatitis B and tetanus, diptheria, and pertussis (Tdap) immunizations, are only given intramuscularly.

Injection Sites

When selecting an IM site, determine that the site is free of pain, infection, necrosis, bruising, and abrasions. Also consider the location of underlying bones, nerves, and blood vessels and the volume of medication you will administer. An IM injection requires a longer and larger-gauge needle to penetrate deep muscle tissue (Box 24.4). The choice of needle length and site of injection must be made based on the size of the muscle, the thickness of adipose tissue at the injection site, the volume to be administered, injection technique, and the depth below the muscle surface to be injected (CDC, 2017). Note that the most common intramuscular injections are immunizations.

Ventrogluteal Muscle

The ventrogluteal muscle is the preferred and safest injection site for all adults, children, and infants, especially for large-volume,

BOX 24.4

Guidelines for Intramuscular (IM) Injections

- Administer adult immunizations and parenteral medications that are in aqueous solutions with a 20- to 25-gauge needle.
- Adults weighing < 60 kg (<130 lb): a ⅝- to 1-inch needle is sufficient to ensure intramuscular injection in the deltoid muscle if the injection is made at a 90-degree angle and the tissue is not bunched.
- Adults weighing 60–70 kg (130–152 lb): a 1-inch needle is sufficient.
- For women who weigh 70–90 kg (152–200 lb) and men who weigh 70–118 kg (152–260 lb), a 1- to 1½-inch needle is recommended.
- For women who weigh > 90 kg (> 200 lb) or men who weigh > 118 kg (>260 lb), a 1½-inch needle is recommended.
- For infants less than 12 months, the anterolateral aspect of the thigh is the recommended site for injection, but the ventrogluteal is equally safe to use if the muscle is well developed. For most infants, a 1-inch needle is sufficient to penetrate the thigh muscle.
- For toddlers aged 12 months to 2 years, the anterolateral thigh muscle or the ventrogluteal site is preferred, and the needle should be at least 1 inch. The deltoid muscle can be used if the muscle mass is adequate. If more than one vaccine is administered, they should be spaced 1 inch apart.
- For children aged 3–10 years, the deltoid muscle is preferred, with the needle length ranging from ⅝ to 1 inch based on technique. The anterolateral thigh can also be used with a needle length of 1 to 1¼ inches.
- For adolescents aged 11–18 years, the deltoid muscle is preferred, but the anterolateral thigh can be used. For injection into the anterolateral thigh, most adolescents will require a 1- to 1½-inch needle.
- The angle of insertion for an IM injection is 90 degrees.
- An adult patient who is well developed tolerates 2 to 5 mL of medication in a larger muscle without severe muscle discomfort (Hopkins and Arias, 2013; Nicoll and Hesby, 2002). Larger volumes of medication (4 to 5 mL), however, are unlikely to be absorbed properly. Children, older adults, and patients who are thin tolerate only 2 mL of an IM injection. Do not give more than 1 mL to small children and older infants, and do not give more than 0.5 mL to smaller infants (Hockenberry and Wilson, 2017).
- The **Z**-track method, a technique for pulling the skin during an injection, is recommended for IM injections (Yilmaz et al., 2016). It prevents leakage of medication into subcutaneous tissues, seals medication in the muscle, and minimizes irritation.
  - To use the **Z**-track method, apply the appropriate-sized needle to the syringe and select an IM site, preferably in a large, deep muscle such as the ventrogluteal.
  - Pull the overlying skin and subcutaneous tissues approximately 2.5 to 3.5 cm (1 to 1½ inches) laterally to the side with the ulnar side of the nondominant hand.
  - Hold the skin in this position until you have administered the injection (Fig. 24.11).
  - After cleaning a site, inject the needle deeply into the muscle.
  - To reduce injection site discomfort, there is no longer any need to aspirate after the needle is injected when administering vaccines (Lilley, 2016).

Adapted from Centers for Disease Control and Prevention (CDC): Vaccine administration, 2017. https://www.cdc.gov/vaccines/hcp/acip-recs/general-recs/administration.html.

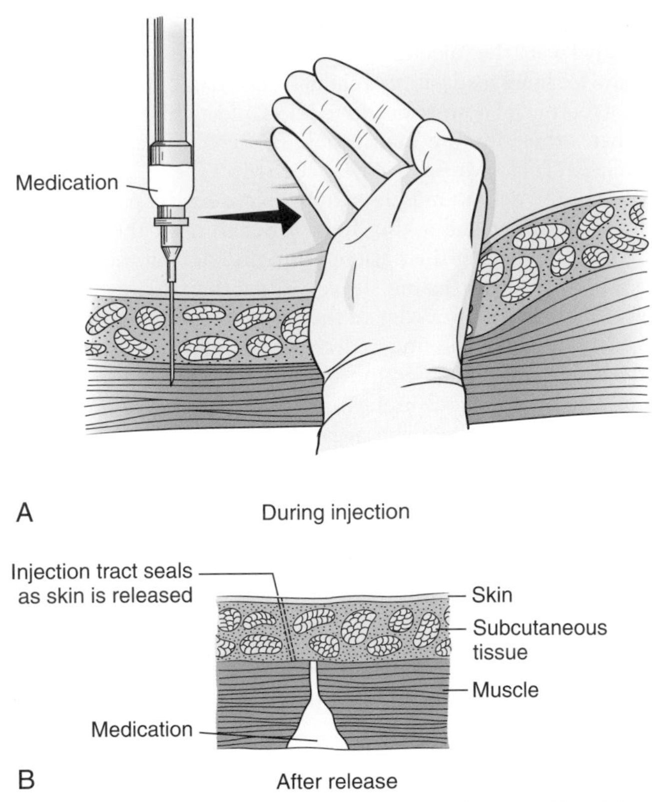

FIG 24.11 (A) Pulling on overlying skin with dorsum of hand during intramuscular (IM) injection moves tissue to prevent later tracking. (B) The Z-track left after injection prevents the deposit of medication through sensitive tissue.

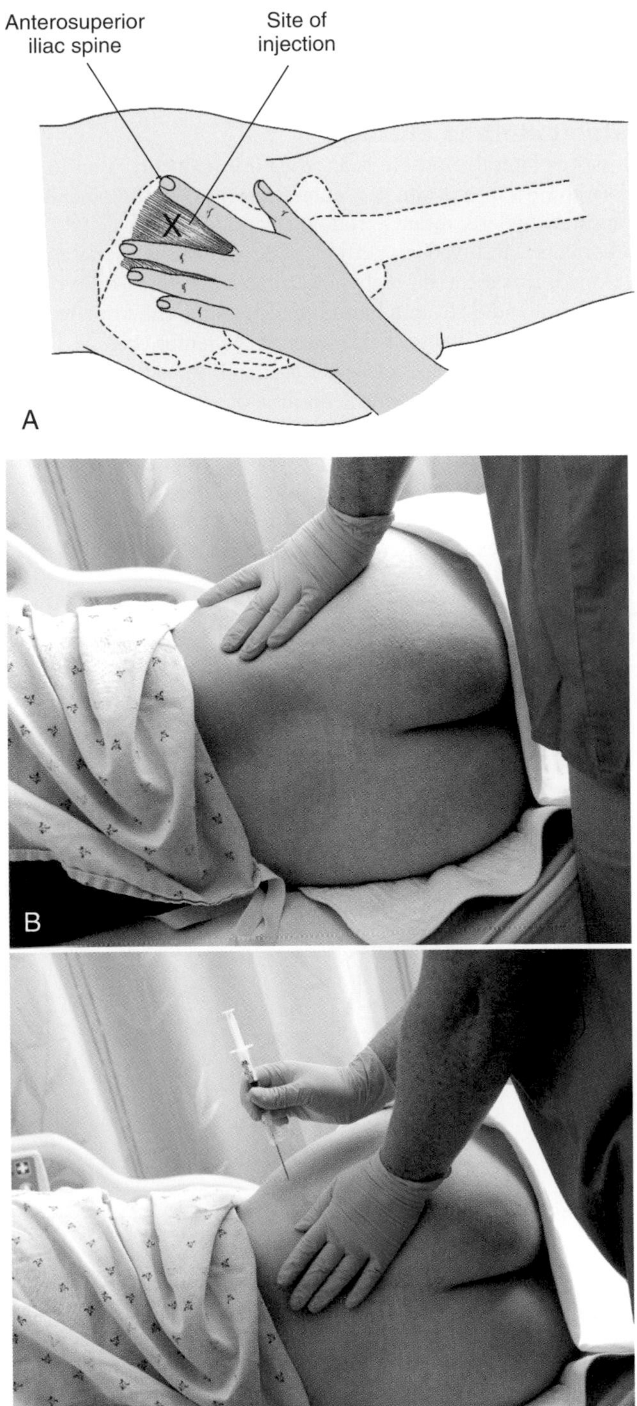

FIG 24.12 (A) Landmarks for ventrogluteal site. (B) Locating ventrogluteal site in patient. (C) Giving intramuscular injection in ventrogluteal muscle using Z-track method.

viscous, and irritating medications (CDC, 2017; Gūnes et al., 2016; Hockenberry and Wilson, 2017; Hopkins and Arias, 2013; Kara et al., 2015). The site involves the gluteus medius, where the thickness of subcutaneous tissue is less than other injection sites and there are relatively fewer nerves and blood vessels (Kara et al., 2015). Furthermore, in this site, the muscles are large and well established, and it is easy to find the muscle limit points (Kara et al., 2015).

The ventrogluteal site is recommended for volumes greater than 2 mL (Hopkins and Arias, 2013; Nicoll and Hesby, 2002). Research shows that injuries such as fibrosis, nerve damage, abscess, tissue necrosis, muscle contraction, gangrene, and pain are associated with all the common IM sites except the ventrogluteal site (Hopkins and Arias, 2013).

One way to locate the ventrogluteal muscle is the "V" method (Kara et al., 2015). First, position a patient in a supine or lateral position with the knee and hip flexed to relax the muscle. Use your right hand for the left hip and your left hand for the right hip. For example, if you are administering the injection into the patient's left hip, place the palm of your right hand over the greater trochanter of the patient's hip with your wrist perpendicular to the femur. Then move your thumb toward the patient's groin and your index finger toward the anterior superior iliac spine. Extend or open your middle finger back along the iliac crest toward the patient's buttock. The index finger, middle finger, and iliac crest form a V-shaped triangle, with the injection site in the center of the triangle (Fig. 24.12A–C; Kara et al., 2015; Kilic et al., 2014).

There has been some evidence to suggest that the "V" technique is not always reliable because of differences in nurses' hand structure and patient's body structure, especially when a patient is obese (Kara et al., 2015; Larkin et al., 2018). Thus the "G" method or geometric method is another option for identifying the correct ventrogluteal site. With a patient in the side-lying position, you reference three bony prominences and draw imaginary lines between the ends of the bones (Kara et al., 2015). You imagine lines drawn from the patient's greater trochanter to the iliac crest, then to the anterosuperior iliac spine, and from the greater trochanter to the anterosuperior iliac spine. Thus a triangle is created by the imaginary lines. After that, draw median lines from every corner of triangle to the opposite side. The convergence point of the three median lines is the center for the triangle, the needle entry point for intramuscular injections (Kaya et al., 2015).

Vastus Lateralis Muscle

The vastus lateralis muscle is another injection site used in adults and is the preferred site for administration of biologicals (e.g., immunizations) to infants, toddlers, and children (CDC, 2017; Hockenberry and Wilson, 2017). The muscle is thick and well developed; it is located on the anterolateral aspect of the thigh. It extends in an adult from a hand breadth above the knee to a hand breadth below the greater trochanter of the femur (Fig. 24.13). Use the middle third of the muscle for injection. The width of the muscle usually extends from the midline of the thigh to the midline of the outer side of the thigh. With young children or cachectic patients, it helps grasp the body of the muscle during injection to ensure that the medication is deposited in muscle tissue. To help relax the muscle, ask the patient to lie flat with the knee slightly flexed and foot externally rotated or assume a sitting position.

Deltoid Muscle

Although the deltoid site is easily accessible, the muscle is not well developed in many adults. There is potential for injury because the axillary, radial, brachial, and ulnar nerves and the brachial artery lie within the upper arm under the triceps and along the humerus (Fig. 24.14). Carefully assess the condition of the deltoid muscle, consult medication references for suitability of medication, and carefully locate the injection site using anatomical landmarks. Use this site for small medication volumes (less than 2 mL); administration of routine immunizations in toddlers, older children, and adults; or when other sites are inaccessible because of dressings or casts (CDC, 2017; Hopkins and Arias, 2013).

Locate the deltoid muscle by fully exposing the patient's upper arm and shoulder and asking him or her to relax the arm at the side or by supporting the patient's arm and flexing the elbow. Do not roll up any tight-fitting sleeve. Allow the patient to sit or lie down. Palpate the lower edge of the acromion process, which forms the base of a triangle in line with the midpoint of the lateral aspect of the upper arm. The injection site is in the center of the triangle, about 3 to 5 cm (1 to 2 inches) below the acromion process (see Fig. 24.14B). You locate the apex of the triangle by placing four fingers across the deltoid muscle, with the top finger along the acromion process. The injection site is three finger widths below the acromion process.

Delegation and Collaboration

The skill of administering IM injections cannot be delegated to nursing assistive personnel (NAP). The nurse directs the NAP about:

- Potential medication side effects and to immediately report their occurrence to the nurse.
- Reporting any change in the patient's condition to the nurse.

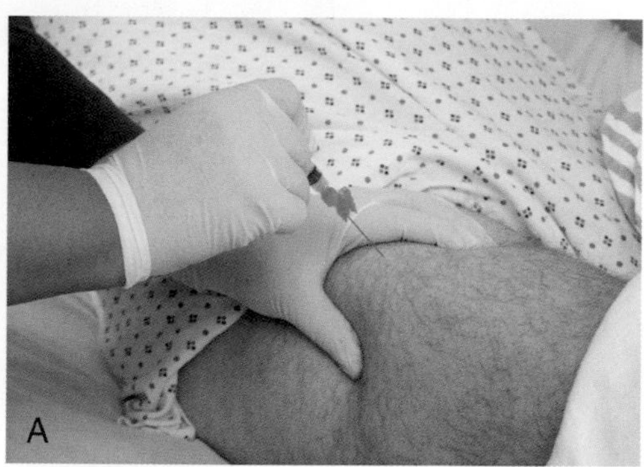

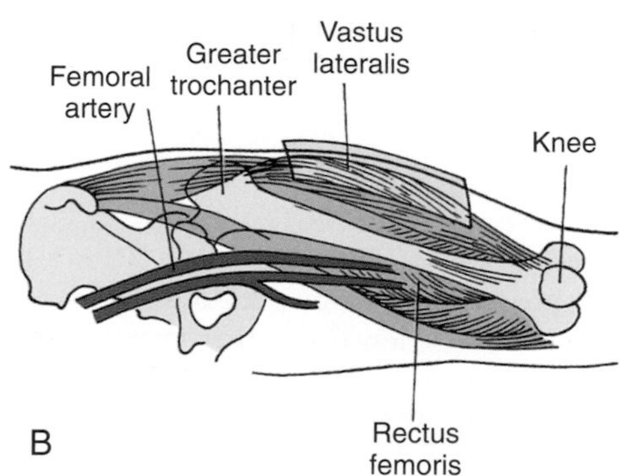

FIG 24.13 (A) Injection into the vastus lateralis muscle. (B) Landmarks for vastus lateralis site.

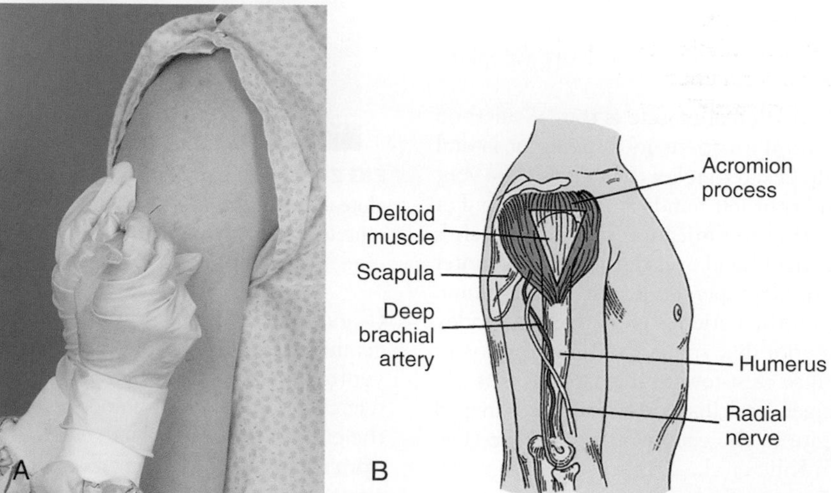

FIG 24.14 (A) Administering intramuscular (IM) injection in deltoid site. (B) Anatomical view of the deltoid muscle.

Equipment

- Proper-size syringe and sharp with engineered sharps injury protection (SESIP) needle:
  - Intramuscular (IM): Syringe 2 to 3 mL for adult, 0.5 to 1 mL for infants and small children
- Needle length typically corresponds to site of injection, age, gender, and size of patient. Refer to the following guidelines for vaccine administration; length needed may vary outside of these guidelines for patients who are smaller or larger than average.

Needle Length for Immunizations (Based on CDC [2017] Guidelines)

Site	Child	Adult
Ventrogluteal	½–1 inch[a]	1½ inches
Vastus lateralis	⅝–1¼ inch	⅝–1 inch
Deltoid	⅝–1 inch	1–1½ inches
Gender—Male	**Gender—Female**	**Needle Length**
Less than 130 pounds	Less than 130 pounds	⅝–1 inch
130–152 pounds	130–152 pounds	1 inch
153–260 pounds	153–200 pounds	1–1½ inches
260+ pounds	200+ pounds	1½ inches
Age Group	**Needle Length**	**Site**
Neonates[b]	⅝ inch (16 mm)[c]	Vastus lateralis
Infants, 1–12 months	1 inch (25 mm)	Vastus lateralis
Toddlers, 1–2 years	1–1¼ inch (25–32 mm) ⅝[c]–1 inch (16–25 mm)	Vastus lateralis[d] Deltoid muscle of arm
Children, 3–10 years	⅝[c]–1 inch (16–25 mm) 1–1¼ inches (25–32 mm)	Deltoid muscle of arm[d] Vastus lateralis
Children, 11–18 years	⅝[c]–1 inch (16–25 mm) 1–1½ inches (25–38 mm)	Deltoid muscle of arm[d] Vastus lateralis
Men and women, <60 kg (130 lb)	1 inch (25 mm)	Deltoid muscle of arm
Men and women, 60–70 kg (130–152 lb)	1 inch (25 mm)	Deltoid muscle of arm
Men, 70–118 kg (152–260 lb)	1–1½ inches (25–38 mm)	Deltoid muscle of arm
Women, 70–90 kg (152–200 lb)	1–1½ inches (25–38 mm)	Deltoid muscle of arm
Men, >118 kg (260 lb)	1½ inches (38 mm)	Deltoid muscle of arm
Women, >90 kg (200 lb)	1½ inches (38 mm)	Deltoid muscle of arm

[a]Recommendation from Hockenberry and Wilson (2017).
[b]First 28 days of life.
[c]If skin is stretched tightly and subcutaneous tissues are not bunched.
[d]Preferred site.

- Needle gauge often depends on length of needle; administer biologic and medication in aqueous solution with a 20- to 25-gauge needle. Use 18- to 21-gauge needles for medications in oil-based solutions.
- Alcohol swab
- Small gauze pad
- Vial or ampule of medication
- Clean gloves
- Medication administration record (MAR) or computer printout
- Puncture-proof container
- *Option:* Eutectic mixture of local anesthetics (EMLA) cream or vapocoolant spray

ASSESSMENT

1. Check accuracy and completeness of each MAR or computer printout with health care provider's written medication order. Check patient's name, medication name and dosage, route of administration, and time of administration. Recopy or reprint any portion of MAR that is difficult to read. *Rationale: The order sheet is the most reliable source and only legal record of medications that patient is to receive. Ensures that patient receives the correct medications (Westbrook et al., 2017). Transcription errors are a source of medication errors (Truitt et al., 2016).*
2. Assess patient's medical and medication history. *Rationale: Determines need for medication or possible contraindications for medication administration.*
3. Assess patient's history of allergies: known type of allergies and normal allergic reaction. *Rationale: Do not prepare medication if there is a known patient allergy.*
4. Review medication reference information for medication action, purpose, normal dose, side effects, time of peak onset, and nursing implications. *Rationale: Allows you to administer medication safely and monitor patient's response to therapy.*

5. Check date of expiration for medication. *Rationale: Dose potency increases or decreases when outdated.*
6. Observe patient's previous verbal and nonverbal responses toward injection. *Rationale: Anticipating patient's anxiety allows you to use distraction to reduce pain awareness.*
7. Perform hand hygiene. Assess for contraindications to IM injections, such as muscle atrophy, reduced blood flow, or circulatory shock. *Rationale: Atrophied muscle absorbs medication poorly. Factors interfering with blood flow to muscles impair drug absorption.*
8. Assess patient's symptoms before initiating medication therapy. *Rationale: Provides information for you to evaluate desired effects of medication.*

Safe Patient Care *Because of the documented adverse effects of IM injections, other routes of medication injection are preferred. Consider contacting health care provider for alternative route of medication administration.*

9. Assess patient's or family caregiver's knowledge, experience, and health literacy. *Rationale: Ensures patient or family caregiver has the capacity to obtain, communicate, process, and understand basic health information (CDC, 2016).*

STEP	RATIONALE
PLANNING	
1. Expected outcomes following completion of procedure:	
• Patient experiences no pain or mild burning at injection site.	Medications may cause minor tissue irritation.
• Patient achieves desired effect of medication with no signs of allergies or undesired effects.	Medication administered without patient injury.
• Patient explains medication purpose, dosage, effects, and side effects to be aware of.	Demonstrates learning.
2. Provide privacy and prepare environment.	Providing privacy and preparing the environment early help the student/nurse think about the need to remove clutter from the over-bed or bedside table.
3. Discuss purpose of each medication, action, and possible adverse effects. Allow patient to ask any questions. Tell patient that injection will cause slight burning or sting.	Patient has right to be informed, and patient's understanding of each medication improves adherence to drug therapy. Helps minimize patient's anxiety.
IMPLEMENTATION	
1. Perform hand hygiene and prepare medication using aseptic technique. Prepare medications for one patient at a time. Keep all pages of MARs or computer printouts for one patient together or look at only one patient's electronic MAR at a time. Check label of medication carefully with MAR or computer printout two times (see Skill 24.1 or Procedural Guideline 24.1) when preparing medication.	Ensures that medication is sterile. Preventing distractions reduces medication preparation errors. Use no-interruption zone (NIZ) when possible (Prakash et al., 2014; Yoder et al., 2015). *These are the first and second checks for accuracy* and ensure that correct medication is administered.
2. Take medication(s) to patient at correct time (see agency policy). Medications that require exact timing include STAT, first-time or loading doses, and one-time doses. Give time-critical scheduled medications (e.g., antibiotics, anticoagulants, insulin, anticonvulsants, immunosuppressive agents) at exact time ordered (no later than 30 minutes before or after scheduled dose). Give non–time-critical scheduled medications within a range of 1 or 2 hours of scheduled dose (ISMP, 2011). During administration, apply seven rights of medication administration.	Hospitals must adopt medication administration policy and procedure for timing of medication administration that considers nature of the prescribed medication, specific clinical application, and patient needs (DHHS, 2011; ISMP, 2011). Time-critical scheduled medications are those for which early or delayed administration of maintenance doses of greater than 30 minutes before or after the scheduled dose may cause harm or result in substantial suboptimal therapy or pharmacological effect. Non–time-critical medications are those for which early or delayed administration within a specified range of either 1 or 2 hours should not cause harm or result in substantial suboptimal therapy or pharmacological effect (DHHS, 2011; ISMP, 2011).
3. Identify patient using at least two identifiers (e.g., name and birthday or name and medical record number) according to agency policy. Compare identifiers with information on patient's MAR or medical record.	Ensures correct patient. Complies with The Joint Commission standards and improves patient safety (TJC, 2019). Some agencies are now using a bar-code system to help with patient identification.
4. At patient's bedside again compare MAR or computer printout with names of medications on medication labels and patient name. Ask patient if he or she has allergies.	*This is the third check for accuracy* and ensures that patient receives correct medication. Confirms patient's allergy history.

STEP	RATIONALE
5. Perform hand hygiene and apply clean gloves. Keep sheet or gown draped over body parts not requiring exposure.	Reduces transmission of infection. Respects patient's dignity while exposing injection site.
6. Select appropriate injection site. Note integrity and size of muscle. Palpate for and avoid areas of tenderness or hardness. Use ventrogluteal if possible. If patient receives frequent injections, rotate sites.	Ventrogluteal is preferred injection site for adults. It is also preferred site for children of all ages (CDC, 2017; Hockenberry and Wilson, 2017; Nicoll and Hesby, 2002; Ogston-Tuck, 2014b).
7. Help patient to comfortable position. Position patient depending on chosen site (e.g., sit, lie flat, on side, or prone).	Reduces strain on muscle and minimizes injection discomfort.

Safe Patient Care *Ensure that medical condition (e.g., circulatory shock, orthopedic surgery) does not contraindicate patient's position for injection.*

STEP	RATIONALE
8. Relocate site using anatomical landmarks.	Injection into correct anatomical site prevents injury to nerves, bone, and blood vessels.
9. Clean site with antiseptic swab. Apply swab at center of site and rotate outward in circular direction for about 5 cm (2 inches).	Mechanical action of swab removes secretions containing microorganisms.
a. *Option:* Apply EMLA cream on injection site at least 1 hour before IM injection or use vapocoolant spray (e.g., ethyl chloride) just before injection.	Decreases pain at injection site.
10. Hold swab or gauze between third and fourth fingers of nondominant hand.	Swab or gauze remains readily accessible for use when withdrawing needle after injection.
11. Remove needle cap or sheath by pulling it straight off.	Preventing needle from touching sides of cap prevents contamination.
12. Hold syringe between thumb and forefinger of dominant hand; hold as dart, palm down.	Quick, smooth injection requires proper manipulation of syringe parts.
13. Administer injection:	
a. Position ulnar side of nondominant hand just below site and pull skin laterally approximately 2.5 to 3.5 cm (1 to 1½ inches). Hold position until medication is injected. With dominant hand inject needle quickly at 90-degree angle into muscle.	Z-track creates zigzag path through tissues that seals needle track to avoid tracking medication. A quick, dartlike injection reduces discomfort. Use Z-track for all IM injections (Hopkins and Arias, 2013; Nicoll and Hesby, 2002; Ogston-Tuck, 2014b; Yilmaz et al., 2016).
b. *Option:* If patient's muscle mass is small, grasp body of muscle between thumb and forefingers.	Ensures that medication reaches muscle mass (CDC, 2017; Hockenberry and Wilson, 2017).
c. After needle pierces skin, while still pulling on skin with nondominant hand, grasp lower end of syringe barrel with fingers of nondominant hand to stabilize it. Move dominant hand to end of plunger. Avoid moving syringe.	Smooth manipulation of syringe reduces discomfort from needle movement. Skin remains pulled until after medication is injected to ensure Z-track administration.
d. Pull back on plunger 5 to 10 seconds. If no blood appears, inject medication slowly at rate of 10 sec/mL (Nicoll and Hesby, 2002).	Aspiration of blood into syringe indicates possible placement of needle into a vein. Slow injection rate reduces pain and tissue trauma and reduces chance of leakage of medication back through needle track (Hockenberry and Wilson, 2017; Nicoll and Hesby, 2002). The CDC (2017) no longer recommends aspiration when administering an immunization.

Safe Patient Care *If blood appears in syringe, remove needle, dispose of medication and syringe properly, and prepare another dose of medication for injection to prevent injection of medication directly into the bloodstream.*

STEP	RATIONALE
e. Once medication is injected, wait 10 seconds, then smoothly and steadily withdraw needle, release skin, and apply gauze gently over site.	Allows time for medication to absorb into muscle before removing syringe. Dry gauze minimizes discomfort associated with alcohol on nonintact skin.
14. Apply gentle pressure to site. Do not massage site. Apply bandage if needed.	Massage damages underlying tissue.
15. Help patient to comfortable position.	Gives patient sense of well-being.
16. Discard uncapped needle or needle enclosed in safety shield and attached syringe into puncture- and leak-proof receptacle.	Prevents injury to patients and health care personnel. Recapping needles increases risk for needlestick injury (OSHA, 2012).

STEP	RATIONALE
17. Be sure nurse call system is in an accessible location within patient's reach.	Ensures patient can call for assistance if needed.
18. Raise side rails (as appropriate) and lower bed to lowest position.	Ensures patient safety.
19. Remove and dispose of gloves and perform hand hygiene.	Reduces transmission of microorganisms.
20. Stay with patient for several minutes and observe for any allergic reactions.	Dyspnea, wheezing, and circulatory collapse are signs of severe anaphylactic reaction.

EVALUATION

STEP	RATIONALE
1. Return to room in 15 to 30 minutes and ask if patient feels any acute pain, burning, numbness, or tingling at injection site.	Continued discomfort may indicate injury to underlying bones or nerves.
2. Inspect site; note any bruising or induration. Apply warm compress to site.	Bruising or induration indicates complication associated with injection. Document findings and notify health care provider.
3. Observe patient's response to medication at times that correlate with onset, peak, and duration of medication.	IM medications are absorbed rapidly. Adverse effects of parenteral medications will develop rapidly. Evaluates effect of medication at key therapeutic times
4. **Use Teach-Back:** "I want to be sure I explained to you the purpose of this IM injection. Explain to me why you are receiving the injection and what you might expect to feel during the injection." Revise your instruction now or develop a plan for revised patient/family caregiver teaching if patient/family caregiver is not able to teach back correctly.	Determines patient's/family caregiver's level of understanding of instructional topic.

Unexpected Outcomes	Related Interventions
1. Patient complains of localized pain or continued burning at injection site, indicating potential injury to nerve or vessels.	• Assess injection site. • Notify patient's health care provider.
2. Patient displays adverse reaction with signs of urticaria, eczema, pruritus, wheezing, and dyspnea.	• Follow agency policy or guidelines for appropriate response to allergic reactions (e.g., administration of antihistamine such as diphenhydramine or epinephrine). • Notify patient's health care provider immediately. • Add allergy information to patient's record.

Recording

- Record medication, dose, route, site, and time and date given.
- Record patient's response to medication and any adverse effects.
- Document your evaluation of patient learning.

Hand-Off Reporting

- Report any undesirable effects from medication to patient's health care provider.

✦ SKILL 24.4 Administering Intradermal Injections

Purpose

Intradermal (ID) injections are typically administered for skin testing (e.g., tuberculosis [TB] screening and allergy tests). Because such medications are potent, you inject them into the dermis, where blood supply is reduced, and drug absorption occurs slowly. A patient may have an anaphylactic reaction if a medication enters the circulation too rapidly. The health care provider may perform skin testing in patients with a history of numerous allergies. Skin testing often requires you to inspect the test site visually; you need to ensure that ID sites are free of lesions and injuries and are relatively hairless. The inner forearm and upper back are ideal locations.

To administer an ID injection, use a tuberculin or small syringe with a short (⅜- to ⅝-inch), fine-gauge (25- to 27-gauge) needle. The angle of insertion for an ID injection is 5 to 15 degrees (Fig. 24.15). Inject only small amounts of medication (0.01 to 0.1 mL) intradermally. If a bleb does not appear or if the site bleeds after needle withdrawal, the medication may have entered subcutaneous tissues. In this situation, skin test results will not be valid.

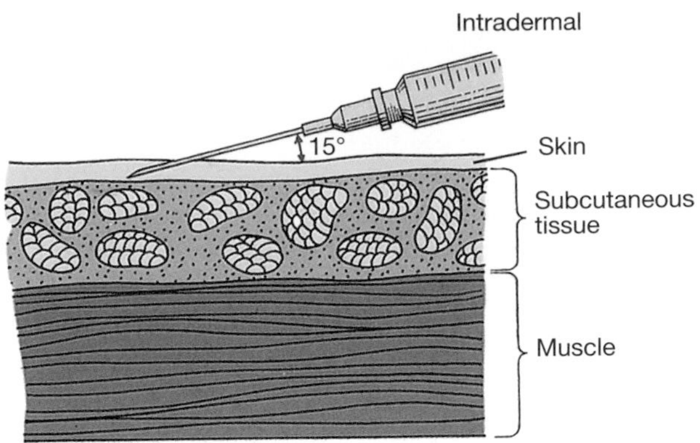

FIG 24.15 Intradermal needle tip inserted into dermis.

Delegation and Collaboration

The skill of administering ID injections cannot be delegated to nursing assistive personnel (NAP). The nurse directs the NAP about:

- Potential medication side effects or allergic response signs and to report their occurrence to the nurse.
- Reporting any change in the patient's vital signs or condition to the nurse.

Equipment

- Syringe: 1-mL tuberculin syringe with preattached 25- to 27-gauge, ⅜- to ⅝-inch needle
- Alcohol swab
- Small gauze pad
- Vial or ampule of medication
- Clean gloves
- Medication administration record (MAR) or computer printout
- Puncture-proof container

ASSESSMENT

1. Check accuracy and completeness of each MAR or computer printout with health care provider's written medication order. Check patient's name, medication name and dosage, route of administration, and time of administration. Recopy or reprint any portion of MAR that is difficult to read. *Rationale: The order sheet is the most reliable source and only legal record of medications that patient is to receive. Ensures that patient receives the correct medications (Westbrook et al., 2017). Transcription errors are a source of medication errors (Truitt et al., 2016).*
2. Review medication reference information about expected reaction/anticipated effects and appropriate time to read site when testing skin with specific allergen or when giving medication. *Rationale: Type of reaction depends on patient's ability to mount a cell-mediated immune response. Knowledge of expected and adverse reactions to skin testing helps you determine for which symptoms to monitor, how frequently, and when to reassess patient.*
3. Assess patient's history of allergies: known type of allergens and normal allergic reaction. *Rationale: You do not administer any medication if there is known patient allergy. Medications are potent and can cause severe anaphylaxis.*
4. Perform hand hygiene. Assess for contraindication to ID injections such as reduced local tissue perfusion. *Rationale: Decreased perfusion reduces absorption of medication.*
5. Assess for history of severe adverse reactions or necrosis that happened after previous ID injection. *Rationale: Prior history of severe reactions increases the risk for future severe reactions.*
6. Check date of expiration for medication. *Rationale: Dose potency increases or decreases when outdated.*
7. Assess patient's or family caregiver's knowledge, experience, and health literacy. *Rationale: Ensures patient or family caregiver has the capacity to obtain, communicate, process, and understand basic health information (CDC, 2016).*

STEP	RATIONALE
PLANNING	
1. Expected outcomes following completion of procedure:	
• Patient experiences very mild burning sensation during injection but no discomfort after injection.	Normal reaction to medication deposited in dermis.
• Small, light-colored bleb approximately 6 mm (¼ inch) in diameter forms at site and gradually disappears. Minimal bruising may be present.	Medication is in dermis and eventually absorbed. Bruising is result of minor bleeding from capillaries.
• Patient can identify signs of skin reaction and their significance.	Demonstrates learning.
2. Provide privacy and prepare environment.	Providing privacy and preparing the environment early help the student/nurse think about the need to remove clutter from the over-bed or bedside table.
3. Discuss purpose of each medication, action, and possible adverse effects. Allow patient to ask any questions. Tell patient that injection will cause slight burning or sting.	Patient has right to be informed, and patient's understanding of each medication improves adherence to drug therapy. Helps minimize patient's anxiety.

STEP	RATIONALE

IMPLEMENTATION

STEP	RATIONALE
1. Perform hand hygiene and prepare medication using aseptic technique. Prepare medications for one patient at a time. Keep all pages of MARs or computer printouts for one patient together or look at only one patient's electronic MAR at a time. Check label of medication carefully with MAR or computer printout two times (see Skill 24.1 or Procedural Guideline 24.1) when preparing medication.	Ensures that medication is sterile. Preventing distractions reduces medication preparation errors. Use no-interruption zone (NIZ) when possible (Prakash et al., 2014; Yoder et al., 2015). *These are the first and second checks for accuracy* and ensure that correct medication is administered.
2. Take medication(s) to patient at correct time (see agency policy). Give non–time-critical scheduled medications within a range of 1 or 2 hours of scheduled dose (ISMP, 2011). During administration, apply seven rights of medication administration.	Hospitals must adopt medication administration policy and procedure for timing of medication administration that considers nature of the prescribed medication, specific clinical application, and patient needs (DHHS, 2011; ISMP, 2011).
3. Identify patient using at least two identifiers (e.g., name and birthday or name and medical record number) according to agency policy. Compare identifiers with information on patient's MAR or medical record.	Ensures correct patient. Complies with The Joint Commission standards and improves patient safety (TJC, 2019). Some agencies are now using a bar-code system to help with patient identification.
4. At patient's bedside again compare MAR or computer printout with names of medications on medication labels and patient name. Ask patient again if he or she has allergies.	*This is the third check for accuracy* and ensures that patient receives correct medication. Confirms patient's allergy history.
5. Perform hand hygiene and apply clean gloves. Keep sheet or gown draped over body parts not requiring exposure.	Reduces transmission of infection.
6. Select appropriate injection site. Note lesions or discolorations of skin. If possible, select site three to four finger widths below antecubital space and one hand width above wrist. If you cannot use forearm, inspect upper back. If necessary, use sites appropriate for subcutaneous injections.	An ID injection site is free of discoloration or hair so that you can see results of skin test and interpret them correctly (WHO, 2015).
7. Help patient to comfortable position. Have him or her extend elbow and support it and forearm on flat surface.	Stabilizes injection site for easy accessibility.
8. Clean site with antiseptic swab. Apply swab at center of site and rotate outward in circular direction for about 5 cm (2 inches). *Option:* Use vapocoolant spray (e.g., ethyl chloride) before injection.	Mechanical action of swab removes secretions containing microorganisms. Decreases pain at injection site.
9. Hold swab or gauze between third and fourth fingers of nondominant hand.	Gauze or swab remains readily accessible when withdrawing needle.
10. Remove needle cap from needle by pulling it straight off.	Preventing needle from touching sides of cap prevents contamination.
11. Hold syringe between thumb and forefinger of dominant hand with bevel of needle pointing up.	Smooth injection requires proper manipulation of syringe parts. With bevel up, you are less likely to deposit medication into tissues below dermis.
12. Administer injection.	
a. With nondominant hand, stretch skin over site with forefinger or thumb.	Needle pierces tight skin more easily.
b. With needle almost against patient's skin, insert it slowly at 5- to 15-degree angle until resistance is felt. Advance needle through epidermis to approximately 3 mm (⅛ inch) below skin surface. You will see bulge of needle tip through skin (see Fig. 24.15).	Ensures that needle tip is in dermis. You will obtain inaccurate results if you do not inject needle at correct angle and depth (WHO, 2015).
c. Inject medication slowly. Normally you feel resistance. If not, needle is too deep; remove and begin again.	Slow injection minimizes discomfort at site. Dermal layer is tight and does not expand easily when you inject solution.

Safe Patient Care *It is not necessary to aspirate because dermis is relatively avascular.*

STEP	RATIONALE
d. While injecting medication, note that small bleb (approximately 6 mm [¼ inch]) resembling mosquito bite appears on skin surface (see illustration).	Bleb indicates that you deposited medication in dermis.

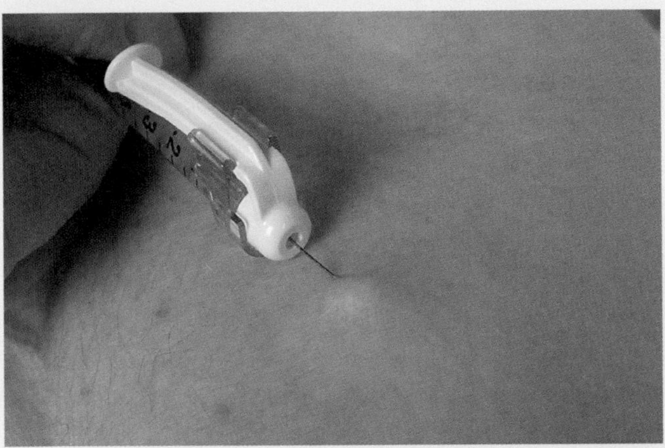

STEP 12d Injection creates small bleb.

STEP	RATIONALE
e. After withdrawing needle, apply alcohol swab or gauze gently over site.	Do not massage site. Apply bandage if needed.
13. Help patient to comfortable position.	Gives patient sense of well-being.
14. Discard uncapped needle or needle enclosed in safety shield and attached syringe into puncture- and leak-proof receptacle.	Prevents injury to patients and health care personnel. Recapping needles increases risk for needlestick injury (OSHA, 2012).
15. Be sure nurse call system is in an accessible location within patient's reach.	Ensures patient can call for assistance if needed.
16. Raise side rails (as appropriate) and lower bed to lowest position.	Ensures patient safety.
17. Remove and dispose of gloves and perform hand hygiene.	Reduces transmission of microorganisms.
18. Stay with patient for several minutes and observe for any allergic reactions.	Dyspnea, wheezing, and circulatory collapse are signs of severe anaphylactic reaction.

EVALUATION

STEP	RATIONALE
1. Return to room in 15 to 30 minutes and ask if patient feels any acute pain, burning, numbness, or tingling at injection site.	Continued discomfort could indicate injury to underlying tissues.
2. Ask patient to discuss implications of skin testing and signs of hypersensitivity.	Patient's ability to recognize signs of skin testing helps ensure timely reporting of results.
3. Inspect bleb. *Option:* Use skin pencil and draw circle around perimeter of injection site. Read TB test site at 48 to 72 hours; look for induration (hard, dense, raised area) of skin around injection site of:	Determines if reaction to antigen occurs; indication positive for tuberculosis or tested allergens. Site must be read at various intervals to determine test results. Pencil marks make site easy to find. You determine results of skin testing at various times, based on type of medication used or type of skin testing completed. Manufacturer directions determine when to read test results.
• 15 mm or more in patients with no known risk factors for tuberculosis.	Degree of reaction varies based on patient condition.
• 10 mm or more in patients who are recent immigrants; injection drug users; residents and employees of high-risk settings; patients with certain chronic illnesses; children less than 4 years of age; and infants, children, and adolescents exposed to high-risk adults.	

STEP	RATIONALE
• 5 mm or more in patients who are human immunodeficiency virus (HIV) positive, have fibrotic changes on chest x-ray film consistent with previous tuberculosis infection, have had organ transplants, or are immunosuppressed.	
4. **Use Teach-Back:** "I want to be sure I explained to you the purpose of TB skin testing and what you might see after the test. Explain to me what the injection site might look like in 2 to 3 days and what that would mean." Revise your instruction now or develop a plan for revised patient/family caregiver teaching if patient/family caregiver is not able to teach back correctly.	Determines patient's/family caregiver's level of understanding of instructional topic.

Unexpected Outcomes	Related Interventions
1. Patient complains of localized pain or continued burning at injection site, indicating potential injury to nerve or vessels.	• Assess injection site. • Notify patient's health care provider.
2. Raised, reddened, or hard zone (induration) forms around ID test site.	• Notify patient's health care provider. • Document sensitivity to injected allergen or positive test if tuberculin skin testing was completed.
3. Patient has adverse reaction with signs of urticaria, pruritus, wheezing, and dyspnea.	• Notify patient's health care provider immediately. • Follow agency policy for appropriate response to drug reactions (e.g., administration of antihistamine such as diphenhydramine or epinephrine). • Add allergy information to patient's record.

Recording

- Record drug, dose, route, site, time, and date.
- Record area of ID injection and appearance of skin.
- Record patient teaching, validation of understanding, and patient's response to medication, including any adverse reaction.

Hand-Off Reporting

- Report any undesirable effects from medication to patient's health care provider.

✦ SKILL 24.5 Administering Medications by Intravenous Bolus

Purpose

In the past nurses, often mixed medications into large volumes of intravenous (IV) fluids (500 to 1000 mL). However, today's safety standards and evidence-based practice no longer support this practice on a routine basis (Gorski, 2018; Infusion Nurses Society [INS], 2016; TJC, 2019). Many patient safety risks, such as incorrect calculation, poor aseptic technique, incorrect labeling, pump programming errors, lack of medication knowledge, and mix-up with another medication, occur when nurses must prepare medications in IV containers on patient care units (Gorski, 2018). There are many current best practices for preparation and administration of IV medication (Box 24.5).

Delegation and Collaboration

The skill of administering medications by IV bolus cannot be delegated to nursing assistive personnel (NAP). The nurse directs the NAP about:

- Potential medication actions and side effects and to immediately report their occurrence to the nurse.
- Reporting any patient complaints of moisture or discomfort around IV insertion site.
- Obtaining any required vital signs and reporting them to the nurse.

Equipment

- Watch with second hand
- Clean gloves
- Antiseptic swab
- Medication in vial or ampule
- Proper-size syringes for medication and saline flush with needless device or SESIP (sharps with engineered sharps injury protection) needle (21 to 25 gauge)
- Intravenous lock: Vial of normal saline flush solution (saline recommended [Alexander et al., 2014]); if agency continues to use heparin flush, the most common concentration is 10 units/mL; check agency policy.
- Medication administration record (MAR) or computer printout
- Puncture-proof container

BOX 24.5

Best Practices for Administration of Intravenous (IV) Solutions and Medications

- Review medication orders for standardized concentrations and dosages of medication.
- Use standardized procedures for ordering, preparing, and administering IV medications.
- Administer solutions and medications prepared and dispensed from the pharmacy or as commercially prepared when possible.
- Never prepare high-alert medications (e.g., heparin, dopamine, dobutamine, nitroglycerin, potassium, antibiotics, or magnesium) on a patient care unit.
- Review medication order for use of standardized infusion concentrations of "high-alert" medications.
- Standardize the storage of IV medications.
- Use the mnemonic CATS PRRR to help remember safety checks for administering IV medications: *C*, compatibilities; *A*, allergies; *T*, tubing correct; *S*, site checked; *P*, pump safety checked; *R*, right rate; *R*, release clamps; *R*, return and reassess the patient.
- Use standardized label practices. Bold patient name, generic drug name, and patient-specific dose.
- Correctly use technology such as intelligent-infusion devices, bar code–assisted medication administration, and electronic medication administration record.

Adapted from Infusion Nurses Society: Infusion nursing standards of practice, *J Intraven Nurs* 34(1S), 2011; Institute for Safe Medication Practices (ISMP): Guidelines for standard order sets, 2010. http://www.ismp.org/tools/guidelines/StandardOrderSets.pdf; Institute for Safe Medication Practices (ISMP): Principles of designing a medication label for intravenous piggyback medication for patient specific, inpatient use, 2016. http://www.ismp.org/Tools/guidelines/labelFormats/Piggyback.asp; The Joint Commission: 2017 National Patient Safety Goals hospital program, 2017. http://www.jointcommission.org/standards_information/npsgs.aspx.

ASSESSMENT

1. Check accuracy and completeness of each MAR or computer printout with health care provider's written medication order. Check patient's name, medication name and dosage, route of administration, and time of administration. Recopy or reprint any portion of MAR that is difficult to read. *Rationale: The order sheet is the most reliable source and only legal record of medications that patient is to receive. Ensures that patient receives the correct medications (Westbrook et al., 2017). Transcription errors are a source of medication errors (Truitt et al., 2016).*
2. Assess patient's medical and medication history. *Rationale: Identifies need for medication.*
3. Review medication reference information for medication action, purpose, side effects, normal dose, time of peak onset, how slowly to give medication, and nursing implications such as need to dilute medication. *Rationale: Knowledge of medication allows you to give it safely and monitor patient's response to therapy.*
4. If you give medication through an existing IV line, determine compatibility of medication with IV fluids and any additives within IV solution. *Rationale: IV medication is not always compatible with IV solution and/or additives, and a new site may need to be initiated (Gorski, 2018).*
5. Perform hand hygiene. Assess condition of IV needle insertion site for signs of infiltration or phlebitis. *Rationale: Do not administer medication if site is edematous or inflamed.*
6. Assess patency of patient's existing IV infusion line or saline lock (see Chapter 28). *Rationale: For medication to reach venous circulation effectively, IV line must be patent, and fluids must infuse easily.*
7. Check patient's history of medication allergies: known allergens and normal allergic response. *Rationale: IV bolus delivers medication rapidly. Allergic response is immediate.*
8. Assess patient's symptoms before initiating medication therapy. *Rationale: Provides information to evaluate desired effects of medication.*
9. Assess patient's or family caregiver's knowledge, experience, and health literacy. *Rationale: Ensures patient or family caregiver has the capacity to obtain, communicate, process, and understand basic health information (CDC, 2016).*

STEP	RATIONALE
PLANNING	
1. Expected outcomes following completion of procedure:	
• Patient experiences no medication side effects or adverse reactions.	Medication administered safely with desired therapeutic effect achieved.
• IV site remains intact, without signs of swelling or inflammation or symptoms of tenderness at site.	Medication infuses without complications to IV site and surrounding tissues.
• Patient explains medication purpose, effects, and side effects.	Demonstrates learning.
2. Provide privacy and prepare environment.	Providing privacy and preparing the environment early help the student/nurse think about the need to remove clutter from the over-bed or bedside table.
3. Discuss purpose of each medication, action, and possible adverse effects. Allow patient to ask any questions. Tell patient that injection will cause slight burning or sting.	Patient has right to be informed, and patient's understanding of each medication improves adherence to drug therapy. Helps minimize patient's anxiety.

STEP	RATIONALE

IMPLEMENTATION

STEP	RATIONALE
1. Perform hand hygiene and prepare medication using aseptic technique. Prepare medications for one patient at a time. Keep all pages of MARs or computer printouts for one patient together or look at only one patient's electronic MAR at a time. Check label of medication carefully with MAR or computer printout two times (see Skill 24.1 or Procedural Guideline 24.1) when preparing medication.	Ensures that medication is sterile. Preventing distractions reduces medication preparation errors. Use no-interruption zone (NIZ) when possible (Prakash et al., 2014; Yoder et al., 2015). *These are the first and second checks for accuracy* and ensure that correct medication is administered.

Safe Patient Care *Some IV medications require dilution before administration. Verify with agency policy or pharmacy if dilution is permitted. If a small amount of medication is given (e.g., less than 1 mL), dilute medication in small amount (e.g., 5 mL) of normal saline or sterile water so that it does not collect in the "dead spaces" (e.g., Y-site injection port, IV cap) of the IV delivery system.*

STEP	RATIONALE
2. Take medication(s) to patient at correct time (see agency policy). Medications that require exact timing include STAT, first-time or loading doses, and one-time doses. Give time-critical scheduled medications (e.g., antibiotics, anticoagulants, insulin, anticonvulsants, immunosuppressive agents) at exact time ordered (no later than 30 minutes before or after scheduled dose). Give non–time-critical scheduled medications within a range of 1 or 2 hours of scheduled dose (ISMP, 2011). During administration, apply seven rights of medication administration.	Hospitals must adopt medication administration policy and procedure for timing of medication administration that considers nature of the prescribed medication, specific clinical application, and patient needs (DHHS, 2011; ISMP, 2011). Time-critical scheduled medications are those for which early or delayed administration of maintenance doses of greater than 30 minutes before or after the scheduled dose may cause harm or result in substantial suboptimal therapy or pharmacological effect. Non–time-critical medications are those for which early or delayed administration within a specified range of either 1 or 2 hours should not cause harm or result in substantial suboptimal therapy or pharmacological effect (DHHS, 2011; ISMP, 2011).
3. Identify patient using at least two identifiers (e.g., name and birthday or name and medical record number) according to agency policy. Compare identifiers with information on patient's MAR or medical record.	Ensures correct patient. Complies with The Joint Commission standards and improves patient safety (TJC, 2019). Some agencies are now using a bar-code system to help with patient identification.
4. At patient's bedside, again compare MAR or computer printout with names of medications on medication labels and patient name. Ask patient if he or she has allergies.	*This is the third check for accuracy* and ensures that patient receives correct medication. Confirms patient's allergy history.
5. Perform hand hygiene and apply clean gloves.	Reduces transmission of infection.
6. IV push (existing IV line):	
a. Select injection port of IV tubing closest to patient. Use needleless injection port.	Follows provisions of Needle Safety and Prevention Act of 2001 (OSHA, 2012.).

Safe Patient Care *Never administer IV medications through tubing that is infusing blood, blood products, or parenteral nutrition solutions.*

STEP	RATIONALE
b. Clean injection port with antiseptic swab. Allow to dry.	Prevents transfer of microorganisms during blunt cannula insertion.
c. Connect syringe to IV line: Insert needleless tip of syringe containing drug through center of port (see illustration).	Prevents introduction of microorganisms. Prevents damage to port diaphragm and possible leakage from site.
d. Occlude IV line by pinching tubing just above injection port (see illustration). Pull back gently on plunger of syringe to aspirate for blood return.	Final check ensures that medication is being delivered into bloodstream.

Safe Patient Care *In the case of smaller-gauge IV needles, blood return sometimes is not aspirated even if IV line is patent. If IV site does not show signs of infiltration and IV fluid is infusing without difficulty, give IV push.*

STEP	RATIONALE
e. Release tubing and inject medication within amount of time recommended by agency policy, pharmacist, or medication reference manual. Use watch to time administrations (see illustration). You can pinch IV line while pushing medication and release it when not pushing medication. Allow IV fluids to infuse when not pushing medication.	Ensures safe medication infusion. Most medications are delivered slowly, between 1 to 10 minutes; for example morphine IV push delivery of 15 mg is recommended over 4 to 5 minutes (Gorski, 2018). Rapid injection of IV drug can be fatal. Allowing IV fluids to infuse while pushing IV drug enables medication to be delivered to patient at prescribed rate (Box 24.6).

STEP	RATIONALE

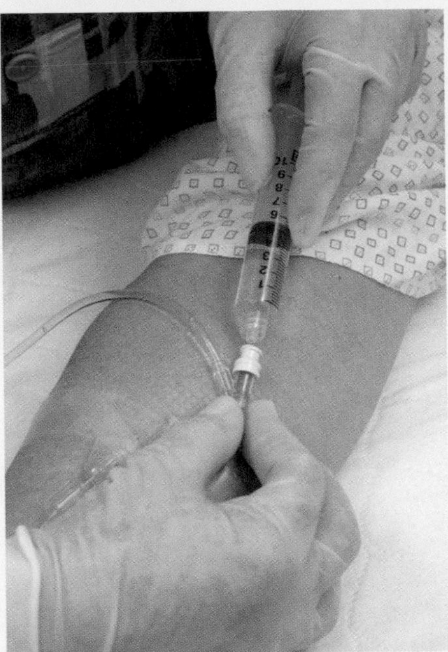

STEP 6c Connect syringe to IV line with needleless blunt cannula tip.

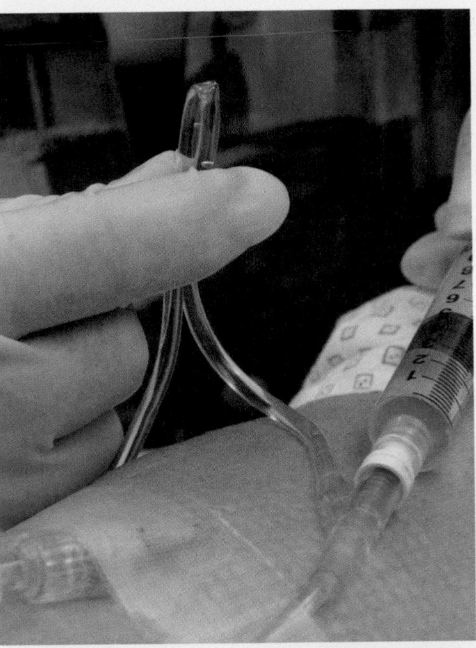

STEP 6d Occlude IV tubing above injection port.

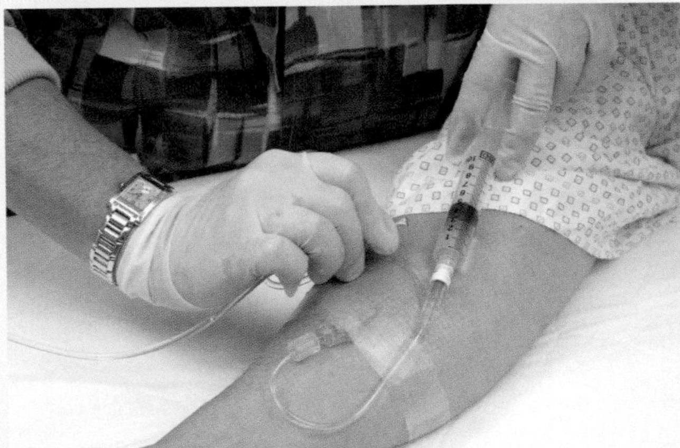

STEP 6e Use watch to time IV push medication.

BOX 24.6

Advantages and Disadvantages of the Intravenous (IV) Push Method

Advantages

- Barriers of absorption are bypassed
- There is rapid onset of medication effects, which is useful in patients experiencing critical or emergent health problems.
- Medications can be prepared quickly and given over a shorter time than by IV piggyback.
- Doses of short-acting medications can be titrated based on a patient's needs and responses to the drug therapy. This is important for infants, children, and older patients.
- Method provides a more accurate dose of medication delivered because no medication is left in intravenously.

Disadvantages

- Not all medications can be delivered by IV push.
- There is higher risk for infusion reactions; some are mild to severe because the medication action peaks quickly.
- When giving medication quickly (e.g., less than 1 minute), there is very little opportunity to stop the injection if an adverse reaction occurs.
- Risk for infiltration and phlebitis is increased, especially if a highly concentrated medication, a small peripheral vein, or a short venous access device is used.
- Hypersensitivity reaction can cause an immediate or delayed systemic reaction to a medication, requiring supportive measures.

STEP	RATIONALE
f. After injecting medication, withdraw syringe and recheck IV fluid infusion rate.	Injection of bolus may alter rate of fluid infusion. Rapid fluid infusion can cause circulatory fluid overload.
g. If IV medication is incompatible with IV fluids, stop IV fluids, clamp IV line, and flush with 10 mL of normal saline or sterile water (see agency policy). Then give newly prepared IV bolus over appropriate amount of time and flush with another 10 mL of normal saline or sterile water at same rate as medication was administered.	Allows IV bolus to be administered without risks associated with IV incompatibilities. Ensure that agency guidelines permit flushing lines with incompatible medications. A new site may need to be initiated.

STEP	RATIONALE
h. If IV line that currently is hanging is a medication, disconnect it and administer IV push medication as outlined in Step 7. Verify agency policy for stopping IV fluids or continuous IV medications. If unable to stop IV infusion, start new IV site (see Chapter 28) and administer medication using IV push (IV lock) method.	Avoids giving patient sudden bolus of medication in existing IV line.
7. IV push (IV lock):	
a. Prepare flush solutions according to agency policy.	
(1) Saline flush method (preferred method): Prepare two syringes filled with 2 to 3 mL of normal saline (0.9%). Many agencies do not provide prefilled normal saline syringes for flushing IV lines.	Normal saline is effective in keeping IV locks patent and is compatible with wide range of medications (Patidar et al., 2014).
(2) Heparin flush method (prepare heparin flush and saline syringe according to agency policy).	
b. Administer medication:	
(1) Clean injection port with antiseptic swab.	Prevents transfer of microorganisms during needle insertion.
(2) Insert needleless tip of syringe with normal saline 0.9% through center of injection port of IV lock (see illustrations).	

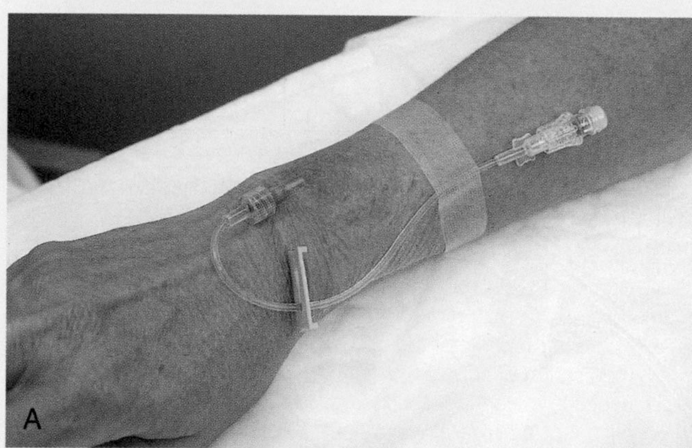
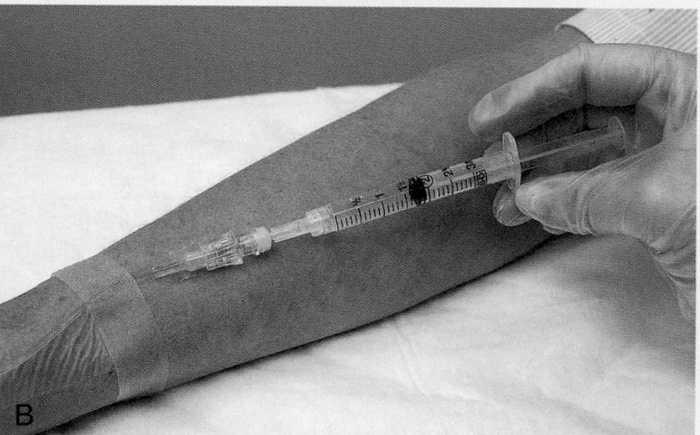

STEP 7b(2) (A) IV catheter with saline lock adapter. (B) Syringe inserted into injection port.

STEP	RATIONALE
(3) Pull back gently on syringe plunger and check for blood return.	Indicates if needle or catheter is in vein.
(4) Flush IV site with normal saline by pushing slowly on plunger.	Clears needle and reservoir of blood. Flushing without difficulty indicates patent IV line.

Safe Patient Care *Carefully observe the area of skin above the IV catheter. Note any puffiness or swelling as the IV site is flushed, which could indicate infiltration into the tissues, requiring removal of catheter.*

STEP	RATIONALE
(5) Remove saline-filled syringe.	
(6) Clean injection port with antiseptic swab.	Prevents transmission of microorganisms.
(7) Insert needleless tip of syringe containing prepared medication through injection port of IV lock.	Allows administration of medication.
(8) Inject medication within amount of time recommended by agency policy, pharmacist, or medication reference manual. Use watch to time administration.	Many medication errors are associated with IV pushes being administered too quickly. Following guidelines for IV push rates promotes patient safety (Box 24.7).
(9) After administering bolus, withdraw syringe.	
(10) Clean injection port with antiseptic swab.	Prevents transmission of microorganisms.
(11) Flush injection port.	
(a) Attach syringe with normal saline and inject flush at same rate that medication was delivered.	Flushing IV line with saline prevents occlusion of IV access device and ensures that all medication is delivered. Flushing IV site at same rate as medication ensures that any medication remaining within IV needle is delivered at the correct rate.

BOX 24.7

Guidelines for Rate of Intravenous (IV) Push Medication Administration

- Verify the rate of administration of IV push medication using agency guidelines or a medication reference manual. The Institute for Safe Medication Practices (ISMP, 2016) has identified the following strategies to reduce harm from rapid IV push medications:
  - Use commercially available or pharmacy-prepared IV push medication whenever possible.
  - Do not dilute IV push medications unless recommended by the manufacturer, agency policy, or reference literature.
  - Administer IV push medications at the rate recommended by the manufacturer, agency policy, or reference literature.
  - Appropriately label clinically prepared syringes.
- Review the amount of medication that a patient will receive each minute, the recommended concentration, and rate of administration. For example, if a patient is to receive 6 mL of a medication over 3 minutes, give 2 mL of the IV bolus medication every minute.
- Some IV medications can only be given safely by IV push when a patient is being continuously monitored for dysrhythmias, blood pressure changes, or other adverse effects. Therefore you can push some medications only in specific areas within a health care agency (e.g., critical care unit). Confirm agency guidelines regarding requirements for special monitoring.

STEP	RATIONALE
8. Help patient to comfortable position.	Gives patient sense of well-being.
9. Discard uncapped needle or needle enclosed in safety shield and attached syringe into puncture- and leak-proof receptacle.	Prevents injury to patients and health care personnel. Recapping needles increases risk for needlestick injury (OSHA, 2012).
10. Be sure nurse call system is in an accessible location within patient's reach.	Ensures patient can call for assistance if needed.
11. Raise side rails (as appropriate) and lower bed to lowest position.	Ensures patient safety.
12. Remove and dispose of gloves and perform hand hygiene.	Reduces transmission of microorganisms.
13. Stay with patient for several minutes and observe for any allergic reactions.	Dyspnea, wheezing, and circulatory collapse are signs of severe anaphylactic reaction.

EVALUATION

1. Observe patient closely for adverse reactions during administration and for several minutes thereafter.	IV medications act rapidly.
2. Observe IV site during injection for sudden swelling and for 48 hours after IV push.	Swelling indicates infiltration into tissues surrounding vein. Signs of infiltration may not occur for 48 hours.
3. Assess patient's status after giving medication to evaluate effectiveness of the medication.	Some IV bolus medications can cause rapid changes in patient's physiological status, thus requiring careful monitoring and assessment and possibly future laboratory testing (e.g., vasopressors and antiarrhythmics require blood pressure and heart rate monitoring, and heparin requires laboratory studies after administration to determine therapeutic levels).
4. **Use Teach-Back:** "I want to be sure I explained to you why you are receiving this IV medication. Can you explain to me what the medication is for and when to call the nurse?" Revise your instruction now or develop a plan for revised patient/family caregiver teaching if patient/family caregiver is not able to teach back correctly.	Determines patient's/family caregiver's level of understanding of instructional topic.

Unexpected Outcomes	Related Interventions
1. Patient develops adverse reaction to medication.	• Stop delivering medication immediately and follow agency policy or guidelines for appropriate response to allergic reaction (e.g., administration of antihistamine such as diphenhydramine or epinephrine) and reporting of adverse drug reactions. • Notify patient's health care provider of adverse effects immediately. • Add allergy information to patient's record.

Unexpected Outcomes	Related Interventions
2. IV medication is incompatible with IV fluids (e.g., IV fluid becomes cloudy in tubing; see agency policy).	• Stop IV fluids and clamp IV line. • Flush IV line with 10 mL of 0.9% sodium chloride or sterile water. • Give newly prepared IV bolus over appropriate amount of time. • Flush with another 10 mL of 0.9% sodium chloride or sterile water at same rate as medication was administered. • Restart IV fluids with new tubing at prescribed rate. • If unable to stop IV infusion, start new IV site (see Chapter 28) and administer medication using IV push (IV lock) method.
3. IV site shows symptoms of infiltration or phlebitis (see Chapter 28).	• Stop IV infusion immediately or discontinue access device and restart in another site. • Determine how much damage IV medication can produce in subcutaneous tissue. • Provide IV extravasation care (e.g., injecting phentolamine around IV infiltration site) as indicated by agency policy, use a medication reference, and consult pharmacist to determine appropriate follow-up care.

Recording

- Record medication administration, including dose, route, date and time administered.
- Record condition of IV site and patient teaching about medication.
- Record patient's response to medication, including any adverse effects.
- Document your evaluation of patient learning.

Hand-Off Reporting

- Report any adverse reactions to patient's health care provider. Patient's response may indicate need for additional medical therapy.

✦ SKILL 24.6 Administering Intravenous Medications by Piggyback and Syringe Pumps

Purpose

One method of administering intravenous (IV) medications involves infusing small volumes (25 to 250 mL) of compatible IV fluids over a desired time period (e.g., 30 to 60 minutes). This method reduces the risk of rapid dose infusion from IV push and provides patient independence. Patients must have an established IV line that is patent by either a continuous infusion or intermittent flushes of normal saline.

Piggyback

A piggyback is a small (25- to 250-mL) IV bag connected to a short tubing line that connects to the upper Y-port of a primary infusion line or to an intermittent venous access such as a saline lock. The IV container that holds the medication is labeled following the IV piggyback medication format of the ISMP (2016). The piggyback tubing is a microdrip or macrodrip system. The set is called a piggyback because the small bag is set higher than the primary infusion bag when administered by gravity. The port of the primary IV line contains a back-check valve that automatically stops the flow of the primary infusion when the piggyback infusion flows, preventing the primary infusion from flowing. After the piggyback solution infuses and the solution within the tubing falls below the level of the primary infusion drip chamber, the back-check valve opens, and the primary infusion begins to flow again.

Volume-Control Administration

Volume-control administration sets (e.g., Volutrol, Buretrol, Pediatrol) are small (50- to 150-mL) containers that attach just below the primary infusion bag or bottle. The set is attached and filled in a manner similar to that used with a regular IV infusion. However, the priming filling of the set is different, depending on the type of filter (floating valve or membrane) within the set. Follow package directions for priming sets.

Mini-Infusion Pump

The mini-infusion pump is battery operated and delivers medication in very small amounts of fluid (5 to 60 mL) within controlled infusion times using standard syringes (Fig. 24.16).

Delegation and Collaboration

The skill of administering IV medications by piggyback, intermittent infusion sets, and mini-infusion pumps cannot be delegated to nursing assistive personnel (NAP). The nurse directs the NAP about:

- Potential medication actions and side effects and to immediately report their occurrence to the nurse.
- Reporting any patient complaints of moisture or discomfort around IV insertion site.
- Reporting any change in patient's condition or vital signs to the nurse.

Equipment

- Adhesive tape *(optional)*
- Antiseptic swab
- Clean gloves
- IV pole
- Medication administration record (MAR) or computer printout
- Puncture-proof container

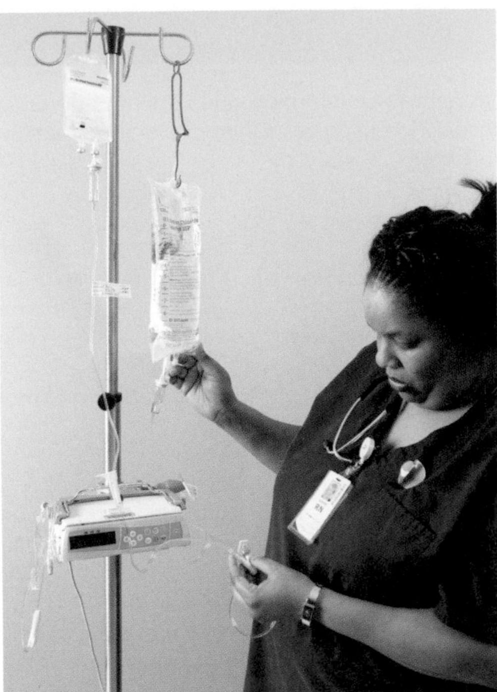

FIG 24.16 Mini-infusion pump.

Piggyback or Mini-Infusion Pump

- Medication prepared in 5- to 250-mL labeled infusion bag or syringe
- Prefilled syringe containing normal saline flush solution (for saline lock only)
- Short microdrip, macrodrip, or syringe IV tubing set, with blunt-end needleless cannula attachment
- Needleless device
- Syringe pump if indicated

Volume-Control Administration Set

- Volutrol or Buretrol
- Infusion tubing with needleless system attachment
- Syringe (1 to 20 mL)
- Vial or ampule of ordered medication

ASSESSMENT

1. Check accuracy and completeness of each MAR or computer printout with health care provider's written medication order. Check patient's name, medication name and dosage, route of administration, and time of administration. Recopy or reprint any portion of MAR that is difficult to read. *Rationale: The order sheet is the most reliable source and only legal record of medications that patient is to receive. Ensures that patient receives the correct medications (Westbrook et al., 2017). Transcription errors are a source of medication errors (Truitt et al., 2016).*
2. Assess patient's medical and medication history. *Rationale: Determines need for medication or possible contraindications for medication administration.*
3. Assess patient's history of allergies: known type of allergens and normal allergic reaction. *Rationale: IV administration of medication may cause rapid response. Allergic response is immediate.*
4. Review medication reference information for medication action, purpose, normal dose, side effects, time and peak of onset, how slowly to give medication, and nursing implications (e.g., need to dilute medication, administer through filter). *Rationale: Allows you to administer medication safely and monitor patient's response to therapy.*
5. If you give medication through existing IV line, determine compatibility of medication with IV fluids and any additional additives within IV solution. *Rationale: IV medication is sometimes not compatible with IV solution and/or additives.*

Safe Patient Care *Never administer IV medications through tubing that is infusing blood, blood products, or parenteral nutrition solutions.*

6. Perform hand hygiene. Assess patency and placement of patient's existing IV infusion line or saline lock (see Chapter 28). *Rationale: Do not administer medication if site is edematous or inflamed.*

Safe Patient Care *If patient's IV site is saline locked, clean the port with alcohol and assess the patency of the IV line by flushing it with 2 to 3 mL of sterile sodium chloride.*

7. Assess patient's symptoms before initiating medication therapy. *Rationale: Provides information to evaluate desired effects of medication.*
8. Assess patient's or family caregiver's knowledge, experience, and health literacy. *Rationale: Ensures patient or family caregiver has the capacity to obtain, communicate, process, and understand basic health information (CDC, 2016).*

STEP	RATIONALE
PLANNING	
1. Expected outcomes following completion of procedure:	
• Patient experiences no adverse reactions.	Medication was administered safely with desired therapeutic effect.
• Medication infuses within desired time frame.	IV line remains patent.
• IV site remains intact, without signs of swelling, inflammation, or the symptom of tenderness at site.	Fluid infuses into vein, not tissues.
• Patient explains medication purpose, dosage, effects and side effects.	Demonstrates learning.
2. Provide privacy and prepare environment.	Providing privacy and preparing the environment early help the student/nurse think about the need to remove clutter from the over-bed or bedside table.

STEP	RATIONALE
3. Discuss purpose of each medication, action, and possible adverse effects. Allow patient to ask any questions. Tell patient that injection will cause slight burning or sting.	Patient has right to be informed, and patient's understanding of each medication improves adherence to drug therapy. Helps minimize patient's anxiety.

IMPLEMENTATION

STEP	RATIONALE
1. Perform hand hygiene and prepare medication using aseptic technique. Prepare medications for one patient at a time. Keep all pages of MARs or computer printouts for one patient together or look at only one patient's electronic MAR at a time. Check label of medication carefully with MAR or computer printout two times (see Skill 24.1 or Procedural Guideline 24.1) when preparing medication.	Ensures that medication is sterile. Preventing distractions reduces medication preparation errors. Use no-interruption zone (NIZ) when possible (Prakash et al., 2014; Yoder et al., 2015). *These are the first and second checks for accuracy* and ensure that correct medication is administered.
2. Take medication(s) to patient at correct time (see agency policy). Medications that require exact timing include STAT, first-time or loading doses, and one-time doses. Give time-critical scheduled medications (e.g., antibiotics, anticoagulants, insulin, anticonvulsants, immunosuppressive agents) at exact time ordered (no later than 30 minutes before or after scheduled dose). Give non–time-critical scheduled medications within a range of 1 or 2 hours of scheduled dose (ISMP, 2011). During administration apply seven rights of medication administration.	Hospitals must adopt medication administration policy and procedure for timing of medication administration that considers nature of the prescribed medication, specific clinical application, and patient needs (DHHS, 2011; ISMP, 2011). Time-critical scheduled medications are those for which early or delayed administration of maintenance doses of greater than 30 minutes before or after the scheduled dose may cause harm or result in substantial suboptimal therapy or pharmacological effect. Non–time-critical medications are those for which early or delayed administration within a specified range of either 1 or 2 hours should not cause harm or result in substantial suboptimal therapy or pharmacological effect (DHHS, 2011; ISMP, 2011).
3. Identify patient using at least two identifiers (e.g., name and birthday or name and medical record number) according to agency policy. Compare identifiers with information on patient's MAR or medical record.	Ensures correct patient. Complies with The Joint Commission standards and improves patient safety (TJC, 2019). Some agencies are now using a bar-code system to help with patient identification.
4. At patient's bedside, again compare MAR or computer printout with names of medications on medication labels and patient name. Ask patient if he or she has allergies.	*This is the third check for accuracy* and ensures that patient receives correct medication. Confirms patient's allergy history.
5. Administer infusion.	
a. Piggyback infusion:	
(1) Connect infusion tubing to medication bag (see Chapter 28). Fill tubing by opening regulator flow clamp. Once tubing is full, close clamp and cap end of tubing.	Filling infusion tubing with solution and freeing air bubbles prevent air embolus. Capping reduces transmission of microorganisms.
(2) Hang piggyback (see illustration) medication bag above level of primary fluid bag. (Use hook to lower main bag.) Primary line continues to infuse.	Height of fluid bag affects rate of flow to patient.

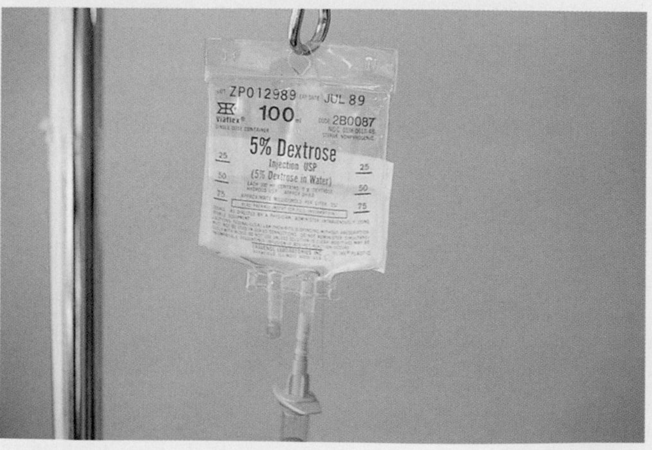

STEP 5a(2) Small-volume minibag for piggyback infusion.

STEP	RATIONALE
(3) Connect tubing of piggyback infusion to appropriate connector on upper Y-port of primary infusion line:	Connection allows IV medication to enter main IV line.
(a) Needleless system: Wipe off needleless port of main IV line with alcohol swab, allow to dry, and insert cannula tip of piggyback infusion tubing (see illustrations).	Use needleless connections to prevent accidental needlestick injuries (INS, 2016; OSHA, 2012).

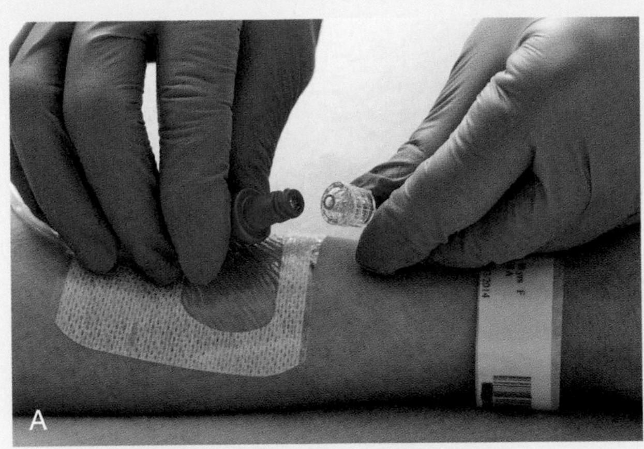
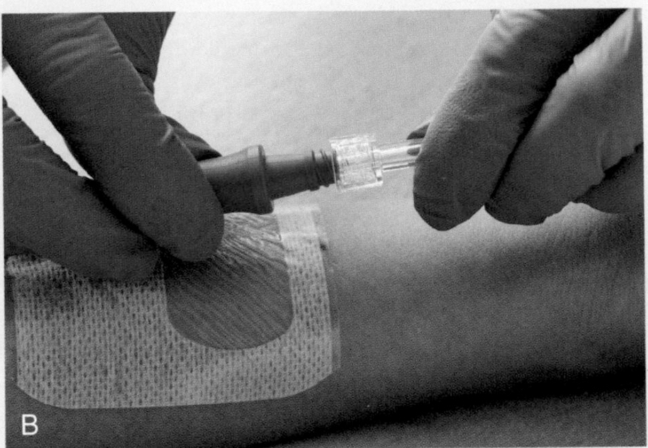

STEP 5a(3)(a) (A) Needleless lock cannula system. (B) Blunt-ended cannula inserts into port and locks.

STEP	RATIONALE
(b) Normal saline lock: Follow Steps 7a(1) through 7b(6) in Skill 24.5 to flush and prepare lock. Wipe off port with alcohol swab, let dry, and insert tip of piggyback infusion tubing via needleless access.	Flushing of lock ensures patency.
(4) Regulate flow rate of medication solution by adjusting regulator clamp or IV pump infusion rate. Infusion times vary. Refer to medication reference or agency policy for safe flow rate.	Provides slow, safe, intermittent infusion of medication and maintains therapeutic blood levels.
(5) Once medication has infused:	
(a) Continuous infusion: Check flow rate of primary infusion. Primary infusion automatically begins after piggyback solution is empty.	Back-check valve on piggyback prevents flow of primary infusion until medication infuses. Checking flow rate ensures proper administration of IV fluids.
(b) Normal saline lock: Disconnect tubing, clean port with alcohol, and flush IV line with 2 to 3 mL of sterile 0.9% sodium chloride. Maintain sterility of IV tubing between intermittent infusions.	
(6) Regulate continuous main infusion line to ordered rate.	Infusion of piggyback sometimes interferes with main line infusion rate.
(7) Leave IV piggyback and tubing in place for future drug administration (see agency policy) or discard it and the uncapped needle or needle enclosed in safety shield of flushing syringe in puncture- and leak-proof container.	Establishing secondary line produces route for microorganisms to enter main line. Repeated changes in tubing increase risk for infection transmission.
b. Volume-control administration set (e.g., Volutrol):	
(1) Fill Volutrol with desired amount of IV fluid (50 to 100 mL) by opening clamp between Volutrol and main IV bag (see illustration).	Small volume of fluid dilutes IV medication and reduces risk of fluid infusing too rapidly.
(2) Close clamp and check to be sure that clamp on air vent Volutrol chamber is open.	Prevents additional leakage of fluid into Volutrol. Air vent allows fluid in Volutrol to exit at regulated rate.
(3) Clean injection port on top of Volutrol with antiseptic swab.	Prevents introduction of microorganisms during needle insertion.
(4) Remove needle cap or sheath and insert needleless syringe or syringe needle through port and inject medication (see illustration). Gently rotate Volutrol between hands.	Rotating mixes medication with solution to ensure equal distribution in Volutrol.

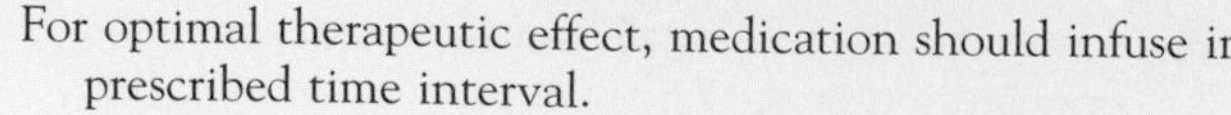

STEP	RATIONALE
(5) Regulate IV infusion rate to allow medication to infuse in time recommended by agency policy, pharmacist, or medication reference manual.	For optimal therapeutic effect, medication should infuse in prescribed time interval.
(6) Label Volutrol with name of medication; dosage; total volume, including diluent; and time of administration following ISMP (2016) safe-medication label format.	Alerts nurses to medication being infused. Prevents other medications from being added to Volutrol.
(7) If patient is receiving continuous IV infusion, check infusion rate after Volutrol infusion is complete.	Ensures appropriate rate of administration.
(8) Dispose of uncapped needle or needle enclosed in safety shield and syringe in puncture- and leak-proof container. Discard supplies in appropriate container.	Prevents accidental needlesticks (OSHA, 2012). Reduces transmission of microorganisms.
c. Mini-infusion administration:	
(1) Connect prefilled syringe to mini-infusion tubing; remove end cap of tubing.	Special tubing designed to fit syringe delivers medication to main IV line.
(2) Carefully apply pressure to syringe plunger, allowing tubing to fill with medication.	Ensures that tubing is free of air bubbles to prevent air embolus.
(3) Place syringe into mini-infusion pump (follow product directions) and hang on IV pole. Be sure that syringe is secured (see illustration).	Secure placement is needed for proper infusion.

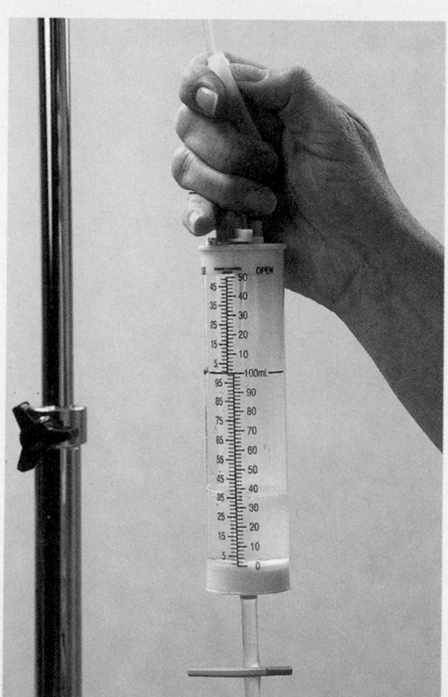

STEP 5b(1) Fill volume-control administration device.

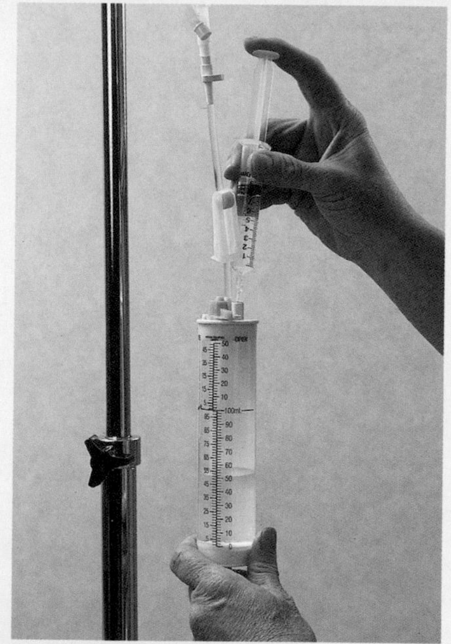

STEP 5b(4) Medication injected into device.

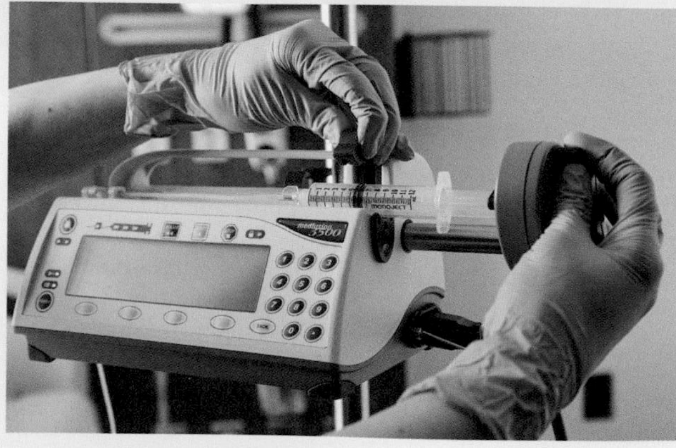

STEP 5c(3) Ensure that syringe is secure after placing it into mini-infusion pump.

STEP	RATIONALE
(4) Connect end of mini-infusion tubing to main IV line or saline lock:	Establishes route for IV medication to enter main IV line.
(a) Existing IV line: Wipe off needleless port on main IV line with alcohol swab, allow to dry, and insert tip of mini-infusion tubing through center of port.	Needleless connections reduce risk for accidental needlestick injuries (OSHA, 2012).
(b) Normal saline lock: Follow Steps 7a(1) through 7b(6) in Skill 24.5 to flush and prepare lock. Wipe off port with alcohol swab, allow to dry, and insert tip of mini-infusion tubing.	
(5) Set pump to deliver medication within time recommended by agency policy, pharmacist, or medication reference manual. Press button on pump to begin infusion.	Pump automatically delivers medication at safe, constant rate based on volume in syringe.
(6) Once medication has infused:	
(a) Main IV infusion: Check flow rate. Infusion automatically begins to flow once pump stops. Regulate infusion to desired rate as needed.	Maintains patent primary IV fluids.
(b) Normal saline lock: Disconnect tubing, clean port with alcohol, and flush IV line with 2 to 3 mL of sterile 0.9% sodium chloride. Maintain sterility of IV tubing between intermittent infusions.	
(c) Dispose of uncapped needle or needle enclosed in safety shield of flushing syringe in puncture- and leak-proof container. Discard supplies in appropriate container	
6. Help patient to comfortable position.	Gives patient sense of well-being.
7. Be sure nurse call system is in an accessible location within patient's reach.	Ensures patient can call for assistance if needed.
8. Raise side rails (as appropriate) and lower bed to lowest position.	Ensures patient safety.
9. Remove and dispose of gloves and perform hand hygiene.	Reduces transmission of microorganisms.

EVALUATION

1. Observe patient for signs or symptoms of adverse reaction.	IV medications act rapidly.
2. During infusion, periodically check infusion rate and condition of IV site.	IV must remain patent for proper drug administration. Infiltration of IV site requires discontinuing infusion.
3. Ask patient to explain purpose and side effects of medication.	Evaluates patient's understanding of instruction.
4. **Use Teach-Back:** "I want to be sure I explained to you the reason for this IV medication. Can you explain to me why you are receiving the medication and what to report to the nurse?" Revise your instruction now or develop a plan for revised patient/family caregiver teaching if patient/family caregiver is not able to teach back correctly.	Determines patient's/family caregiver's level of understanding of instructional topic.

Unexpected Outcomes	Related Interventions
1. Patient develops adverse or allergic reaction to medication.	• Stop medication infusion immediately. • Follow agency policy or guidelines for appropriate response to allergic reaction (e.g., administration of antihistamine such as diphenhydramine or epinephrine) and reporting of adverse medication reactions. • Notify patient's health care provider of adverse effects immediately. • Add allergy information to patient record per agency policy.
2. Medication does not infuse over established time frame.	• Determine reason (e.g., improper calculation of flow rate, poor positioning of IV needle at insertion site, infiltration). • Take corrective action as indicated by agency policy or health care provider.

Unexpected Outcomes	Related Interventions
3. IV site shows signs of infiltration or phlebitis (see Chapter 28).	• Stop IV infusion and discontinue access device. • Treat IV site as indicated by agency policy. • Insert new IV catheter if therapy continues. • For infiltration, determine how harmful IV medication is to subcutaneous tissue. Provide IV extravasation care (e.g., injecting phentolamine around IV infiltration site) as indicated by agency policy or consult pharmacist to determine appropriate follow-up care.

Recording

- Immediately record medication, dose, route, infusion rate, and date and time administered.
- Record volume of fluid in medication bag or syringe pump as fluid intake.
- Record patient's response to medication and any adverse effects.
- Document your evaluation of patient learning.

Hand-Off Reporting

- Report any adverse reactions to patient's health care provider.

✦ SKILL 24.7 Administering Medications by Continuous Subcutaneous Infusion

Purpose

The continuous subcutaneous infusion (CSQI or CSCI) route of medication administration is used for selected medications (e.g., opioids, insulin [Fig. 24.17]). The route is also effective with medications to stop preterm labor (e.g., terbutaline [Brethine]) and to treat pulmonary hypertension (e.g., treprostinil sodium [Remodulin]). One factor that determines the infusion rate of CSQI is the rate of medication absorption. Most patients can absorb 1 to 2 mL/hr of medication or 62 mL/hr of fluid, but the rate of absorption is more dependent on osmotic pressure than rate of administration (Alexander et al., 2014; Arthur, 2015; Caccialanza et al., 2016).

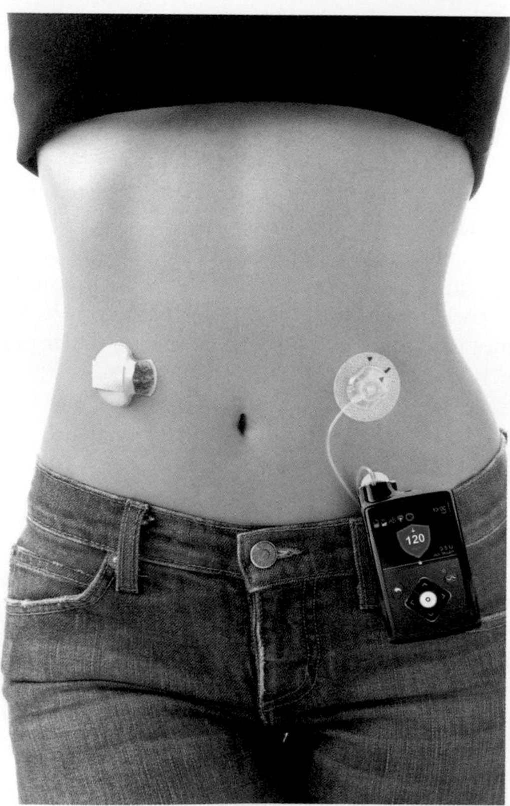

FIG 24.17 MiniMed Paradigm REAL-Time Insulin CSQI Pump and Continuous Glucose Monitoring System. *(Courtesy Medtronic MiniMed, Northridge, CA.)*

The CSQI route requires a computerized pump with safety features, including lockout intervals and warning alarms. Ideally, medication pumps are individualized based on the medication being delivered and the patient's needs. You also need to consider the availability and cost of the pump and its supplies. When possible, have patients select the pump that fits their individual and home needs and is easiest to use.

Delegation and Collaboration

The skill of administering CSQI medications cannot be delegated to nursing assistive personnel (NAP). The nurse directs the NAP about:

- Potential medication side effects or reactions and to immediately report their occurrence to the nurse.
- Reporting complications (e.g., leaking, redness, discomfort) at the CSQI needle insertion site to the nurse.
- Obtaining any required vital signs and reporting them to the nurse.

Equipment

Initiation of CSQI

- Clean gloves
- Alcohol swab
- Antibacterial skin preparation such as chlorhexidine
- Small-gauge (25- to 27-gauge) winged intravenous (IV) catheter with attached tubing or CSQI-designed catheter (e.g., Sof-Set)
- Infusion pump
- Occlusive, transparent dressing
- Tape
- Medication in appropriate syringe or container
- Medication administration record (MAR) or computer printout

Discontinuing CSQI

- Clean gloves
- Small, sterile gauze dressing

- Tape or adhesive bandage
- Alcohol swab and chlorhexidine *(optional)*
- Puncture-proof container

ASSESSMENT

1. Check accuracy and completeness of each MAR or computer printout with health care provider's written medication order. Check patient's name, medication name and dosage, route of administration, and time of administration. Recopy or reprint any portion of MAR that is difficult to read. *Rationale: The order sheet is the most reliable source and only legal record of medications that patient is to receive. Ensures that patient receives the correct medications (Westbrook et al., 2017). Transcription errors are a source of medication errors (Truitt et al., 2016).*
2. Assess patient's medical and medication history. *Rationale: Determines need for medication or possible contraindications for medication administration.*
3. Assess patient's history of allergies: known type of allergens and normal allergic reaction. *Rationale: CSQI administration of medications may cause rapid response. Allergic response is immediate.*
4. Collect drug reference information necessary to administer drug safely, including action, purpose, side effects, normal dose, time of peak onset, how slowly to give medication, and nursing implications. *Rationale: Knowledge of medication allows you to give medication safely and monitor patient's response to therapy.*
5. Assess patient's previous verbal and nonverbal response to needle insertion. *Rationale: Anticipating patient's anxiety allows you to use distraction to reduce pain awareness.*
6. If an analgesic is being administered, assess patient's pain severity using a scale from 0 to 10, with 0 being no pain and 10 being the worst pain ever experienced. *Rationale: Provides an objective measure of pain severity.*
7. Assess for contraindications to CSQI (e.g., thrombocytopenia or reduced local tissue perfusion). *Rationale: Any existing coagulation disorder contraindicates heparin infusion. Reduced tissue perfusion interferes with medication absorption and distribution.*
8. Perform hand hygiene. Assess adequacy of patient's adipose tissue to determine appropriate infusion site. *Rationale: Physiological changes of aging or patient illness influence amount of subcutaneous tissue, which affects choice of catheter insertion site.*
9. Assess patient's symptoms before initiating medication therapy. Determine severity of pain (if using analgesia) or measure blood glucose level (if using insulin). *Rationale: Provides information to evaluate desired effects of CSQI medication.*
10. Assess patient's or family caregiver's knowledge, experience, and health literacy. *Rationale: Ensures patient or family caregiver has the capacity to obtain, communicate, process, and understand basic health information (CDC, 2016).*

STEP	RATIONALE
PLANNING	
1. Expected outcomes following completion of procedure:	
• Needle insertion site remains free from infection.	Risk for infection at needle insertion site is potential complication of CSQI therapy.
• Patient achieves desired effect of medication with no signs of adverse reactions.	Medication is delivered safely with desired therapeutic effect achieved.
• Patient explains medication purpose, dosage, effects and side effects of medication.	Demonstrates learning.
2. Provide privacy and prepare environment.	Providing privacy and preparing the environment early help the student/nurse think about the need to remove clutter from the over-bed or bedside table.
3. Discuss purpose of each medication, action, and possible adverse effects. Allow patient to ask any questions. Tell patient that injection will cause slight burning or sting.	Patient has right to be informed, and patient's understanding of each medication improves adherence to drug therapy. Helps minimize patient's anxiety.
IMPLEMENTATION	
1. Review manufacturer directions for pump.	Ensures proper use of equipment.
2. Perform hand hygiene and prepare medication using aseptic technique. Prepare medications for one patient at a time. Keep all pages of MARs or computer printouts for one patient together or look at only one patient's electronic MAR at a time. Check label of medication carefully with MAR or computer printout two times (see Skill 24.1 or Procedural Guideline 24.1) when preparing medication.	Ensures that medication is sterile. Preventing distractions reduces medication preparation errors. Use no-interruption zone (NIZ) when possible (Prakash et al., 2014; Yoder et al., 2015). *This is the first check for accuracy* and ensures that correct medication is administered.
3. Obtain and program medication administration pump. Place syringe in pump.	Ensures that medication dose administered is accurate.
4. Read label on prefilled syringe and compare with MAR or computer printout.	*This is the second check for accuracy.*

STEP	RATIONALE
5. Identify patient using at least two identifiers (e.g., name and birthday or name and medical record number) according to agency policy. Compare identifiers with information on patient's MAR or medical record.	Ensures correct patient. Complies with The Joint Commission standards and improves patient safety (TJC, 2019). Some agencies are now using a bar-code system to help with patient identification.
6. At patient's bedside, again compare MAR or computer printout with names of medications on medication labels and patient name. Ask patient if he or she has allergies.	*This is the third check for accuracy* and ensures that patient receives correct medication. Confirms patient's allergy history.
7. Position patient supine.	Respects patient's dignity.
8. Initiate CSQI:	
a. Be sure that patient is comfortable, sitting or lying down.	Eases pain associated with insertion of needle.
b. Perform hand hygiene and apply clean gloves. Select appropriate injection site free of irritation and away from bony prominences and waistline. Most common sites used are subclavicular and abdomen.	Ensures proper medication absorption.
c. Clean injection site with alcohol using circular motion, followed by antiseptic, using straight cleaning strokes. Allow both agents to dry.	Reduces risk for infection at insertion site.
d. Hold needle in dominant hand and remove needle guard.	Prepares needle for insertion.
e. Gently pinch or lift up skin with nondominant hand.	Ensures that needle will enter subcutaneous tissue.
f. Gently and firmly insert needle at 45- to 90-degree angle (see illustration). Some shorter prepackaged needles (e.g., Sof-Set, Subcutaneous-Set) are inserted at a 90-degree angle. Refer to manufacturer directions.	Decreases pain related to insertion of needle.
g. Release skinfold and apply tape over "wings" of needle.	Secures needle.

Safe Patient Care *Some cannulas have a sharp needle covered with a plastic catheter. In this case, remove the needle and leave the plastic catheter in the skin.*

STEP	RATIONALE
h. Place occlusive, transparent dressing over insertion site (see illustration).	Protects site from infection and allows you to assess site during medication infusion.
i. Attach tubing from needle to tubing from infusion pump and turn pump on.	Allows you to administer medication.
j. Dispose of any sharps in appropriate leak- and puncture-proof container. Discard used supplies.	Prevents accidental needlestick injuries and follows CDC guidelines for disposal of sharps (OSHA, 2012).
k. Help patient to comfortable position.	Gives patient sense of well-being.
l. Inspect site before leaving patient and instruct patient to inform you if site becomes red or begins to leak.	Initiate new site with new needle whenever erythema or leaking occurs. If site is free from complications, rotate needle every 2 to 7 days (Alexander et al., 2014; Arthur, 2015; INS, 2016).
m. Be sure nurse call system is in an accessible location within patient's reach.	Ensures patient can call for assistance if needed.

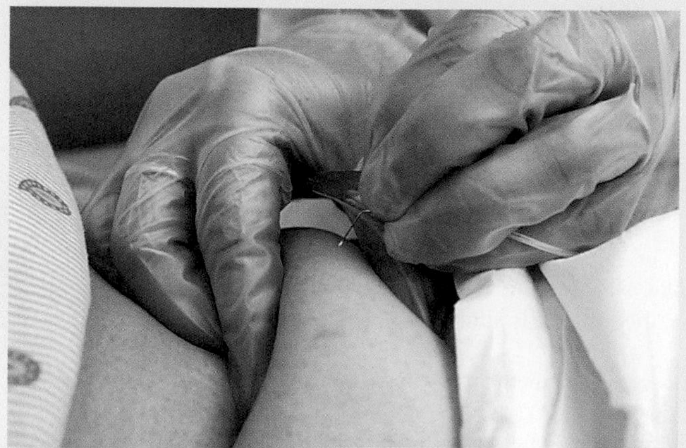
STEP 8f Insert butterfly needle into subcutaneous tissue of abdomen.

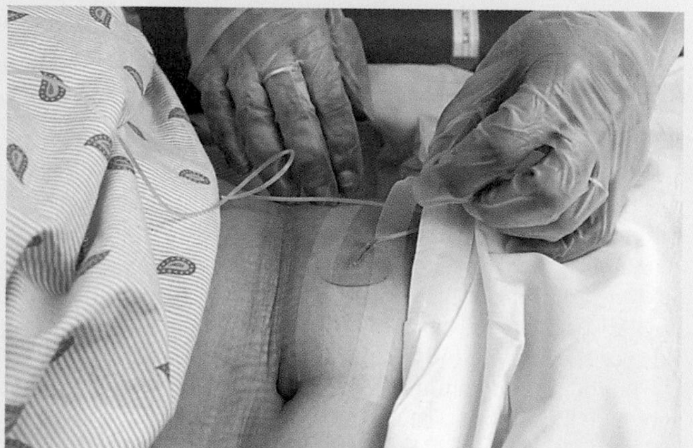
STEP 8h Place occlusive, transparent dressing over insertion site.

STEP	RATIONALE
n. Raise side rails (as appropriate) and lower bed to lowest position.	Ensures patient safety.
o. Remove gloves and perform hand hygiene.	Reduces transmission of microorganisms.
p. Stay with patient for several minutes and observe for any allergic reactions.	Dyspnea, wheezing, and circulatory collapse are signs of severe anaphylactic reaction.
9. Discontinue CSQI:	
a. Verify order and establish alternative method for medication administration if applicable.	If medication will be required after discontinuing CSQI, a different medication and/or route is often necessary to continue to manage patient's illness or pain.
b. Stop infusion pump.	Prevents medication from spilling.
c. Perform hand hygiene and apply clean gloves.	Follows CDC recommendations to prevent accidental exposure to blood and body fluids (OSHA, 2012).
d. Remove dressing without dislodging or removing needle. Discard properly.	Exposes needle.

Safe Patient Care *If site is infected, clean it with alcohol and antiseptic. Apply triple antibiotic cream to site if it is excoriated (abraded).*

STEP	RATIONALE
e. Remove tape from wings of needle and pull needle out at same angle at which it was inserted.	Minimizes patient discomfort.
f. Apply gentle pressure at site until no fluid leaks out of skin.	Dressing adheres to site if skin remains dry.
g. Apply small sterile gauze dressing or adhesive bandage to site.	Prevents bacterial entry into puncture site.
h. Help patient to comfortable position.	Gives patient sense of well-being.
i. Be sure nurse call system is in an accessible location within patient's reach.	Ensures patient can call for assistance if needed.
j. Raise side rails (as appropriate) and lower bed to lowest position.	Ensures patient safety.
k. Dispose of uncapped needles and syringes in puncture- and leak-proof container.	Prevents accidental needlestick injuries and follows CDC guidelines for disposal of sharps (OSHA, 2012).
l. Remove and dispose of gloves and perform hand hygiene.	Reduces transmission of microorganisms.

EVALUATION

1. Evaluate patient's response to medication.	Determines effect of therapy. Decreased or absent response to medication may indicate that patient is not receiving medication into subcutaneous tissue (e.g., pump malfunction, medication leaking at site).
2. Assess site at least every 4 hours for redness, pain, drainage, or swelling.	Indicates infection at insertion site.
3. **Use Teach-Back:** "I want to be sure you understand your continuous infusion into your skin and the medication you are receiving. Tell me in your own words why you have a continuous infusion to receive your medication." Revise your instruction now or develop a plan for revised patient/family caregiver teaching if patient/family caregiver is not able to teach back correctly.	Determines patient's/family caregiver's level of understanding of instructional topic.

Unexpected Outcomes	Related Interventions
1. Patient complains of localized pain or burning at insertion site, or site appears red or swollen or is leaking, indicating potential infection or needle dislodgement.	• Remove needle and place new needle in different site. • Continue to monitor original site for signs of infection and notify health care provider if you suspect infection.
2. Patient displays signs of allergic reaction to medication.	• Stop delivering medication immediately and follow agency policy or guidelines for appropriate response to allergic reaction (e.g., administration of antihistamine such as diphenhydramine or epinephrine) and reporting of adverse drug reactions. • Notify patient's health care provider of adverse effects immediately. • Add allergy information to medical record.

Unexpected Outcomes	Related Interventions
3. CSQI becomes dislodged.	• Stop infusion, apply pressure at site until no fluid leaks out of skin, cover site with gauze dressing or adhesive bandage, and initiate new site. • Assess patient to determine effects of not receiving medication (e.g., assess patient's pain level using age-appropriate pain scale, obtain blood glucose level).

Recording

- After initiating CSQI, immediately chart medication, dose, infusion rate, route, site, time, date, and type of medication pump.
- If medication is an opioid, follow agency policy to document waste.
- Record patient's response to medication and appearance of site every 4 hours.
- Document your evaluation of patient learning.

Hand-Off Reporting

- Report any adverse effects from medication or infection at insertion site to patient's health care provider. Patient's condition often indicates need for additional medical therapy.

SPECIAL CONSIDERATIONS

Patient-Centered Care

- Research shows that ethnicity, genetics, and culture influence drug response, pharmacokinetics, and pharmacodynamics, as well as patient adherence and education (Burchum and Rosenthal, 2016; Tantisira et al., 2015).
- Knowledge about variations in therapeutic dose and adverse effects is essential in administering medications to different ethnic groups. Some patients experience a therapeutic response at different dosages than recommended and require careful monitoring.
- Good communication skills enable you to communicate and educate diverse patient populations. For example, if a patient's culture values patience and modesty, make your questions specific, and take time when assessing the patient's knowledge about adverse drug effects.
- Cultural assessment also yields information about dietary preferences, tobacco and alcohol use, and use of herbal remedies that affect drug action and response.
- Cultural context is essential in planning education for patients and families (Burchum and Rosenthal, 2016).

Patient Education

- Instruct a patient not to squeeze medication out of an injection site.
- Patients should wear medical identification bands listing all allergies.
- Patients who self-administer injections containing insulin or heparin at home must be able to handle equipment, store medications properly, and administer injections correctly. Provide necessary education and ensure return demonstration for patients and family caregivers.

Age-Specific

Pediatric

- Children can be anxious or afraid of needles. Assistance with properly positioning and holding the child is sometimes necessary. Distraction such as blowing bubbles and pressure at the injection site before giving the injection helps reduce the child's anxiety.
- Children with ongoing exposure to high-risk individuals (e.g., HIV-infected, homeless, incarcerated) should be tested for tuberculosis every 2 to 3 years (Hockenberry and Wilson, 2017).
- The therapeutic dose of IV push medications for infants and children is often small and difficult to prepare accurately even with a tuberculin syringe. Infuse these medications slowly and in small volumes because of the risk for fluid-volume overload (Hockenberry and Wilson, 2017). To maintain pediatric safety, carefully follow agency guidelines when administering IV bolus medication.
- Insulin pumps offer flexibility for adolescents, placing the responsibility of diabetes management on the child. Extensive child and family education is needed in using CSQI (Hockenberry and Wilson, 2017).
- Clean and rotate sites in children every 48 to 72 hours or at the first sign of inflammation (Hockenberry and Wilson, 2017).

Gerontological

- The renal and metabolic systems do not function as efficiently in older patients because of the aging process. To reduce the risk of adverse effects of IV push medications, administer them over longer periods of time.
- Altered pharmacokinetics of medications and the effects of polypharmacy place older adults at risk for medication toxicity. Carefully monitor the response of older adults to IV medication therapy (Touhy and Jett, 2018).
- Hypodermoclysis (the subcutaneous infusion of fluids) is an easy-to-use, safe, and cost-effective alternative to IV hydration for older adults (Touhy and Jett, 2018).

Home Care

- Improper disposal of used needles and sharps in the home setting poses a health risk to the public and waste workers. Several options for safe sharps disposal at home exist, including allowing patients to transport their own sharps containers from home to collection sites (e.g., doctor's office, a hospital, or a pharmacy); mailing their used syringes to a collection site (mail-back programs); syringe exchange programs; and special devices that destroy the needle on the syringe, rendering it safe for disposal (see Chapter 32).
- IV push medications are frequently given in the home. Nurses, pharmacists, and health care providers need to collaborate closely in the care of these patients. Patients and families who are independently responsible for managing IV medications need to understand all aspects of administration safety. Adequate eyesight and manual dexterity are necessary to manipulate a syringe. Patients and family caregivers need to understand the venous access device, the rate at which to give medications, and how to flush the access device. Patients need to store medications safely, dispose of IV supplies appropriately, and know whom to contact in case of an emergency.

- Patients in the home using CSQI need a responsible family caregiver if available. Educate the patient or family caregiver about the desired effect of the medication, side effects and adverse effects of the medication, operation of the pump, how to evaluate the effectiveness of the medication, when and how to assess and rotate insertion sites, and when to call a health care provider for problems. Patients need to know where and how to obtain and dispose of all required supplies.
- Patients managing CSQI at home may use an antibacterial soap (e.g., Hibiclens, pHisoHex) instead of alcohol and chlorhexidine to cleanse the insertion site.

✦ PRACTICE REFLECTIONS

Consider a time when you were caring for patients who required a variety of routes for administering IV medication.

1. What might be the safety issues associated with these different routes?
2. How might you ensure you are correctly assessing for medication compatibility, rate of infusion, and route of administration?
3. How would you ensure the patient or family caregiver clearly understood the need for these different routes?

✦ CLINICAL REVIEW QUESTIONS

1. Place the steps of administering an intradermal injection in the correct order.
   1. Inject medication slowly.
   2. Note the presence of a bleb.
   3. Advance needle through epidermis to 3 mm.
   4. Using nondominant hand, stretch skin over site with forefinger.
   5. Insert needle at a 5- to 15-degree angle into the skin until resistance is felt.
   6. Cleanse site with antiseptic swab.
2. A patient with diabetes is receiving insulin using an insulin pump. Place the steps of discontinuing the insulin pump in the correct order.
   1. Perform hand hygiene and apply clean gloves.
   2. Stop infusion pump.
   3. Remove dressing and discard properly.
   4. Apply gentle pressure to site until no fluid is leaking from skin.
   5. Verify order and establish an alternative route for medication if applicable.
   6. Apply small sterile gauze dressing to site.
   7. Remove tape from wings of needle and pull needle out.
3. You are administering an IV push medication to a patient who has a compatible IV fluid running through intravenous tubing. Place the following steps in the appropriate order.
   1. Release tubing and inject medication within amount of time recommended by agency policy, pharmacist, or medication reference manual. Use watch to time administration.
   2. Select injection port of IV tubing closest to patient. Whenever possible, injection port should accept a needleless syringe. Use IV filter if required by medication reference or agency policy.
   3. After injecting medication, release tubing, withdraw syringe, and recheck fluid infusion rate.
   4. Connect syringe to port of IV line. Insert needleless tip or small-gauge needle of syringe containing prepared drug through center of injection port
   5. Clean injection port with antiseptic swab. Allow to dry.
   6. Occlude IV line by pinching tubing just above injection port. Pull back gently on syringe plunger to aspirate blood return.

Answers and Rationales for Clinical Review Questions can be found on the Evolve website.

REFERENCES

Akbari Sari A, et al: Slow versus fast subcutaneous heparin injections for preventing bruising and site-pain intensity, *Cochrane Database Syst Rev* 18(7), 2014.

Alexander M, et al: *Core curriculum for infusion nursing*, ed 4, Philadelphia, 2014, Lippincott Williams & Wilkins.

Arthur A: Innovations in subcutaneous infusions, *J Infus Nurs* 38(3):179–187, 2015.

Bravo K, Cochran G: Nursing strategies to increase medication safety in inpatient settings, *J Nurs Care Qual* 31(4):335, 2016.

Burchum J, Rosenthal L: *Lehne's pharmacology for nursing care*, ed 9, St. Louis, 2016, Saunders.

Caccialanza R, et al: Subcutaneous infusion of fluids for hydration or nutrition: a review, *JPEN J Parenter Enteral Nutr* 2:2016.

Centers for Disease Control and Prevention (CDC): Vaccine administration: epidemiology and prevention of vaccine-preventable diseases, 2015. http://www.cdc.gov/vaccines/pubs/pinkbook/vac-admin.html.

Centers for Disease Control and Prevention (CDC): What is health literacy, 2016. https://www.cdc.gov/healthliteracy/learn/index.html.

Centers for Disease Control and Prevention (CDC): Vaccine administration, 2017. https://www.cdc.gov/vaccines/hcp/acip-recs/general-recs/administration.html.

Department of Health and Human Services: Centers for Medicare & Medicaid (DHHS): *Updated guidance on medication administration, Hospital Appendix A of State Operations Manual*, Baltimore, 2011, Department of Health and Human Services.

Diggle D: Are you FIT for purpose? The importance of getting injection technique right, *J Diabetes Nurs* 18:50–57, 2014.

Gorski LA: *Phillip's manual of IV therapeutics: evidence-based practice for infusion therapy*, Philadelphia, 2018, FA Davis, p 7.

Gunes UY, et al: Is the ventrogluteal site suitable for intramuscular injections in children under the age of three?, *J Adv Nurs* 71(1):127, 2016.

Gülnar E, Çalışkan N: Ventrogluteal intramuscular injection for nurse examination of knowledge for practice, *DEUHYO* 7(2):70–77, 2014.

Hibbard P, et al: Approach to immunizations in healthy adults, UpToDate, 2017. https://www.uptodate.com/contents/approach-to-immunizations-in-healthy-adults.

Hirsch LJ, et al: Glycemic control, reported pain and leakage with a 4 mm x 32 G pen needle in obese and non-obese adults with diabetes: a post hoc analysis, *Curr Med Res Opin* 28(8):1305, 2012.

Hockenberry MJ, Wilson D: *Wong's essentials of pediatric nursing*, ed 10, St. Louis, 2017, Mosby.

Holliday R, et al: Body mass index: a reliable predictor of subcutaneous fat thickness and needle length for ventral gluteal intramuscular injections, *Am J Ther* 8, 2016.

Hopkins U, Arias C: Large-volume IM injections: a review of best practices, Oncol Nurse Advisor 32, 2013. http://www.oncologynurseadvisor.com/chemotherapy/large-volume-im-injections-a-review-of-best-practices/article/281208/.

Infusion Nurses Society (INS): Infusion therapy standards of practice, *J Infus Nurs* 39(1 Suppl):S1, 2016.

Institute for Safe Medication Practices (ISMP): Acute care guidelines for timely administration of scheduled medications. 2011. http://www.ismp.org/Tools/guidelines/acutecare/tasm.pdf.

Institute for Safe Medication Practices (ISMP): ISMP Medication Safety Alert: independent double checks: undervalued and misused: selective use of this strategy can play an important role in medication safety, 2013. http://www.ismp.org/NEWSLETTERS/acutecare/showarticle.aspx?id=51.

Institute for Safe Medication Practices (ISMP): ISMP's list of error-prone abbreviations, symbols, and dose designations, 2015. https://www.ismp.org/tools/errorproneabbreviations.pdf.

Institute for Safe Medication Practices (ISMP): Principles of designing a medication label for intravenous piggyback medication for patient specific inpatient use, 2016. https://www.ismp.org/tools/guidelines/labelFormats/IVPB.asp.

Joo G, et al: The effect of different methods of intravenous injection on glass particle contamination from ampules, *Springerplus* 5:15, 2016.
Kara D, et al: Using ventrogluteal site in intramuscular injections is a priority or an alternative?, *Int J Caring Sciences* 8(2):507–513, 2015.
Kaya N, et al: The reliability of site determination methods in ventrogluteal area injection: a cross-sectional study, *Int J Nurs Stud* 52:355–360, 2015.
Kilic E, et al: Comparing applications of intramuscular injections to dorsogluteal or ventrogluteal regions, *J Exp Integr Me* 4(3):171–174, 2014.
Larkin T, et al: Comparison of the V and G methods for ventrogluteal site identification: muscle and subcutaneous fat thickness and considerations for successful intramuscular injection, *Int J Ment Health Nurs* 27(2):631–641, 2018.
Levitsky L, et al: Management of type 1 diabetes mellitus in children and adolescents, UpToDate, 2017. https://www.uptodate.com/contents/management-of-type-1-diabetes-mellitus-in-children-and-adolescents.
Lilley LL, et al: *Pharmacology and the nursing process*, ed 8, St. Louis, 2016, Mosby.
McCulloch D, et al: General principles of insulin therapy in diabetes mellitus. UpToDate, 2017. http://www.uptodate.com/contents/general-principles-of-insulin-therapy-in-diabetes-mellitus.
Nicoll L, Hesby A: Intramuscular injection: an integrative research review and guideline for evidence-based practice, *Appl Nurs Res* 16(2):159, 2002.
Occupational Safety and Health Administration (OSHA): Bloodborne pathogens and needlestick injuries, 77 FR 19934, 2012. https://www.osha.gov/FedReg_osha_pdf/FED20120403.pdf.
Ogston-Tuck S: Subcutaneous injection technique: an evidence based approach, *Nurs Stand* 29(3):53–58, 2014a.
Ogston-Tuck S: Intramuscular injection technique: an evidence based approach, *Nurs Stand* 29(4):55, 2014b.
Patidar A, et al: Comparative efficacy of heparin saline and normal saline flush for maintaining patency of peripheral intravenous lines: a randomized control trial, *IJHSR* 4(3):159–166, 2014.
Prakash V, et al: Mitigating errors caused by interruptions during medication verification and administration: interventions in a simulated ambulatory chemotherapy setting, *BMJ Qual Saf* 23(11):884, 2014.
Royal College of Nursing (RCN): *Infusion therapy standards: rapid evidence review*, London, 2016, Royal College of Nursing.
Sepah Y, et al: Aspiration in injections: should we continue or abandon the practice?, *F1000Res* 3:157, 2017. http://doi.org/10.12688/f1000research.1113.3.
Tantisira K: Overview of pharmacogenomics, UpToDate, 2015. available at http://www.uptodate.com/contents/overview-of-pharmacogenomics.
The Joint Commission (TJC): *2019 National Patient Safety Goals*, Oakbrook Terrace, IL, 2019, The Commission. http://www.jointcommission.org/standards_information/npsgs.aspx.
Touhy TA, Jett KF: *Ebersole and Hess' gerontological nursing & healthy aging*, ed 5, St. Louis, 2018, Mosby.
Truitt E, et al: Effect of the implementation of barcode technology and an electronic medication administration record on adverse drug events, *Hosp Pharm* 51(6):474–483, 2016.
Westbrook JI, et al: Effectiveness of a 'do not interrupt' bundled intervention to reduce interruptions during medication administration: a cluster randomised controlled feasibility study, *BMJ Qual Saf* 0:1–9, 2017.
World Health Organization (WHO): Tuberculosis fact sheet, 2015. http://www.who.int/mediacentre/factsheets/fs104/en/.
World Health Organization (WHO): WHO guideline on the use of safety-engineered for intramuscular, intradermal, and subcutaneous injection in health care settings, 2016, World Health Organization.
Yilmaz D, et al: The effect of the Z-track technique on pain and drug leakage in intramuscular injections, *Clin Nurse Spec* 30(6):E7–E12, 2016.
Yoder M, et al: The effect of a safe zone on nurse interruptions, distractions, and medication administration errors, *J Infus Nurs* 38(2):140, 2015.

25 Wound Care and Irrigation

SKILLS AND PROCEDURES

EVOLVE WEBSITE/RESOURCES LIST

http://evolve.elsevier.com/Perry/nursinginterventions
Audio Glossary • Checklists • Clinical Review Questions • Answers and Rationales for Clinical Review Questions • Video Clips

INTRODUCTION

Proper wound care promotes wound healing that results in an intact skin layer (Fig. 25.1). Wound healing is extremely complex, involving a series of physiological processes among cells and tissues. The location, severity, and extent of a surgical wound or an injury and the tissue layers involved all affect the wound-healing process (Doughty and Sparks-Defriese, 2016). Likewise, the rate of healing depends on numerous internal and external factors (Box 25.1). Effective wound management requires you to understand the processes of wound healing, the factors that interfere with healing, and how to perform a comprehensive wound assessment.

Assessment of a wound provides you with information needed to recognize changes in a wound so that you can institute appropriate wound care measures. The wound assessment is the foundation for the wound plan of care and helps to determine wound-healing progress or deterioration.

A partial-thickness wound (loss of the epidermis and superficial dermal layers) heals by regeneration. However, a full-thickness wound (total loss of epidermis and dermis and in some cases as deep as the muscle layer or bone) heals by scar formation. In a full-thickness wound, healing occurs in four phases (Box 25.2). Collagen deposition begins during inflammation and peaks during proliferation. It is important for nurses to assess for the presence of this new tissue, called the "healing ridge" (Fig. 25.2). This "healing ridge" is composed of newly formed collagen, and you can usually feel it along the edges of an intact surgical suture line by days 5 to 9 (Doughty and Sparks-Defriese, 2016). Types of healing are primary, secondary, and tertiary intention (Fig. 25.3). Healing by primary intention occurs when the wound edges of a clean surgical incision are approximated together. Wounds left open and allowed to heal by scar formation are classified as healing by secondary intention. Healing by tertiary intention is often called delayed primary intention. It occurs when wounds are not closed immediately but left open for several days to allow edema or infection to diminish. The wound edges are then stapled or sutured closed. The type of wound and the manner in which it heals dictate the types of treatment and wound support required.

PRACTICE STANDARDS

- Berrios-Torres et al., 2017: Centers for Disease Control and Prevention guideline for the prevention of surgical site infection
- National Pressure Ulcer Advisory Panel (NPUAP), European Pressure Ulcer Advisory Panel (EPUAP), and Pan Pacific Pressure Injury Alliance (PPPIA), 2016: Prevention and treatment of pressure ulcers: Quick reference guide
- The Joint Commission (TJC), 2019: National Patient Safety Goals—Patient identification

EVIDENCE-BASED PRACTICE

Prevention of Surgical Site Infection

Research supports pre- and intraoperative intervention to reduce the risk for surgical site infection (SSI). Preoperative shaving is not a standard of practice; the use of razors before surgery increases the incidence of wound infection compared with clipping, depilatory use, or no hair removal at all (Berrios-Torres et al., 2017; Institute for Healthcare Improvement [IHI], 2014). Razors cause small skin cuts that may serve as a portal for skin bacteria to enter the skin and contribute to an SSI. There is little evidence to support hair removal, and it may be unnecessary for many procedures. When hair must be removed to perform a procedure safely, use clippers rather than shaving with a razor because this results in fewer SSIs (IHI, 2014).

Evidence-based interventions for hair removal before surgery or when providing wound care include the following:

- Use clippers for hair removal, and train staff members in proper use (IHI, 2012, 2014).

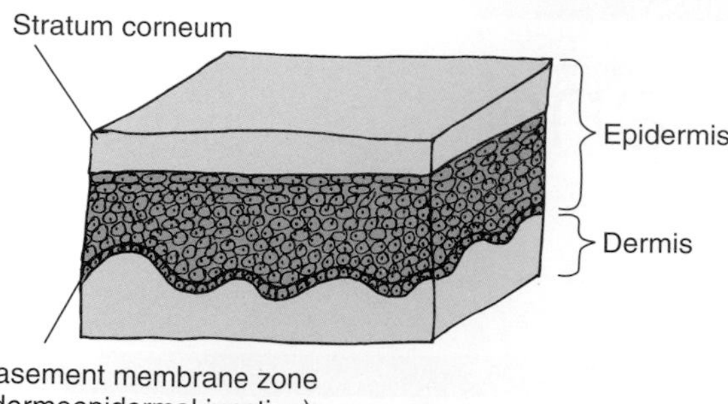

FIG 25.1 Diagram of layers of the skin and subcutaneous tissue.

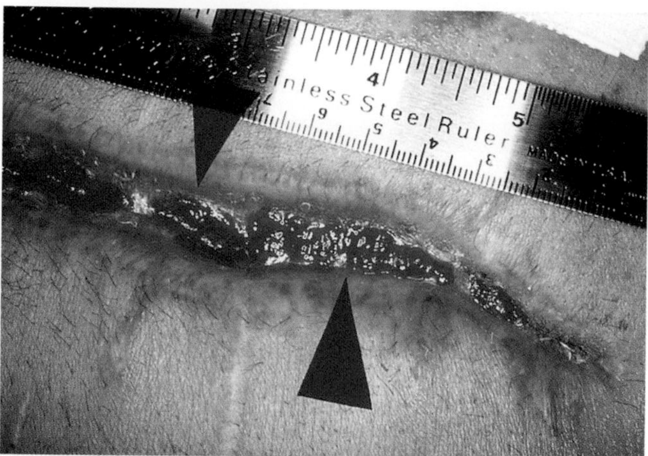

FIG 25.2 Surgical wound with epithelialization occurring; epithelial healing ridge is apparent. *(From Bryant RA, Nix DP: editors:* Acute and chronic wounds current management concepts, *ed 3, St. Louis, 2007, Mosby.)*

BOX 25.1

Factors That Influence Wound Healing

- With increasing age, there is a reduction in collagen deposition, which is thought to contribute to the development of dermal atrophy and poor wound healing (Baranoski et al., 2015b).
- Inadequate nutrition, including proteins, carbohydrates, lipids, vitamins, and minerals, impairs wound healing, resulting in severe alterations such as dehiscence (Stotts, 2016).
- Obesity results in a higher risk for incidence of wound complications, such as surgical site infection and wound dehiscence. Fat tissue has less vascularization, which decreases transport of nutrients and cellular elements required for healing (Gallagher, 2016).
- A hematocrit value less than 20% and a hemoglobin value less than 10 g/100 mL negatively influence tissue repair because of decreased oxygen delivery. Oxygen release to tissue is reduced in smokers and in patients with peripheral vascular diseases.
- Diabetes causes impaired wound healing from reduced collagen synthesis and deposition, decreased wound strength, and impaired leukocyte (white blood cell) function.
- Wound infection prolongs the inflammatory response, and the microorganisms use nutrients and oxygen that are intended for repair.
- Long-term steroid therapy, chemotherapy, or the use of immunosuppressive medications may diminish the inflammatory response and reduce the healing potential.
- An open wound must be maintained in a moist environment, and a closed wound must be protected from microorganisms and stress.

BOX 25.2

Phases of Wound Healing (Full-Thickness Wounds)

Hemostasis

Blood vessels constrict; clotting factors activate coagulation to stop bleeding. Clot formation seals disrupted vessels so that blood loss is controlled and acts as a temporary bacterial barrier. Growth factors are released, attracting cells needed to begin tissue repair.

Inflammatory Phase

Vasodilation occurs, with leakage of plasma and blood cells into the wound, observed as edema, erythema, and exudate. Leukocytes (white blood cells) arrive in the wound to begin cleanup. Macrophages appear and regulate the wound repair. The purpose of inflammation is to ensure a clean wound bed in a noncomplicated wound.

Proliferative/Phase

New capillaries are created, restoring the delivery of oxygen and nutrients to the wound bed. At the same time, new granulation tissue forms. Collagen is synthesized and begins to provide strength and structural integrity to a wound. Contraction reduces the size of the wound. Epithelial resurfacing (construction of new epidermis) begins to cover the wound.

Maturation/Remodeling Phase

Collagen is remodeled to become stronger and provide tensile strength to the wound. This phase begins around day 21 after wounding and continues beyond 1 year. Outer appearance in an uncomplicated wound is that of a well-healed scar.

Data from Doughty DB, Sparks-Defriese B: Wound healing physiology. In Bryant RA, Nix DP, editors: *Acute and chronic wounds: current management concepts,* ed 5, St. Louis, 2016, Mosby.

- Educate patients not to shave preoperatively or when doing wound care (IHI, 2012).
- Instruct patient to shower or bathe (full body) with soap or an antiseptic agent at least on the night before surgery. **NOTE:** Some patients may be instructed to shower and/or bathe multiple times before surgery (Berrios-Torres et al., 2017).
- The is no evidence to support the use of chlorhexidine showering/bathing compared with standard antiseptic agents in minimal-risk patients (Franco et al., 2017).
- Skin preparation in the operating room includes an alcohol-based agent (Berrios-Torres et al., 2017).

SAFETY GUIDELINES

- Safety is a priority when performing a wound assessment or wound irrigation, when emptying a wound collection device, and during removal of staples or stitches because of the risk for infection.
- The loss of intact skin places a patient at risk for infection. It is important to use proper infection control practices to reduce the risk of infection when measuring a wound. Handwashing before and after wound care and the use of gloves (per agency policy, either sterile or clean) are employed when measuring wounds, when performing wound irrigation, when emptying a wound collection device, and during the removal of staples and stitches.
- Place a wound measurement guide or cotton-tipped applicator over a wound during measurement so as not to cause wound trauma.
- Perform wound irrigation by gently introducing the ordered fluid into the wound to prevent tissue injury.
- When removing staples or stitches, use the correct instruments to prevent trauma to the newly healed incision.

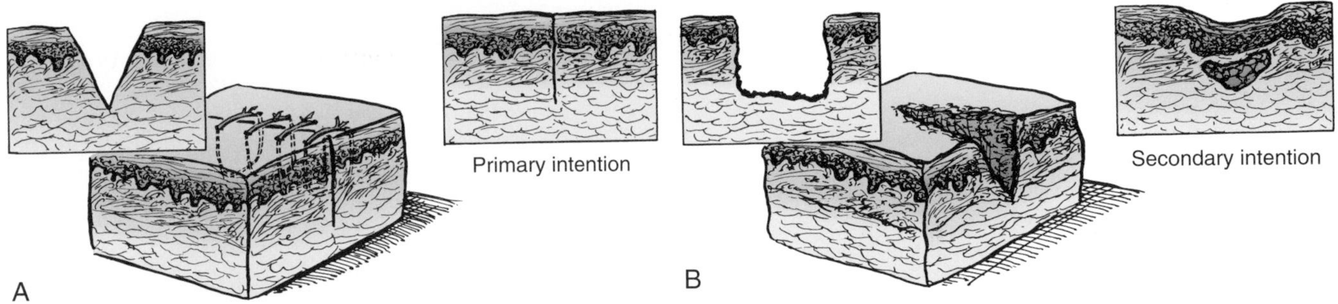

FIG 25.3 (A) Wound healing by primary intention, such as with a surgical incision. Wound-healing edges are pulled together and approximated with sutures, staples, or adhesive, and healing occurs by connective tissue deposition. (B) Wound healing by secondary intention. Wound edges are not approximated, and healing occurs by granulation tissue formation and contraction of the wound edges. (*Used with permission from Bryant RA, editor:* Acute and chronic wounds: nursing management, *ed 2, St. Louis, 2000, Mosby.)*

PROCEDURAL GUIDELINE 25.1 *Performing a Wound Assessment*

Purpose

Wound assessment provides the baseline for planning and evaluating the wound care plan. Normal wound healing occurs in an organized fashion, and evaluating the wound status provides an ongoing assessment of the progress of wound healing and helps to determine wound treatments. Acute care settings generally require wound assessment daily or with each dressing change. Long-term care facilities may require an initial admission wound assessment and weekly assessment for chronic wounds. Check agency policy for frequency of wound assessment and specific wound assessment tool.

The frequency of routine wound assessment depends on a patient's overall condition, policy of the health care setting, type of dressings used, and overall patient goals (Nix, 2016). Wound size may increase in a wound with necrotic tissue. Removal of the necrotic tissue may result in a larger wound and is an expected finding. An increase in the amount and consistency of the drainage and new presence of odor may indicate a wound infection, and a wound culture is often necessary to support appropriate antibiotics.

The following parameters are included in a wound assessment:

- *Location:* Note the anatomical position of the wound.
- *Type of wound:* If possible, note the etiology of the wound (i.e., surgical, pressure, trauma).
- *Extent of tissue involvement:* A full-thickness wound involves both the dermis and epidermis. A partial-thickness wound involves only the epidermal layer. If it is a pressure injury, use the staging system of the National Pressure Ulcer Advisory Panel (NPUAP, 2016; NPUAP, EPUAP, PPPIA, 2016) (see Chapter 26).
- *Type and percentage of tissue in wound base:* Describe the type of tissue (i.e., granulation, slough, and eschar) and the approximate amount.
- *Wound dimensions:* Follow agency policy to measure wound width, length, and depth.
- *Wound drainage/exudate:* Describe the amount, color, and consistency. Serous drainage is clear like plasma; sanguineous or bright red drainage indicates fresh bleeding; serosanguinous drainage is pink; and purulent drainage is thick and can be yellow, pale green, or white.
- *Odor:* Note the presence or absence of odor, which may indicate infection.
- *Wound edge:* The rim of the wound provides information regarding epithelialization. Ideally, the wound edge should be attached, moist, and flush with the wound base so that epithelialization can occur (Nix, 2016).
- *Periwound area:* Assess the color, temperature, and integrity of the skin.
- *Pain:* Use a validated pain assessment scale to evaluate pain.

Delegation and Collaboration

The skill of wound assessment cannot be delegated to nursing assistive personnel (NAP). It is the nurse's responsibility to assess and document wound characteristics. The nurse directs the NAP to:

- Report drainage from the wound that is present on sheets or as strike-through from the dressing to nurse for further assessment.
- Report the presence of odor around the wound.
- Report any dressing that is no longer adherent.

Equipment

Protective equipment: clean gloves, gown, and goggles if splash/spray risk exists; agency tool to document assessment; measuring guide; cotton-tipped applicator; dressing supplies as ordered; disposable waterproof biohazard bag

Procedural Steps

1. Identify patient using at least two identifiers (e.g., name and birthday or name and medical record number) according to agency policy (TJC, 2019).
2. Examine the medical record for the last wound assessment to use as a comparison for this wound assessment. Review the record to determine the etiology of the wound.
3. Determine agency-approved wound assessment tool and review the frequency of assessment. Examine the previous wound assessment to use as comparison for this assessment.
4. Assess comfort level or pain on a scale of 0 to 10 and identify if symptoms of anxiety are present. Offer pain medication as indicated (preferably 30 minutes before full assessment).

Continued

PROCEDURAL GUIDELINE 25.1 *Performing a Wound Assessment—cont'd*

5. Perform hand hygiene. Close room door or bed curtains and position patient.
   a. Position comfortably to permit observation of wound in well-lighted room.
   b. Expose only the area of the wound.
6. Explain procedure of wound assessment to patient.
7. Form a cuff on waterproof biohazard bag and place near bed.
8. Apply clean gloves and remove soiled dressings.
9. Examine dressings for quality of drainage (color, consistency), presence or absence of odor, and quantity of drainage (note if dressings were saturated, slightly moist, or had no drainage). Discard dressings in waterproof biohazard bag. Discard gloves.
10. Perform hand hygiene and apply clean gloves.
11. Inspect wound and determine type of wound healing (e.g., primary or secondary intention).
12. Use agency-approved assessment tool and assess the following:
    a. Wound healing by primary intention (surgical wound):
       (1) Assess anatomical location of wound on body.
       (2) Note if incisional wound margins are approximated or closed together. The wound edges should be together with no gaps.
       (3) Observe for presence and character of drainage. A closed incision should not have any drainage.
       (4) Look for evidence of infection (presence of erythema, odor, or wound drainage).
       (5) Lightly palpate along incision to feel a healing ridge (see Fig. 25.2). The ridge will appear as an accumulation of new tissue presenting as firmness beneath the skin, extending to about 1 cm (½ inch) on each side of the wound between 5 and 9 days after the incision had been created. This is an expected positive sign (Doughty and Sparks-Defriese, 2016).
    b. Wound healing by secondary intention (e.g., pressure injury or contaminated surgical or traumatic wound):
       (1) Assess anatomical location of wound.
       (2) Assess wound dimensions: Measure size of wound (including length, width, and depth) using a centimeter measuring guide. Measure length by placing a ruler above wound at the point of greatest length (or head to foot). Measure width from side to side (Nix, 2016; see illustration). Measure depth by inserting cotton-tipped applicator in area of greatest depth and placing a mark on applicator at skin level. Discard measuring guide and cotton-tipped applicator in a biohazard bag.
       (3) Assess for undermining: Use cotton-tipped applicator to gently probe wound edges. Measure depth and note location using the face of a clock as a guide. The 12 o'clock position (top of wound) would be the head of patient, and the 6 o'clock position would be the bottom of the wound toward patient's feet. Document the number of centimeters that area extends from wound edge (e.g., underneath intact skin).
       (4) Assess extent of tissue loss: If wound is a pressure injury (see Chapter 26), determine the deepest viable tissue layer in wound bed and determine stage. If necrotic tissue does not allow visualization of base of wound, the stage cannot be determined. If the wound is not a pressure injury, determine if there is partial-thickness loss (epidermis and part of the dermis) or full-thickness loss (loss of both the epidermis and the dermis). If it is a pressure injury, use the staging system of the National Pressure Ulcer Advisory Panel (NPUAP, 2016; NPAUP, EPUAP, PPPIA, 2016) (see Chapter 26).
       (5) Observe tissue type, including percentage of granulation, slough, and necrotic tissue.
       (6) Note presence of exudate: amount, color, consistency and odor. Indicate amount of exudate by using part of dressing saturated (completely or partially saturated) or in terms of quantity (e.g., scant, moderate, or copious).
       (7) Note if wound edges are rounded toward wound bed; this may be an indication of delayed wound healing. Describe presence of epithelialization at wound edges (if present) because this indicates movement toward healing.

Safe Patient Care *Compare the wound assessment to previous assessment and determine progress toward healing. If there is no movement toward healing or if you notice deterioration, consider a wound care consultation. Lack of wound healing is often related to infection. Notify health care provider and wound, ostomy, continence nurse or wound care team.*

13. Inspect the periwound skin, including color, texture, and temperature, and describe skin integrity (e.g., open macerated areas, blistering). Periwound assessment provides clues about the effectiveness of wound treatment and possible wound extension (Nix, 2016).
14. Apply dressings per order. Place time, date, and initials on new dressing.
15. Reassess patient's pain and level of comfort, including pain at wound site, using a scale of 0 to 10, after dressing is applied.
16. Discard biohazard bag, soiled supplies, and gloves per agency policy. Perform hand hygiene.
17. Record wound assessment findings and compare assessment with previous wound assessments to monitor wound healing.

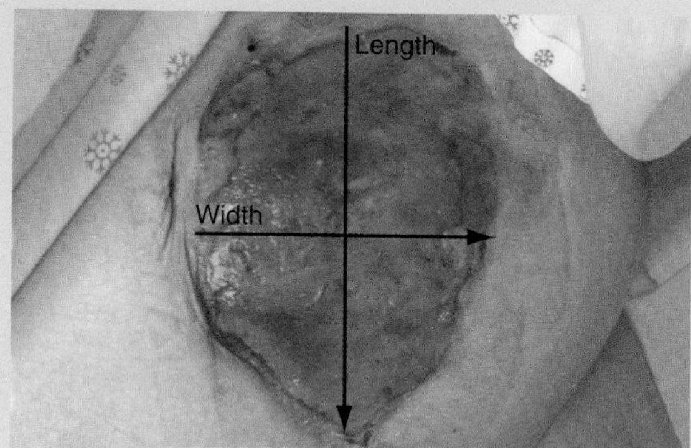

STEP 12b(2) Measuring wound length and width.

✦ SKILL 25.1 Performing a Wound Irrigation

Purpose

Wound irrigation cleanses and irrigates surgical wounds or chronic wounds such as pressure injuries by removing debris from a wound surface, decreasing bacterial counts, and loosening and removing necrotic tissue (Ramundo, 2016). If a patient has a deep wound with a narrow opening, attach a soft catheter (a rubber catheter that is flexible and can easily be introduced into the wound without causing trauma) to the syringe for wound irrigation. Irrigation should not cause tissue injury or discomfort.

Solutions used for irrigations include sterile normal saline, sterile warm water, and commercially available wound cleansers. Typically, you use sterile technique for cleansing and irrigating surgical wounds and clean technique for certain chronic wounds, such as a pressure injury that has not shown evidence of healing over a 2-week period.

Delegation and Collaboration

The skill of wound irrigation cannot be delegated to nursing assistive personnel (NAP) unless it is a chronic wound. It is the nurse's responsibility to assess and document wound characteristics. The nurse directs the NAP to:

- Notify the nurse when the wound is exposed so that an assessment can be completed.
- Report to the nurse patient's pain, presence of blood, and drainage.

Equipment

- Irrigation/cleansing solution per order (volume 1.5 to 2 times the estimated wound volume)
- Irrigation delivery system (per order), depending on amount of desired pressure: sterile irrigation 35-mL syringe with sterile soft angiocatheter or 19-gauge needle (Wound Ostomy and Continence Nurses Society [WOCN], 2016) or handheld shower
- Protective equipment: sterile and clean gloves, gown, and goggles if splash or spray risk exists
- Waterproof underpad if needed
- Dressing supplies
- Disposable waterproof biohazard bag
- Wound assessment supplies (see Procedural Guideline 25.1)

ASSESSMENT

1. Identify patient using at least two identifiers (e.g., name and birthday or name and medical record number) according to agency policy. *Rationale: Ensures correct patient. Complies with The Joint Commission standards and improves patient safety (TJC, 2019).*
2. Review health care provider's order for irrigation of open wound and type of solution to be used. *Rationale: Open-wound irrigation requires medical order, including type of solution(s) to use.*
3. Assess patient's level of comfort using pain scale of 0 to 10. *Rationale: Provides baseline to determine tolerance to procedure.*
4. Review medical record for sign and symptoms related to patient's open wound. *Rationale: Provides ongoing data to indicate change in wound status (Nix, 2016).*
   a. Extent of impairment of skin integrity, including size of wound.
   b. Number of drains present. *Rationale: Awareness of drain position facilitates safe dressing removal and determines need for special dressings.*
   c. Drainage, including amount, color, consistency, and any odor noted. *Rationale: Ongoing data; drainage should decrease in healing wound. When drainage increases, it is often related to infection (Doughty and Sparks-Defriese, 2016).*
   d. Wound tissue color. *Rationale: Color represents type of tissue present in the wound. Red tissue indicates healthy tissue; white, brown, or black tissue is devitalized tissue. Proper selection of wound care products on basis of wound color facilitates removal of necrotic tissue and promotes new tissue growth (Nix, 2016).*
   e. Culture reports. *Rationale: Infected wound is colonized with bacteria. Culture reports identify type of bacteria and proper treatment. Ongoing wound cultures document resolution of infectious process (Stotts, 2016).*
5. Assess patient for history of allergies to antiseptics, solutions, medications, tapes, or dressing material. *Rationale: Known allergies suggest applying sample of prescribed wound treatment as skin test before flushing wound with large volume of solution or selecting different tape or dressing material.*
6. Assess patient's and family caregiver's understanding of need for irrigation and signs of wound infection. *Rationale: Determines extent of instruction required.*
7. Assess patient's or family caregiver's knowledge, experience and health literacy level. *Rationale: Ensures patient has the capacity to obtain, communicate, process, and understand basic health information (Centers for Disease Control and Prevention [CDC], 2016).*

STEP	RATIONALE
PLANNING	
1. Expected outcomes following completion of procedure:	
• Patient states acceptable level of comfort on pain scale of 0 to 10 after wound irrigation.	Premedication, gently administered irrigation, and repositioning patient ensure comfort.
• Wound begins to demonstrate signs of healing; wound is free of excessive drainage, exudate, and inflammation.	Healing progresses in absence of debris and in a protective environment.
• Skin integrity is maintained; no redness, edema, or inflammation noted in surrounding tissue.	No further skin and tissue damage has resulted from wound irrigation.
• Patient is able to describe signs of wound healing and infection.	Demonstrates learning.

STEP	RATIONALE
2. Perform hand hygiene. Administer analgesic at least 30 minutes before starting wound irrigation procedure.	Promotes pain control and permits patient to move more easily and be positioned to facilitate wound irrigation (Krasner, 2016).
3. Gather appropriate supplies for wound irrigation and dressing.	Ensures an organized procedure.
4. Explain procedure to patient and family caregiver. Describe signs of healing and infection during irrigation.	Promotes cooperation and reduces anxiety.
5. Close room door or bed curtains, perform hand hygiene, and position patient.	Maintains privacy; frequent hand hygiene reduces microorganisms.
a. Position comfortably to permit gravitational flow of irrigating solution over wound and into collection receptacle (see illustration).	Directing solution from top to bottom of wound and from clean to contaminated area prevents further infection. Position also avoids fluid retention in the wound as the flow of the irrigant moves away from the wound.

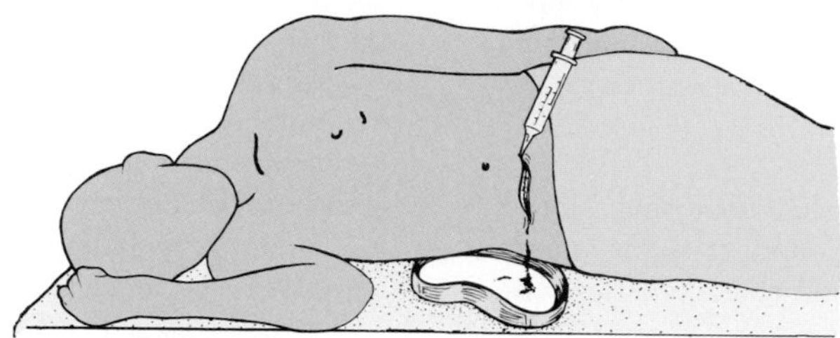

STEP 5a Patient position for wound irrigation.

STEP	RATIONALE
b. Position patient so that wound is vertical to collection basin. Irrigant should be room temperature.	Room-temperature solution increases comfort and reduces vascular constriction response in tissues.
c. Place padding or extra towel on bed under area where irrigation will take place.	Protects bedding from becoming wet.

IMPLEMENTATION

STEP	RATIONALE
1. Perform hand hygiene.	While cleaning wound, use meticulous hand hygiene and proper infection control procedures before and after removing soiled dressings to limit risk for health care–acquired infection (Jaszarowski and Murphree, 2016).
2. Form a cuff on waterproof biohazard bag and place near bed.	Cuffing helps to maintain large opening, thereby permitting placement of contaminated dressings without touching bag itself.
3. Apply gown, mask, goggles as indicated; apply clean gloves and remove old dressing.	Reduces transmission of microorganisms. Protects from splashes or sprays of blood and body fluids.
4. Discard old dressing and gloves in biohazard bag. Perform hand hygiene.	Reduces transmission of microorganisms.
5. Apply clean or sterile gloves (check agency policy). Perform wound assessment and examine recent charted assessment of patient's open wound (see Procedural Guideline 25.1).	Provides ongoing wound-healing data. Use sterile precautions when sterile gloves are needed.
6. Expose area near wound only.	Provides privacy and prevents chilling of patient.
7. Irrigate wound with wide opening:	The cleansing solution is introduced directly into the wound with a syringe, a syringe and catheter, or a pulsed lavage device.
a. Fill 35-mL syringe with irrigation solution.	Irrigating wound uses mechanical force from pushing syringe, which helps with separation and removal of necrotic debris and surface bacteria (Jaszarowski and Murphree, 2016). Flushing wound helps remove debris and facilitates healing by secondary intention.
b. Attach 19-gauge angiocatheter.	The 35-mL syringe with a 19-gauge angiocatheter will facilitate optimum pressure for cleansing and removing debris with minimal risk for tissue injury (Ramundo, 2016). Irrigation pressures delivered between 4 and 15 psi with 19-gauge catheter are most effective (WOCN, 2016).

STEP	RATIONALE
Safe Patient Care *Pulsatile high-pressure lavage is an alternative to using the 35-mL syringe and the 19-gauge angiocatheter. A pulsatile lavage machine combines intermittent high-pressure lavage with suction to loosen necrotic tissue and facilitate removal by other methods of debridement (Ramundo, 2016).*	
c. Hold syringe tip 2.5 cm (1 inch) above upper end of wound and over area being cleaned.	Prevents syringe contamination. Careful placement of syringe prevents unsafe pressure of flowing solution.
d. Using continuous pressure, flush wound; repeat Steps 7a to 7d until solution draining into basin is clear.	Clear solution indicates removal of all debris.
8. Irrigate deep wound with very small opening:	
a. Attach soft catheter to filled 35-mL irrigation syringe.	Catheter permits direct flow of irrigant into wound. Expect wound to take longer to empty when opening is small.
b. Gently insert tip of catheter into opening about 1.3 cm (0.5 inch).	Prevents tip from touching fragile inner wall of wound.
Safe Patient Care *Do not force catheter into the wound because this will cause tissue damage.*	
c. Using slow, continuous pressure, flush wound.	Use of slow mechanical force of stream of solution loosens particulate matter on wound surface and promotes healing (Ramundo, 2016).
Safe Patient Care *Pulsatile high-pressure lavage is often the irrigation of choice for necrotic wounds. Pressure settings should be set per provider order, usually between 4 and 15 psi, and should not be used on skin grafts or exposed blood vessels, muscle, tendon, or bone. Use with caution if patient has coagulation disorder or is taking anticoagulants (Ramundo, 2016).*	
d. While keeping catheter in place, pinch it off just below syringe.	Avoids contamination of sterile solution.
e. Remove and refill syringe. Reconnect to catheter and repeat until solution draining into basin is clear.	Clear solution indicates removal of all debris.
9. Clean wound with handheld shower:	
a. With patient seated comfortably in shower chair or standing if condition allows, adjust spray to gentle flow; make sure that water is warm.	Useful for patients able to shower with help or independently. May be accomplished at home.
b. Shower for 5 to 10 minutes with shower head 30 cm (12 inches) from wound.	Ensures that wound is cleaned thoroughly.
10. When indicated, obtain cultures (see Chapter 9) after cleaning with nonbacteriostatic saline.	WOCN (2016) recommends using quantitative bacterial cultures (tissue biopsy or swab cultures). Most common type of wound cultures are swab technique, aspirated wound fluid, or tissue biopsy.
Safe Patient Care *Obtain a wound culture if there is inflammation around the wound, purulent odor or drainage, new drainage, or patient is febrile.*	
11. Dry wound edges with gauze; dry patient after shower.	Prevents maceration of surrounding tissue from excess moisture.
12. Remove and dispose of gloves. Perform hand hygiene. Apply clean or sterile gloves (see agency policy). Apply appropriate dressing and label with time, date, and nurse's initials.	Reduces transmission of microorganisms. Maintains protective barrier and healing environment for wound.
13. Remove mask, goggles, and gown.	Prevents transfer of microorganisms.
14. Dispose of equipment and soiled supplies; remove and dispose of gloves. Perform hand hygiene.	Reduces transmission of microorganisms.
15. Help patient to comfortable position.	
16. Raise side rails (as appropriate) and lower bed to lowest position.	Provides for patient safety and reduces the risk for falls.
17. Be sure nurse call system is in an accessible location within patient's reach; instruct patient in use.	Assists patient or family member in calling for assistance.

STEP	RATIONALE
EVALUATION	
1. Have patient rate level of comfort on scale of 0 to 10.	Patient's pain should not increase as result of wound irrigation.
2. Monitor type of tissue in wound bed.	Identifies wound-healing progress and determines type of wound cleaning and dressing needed.
3. Inspect dressing periodically (see agency policy).	Determines patient's response to wound irrigation and need to modify plan of care.
4. Evaluate periwound skin integrity.	Determines if extension of wound has occurred or signs of infection are present (warm red periwound skin).
5. Observe for presence of retained irrigant.	Retained irrigant is medium for bacterial growth and subsequent infection.
6. **Use Teach-Back:** "I want to be sure that I explained how to irrigate your wound. You are going to be doing this at home; please show me how you will irrigate the wound with this syringe." Revise your instruction now or develop a plan for revised patient/family caregiver teaching if patient/family caregiver is not able to teach back correctly.	Determines patient's/family caregiver's level of understanding of instructional topic.

Unexpected Outcomes	Related Interventions
1. Bleeding or serosanguinous drainage appears.	• Flush wound during next irrigation using less pressure. • Notify health care provider of bleeding.
2. Increased pain or discomfort occurs.	• Decrease force of pressure during wound irrigation. • Assess patient for need for additional analgesia before wound care.
3. Suture line opening extends.	• Notify health care provider. • Reevaluate amount of pressure to use for next wound irrigation.

Recording

- Record wound assessment before and after irrigation, amount and type of solution used, irrigation device used, patient tolerance of the procedure, and type of dressing applied after irrigation.
- Document your evaluation of patient learning.

Hand-Off Reporting

- Report the location of the wound irrigated; discuss the type of solution used and the quality of the return irrigation and the last time the wound was irrigated.
- Immediately report to attending health care provider any evidence of fresh bleeding, sharp increase in pain, retention of irrigant, or signs of shock.

✦ SKILL 25.2 Managing Wound Drainage Evacuation

Purpose

A wound drainage device is used to collect, measure, and document wound drainage and the wound-healing process. Wound drainage is facilitated when a surgeon inserts a drain directly through the suture line into the wound or through a small stab wound near the surgical site. Jackson-Pratt and Hemovac drains are portable drainage self-contained suction devices that are connected to a drainage tube within the wound and provide constant low-pressure suction to remove and collect drainage. A Jackson-Pratt drain (Fig. 25.4) is used for small amounts of drainage (100 to 200 mL per 24 hours). A Hemovac or ConstaVac drainage system is used for larger amounts of drainage (500 mL per 24 hours).

Delegation and Collaboration

The assessment of wound drainage and maintenance of drains and the drainage system cannot be delegated to nursing assistive personnel (NAP). However, you may delegate emptying a closed drainage container or pouch, measuring the amount of drainage, and reporting the amount on the patient's intake and output (I&O) record to NAP. The nurse directs the NAP by:

- Discussing any increase in frequency of emptying the drain other than once a shift.
- Instructing to report to the nurse any change in amount, color, or odor of drainage.
- Reviewing the I&O procedure.

Equipment

- Graduated measuring cylinder
- Alcohol wipes
- Split gauze sponges (for drain site)
- Dressing materials (for surgical incision)
- Nonallergenic tape
- Clean gloves

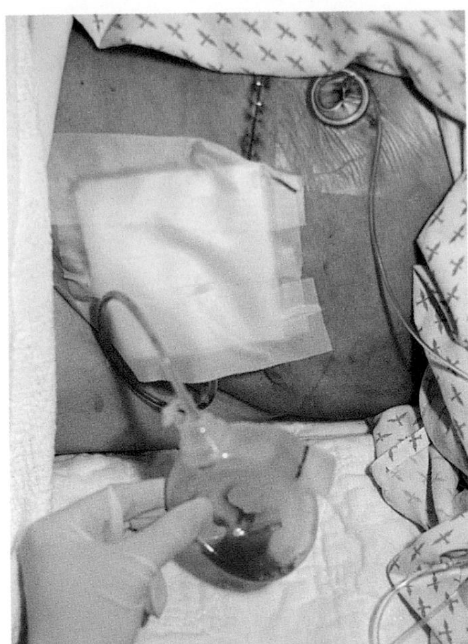

FIG 25.4 Jackson-Pratt drainage tube and reservoir.

- Safety pin(s)
- Protective equipment: goggles, mask, and gown if risk of spray from drain is present
- Disposable drape or barrier
- *Option:* Normal saline for cleansing tube insertion site

ASSESSMENT

1. Identify patient using at least two identifiers (e.g., name and birthday or name and medical record number) according to agency policy. *Rationale: Ensures correct patient. Complies with The Joint Commission standards and improves patient safety (TJC, 2019).*
2. Review medical record to identify presence, location, and purpose of closed wound drain and drainage system as patient returns from surgery. *Rationale: Drainage tubing is usually placed near wound through small surgical incision.*
3. Perform hand hygiene. Apply clean gloves if there is a risk of contacting drainage. Assess for drainage on patient's dressing. Identify number of wound drain tubes and what each one will be draining. Check if each drain tube is labeled with a number or source. Label if necessary. *Rationale: Assigning labeling system to each drain helps with consistent documentation when patient has multiple drainage tubes.*
4. Inspect system to determine presence of one straight tube or Y-tube arrangement with two tube insertion sites. *Rationale: Allows nurse to plan skin care and identifies quantity of sterile dressing supplies needed.*
5. Inspect system to ensure proper functioning. Complete systematic inspection includes insertion site, drainage moving through tubing in direction of reservoir, patency of drainage tubing, airtight connection sites, and presence of any leaks or kinks in system. Remove and dispose of gloves. Perform hand hygiene. *Rationale: Properly functioning system maintains suction until reservoir is filled or drainage is no longer being produced or accumulated. Tension on drainage tubing increases injury to skin and underlying muscle.*
6. Determine if drain tube needs self-suction, wall suction, or no suction by checking health care provider's orders. *Rationale: Some drain tubes such as Hemovac can be used with self-suction or wall suction.*
7. Identify type of drainage containers available. *Rationale: Determines frequency for emptying drainage.*
8. Assess patient's or family caregiver's knowledge, experience, and health literacy level. *Rationale: Ensures patient has the capacity to obtain, communicate, process, and understand basic health information (CDC, 2016).*
9. Assess patient's level of understanding of purpose of drainage system and precautions to take to avoid accidental removal. *Rationale: Determines extent of instruction required.*

STEP	RATIONALE

PLANNING

Step	Rationale
1. Expected outcomes following completion of procedure:	
• Wound healing continues.	Patient is comfortable, and wound drainage is collected.
• Vacuum is reestablished.	Suction system is intact.
• Tubing is patent.	Fluid is draining away from wound area.
• Patient describes precautions to avoid inadvertent drain removal.	Demonstrates learning.
2. Close room door or bedside curtains.	Ensures privacy.
3. Explain procedure to patient.	Promotes patient's cooperation and reduces anxiety.

IMPLEMENTATION

Step	Rationale
1. Perform hand hygiene and apply clean gloves.	Reduces transmission of microorganisms.
2. Place open specimen container or graduated measuring cylinder on bed between you and patient.	Permits measuring and discarding of wound drainage.
3. Empty Hemovac or ConstaVac:	When a drainage device is more than half full, it should be emptied, and the volume of the exudate measured.
a. Maintain asepsis while opening plug on port indicated for emptying drainage reservoir.	Vacuum will be broken, and reservoir will pull air in until chamber is fully expanded.

STEP	RATIONALE
(1) Tilt suction container in direction of plug.	Drains fluid toward plug.
(2) Slowly squeeze two flat surfaces together, tilting toward measuring container.	Prevents splashing of contaminated drainage. Squeezing empties reservoir of drainage.
b. Drain all contents into measuring container (see illustration).	Contents counted as fluid output. When wound drainage accumulates in a wound bed, it interferes with wound healing.
c. Hold uncovered antiseptic swab in dominant hand. Place suction device on flat surface with open outlet facing upward; continue pressing downward until bottom and top are in contact (see illustration).	Cleaning plug reduces transmission of microorganisms into drainage evacuation.
d. Holding surfaces together with one hand and using antiseptic swab, quickly clean opening, plug with other hand, and immediately replace plug; secure suction device on patient's bed.	Compression of surface of Hemovac creates vacuum.
e. Check device for reestablishment of vacuum, patency of drainage tubing, and absence of stress on tubing.	Facilitates wound drainage and prevents tension on drainage tubing.
4. Empty Hemovac with wall suction:	Empties drainage and reestablishes suction to wound bed.
a. Turn off suction.	
b. Disconnect suction tubing from Hemovac port.	Allows port to be opened.
c. Empty Hemovac as described in Steps 3a and 3b.	
d. Use an antiseptic swab to clean port opening and the end of the suction tubing. Reconnect tubing to port.	Cleaning plug reduces transmission of microorganisms.
e. Set suction level as prescribed or on low if health care provider does not specify suction level.	Reestablishes wound suction.
5. Empty Jackson-Pratt suction drain:	
a. Open port on top of bulb-shaped reservoir (see illustration).	Breaks vacuum for drain.
b. Tilt bulb in direction of port and drain toward opening. Empty drainage from device into measuring container (see illustration). Clean end of emptying port and plug with antiseptic wipe.	Reduces transmission of microorganisms.
c. Compress bulb over drainage container. While compressing bulb, replace plug immediately.	Reestablishes vacuum.
6. Place and secure drainage system below site with safety pin on patient's gown. Be sure that there is slack in tubing from reservoir to wound.	Pinning drainage tubing to patient's gown prevents tension or pulling on tubing and insertion site.

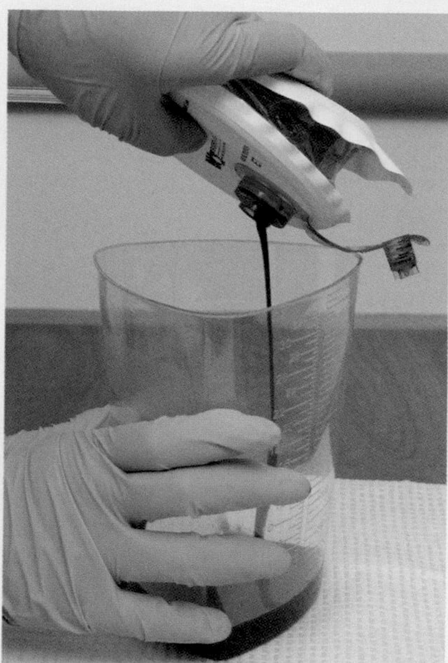

STEP 3b Hemovac contents drained into measuring container.

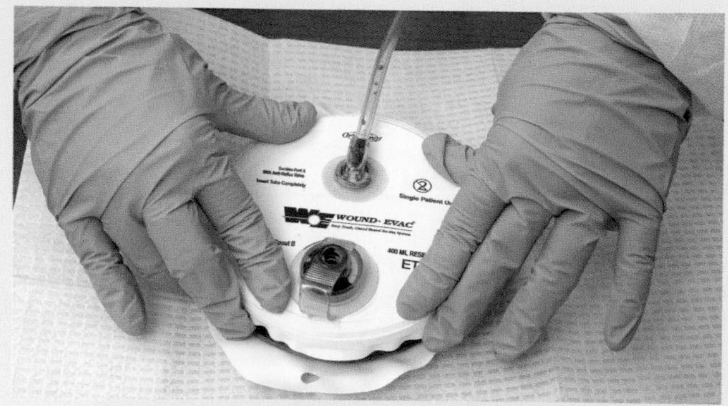

STEP 3c Hemovac compressed to create suction.

STEP	RATIONALE
7. Note characteristics of drainage in measuring container; measure volume and discard by flushing in commode.	Contents count as fluid output.
8. Discard soiled supplies and remove and dispose of gloves. Perform hand hygiene.	Reduces transmission of microorganisms.
9. Apply clean gloves. Proceed with dressing change (see Chapter 27) around drain site and inspection of skin if indicated or ordered. Split gauze sponge dressings are often used around drain tubes (see illustration) and taped in place.	Prevents entrance of bacteria into surgical wound.
10. Discard contaminated materials and remove gloves. Perform hand hygiene.	Reduces transmission of microorganisms.
11. Assist patient to comfortable position.	Promotes patient comfort.
12. Raise side rails (as appropriate) and lower bed to lowest position.	Provides for patient safety and reduces the risk for falls.
13. Be sure nurse call system is in an accessible location within patient's reach; instruct patient in its use.	Provides patient or family member a resource to call for assistance.

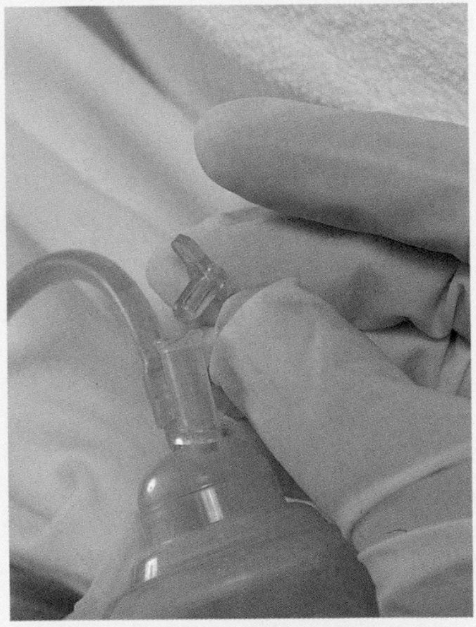

STEP 5a Opening port of Jackson-Pratt device.

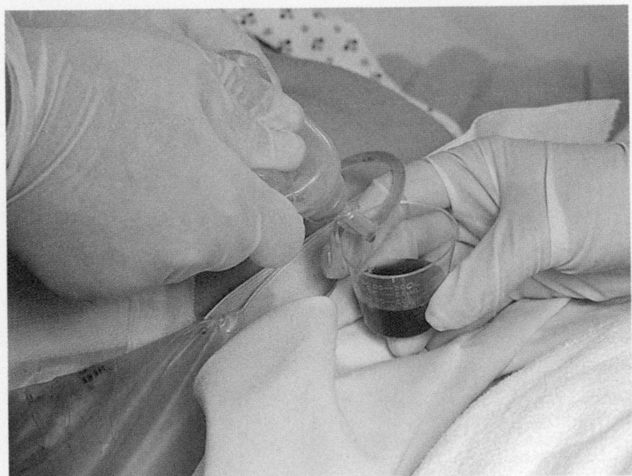

STEP 5b Emptying contents from Jackson-Pratt drainage device.

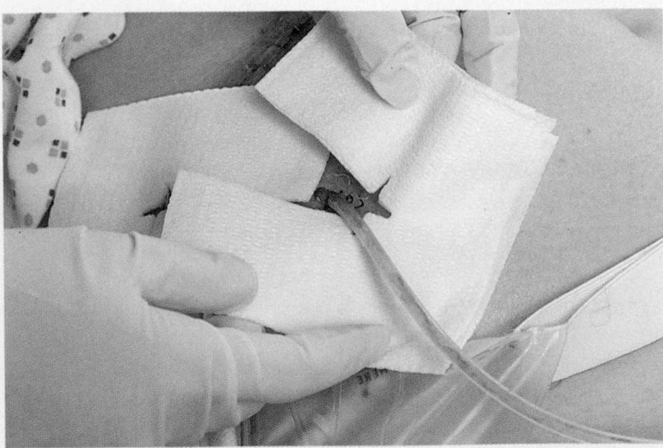

STEP 9 Applying split gauze sponge dressing around Jackson-Pratt drain tube.

STEP	RATIONALE

EVALUATION

1. Observe for drainage in suction device.

Indicates presence of vacuum, patency of tubing, and functioning of drainage suction device.

Safe Patient Care *Inspect for clots or cellular debris. Clots or large collections of debris may block drainage flow. The Y-site in the drainage tubing is especially prone to clogging.*

2. Inspect wound for drainage or collection of drainage fluid under skin, causing seroma.

Drainage should not be significant under suture line. May indicate inadequate functioning of drainage suction device.

3. Measure drainage from drainage system, and record on I&O form every 8 to 12 hours and as needed for large drainage volume.

Determines status of wound healing. Collect diagnostic specimen in presence of unexpected purulence or pungent odor, report findings to health care provider, and record in progress note.

4. **Use Teach-Back:** "I want to be sure I explained clearly why it is important not to pull on your drain. Tell me what can happen if you pull the drain out accidentally." Revise your instruction now or develop a plan for revised patient/family caregiver teaching if patient/family caregiver is not able to teach back correctly.

Determines patient's/family caregiver's level of understanding of instructional topic.

Unexpected Outcomes	Related Interventions
1. Site where tube exits becomes infected.	• Notify health care provider about presence of signs of infection: purulent drainage, odor, reddened site, increased white blood cell count, and temperature elevation. • Use aseptic technique when changing dressings.
2. Bleeding appears in or around drainage collector.	• Determine amount of bleeding and notify health care provider if excessive. • Assess for tension on patient's drainage tubing. • Secure tubing to prevent pulling and pain.
3. Patient experiences pain.	• Assess patient's level of pain. • Medicate patient. • Stabilize drainage tubing to reduce tension and pulling against incision. • Notify health care provider if signs of wound infection are present.
4. Drainage suction device is not accumulating drainage.	• Assess drainage tubing for clots. • Assess drainage system for air leaks or kinks. • Notify health care provider.

Recording

- Record type of drainage device, results from emptying wound drainage system, and dressing change in progress notes and I&O record. Note characteristics of insertion site and drainage. Record patient's level of comfort.
- Document your evaluation of patient learning.

Hand-Off Reporting

- Report the number and location of drains; describe the color, consistency, and odor of the drainage if present; and report the output.
- Report to health care provider unexpected increase in drainage from a drain.

✦ SKILL 25.3 Removing Sutures and Staples

Purpose

Sutures are used to close a surgical incision both within tissue layers in deep wounds and for the outer skin layer. The choice of suture technique depends on the type and anatomical location of a wound, the thickness of the skin, the degree of tension, and the desired cosmetic effect (Whitney, 2016). Deep sutures are a material that is absorbed or an inert wire that remains indefinitely. Nonabsorbable sutures (sutures that require removal) are available in silk, cotton, Prolene, wire, nylon, and Dacron. Removable skin sutures are interrupted or continuous. Interrupted sutures are separate stitches, each with its own knot (Fig. 25.5A). A continuous suture is one long "thread" that spirals along the entire suture line at evenly spaced intervals. The surface appearance is very similar to a line of interrupted sutures except that each section crossing the incision line does not have a knot (see Fig. 25.5B). Another type of continuous stitch is a blanket continuous suture. This suture spirals along the incision, with each turn pulled over to one side. The suture is looped around the thread of the previous stitch before making the next turn in the spiral (see Fig. 25.5C). When appearance and

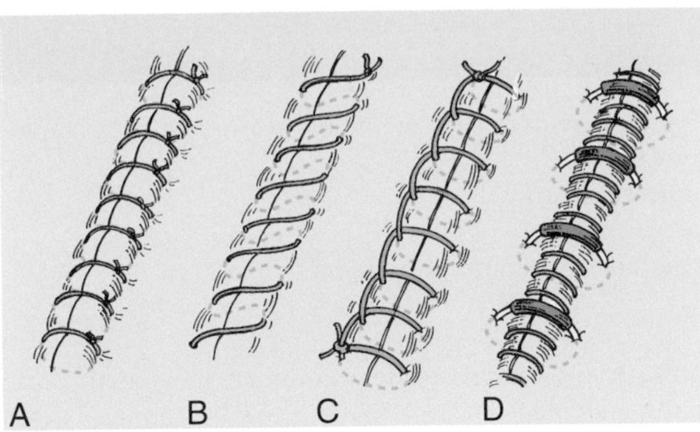

FIG 25.5 Sutures. (A) Interrupted. (B) Continuous. (C) Blanket continuous. (D) Retention.

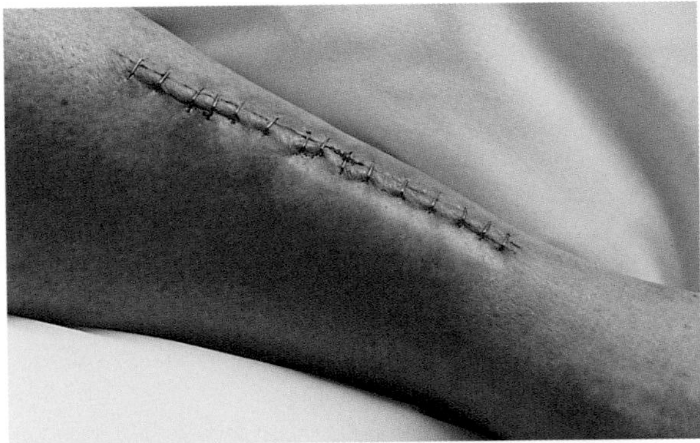

FIG 25.6 Suture line secured with staples.

minimal scarring are important, very fine Dacron or subcutaneous sutures beneath the skin are used. An obese patient with abdominal surgery may have retention sutures covered with rubber tubing to provide greater strength (see Fig. 25.5D).

Staples are made of stainless steel, are quick to use, and provide ample strength. They are used for skin closure of abdominal incisions and orthopedic surgery when appearance of the incision is not critical (Fig. 25.6). The time of removal is based on the stage of incisional healing and extent of surgery.

Delegation and Collaboration

The skill of staple and/or suture removal cannot be delegated to nursing assistive personnel (NAP). The nurse directs the NAP to:

- Report to the nurse drainage, bleeding, or swelling at the incision site or an elevation in patient's temperature.
- Report to the nurse patient's complaints of pain.
- Provide special hygiene practices following suture removal.

Equipment

- Disposable waterproof biohazard bag
- Sterile suture removal set (forceps and scissors) or sterile staple extractor
- Sterile antiseptic swabs
- Gauze pads
- Steri-Strips or butterfly adhesive strips
- Clean gloves (*optional:* sterile gloves)

ASSESSMENT

1. Identify patient using at least two identifiers (e.g., name and birthday or name and medical record number) according to agency policy. *Rationale: Ensures correct patient. Complies with The Joint Commission standards and improves patient safety (TJC, 2019).*
2. Review patient's medical record for the following information:
   a. Check health care provider's order. *Rationale: Health care provider's order is required for removal of sutures. Agency policy determines which health care providers may remove sutures and staples.*
   b. Review specific directions related to suture or staple removal. *Rationale: Indicates specifically which sutures are to be removed (e.g., every other suture).*

Safe Patient Care *Sutures and staples generally are removed within 7 to 10 days after surgery if healing is adequate. Retention sutures are left in place longer (14 days or more). Sutures and staples must remain in place long enough to ensure initial wound closure. If any sign of suture line separation is evident during the removal process, the remaining sutures are left in place, and a description is documented and reported to the health care provider.*

   c. Determine history of conditions that may pose risk for impaired wound healing: advanced age, cardiovascular disease, diabetes, immunosuppression, radiation, obesity, smoking, poor nutrition, and infection. *Rationale: Preexisting health disorders affect speed of healing and sometimes result in dehiscence.*
3. Assess patient for history of allergies. *Rationale: Determines if patient is sensitive to antiseptic or latex.*
4. Assess patient's comfort level on pain scale of 0 to 10. *Rationale: Provides baseline of patient's comfort level to determine response to therapy.*
5. Assess patient's or family caregiver's knowledge, experience, and health literacy level. *Rationale: Ensures patient has the capacity to obtain, communicate, process, and understand basic health information (CDC, 2016).*
6. Assess patient's or family caregiver's knowledge of wound care and observations to make. *Rationale: Determines extent of instruction required.*

Safe Patient Care *If wound edges are separated or signs of infection are present, the wound has not healed properly. Notify the health care provider because sutures or staples may need to remain in place and/or other wound care initiated.*

STEP	RATIONALE
PLANNING	
1. Expected outcomes following completion of procedure:	
• All suture material or staples are removed.	Removes source of infection or irritation from retained sutures.
• Suture line is intact.	Wound is healing and does not require protective dressings.

STEP	RATIONALE
• Patient states acceptable level of comfort on scale of 0 to 10 following removal of sutures or staples.	Some patients require pain medicine before suture or staple removal.
• Patient or family caregiver is able to describe wound care following staple/suture removal.	Demonstrates learning.
2. Explain to patient how you will remove staples or sutures and that removal is usually not painful, but patient may feel pulling or tugging of skin.	Gains patient cooperation and reduces anxiety.
3. Administer prescribed analgesic if needed at least 30 minutes before procedure.	Promotes patient comfort to help minimize movement during suture removal.

Safe Patient Care *For patient who is highly anxious or who has an extensive wound, consider need to administer analgesic 30 minutes before suture removal.*

4. Position patient comfortably while exposing suture line. Ensure that direct lighting is on staple/suture line.	Aids visibility and correct placement of forceps or extractor during removal process, ultimately reducing soft tissue injury.
5. Close curtains or room door.	Provides privacy.

IMPLEMENTATION

1. Perform hand hygiene.	Reduces transmission of microorganisms.
2. Form a cuff on waterproof biohazard bag and place near bed within easy reach.	Provides for easy disposal of contaminated dressings and prevents passing items over sterile work area.
3. Prepare materials needed for staple/suture removal: a. Open sterile staple/suture removal kit. b. Open sterile antiseptic swabs and place on inside surface of kit. c. Obtain gloves (sterile gloves if policy indicates).	Ensures an organized procedure.
4. Apply clean gloves. Carefully remove dressing or inspect uncovered wound. Discard dressing in prepared refuse bag. Inspect incision for healing ridge and skin integrity of suture line for uniform closure of wound edges, normal color, and absence of drainage and inflammation (see illustration). Palpate around suture line gently, look for expression of drainage, and note any tenderness. Remove and dispose of gloves following assessment.	Reduces transmission of infection. Indicates adequate wound healing for support of internal structures without continued need for sutures or staples (Whitney, 2016).

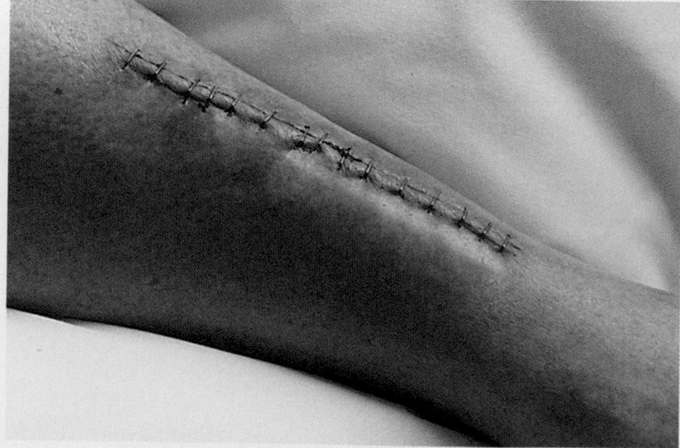

STEP 4 Suture line secured with staples.

5. Perform hand hygiene. Apply clean or sterile gloves as required by agency policy.	Reduces transmission of infection.
6. Clean sutures or staples and healed incision with antiseptic swabs. Start at sides next to incision and then wipe across suture line using new antiseptic swab for each swipe.	Removes surface bacteria from incision and sutures or staples.

STEP	RATIONALE
7. Remove staples:	
a. Place lower tip of staple extractor under first staple. As you close handles, upper tip of extractor depresses center of staple, causing both ends of staple to be bent upward and simultaneously exit their insertion sites in dermal layer (see illustration).	Avoids excess pressure to suture line and secures smooth removal of each staple.
b. Carefully control staple extractor.	Avoids pressure on suture line and patient discomfort.
c. As soon as both ends of staple are visible, move it away from skin surface (see illustration) and continue until staple is over refuse bag.	Prevents scratching tender skin surface with sharp, pointed ends of staple for comfort and infection control.
d. Release handles of staple extractor, allowing staple to drop into refuse bag.	Avoids contaminating sterile field with used staples.
e. Repeat Steps 7a to 7d until all staples are removed.	
8. Remove interrupted sutures:	
a. Place gauze few inches from suture line. Hold scissors in dominant hand and forceps (clamp) in nondominant hand.	Gauze serves as receptacle for removed sutures. Placement of scissors and forceps allows for efficient suture removal.

Safe Patient Care *Placement of scissors and forceps is very important. Avoid pinching the skin around the wound when lifting the suture. Likewise, avoid cutting the skin around the wound by accident when snipping the suture.*

STEP	RATIONALE
b. Grasp knot of suture with forceps and gently pull up knot while slipping tip of scissors under suture near skin (see illustration).	Releases suture.
c. Snip suture as close to skin as possible at end distal to knot.	

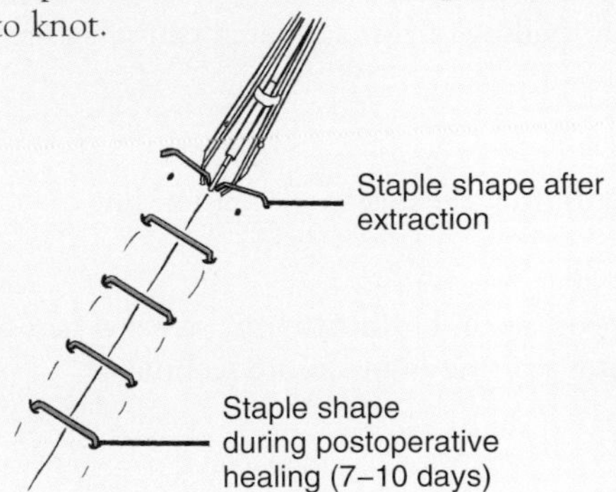

STEP 7a Staple extractor placed under staple.

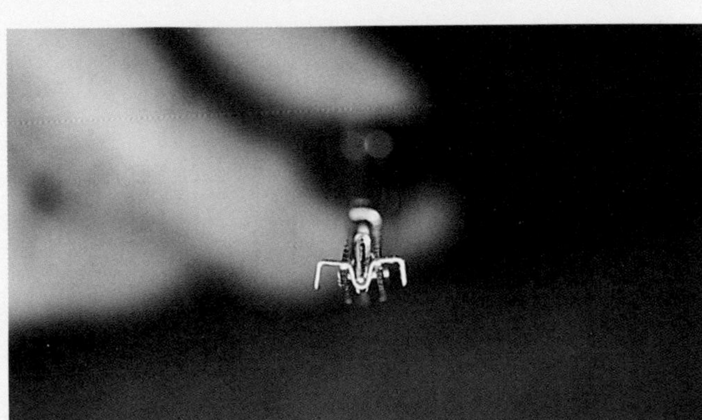

STEP 7c Metal staple removed by extractor.

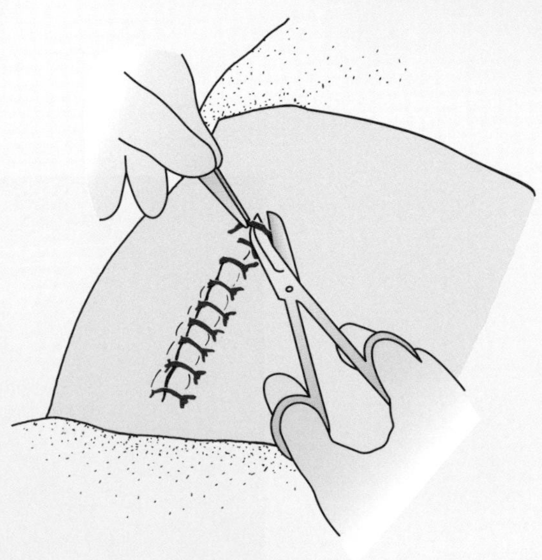

STEP 8b Removal of intermittent suture. Nurse cuts suture as close to skin as possible, away from knot.

STEP	RATIONALE

Safe Patient Care *Never snip both ends of suture; there will be no way to remove the part of the suture situated below the surface.*

STEP	RATIONALE
d. Grasp knotted end with forceps, and in one continuous smooth action, pull suture through from the other side (see illustration). Place removed suture on gauze.	Smoothly removes suture without additional tension to suture line.

Safe Patient Care *Never pull exposed surface of any suture into tissue below epidermis. The exposed surface of any suture is considered contaminated.*

STEP	RATIONALE
e. Repeat Steps 8a to 8d until you have removed every other suture.	
f. Observe incisional integrity. Based on observations of wound response to suture removal and health care provider's original order, determine whether remaining sutures will be removed at this time. If so, repeat Steps 8a to 8d until you have removed all sutures.	Determines status of wound healing and if suture line will remain closed after all sutures are removed.
g. If any doubt, stop and notify health care provider.	
9. Remove continuous and blanket stitch sutures:	
a. Place sterile gauze a few inches from suture line. Grasp scissors in dominant hand and forceps in nondominant hand.	Gauze serves as receptacle for removed sutures. Placement of scissors and forceps allows for efficient suture removal.
b. Snip first suture close to skin surface at end distal to knot.	Releases suture.
c. Snip second suture on same side.	Releases interrupted sutures from knot.
d. Grasp knotted end and gently pull with continuous smooth action, removing suture from beneath skin. Place suture on gauze compress.	Smoothly removes sutures without additional tension to suture line. Prevents pulling of contaminated part of suture through skin.
e. Repeat Steps 9a to 9d in consecutive order until entire suture line is removed.	
10. Inspect incision to make sure that all sutures are removed and identify any trouble areas. Gently wipe suture line with antiseptic swab to remove debris and clean incision.	Reduces risk for further separation of incision line.
11. Apply Steri-Strips if *any* separation greater than two stitches or two staples in width is apparent to maintain contact between wound edges.	Steri-Strips support wound by distributing tension across wound and eliminates scarring from closure technique.
a. Cut Steri-Strips to allow strips to extend 4 to 5 cm (1½ to 2 inches) on each side of incision.	
b. Remove from backing and apply across incision (see illustration).	

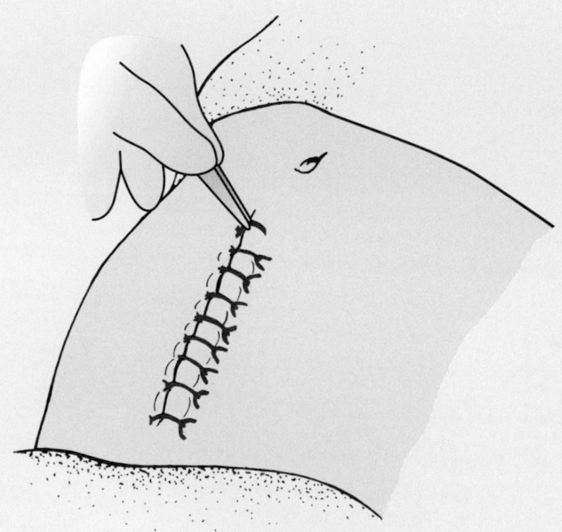

STEP 8d Nurse removes suture and never pulls contaminated stitch through tissues.

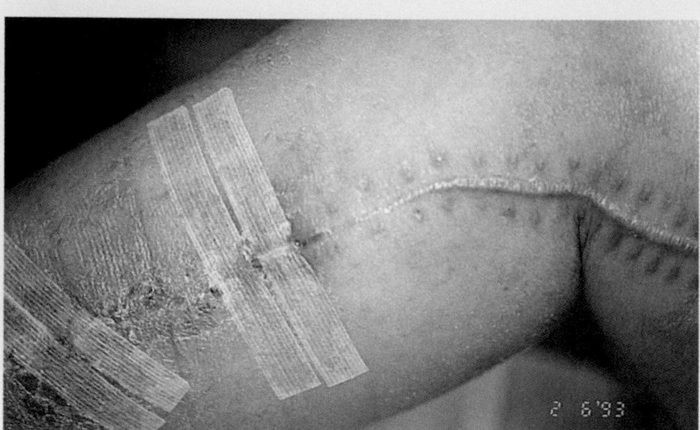

STEP 11b Steri-Strips over incision.

STEP	RATIONALE
c. Instruct patient to take a shower rather than soak in bathtub according to health care provider's preference.	Steri-Strips are not removed; strips loosen over time (5 to 7 days), and they are allowed to fall off gradually.
12. Remove and discard gloves. Perform hand hygiene and apply new pair of gloves. Reapply new dressing only if ordered. Instruct patient about applying own dressing if needed at home.	Healing by primary intention eliminates need for dressing.
13. Discard all contaminated materials and remove and dispose of gloves.	Reduces transmission of infection.
14. Dispose of sharps (disposable staple extractor and/or scissors) in designated sharps disposal bin and perform hand hygiene.	Reduces transmission of infection. Provides a safe environment because instruments are sharp and contaminated.
15. Help patient to comfortable position.	Promotes patient comfort.
16. Raise side rails (as appropriate) and lower bed to lowest position.	Provides for patient safety and reduces the risk for falls.
17. Be sure nurse call system is in an accessible location within patient's reach; instruct patient in use.	Provides patient or family member a resource to call for assistance.

EVALUATION

1. Assess sites where staples/sutures were removed; inspect condition of incision and surrounding skin. Look for any pieces of removed suture left behind.	Ensures that sources of infection have been removed and incision line is intact.
2. Determine if patient has pain along incision.	Determines comfort level and can indicate if suture material remains in skin.
3. **Use Teach-Back:** "I want to be sure that I have adequately explained the signs of a wound or incision infection before you are discharged. Tell me the signs of infection and what you need to tell your health care provider if this happens." Revise your instruction now or develop a plan for revised patient/family caregiver teaching if patient/family caregiver is not able to teach back correctly.	Determines patient's/family caregiver's level of understanding of instructional topic.

Unexpected Outcomes	Related Interventions
1. Retained suture is present.	• Notify health care provider. • Instruct patient to notify health care provider if signs of suture line infection develop following discharge from agency.
2. Patient experiences wound separation or drainage secondary to healing problems.	• Leave remaining sutures or staples in place. • Place Steri-Strip closures across suture line. • Notify health care provider.

Recording

- Record condition of wound, number of sutures removed, and patient's response in progress note.
- Document your evaluation of patient learning.

Hand-Off Reporting

- Report the location and appearance of the wound/incision where the sutures/staples were removed. Provide information on patient's response when sutures/staples were removed.
- Notify health care provider immediately of any of the following findings: suture line separation, evisceration, bleeding, or new purulent drainage.

✦ SKILL 25.4 Negative-Pressure Wound Therapy

Purpose

Negative-pressure wound therapy (NPWT) is the application of subatmospheric (negative) pressure to a wound through suction and is used to facilitate healing of more complicated wounds and to collect wound exudate (Netsch et al., 2016). NPWT assists and accelerates wound healing by generating negative pressure at the wound surface, which removes wound exudate, stimulates granulation tissue, reduces the bacterial burden in the wound, contracts the wound bed, and provides a moist wound environment. NPWT is available in several different forms and includes a wound filler dressing, suction catheter, transparent adhesive dressing, suction source, and collection container (Fig. 25.7). Wounds managed by NPWT include large acute (surgical) and traumatic

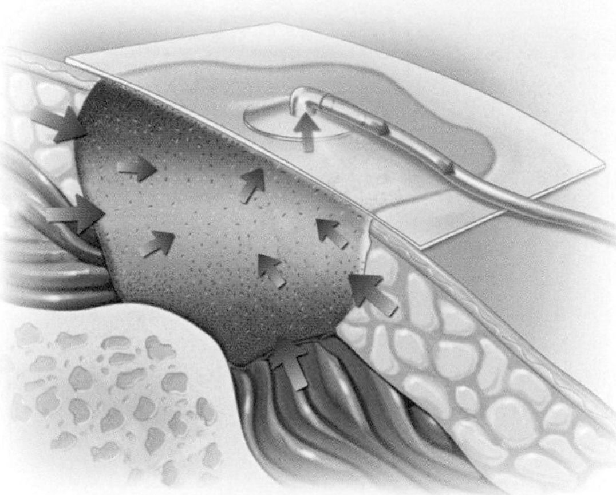

FIG 25.7 Wound NPWT in place. This is a wound vacuum-assisted closure (VAC) system using negative pressure to remove fluid from the area surrounding the wound, reducing edema and improving circulation to the area. *(Courtesy KCI, San Antonio, TX.)*

wounds, surgical dehiscence, pressure ulcers, surgical flaps, and compromised flaps.

Delegation and Collaboration

The skill of NPWT cannot be delegated to nursing assistive personnel (NAP). The nurse directs the NAP to:

- Use caution in positioning or turning patient to avoid tubing displacement.
- Report any change in dressing shape or integrity to the nurse.
- Report any change in patient's temperature or comfort level to the nurse.
- Report any wound fluid leakage around the edges of the adhesive drape.

Equipment

- NPWT unit
- NPWT dressing (gauze or foam, depending on manufacturer's recommendations; transparent dressing, adhesive drape)
- NPWT suction device
- Tubing for connection between NPWT unit and NPWT dressing
- 3 pairs gloves, clean and sterile
- Sterile scissors
- Skin preparation/skin barrier protectant/hydrocolloid dressing/skin barrier
- Protective equipment: gown, mask, and goggles if splashing is a risk
- Waterproof, disposable trash biohazard bag

ASSESSMENT

1. Identify patient using at least two identifiers (e.g., name and birthday or name and medical record number) according to agency policy. *Rationale: Ensures correct patient. Complies with The Joint Commission standards and improves patient safety (TJC, 2019).*
2. Review health care provider's orders for NPWT and frequency of dressing change, amount of negative pressure, type of foam or gauze to use, and pressure cycle (intermittent or continuous). *Rationale: Determines frequency of dressing change, negative-pressure setting, and special instructions. Health care provider's order is also necessary for reimbursement.*
3. Review medical record for most current signs and symptoms related to condition of patient's wound. *Rationale: Provides baseline to compare your findings with previous dressing change assessments and reflects wound-healing progress.*
4. Assess patient's level of comfort on pain scale of 0 to 10. *Rationale: Serves as baseline to measure response to dressing therapy.*
5. Perform hand hygiene. Apply clean gloves. Assess location, appearance, and size of wound (see Procedural Guideline 25.1). Remove and dispose of gloves. Perform hand hygiene. *Rationale: Provides information regarding status of wound healing, presence of complications, and proper type of supplies and help needed.*
6. Assess patient's or family caregiver's knowledge, experience, and health literacy level. *Rationale: Ensures patient has the capacity to obtain, communicate, process, and understand basic health information (CDC, 2016).*
7. Assess patient's and family caregiver's knowledge of purpose of dressing and whether they will participate in dressing wound. *Rationale: Identifies patient's learning needs. Prepares patient and family caregivers if dressing will need to be changed at home.*

STEP	RATIONALE
PLANNING	
1. Expected outcomes following completion of procedure:	
• Patient's wound shows evidence of healing as wound decreases in size with less drainage, redness, or swelling.	Dressing is effective in promoting healing and preventing infection.
• Patient reports acceptable level of comfort on scale of 0 to 10 during and after dressing changes.	Analgesic and comfort measures effective in controlling pain.
• Dressing remains intact with airtight seal and prescribed negative pressure.	Dressing is applied correctly and maintains negative pressure.
• Patient or family caregiver demonstrates correct method of dressing changes.	Indicates that patient and family caregiver learning has occurred.
2. Close room door or cubicle curtains.	Provides for patient privacy and reduces transmission of organisms.
3. Administer prescribed analgesic as needed 30 minutes before dressing change.	Removal of NWPT before new application can be painful. Comfortable patient will be less likely to move suddenly, causing wound or supply contamination.
4. Position patient comfortably and drape to expose only wound site.	Promotes patient's cooperation and completion of procedure smoothly.

STEP	RATIONALE
5. Explain procedure to patient and family caregiver, instructing not to touch wound or sterile supplies.	Relieves anxiety and promotes understanding of healing process. Prevents contamination of sterile supplies.

IMPLEMENTATION

STEP	RATIONALE
1. Form a cuff on top of disposable waterproof biohazard bag and place within reach of work area.	Cuff prevents accidental contamination of top of outer bag.
2. Perform hand hygiene and apply clean gloves. If risk for spray exists, apply protective gown, goggles, and mask.	Reduces transmission of infectious organisms from soiled dressings to nurse's hands.
3. Follow manufacturer directions for removal and replacement because each NPWT unit varies slightly with approach. Turn off NPWT unit by pushing therapy on/off button.	Deactivates therapy and allows for proper drainage of fluid in drainage tubing.
a. Keeping tube connectors attached to NPWT unit, raise tubing connectors; disconnect tubes from one another and drain fluids into drainage collector.	Prevents backflow of any drainage in tubing back into wound.
b. Before draining, tighten clamp on canister tube and disconnect canister and dressing tubing at connection points.	Prevents drainage from exiting tubing when removed.
4. Remove transparent film by gently stretching and slowly pull away from skin.	Prevents injury to wound tissue. Protects periwound skin breakdown from transparent adhesive.
5. Remove old dressing one layer at a time and discard in bag. Observe drainage on dressing. Use caution to avoid tension on any drains that are present. Remove gloves and dispose.	Determines type and amount of dressings needed for replacement. Prevents accidental removal of drains.
6. Perform hand hygiene and conduct a wound assessment (see Procedural Guideline 25.1). Apply clean gloves if there is a risk of contacting drainage. Observe surface area and tissue type, color, odor, and drainage within wound. Measure length, width, and depth of wound as ordered.	Measurement of wound is necessary to assess wound healing progression and justify continuation of NPWT for third-party payers (Netsch et al., 2016). Determines condition of wound and need for replacement of dressing.

Safe Patient Care *This is a time when a wound care nurse or physician might debride the wound. Debridement of eschar or slough, if present, should be performed for removal of devitalized tissue to prepare the wound bed (Netsch et al., 2016).*

STEP	RATIONALE
7. Remove and discard gloves in waterproof bag (if worn) and perform hand hygiene. Avoid having patient see old dressing because sight of wound drainage may be upsetting.	Lessens patient anxiety during procedure.
8. Clean wound.	Irrigation removes wound debris and cleans wound bed.
a. Apply sterile or clean gloves, depending on agency policy and wound status.	Cleaning periwound is essential for airtight seal.
b. If ordered, irrigate wound with normal saline or other solution ordered by health care provider (see Skill 25.1). Gently blot periwound with gauze to dry thoroughly.	Cleanses wound of debris and exudate.

Safe Patient Care *Health care providers may order wound cultures routinely. However, when drainage looks purulent or has a foul odor or if there is a change in amount or color, obtain wound culture. This may be an indication that NPWT may need to be discontinued (Martindell, 2012).*

STEP	RATIONALE
9. Apply skin protectant, barrier film, solid skin barrier sheet, or hydrocolloid dressing to periwound skin.	Maintains airtight seal needed for NPWT wound therapy (Netsch et al., 2016). Protects periwound skin from moisture-associated skin damage (Martindell, 2012).
10. Fill any uneven skin surfaces (e.g., creases, scars, and skinfolds) with skin-barrier product (e.g., paste, strip).	Further helps to maintain airtight seal (Netsch et al., 2016).
11. Remove and discard gloves. Perform hand hygiene.	Prevents transmission of microorganisms.
12. Depending on type of wound, apply sterile or new clean gloves (see agency policy).	Fresh sterile wounds require sterile gloves. Chronic wounds require clean technique (WOCN, 2016).
13. Apply NPWT.	
a. Prepare NPWT filler dressing. Consult with wound care expert for appropriate type.	Filler dressing depends on NPWT used and can include foam or gauze dressings with or without antimicrobials such as silver. Type of dressing may be adjusted based on undermining, tunneling, or sinus tracts present (Netsch et al., 2016).

STEP	RATIONALE
(1) Measure wound and select appropriate-size dressing.	Black polyurethane (PU) foam has larger pores and is most effective in stimulating granulation tissue and wound contraction; soft foam is denser, with smaller pores, and is used when growth of granulation tissue needs to be restricted (Martindell, 2012; Netsch et al., 2016).
(2) Using sterile scissors, cut filler gauze dressing or foam to wound size, making sure to fit exact size and shape of wound, including tunnels and undermined areas.	Proper size of dressing maintains negative pressure to entire wound (Netsch et al., 2016).

Safe Patient Care *In some instances, an antimicrobial product such as silver-impregnated gauze or topical antibiotic is ordered. These products help reduce the bioburden of the wound.*

STEP	RATIONALE
b. Place filler dressing in wound following manufacturer instructions. Be sure that filler dressing is in contact with entire wound base, margins, and tunneled and undermined areas. Count number of filler dressings and document in patient's chart.	Creates seal that will maintain negative pressure to entire wound. Edges of dressing must be in direct contact with patient's skin. Dressing count provides the number of filler dressings that should be removed at the next dressing change.
c. Place suction device per manufacturer instructions.	
d. Apply NPWT transparent dressing over foam or gauze filler dressing.	
(1) Trim dressing to cover wound and dressing so that it will extend onto periwound skin approximately 2.5 to 5 cm (1 to 2 inches).	Prepares dressing for appropriate size of the wound.
(2) Apply transparent dressing, keeping it airtight and wrinkle-free (see illustration).	Airtight and wrinkle-free dressing maintains a negative-pressure environment. A snug and tight application of the dressing must be applied to ensure an airtight seal (Box 25.3).
(3) Secure tubing to transparent film, aligning drainage holes to ensure occlusive seal. Do not apply tension.	Excessive tension may compress foam dressing and impede wound healing. It also produces shear force on periwound area (Kinetic Concepts International, 2013).

BOX 25.3

Maintaining an Airtight Seal With Negative-Pressure Wound Therapy

To avoid loss of suction (negative pressure), the wound and dressing must stay sealed after therapy is initiated. Problem seal areas include wounds around joints; near skin creases and folds; and near moisture, such as diaphoresis, wound drainage, and urine or stool. The following points may help to maintain an airtight seal:

- Clip hair on skin around wound (check agency policy).
- Fill uneven skin surfaces with a skin-barrier product such as paste or strips.
- Make sure that periwound skin surface is completely dry.
- Cut transparent film to extend 2.5 to 5 cm (1 to 2 inches) beyond wound perimeter.
- Frame periwound area with skin sealant, solid skin barrier, or hydrocolloid dressing.
- Cut or mold transparent dressing to fit wound.
- Avoid wrinkles when applying transparent film.
- Identify any air leaks with a stethoscope and repair them with the transparent dressing.
- Use only one or two additional layers for large leaks. Multiple layers reduce moisture vapor transmission and cause maceration of wound.

Data from Netsch DS: Refractory wounds. In Wound Ostomy and Continence Nurses Society: *Core curriculum: wound management*, Philadelphia, 2016, Wolters Kluwer; Netsch DS et al: Negative-pressure wound therapy. In Bryant RA, Nix DP, editors: *Acute and chronic wounds: current management concepts*, ed 5, St. Louis, 2016, Mosby.

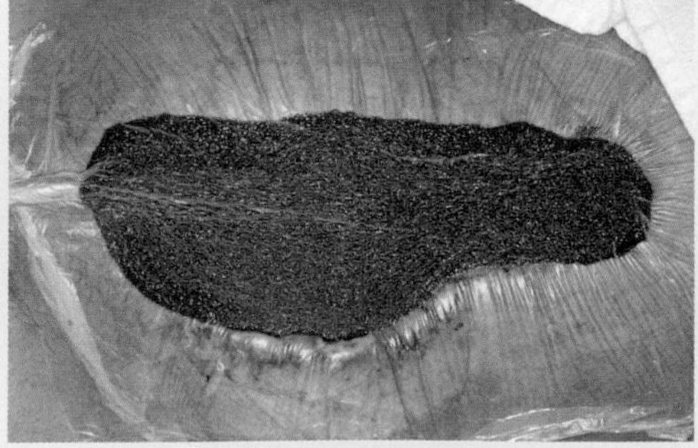

STEP 13d(2) Foam wound filler; transparent dressing over existing wound.

STEP	RATIONALE
(4) Secure tubing several centimeters away from dressing, avoiding pressure points.	Drainage tubes over bony pressure prominences can cause medical device–related pressure injuries (Netsch et al., 2016; Pittman et al., 2015).
14. After wound is completely covered, connect tubing from dressing to tubing from canister and NPWT unit and set at ordered suction level.	Intermittent or continuous negative pressure varies from −75 mm Hg to −125 mm Hg, depending on the device and the characteristics of the wound (Netsch et al., 2016; WOCN, 2016).
a. Remove canister from sterile packing and push unit until you hear click. **NOTE:** An alarm sounds if canister is not properly engaged.	
b. Connect dressing tubing to canister tubing (follow manufacturer's instructions). Make sure that both clamps are open.	
c. Place on level surface or hang from foot of bed. **NOTE:** Unit alarms and deactivates therapy if it is tilted beyond 45 degrees.	
d. Press power button (commonly this is a green-lit button) and set pressure as ordered.	
15. Inspect NPWT system.	
a. Verify that the system is on. This is different for each type of NPWT unit. For example, on some units the display screen shows "Therapy On." Check agency policy and procedure for specific information.	
b. Verify that all clamps are open and that all tubing is patent.	
c. Examine system to be sure that seal is intact and that therapy is working.	Negative pressure is achieved when a tight seal is present (Netsch et al., 2016).
d. If a leak is present, use strips of transparent dressing to patch areas around edges of wound.	
16. Record initials, date, and time on new dressing.	Provides reference for next dressing change.
17. Help patient to comfortable position. Patients may ambulate with NPWT.	Enhances patient comfort and relaxation.
18. Discard gloves and dispose of any dressing material. Perform hand hygiene.	Prevents transmission of microorganisms.
19. Raise side rails (as appropriate) and lower bed to lowest position.	Provides for patient safety and reduces the risk for falls.
20. Be sure nurse call system is in an accessible location within patient's reach; instruct patient in use.	Provides patient or family member a resource to call for assistance.

EVALUATION

1. Inspect condition of wound on ongoing basis; note drainage and odor.	Determines status of wound healing.
2. Ask patient to rate pain using scale of 0 to 10.	Determines patient's level of comfort following procedure.
3. Verify airtight dressing seal and correct negative-pressure setting.	Determines effective negative pressure being applied.
4. Measure wound drainage output in canister on regular basis.	Monitors fluid balance and wound drainage.
5. **Use Teach-Back:** "I want to be sure I explained clearly what your wound should look like as it is healing and the signs of infection before you are discharged. Explain to me what your wound will look like as it begins to heal." Revise your instruction now or develop a plan for revised patient/family caregiver teaching if patient/family caregiver is not able to teach back correctly.	Determines patient's/family caregiver's level of understanding of instructional topic.

Unexpected Outcomes	Related Interventions
1. Wound appears inflamed and tender, drainage has increased, and odor is present.	• Notify health care provider. • Obtain wound culture.

Unexpected Outcomes	Related Interventions
2. Patient reports increase in pain.	• Patient may need more analgesia. • Instill normal saline to moisten filler dressings to allow loosening from granulation tissue. • If using black foam, switch to polyvinyl alcohol (PVA) white soft foam. • Decrease pressure setting. • Change from intermittent to continuous cycling. • Change type of NPWT system.
3. Negative-pressure seal has broken.	• Take preventive measures (see Box 25.3).
4. Wound hemorrhages.	• Stop NPWT immediately and notify health care provider.
5. Patient or family caregiver is unable to perform dressing change.	• Provide additional teaching and support. • Obtain services of home care agency.

Recording

- Record appearance and condition of wound, characteristics and amount of drainage, placement of NPWT, negative-pressure setting, and patient's response.

Hand-Off Reporting

- Report on the location of NPWT, time of dressing change if done, and any interventions, such as reinforcement of dressing.
- Discuss whether the patient or caregiver is participating in changing the NPWT dressing.
- Report brisk, bright bleeding; evidence of poor wound healing; and signs of possible wound infection to health care provider.

SPECIAL CONSIDERATIONS

Patient-Centered Care

- Determine what effect a chronic wound and subsequent wound care may have from the patient's cultural perspective.
- Be sensitive to patient's cultural beliefs and practices and determine if skin substitutes used to treat chronic or severe wounds might be unacceptable.

Patient Education

- The patient and family caregiver should be instructed to immediately contact the health care team if the wound drainage system becomes dislodged.
- Instruct how to change dressings around drainage tube. Ask patient or family caregiver to record the amount of drainage and bring the record to the health care provider at the next outpatient visit.
- Instruct patient to examine the area where the sutures were removed checking for any separation of the incision edges.
- If patient is using NPWT at home, instruct patient and family caregiver how to determine if the battery life of the device is adequate and demonstrate how to recharge.

Age-Specific

Pediatric

- Neonatal skin is immature and easily damaged by pressure irrigation. Check that products are approved for this patient population.
- NPWT is not appropriate for fragile neonatal skin.

Gerontological

- A 20% loss in dermal thickness occurs with aging. The skin is less resilient, and wound irrigation can easily result in skin tears and other trauma (Baranoski et al., 2015a).
- There may be a higher risk for dehiscence after sutures are removed because of delayed healing of aging skin.

Home Care

- Assess patient's home environment to determine adequacy of facilities for performing wound care and storing supplies.
- Provide support for patient and caregiver during the wound-healing process. Chronic wounds do not heal properly and do not close in a timely manner (Doughty and Sparks-Defriese, 2016).
- Provide community resources for patient and family caregiver for obtaining supplies and properly disposing of contaminated products.

✦ PRACTICE REFLECTIONS

Reflect on a scenario where you care for a patient with a chronic wound. You care for him in the hospital and follow the patient into the home setting.

1. What parameters would you include in a wound assessment? How might the parameters in a hospital setting differ from those in the home? Include information about how to objectively assess the wound.
2. What issues might you encounter if the patient is an older adult?
3. What challenges might you encounter in the home?

✦ CLINICAL REVIEW QUESTIONS

1. The health care provider has written an order to remove the staples from an abdominal incision. List the following steps in the correct sequence for staple removal.
   1. Assess and verify healing ridge.
   2. Apply Steri-Strips over incision.
   3. Explain procedure to patient.
   4. Clean sutures or staples and healed incision with antiseptic swabs.
   5. Remove staples.

2. Indications of new tissue growth include which of the following? (Select all that apply.)
   1. Inflammation around perimeter of wound
   2. Red, moist wound tissue
   3. Reduced wound size
   4. Brown-tinged tissue
   5. Scar formation
3. Correct principles of practice for a wound irrigation include which of the following? (Select all that apply.)
   1. Use a 35-mL syringe.
   2. Use a 17-gauge angiocatheter, which has minimal risk for tissue injury.
   3. Place irrigation catheter tip 2.5 (1 inch) above the upper end of the wound.
   4. Use intermittent pressure to irrigate the wound.
   5. Insert tip of catheter 1.3 cm (0.5 inch) in a deep wound.

Answers and Rationales for Clinical Review Questions can be found on the Evolve website.

REFERENCES

Baranoski S, et al: Skin: an essential organ. In Baranoski S, Ayello EA, editors: *Wound care essentials: practice principles*, ed 4, Philadelphia, 2015a, Lippincott Williams & Wilkins.

Baranoski S, et al: Wound assessment. In Baranoski S, Ayello EA, editors: *Wound care essentials: practice principles*, ed 4, Philadelphia, 2015b, Lippincott Williams & Wilkins.

Berrios-Torres SI, et al: Centers for Disease Control and Prevention guideline for the prevention of surgical site infection, *JAMA Surg* 152(8):784–2017, 2017.

Centers for Disease Control and Prevention: What is health literacy, 2016. https://www.cdc.gov/healthliteracy/learn/index.htmlde.

Doughty DB, Sparks-Defriese B: Wound healing physiology. In Bryant RA, Nix DP, editors: *Acute and chronic wounds: current management concepts*, ed 5, St. Louis, 2016, Mosby.

Franco LM, et al: Preoperative bathing of the surgical site with chlorohexidine for infection prevention: systematic review with meta-analysis, *Am J Infect Control* 45(4):343, 2017.

Gallagher S: Skin care needs of the obese patient. In Bryant RA, Nix DP, editors: *Acute and chronic wounds: current management concepts*, ed 5, St. Louis, 2016, Mosby.

Institute for Healthcare Improvement: How to prevent surgical site infection, 2012. http://www.ihi.org/resources/Pages/Tools/HowtoGuidePreventSurgicalSiteInfection.aspx.

Institute for Healthcare Improvement (IHI): Surgical site infection, 2014. http://www.ihi.org/topics/ssi/pages/default.aspx.

Jaszarowski KA, Murphree RW: Wound cleansing and dressing selection. In Wound Ostomy and Continence Nurses Society, editor: *Core curriculum: wound management*, Philadelphia, 2016, Wolters Kluwer.

Kinetic Concepts International (KCI): *VAC therapy for wounds, product information*, San Antonio, TX, 2013, Kinetic Concepts International (KCI).

Krasner DL: Wound pain: impact and assessment. In Bryant RA, Nix DP, editors: *Acute and chronic wounds: current management concepts*, ed 5, St. Louis, 2016, Mosby.

Martindell D: The safe use of negative-pressure wound therapy, *Am J Nurs* 112(6):61, 2012.

National Pressure Ulcer Advisory Panel (NPUAP): National Pressure Ulcer Advisory Panel announces a change in terminology from pressure ulcer to pressure injury and updates the stages of pressure injury, April 2016. https://www.npuap.org/national-pressure-ulcer-advisory-panel-npuap-announces-a-change-in-terminology-from-pressure-ulcer-to-pressure-injury-and-updates-the-stages-of-pressure-injury/.

National Pressure Ulcer Advisory Panel (NPUAP), European Pressure Ulcer Advisory Panel (EPUAP), and Pan Pacific Pressure Injury Alliance (PPIA): Prevention and treatment of pressure ulcers: Quick reference guide, January 2016. http://www.npuap.org/wp-content/uploads/2014/08/Quick-Reference-Guide-DIGITAL-NPUAP-EPUAP-PPPIA-Jan2016.pdf.

Netsch DS, et al: Negative pressure wound therapy. In Bryant RA, Nix DP, editors: *Acute and chronic wounds: current management concepts*, ed 5, St. Louis, 2016, Mosby.

Nix DP: Skin and wound inspection and assessment. In Bryant RA, Nix DP, editors: *Acute and chronic wounds: current management concepts*, ed 5, St. Louis, 2016, Mosby.

Pittman J, et al: Medical device–related hospital-acquired pressure ulcers, *J Wound Ostomy Continence Nurs* 42(2):151, 2015.

Ramundo J: Wound debridement. In Bryant RA, Nix DP, editors: *Acute and chronic wounds: current management concepts*, ed 5, St. Louis, 2016, Mosby.

Stotts NA: Wound infection: diagnosis and management. In Bryant RA, Nix DP, editors: *Acute and chronic wounds: current management concepts*, ed 5, St Louis, 2016, Mosby.

The Joint Commission (TJC): *2019 National Patient Safety Goals*, Oakbrook Terrace, IL, 2019, The Commission. http://www.jointcommission.org/standards_information/npsgs.aspx.

Whitney JD: Surgical wounds and incision care. In Bryant RA, Nix DP, editors: *Acute and chronic wounds: current management concepts*, ed 5, St. Louis, 2016, Mosby.

Wound Ostomy and Continence Nurses Society (WOCN): *Guideline for prevention and management of pressure ulcers (injuries)*, Mount Laurel, NJ, 2016, WOCN.

26 Pressure Injury Prevention and Care

SKILLS AND PROCEDURES

EVOLVE WEBSITE/RESOURCES LIST

http://evolve.elsevier.com/Perry/nursinginterventions

Audio Glossary • Case Studies • Checklists • Clinical Review Questions • Answers and Rationales for Clinical Review Questions • Video Clips

INTRODUCTION

A pressure injury is localized damage to the skin and underlying soft tissue, usually occurring over a bony prominence or related to pressure from a medical device. Pressure injuries present a significant health care threat to patients with restricted mobility or chronic disease and to older patients (Pieper, 2016). Understanding of the impact, etiology, and classification of pressure injuries is key to planning care for the population that is vulnerable to the development of pressure injuries.

PRESSURE INJURY ETIOLOGY

A pressure injury can present as intact skin or an open ulcer because of intense and/or prolonged pressure or pressure in combination with shear. The tolerance of soft tissue for pressure and shear may also be affected by microclimate, nutrition, perfusion, co-morbidities, and the condition of the soft tissue (National Pressure Ulcer Advisory Panel [NPUAP], 2014a). Pressure injuries can occur when patients are in bed or sitting or when an external source such as a cast edge applies unrelieved pressure to the skin (Ayello et al., 2015). Pressure points over bony prominences are where pressure injuries can develop in sitting and lying positions (Fig. 26.1).

Three pressure-related forces lead to the development of a pressure injury: (1) intensity of pressure (how much pressure is applied), (2) duration of pressure (how long pressure is applied), and (3) tissue tolerance (the ability of skin and its supporting structures to endure pressure without adverse effects). The intensity of the pressure must compress the blood flow to the skin. Both low pressure over a prolonged period and high pressure over a short period can create a pressure injury. The greater the pressure and the longer pressure is applied, the greater the likelihood that a pressure injury will develop. Special mattresses and support surfaces help reduce or redistribute this pressure (see Procedural Guideline 26.1). The third factor, tissue tolerance, refers to the ability of the tissue to react to the pressure.

Three external factors (i.e., shear, friction, and moisture) make the tissues less tolerant to pressure (Pieper, 2016). Shear is a parallel force that stretches tissue and blood vessels, such as when the head of the bed is elevated more than 30 degrees, and shear force occurs in the sacrococcygeal region (Fig. 26.2). The sliding of the body transmits pressure to the sacrum and the deep fascia, the skin over the sacrum sticks to the bed sheets, but the bony structure slides down, occluding the blood vessels and causing deep tissue injury. Friction, the rubbing of the tissue against a surface, abrades the top layer of skin (epidermis), which makes tissue susceptible to pressure injury. Skin moisture (most often from fecal and urinary incontinence) softens skin, creating the risk for skin breakdown. Other factors related to pressure injury development include poor nutrition; advanced age; medical conditions causing poor tissue perfusion (e.g., low blood pressure, smoking, elevated temperature, anemia); and psychosocial status, in particular, stress-induced cortisol secretion (Pieper, 2016; Ratliff et al., 2017; Wound Ostomy and Continence Nurses Society [WOCN], 2016).

WOUND HEALING

You have an important role in wound healing, supporting patients by providing the appropriate wound-healing environment. A comprehensive wound assessment provides the information needed for planning wound care for a patient. To provide appropriate wound care, you must understand the process of wound healing. The physiology of wound healing occurs via two mechanisms: (1) regeneration (i.e., replacement of damaged or lost tissue with more of the same as occurs in partial-thickness wounds) or (2) connective tissue repair in wounds with tissue loss where scar formation replaces lost tissue, such as in full-thickness wounds (Doughty and Sparks, 2016).

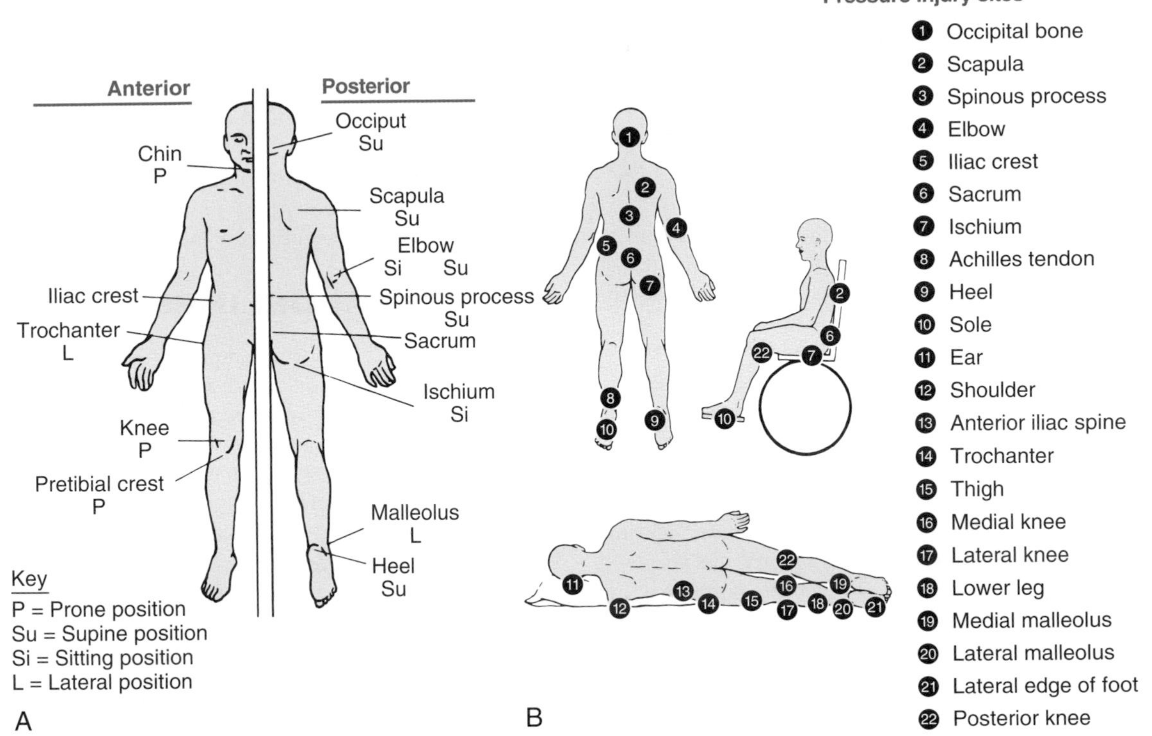

FIG 26.1 (A) Bony prominences most frequently underlying pressure injuries. (B) Pressure injury sites. *(Courtesy San Diego Veterans Administration Medical Agency.)*

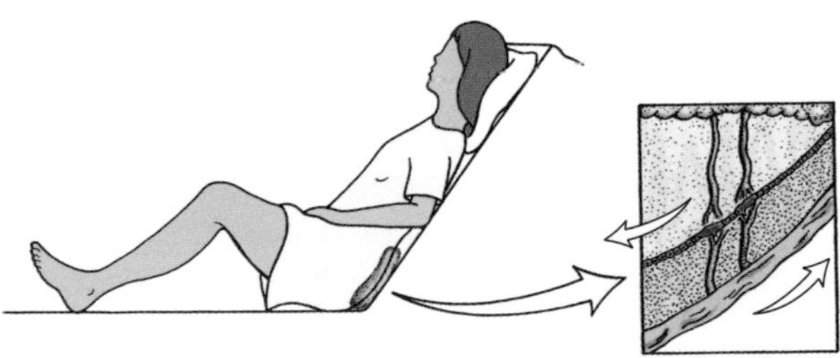

FIG 26.2 Shear exerted in the sacral area.

Wound healing is a process that requires specific nutrients to fuel healing (Stotts, 2016). Infection prolongs the inflammatory phase, which prevents epithelialization. Medications such as steroids slow the inflammatory process, making wounds more prone to infection and delayed healing (Table 26.1). High levels of stress increase cortisol levels, which reduce the number of lymphocytes and decrease the inflammatory response.

PRACTICE STANDARDS

- National Pressure Ulcer Advisory Panel (NPUAP), 2014b: Pressure ulcer treatment recommendations: clinical practice guidelines—Assessment of pressure injury risk factors and prevention strategies
- Qaseem et al. and Clinical Guidelines Committee of the American College of Physicians, 2015: Risk assessment and prevention of pressure ulcers: a clinical practice guideline from the American College of Physicians—Support surface guidelines
- The Joint Commission (TJC), 2019: National Patient Safety Goals—Patient identification

TABLE 26.1

Factors That Delay Wound Healing

Factor	Rationale
Advanced age	Aging affects all phases of wound healing. The most significant change includes a diminished inflammatory response.
Obesity	Fatty subcutaneous tissue is less vascular.
Diabetes mellitus	Vascular changes reduce blood flow to peripheral tissues; leukocyte malfunction results from hyperglycemia, resulting in high risk for infection.
Inadequate blood supply	Vascular changes decrease delivery of oxygen and nutrients.
Nutritional deficiencies	Inadequate nutrition slows healing because of lack of nutrients (vitamin C, protein, zinc) needed for wound healing (Stotts, 2016).
Corticosteroid drugs	Immunosuppression decreases the inflammatory response and collagen synthesis.
Chemotherapy	Chemotherapy interferes with leukocyte (white blood cell) production and immune response.
Infection	Infection increases inflammatory response and tissue destruction.
Smoking	Smoking impedes blood flow from vasoconstriction.
Poor general health	When health is poor, factors needed for wound healing are absent.

- Wound, Ostomy, and Continence Nurses Society (WOCN), 2016: Guideline for prevention and management of pressure ulcers—Assessment for pressure injuries and prevention strategies

EVIDENCE-BASED PRACTICE

Pressure-Mapping Devices Along With Position Changes

Repositioning at-risk patients may help to prevent the development of a pressure injury, and in a patient with a pressure injury, it may reduce pressure and thus support healing. Repositioning reduces the duration of pressure on high-risk areas such as the sacrum, heels, and trochanter. Repositioning frequency should be done on an individualized, regular schedule for each patient. However, there is a lack of agreement on the frequency of patient repositioning as well as the best position to redistribute pressure (Berlowitz et al., 2018a).

A method to determine pressure at the skin/surface interface could provide feedback on the optimal body position. A continuous bedside pressure-mapping (CBPM) device might provide real-time feedback of optimal body position by displaying pressure images at a patient's bedside, allowing off-loading of high-pressure areas and possibly preventing pressure injury formation. Evidence-based practice guidelines for the prevention of pressure injuries include the following:

- Individualized repositioning of patients may prevent pressure injury formation (Berlowitz et al., 2018a).
- Patients should be placed at an angle no greater than 30 degrees when positioned on their side to avoid pressure over the greater trochanter and other bony prominences.
- The head of the bed should not be elevated greater than 30 degrees to prevent sliding and friction injuries.
- Use of a pressure-mapping system assists nurses in targeting at-risk patients and in developing an individualized repositioning schedule (Hultin et al., 2017).
- Use of a pressure-mapping system reduces peak interface systems and assists in preventing pressure injuries (Hultin et al., 2017).
- The use of a pressure-mapping system may provide a reduction in the development of pressure injury and increase staff awareness of pressure injury interventions (Hultin et al., 2017).

SAFETY GUIDELINES

Preventing skin breakdown and pressure injuries is essential for safe patient care. Preventing injuries to a patient's skin protects the patient's overall level of health, independence, and optimal functioning. Safety guidelines for the prevention of pressure injuries include the following:

- Routinely perform skin assessment and position the patient in bed to provide privacy and to assess the skin adequately; when turning the patient onto the side, be sure that the side rail is up on the side of the bed to which the patient is turned to prevent falls.
- Use an individualized approach based on risk assessment to reposition patients to reduce pressure injury (Berlowitz et al., 2018a).
- Minimize friction and shear when repositioning patients.
- Provide prompt hygiene for patients with draining wounds or who are incontinent; this reduces prolonged skin moisture from urine, feces, and wound drainage (Ayello, 2017).
- Routinely assess existing pressure injuries to monitor wound healing.

✦ SKILL 26.1 Risk Assessment, Skin Assessment, and Prevention Strategies

Purpose

The use of a skin assessment tool for daily risk assessment aids in identifying factors that place a patient at risk for skin breakdown (Chaboyer et al., 2017). Risk assessment allows you to plan appropriate interventions to reduce or prevent skin breakdown. In addition to the risk assessment tool, a daily skin inspection, including an examination of pressure points, is essential. One assessment scale is the Braden Scale for Predicting Pressure Sore Risk (Table 26.2). Use an agency-approved assessment scale on a patient's admission to a health care agency and at scheduled intervals to assess pressure injury risk or presence.

Delegation and Collaboration

The skill of pressure injury risk assessment cannot be delegated to nursing assistive personnel (NAP). The nurse instructs the NAP to:

- Frequently change the patient's position and specific positions individualized for the patient.
- Report any redness or break in the patient's skin.
- Report any abrasion from medical devices.

Equipment

- Risk assessment tool (see agency policy)
- Positioning aids (see Chapter 17)
- Clean gloves

ASSESSMENT

1. Identify patient using at least two identifiers (e.g., name and birthday or name and medical record number) according to agency policy. *Rationale: Ensures correct patient. Complies with The Joint Commission standards and improves patient safety (TJC, 2019).*
2. Review medical record to assess patient's risk for pressure injury formation. *Rationale: Determines need to administer preventive care and identifies specific factors that place patient at risk (Haesler, 2017; NPUAP et al., 2014a).*
   a. Paralysis or immobilization caused by restrictive devices. *Rationale: Patient is unable to turn or reposition independently to relieve pressure.*
   b. Presence of medical device such as nasogastric (NG) tube, oxygen equipment, artificial airways, drainage tubing, or mechanical devices (Doughty and McNichol, 2016b). *Rationale: Medical devices have potential to exert pressure on patient's nares or ears or on tissue adjacent to devices such as artificial airways and drainage tubes (Pittman et al., 2015).*
      (1) If not medically contraindicated, remove medical device to observe and palpate skin and tissues under and around each medical device. *Rationale: Pressure area assumes same configuration as medical device (Schallom et al., 2015; WOCN, 2016).*

TABLE 26.2

Braden Scale for Predicting Pressure Sore Risk[a]

	1	2	3	4
Sensory Perception	**1. Completely Limited**	**2. Very Limited**	**3. Slightly Limited**	**4. No Impairment**
Ability to respond meaningfully to pressure-related discomfort	Unresponsive (does not moan, flinch, or grasp) to painful stimuli because of diminished level of consciousness or sedation *Or* Limited ability to feel pain over most of body surface	Responds only to painful stimuli; cannot communicate discomfort except by moaning or restlessness *Or* Has a sensory impairment that limits the ability to feel pain or discomfort over ½ of body	Responds to verbal commands but cannot always communicate discomfort or need to be turned *Or* Has some sensory impairment that limits ability to feel pain or discomfort in one or two extremities	Responds to verbal commands; has no sensory deficit that would limit ability to feel or voice pain or discomfort
Moisture	**1. Constantly Moist**	**2. Very Moist**	**3. Occasionally Moist**	**4. Rarely Moist**
Degree to which skin is exposed to moisture	Skin kept moist almost constantly by perspiration, urine; dampness detected every time patient is moved or turned	Skin often but not always moist; must change linens at least once a shift	Skin occasionally moist, requiring an extra linen change approximately once a day	Skin usually dry; must change linens only at routine intervals
Activity	**1. Bedfast**	**2. Chairfast**	**3. Walks Occasionally**	**4. Walks Frequently**
Degree of physical activity	Confined to bed	Ability to walk severely limited or nonexistent; cannot bear own weight and/or must be assisted into chair or wheelchair	Walks occasionally during day but for very short distances, with or without assistance; spends majority of each shift in bed or chair	Walks outside room at least twice a day and inside room at least once every 2 hours during waking hours
Mobility	**1. Completely Immobile**	**2. Very Limited**	**3. Slightly Limited**	**4. No Limitation**
Ability to change and control body position	Does not make even slight changes in body or extremity position without assistance	Makes occasional slight changes in body or extremity position but unable to make frequent or significant changes independently	Makes frequent although slight changes in body or extremity position independently	Makes major and frequent changes in position without assistance
Nutrition	**1. Very Poor**	**2. Probably Inadequate**	**3. Adequate**	**4. Excellent**
Usual food intake pattern	Never eats a complete meal; rarely eats more than ⅓ of any food offered; eats 2 servings or less of protein (meat or dairy products) per day; takes fluids poorly; does not take a liquid dietary supplement *Or* Is NPO and/or maintained on clear liquids or IV fluids for more than 5 days	Rarely eats a complete meal and generally eats only about ½ of any food offered; protein intake includes only 3 servings of meat or dairy products per day; occasionally takes a dietary supplement *Or* Receives less than optimum amount of liquid diet or tube feeding	Eats over half of most meals; eats a total of 4 servings of protein (meat, dairy products) each day; occasionally refuses a meal but usually takes a supplement if offered *Or* Is on a tube feeding or TPN regimen that probably meets most nutritional needs	Eats most of every meal; never refuses a meal; usually eats a total of 4 or more servings of meat and dairy products; occasionally eats between meals; does not require supplementation
Friction and Shear	**1. Problem**	**2. Potential Problem**	**3. No Apparent Problem**	
	Requires moderate to maximum assistance in moving; complete lifting without sliding against sheets impossible; frequently slides down in bed or chair, requiring frequent repositioning with maximum assistance; spasticity, contractures, or agitation leads to almost constant friction	Moves feebly or requires minimum assistance; during a move skin probably slides to some extent against sheets, chair, restraints, or other devices; maintains relatively good position in chair or bed most of the time but occasionally slides down	Moves in bed and chair independently and has sufficient muscle strength to lift up completely during move; maintains good position in bed or chair	
				Total Score

Adapted from Barbara Braden, PhD, RN, Creighton University School of Nursing, Omaha, NE.

IV, Intravenous; *NPO*, nothing by mouth; *TPN*, total parenteral nutrition.

[a]Score patient in each of the six subscales. Maximum score is 23, indicating little or no risk. A score of ≤16 indicates "at risk"; ≤9 indicates very high risk.

c. Sensory loss (e.g., hemiplegia, spinal cord injury). *Rationale: Patient is unable to feel discomfort from pressure and does not independently change position.*
d. Circulatory disorders (e.g., peripheral vascular diseases, vascular changes from diabetes mellitus, neuropathy). *Rationale: These disorders reduce perfusion of tissue layers of skin.*
e. Fever. *Rationale: Increases metabolic demands of tissues. Accompanying diaphoresis leaves skin moist.*
f. Anemia. *Rationale: Decreased hemoglobin level reduces oxygen-carrying capacity of blood and amount of oxygen available to tissues.*
g. Malnutrition. *Rationale: Inadequate nutrition leads to weight loss, muscle atrophy, and reduced tissue mass. Nutrient deficiencies result in impaired or delayed healing (Stotts, 2016).*
h. Fecal or urinary incontinence. *Rationale: Skin becomes exposed to moist environment that contains bacteria. Excessive moisture macerates skin (Ayello, 2017; Berlowitz et al., 2018b).*
i. Heavy sedation and anesthesia. *Rationale: Sedation alters sensory perception, and patient does not perceive pressure and change position.*
j. Age. *Rationale: Neonates and very young children are at high risk, with the head being most common site of pressure injury occurrence (WOCN, 2016). There is loss of dermal thickness in older adults, impairing ability to distribute pressure (Pieper, 2016).*
k. Dehydration. *Rationale: Results in decreased skin elasticity and turgor.*
l. Edema. *Rationale: Edematous tissues are less tolerant of pressure, friction, and shear.*
m. Existing pressure injuries. *Rationale: Limit surfaces available for position changes, placing available tissues at increased risk.*
n. History of pressure injury. *Rationale: Tensile strength of skin from previously healed pressure injury is 80% or less; therefore, this area cannot tolerate pressure as much as undamaged skin (Doughty and Sparks, 2016).*

3. Select agency-approved risk assessment tool such as the Braden Scale or Norton Scale. Perform risk assessment when patient enters health care setting and repeat on regularly scheduled basis or when there is significant change in patient's condition (WOCN, 2016). *Rationale: Valid and reliable risk assessment tools evaluate patient's risk for developing a pressure injury. Identifying risk factors that contribute to the potential for skin breakdown allows you to target specific interventions for decreasing risk for skin breakdown.*

Safe Patient Care *In acute care settings, perform initial assessment within 8 hours of admission and reassess every 24 hours or as patient condition changes; in critical care areas, perform assessment on admission and reassess every 24 hours or as patient condition changes; and in long-term and home care settings, perform assessment on admission. In long-term care settings, reassess weekly and then according to agency standards or when patient condition changes. In home care setting, reassess every registered nurse visit.*

4. Obtain risk score (see Tables 26.2) and evaluate its meaning based on patient's unique characteristics. When using the Braden scale, there are risk scores identified for specific patient populations. Patients at moderate risk include intensive care patients ≤14; older adults ≤14 (Alderden et al., 2017). *Rationale: Risk cutoff score depends on instrument used. Score involves identifying risk factors that contributed to it and minimizing these specific deficits (Alderden et al., 2017; Ayello et al., 2015).*
5. Close room or pull curtains around bed. *Rationale: Maintains patient privacy.*
6. Perform hand hygiene. Assess condition of patient's skin over regions of pressure (see Fig. 26.1). Apply gloves as needed with open and/or draining wounds. *Rationale: Body weight against bony prominences places underlying skin at risk for the development of skin injuries.*
   a. Inspect for skin discoloration (see Box 26.2 for patients with darkly pigmented skin) and tissue consistency (firm or boggy feel) and/or palpate for abnormal sensations (Nix, 2016). *Rationale: Indicates that tissue was under pressure; hyperemia is a normal physiological response to hypoxemia in tissues.*
   b. Palpate discolored area on skin and under and around medical devices, release your fingertip, and look for blanching. If an area of redness blanches (lightens in color) on palpation, this indicates normal reactive hyperemia; tissue is not at risk for the development of an injury. *Rationale: Tissue that does not blanch when palpated indicates abnormal reactive hyperemia; indication of possible ischemic injury.*
   c. Inspect for pallor and mottling. *Rationale: Persistent hypoxia in tissues that were under pressure; an abnormal physiological response.*
   d. Inspect for absence of superficial skin layers. *Rationale: Represents early pressure injury formation; usually a partial-thickness wound that may have resulted from friction and/or shear.*
   e. Inspect for changes in skin temperature, edema, and tissue consistency, especially in individuals with darkly pigmented skin. *Rationale: Localized heat, edema, and induration have been identified as warning signs for pressure injury development. Because it is not always possible to observe changes in skin color on darkly pigmented skin, these additional signs should be considered in assessment (NPUAP, 2016; NPUAP et al., 2014a).*
   f. Inspect for wound drainage. *Rationale: Wound drainage increases risk for skin breakdown because it is caustic to skin and underlying tissues.*
7. Assess skin and tissue around and beneath medical devices every nursing shift for additional areas of potential pressure injury resulting from medical devices (Black et al., 2015; Haesler, 2017; Table 26.3). *Rationale: Patients at high risk have multiple sites for pressure necrosis from medical devices in areas other than bony prominences (Chaboyer et al., 2017; Makic, 2015). Pressure points around medical devices (e.g., oxygen cannula and masks, drainage tubing [e.g., Jackson-Pratt, Hemovac]) can cause pressure injury to underlying tissue and become full-thickness pressure injuries (Black et al., 2015; Pittman et al., 2015; Schallom et al., 2015).*
   a. Nares: NG tube, oxygen cannula. *Rationale: Pressure to nares occurs from tape and other materials used to secure NG tube.*
   b. Ears: oxygen cannula, pillow. *Rationale: Oxygen equipment is a significant risk for pressure injuries (Padula et al., 2017). Patients' ears and tips of nares are at risk for pressure injuries from nasal cannula (Black et al., 2015; Schallom et al., 2015).*
   c. Tongue and lips: oral airway, endotracheal (ET) tube. *Rationale: Pressure can result from artificial airway and*

TABLE 26.3

Strategies to Prevent Medical and Immobilization Device–Related Pressure Injuries

Device	Pressure Areas	Prevention Strategies*
Nasogastric tubes	Nares Skin on nasal bridge	Secure tube using pressure-relieving techniques, which direct the pressure from the tube away from the nares (see Chapters 13 and 20). Reposition tube.
Endotracheal tubes	Lips Tongue	Reposition tube into different locations within mouth and ensure depth of tube does not change (Bryant and Nix, 2016b) (see Chapter 16).
Nasotracheal tube	Nose/nasal bridge Nares	Change stabilizer every other day, sooner if loose or leaking (Bryant and Nix, 2016b) (see Chapter 16). Reposition.
Tracheostomy tubes and tapes	Front of neck and stoma site	Remove securing device daily (see Chapter 16). Increase stoma care. Use commercially available foam or collar-type adjustable straps instead of ties or twill (Bryant and Nix, 2016b).
Oxygen cannula and tubing	Ears Nose	Use commercially available foam ear protectors (Bryant and Nix, 2016b). Periodically remove cannula to relieve pressure and inspect for pressure injury (Schallom et al., 2015).
Oxygen mask	Forehead Nose/nasal bridge	Consider masks with gel borders. Apply the minimum tension to mask straps to create the seal. Refit mask if edema on face changes.
Noninvasive positive-pressure ventilation (NIPPV)/bi-level positive airway pressure (BiPAP)	Forehead Nose/nasal bridge	Apply protective dressing or liquid skin barrier to bridge of nose or forehead prior to application of device. If appropriate, remove mask periodically for a few minutes.
Drainage tubing	Area immediately next to drainage tube Adjacent area during patient position changes	Apply appropriate dressing around drainage tube insertion site. Check tubing placement with each position change. Instruct patient not to lie on the tubing (Pittman et al., 2015).
Indwelling catheter	Thighs Female: urethra, labia Male: tip of penis	Provide meticulous perineal care (see Chapter 11). Anchor and secure catheter to reduce pressure.
Orthopedic devices	All areas where device contacts the patient's skin and tissues	When possible and not contraindicated, inspect under the device twice a day (Bryant and Nix, 2016b).
Neck collar	Neck and occipital region Scalp	Remove hard collars as soon as possible and replace with softer collar (Black et al., 2015). Inspect scalp daily.
Compression stockings	Calf Behind knee Heel Toes	Verify proper fit (see Chapter 18). To reduce pressure and risk of injury to skin and underlying tissue, remove stockings twice daily (at least once per shift) for at least 1 hour (Black et al., 2015).
Immobilization devices	Wrists Ankles	Apply dressing between immobilizer and patient's skin (Black et al., 2015). Verify that there is some space between immobilizer and patient's skin. With assistive personnel present, remove restraints one at a time to inspect skin.

*In addition to routine inspection and cleaning of skin under and around medical device.

materials used to secure airway (Black et al., 2015; Padula et al., 2017).

d. Forehead: pulse oximetry device. *Rationale: Adhesive can cause skin blistering.*

e. Drainage or other tubing. *Rationale: Stress and pressure against tissue at exit site or from tubing lying under any part of patient's body can cause skin injury (Black et al., 2015).*

f. Indwelling urethral (Foley) catheter. *Rationale: For female patients, catheter can place pressure on labia, especially when edematous. For male patients, pressure from catheter not properly anchored can put pressure on tip of penis and urethra (Black et al., 2015).*

g. Orthopedic and positioning devices such as casts, neck collars, splints. *Rationale: Applied devices have potential to cause pressure to underlying and adjacent skin and tissue (Black et al., 2015).*

h. Compression stockings. *Rationale: Compression stockings have potential to cause pressure, especially if they fit poorly or are rolled down (Black et al., 2015).*

i. Immobilization device and restraints. *Rationale: Pressure points can occur if the device is too tight or poorly placed or if the patient strains against the device.*

j. Remove and dispose of gloves (if worn) and perform hand hygiene.

8. Observe patient for preferred positions when in bed or chair. *Rationale: Preferred positions result in weight of body being placed on certain bony prominences. Presence of contractures may result in pressure exerted in unexpected places.*
9. Observe ability of patient to initiate and help with position changes. *Rationale: Potential for pressure, friction, and shear increases when patient is completely dependent on others for position changes.*
10. Assess patient's or family caregiver's knowledge, experience, and health literacy level. *Rationale: Ensures patient has the capacity to obtain, communicate, process, and understand basic health information (Centers for Disease Control and Prevention [CDC], 2016).*
11. Assess patient's and family caregiver's understanding of what a pressure injury is and the individual risks for patient to develop pressure injuries. *Rationale: Determines baseline knowledge for pressure injury risk and identifies areas for patient teaching.*

STEP	RATIONALE
PLANNING	
1. Expected outcomes following completion of procedure:	
• Risk factors are identified.	Establishes baseline for future assessment.
• Patient experiences no change from baseline skin assessment.	Prevention guidelines prevent occurrence or worsening of pressure injury.
• Skin is intact, with no evidence of erythema or no signs of breakdown.	Prevention strategies reduce risk factors.
• Patient and family caregiver learn patient's personal risk factors for pressure injury.	Demonstrates learning.
2. Explain procedure(s) and purpose to patient and family caregiver.	Relieves anxiety and provides opportunity for education.
3. Provide privacy and prepare environment.	Ensures patient comfort and safety.
IMPLEMENTATION	
1. Perform hand hygiene. If patient has open, draining wounds, apply clean gloves.	Use of standard precautions prevents accidental exposure to body fluids.
2. Following initial assessment, continue to inspect skin at least once a day.	
a. Observe patient's skin; pay special attention to bony prominences and areas around and under medical devices and tubes. If you find reddened area, gently press area with gloved finger to check for blanching. If area does not blanch, suspect tissue injury and recheck in 1 hour. Any discoloration may vary from pink to a deep red.	Routine skin inspection is fundamental to risk assessment and in selecting interventions to reduce risk (Haesler, 2017; WOCN, 2016). Persistent redness when lightly pigmented skin is pressed can indicate tissue injury. If area of redness blanches (lightens in color), it indicates that skin is not at risk for breakdown.

Safe Patient Care *Do not massage reddened areas because doing so may cause additional tissue trauma. Reddened areas indicate blood vessel damage, and massaging can further damage the vessel (Bryant and Nix, 2016a).*

STEP	RATIONALE
b. If patient has darkly pigmented skin, look for color changes that differ from his or her normal skin color.	Darkly pigmented skin may not blanch. A change in color may occur at the site of pressure; this change in color differs from patient's usual skin color (NPUAP et al., 2014a; see Box 26.2).
3. Each shift, check all treatment and assistive devices (e.g., catheters, feeding tubes, casts, braces) for potential pressure points.	Pressure from these devices increases risk on bony prominences and other areas.
a. Verify that device is correctly sized, positioned, and secured.	Incorrect size, placement, and securing of medical device can cause excessive pressure and rubbing by device on underlying skin (Makic, 2015).
b. Consider protecting underlying at-risk skin with a protective dressing (e.g., silicone, hydrocolloid).	Dressings absorb moisture from body and reduce pressure to underlying skin (Black et al., 2015; Makic, 2015).

Safe Patient Care *Inspect skin around and beneath orthopedic devices (e.g., cervical collar, braces, or cast). Note any abrasions or warmth in areas where devices can rub against the skin (Pittman et al., 2015; Schallom et al., 2015).*

STEP	RATIONALE
4. Remove and dispose of gloves; perform hand hygiene.	Reduces transmission of microorganisms.
5. Review patient's pressure injury risk assessment score.	Risk scores aid in identifying interventions to lessen or eliminate present risk factors.
6. If immobility, inactivity, or poor sensory perception is a risk factor(s) for patient, consider one of the following interventions (NPUAP et al., 2014a; WOCN, 2016):	Immobility and inactivity reduce patient's ability or desire to independently change position. Poor sensory perception decreases patient's ability to feel sensation of pressure or discomfort.
a. Reposition patient on scheduled basis and frequently assess individual's skin condition to help identify early signs of pressure injury. If skin changes occur, reevaluate the plan.	Reduces duration and intensity of pressure. Some patients may require more frequent repositioning.
b. When patient is in side-lying position in bed, use 30-degree lateral position (see illustration). Avoid 90-degree lateral position.	Reduces direct contact of trochanter with support surface.
c. When needed, use pillow bridging (see illustration).	Use of pillows prevents direct contact between bony prominences.
d. Place patient (when lying in bed) on pressure-redistribution surface.	Reduces amount of pressure exerted on tissues.
e. Place patient (when in chair) on pressure-redistribution device and shift points under pressure at least every hour.	Reduces amount of pressure on sacral and ischial areas.
7. If friction and shear are identified as risk factors, consider the following interventions:	Friction and shear damage underlying skin.

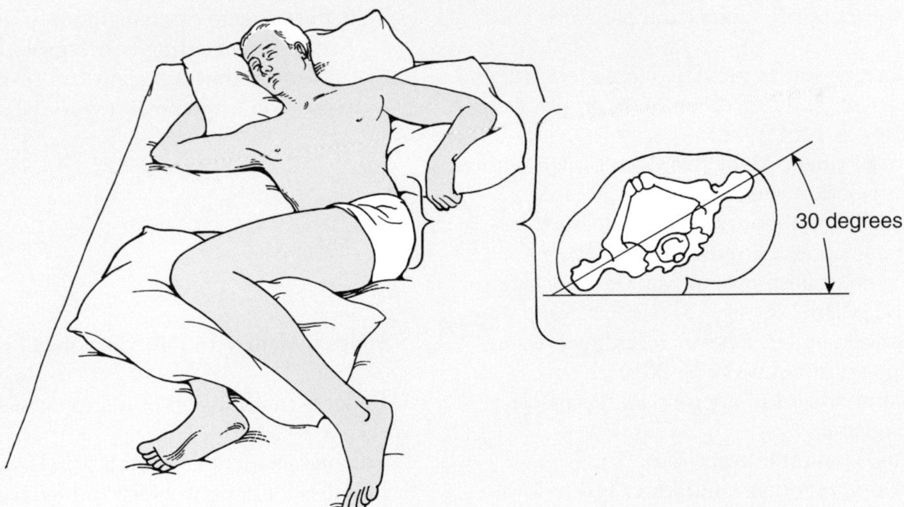

STEP 6b Thirty-degree lateral position with pillow placement.

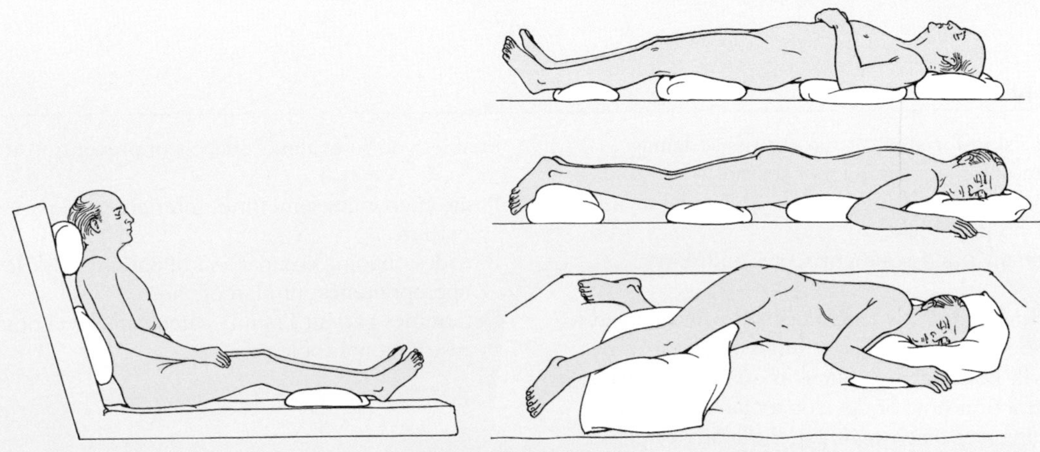

STEP 6c Pillow bridging.

STEP	RATIONALE
a. Use safe patient handling guidelines to reposition patient. For example, use slide board to transfer patient from bed to stretcher.	Proper repositioning of patient prevents creating shear from dragging patient along sheets. Slide board provides slippery surface to reduce friction. Use lift team when appropriate.
b. Ensure that heels are free from surface of bed by using a pillow under calves to elevate heels or use a heel-suspension device; knees should be in 5- to 10-degree flexion (Baath et al., 2016; WOCN, 2016).	"Floating" heels from bed surface off-load the heel completely and redistribute the weight of the leg along the calf without applying pressure on the Achilles tendon (Baath et al., 2016).
c. Maintain head of the bed (HOB) at 30 degrees or lower or at the lowest degree of elevation consistent with patient's condition (do not lower HOB if patient is at risk for aspiration; WOCN, 2016).	Decreases potential for patient to slide toward foot of bed and incur shear injury.
8. If patient receives low score on moisture subscale, consider one of the following interventions:	Continual exposure of body fluids on patient's skin increases risk for skin breakdown and pressure injury development.
a. Apply clean gloves. Clean and dry the skin as soon as possible after each incontinent episode (WOCN, 2016). Apply moisture barrier ointment to perineum and surrounding skin after each incontinent episode.	Protects skin from fecal or urinary incontinence. Friction and shear are enhanced in the presence of moisture.
b. If skin is denuded, use protective barrier paste after each incontinent episode.	Provides barrier between skin and stool/urine, allowing for healing.
c. If moisture source is from wound drainage, consider frequent dressing changes, skin protection with protective barriers, or collection devices.	Removes frequent exposure of the skin to wound drainage.
9. If friction and shear are risk factors and patient is chair-bound:	Relief of pressure by changing from lying to sitting position is insufficient if sitting lasts a prolonged time. The maximum amount of time a patient can sit before there is a need to reposition is unknown (WOCN, 2016).
a. Tilt patient's chair seat to prevent sliding forward, and support arms, legs, and feet to maintain proper posture (NPUAP et al., 2014b).	
b. Limit amount of time patient spends in a chair without pressure redistribution (NPUAP et al., 2014b).	
c. For patients who can reposition themselves while sitting, encourage pressure redistribution every 15 minutes using chair push-ups, forward lean, or side to side (WOCN, 2016).	
10. Educate patient and family caregiver regarding pressure injury risk and prevention (WOCN, 2016).	Helps to adhere to interventions to reduce pressure injury risk.
11. Remove gloves and discard in appropriate receptacle. Perform hand hygiene.	Reduces transmission of microorganisms.
12. Assist patient to a comfortable position.	Enhances patient comfort and relaxation.
13. Raise side rails (as appropriate) and lower bed to lowest position.	Provides for patient safety and reduces the risk for falls.
14. Place nurse call system accessible within reach; instruct patient in use.	Ensures patient can call for assistance if needed.

EVALUATION

1. Observe patient's skin for areas at risk for tissue damage, noting change in color, appearance, or texture.	Enables you to evaluate success of prevention techniques.
2. Observe tolerance of patient for position change by measuring level of comfort on pain scale.	Position changes sometimes interfere with patient's sleep and rest pattern.
3. Compare subsequent risk assessment scores and skin assessments.	Provides ongoing comparison of patient's risk level to facilitate appropriateness of plan of care.
4. **Use Teach-Back:** "I want you to understand why we need to assess your skin on an ongoing basis. Tell me in your own words why we will be checking your skin on a regular basis." Revise your instruction now or develop a plan for revised patient/family caregiver teaching if patient/family caregiver is not able to teach back correctly.	Determines patient's/family caregiver's level of understanding of instructional topic.

Unexpected Outcomes	Related Interventions
1. Skin becomes mottled, reddened, purplish, or bluish.	• Refer patient to wound, ostomy, and continence (WOC) nurse; dietitian; clinical nurse specialist (CNS); nurse practitioner (NP); and/or physical therapist as necessary. Reevaluate position changes and bed surface.
2. Areas under pressure develop persistent discoloration, induration, or temperature changes.	• Refer patient to WOC nurse, dietitian, CNS, NP, and/or physical therapist as necessary. • Modify patient's positioning and turning schedule.

Recording

- Record patient's risk and skin assessments, turning intervals, pressure-redistribution support surface, moisture-protection, and other interventions.
- Report need for additional consultations (if indicated) for high-risk patient.
- Document your evaluation of patient learning.

Hand-Off Reporting

Report to health care provider results of the skin assessment, with emphasis on the areas of potential or actual skin impairment. Report on strategies shown to be useful.

PROCEDURAL GUIDELINE 26.1 *Selection of a Pressure-Redistribution Support Surface*

Purpose

A support surface is a special bed or device placed over or used as a bed mattress for pressure redistribution. It is designed for the management of tissue loads to prevent pressure injuries and to provide an environment conducive to pressure injury healing (Nix and Mackey, 2016; NPUAP, 2014b). Individuals at risk for pressure injury development or those with pressure injuries should be placed on a support surface based on current clinical guidelines (Qaseem et al., 2015).

Delegation and Collaboration

The selection of a pressure-redistribution support device cannot be delegated to nursing assistive personnel (NAP).

Equipment

Pressure injury risk assessment tool (see agency policy; see Skill 26.1); body chart, tape measure, and/or camera to document existing areas of impaired skin integrity; documentation form or electronic health record; proper support surface (McNichol et al., 2015); skin-care products

Procedural Steps

1. Assess patient's risk for skin breakdown using a risk assessment tool (e.g., Braden Scale score of 18 or less indicates patient is at risk; see Skill 26.1).
2. Perform hand hygiene. Assess patient's existing pressure injuries, including location, stage, areas of blistering, abnormal reactive hyperemia, and abrasion.
3. Consider patient weight and weight distribution and the following risk factors/co-morbidities: advanced age, fever, poor dietary intake of protein, diastolic pressure less than 60 mm Hg, hemodynamic instability, generalized edema, and anemia (WOCN, 2016).
4. Assess patient's level of comfort using a pain scale of 0 to 10.
5. Determine the need for a pressure-reduction surface from assessment data.
6. Identify patient factors when selecting an appropriate surface (Fig. 26.3):
   a. Does patient need pressure redistribution (e.g., you cannot reposition the patient, or there is an existing pressure injury)?
   b. Is the surface needed for short- or long-term care? A short-term surface is usually needed for an acute illness and hospitalization. A long-term surface is usually needed for extended or home care.
   c. What is the potential comfort level achieved by the surface? If patient is sensitive to noise, a device with a loud motor will increase his or her discomfort.
   d. Are patient and family caregivers cooperative and adherent to repositioning? In addition, are they aware that a support surface should never replace repositioning? Is adequate help available for repositioning? In a home setting, a support surface is often necessary when the family caregiver or patient is unable to reposition independently or needs help with repositioning.
   e. Does the support surface have a potential to interfere with patient's independent functioning? The height of the overlay and its soft edge may affect a patient's ability to transfer, and a high-air-loss bed may not be appropriate for a patient who needs to get in and out of bed frequently.
   f. What are patient's financial limitations, and is the device covered by insurance?
   g. If patient is using the device in the home, what are the environmental limitations? Will the home and existing electrical service accommodate the surface selected? Can the family caregivers in the home manage the surface?
   h. How durable is the product? Is the surface easily subjected to puncture? How easily can the surface be cleaned?

Continued

PROCEDURAL GUIDELINE 26.1 *Selection of a Pressure-Redistribution Support Surface—cont'd*

i. Does patient need pressure-redistribution surfaces in a chair/wheelchair? Has the family caregiver been instructed on appropriate inflation of the device?

7. Place "at-risk" patients on a pressure-reduction surface and high-specification foam mattress and not on a standard hospital mattress (NPUAP, 2014b; WOCN, 2016).

8. Check agency policy regarding implementing a support surface.

a. Obtain a health care provider's order. This may be required for a patient to obtain third-party reimbursement.

b. Consult with agency case manager or social worker to help with patient's financial eligibility and terms and

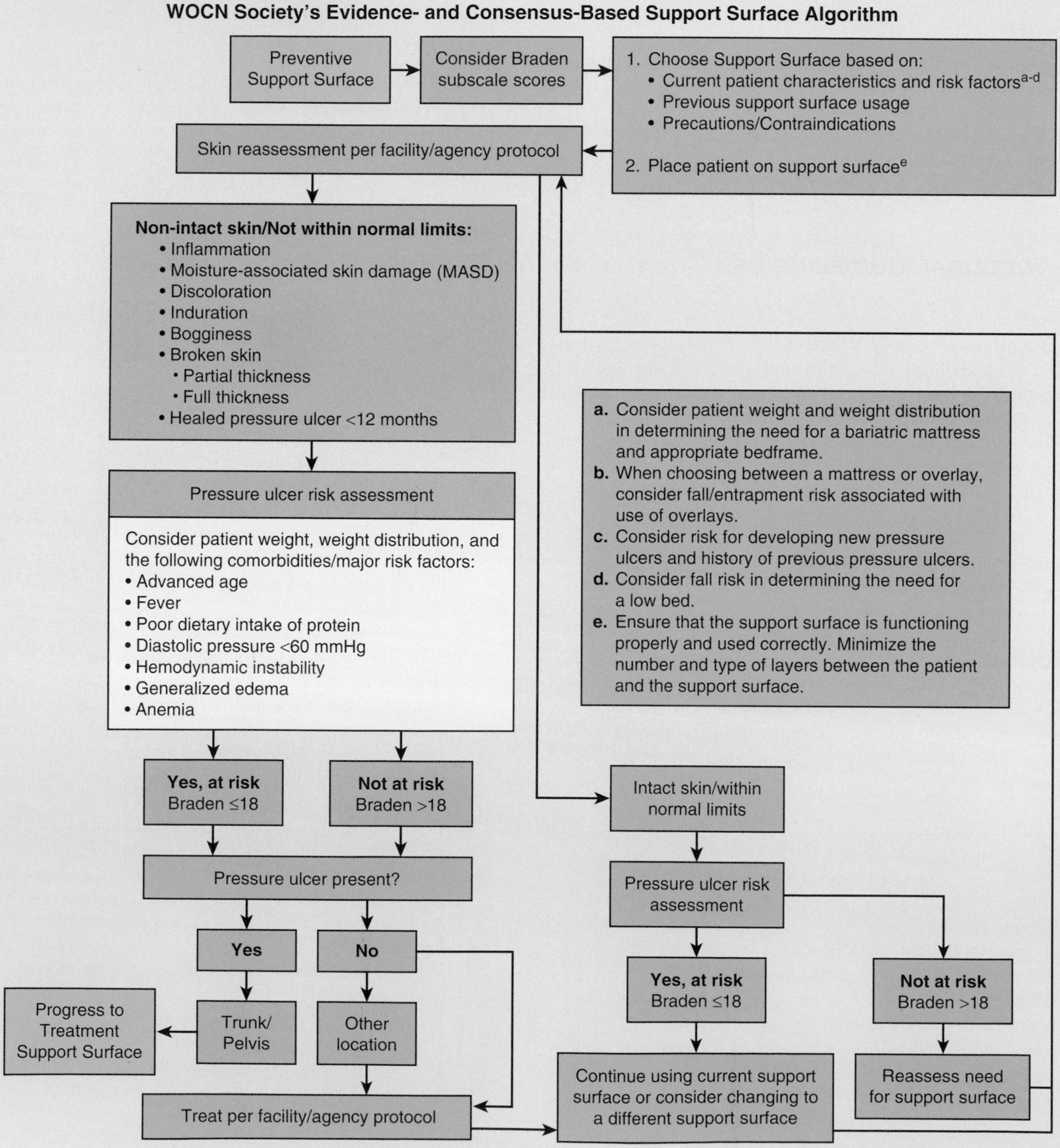

WOCN Society's Evidence- and Consensus-Based Support Surface Algorithm

Preventive Support Surface → Consider Braden subscale scores →

1. Choose Support Surface based on:
   - Current patient characteristics and risk factors[a-d]
   - Previous support surface usage
   - Precautions/Contraindications
2. Place patient on support surface[e]

→ Skin reassessment per facility/agency protocol

Non-intact skin/Not within normal limits:
- Inflammation
- Moisture-associated skin damage (MASD)
- Discoloration
- Induration
- Bogginess
- Broken skin
  - Partial thickness
  - Full thickness
- Healed pressure ulcer <12 months

Pressure ulcer risk assessment

Consider patient weight, weight distribution, and the following comorbidities/major risk factors:
- Advanced age
- Fever
- Poor dietary intake of protein
- Diastolic pressure <60 mmHg
- Hemodynamic instability
- Generalized edema
- Anemia

Yes, at risk Braden ≤18 | **Not at risk** Braden >18

Pressure ulcer present?

Yes → Trunk/Pelvis → Progress to Treatment Support Surface

No → Other location → Treat per facility/agency protocol

Intact skin/within normal limits → Pressure ulcer risk assessment

Yes, at risk Braden ≤18 → Continue using current support surface or consider changing to a different support surface

Not at risk Braden >18 → Reassess need for support surface

a. Consider patient weight and weight distribution in determining the need for a bariatric mattress and appropriate bedframe.
b. When choosing between a mattress or overlay, consider fall/entrapment risk associated with use of overlays.
c. Consider risk for developing new pressure ulcers and history of previous pressure ulcers.
d. Consider fall risk in determining the need for a low bed.
e. Ensure that the support surface is functioning properly and used correctly. Minimize the number and type of layers between the patient and the support surface.

FIG 26.3 Flow diagram for ordering specialty beds. (*From McNichol L et al.: Identifying the right surface for the right patient at the right time: generation and content validation of an algorithm for support surface selection,* J Wound Ostomy Continence Nurs *42(1), 2015.*)

TABLE 26.4

Support Surfaces

Category and Mechanism of Action	Indications for Use	Advantages	Disadvantages
Support Surfaces and Overlays			
Foam Overlay (Available as an Overlay or in a Full Mattress)			
Reduces pressure; the cover (top) can reduce friction and shear; base height of 7.5–10 cm (3–4 inches); see manufacturer guidelines regarding amount of body weight supported	Use for moderate- to high-risk patients	One-time charge No setup fee Cannot be punctured Available in various sizes (e.g., bed, chair, operating room table) Little maintenance Does not need electricity	Elevated body temperature Hot and may trap moisture Limited life span Plastic protective sheet needed for incontinent patients or patients with draining wounds Not indicated for those with existing stage 3 or 4 pressure injuries
Water Overlay (Available as an Overlay or in a Full Mattress)			
Redistributes pressure and pressure points because surface provides flotation by redistributing patient's weight evenly over entire support surface	Use for high-risk patients	Readily available Some control over motion sensations Easy to clean	Easily punctured Heavy Fluid motion may make procedures (e.g., dressing changes, CPR) difficult Maintenance needed to prevent microorganism growth Patient transfers out of bed are difficult Difficult to raise and lower head of bed
Gel Overlay			
Redistributes pressure because surface provides flotation by redistributing patient's weight evenly over entire support surface	Use for moderate- to high-risk patients Use for patients who are wheelchair dependent	Low maintenance Easy to clean Multiple-patient use Impermeable to needle punctures	Heavy Expensive Lacks airflow for moisture control Variable friction control
Nonpowered Air-Filled Overlay			
Redistributes pressure by lowering mean interface pressure between patient's tissue and overlay	Use for moderate- to high-risk patients Use for patients who can reposition themselves	Easy to clean Multiple-patient use Low maintenance Potential repair of some air-filled products Durable	Damaged by punctures from needles and sharps Requires routine monitoring to determine adequate inflation pressure Patient transfers out of bed can be difficult
Low-Air-Loss Overlay (Available as an Overlay or in a Full Mattress)			
Maintains constant and slight air movement against patient's skin; redistributes pressure, assists in managing the heat and humidity (microclimate) of the skin	Use for moderate- to high-risk patients	Easy to clean Maintains constant inflation Deflates to facilitate transfer and CPR Moisture control Fabric covering overlay is air permeable, bacteria impermeable, and waterproof Reduces shear and friction Setup provided by manufacturer	Damaged by needles and sharps Can be noisy Requires electricity, some are available with short backup battery In home may need to purchase backup generator in case of loss of electrical power
Specialty Beds			
Air-Fluidized Bed			
Bedframe contains silicone-coated beads and provides pressure redistribution by the fluid-like medium that is created by forcing air through beads, resulting in immersion and envelopment of the patient	Use for high-risk patients Use for patients with stage 3 or 4 pressure injuries or burns	Less frequent turning or repositioning Improved patient comfort Becomes firm for CPR or other treatments when device is turned "off" Reduces shear, friction, and edema to site May facilitate management of copious wound drainage or incontinence Setup provided by manufacturer	Continuous circulation of warm, dry air may increase patient risk for dehydration Possible increase in room temperature Patient may experience disorientation Patient transfer difficult Heavy Expensive May not be wide enough for use with obese patients or patients with contractures Patient cannot lie prone because of risk of suffocation

Continued

TABLE 26.4
Support Surfaces—cont'd

Category and Mechanism of Action	Indications for Use	Advantages	Disadvantages
Low–Air-Loss Bed			
Bedframe with series of connected air-filled pillows; the flow of air controls the amount of pressure in each pillow and assists in managing the heat and humidity (microclimate) of the patient's skin; redistributes pressure	Use for patients who need pressure redistribution, those who cannot be repositioned frequently, or those who have skin breakdown on more than one surface Contraindicated in patients with unstable spinal column	Can raise and lower head and foot of bed Easy transfer in and out of bed Setup provided by manufacturer	Portable motor can be noisy Bed surface material slippery; patients can easily slide down mattress or out of bed when being transferred
Kinetic Therapy Bed			
Provides continuous passive motion to promote mobilization of pulmonary secretions and low air loss and provides pressure redistribution	Used primarily to facilitate pulmonary hygiene in patients with acute respiratory conditions Should not be used when the patient is hemodynamically unstable	Reduces pulmonary complications associated with restricted mobility	Does not reduce shear or moisture Cannot be used with cervical or skeletal traction Possible motion sickness initially

Data from Doughty D, McNichol L: *Wound, Ostomy and Continence Nurses Society (WOCN): Core curriculum: wound management,* Philadelphia, 2016, Wound, Ostomy, and Continence Society; Wound, Ostomy and Continence Nurses Society (WOCN): *Guideline for prevention and management of pressure ulcers, WOCN clinical practice guideline series,* ed 2, Mt. Laurel, NJ: 2016, Author.

CPR, Cardiopulmonary resuscitation.

PROCEDURAL GUIDELINE 26.1 *Selection of a Pressure-Redistribution Support Surface—cont'd*

length of third-party reimbursement for the surface for home care support surface usage.

   c. Consult with agency home care or discharge planning if the device is anticipated for long-term use. Specific procedures and evaluations are needed for continuity of surface when patient is transferred to extended care or discharged home.

9. Choose the appropriate surface (Table 26.4).
   a. Pressure-redistribution devices redistribute the pressure/load over the patient's body to reduce the overall pressure and avoid areas of localized pressure (WOCN, 2016). Surfaces providing pressure redistribution include therapeutic mattress replacements, nonpowered and powered (e.g., moving) surfaces, low-air-loss beds and mattresses, and air-fluidized beds (Berlowitz et al., 2018; Doughty and McNichol, 2016a). Pressure-redistribution surfaces are also used in the operating room for individuals who are at high risk or for lengthy procedures (Broome et al., 2015).
   b. Use a nonpowered support surface if patient can assume a variety of positions without bearing weight on a pressure injury without bottoming out. Bottoming out makes the support surface ineffective because it is inadequate for patient's weight, and the body sinks too deeply into the surface.

Safe Patient Care *Hand checks are a satisfactory but subjective method for assessing for "bottoming out" of static air overlay mattresses. According to the NPUAP (2014b), the hand-check method is inappropriate for replacement mattresses and integrated bed systems (bedframe and support surfaces) (Call et al., 2015; WOCN, 2016).*

   c. Select a powered support surface when patient cannot assume a variety of positions without bearing weight on a pressure injury, if patient fully compresses the nonpowered support surface, or if the pressure injury does not show evidence of healing. Alternating or powered mattresses are associated with lower incidence of pressure injuries compared with standard mattresses (Berlowitz et al., 2018; Doughty and McNichol, 2016a).
   d. High-specification foam is effective in decreasing the incidence of pressure injuries in fairly high-risk patients, including older adults and patients with fractures of the neck and femur (Doughty and McNichol, 2016a; McInnes et al., 2015; WOCN, 2016).
   e. Patients with stage 3 or 4 pressure injuries on multiple turning surfaces often benefit from an air-fluidized bed (Doughty and McNichol, 2016a).
   f. When excess moisture is a potential risk, a support surface that provides airflow is important in drying the skin and reducing the incidence of pressure injuries (NPUAP, 2014b; WOCN, 2016).
10. Perform hand hygiene. Position patient onto surface. Avoid applying shear or friction when positioning patient. Observe for side effects associated with specific pressure-reducing surface (e.g., nausea, dizziness).
11. Assist patient to comfortable position and raise side rails (as appropriate) and lower bed to lowest position.
12. Place nurse call system within accessible reach; instruct patient in use.
13. Document pressure injury risk assessment and skin assessment, the support surface selected, and patient response to the surface (see specific skills for recording and reporting details).

✦ SKILL 26.2 Treatment of Pressure Injuries and Wound Management

Purpose

A wound environment conducive to healing is achieved by using topical wound therapy with the following objectives: control or eliminate causative factors, provide systemic support to reduce existing and potential cofactors, prevent and manage infection, cleanse the wound, remove nonviable tissue, maintain appropriate level of moisture, eliminate dead space, control odor, eliminate or minimize pain, and protect the periwound skin (Armstrong et al., 2018; Bryant and Nix, 2016b). The cause of a wound must be determined before wound therapy is instituted. For example, if the contributing causes of a pressure injury (pressure, shear, friction, moisture) are not addressed, the tissue damage continues, and healing does not occur. The choice of topical treatment (dressings and solutions) is dictated by these objectives.

Delegation and Collaboration

The skill of treating pressure injuries and dressing changes cannot be delegated to nursing assistive personnel (NAP). The nurse instructs the NAP to:

- Report immediately to the nurse pain, fever, or any wound drainage.
- Report immediately to the nurse any change in skin integrity.
- Report any potential contamination to existing dressing such as patient incontinence or dislodgement of the dressing.

Equipment

- Clean gloves
- Sterile gloves *(optional)*
- Goggles and cover gown (if splash is a risk)
- Plastic bag for dressing disposal
- Wound-measuring device
- Cotton-tipped applicators
- Normal saline or cleansing agent (as ordered)
- Topical agent or solution (as ordered)
- Dressings
- Hypoallergenic tape if needed
- Irrigating syringe *(optional)*

ASSESSMENT

1. Identify patient using at least two identifiers (e.g., name and birthday or name and medical record number) according to agency policy. *Rationale: Ensures correct patient. Complies with The Joint Commission standards and improves patient safety (TJC, 2019).*
2. Review accuracy of health care provider's order. *Rationale: Ensures administration of proper medication and treatment.*

Safe Patient Care *Verify that the order is consistent with established wound care guidelines and outcomes for a patient. If the order is not consistent with guidelines or varies from the identified outcome for a patient, review with the health care team.*

3. Assess patient's level of comfort on pain scale of 0 to 10. If patient is in pain, determine if prn pain medication has been ordered and administer. *Rationale: Dressing change should not be traumatic for patient; evaluate wound pain before, during, and after wound care management (Hopf et al., 2016).*
4. Determine if patient has allergies to topical agents. *Rationale: Topical agents could contain elements that cause localized skin reactions.*
5. Close room door and bedside curtains. *Rationale: Provides privacy.*
6. Position patient to allow dressing removal and position plastic bag for dressing disposal. *Rationale: Provides an accessible area for dressing change. Proper disposal of old dressing promotes proper handling of contaminated waste.*
7. Perform hand hygiene and apply clean gloves. Remove and discard old dressing. *Rationale: Reduces transmission of microorganisms and prevents accidental exposure to body fluids.*
8. Assess patient's wounds using the following wound parameters and continue ongoing wound assessment per agency policy. NOTE: This may be done during wound care procedure. *Rationale: Determines effectiveness of wound care and guides treatment plan of care (WOCN, 2016).*
   a. **Wound location.** Describe body site where wound is located.
   b. **Stage of wound for pressure injuries.** Describe extent of tissue destruction (Box 26.1). *Rationale: Staging is based on depth of tissue destruction (Edsberg et al., 2016). Wounds are documented as unstageable if wound base is not visible (NPUAP, 2016; NPUAP et al., 2014a).*
   c. **Wound size.** Length, width, and depth of wound are measured per agency protocol. Use disposable measuring guide for length and width. Use cotton-tipped applicator to assess depth (see illustration). *Rationale: Injury size changes as healing progresses; therefore, longest and widest areas of wound change over time. Measuring width and length by measuring consistent areas provides consistent measurement (Nix, 2016).*
   d. **Presence of undermining, sinus tracts, or tunnels.** Use sterile cotton-tipped applicator to measure depth and, if needed, a gloved finger to examine wound edges. *Rationale: Wound depth determines amount of tissue loss.*
   e. **Condition of wound bed.** Describe type and percentage of tissue in wound bed. *Rationale: Approximate percentage of each type of tissue in wound provides critical information on progress of wound healing and choice of dressing. Wound with high percentage of black tissue requires debridement;*

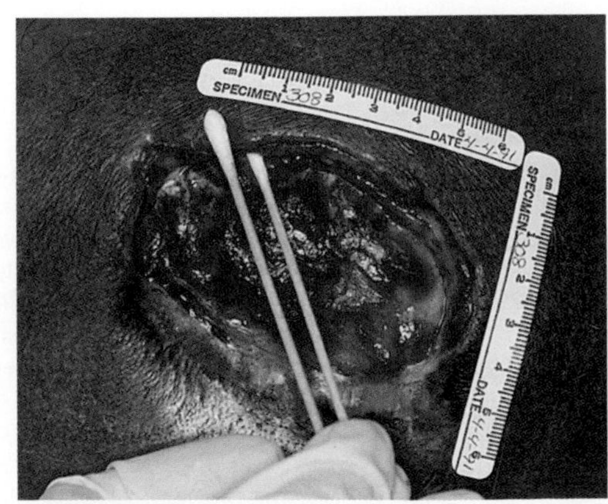

STEP 8c Measuring wound width, length, and undermining of skin.

BOX 26.1

Staging of Pressure Injuries

Stage 1

Pressure Injury: Nonblanchable Erythema of Intact Skin

Intact skin with a localized area of nonblanchable erythema, which may appear differently in darkly pigmented skin. Presence of blanchable erythema or changes in sensation, temperature, or firmness may precede visual changes. Color changes do not include purple or maroon discoloration; these may indicate deep tissue pressure injury.

Lightly Pigmented

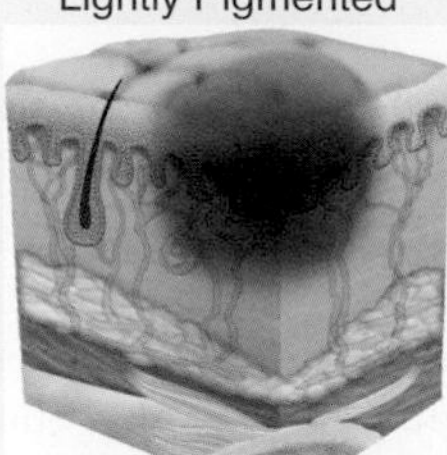

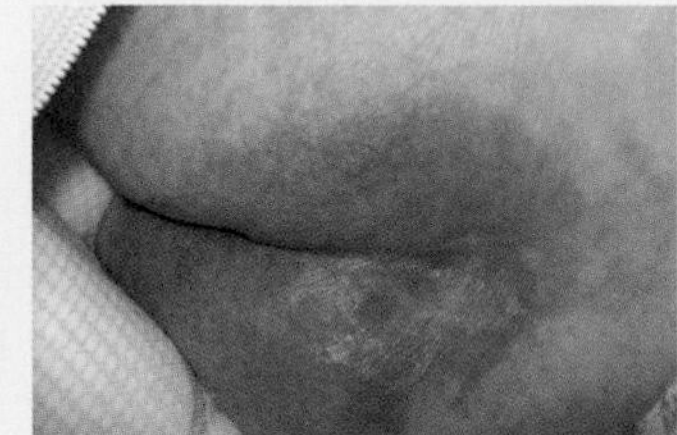

Darkly Pigmented

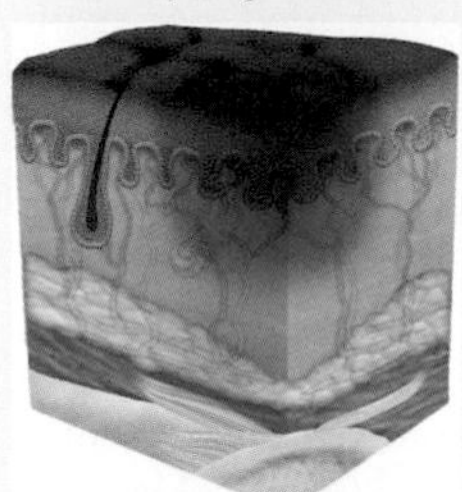

Stage 2

Pressure Injury: Partial-Thickness Skin Loss With Exposed Dermis

Partial-thickness loss of skin with exposed dermis, in which the wound bed is viable, pink or red, and moist and may also present as an intact or ruptured serum-filled blister. Adipose (fat) and deeper tissues are not visible. Granulation tissue, slough, and eschar are not present. These injuries commonly result from adverse microclimate and shear in the skin over the pelvis and shear in the heel. This stage should not be used to describe moisture-associated skin damage (MASD), including incontinence-associated dermatitis (IAD), intertriginous dermatitis (ITD), medical adhesive–related skin injury (MARSI), or traumatic wounds (skin tears, burns, abrasions).

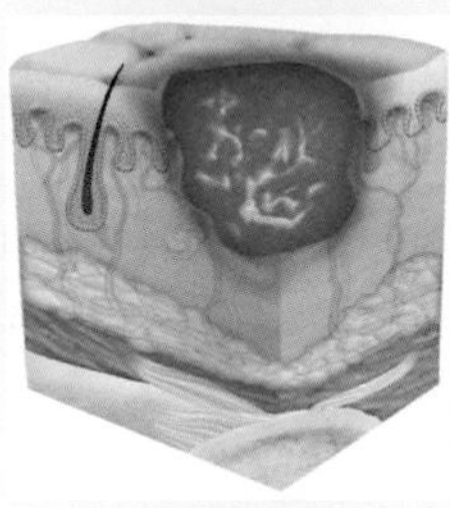

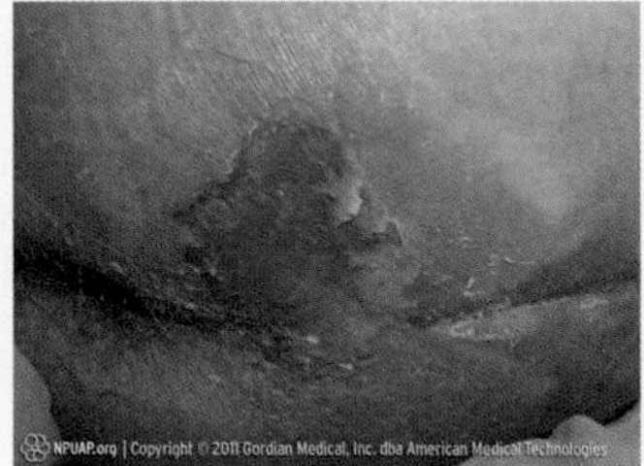

Stage 3

Pressure Injury: Full-Thickness Skin Loss

Full-thickness loss of skin, in which adipose (fat) is visible in the injury and granulation tissue and epibole (rolled wound edges) are often present. Slough and/or eschar may be visible. The depth of tissue damage varies by anatomical location; areas of significant adiposity can develop deep wounds. Undermining and tunneling may occur. Fascia, muscle, tendon, ligament, cartilage, and/or bone are not exposed. If slough or eschar obscures the extent of tissue loss, this is an unstageable pressure injury.

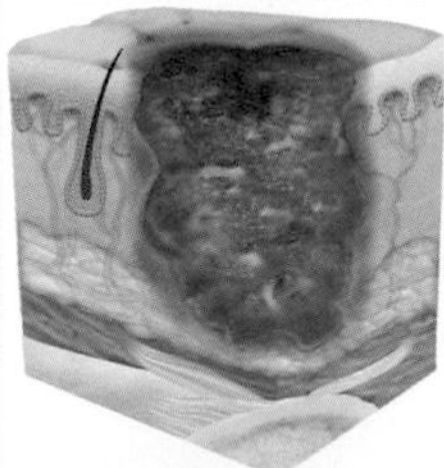

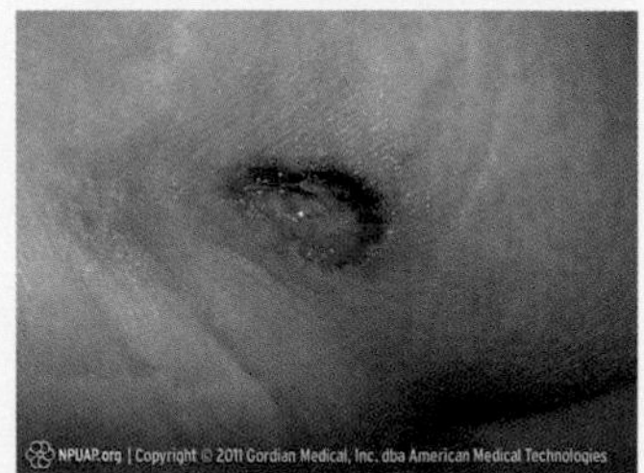

Stage 4

Pressure Injury: Full-Thickness Skin and Tissue Loss

Full-thickness skin and tissue loss with exposed or directly palpable fascia, muscle, tendon, ligament, cartilage, or bone in the injury. Slough and/or eschar may be visible. Epibole (rolled edges), undermining, and/or tunneling often occur. Depth varies by anatomical location. If slough or eschar obscures the extent of tissue loss, this is an unstageable pressure injury.

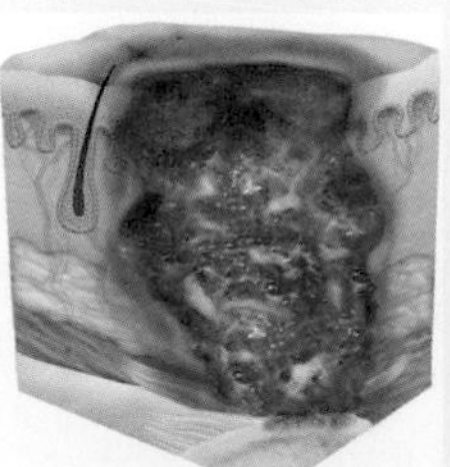

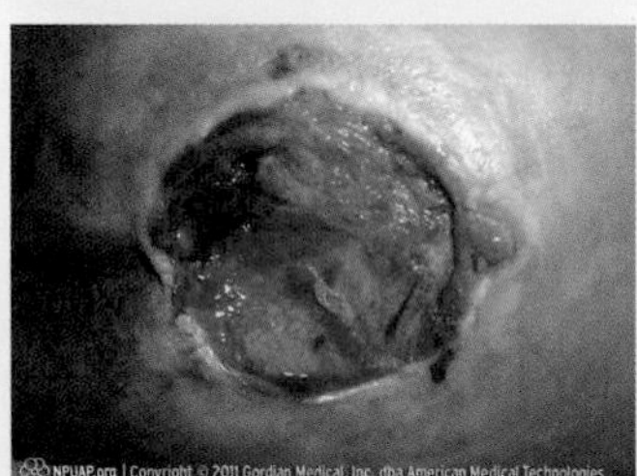

Deep Tissue Pressure Injury

Persistent Nonblanchable Deep Red, Maroon, or Purple Discoloration

Intact or nonintact skin with localized area of persistent nonblanchable deep red, maroon, or purple discoloration or epidermal separation revealing a dark wound bed or blood-filled blister. Pain and temperature change often precede skin-color changes. Discoloration may appear differently in darkly pigmented skin. This injury results from intense and/or prolonged pressure and shear forces at the bone–muscle interface. The wound may evolve rapidly to reveal the actual extent of tissue injury or may resolve without tissue loss. If necrotic tissue, subcutaneous tissue, granulation tissue, fascia, muscle, or other underlying structures are visible, this indicates a full-thickness pressure injury (unstageable, stage 3 or 4). Do not use deep tissue pressure injury (DTPI) to describe vascular, traumatic, neuropathic, or dermatological conditions.

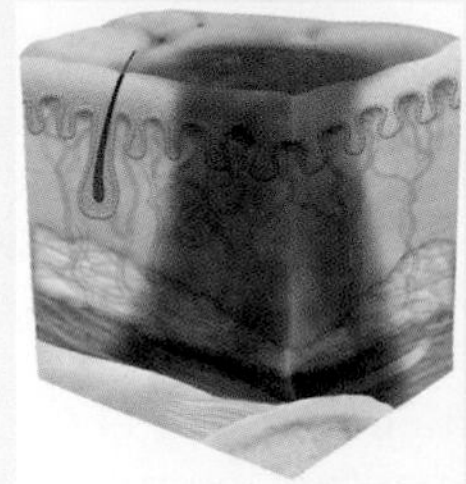

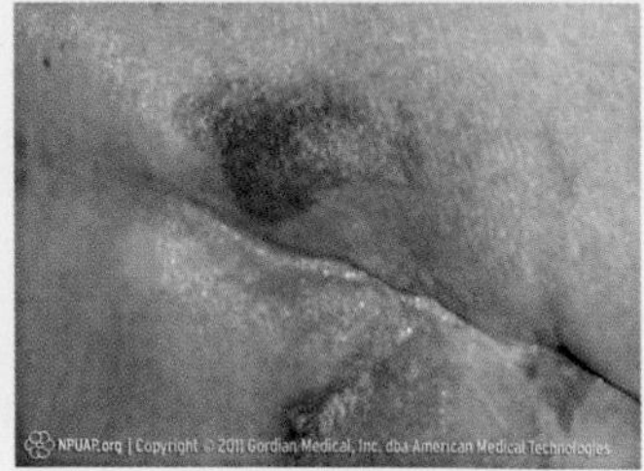

BOX 26.1

Staging of Pressure Injuries—cont'd

Unstageable Pressure Injury

Obscured Full-Thickness Skin and Tissue Loss

Full-thickness skin and tissue loss in which the extent of tissue damage within the injury cannot be confirmed because it is obscured by slough or eschar. If slough or eschar is removed, a stage 3 or 4 pressure injury will be revealed. Stable eschar (i.e., dry, adherent, intact without erythema or fluctuance) on the heel or ischemic limb should not be softened or removed.

Dark Eschar

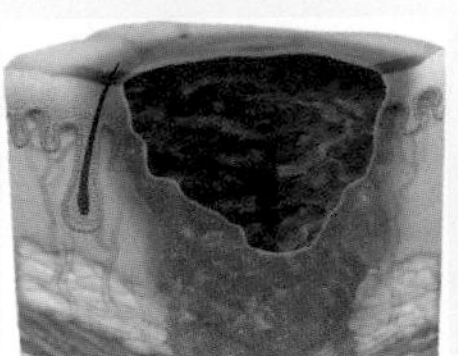

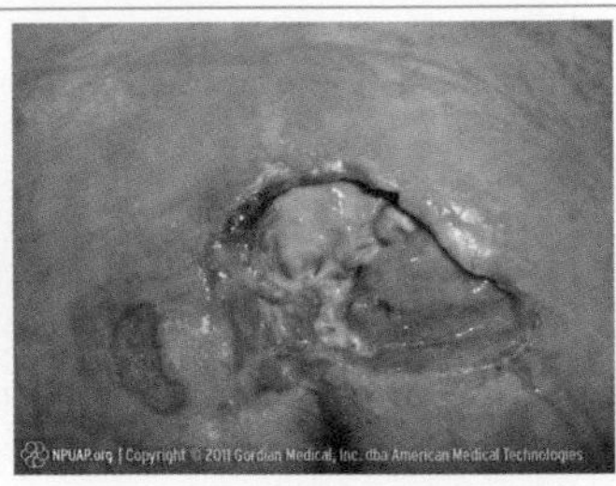

Slough Eschar

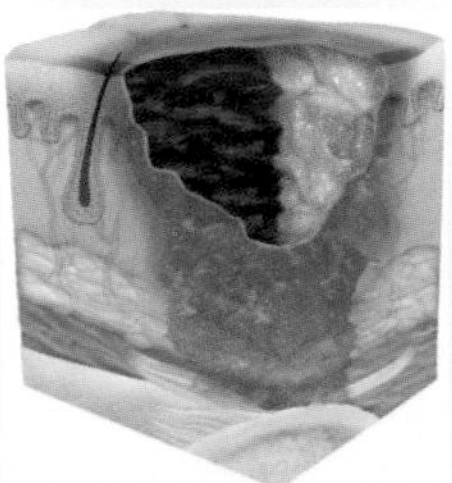

Used with permission of the National Pressure Ulcer Advisory Panel, (NPUAP), European Pressure Ulcer Advisory Panel (EPUAP), and Pan Pacific Pressure Injury Alliance (PPPIA): *Prevention and treatment of pressure ulcers: quick reference guide,* July 22, 2016.

BOX 26.2

Skin Assessment of Pressure Injuries: Patients With Darkly Pigmented Skin

- Patients with darkly pigmented skin cannot be assessed for pressure injury risk by examining only skin color. Changes in sensation, temperature, or tissue consistency may precede visual skin changes (Ratliff et al., 2017; WOCN, 2016).
- Use natural lighting, but note that visual inspection techniques to identify pressure injuries are ineffective in darkly pigmented skin. Skin inspection techniques for individuals with darkly pigmented skin must include assessment of temperature, edema, and changes in tissue consistency as compared with the surrounding skin (WOCN, 2016).
- Assess localized skin color changes. Any of the following may appear:
  - Color remains unchanged when pressure is applied.
  - Color changes occur at site of pressure, which differ from patient's usual skin color.
  - If patient previously had a pressure injury, that area of skin may be lighter than original color.
  - Localized area of skin may be purple/blue or violet instead of red. Purple or maroon discoloration may indicate deep tissue injury (WOCN, 2016).
- Circumscribed area of intact skin may be warm to touch. As tissue changes color, intact skin will feel cool to touch. **NOTE:** Gloves may decrease sensitivity to changes in skin temperature.
- Localized heat (inflammation) is detected by making comparisons to surrounding skin.
- Localized area of warmth eventually will be replaced by area of coolness, which is a sign of tissue devitalization.
- Edema may occur with induration of more than 15 mm in diameter and may appear taut and shiny.
- Palpate tissue consistency in surrounding tissues to identify any changes in tissue consistency between area of injury and normal tissue.
- Patient complains of discomfort at a site that is predisposed to pressure injury development (e.g., bony prominence, under medical devices).

Adapted from Nix DP: Skin and wound inspection and assessment. In Bryant RA, Nix DP, editors: *Acute and chronic wounds: current management concepts*, ed 5, St. Louis, 2016, Mosby; Wound Ostomy and Continence Nurses Society (WOCN): *Guideline for prevention and management of pressure ulcers, WOCN clinical practice guideline series*, Mt. Laurel, NJ, 2016, WOCN Society.

yellow tissue or slough tissue may indicate presence of infection or colonization; and granulation tissue indicates that wound is moving toward healing.

f. **Volume of exudate.** Describe amount, characteristics, odor, and color. *Rationale: Amount and type of exudate may indicate type and frequency of dressing changes (Bates-Jensen, 2016).*

g. **Condition of periwound skin.** Examine skin for breaks, dryness, and presence of rash, swelling, redness, or warmth. Modify assessment based on patient's skin color (Box 26.2). *Rationale: Impaired skin condition at edge of injury indicates progressive tissue damage.*

h. **Wound edges.** Examine edges for condition of tissue. *Rationale: Provides information regarding epithelialization, chronicity, and etiology.*

9. Assess periwound skin; check for maceration, redness, denuded tissue. *Rationale: Maceration on periwound skin shows need to alter choice of wound dressing. Skin condition determines if skin barrier needed.*

10. Remove gloves and discard in appropriate receptacle. Perform hand hygiene. *Rationale: Reduces transmission of microorganisms.*

Safe Patient Care *Repeated hand hygiene will be necessary as you assess other pressure areas. Different organisms contaminate different wounds.*

11. Assess for factors affecting wound healing: poor perfusion, immunosuppression, or preexisting infection. *Rationale: Factors affect treatment and wound healing.*
12. Assess patient's nutritional status (see Chapter 13). Clinically significant malnutrition is present if (1) serum albumin level is less than 3.5 g/dL, (2) lymphocyte count is less than 1800/mm^3, or (3) body weight decreases more than 15% (see illustration; WOCN, 2016). *Rationale: Delayed wound healing occurs in poorly nourished patients.*

Safe Patient Care *When you suspect malnutrition, obtain a nutritional consultation to modify patient's diet to promote wound healing.*

13. Assess patient's or family caregiver's knowledge, experience, and health literacy level. *Rationale: Ensures patient has the capacity to obtain, communicate, process, and understand basic health information (CDC, 2016).*
14. Assess patient's and family caregiver's understanding of prevention, treatment, and factors contributing to recurrence of pressure injuries (WOCN, 2016). *Rationale: Patient and family caregiver need to partner with health care providers to prevent further skin breakdown.*

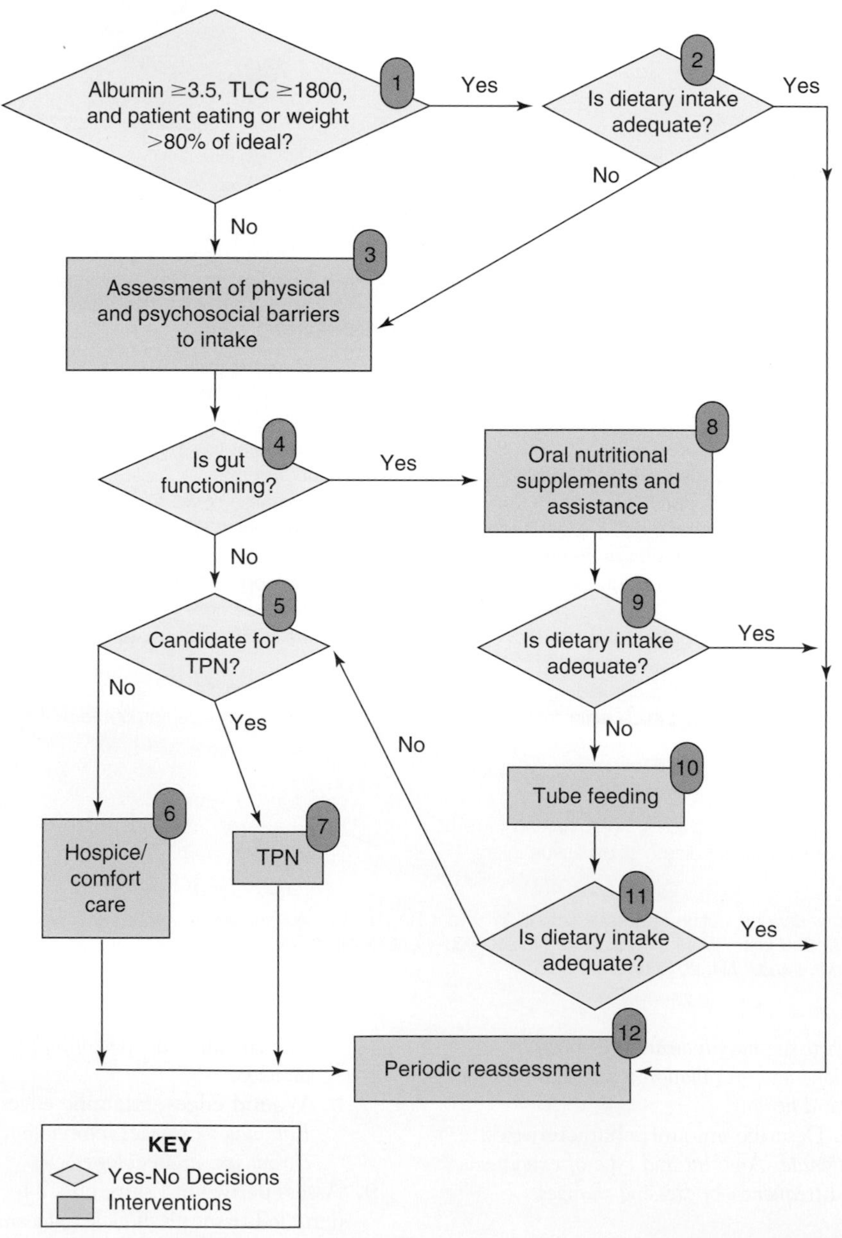

STEP 12 Nutritional assessment and support. *TLC*, Total lymphocyte count; *TPN*, total parenteral nutrition. *(From Bergstrom N et al:* Treatment of pressure injuries, *AHCPR Pub. No. 95-0652, Rockville, MD, 1994, Agency for Health Care Policy and Research, Public Health Service, US Department of Health and Human Services.)*

STEP	RATIONALE
PLANNING	
1. Expected outcomes following completion of procedure:	
• Wound drainage decreases.	Reflects decrease in inflammatory process and progress toward healing.
• Granulation tissue is present in wound base.	Evidence that wound is healing.
• Skin surrounding injury remains healthy and intact.	No additional damage is evident; dressing is appropriate to contain wound drainage.
• Nutritional intake meets caloric and nutrient targets.	Nutritional therapy provides adequate protein to support wound healing.
• Patient's overall skin remains intact and without further breakdown.	Patient remains at risk for further breakdown while existing injury heals.
• Patient or family caregiver able to describe signs of wound healing and wound deterioration.	Demonstrates learning.
2. Explain procedure to patient and family caregiver.	Preparatory explanations relieve anxiety, correct any misconceptions about injury and its treatment, and offer an opportunity for patient and family caregiver education.
3. Prepare the following equipment and supplies:	
a. Normal saline or other wound-cleaning agent in sterile solution container and gloves	Used to clean injury surface before applying topical agents and new dressing.
Safe Patient Care *Use only noncytotoxic agents to clean pressure injuries.*	
b. Prescribed topical agent:	
(1) Enzyme debriding agents. (Follow specific manufacturer directions for frequency of application.) *Or*	Enzymes debride dead tissue to clean injury surface. Enzymes are not applied to healthy tissue.
(2) Topical antibiotics	Topical antibiotics decrease bioburden of wound and should be considered for use if no healing is noted after 2 to 4 weeks of optimal care (WOCN, 2016).
c. Appropriate dressing based on pressure injury characteristics, principles of wound management, and patient care setting. Dressing options include (Table 26.5):	Dressing should maintain moist environment for wound while keeping surrounding skin dry (Bryant and Nix, 2016b).
(1) Gauze—Apply as moist dressing, a dry cover dressing when using enzymes or topical antibiotics, or a means to deliver solution to wound.	Gauze delivers moisture to wound and is absorptive.
(2) Transparent film dressing—Apply over superficial injuries with minimal or no exudate and skin subjected to friction.	Maintains moist environment and offers intact skin protection.
(3) Hydrocolloid dressing	Maintains moist environment to facilitate wound healing while protecting wound base.
(4) Hydrogel—available in sheet or in tube	Maintains moist environment to facilitate wound healing.
(5) Calcium alginate	Highly absorbent of wound exudate in heavily draining wounds.
(6) Foam dressings	Protective and prevents wound dehydration; also absorbs moderate to large amounts of drainage. Foam dressings (e.g., Allevyn) can be used in the prevention of pressure injury in high-risk patients or those undergoing long surgeries (Byrne et al., 2016).
(7) Silver impregnated dressings/gels	Controls bacterial burden in wound.
(8) Wound fillers	Fills shallow wounds, hydrates, and absorbs.
d. Hypoallergenic tape or adhesive dressing sheet	Used to secure nonadherent dressing. Prevents skin irritation and tearing.

TABLE 26.5

Dressings by Pressure Injury Stage

Pressure Injury Stage	Pressure Injury Status	Dressing	Comments*	Expected Change	Adjuvants
1	Intact	None Transparent dressing Hydrocolloid	Allows visual assessment. Protects from shear. Do not use transparent dressing in presence of excessive moisture. Hydrocolloid does not allow visual assessment.	Resolves slowly without epidermal loss over 7 to 14 days	Turning schedule. Support hydration. Nutritional support. Use pressure-redistribution bed or chair cushion.
2	Clean	Composite film Hydrocolloid Hydrogel covered with foam or gauze dressing	Limits shear. Change when seal of dressing breaks; maximal wear time 7 days. Provides moist environment.	Heals through re-epithelialization	See previous stage. Manage incontinence.
3	Clean	Hydrocolloid Hydrogel covered with foam dressing	Change when seal of dressing breaks; maximum wear time 7 days. Apply over wound to protect and absorb moisture.	Heals through granulation and reepithelialization	See previous stages. Evaluate pressure-redistribution needs.
		Calcium alginate	Use when there is significant exudate. Cover with secondary dressing.		
		Gauze	Use with normal saline or other prescribed solution. Wring out excess solution; unfold to make contact with wound. Cover with dry dressing tape in place.		
4	Clean	Hydrogel covered with foam dressing	See stage 3: clean.	Heals through granulation, scar tissue development, and reepithelialization	Surgical consultation may be necessary for closure. See stages 1, 2, and 3.
		Calcium alginate	Used with significant exudate; must cover with secondary dressing.		
		Gauze	See stage 3: clean.		
Unstageable	Wound covered with eschar	Adherent film	Facilitates softening of eschar.	Eschar lifts at edges as healing progresses.	See previous stages. Surgical consultation may be considered for debridement.
		Gauze plus ordered solution	Delivers solution and may soften the eschar.		May be considered for slow debridement.
		Enzymes	Breaks down eschar, providing debridement.	Eschar loosens over time.	
		None	If eschar is dry and intact and debridement is not part of the plan of care, no dressing is used, allowing eschar to act as physiological cover.		

*As with all occlusive dressings, wounds should not be clinically infected.

STEP	RATIONALE
IMPLEMENTATION	
1. Assemble remaining supplies at bedside. Close room door or bedside curtains.	Organizes procedure and maintains patient privacy.
2. Perform hand hygiene and apply clean gloves. Open sterile packages and topical solution containers (see Chapter 5). Keep dressings sterile. Wear goggles, mask, and moisture-proof cover gown if potential for contamination from spray exists when cleaning wound.	Reduces transmission of microorganisms.
3. Remove bed linen and arrange patient's gown to expose wound and surrounding skin. Keep remaining body parts draped.	Prevents unnecessary exposure of body parts.
4. Moisten gauze in cleaning solution. Clean wound thoroughly with normal saline or prescribed wound-cleaning agent moving from least contaminated to most contaminated area. For deep injuries, clean with saline delivered with irrigating syringe as ordered. Remove gloves and discard.	Cleaning wound removes wound exudate and/or dressing residue and reduces surface bacteria.
5. Perform hand hygiene and apply clean or sterile gloves (refer to agency policy).	Maintains aseptic technique during cleaning, measuring, and applying dressings.
6. Apply topical agents to wound using cotton-tipped applicators or gauze as ordered:	
a. Enzymes	Follow manufacturer directions for method and frequency of application. Be aware of which solutions inactivate enzymes and avoid their use in wound cleaning.
(1) Apply small amount of enzyme debridement ointment directly to necrotic areas. *Do not apply enzyme to surrounding skin.*	Thin layer absorbs and acts more effectively than thick layer. Excess medication irritates surrounding skin (Bryant and Nix, 2016b). Proper distribution of ointment ensures effective action.
Safe Patient Care *If using an enzymatic debriding agent, do not use wound-cleaning agents with metals.*	
(2) Place moist gauze dressing directly over wound followed by a dry dressing and tape in place. Follow specific manufacturer recommendation for type of dressing material to use to cover a pressure injury when using enzymes. Tape dressing in place.	Protects wound and prevents removal of ointment during turning or repositioning.
b. Antibacterials (e.g., bacitracin, metronidazole, and silver sulfadiazine).	Reduces bacterial growth.
7. Apply prescribed wound dressing:	
a. Hydrogel:	Hydrogel dressings are designed to hydrate and bring moisture to wound (Bryant and Nix, 2016b).
(1) Cover surface of wound with thick layer of amorphous hydrogel or cut sheet to fit wound base.	Provides moist environment to facilitate wound healing.
(2) Apply secondary dressing such as dry gauze; tape in place.	Holds hydrogel against wound surface because amorphous hydrogel (in tube) or sheet form does not adhere to wound and requires secondary dressing to hold it in place.
(3) If using impregnated gauze, pack loosely into wound; cover with secondary gauze dressing and tape.	A loosely packed dressing delivers gel to wound base and allows any wound debris to be trapped in gauze.
b. Calcium alginate:	Alginate dressings absorb serous fluid or exudate, forming a nonadhesive hydrophilic gel, which conforms to shape of wound (Bryant and Nix, 2016b). Use in heavily draining wounds.
(1) Lightly pack wound with alginate using sterile cotton-tipped applicator or gloved finger.	The dressing swells and increases in size; tight packing can compromise blood flow to the tissues.
(2) Apply secondary dressing and tape in place.	
c. Transparent film dressing; hydrocolloid; and foam dressings (see Chapter 27).	

STEP	RATIONALE

Safe Patient Care *Use transparent dressings for autolytic debridement of noninfected superficial pressure injuries. A hydrocolloid dressing protects skin from friction and/or provides moisture to the wound. Some brands have custom shapes available for specific anatomical parts such as heels, elbows, and sacrum.*

STEP	RATIONALE
8. Reposition patient comfortably off wound/pressure injury.	Eliminates pressure over wound.
9. Remove and dispose of gloves. Dispose of soiled supplies in appropriate receptacle. Perform hand hygiene.	Reduces transmission of microorganisms.
10. Assist patient to comfortable position.	Enhances patient comfort and relaxation.
11. Raise side rails (as appropriate) and lower bed to lowest position	Provides for patient safety and reduces the risk for falls.
12. Place nurse call system within accessible reach; instruct patient in use.	Ensures patient can call for assistance if needed.

EVALUATION

STEP	RATIONALE
1. Observe skin surrounding wound/injury for inflammation, edema, and tenderness.	Determines progress of wound healing.
2. Inspect dressings and exposed injuries, observing for drainage, foul odor, and tissue necrosis. Monitor patient for signs and symptoms of infection: fever and elevated white blood cell (WBC) count.	Injuries can become infected.
3. Compare subsequent injury measurements, using one of the scales designed to measure wound healing such as PUSH Tool or Bates Wound Assessment Tool (BWAT).	Allows comparison of serial measurements to evaluate wound healing. Provides standard method of data collection that demonstrates injury progress or lack thereof.
4. **Use Teach-Back:** "I want to be sure that you understand why we measure and assess your pressure injury on an ongoing basis. Can you tell me why we want to measure the injury and look at the tissue type and surrounding skin?" Revise your instruction now or develop a plan for revised patient/family caregiver teaching if patient/family caregiver is not able to teach back correctly.	Determines patient's/family caregiver's level of understanding of instructional topic.

Unexpected Outcomes	Related Interventions
1. Skin surrounding injury becomes macerated.	• Reduce exposure of surrounding skin to topical agents and moisture. • Select dressing that has increased moisture-absorbing capacity.
2. Injury becomes deeper, with increased drainage and/or development of necrotic tissue.	• Review current wound care management. • Consult with interprofessional team regarding changes in wound care regimen. • Obtain wound cultures (see Chapter 9).
3. Pressure injury extends beyond original margins.	• Monitor for systemic signs and symptoms of poor wound healing such as abnormal laboratory results (WBC count, levels of hemoglobin/hematocrit, serum albumin, serum prealbumin, total proteins), weight loss, and fluid imbalances. • Assess and revise current turning schedule. • Consider alternate pressure-redistribution devices.

Recording

- Record appearance and condition of the wound, type of topical agent or dressing used, presence of pain and how addressed, and patient's response in medical record.
- Document your evaluation of patient learning.

Hand-Off Reporting

- Report any deterioration in wound appearance to the health care provider. Describe the location of the wound; type and percentage of wound tissue; presence or absence of wound drainage; odor; type, and quantity of dressings used; the location of the dressings (for the next dressing change); and patient's response.

SPECIAL CONSIDERATIONS

Patient-Centered Care

- Be mindful that patients with dark skin may need a close examination for skin color changes (see Box 26.2). Also, let patients and family caregivers help identify skin color changes (as appropriate). The patient and family caregiver are familiar with bodily changes and are an important resource in your assessment.

- When assessing the patient's skin for the presence of skin issues, a change in tissue may be noted only by touching the skin to note temperature changes. It is important to educate the patient and family caregiver why touch is important when assessing the skin.
- Describe what you are doing when you gently palpate areas of the skin or apply treatments to wounds.

Patient Education

- When assessing a patient for pressure injury risk, describe to the patient and family caregivers the importance of determining possible risk factors. Informing them of the need to identify risk factors educates them on the increased risk for pressure injury development.
- Describe to patient and family caregivers what interventions will be instituted for prevention and treatment, and instruct family caregiver as appropriate.

Age-Specific

Pediatric

- Immature skin in a pediatric patient is susceptible to skin tears.
- Moist skin covered with a diaper may soften, causing skin breakdown. Reinforce wound dressings in the diaper zone with water-resistant tape. Carefully remove this tape to avoid skin stripping.

Gerontological

- In an older adult, the epidermal-dermal junction becomes flatter, putting the patient at increased risk for epidermal damage.
- Pressure injuries in an older adult have a slower and less intense inflammatory reaction; closely monitor older patients with wounds.

Home Care

- Evaluate the home environment for the use of a pressure-redistribution support surface (including a wheelchair). The bed at home for a bed-bound patient should have the appropriate type of support surface.
- Ensure that patient and family caregiver know how to use the wound products chosen.
- Choose a dressing that does not require multiple dressing changes in a 24-hour period. This decreases the amount of time that the family caregiver will need to devote to the wound management program and increases compliance.

✦ PRACTICE REFLECTIONS

Consider caring for a patient who has undergone spinal surgery, is bed bound, has no sensation in the lower extremities, and has limited ability to move. What information would you consider when planning the care for this patient at risk for skin breakdown.

1. What information is needed to consider the type of support surface for this patient?
2. What are some of the interventions you might plan to help reduce the risk factors for pressure injury occurrence?
3. Did you consider the use of products to address incontinence issues?
4. List two products that you might use.

✦ CLINICAL REVIEW QUESTIONS

1. Which of the following place a patient at risk for pressure injury? (Select all that apply.)
   1. Draining abdominal wound
   2. Hemiparesis
   3. Prior pressure injury
   4. Independently moves up in bed
   5. Artificial airway
2. You need to determine a patient's need for a support surface. What factors will you use to determine whether an air-fluidized surface would be appropriate? (Select all that apply.)
   1. Stage 3 or 4 pressure injury
   2. Prevention of development of a pressure injury
   3. High-risk patient who does not tolerate frequent repositioning.
   4. Obese patient (body mass index [BMI] greater than 35)
   5. Braden risk assessment score of 22
3. Match the dressing selection with pressure injury stage.

1. Stage 1	a. Transparent
2. Stage 2	b. Hydrocolloid
3. Stage 3	c. Hydrogel with foam
4. Stage 4	d. Calcium alginate
5. Unstageable	e. Gauze
	f. Adherent film
	g. Enzymes

Answers and Rationales for Clinical Review Questions can be found on the Evolve website.

REFERENCES

Alderden J, et al: Midrange Braden subscale scores are associated with increased risk for pressure injury development among critical care patients, *J Wound Ostomy Continence Nurs* 44(5):420, 2017.

Armstrong D, et al: Basic principles of wound management, *UpToDate* 2018. https://www.uptodate.com/contents/basic-principles-of-wound-management.

Ayello EA: CMS MDS 3.0 Section M Skin conditions in long-term care: pressure ulcers, skin tears, and moisture-associated akin damage data update, *Adv Skin Wound Care* 30(9):415, 2017.

Ayello EA, et al: Pressure ulcers. In Baranoski S, Ayello EA, editors: *Wound care essentials: practice principles*, ed 4, Philadelphia, 2015, Lippincott Williams & Wilkins.

Baath C, et al: Prevention of heel pressure ulcers among older patients from ambulance care to hospital discharge: a multi centre randomized controlled trial, *Appl Nurs Res* 30:170, 2016.

Bates-Jensen BM: Assessment of the patient with a wound. In *Core curriculum: wound management*, Philadelphia, PA, 2016, Wolters Kluwer.

Berlowitz D, et al: Prevention of pressure-induced skin and soft tissue injury, *UpToDate* 2018a. https://www.uptodate.com/contents/prevention-of-pressure-induced-skin-and-soft-tissue-injury.

Berlowitz D, et al: Epidemiology, pathogenesis, and risk assessment of pressure-induced skin and soft tissue injury, *UpToDate* 2018b. https://www.uptodate.com/contents/epidemiology-pathogenesis-and-risk-assessment-of-pressure-induced-skin-and-soft-tissue-injury.

Black J, et al: Use of wound dressings to enhance prevention of pressure ulcers caused by medical devices, *Int Wound J* 12:322, 2015.

Broome C, et al: Nursing care of the super bariatric patient: challenges and lessons learned, *Rehabil Nurs* 40:92, 2015.

Bryant RA, Nix DP: Developing and maintaining a pressure ulcer prevention program. In Bryant RA, Nix DP, editors: *Acute and chronic wounds: current management concepts*, ed 5, St. Louis, 2016a, Mosby.

Bryant RA, Nix DP: Principles of wound healing and topical management. In Bryant RA, Nix DP, editors: *Acute and chronic wounds: current management concepts*, ed 5, St. Louis, 2016b, Mosby.

Byrne J, et al: Prophylactic sacral dressing for pressure ulcer prevention in high-risk patients, *Am J Crit Care* 25(3):228–234, 2016.

Call E, et al: Hand check method: is it an effective method to monitor support surfaces for bottoming out?, A National Pressure Ulcer Advisory Position Statement 2015. http://www.npuap.org/wp-content/uploads/2012/01/Hand-Check-Position-Statement-June-2015.pdf.

Centers for Disease Control and Prevention: What is health literacy, 2016. https://www.cdc.gov/healthliteracy/learn/index.html.

Chaboyer W, et al: Adherence to evidence-based pressure injury prevention guidelines in routine clinical practice: a longitudinal study, *Int Wound J* 14:1290, 2017.

Doughty D, McNichol L: *Wound, Ostomy, and Continence Nurses Society (WOCN) Core curriculum: wound management*, Philadelphia, 2016a, Wound, Ostomy, and Continence Society.

Doughty DB, McNichol LL: General concepts related to skin and soft tissue injury caused by mechanical factors. In *Core curriculum: wound management*, Philadelphia, PA, 2016b, Wolters Kluwer.

Doughty DB, Sparks B: Wound-healing physiology. In Bryant RA, Nix DP, editors: *Acute and chronic wounds: current management concepts*, ed 5, St. Louis, 2016, Mosby.

Edsberg LE, et al: Revised National Pressure Ulcer Advisory Panel Pressure injury staging system revised pressure injury staging system, *J Wound Ostomy Continence Nurs* 43(6):585, 2016.

Haesler E: Evidence summary pressure injuries preventing medical device related pressure injuries, *Wound Pract Res* 25(4):214, 2017.

Hopf H, et al: Managing wound pain. In Bryant RA, Nix DP, editors: *Acute and chronic wounds: current management concepts*, ed 5, St. Louis, 2016, Mosby.

Hultin L, et al: Pressure mapping in elderly care: a tool to increase pressure injury knowledge and awareness among staff, *J Wound Ostomy Continence Nurs* 44(2):142, 2017.

Makic MB: Medical device–related pressure ulcers and intensive care, *J Perianesth Nurs* 30(4):336, 2015.

McInnes E, et al: Support surfaces for pressure ulcer prevention, *Cochrane Database Syst Rev* (9):CD001735, 2015.

McNichol L, et al: Identifying the right surface for the right patient at the right time: generation and content validation of an algorithm for support surface selection, *J Wound Ostomy Continence Nurs* 42(1):19, 2015.

National Pressure Ulcer Advisory Panel (NPUAP): NPUAP announces a change in terminology from pressure ulcer to pressure injury and updates the stages of pressure injury, 2016. http://www.npuap.org/national-pressure-ulcer-advisory-panel-npuap-announces-a-change-interminology-from-pressure-ulcer-to-pressure-injury-and-updates-the-stages-of-pressure-injury.

National Pressure Ulcer Advisory Panel (NPUAP), European Pressure Ulcer Advisory Panel (EPUAP) and Pan Pacific Pressure Injury Alliance (PPPIA): Haesler Emily, editor: *Prevention and treatment of pressure ulcers: quick reference guide*, Perth, Australia, 2014a, Cambridge Media.

National Pressure Ulcer Advisory Panel (NPUAP) Support Surfaces Standard Initiative: *Pressure ulcer treatment recommendations: clinical practice guidelines*, Washington, DC, 2014b, National Pressure Ulcer Advisory Panel.

Nix DP: Skin and wound inspection and assessment. In Bryant RA, Nix DP, editors: *Acute and chronic wounds: current management concepts*, ed 5, St. Louis, 2016, Mosby.

Nix D, Mackey DM: Support surfaces. In Bryant RA, Nix DP, editors: *Acute and chronic wounds: current management concepts*, ed 5, St. Louis, 2016, Mosby.

Padula CA, et al: Prevention of medical device-related pressure injuries associated with respiratory equipment use in a critical care unit, *J Wound Ostomy Continence Nurs* 44(2):138, 2017.

Pieper B: Pressure ulcers: impact, etiology and classification. In Bryant RA, Nix DP, editors: *Acute and chronic wounds: current management concepts*, ed 5, St. Louis, 2016, Mosby.

Pittman J, et al: Medical device–related hospital-acquired pressure ulcers, *J Wound Ostomy Continence Nurs* 42(2):151, 2015.

Qaseem A, et al: Risk assessment and prevention of pressure ulcers: a clinical practice guideline from the American College of Physicians, *Ann Intern Med* 162(5):359–369, 2015.

Ratliff CR, et al: WOCN 2016 guideline for prevention and management of pressure injuries (ulcers): an executive summary, *J Wound Ostomy Continence Nurs* 44(3):241, 2017.

Schallom M, et al: Pressure ulcer incidence in patients wearing nasal-oral versus full-face noninvasive ventilation masks, *Am J Crit Care* 24(4):349, 2015.

Stotts NA: Nutritional assessment and support. In Bryant RA, Nix DP, editors: *Acute and chronic wounds: current management concepts*, ed 5, St. Louis, 2016, Mosby.

The Joint Commission (TJC): *2019 National Patient Safety Goals*, Oakbrook Terrace, IL, 2019, The Commission. http://www.jointcommission.org/standards_information/npsgs.aspx.

Wound Ostomy and Continence Nurses (WOCN) Society: Guideline for prevention and management of pressure ulcers. In *WOCN clinical practice guidelines series*, Mount Laurel, NJ, 2016, The Society.

27 Dressings, Bandages, and Binders

SKILLS AND PROCEDURES

EVOLVE WEBSITE/RESOURCES LIST

http://evolve.elsevier.com/Perry/nursinginterventions

Audio Glossary • Checklists • Clinical Review Questions • Answers and Rationales for Clinical Review Questions

INTRODUCTION

The use of dressings, bandages, and binders requires an understanding of wound healing and factors that influence wound healing. Dressings are an important part of wound healing because of their ability to control moisture, debride dead tissue, and protect a wound. Numerous dressings and wound care products are available for managing acute and chronic wounds (Table 27.1). The type and condition of a wound bed, surrounding periwound, and type and amount of drainage determine the type of dressing to use (Box 27.1).

PRACTICE STANDARDS

- Centers for Disease Control and Prevention, 2017: Guideline for prevention of surgical site infection—Aseptic principles for wound care
- National Pressure Ulcer Advisory Panel (NPUAP) and European Pressure Ulcer Advisory Panel (EPUAP), 2014: New 2014 prevention and treatment of pressure ulcers: clinical practice guidelines—Assessment of pressure injury risk factors and prevention strategies
- The Joint Commission (TJC), 2019: National Patient Safety Goals—Patient identification

EVIDENCE-BASED PRACTICE

Management of Chronic Wounds

Management of chronic wounds is a challenge for the entire health care team. Chronic wounds are those wounds that fail to move past the inflammatory phase of wound healing (Evans et al., 2018; Munro, 2017). These wounds often have bacterial bioburden and slough. The tissue, inflammation/infection, moisture, and edge of wound (TIME) framework provides an organized approach to wound healing (Chamanga et al., 2015; Munro, 2017). Infection is the most frequent complication in nonhealing wounds; this factor alone increases health care cost, increases length of stay in health care agencies, and impacts patients' independence and quality of life (Barrett, 2017). Management of chronic wounds includes the following:

- Wounds require consistent monitoring as their dressing needs change over time (Evans et al., 2018).
- Wound cleansing with topical antimicrobial agents reduces the bioburden in chronic wounds and improves wound healing (Evans et al., 2018).
- Enzymatic debriding agents applied directly to a wound bed act by digesting collagen in necrotic tissue (Evans et al., 2018; Ramundo, 2016).
- Hydrogel dressings have been identified as the dressing of choice for early debridement in chronic wounds. This is followed by low-adherent, moisture-retention dressings for the granulation stage and low-adherent dressings for the epithelialization phase (Armstrong et al., 2018).
- Polyurethane film dressings are effective in reducing infection in chronic wounds and surgical sites (Arroyo et al., 2015).
- Multilayered soft silicone foam dressings are effective in preventing pressure injuries adjacent to chronic wounds (Santamaria et al., 2015).
- Silicone or foam dressings on skin around drainage tubes, wound irrigation systems, nasoenteral tubes, and other devices reduce the risk for medical device–related pressure injuries and resultant chronic wounds (Pittman et al., 2015).
- A moist environment promotes wound healing; a wound that is left open to air is likely to become dry and painful (Doughty and Sparkes-DeFriese, 2016).

SAFETY GUIDELINES

Many wounds are colonized or contaminated with low levels of bacteria. Know the cause and type of wound to ensure the proper

TABLE 27.1

Comparison of Wound Care Products

Product Category	Indications for Use	Contraindications	Advantages	Disadvantages	Frequency of Change (per Manufacturer Recommendations)
Gauze Dressings					
Cotton or synthetic material; woven or nonwoven construction	Protection of surgical incision Mechanical debridement (damp-to-dry) Secondary dressing for other wound products Packing wounds	Granulating wounds as primary treatment	Available in many sizes and forms Sterile and nonsterile	Moisture evaporates quickly, and dressing dries out Lint fibers may be left in wound and increase risk of infection Requires frequent dressing changes	Usually change 2 or 3 times per day as needed.
Transparent Films					
Adhesive membrane dressings; waterproof, impermeable to fluids and bacteria; allow oxygen and moisture vapor exchange	Shallow wounds Dry to minimally exudative wound Promote autolytic debridement Stage 1 or 2 pressure injuries As a secondary dressing to other products, such as alginates and foam Selected to allow a 2.5-cm (1-inch) perimeter of intact surrounding skin	Not recommended for acutely infected wounds Third-degree burns	Easy to apply and remove without damage to underlying tissue Permit viewing of wound Create second skin; protect from friction Waterproof Create moist wound that softens thin slough and eschar Protective shield to external fluids and bacteria	May cause skin maceration May not adhere to moist areas May cause skin stripping if improperly removed	Change every 3 or 4 days or as needed. If using to facilitate autolytic debridement, change every 24 hours. Change when exudate extends beyond the edges of the wound on to periwound skin.
Hydrocolloids					
Adhesive dressings that contain gel-forming agents; mold to body contours, considered semiocclusive dressings	Partial- or full-thickness wound; shallow Minimal to moderate exudating wounds Clean stage 2 and noninfected shallow stage 2 to 4 pressure injuries Can be used in combination with absorbent powder or alginate	Third-degree burns, acutely infected wounds; arterial or diabetic ulcers (use with caution) Wounds with dry eschar Use with caution in persons with diabetes or arterial disease	Available in many sizes Promote autolytic debridement of necrotic tissue Reduce pain Impermeable to fluids/bacteria Thermal insulator Easy to apply and remove	Potential for periwound maceration if dressing left in place too long Drainage (gelatinous mass) under dressing often mistaken for pus/infection Adhesive possibly too aggressive for fragile skin	Change times a week or every 2 to 5 days.
Hydrogel					
Glycerin- or water-based dressings designed to maintain clean, moist wound; may also absorb small amount of exudate	Partial- or full-thickness wound; shallow or deep Dry to lightly exudative wound with or without clean granular wound base Shallow or deep wounds Wounds with undermining Necrotic wounds	Third-degree burns Wounds with heavy exudate	Nonadherent Cool and soothing Decrease pain Facilitates autolysis Conform to wound	Potential for maceration or candidiasis of periwound area	Change daily if adhesive sheets or wound fillers are not used. Change adhesive covers up to 3 times per week.

TABLE 27.1

Comparison of Wound Care Products—cont'd

Product Category	Indications for Use	Contraindications	Advantages	Disadvantages	Frequency of Change (per Manufacturer Recommendations)
Alginates					
Highly absorbent, nonwoven material that forms gel when exposed to wound drainage; fibrous product derived from brown seaweed	Moderate to heavily exudating wounds; shallow or deep Full-thickness wounds without depth Leg ulcers, donor sites, traumatic wounds	Third-degree burns Dry necrotic wounds Wounds covered with eschar Used in combination with hydrogels	Nonadhering, nonocclusive Hemostatic properties May be packed into tunneled areas Promote autolytic debridement in exudating wounds Highly absorbent	More expensive than gauze or gauze packing strips Not practical for large wounds Gelled material may be mistaken for purulence	Change daily or as often as needed, usually every 24 to 48 hours.
Foam Dressings					
Absorbent, nonadherent polyurethane or film-coated layer used to protect wounds and maintain moist healing environment	Moderate to heavily exudating wounds Partial- and full-thickness wounds; shallow and deep Stage 2 to 4 pressure injuries	Ischemic wound with dry eschar Third-degree burns Ischemic wounds with dry eschar	Highly absorbent while maintaining moist wound environment Often used as secondary dressing along with films and absorbers Many nonadherent to wound bed	Nonadhesive foams require secondary dressing Maceration of periwound may occur if dressing left on too long	Change every 24 hours or as needed.

Modified from Bryant RA, Nix DP: Principles of wound healing and topical management. In Bryant RA, Nix DP: *Acute and chronic wounds: nursing management*, ed 5, St. Louis, 2016, Mosby.

BOX 27.1

Characteristics and Outcomes of an Ideal Dressing

Characteristics

- Is nontraumatic and able to absorb exudate and keeps wound bed moist and surrounding periwound tissues dry and intact
- Appropriate for infected wounds
- Can be removed without trauma, pain, or leaving dressing fragments in the wound
- Conforms to the body part for ease of movement
- Maintains stable physiological wound environment
- Easy to apply and remove with easy-to-follow patient/family instructions
- Cost-effective

Outcomes

- Reduces volume of exudate and amount of necrotic tissue
- Resolves or prevents periwound erythema
- Reduces wound dimensions or depth of sinus tract
- Reduces pain intensity during dressing changes

Data from Doughty DB, McNichol LL, editors: Wound Ostomy and Continence Nurses Society *Core Curriculum: Wound Management*, Philadelphia, 2016, Wolters Kluwer; Bryant RA, Nix DP: Principles of wound healing and topical management. In Bryant RA, Nix DP: *Acute and chronic wounds: nursing management*, ed 5, St. Louis, 2016, Mosby.

TABLE 27.2

Types of Wound Drainage

Serous Appearance: Clear, watery plasma	**Purulent** Appearance: Thick yellow, green, tan, or brown
Serosanguineous Appearance: Pale, red, watery—mixture of serous and sanguineous	**Sanguineous** Appearance: Bright red—indicates active bleeding

treatment plan is in place and healing outcomes are achieved (see Box 27.1). For safe and effective wound care management, follow these guidelines:

- Know the expected amount and type of wound drainage (Table 27.2). Wounds with a large amount of drainage usually require more frequent dressing changes or need more absorptive dressings.
- Identify appropriate wound-cleansing agents. Because no agent is ideal for every situation, verify the type and frequency of cleansing agent used (CDC, 2017).
- Determine if wound-drainage devices are present in the wound to prevent their accidental dislocation when you remove the old dressing.
- Verify that wound-drainage devices do not cause pressure on adjacent skin, which can result in a medical-device pressure injury (MDPI) (Kayser et al., 2018).

- A wound is an alteration in skin integrity that increases a patient's risk for infection. Perform hand hygiene before and after a dressing change.
- Wear personal protective equipment (PPE), such as gloves, mask, gown, and goggles, as indicated and if risk of splashing exists. Follow isolation protocols to prevent the spread of infection.
- Dispose of contaminated dressings and supplies properly (see agency policy).

✦ SKILL 27.1 Applying a Gauze Dressing (Dry and Damp-to-Dry)

Purpose

A dry gauze dressing protects a wound from injury, prevents the introduction and spread of bacteria, reduces discomfort, and speeds healing (Fig. 27.1). These dressings are commonly used for abrasions and nondraining postoperative incisions. Telfa gauze dressings contain a shiny, nonadherent surface on one side that does not stick to wounds. Drainage passes through the nonadherent surface to the outer gauze dressing (see Table 27.1).

Damp-to-dry dressings (also called *wet-to-dry* or *moist-to-dry*) are gauze moistened with an appropriate solution. When other forms of moisture-retentive dressings are not available, moist gauze is effective to mechanically debride a wound to promote wound healing (Bryant and Nix, 2016).

Recent advances in wound care have created several new debriding products used for debriding necrotic wounds. Autolytic debriding products are applied to wounds to allow enzymes to self-digest dead tissue. Enzymatic debriding agents applied directly to a wound bed act by digesting collagen in necrotic tissue (NPUAP and EPUAP, 2014; Ramundo, 2016). Both autolytic and enzymatic products are often used in combination with moist gauze but may also come as prepackaged dressings that do not require any additional gauze (see Table 27.1).

Delegation and Collaboration

The skill of applying dry and damp-to-dry dressings can be delegated to nursing assistive personnel (NAP) if the wound is chronic (see agency policy and Nurse Practice Act). The nurse is responsible for wound assessments, care of acute new wounds, wound care requiring sterile technique, and evaluation of wound healing. The nurse directs the NAP about:

- Any unique modifications of the dressing change, such as the need for use of special tape or taping techniques to secure the dressing.
- Reporting pain, fever, bleeding, or wound drainage to the nurse immediately.

Equipment

- Clean and sterile gloves
- Sterile dressing set including scissors and forceps (check agency policy; Fig. 27.2)
- Sterile drape *(optional)*
- Necessary dressings: fine-mesh gauze, 4 × 4–inch gauze, abdominal (ABD) pads
- Sterile basin *(optional)*
- Antiseptic ointment (as prescribed)
- Wound cleanser (as prescribed)
- Sterile normal saline (or prescribed solution)
- Debriding gel as ordered
- Tape (include nonallergenic tape as necessary), Montgomery ties, or DuoDerm as needed (include nonallergic tape if necessary)
- Skin barrier (optional if using Montgomery ties)
- Measuring device: cotton-tipped applicator, measuring guide, camera
- Adhesive remover, scissors, or hair clipper *(optional)*
- Protective waterproof underpad
- Biohazard bag
- Personal protective equipment (PPE) (e.g., gown, goggles, mask) if needed
- Additional lighting if needed (e.g., flashlight, treatment light)

ASSESSMENT

1. Identify patient using at least two identifiers (e.g., name and birthday or name and medical record number) according to agency policy. *Rationale: Ensures correct patient. Complies with The Joint Commission standards and improves patient safety (TJC, 2019).*
2. Assess patient for allergies, especially antiseptics, tape, or latex. *Rationale: Reduces risk for localized or systemic allergic*

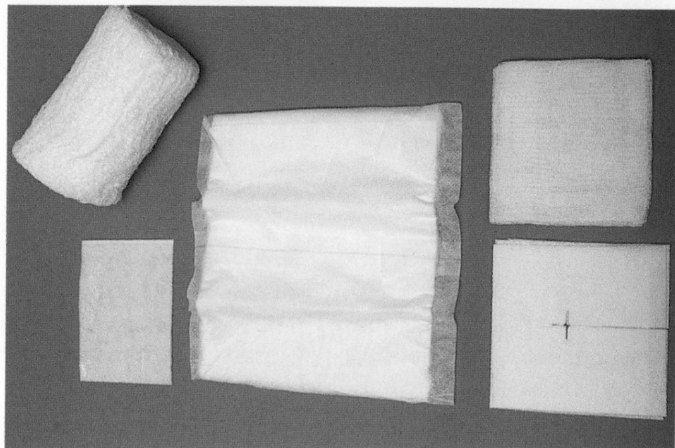

FIG 27.1 Types of gauze dressings: 4 × 4, split, roll, and abdominal (ABD) pad.

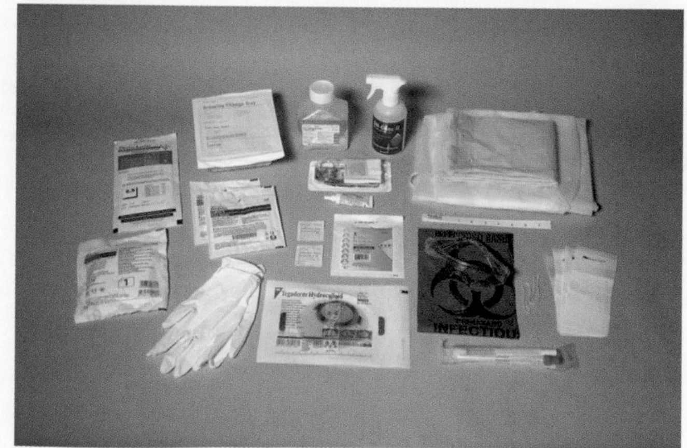

FIG 27.2 Dressing set with personal protective equipment (PPE) and wound cleansers.

reactions to supplies. Order needed in most agencies for dressing change.

3. Ask patient to rate level of pain using a pain scale of 0 to 10 and assess character of pain. Administer prescribed analgesic as needed 30 minutes before dressing change. *Rationale: Superficial wounds with multiple exposed nerves may be intensely painful, whereas deeper wounds with destruction of dermis should be less painful (Krasner, 2016). A comfortable patient is less likely to move suddenly, causing wound or supply contamination. Serves as baseline to measure response to dressing therapy.*
4. Assess need, readiness, and willingness for patient or family caregiver to participate in dressing wound. *Rationale: Identifies areas for patient education to prepare patient or family caregiver if dressing must be changed at home.*
5. Review medical orders for type of dressing and cleansing agent. *Rationale: Indicates types of dressing supplies needed.*
6. Identify patients at risk for wound-healing problems, including aging, premature infant, obesity, diabetes mellitus, circulation disorders, nutritional deficit, immunosuppression, radiation therapy, high levels of stress, and use of steroids. *Rationale: Physiological changes resulting from aging, chronic illness, poor nutrition, medications that affect wound healing, and cancer treatments have potential to affect wound healing (Doughty and Sparks-DeFriese, 2016).*
7. Perform hand hygiene and apply clean gloves as needed. *Rationale: Reduces transmission of microorganisms.*
8. Assess size, location, and condition of wound. Remove gloves if worn and perform hand hygiene. Review previous nurses' notes in electronic health record (EHR) or chart. *Rationale: Helps to plan for proper dressing type and securement of supplies needed and if help is needed during dressing procedure.*
9. Assess patient's and family caregiver's knowledge, experience, and health literacy level. *Rationale: Ensures patient and family caregiver have the capacity to obtain, communicate, and understand basic health information (Centers for Disease Control and Prevention [CDC], 2016).*

STEP	RATIONALE
PLANNING	
1. Expected outcomes following completion of procedure:	
• Patient's wound shows evidence of healing by decrease in size and reduced drainage, redness, or swelling.	Indicates that wound is healing appropriately.
• Patient reports pain less than previous assessment after dressing change.	Indicates that patient has appropriate analgesia.
• Dressing remains clean, dry, and intact.	Indicates that proper application and securement are used for dressing.
• Patient or family caregiver explains purpose of dressing and method of dressing application.	Indicates understanding and that learning has occurred.
2. Provide privacy and prepare environment.	Providing privacy and preparing the environment early promote comfort and safety of patient.
3. Position patient comfortably and drape to expose only wound site. Instruct patient not to touch wound or sterile supplies.	Draping provides access to wound while minimizing exposure. Dressing supplies become contaminated when touched by patient's hand.
4. Obtain specific dressing equipment and organize workspace.	Facilitates a smooth and organized dressing change
5. Place disposable biohazard bag within reach of work area.	Ensures easy disposal of soiled dressings.
Perform hand hygiene and apply clean gloves. Apply gown, goggles, and mask if risk for splashing exists.	Use of PPE reduces transmission of microorganisms.
6. Explain procedure to patient and/or family caregiver.	Decreases patient's anxiety.
IMPLEMENTATION	
1. Gently remove tape, bandages, or ties: use nondominant hand to support dressing and, with your dominant hand, pull tape parallel to skin and toward dressing. If dressing is over hairy area, remove in direction of hair growth. Get patient permission to clip or shave area (check agency policy). Remove any adhesive from skin.	Pulling tape toward dressing reduces stress on suture line or wound edges, irritation, and discomfort.
2. With gloved hand or forceps remove dressing one layer at a time, observing appearance of drainage on dressing. Carefully remove outer secondary dressing first; then remove inner primary dressing that is in contact with wound bed. If drains are present, slowly and carefully remove dressings (see illustration), and avoid tension on any drainage devices. Keep soiled undersurface from patient's sight.	Purpose of primary dressing is to remove necrotic tissue and exudate. Appearance of drainage may be upsetting to patient. Avoids accidental removal of drain.

STEP	RATIONALE
a. If bottom layer of damp-to-dry dressing adheres to wound, gently free dressing while alerting patient of discomfort.	Damp-to-dry dressing should debride wound (Bryant and Nix, 2016).
b. If dry dressing adheres to wound that is not to be debrided, moisten with normal saline and remove.	Prevents injury to wound surface and periwound during dressing removal.
3. Inspect wound and periwound for appearance, color, size (length, width, and depth), drainage, edema, presence and condition of drains, approximation (wound edges are together), granulation tissue, or odor (see Chapter 25). Use measuring guide or ruler to measure size of wound (see Chapter 25). Gently palpate wound edges for bogginess or patient report of increased pain.	Assesses condition of wound and periwound condition. Indicates status of healing.
4. Fold dressings with drainage contained inside and remove gloves inside out. With small dressings remove gloves inside out over dressing (see illustrations). Dispose of gloves and soiled dressing according to agency policy. Cover wound lightly with sterile gauze pad. Perform hand hygiene.	Contains soiled dressings, prevents contact of nurse's hands with drainage, and reduces cross-contamination.
5. Describe appearance of wound and any indicators of wound healing to patient.	Wounds may be unsettling and frightening to patients. It helps patient to know that wound appearance is as expected and whether healing is taking place.
6. Create sterile field with sterile dressing tray or individually wrapped sterile supplies on over-bed table (see Chapter 5). Pour any prescribed solution into sterile basin.	Sterile dressings remain sterile while on or within sterile surface. Preparation of all supplies before dressing change prevents break in technique during dressing change.

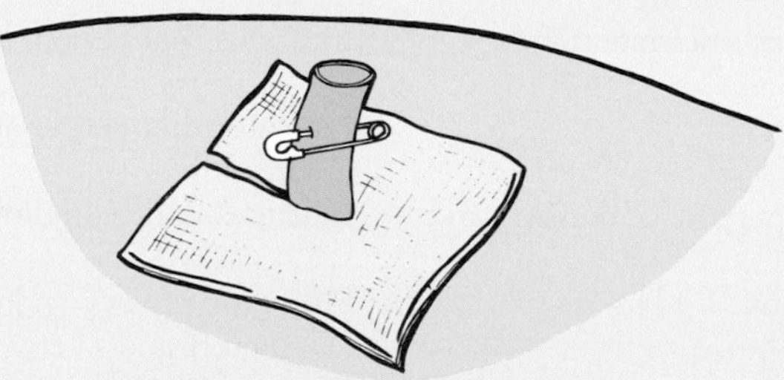

STEP 2 Penrose drain with split gauze.

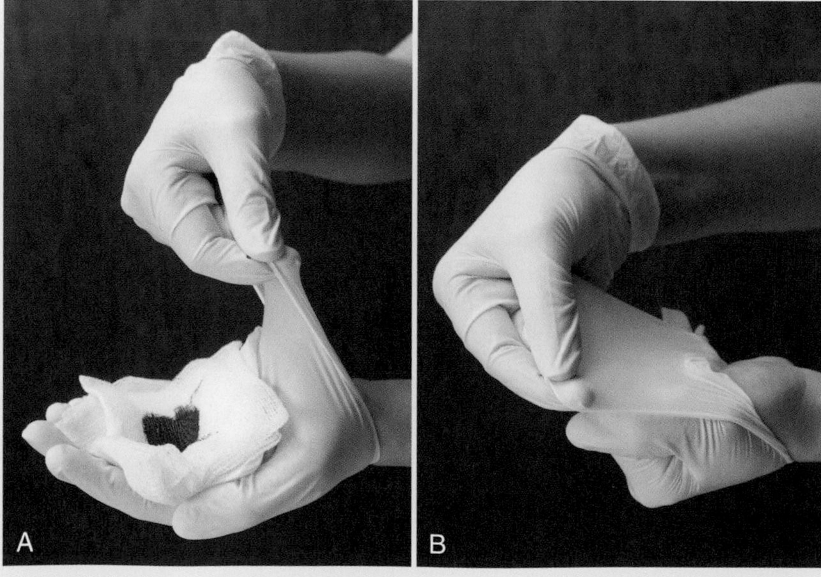

STEP 4 (A and B) Dispose of soiled dressings by placing in gloved hand and pulling glove off over dressing and then off hand.

STEP	RATIONALE
7. Clean wound (see Chapter 25):	
a. Apply clean gloves. Use gauze or cotton ball moistened in saline or antiseptic swab (per health care provider order) for each cleaning stroke or spray wound surface with wound cleaner.	Prevents transfer of organisms from previously cleaned area.
b. Clean from least to most contaminated area (see Chapter 25; see illustration).	Cleaning in this direction prevents introduction of organisms into wound.
c. Clean around any drain (if present), using circular strokes starting near drain and moving outward and away from insertion site (see illustration; see Chapter 25).	Correct aseptic technique in cleaning prevents contamination.
8. Use sterile dry gauze to blot wound bed in same manner as in Step 7.	Drying reduces excess moisture, which could eventually harbor microorganisms.
9. Apply antiseptic ointment (if ordered) with sterile cotton-tipped applicator or gauze, using same technique to apply as for cleaning. Dispose of gloves. Perform hand hygiene.	Helps reduce growth of microorganisms.
10. Apply dressing (see agency policy):	
a. Dry sterile dressing:	Dry dressings are not appropriate for debriding wounds. In the presence of drainage, a dry dressing may adhere to the wound bed and surrounding tissue, causing pain and trauma on removal. Dry dressings have the disadvantage of moisture evaporating quickly, which can cause a dressing to dry out. As a result, frequent dressing changes are usually needed, and there are increased infection rates when compared with semiocclusive dressings (Bryant and Nix, 2016).
(1) Apply clean gloves (see agency policy).	Some agencies or condition of wounds may require sterile gloves.
(2) Apply loose woven gauze as contact layer (see illustration).	Promotes proper absorption of drainage.
(3) If drain is present, apply precut, split 4 × 4–inch gauze around drain.	Secures drain and promotes drainage absorption at site.
(4) Apply additional layers of gauze as needed.	Ensures proper coverage and optimal absorption.
(5) Apply thicker woven pad (e.g., Surgipad, abdominal [ABD] pad; see illustration).	This dressing is used on postoperative wounds when there is excessive drainage.
b. Damp-to-dry dressing:	A damp-to-dry dressing has a moist contact dressing layer that touches the wound surface. The moistened gauze increases the absorptive ability of the dressing to collect exudate and wound debris.
(1) Apply sterile gloves (see agency policy).	Reduces transmission of infection.

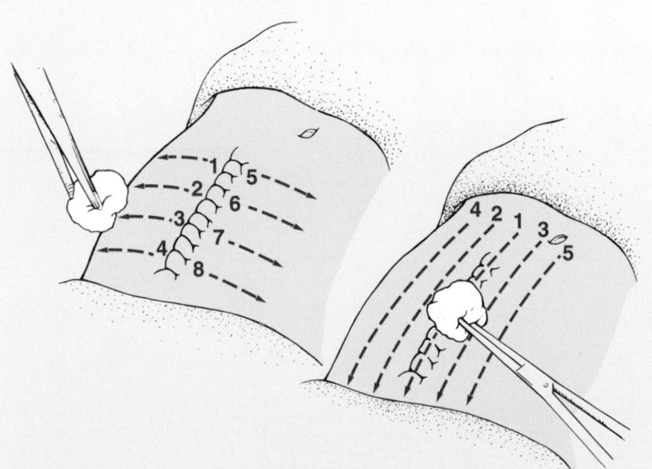

STEP 7b Methods for cleaning a wound; cleaning from least to most contaminated.

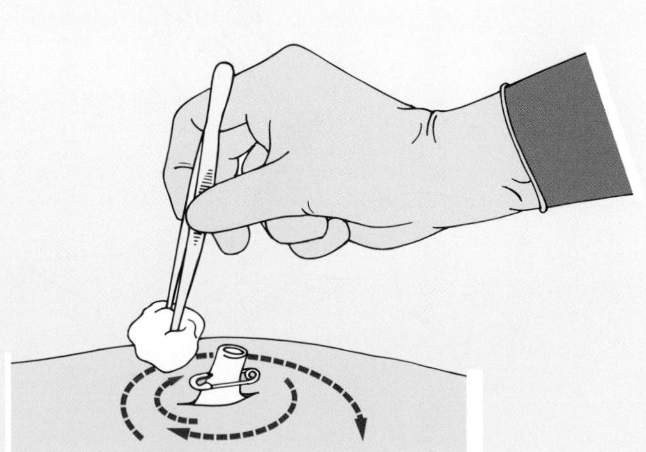

STEP 7c Cleaning around a drain site.

STEP	RATIONALE
(2) Place fine-mesh or loose 4 × 4–inch gauze in container of prescribed sterile solution. Wring out excess solution.	Damp gauze absorbs drainage and, when allowed to dry, traps debris.

Safe Patient Care *If using "packing strips," use sterile scissors to cut the amount of dressing that you will use to pack the wound. Do not let the packing strip touch the outside of the bottle. Place packing strip in container of prescribed sterile solution. Wring out excess solution.*

STEP	RATIONALE
(3) Apply damp fine-mesh or open-weave gauze as single layer directly onto wound surface. If wound is deep, gently pack gauze into wound with sterile gloved hand or forceps until all wound surfaces are in contact with gauze, including dead spaces from sinus tracts, tunnels, and undermining (see illustration A). Be sure that gauze does not touch periwound skin (see illustration B).	Inner gauze should be damp, not dripping wet, to absorb drainage and adhere to debris. When packing a wound, gauze should conform to base and side of wound (Bryant and Nix, 2016). Wound is loosely packed to facilitate wicking of drainage into absorbent outer layer of dressing. Moisture that escapes dressing often macerates the periwound area.

Safe Patient Care *Be sure to count how many pieces of gauze are packed in the wound, especially deep wounds. This ensures that all gauze from previous dressing change are removed from the wound.*

Safe Patient Care *When packing the wound, do not overpack or underpack it (Armstrong et al., 2018; Bryant and Nix, 2016). Packing should fill the wound but should not be above the level of the skin.*

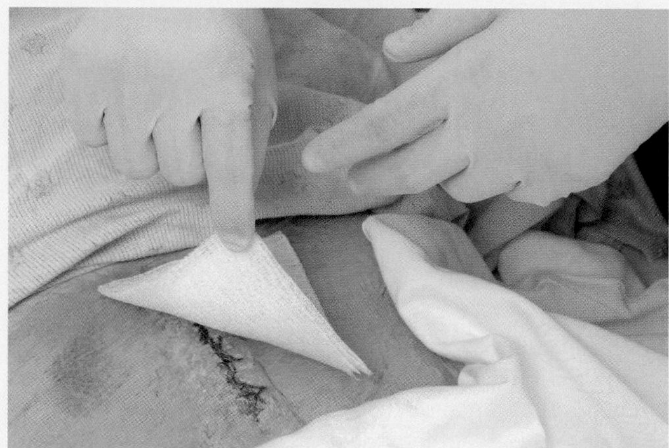

STEP 10a(2) Placing dry gauze dressing over simple wound.

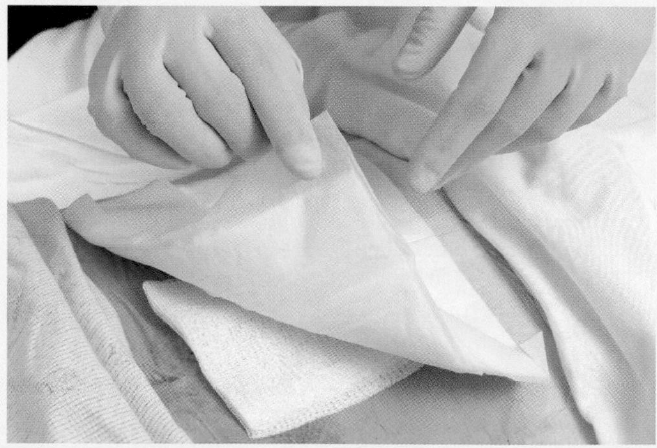

STEP 10a(5) Placing abdominal (ABD) pad over gauze dressing.

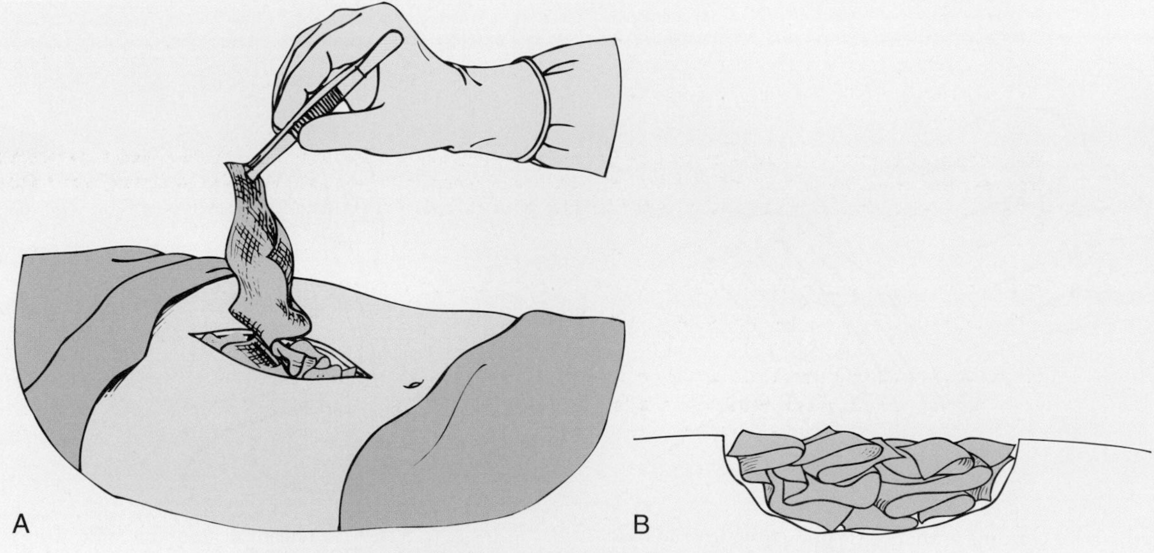

STEP 10b(3) (A) Packing wound with fine-mesh gauze. (B) Cross-section of deep wound packed loosely with gauze roll.

STEP	RATIONALE
(4) Apply dry sterile 4 × 4–inch gauze over moist gauze.	Dry layer pulls moisture from wound.
(5) Cover with ABD pad, Surgipad, or gauze.	Protects wound from entrance of microorganisms.
11. Secure dressing.	
a. *Tape:* Apply tape 2.5 to 5 cm (1 to 2 inches) beyond dressing. Use nonallergenic tape when necessary.	Supports wound and ensures placement and stability of dressing.
b. Montgomery ties (see illustrations):	Prevents skin irritation. Ties allow for repeated dressing changes without removal of tape.
(1) Be sure that skin is clean. Application of skin barrier is recommended (see Chapter 26).	Skin barrier (stomahesive) protects intact skin from stretch and tension of adhesive tape.
(2) Expose adhesive surface of tape ends.	
(3) Place ties on opposite sides of dressing over skin or skin barrier.	
(4) Secure dressing by lacing ties across dressing snugly enough to hold it secure but without placing pressure on skin.	
c. For protective window:	A protective window is an alternative to Montgomery ties for smaller wounds. There is less skin irritation by placing tape on window strips.
(1) Cut strip of stomahesive or hydrocolloid pad into four 1-cm (½-inch) strips.	
(2) Use skin barrier to wipe periwound areas of skin where strips will be applied.	
(3) Apply adhesive strips dressing to frame a "window" around the wound, one strip on each side, one on the top, and one on the bottom of the wound (see illustrations).	
(4) Apply dressing inside window; secure tape ends to adhesive strips (see illustration).	

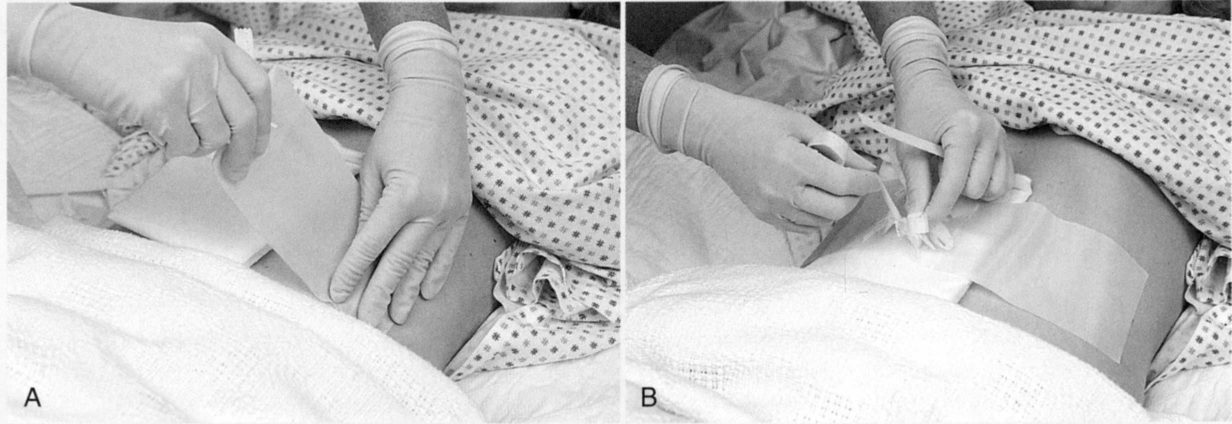

STEP 11b Montgomery ties. (A) Each tie is placed at side of gauze dressing. (B) Securing ties encloses dressing.

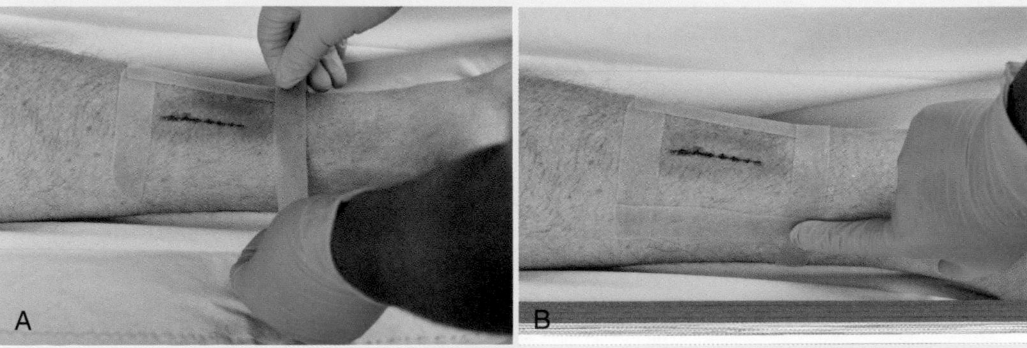

STEP 11c(3) Apply adhesive strips to frame a "window" around wound using four strips.

STEP	RATIONALE
d. For dressing extremity, secure with roller gauze (see illustration) or elastic net.	Roller gauze conforms to contour of foot or hand.
12. Dispose of all dressing supplies. Remove cover gown and goggles; remove gloves inside out; dispose of them according to agency policy. Perform hand hygiene.	Reduces transmission of microorganisms. Clean environment enhances patient comfort.
13. Label tape over dressing with your initials and date dressing is changed.	Provides timeline for when next dressing change is to be scheduled.
14. Help patient to comfortable position.	Promotes patient's sense of well-being.
15. Be sure nurse call system is in an accessible location within patient's reach.	Ensures patient can call for assistance if needed.
16. Raise side rails (as appropriate) and lower bed to lowest position.	Ensures patient safety.
17. Perform hand hygiene.	Reduces transmission of microorganisms.

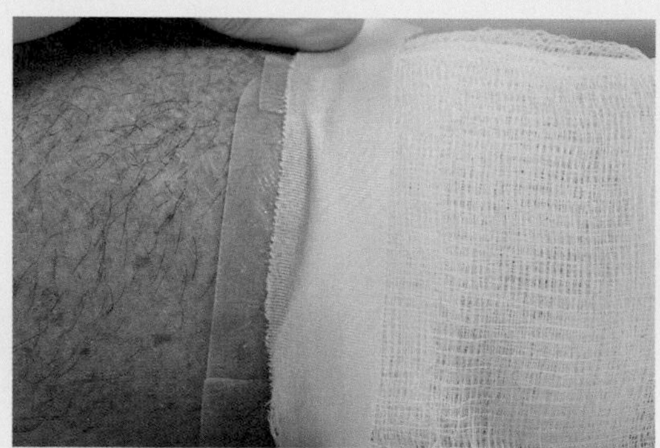

STEP 11c(4) Apply dressing; secure tape ends to adhesive strips.

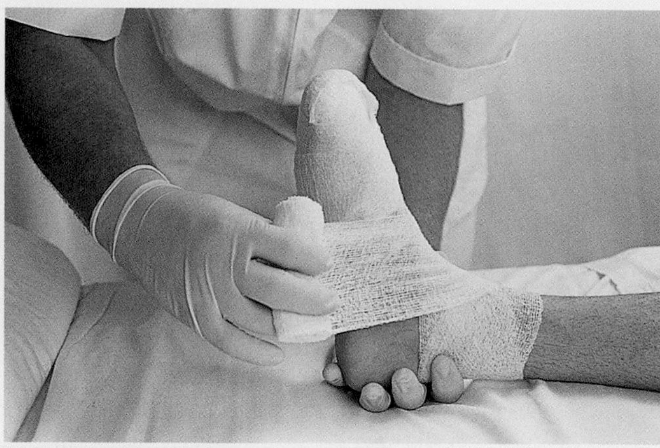

STEP 11d Wrap roller gauze around extremity to secure dressing.

EVALUATION

1. Observe appearance of wound for healing: measure size of wound; observe amount, color, and type of drainage and periwound erythema or swelling.	Determines rate of healing.
2. Ask patient to rate pain using a scale of 0 to 10.	Increased pain is often indication of wound complications such as infection or result of dressing pulling tissue.
3. Inspect condition of dressing at least every shift.	Determines status of wound drainage.
4. **Use Teach-Back:** "I want to be sure I explained why and how often you need to continue these dressing changes when you go home tomorrow. Tell me why it is important to change your dressing and how often you will do this." Revise your instruction now or develop a plan for revised patient/family caregiver teaching if patient/family caregiver is not able to teach back correctly.	Determines patient's and family caregiver's level of understanding of instructional topic.

TABLE 27.3
Problems Associated With Wounds Requiring Debridement

Problem	Nursing Interventions
Solutions used may be irritating to healthy skin around wound.	Protect healthy skin with protective barrier such as stomahesive or apply topical ointments such as zinc oxide. If zinc oxide is used, it should be removed with mineral oil. Avoid scrubbing the skin because scrubbing can cause harm to the epithelial layer.
Wound becomes excessively dry.	A continually moist dressing (with a health care provider's order) might be tried. Eliminate fine-mesh gauze and lightly pack wound with fluffy gauze dampened with prescribed solution.
Wound is deep, and retention of dressing in cavity is suspected.	Irrigate wound copiously with prescribed solution to loosen dressing for removal. Use continuous "ribbon" or strip of gauze to dress deep wounds.
Wound drainage is damaging healthy tissue.	Protect healthy tissue with skin barrier such as a hydrocolloid. Wounds with large amounts of drainage may benefit from occlusive drainage collection device.
Patient's skin is irritated by tape.	Use hydrocolloid under tape, Montgomery ties as needed, fabric tape that has multidirectional stretch; secure dressing with binder or wrap with roll gauze if on extremity.

Unexpected Outcomes	Related Interventions
1. Wound appears inflamed and tender, drainage is evident, and/or odor is present.	• Monitor patient for signs of infection (e.g., fever, increased white blood cell count). • Notify health care provider. • Obtain wound cultures as ordered. • If there is yellow, tan, or brown necrotic tissue, notify health care provider to determine need for debridement (Table 27.3).
2. Wound bleeds during dressing change.	• Observe color and amount of bloody drainage. If excessive, may need to apply direct dressing. • Inspect area along dressing and directly underneath patient to determine amount of bleeding. • Obtain vital signs as needed. • Notify health care provider.
3. Patient reports sensation that "something has given way under the dressing."	• Observe wound for increased drainage or dehiscence (partial or total separation of wound layers) or evisceration (total separation of wound layers and protrusion of viscera through wound opening). • If dehiscence or evisceration occurs, protect wound. Cover with sterile moist dressing. • Instruct patient to lie still. • Stay with patient to monitor vital signs. • Notify health care provider.

Recording

- Record size and appearance of wound, characteristics of drainage, presence of necrotic tissue, type of dressings applied, response to dressing change, and level of comfort.
- Document your evaluation of patient learning.

Hand-Off Reporting

- Report any unexpected appearance of wound drainage, bright red bleeding.
- Report any change in wound integrity (e.g., dehiscence or evisceration).

✦ SKILL 27.2 Applying a Pressure Bandage

Purpose

A pressure bandage is a temporary treatment to control excessive, sudden, unanticipated bleeding. Hemorrhage may occur during or after diagnostic interventions (e.g., cardiac catheterization, arterial puncture, organ biopsy), surgery, or a life-threatening occurrence related to trauma (e.g., stabbing, gunshot wound). Pressure dressings are essential for stopping the flow of blood and promoting clotting at the site (hemostasis) until definitive action can be taken. Given the emergent nature of an acute bleeding episode, the aseptic techniques considered essential in most dressing applications are secondary to the goal of halting the bleeding.

Delegation and Collaboration

The skill of applying a pressure dressing in an emergency cannot be delegated to nursing assistive personnel (NAP). If application requires more than one person, the NAP can assist. The nurse directs the NAP to:

- Assist the nurse as directed.
- Observe the pressure dressing during care activities to make sure that it remains in place and that there is no visible bleeding from the site.
- Observe underneath patient for bleeding after dressing has been applied.

Equipment

- Necessary dressings: fine-mesh gauze, roller gauze, hemostatic dressing (per agency policy), abdominal (ABD) pad, roller gauze
- Adhesive tape, hypoallergenic if necessary
- Adhesive remover *(optional)*
- Clean gloves (if available)
- Personal protective equipment (PPE) (e.g., gown, goggles, mask) as needed
- Equipment for vital signs

ASSESSMENT

1. If situation permits, identify patient using two identifiers (e.g., name and birthday or name and medical record number) according to agency policy. *Rationale: Ensures correct patient. Complies with The Joint Commission standards and improves patient safety (TJC, 2019).*
2. Perform hand hygiene. Anticipate patients at risk for unexpected bleeding. Perform frequent assessments (wearing clean gloves as needed) in patients with traumatic injury, arterial puncture, donor graft site, postoperative incision, wounds after surgical debridement, and history of bleeding disorder. *Rationale: Familiarity with conditions associated with unexpected bleeding allows you to rapidly respond to bleeding.*
3. Look for visible presence of blood, blood pulsating from arterial site. *Rationale: These are signs of hemorrhage.*
4. Assess patient for allergies to antiseptics, tape, or latex. If patient is nonresponsive and no history is available, use nonlatex or nonallergenic supplies. *Rationale: Prevents localized or systemic allergic reaction.*
5. Quickly assess patient's anxiety level. *Rationale: Determines need for education and positive reinforcement during procedure.*
6. Assess patient's baseline vital signs before onset of hemorrhage. *Rationale: If data are available, baseline vital signs indicate status of circulatory function.*
7. If possible, assess patient's or family caregiver's knowledge, experience, and health literacy level. *Rationale: Ensures patient and family caregiver have the capacity to obtain, communicate, process, and understand basic health information (CDC, 2016).*

STEP	RATIONALE
PLANNING	
1. Expected outcomes following completion of procedure:	
• Patient shows cessation of bleeding and no evidence of hematoma formation.	Hemostasis is achieved.
• Patient maintains stable blood pressure and heart rate.	Hemodynamic stability is achieved with minimal blood loss.
• Distal circulation is maintained with intact pulses (distal to site of injury).	Pressure does not impair arterial perfusion.
IMPLEMENTATION	
Phase I: Immediate Action—First Nurse	
1. Perform hand hygiene and apply clean gloves. Identify external bleeding site. You will need to turn patient to observe underneath patients with large ABDs in place. **NOTE:** Wounds to groin area also can result in large amounts of blood loss, which is not always visible.	Quick identification of location increases response time to stop bleeding. Maintaining asepsis and privacy are considered only if time and severity of blood loss permit.
2. Use hands to apply immediate manual pressure to bleeding site.	Hemostasis maintained as supplies are prepared. Bandage must be secured quickly. Situation could be life threatening.
3. Seek help.	Additional support needed to insert intravenous catheter, prepare dressings, and prepare for emergency transport to operating room.
Phase II: Applying Pressure Bandage—Second Nurse	
4. Perform hand hygiene and apply clean gloves. Quickly confirm source of bleeding. • *Arterial bleeding* is bright red and gushes forth in waves, related to patient's heart rate; if vessel is very deep, flow is steady. • *Venous bleeding* is dark red and flows smoothly. • *Capillary bleeding* is oozing of dark red blood; self-sealing controls this bleeding.	Determines method of application and supplies to use.
5. Elevate affected body part (e.g., extremity) if possible.	Helps slow rate of bleeding.

STEP	RATIONALE
6. First nurse continues to apply direct pressure as second nurse unwraps roller bandage and places within easy reach. Second nurse quickly cuts three to five lengths of adhesive tape and places them within reach; *do not clean wound.*	Pressure dressing controls bleeding temporarily. Preparation allows for securing pressure bandage quickly.
7. In simultaneous coordinated actions:	
a. Rapidly cover bleeding area with multiple thicknesses of gauze compresses. First nurse slips fingers out as other nurse exerts adequate pressure to continue controlling bleeding (see illustrations).	Gauze is absorbent. Layers provide bulk against which local pressure can be applied to bleeding site.

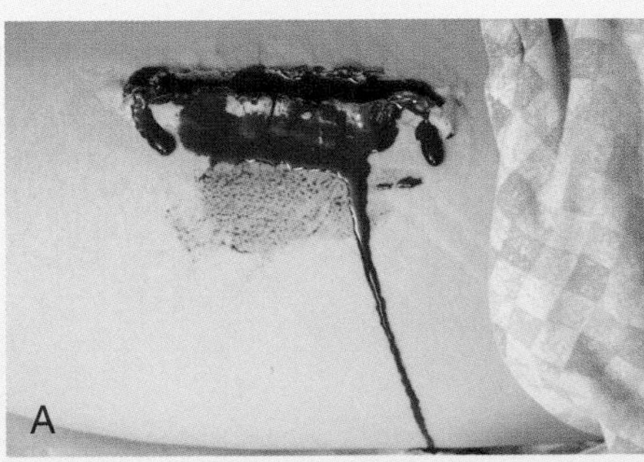

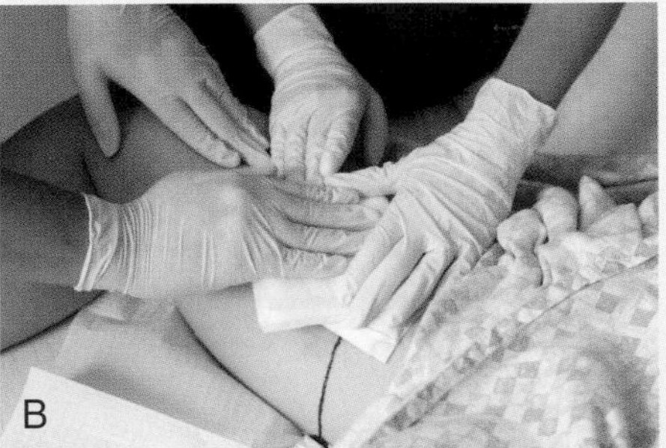

STEP 7a (A) Bleeding wound. (B) Nurses apply pressure dressing.

STEP	RATIONALE
b. Place adhesive strips 7 to 10 cm (3 to 4 inches) beyond width of dressing with even pressure on both sides of fingers as close as possible to central bleeding source. Secure tape on distal end, pull tape across dressing, and keep firm pressure as proximate end of tape is secured.	Tape exerts downward pressure, promoting hemostasis. To ensure blood flow to distal tissues and prevent tourniquet effect, adhesive tape must not be continued around entire extremity.
c. Remove fingers temporarily and quickly cover center of area with third strip of tape.	Provides pressure to source of bleeding.
d. Continue reinforcing area with tape as each successive strip is overlapped on alternating sides of center strip. Keep applying pressure.	Prevents tape from loosening.
e. When pressure bandage is on extremity, apply roller gauze: apply two circular turns tautly with even pressure on both sides of fingers. Compress over bleeding site. Simultaneously remove finger pressure and apply roller gauze over center. Continue with figure-eight turns. Secure end with two circular turns and strip of adhesive (see Procedural Guideline 27.2).	Roller gauze acts as pressure bandage, exerting more even pressure over extremity.

Safe Patient Care *Start pressure bandage from distal to proximal, working toward the heart. If bleeding continues, contact health care provider.*

STEP	RATIONALE
8. Once bandage applied, remove and dispose of gloves and perform hand hygiene.	Reduces transmission of infection.

EVALUATION

STEP	RATIONALE
1. Observe dressing for control of bleeding.	Effective pressure bandage controls bleeding without blocking distal circulation.
2. Evaluate adequacy of circulation (distal pulse, skin characteristics).	Determines level of perfusion to distal body parts.
3. Estimate volume of blood loss (e.g., count number of dressings used, weigh saturated dressing).	Helps to determine blood and fluid replacement needs.
4. Monitor vital signs.	Identifies patient's response to blood loss and early stages of hypovolemic shock.

Unexpected Outcomes	Related Interventions
1. There is continued bleeding. Fluid and electrolyte imbalance, tissue hypoxia, confusion, hypovolemic shock, and cardiac arrest develop.	• Notify health care provider. • Reinforce or adjust pressure dressing. • Initiate intravenous (IV) therapy per order. • Place patient in Trendelenburg's position; provide covers for warmth. • Monitor vital signs every 5 to 15 minutes (apical pulse, distal pulses, and blood pressure).
2. Pressure dressing is too tight and occludes circulation.	• Inspect areas distal to pressure dressing to ensure that circulation has not been occluded. • Adjust dressing as needed.

Recording

- Record location of bleeding, assessment findings, application of pressure dressing, and patient's response.

Hand-Off Reporting

- Report immediately to health care provider present status of patient's bleeding control; time bleeding was discovered; estimated blood loss; nursing interventions (including effectiveness of applied pressure dressing); apical and distal pulses, blood pressure, mental status, signs of restlessness; and the need for health care provider to attend to patient immediately.

PROCEDURAL GUIDELINE 27.1 *Applying a Transparent Dressing*

Purpose

A transparent film dressing is a clear, adherent, nonabsorptive, polyurethane sheet that is impermeable to fluids and bacteria (Bryant and Nix, 2016). Once it is applied, a moist exudate forms over the wound surface, which prevents tissue dehydration and allows for rapid, effective healing by speeding epithelial cell growth. The dressings are appropriate for prophylaxis on high-risk intact skin (e.g., high-friction areas), superficial wounds with minimal or no exudate, and eschar-covered wounds when autolysis is indicated and safe. A transparent dressing is more effective and more cost-efficient than a hydrocolloid dressing in preventing pressure injuries (Dutra et al., 2016). The synthetic permeable membrane acts as a temporary second skin, adheres to undamaged skin to contain exudate, minimizes wound contamination, and allows a wound to "breathe" (Armstrong et al., 2018; Dutra et al., 2015: NPUAP and EPUAP, 2014).

Delegation and Collaboration

The skill of applying a transparent dressing for select wounds (e.g., stage 1 pressure injury) can be delegated to nursing assistive personnel (NAP) (refer to agency policy). The assessment of the wound and care of sterile or new acute wounds cannot be delegated to NAP. The nurse directs the NAP about:

- Explaining how to adapt the skill for a specific patient.
- Reporting any signs of bleeding, drainage, infection, or poor wound healing immediately to the nurse.

Equipment

Sterile gloves *(optional)*; dressing set *(optional)*; sterile saline or other cleansing agent (as ordered); clean gloves; cotton swabs; biohazard bag for disposal; transparent dressing (size as needed); sterile 4 × 4–inch gauze pads; skin-preparation materials *(optional)*; personal protective equipment (PPE) as needed

Procedural Steps

1. Identify patient using at least two identifiers (e.g., name and birthday or name and medical record number) according to agency policy (TJC, 2019).
2. Expose wound site, minimizing exposure. Instruct patient not to touch wound or sterile supplies. Assess patient's pain severity using scale of 0 to 10.
3. Perform hand hygiene and apply clean gloves if needed. Apply PPE (e.g., gown, mask, goggles) as needed.
4. Remove old dressing by stretching film in direction parallel to wound rather than pulling.
5. Dispose of soiled dressing in waterproof bag, remove gloves by pulling them inside out, dispose of them in waterproof bag, and perform hand hygiene.
6. Prepare dressing supplies. **Use sterile supplies for new wounds (check agency policy).**
7. Pour saline or prescribed solution over 4 × 4–inch sterile gauze pads.
8. Apply clean or sterile gloves (check agency policy).
9. Clean wound and periwound area gently with 4 × 4–inch sterile gauze pads moistened in sterile saline or spray with wound cleaner. Clean from least to most contaminated area (see Skill 27.1).
10. Pat skin around wound; dry thoroughly with dry 4 × 4–inch sterile gauze pads.
11. Inspect wound for tissue type, color, odor, and drainage; measure size if indicated (see Chapter 25).

Safe Patient Care *If patient has thin or fragile skin, use a skin barrier on the skin around a wound before dressing application to protect patient's skin from further injury (Bryant and Best, 2016).*

12. Remove gloves and perform hand hygiene.

Safe Patient Care *If wound has a large amount of drainage, choose another dressing that can absorb drainage.*

PROCEDURAL GUIDELINE 27.1 ***Applying a Transparent Dressing—cont'd***

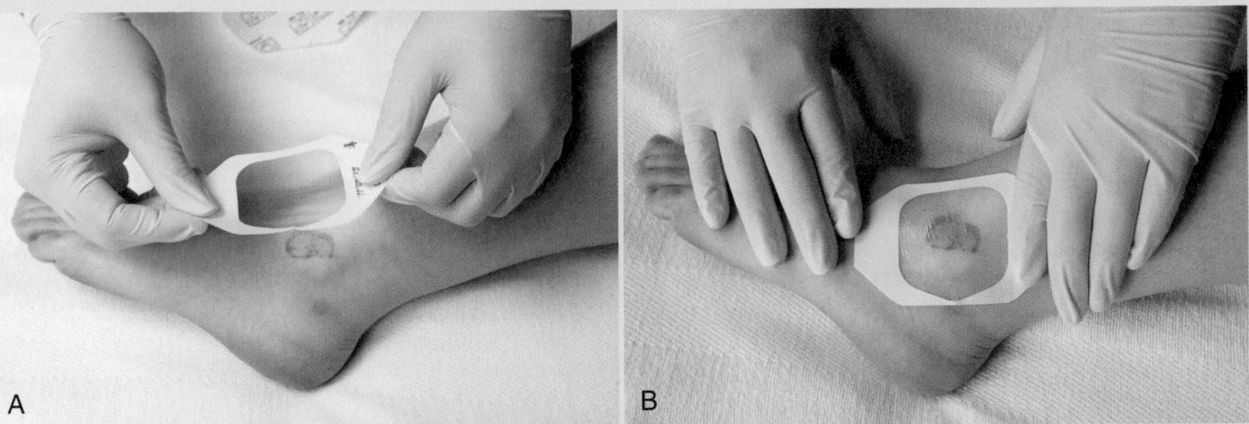

STEP 13b (A) Transparent dressing placed over small wound on ankle. (B) Place film smoothly without stretching.

13. Apply clean gloves and apply transparent dressing according to manufacturer directions. ***Do not stretch film during application, and avoid wrinkles.***
    a. Remove paper backing, taking care not to allow adhesive areas to touch one another.
    b. Place film smoothly over wound without stretching (see illustrations).
    c. Use your fingers to smooth and adhere dressing.
    d. Label dressing with date, your initials, and time of dressing change on outer label of dressing (see illustration).
14. Help patient to comfortable position. Be sure nurse call system is in an accessible location within patient's reach.
15. Raise side rails (as appropriate) and lower bed to lowest position.
16. Discard soiled dressing materials properly. Remove gloves by pulling them inside out and discard in prepared bag. Perform hand hygiene.

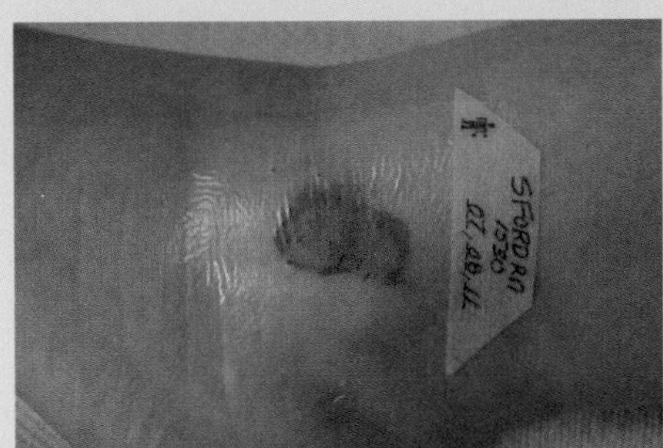

STEP 13d Transparent dressing correctly labeled.

17. Evaluate appearance of wound, amount of drainage, and measure size of wound routinely.
18. Inspect periwound areas.
19. Ask patient to rate pain using scale of 0 to 10.
20. Record appearance of wound, presence and characteristics of drainage, pain level, and presence of odor.

✦ SKILL 27.3 Applying Hydrocolloid, Hydrogel, Foam, or Alginate Dressings

Purpose

A hydrocolloid dressing is a formulation of elastomeric adhesive and gelling agents. It promotes significantly better wound-healing outcomes compared with conventional gauze (Armstrong et al., 2018; Bryant and Nix, 2016). Hydrocolloid dressings absorb drainage and hydrate and debride wounds. When the dressing is in contact with wound, exudate is absorbed into the dressing, and a gel forms next to the wound surface.

Hydrogel dressings are glycerin-based or water-based dressings that hydrate wounds, promoting moist wound healing and autolysis (Bryant and Nix, 2016). These dressings are similar to hydrocolloids and come in the form of sheets, amorphous gels, and impregnated gauze.

Foam dressings absorb exudate in superficial or deep wounds, protect friable periwound skin, provide autolytic debridement, and pad high-trauma areas. Foam dressings are used to manage chronic and infected wounds. In addition, multilayered foam dressings add in preventing heel and sacral pressure injuries (Santamaria et al., 2015).

Alginate dressings are manufactured from natural substances (seaweed) and are known for their absorptive properties, forming a gel over the wound surface to contain exudate. This dressing may come as a sheet or rope that can be packed into a wound that has moderate to heavy drainage. An alginate dressing creates a moist environment and promotes autolysis, granulation, and epithelialization of the wound bed (Bryant and Nix, 2016).

Delegation and Collaboration

The skill of applying a hydrocolloid, hydrogel, foam, or alginate dressing cannot be delegated to nursing assistive personnel (NAP). The nurse directs the NAP to:

- Help position patient during dressing application.
- Immediately report to the nurse any pain, fever, bleeding, wound drainage, or slippage of dressing.

Equipment

- Clean gloves
- Sterile gloves *(optional)*
- Dressing kit *(optional)* (items will vary):
  - Sterile scissors
  - Sterile drape
  - Face mask
  - Sterile gloves
  - Tape measure
  - Tape (nonallergenic paper or adhesive)
  - 4 × 4 gauze squares
  - Dressing change label
  - Antiseptic swabs
- Necessary primary dressings: hydrocolloid, hydrogel, foam, or alginate
- Secondary dressing of choice
- Montgomery ties
- Sterile saline or other cleansing solution (as ordered) or irrigating solution
- Skin barrier wipe
- Biohazard bag
- Adhesive remover
- Debriding gel (as ordered)
- Additional personal protective equipment (PPE) (when splashing is a risk)

ASSESSMENT

1. Identify patient using at least two identifiers (e.g., name and birthday or name and medical record number) according to agency policy. *Rationale: Ensures correct patient. Complies with The Joint Commission standards and improves patient safety (TJC, 2019).*
2. Assess for presence of allergies, especially antiseptics, tape, or latex. *Rationale: Prevents localized or systemic reaction to supplies.*
3. Perform hand hygiene and apply clean gloves as needed. Inspect location, size, and condition of wound. *Rationale: Prevents transmission of microorganisms. Determines supplies and help needed.*
4. Ask patient to rate pain using pain scale of 0 to 10 and assess character of pain. Administer prescribed analgesic as needed 30 minutes before dressing change. *Rationale: Patient may require pain medication before dressing change. Allows for peak effect of drug during procedure.*
5. Review health care provider's orders for frequency and type of dressing change. Do not use alginate or absorptive dressings on nonexudative wounds. *Rationale: Indicates type of dressing or application to use.*
6. Review previous nurses' notes in electronic health record (EHR) or chart. Note possible need to use customized shape or size of dressing to fit difficult body parts (e.g., sacrum, heels, or elbows). *Rationale: Customized shapes aid in patient-centered dressing selection and better dressing adherence.*
7. Assess patient's and family caregiver's knowledge, experience, and health literacy level. *Rationale: Ensures patient and family caregiver have the capacity to obtain, communicate, process, and understand basic health information (CDC, 2016).*

STEP	RATIONALE
PLANNING	
1. Expected outcomes following completion of procedure:	
• Patient's wound shows evidence of healing as it becomes smaller in size/depth with less drainage, redness, or swelling.	Dressing effective in promoting healing.
• Patient reports pain less than previously assessed level (scale of 0 to 10) during and after dressing change.	Pain control achieved during dressing removal and reapplication.
• Dressing remains clean, dry, and intact.	Dressing applied correctly.
• Patient or family caregiver explains procedure correctly.	Indicates that learning has occurred.
2. Close room door or curtain.	Provides privacy.
3. Gather and organize dressing supplies and kit on overbed table.	Ensures an organized dressing change procedure.
4. Place biohazard bag within reach of area. Fold top of bag to make a cuff.	Ensures easy disposal of soiled dressings. Do not reach across sterile field.
5. Position patient comfortably to allow access to dressing site.	Facilitates application of dressing.
6. Explain procedure to patient or family caregiver.	Relieves anxiety and promotes understanding of healing process.
IMPLEMENTATION	
1. Perform hand hygiene, apply clean gloves. Apply appropriate PPE as needed if there is risk for splashing.	Reduces transmission of infectious organisms.
2. Drape patient to expose wound site. Instruct patient not to touch wound or sterile supplies.	Draping provides access to wound while minimizing exposure. Dressing supplies become contaminated when touched by patient.
3. Using nondominant hand, gently remove tape, bandages, or ties of existing dressing. Pull tape parallel to skin and toward dressing. If dressing is over hairy areas, remove tape in direction of hair growth and get patient's permission to clip area before applying new dressing (check agency policy). Remove any adhesive from skin.	Pulling tape toward dressing reduces stress on wound edges, irritation, and discomfort.

STEP	RATIONALE
4. With gloved hand or forceps, remove old dressing one layer at a time. Note amount and character of drainage (see illustration). Use caution to avoid tension on any drains.	Reduces irritation and possible injury to skin. Prevents accidental removal of drain.

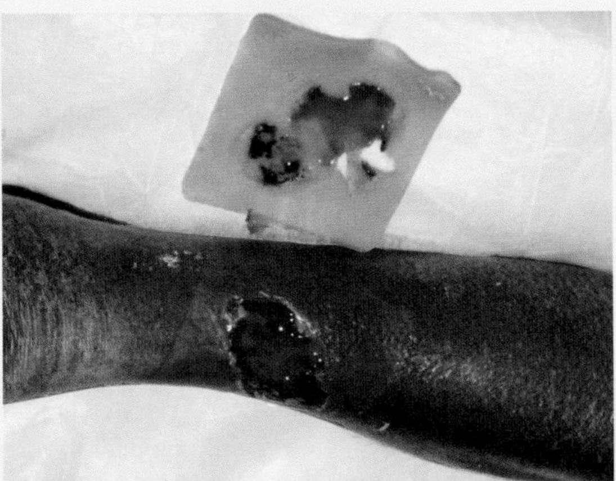

STEP 4 Hydrocolloid dressing after removal from venous injury. Purulent-appearing exudate is present on dressing and wound. This is expected with autolysis under the dressing and is not evidence of infection. *(From Bryant R, Nix D:* Acute and chronic wounds: current management concepts, *ed 5, St. Louis, 2016, Mosby.)*

Safe Patient Care *Check removal directions for specific brand of dressing used. Some brands need to have old dressing soaked, irrigated, or moistened for removal. If necessary, use adhesive remover to ease off dressing, but avoid contact of adhesive remover with the wound. Adhesive remover will also remove adhesive residue on periwound area.*

STEP	RATIONALE
5. Fold dressings with drainage contained inside and remove gloves inside out. With small dressings, remove gloves inside out to enclose dressing (see Skill 27.1). Dispose of gloves and soiled dressing according to agency policy. Cover wound lightly with a sterile 4 × 4–inch gauze pad. Perform hand hygiene.	Contains soiled dressings; prevents contact of nurse's hands with drainage; reduces cross-contamination.

Safe Patient Care *Hydrocolloid dressings interact with wound fluids and form a soft whitish-yellowish gel, which is sometimes hard to remove and may have a faint odor. A residual gel substance occurs in wound beds with some absorption dressings. This gel promotes a moist environment and facilitates autolytic, enzymatic debridement, and wound healing. This is a normal occurrence; do not confuse these findings with pus or purulent exudate, wound infection, or wound deterioration (Bryant and Nix, 2016).*

STEP	RATIONALE
6. Prepare sterile field with drape in sterile dressing kit or individually wrapped sterile drape. Use inside of dressing kit as a sterile work area (see Chapter 5). Pour prescribed solution into sterile bowl.	Creates sterile work area.
7. Remove gauze cover over wound.	Reduces introduction of organisms into wound.
8. Clean wound:	Cleaning and irrigating effectively remove residual dressing gel without injuring newly formed delicate granulation tissue in healing wound bed.
a. Perform hand hygiene. Apply clean gloves. Sterile gloves are optional (see agency policy). Use 4 × 4–inch gauze cotton ball moistened in saline or an antiseptic swab (per health care provider order) for each cleaning stroke. *Option:* Spray wound surface with wound cleaner (see Chapter 25).	
b. Clean from least contaminated to most contaminated.	Cleaning in this direction prevents introduction of organisms into noncontaminated areas.
c. Clean around any drain, using circular stroke starting near drain and moving outward away from insertion site (see Skill 27.1).	
9. Use sterile dry gauze to blot dry wound bed and on skin around wound.	Dressing will not adhere to damp surface. Periwound maceration can enlarge wound and impede healing.
10. Inspect appearance and condition of wound (see Chapter 25). Measure wound size and de pth.	Appearance and measurement indicate state of wound healing.

STEP	RATIONALE

Safe Patient Care *When inspecting a wound be aware of subtle signs of infection: increased or altered exudate; friable, bright red granulation tissue; increased odor; increase pain; localized edema. Any combination of two or more is indicative of a local wound infection, which can be managed with local measures, such as topical antimicrobials or antimicrobial dressings in addition to effective debridement (Swanson et al., 2015).*

STEP	RATIONALE
11. Remove gloves and perform hand hygiene. Apply clean gloves. Sterile gloves are optional (see agency policy).	Reduces transmission of microorganisms.
12. Apply dressing (see manufacturer directions).	Ensures proper application of dressing. Different brands of dressings require different application techniques.
a. **Hydrocolloid dressings:**	
(1) Select proper size wafer, allowing dressing to extend onto intact periwound skin at least 2.5 cm (1 inch; Bryant and Nix, 2016; see illustration). Do not stretch dressing; avoid wrinkles and tenting.	Hydrocolloid design prevents shear and friction from loosening edges and circumvents need for tape along dressing borders (Bryant and Nix, 2016).
(2) For deep wound, apply hydrocolloid granules, impregnated gauze, or paste before the wafer.	Functions as filler material to ensure contact with all wound surfaces. The cushioning effect of a hydrocolloid adhesive dressing diminishes pain and protects the wound and periwound skin.
(3) Remove paper backing from adhesive side and place over wound. Do not stretch and avoid wrinkles or tenting. Hold dressing in place for 30 to 60 seconds after application.	Molds dressing at body temperature (Bryant and Nix, 2016).
(4) If cut from larger piece, tape edges with nonallergenic tape to avoid rolling or adherence to clothing.	

Safe Patient Care *Edges may be notched to help mold around wound. Consider using custom shapes to better conform to certain parts of the body, such as heels, elbows, and sacrum.*

STEP	RATIONALE
b. **Hydrogel dressings:**	
(1) Apply skin barrier wipe to surrounding skin that will come in contact with any adhesive or gel.	Protects periwound skin. Because of high water content of gels, care must be taken to protect periwound skin through use of skin barrier (Bryant and Nix, 2016).
(2) Apply gel or gel-impregnated gauze directly into wound, spreading evenly over wound bed (see illustration). Fill wound cavity with gel about ⅓- to ½ full or pack gauze loosely, including any undermined or tunneled areas. Cover with moisture-retentive dressing or hydrocolloid wafer. *Option:* Hydrogel sheets composed of water should be cut to size of wound *only*.	Hydrogels hydrate and facilitate autolytic debridement of wounds. Filling wound cavity partially full allows for expansion with absorption of exudate (Bryant and Nix, 2016).

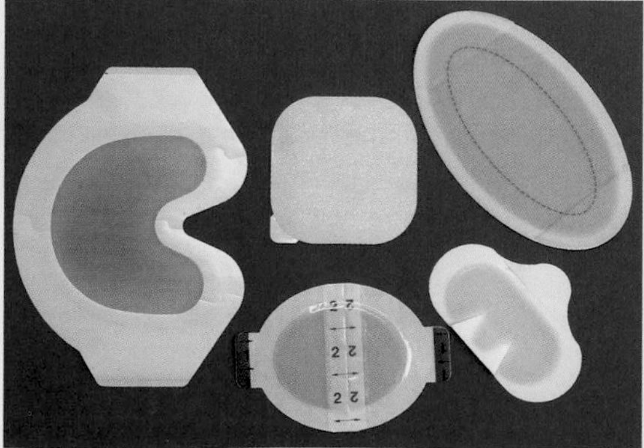

STEP 12a(1) Variety of sizes and shapes of hydrocolloid dressings. *(Courtesy Bonnie Sue Rolstad.)*

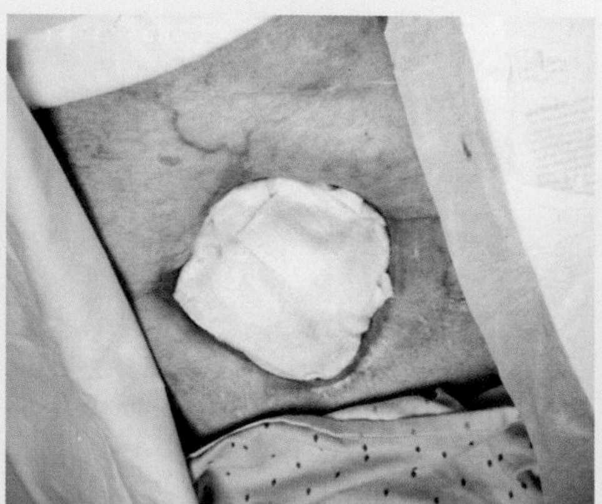

STEP 12b(2) Hydrogel-impregnated gauze used to maintain moist wound bed and fill dead space in this deep abdominal wound with undermining. *(From Bryant R, Nix D:* Acute and chronic wounds: current management concepts, *ed 5, St. Louis, 2016, Mosby.)*

STEP	RATIONALE
(3) Cut hydrogel sheet containing glycerin so that it extends 2.5 cm (1 inch) out on to intact periwound skin. Cover with secondary moisture-retentive dressing if needed.	Protects skin around wound from maceration. The gel dressings are nonadherent and must be covered with a secondary dressing to hold them in place.
(4) Secure dressing with nonallergenic tape if secondary dressing is not self-adhering.	
c. **Foam dressings:**	These dressings provide a moist, warm wound-healing environment and are effective in managing wound exudate (Bryant and Nix, 2016).
(1) Know removal and application characteristics of specific brand of foam dressing (e.g., foam dressings containing an antimicrobial substance).	Foam dressings collect moderate to heavy wound exudate; however, some foam dressings contain an antimicrobial substance to reduce risk for bacterial colonization in wounds (Barrett, 2017)
(2) Apply skin barrier wipe to surrounding skin that will come in contact with thin foam dressing adhesive.	Protects periwound skin from maceration or irritation from adhesive.
(3) Cut foam sheet to extend 2.5 cm (1 inch) out onto intact periwound skin. (Verify which side of foam dressing should be placed toward wound bed and which side should be facing away from it; check product instructions.)	Ensures proper absorption and keeps wound exudate away from wound bed (Bryant and Nix, 2016).
(4) Cut foam to fit around drain or tube.	Some foam dressings are designed to fit around tubes such as a tracheostomy.
(5) Cover with secondary dressing as necessary.	Some foam must be covered with secondary dressing (Bryant and Nix, 2016).
d. **Alginate dressings:**	
(1) Cut sheet or rope to fit size of wound or loosely pack into wound space (see illustration), filling ½ to ⅔ full.	Highly absorptive product expands with absorption of serous fluid or exudate (Bryant and Nix, 2016).
(2) Apply secondary dressing such as transparent film (see illustration; see Procedural Guideline 27.1), foam, or hydrocolloid.	Secondary dressing prohibits drainage on bed linens and clothing.
13. Label dressing with your initials and date dressing changed.	Provides timeline for next dressing change.
14. Help patient return to a comfortable position.	Enhances patient comfort and relaxation.
15. Be sure nurse call system is in an accessible location within patient's reach.	Ensures patient can call for assistance if needed.
16. Raise side rails (as appropriate) and lower bed to lowest position.	Ensures patient safety.
17. Discard soiled dressing materials properly. Remove gloves by pulling them inside out and discard in prepared bag. Perform hand hygiene.	Reduces transfer of microorganisms.

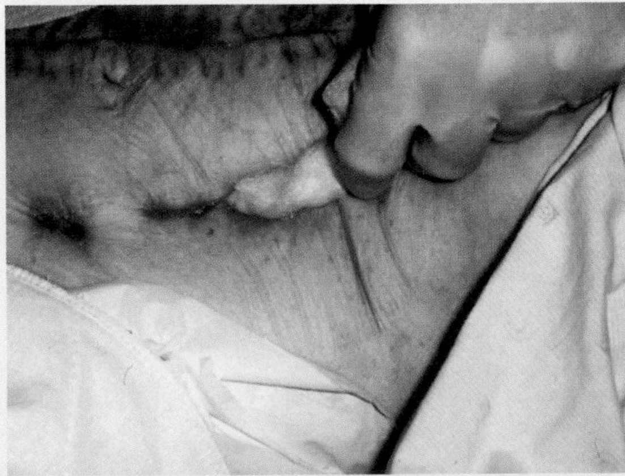

STEP 12d(1) Alginate dressing applied to fill dead space and absorb exudate in full-thickness abdominal wound. *(From Bryant R, Nix D: Acute and chronic wounds: current management concepts, ed 5, St. Louis, 2016, Mosby.)*

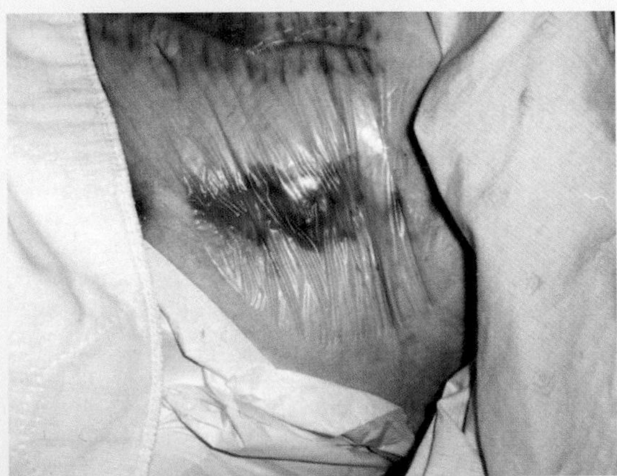

STEP 12d(2) Alginate dressing secured with secondary transparent dressing. *(From Bryant R, Nix D: Acute and chronic wounds: current management concepts, ed 5, St. Louis, 2016, Mosby.)*

STEP	RATIONALE
EVALUATION	
1. Inspect appearance of wound: measure size of wound, observe amount and color of drainage; observe presence of periwound edema or erythema. Palpate around wound for tenderness.	Determines status of wound healing.
2. Evaluate patient's level of comfort.	Documents patient's level of comfort after procedure.
3. Inspect condition of dressing at least every shift or as ordered.	Determines integrity of wound dressing.
4. **Use Teach-Back:** "I want to be sure I explained why I need to use a foam dressing for your wound. Tell me why this foam dressing material is the best option for your wound." Revise your instruction now or develop a plan for revised patient/family caregiver teaching if patient/family caregiver is not able to teach back correctly.	Determines patient's and family caregiver's level of understanding of instructional topic.

Unexpected Outcomes	Related Interventions
1. Wound develops more necrotic tissue and increases in size.	• In rare instances, some wounds do not tolerate hypoxia induced by hydrocolloid dressings. Discontinue use in these patients. Notify health care provider. • Evaluate appropriateness of wound care protocol. • Evaluate for other factors impairing wound healing.
2. Dressing does not stay in place.	• Evaluate size of dressing used for adequate margin (2.5 to 3.75 cm [1 to 1½ inches]) or dry skin more thoroughly before reapplication. • Consider custom shapes for difficult body parts. "Picture frame" edges of hydrocolloid dressing using tape. • Dressing may be secured with roll gauze, tape, transparent dressing, or dressing sheet.
3. Periwound skin is macerated.	• Assess moisture control property of dressing or application technique. May need new type of dressing.

Recording

- Record appearance, color, and size of wound; characteristics of drainage; presence of necrotic tissue; type of dressings applied; patient's response to dressing change; and level of comfort in nurses' notes.
- Document your evaluation of patient learning.

Hand-Off Reporting

- Report any unexpected appearance of wound drainage, bright red bleeding, or evidence of wound dehiscence or evisceration.
- Report any change in exudate, bleeding, odor, pain, or localized edema.
- Report any change in wound management.

PROCEDURAL GUIDELINE 27.2 *Applying Gauze and Elastic Bandages*

Purpose

Gauze and elastic bandages secure or wrap hard-to-cover areas of the body such as dressings on extremities and amputation stumps. Gauze bandages are lightweight and inexpensive, mold easily around body contours, and permit air circulation to prevent skin maceration. Elastic bandages apply compression to a body part. Elastic bandages are a secondary dressing, providing protection, pressure, immobilization, and anchoring of underlying dressings or splints. They are available in rolls of various widths and materials, including gauze, elastic, webbing, elasticized knit, and muslin. Elastic compression to a lower extremity prevents edema by promoting the return of blood from the peripheral to the central circulation. Select a bandage based on the size and shape of the body part to be bandaged. For example, a gauze or elastic bandage on a wrist or ankle would be smaller than a bandage for the upper leg or thigh.

Delegation and Collaboration

The skill of applying an elastic bandage for compression cannot be delegated to nursing assistive personnel (NAP). A nurse assesses the condition of any wound or dressing before applying a bandage. The skill of applying bandages to secure nonsterile dressings can be delegated to NAP (refer to agency policy). The nurse directs the NAP about:

- Modifying the bandage application, such as with special taping.
- Reviewing what to observe and report back to the nurse (e.g., patient's complaint of pain, numbness, or tingling after

PROCEDURAL GUIDELINE 27.2 *Applying Gauze and Elastic Bandages—cont'd*

application or changes in patient's skin color or temperature).

Equipment

Correct width and number of gauze or elastic bandages; clips or adhesive tape; clean gloves if wound drainage is present; *Option:* pillow

Procedural Steps

1. Identify patient using at least two identifiers (e.g., name and birthday or name and medical record number) according to agency policy (TJC, 2019).
2. Review patient's medical record for specific orders related to application of gauze or elastic bandage. Note area to be covered, type of bandage required, frequency of change, and previous response to treatment.
3. Assess patient's level of comfort (pain scale of 0 to 10). Administer prescribed analgesic as needed before dressing change.
4. Perform hand hygiene. Observe adequacy of circulation by palpating temperature of skin and pulses, presence of edema, and sensation (distal to area to be bandaged). Observe skin color and movement of body part to be wrapped. **NOTE:** Impaired circulation may result in pain, coolness to touch when compared with the opposite side of the body, cyanosis or pallor of skin, diminished or absent pulses, edema or localized pooling, and numbness and/or tingling of body part.
5. Apply clean gloves (if drainage or break in skin is present). Inspect skin of area to be bandaged for alterations in integrity as indicated by presence of abrasion, discoloration, or chafing. Pay close attention to areas over bony prominences.
6. Inspect the condition of any wound for appearance, size, and presence and character of drainage and be sure that it is covered with a proper dressing. If not, reapply dressing (check agency policy for type of gloves to use). Remove and dispose of clean gloves and perform hand hygiene.
7. Assess for size of bandage:
   a. *Gauze or basic elastic bandage to secure a dressing:* Assess size of area to be covered. Each successive roll of gauze/elastic should overlap previous layer. Use smaller widths for upper extremities, larger widths for lower extremities.
   b. *Elastic bandage to provide simple compression:* Assess circumference of lower extremity before or shortly after patient gets out of bed in the morning or after patient has been in bed for at least 15 minutes. Select width that will cover and overlap without bulkiness.
8. Identify patient's and family caregiver's present knowledge and literacy level and ability to manipulate bandage if bandaging will be continued at home.
9. Close room door or curtains. Position patient comfortably in an anatomically correct supine position in bed.
10. Perform hand hygiene and apply clean gloves if drainage is present.
11. Apply gauze or elastic bandage to secure dressings:
    a. Elevate dependent extremity for 15 minutes before applying elastic bandage to promote venous return.
    b. Make sure that primary dressing over wound is securely in place.
    c. Begin elastic bandage application at the distal body part. Hold roll of bandage in your dominant hand and use other hand to lightly hold beginning layer.
    d. Apply even tension during application and begin with two circular turns to anchor bandage. Continue to maintain even tension and transfer roll to dominant hand as you wrap bandage (see illustration).
    e. Apply bandage from distal point toward proximal boundary (see illustration), using appropriate turns to cover various shapes of body parts (Table 27.4). Roll gauze, overlapping each layer by one-half to two-thirds the width of the bandage.
    f. Double check your tension and ensure that bandage is snug but not tight and that primary dressing or splint is positioned correctly. A tight bandage may cause numbness and tingling from impaired circulation and/or pressure on peripheral nerves.
    g. While unrolling an elastic bandage, stretch bandage slightly. Explain to patient that smooth, even pressure will be applied to improve circulation, reduce swelling, immobilize body part, and provide pressure.

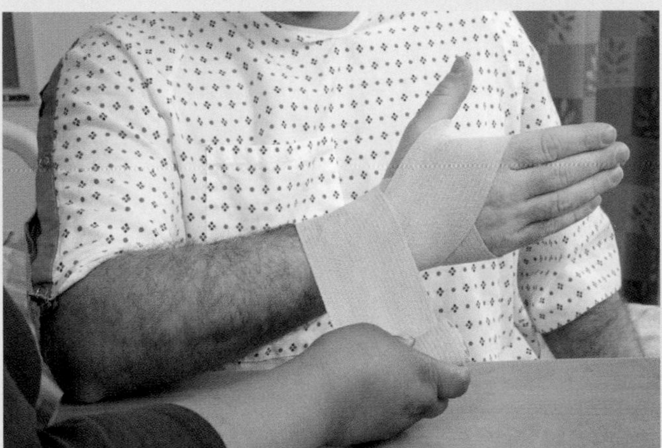

STEP 11d Hold elastic bandage in dominant hand and apply with circular turns.

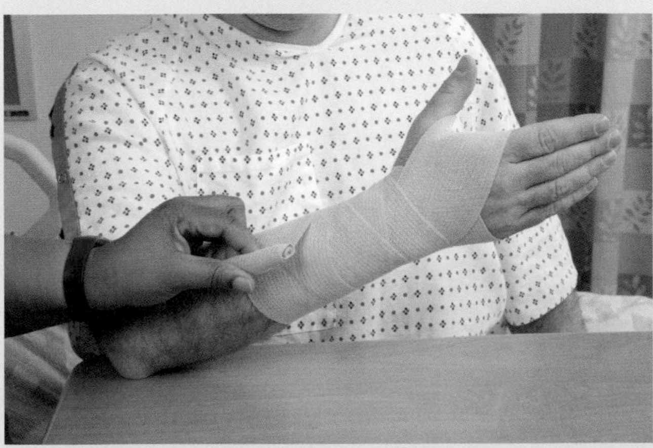

STEP 11e Apply bandage from distal to proximal.

Continued

TABLE 27.4
Types of Bandage Turns

Type	Description	Purpose or Use
Circular Turns	Bandage turn overlapping previous turn completely	Anchors bandage at first and final turn; covers small part (finger, toe)
Spiral Turns	Bandage ascending body part with each turn overlapping previous one by ½ or ⅔ width of bandage	Covers cylindrical body parts such as wrist or upper arm
Spiral-Reverse Turns	Turn requiring twist (reversal) of bandage halfway through each turn	Covers cone-shaped body parts such as the forearm, thigh, or calf; useful with non-stretch bandage material, such as gauze or flannel
Figure-Eight Turns	Oblique overlapping turns alternately ascending and descending over bandaged part, each turn crossing previous one to form figure eight	Covers joints; applies low-grade pressure for venous return; snug fit provides excellent immobilization

PROCEDURAL GUIDELINE 27.2 *Applying Gauze and Elastic Bandages—cont'd*

h. End bandage with two circular turns; secure end of gauze or elastic bandage to outside layer of bandage, not skin, with tape or clips (see illustration).

Safe Patient Care *Keep toes or fingertips uncovered and visible for follow-up circulatory assessment, except in cases in which toes or fingers are treated because of wounds.*

12. Apply elastic bandage over stump (see illustrations):
a. Elevate stump with pillow or support it with the help of another person.

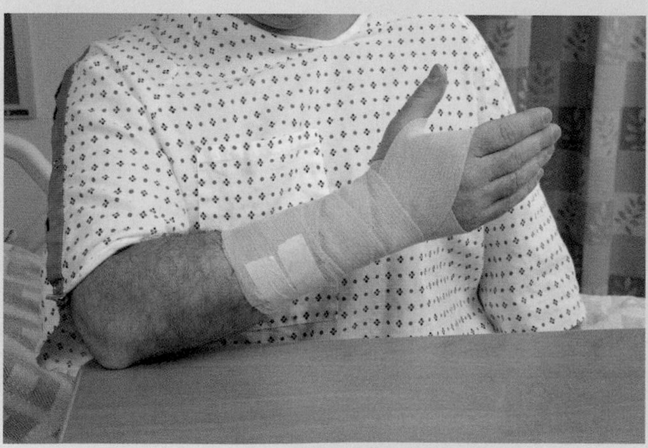

STEP 11h Secure with tape or closure device.

b. Secure bandage by wrapping it twice around proximal end of stump or person's waist (depending on size of stump)
c. Make half turn with bandage perpendicular to its edge.
d. Bring body of bandage over distal end of stump.
e. Continue to fold bandage over stump, wrapping from distal to proximal points.
f. Secure with metal clips, Velcro if provided, or tape.

13. Remove and dispose of gloves if worn and perform hand hygiene. Help patient to comfortable position.
14. Be sure nurse call system is in an accessible location within patient's reach.
15. Raise side rails (as appropriate) and lower bed to lowest position.
16. Assess degree of tightness of bandage, wrinkles, looseness, and presence of drainage.
17. Evaluate distal circulation when bandage application is complete, at least twice during next 8 hours, and then at least every shift.
a. Observe skin color for pallor or cyanosis.
b. Palpate skin for warmth.
c. Palpate distal pulses and compare bilaterally.
d. Ask patient to rate any pain on scale of 0 to 10 and to describe any numbness, tingling, or other discomfort to evaluate for neurological and vascular changes.
18. Observe mobility of extremity.
19. Record patient's level of comfort, circulation status, type of bandage applied, presence of swelling, and range of motion at baseline and after bandage application on flow sheet in nurses' notes in electronic health record (EHR) or chart.
20. Report any changes in neurological or circulatory status to health care provider.

PROCEDURAL GUIDELINE 27.2 *Applying Gauze and Elastic Bandages—cont'd*

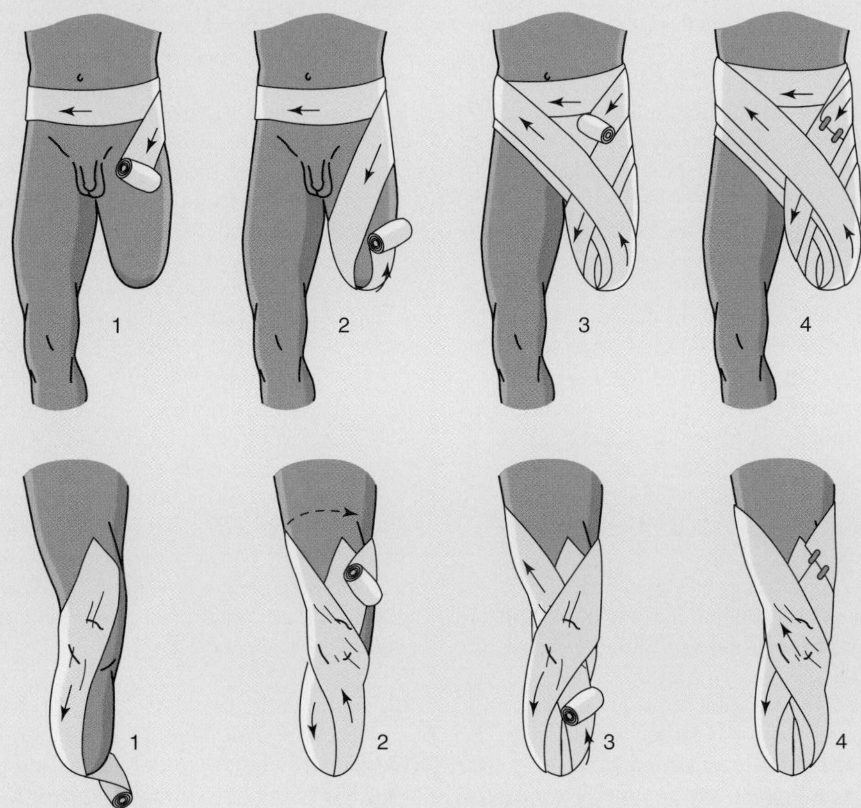

STEP 12 (Top) Correct method for bandaging midthigh amputation stump. Note that bandage must be anchored around patient's waist. (Bottom) Correct method for bandaging midcalf amputation stump. Note that bandage need not be anchored around waist. *(From Monahan F et al:* Phipps' medical-surgical nursing: health and illness perspectives, *ed 8, St. Louis, 2006, Mosby.)*

PROCEDURAL GUIDELINE 27.3 *Applying a Binder*

Purpose

Binders are bandages made of a material specially designed for a specific body part and are usually made of elastic or cotton. The most common type is the abdominal binder. An abdominal binder supports large abdominal incisions that are vulnerable to tension or stress as a patient moves or coughs (Fig. 27.3). Some research demonstrates the benefits of abdominal binders following major abdominal surgery, such as improved postoperative mobility and pain control (Arici et al., 2016; Mizell et al., 2018; Nahabedian et al., 2018). In addition, abdominal binders provide a noninvasive intervention for enhancing recovery of walk performance, controlling pain, and reducing stress on the abdominal muscles (Gallagher, 2016; Giller et al., 2016).

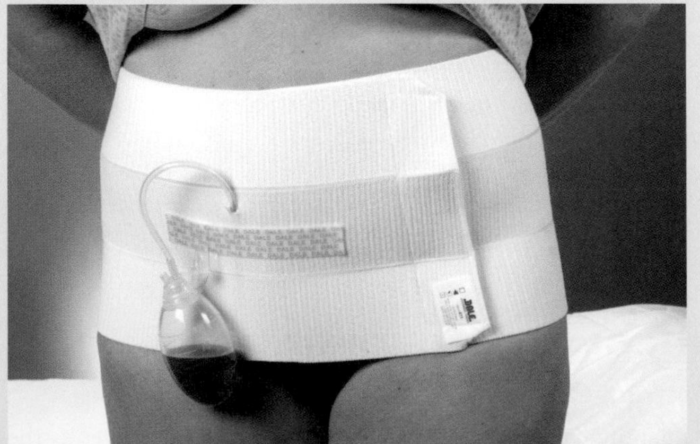

FIG 27.3 Abdominal binder with Velcro closures. *(Courtesy Dale Medical Products, Plainsville, MA.)*

Delegation and Collaboration

The skill of applying a binder can be delegated to nursing assistive personnel (NAP). A nurse assesses the condition of any incision, the skin, and patient's ability to breathe before binder application. The nurse directs the NAP about:

Continued

PROCEDURAL GUIDELINE 27.3 *Applying a Binder—cont'd*

- How to modify the skill, such as special wrapping or manner of securing the binder.
- Reporting patient's complaint of pain, numbness, tingling, or difficulty breathing after applying abdominal binder or any changes in patient's skin color or temperature.

Equipment

Clean gloves if wound drainage present; gauze bandage as needed; correct type and size of binder; closures for cloth binder

Procedural Steps

1. Identify patient using at least two identifiers (e.g., name and birthday or name and medical record number) according to agency policy (TJC, 2019).
2. Review medical record for order for binder (check agency policy).
3. Observe patient who needs support of thorax or abdomen; observe ability to breathe deeply, cough effectively, and turn or move independently.
4. Perform hand hygiene, apply clean gloves as needed. Inspect skin for actual or potential alterations in integrity. Observe for irritation, abrasion, and skin surfaces that rub against one another.
5. Inspect any surgical dressing for intactness, presence of drainage, and coverage of incision. Change any soiled dressing before applying binder (using clean gloves). Remove and dispose of gloves and perform hand hygiene.
6. Determine patient's level of pain using scale of 0 to 10. Administer prescribed analgesic 30 minutes before dressing change.
7. Gather necessary data regarding size of patient and appropriate binder to use (see manufacturer guidelines) to ensure proper fit.
8. Assess patient's or family caregiver's knowledge, experience, and health literacy.
9. Close room door or curtains.
10. Perform hand hygiene and apply clean gloves (if likely to contact wound drainage).
11. Apply abdominal binder:
    a. Position patient in supine position with head slightly elevated and knees slightly flexed.
    b. Help patient roll on side away from you toward raised side rail while firmly supporting abdominal incision and dressing with hands. Fanfold far side of binder toward midline of binder.
    c. Place binder flat on bed, right side up. Fanfold far side of binder toward midline of binder so patient can roll over with minimal effort.
    d. Place fanfolded ends of binder under patient.
    e. Instruct patient or help him or her roll over folded binder. For overweight patients consider asking nurse colleague to help.
    f. Unfold and stretch ends out smoothly on far side of bed. Then stretch out ends on near side of bed.
    g. Instruct patient to roll back into supine position.
    h. Adjust binder so supine patient is centered over binder, using symphysis pubis and costal margins as lower and upper landmarks.
    i. If patient is very thin, pad iliac prominences with gauze bandage.
    j. Close binder. Pull one end of binder over center of patient's abdomen. While maintaining tension on that end of binder, pull opposite end of binder over center and secure with Velcro closure tabs or metal fasteners. Provides continuous wound support and comfort.

Safe Patient Care *After binder is in place, assess patient's ability to breathe deeply and cough effectively. When applied correctly, an abdominal binder over midline abdominal incisions should not affect the patient's pulmonary function.*

12. Assess patient's comfort level and adjust binder as necessary. Ask patient to rate pain on scale of 0 to 10.
13. Remove and dispose of gloves and perform hand hygiene.
14. Help patient to comfortable position.
15. Be sure nurse call system is in an accessible location within patient's reach.
16. Raise side rails (as appropriate) and lower bed to lowest position.
17. Remove binder and surgical dressing to assess skin and wound characteristics at least every 8 hours.
18. Evaluate patient's ability to ventilate properly, including deep breathing and coughing, every 4 hours to determine presence of impaired ventilation and potential pulmonary complications.
19. Record baseline and post-binder condition of skin, circulation, integrity of underlying dressing, and patient's comfort level in nurses' notes in the electronic health record (EHR) or chart. Also record type of bandage applied.
20. Report any complications (e.g., pain, skin irritation, impaired ventilation). Report reduced ventilation (e.g., pulse oximetry, pulmonary function tests), change in incision, or change in drainage to health care provider immediately.

SPECIAL CONSIDERATIONS

Patient-Centered Care

- Identify patient's specific cultural or spiritual practices as they relate to the management of wounds. Open a discussion with your patient and family caregiver by asking if there are any special considerations to be aware of before proceeding with wound care.
- Identify individual measures to minimize a patient's discomfort during a dressing change by understanding his or her values and beliefs about pain management.

Patient Education

- Take time during wound dressing changes to teach the patient and family caregiver about wound care, how to perform a dressing change, how to evaluate if the dressing change is performed correctly, and when to contact the health care provider.
- When a transparent dressing is used, explain to patient and family caregiver that collection of wound fluid under dressing is not "pus" but normal interaction of body fluids with dressing.

Age-Specific

Pediatric

- Children may be fearful of dressing changes, especially if a child had a bad experience with a wound treatment or dressing change in the past. To avoid long-term fear and distress over dressing changes, look for ways to help a child cope. Allow the child to pick a distraction to use during the dressing change (e.g., playing a video game, listening to music; Hockenberry et al., 2017).

Gerontological

- Consider risk factors in older-adult patients for impaired skin integrity, such as sensory impairment, dry and dehydrated skin, or impaired nutritional status, that will affect wound healing (Touhy and Jett, 2018).
- Avoid early and frequent removal of a hydrocolloid dressing to reduce injury to surrounding intact skin.
- Adhesive tape may be too irritating to older adults' skin and cause skin tears. Use paper tape, nonallergenic tape, or wraps or mesh to avoid tape contacting a patient's skin (Touhy and Jett, 2018).

Home Care

- Some wounds may be cleansed in the shower. Have patient verify this practice with health care provider before discharge.
- Clean, instead of sterile, dressings may be used in the home.
- Inform patient and family caregiver how to obtain additional wound care supplies and how to properly dispose of soiled dressings.

✦ PRACTICE REFLECTIONS

A 45-year-old man is being discharged from the health care agency with an open surgical wound. For the past 3 days, damp-to-dry dressings were applied.

1. Think about a discussion you will have with the patient and his wife to evaluate their understanding of the dressing-change process.
2. What information do you need from the patient and his wife to ensure they understand how to dispose of contaminated dressing materials safely in the home?
3. The patient is scheduled for a follow-up visit with the surgeon in 1 week. Because they will be managing the wound for a week, what information will they need to evaluate wound healing or changes in wound status and to know when to contact the health care provider prior to the scheduled appointment?

✦ CLINICAL REVIEW QUESTIONS

1. The patient has a damp-to-moist dressing over a draining surgical wound. The nurse instructs the NAP to report which of the following patient findings to the nurse? (Select all that apply.)
   1. Increase in pain
   2. Increased fever
   3. Degree of wound healing
   4. Changes in amount of wound exudate or color
   5. Patient report of "opening of incision"
2. The health care provider has ordered moist-to-dry dressing changes twice a day for the patient using normal saline. Place the following procedural steps in order.
   1. Clean the wound with saline-moistened gauze.
   2. Remove the old dressing.
   3. Inspect appearance and condition of wound; measure wound size.
   4. Cover wound with 4 × 4–inch sterile gauze and an ABD pad.
   5. Loosely pack the wound with saline-moistened gauze.
   6. Blot the wound dry.
   7. Fasten dressing using nonallergenic tape.
3. Wounds with large amount of exudate (drainage) require absorptive dressing materials. Which dressing materials facilitate exudate absorption while promoting wound healing? (Select all that apply.)
   1. Alginate
   2. Foam
   3. Hydrocolloid
   4. Hydrogel
   5. Transparent

Answers and Rationales for Clinical Review Questions can be found on the Evolve website.

REFERENCES

Arici A, et al: The effect of using an abdominal binder on postoperative gastrointestinal function, mobilization, pulmonary function, and pain in patients undergoing major abdominal surgery: a randomized controlled trial, *Int J Nurs Stud* 62:108, 2016.

Armstrong D, et al: Basic principles of wound management, *UpToDate* 2018. https://www.uptodate.com/contents/basic-principles-of-wound-management.

Arroyo AA, et al: Open label clinical trial comparing the clinical and economic effectiveness of using a polyurethane film surgical dressing with gauze surgical dressings in the care of post-operative surgical wounds, *Int Wound J* 12:285, 2015.

Barrett S: Wound-bed preparation: a vital step in the healing process, *Br J Nurs* 26(12):S24, 2017.

Bryant RA, Best M: Management of draining wounds and fistulas. In Bryant RA, Nix DP, editors: *Acute and chronic wounds: current management concepts*, ed 5, St. Louis, 2016, Mosby.

Bryant RA, Nix DP: Principles of wound healing and topical management. In Bryant RA, Nix DP, editors: *Acute and chronic wounds: current management concepts*, ed 5, St. Louis, 2016, Mosby.

Centers for Disease Control and Prevention (CDC): What is health literacy? 2016. https://www.cdc.gov/healthliteracy/learn/index.html.

Centers for Disease Control and Prevention (CDC): Guideline for the prevention of surgical site infection, *JAMA Surg* 152(8):784, 2017.

Chamanga ET, et al: Chronic wound bed preparation using a cleansing solution, *Br J Nurs* 24(12):S30, 2015.

Doughty D, Sparks-DeFriese B: Wound-healing physiology. In Bryant RA, Nix DP, editors: *Acute and chronic wounds: nursing management*, ed 5, St. Louis, 2016, Mosby.

Dutra RAA, et al: Using transparent polyurethane film and hydrocolloid dressings to prevent pressure ulcers, *J Wound Care* 24(6):268, 2015.

Dutra RAA, et al: Cost comparison of pressure ulcer preventive dressings: hydrocolloid dressings versus transparent polyurethane film, *J Wound Care* 25(11):635, 2016.

Evans K, et al: Overview of treatment of chronic wounds, *UpToDate* 2018. https://www.uptodate.com/contents/overview-of-treatment-of-chronic-wounds.

Gallagher S: Skin care of obese patients. In Bryant RA, Nix DP, editors: *Acute and chronic wounds: current management concepts*, ed 5, St. Louis, 2016, Mosby.

Giller CM, et al: A randomized controlled trial of abdominal binders for the management of postoperative pain and distress after cesarean delivery, *Int J Gynaecol Obstet* 133:188, 2016.

Hockenberry M, et al: *Wong's essentials of pediatric nursing*, ed 10, St. Louis, 2017, Elsevier.

Kayser S, et al: Prevalence and analysis of medical device-related pressure injuries: results from the international pressure ulcer prevalence survey, *Adv Skin Wound Care* 31(6):276, 2018.

Krasner DL: Wound pain: impact and assessment. In Bryant RA, Nix DP, editors: *Acute and chronic wounds: current management concepts*, ed 5, St. Louis, 2016, Mosby.

Mizell J, et al: Complications of abdominal surgical incisions, *UpToDate* 2018. https://www.uptodate.com/contents/complications-of-abdominal-surgical-incisions#!

Munro G: Causes and consideration with chronic wounds: a narrative review of the evidence, *Wound Pract Res* 25(2):88, 2017.

Nahabedian M, et al: Rectus abdominis diastasis, *UpToDate* 2018. https://www.uptodate.com/contents/rectus-abdominis-diastasis.

National Pressure Ulcer Advisory Panel (NPUAP), European Pressure Ulcer Advisory Panel (EPUAP): New 2014 prevention and treatment of pressure ulcers: clinical practice guidelines, 2014. http://www.npuap.org/resources/educational-and-clinical-resources/prevention-and-treatment-of-pressure-ulcers-clinical-practice-guideline.

Pittman J, et al: Medical device related hospital-acquired pressure ulcers, *J Wound Ostomy Continence Nurs* 42(2):151, 2015.

Ramundo JM: Wound debridement. In Bryant RA, Nix DP, editors: *Acute and chronic wounds: nursing management*, ed 5, St. Louis, 2016, Mosby.

Santamaria N, et al: A randomized controlled trial of the effectiveness of soft silicone multi-layered foam dressings in the prevention of sacral and heel pressure ulcers in trauma and critically ill patients: the border trial, *Int Wound J* 12(3):302, 2015.

Swanson T, et al: Ten top tips: identification of wound infection in a chronic wound, *Wounds Int* 6(2):22, 2015.

The Joint Commission (TJC): *2019 National Patient Safety Goals*, Oakbrook Terrace, IL, 2019, The Commission. http://www.jointcommission.org/standards_information/npsgs.aspx.

Touhy TA, Jett K: *Ebersole and Hess' gerontological nursing and healthy aging*, ed 5, St. Louis, 2018, Elsevier.

28 Intravenous and Vascular Access Therapy

SKILLS AND PROCEDURES

EVOLVE WEBSITE/RESOURCES LIST

http://evolve.elsevier.com/Perry/nursinginterventions

Audio Glossary • Checklists • Clinical Review Questions • Answers and Rationales for Clinical Review Questions • Video Clips

INTRODUCTION

Intravenous therapy provides access to the vascular system to deliver solutions and medications and to infuse blood or blood products. Knowledge, critical thinking, and strict adherence to standards of practice are required for initiation of infusion therapy and during the course of treatment. Assessment of a patient's anatomy and physiology of the circulatory system, fluid and electrolyte balance, disease pathophysiology, type and duration of prescribed therapy, allergies, and response to illness plays a key role in decision making to ensure safe delivery of infusion solutions or medications. Successful intravenous (IV) therapy depends on nursing skill, knowledge, and competence; patient preparation; site selection; catheter selection; and catheter insertion. The goal of IV therapy is to maintain and prevent fluid and electrolyte imbalances, administer continuous or intermittent medications (e.g., antibiotics and analgesics), and replenish blood volume (Gorski, 2018).

PRACTICE STANDARDS

- American Association of Blood Banks (AABB), 2017: Technical manual—Regulations for the administration of blood and blood components; mandates use of bar-code system to reduce human error
- Centers for Disease Control and Prevention (CDC), 2011: Guidelines for the prevention of intravascular catheter-related infections
- Infusion Nurses Society (INS), 2016a: Infusion therapy standards of practice
- Occupational Safety and Health Administration (OSHA), 2012: Bloodborne pathogens standards
- The Joint Commission, 2019: National Patient Safety Goals—Patient identification
- U.S. Food and Drug Administration (FDA), 2015: Requirements for blood and blood components intended for transfusion or for further manufacturing use, final rule—Regulations for the collection of blood and blood components used for transfusion

EVIDENCE-BASED PRACTICE

Reducing Complications in Infusion Therapy

Infusion therapy is practiced in health care settings spanning from hospital to home. It is expected that the nurse providing infusion therapy understands and implements evidence-based practice and complies with laws, rules regulations, standards, and policies to keep up with role changes, understand new products and technology, and prevent complications (Infusion Nurses Society [INS], 2016a). Guidelines include the following:

- Passive disinfection caps, which contain a sponge saturated with a disinfecting agent (usually isopropyl alcohol) and are placed on the end of the needleless connector in between intermittent infusions, protect the end and require less disinfection time or do not require disinfection prior to access (INS, 2016a). These caps have been shown to reduce intraluminal contamination and significantly reduce the rates of central line–associated bloodstream infection (CLABSI) (INS, 2016a; Kamboj et al., 2015).
- Compared with all other dressing types, the use of dressings impregnated with chlorhexidine gluconate (CHG), in a patch or in a whole dressing, is more effective in reducing the incidence of bloodstream infections related to central vascular access devices (CVADs; Oncology Nurses Society [ONS], 2017).
- Primary and secondary continuous administration sets used to administer solutions other than lipid, blood, or blood products should be changed no more often than every 96 hours or according to agency policy. Blood transfusion administration sets and filters should be changed after each unit or every 4 hours; however, if more than 1 unit is to be

infused in 4 hours, then the set can be used for a 4-hour period (INS, 2016a, 2016b).
- Remove venous access devices (VADs) upon unresolved complication, discontinuation of infusion therapy, or when no longer necessary for the plan of care (Helton et al., 2016; INS, 2016a).
- Electronic identification systems, including bar-code technology and embedded radiofrequency-emitting chips, help reduce errors in the identification process between a patient and the compatible blood unit (American Association of Blood Banks [AABB], 2017).

SAFETY GUIDELINES

Clinician competence is required for the use, placement, and management of VADs; the use of infusion equipment; and in all aspects of administering infusion therapy (INS, 2016a). Safety guidelines include the following:

- Conduct a complete history and physical assessment, including vital signs, and review laboratory findings before initiating any solutions or medications. Consider prolonged environmental conditions that affect a patient's fluid status (e.g., exposure to hot, humid weather), leading to fluid and electrolyte imbalances, particularly in the infant, older adult, and chronically ill.
- Know the indications for prescribed therapy before initiating IV therapy. Obtain and review the health care provider's order to ensure appropriateness of prescribed solution or medication for patient's age, health status, medical diagnosis, allergy status, acuity, VAD type and tip location, dose, frequency, and route of administration (INS, 2016b).
- Reduce risk for administration-set misconnections by tracing the path between the IV container and the patient, labeling administration sets near the patient connection and solution container, routing tubing with different purposes in different directions, and providing education for patient/caregivers and nursing assistive personnel (NAP) to seek assistance with connecting or disconnecting devices or infusions (The Joint Commission [TJC], 2014).
- Utilize electronic identification systems during pretransfusion and patient identification to prevent transfusion reactions, serious injury, or patient death associated with unsafe administration of blood products. Unsafe administration includes, but is not limited to, hemolytic reactions and administering (1) blood or blood products to the wrong patient, (2) the wrong type of blood product, or (3) blood or blood products that have been improperly stored or handled (National Quality Forum [NQF], 2011).
- Maintain the sterility of a patent IV system by utilizing INS standards (Box 28.1).
- Know and implement the standard precautions for infection control and the Occupational Safety and Health Administration (OSHA) standards for occupational exposure to bloodborne pathogens (Box 28.2).

BOX 28.1

INS Standards to Decrease Intravascular Infection Related to Intravenous Therapy

- Perform hand hygiene before placing and before providing any VAD-associated interventions.
- Assess the VAD catheter–skin junction site and surrounding area for redness, tenderness, swelling, and drainage by visual inspection and palpating through the intact dressing. Assess short-peripheral catheters minimally at least every 4 hours or more if clinically indicated, and daily for outpatient or home care patients. CVADs should be assessed at least daily.
- Change the dressing immediately to assess, cleanse, and disinfect the site in the event of drainage, tenderness, other signs of infection or if dressing becomes loosened or dislodged.
- Perform dressing changes at frequency based on the type of catheter and dressing. Short-peripheral catheter dressings are changed if the dressing becomes damp, loosened, and/or visibly soiled or if there is blood or drainage under the dressing, and at least every 5 to 7 days. Change CVAD dressings at least every 5 to 7 days for TSM dressings and at least every 2 days for gauze dressings that cover a catheter site or are under a TSM.
- Use approved antiseptic agents prior to venipuncture and when performing skin antisepsis. The preferred skin antiseptic is > 0.5% chlorhexidine in alcohol solution. Tincture of iodine, an iodophors (povidone-iodine), or 70% alcohol may be used if chlorhexidine solution is contraindicated.
- Allow skin antiseptic to fully dry prior to dressing placement; for alcoholic chlorhexidine solutions, allow to dry for at least 30 seconds; for iodophors, allow at least 1½ to 2 minutes.
- Use catheter stabilization device that allows visual inspection of access site.
- Vigorously scrub needleless connectors with an approved antiseptic prior to each access using mechanical friction for at least 5 seconds. Disinfect before each access when multiple accesses are required.
- Change needleless connectors using aseptic no-touch technique no more frequently than 96-hour intervals.
- Use passive disinfection caps (e.g., isopropyl alcohol).
- Change administration sets based on solution administered, frequency of the infusion, and immediately upon suspected contamination or when integrity has been compromised.

CVAD, Central vascular access device; *INS,* Infusion Nurses Society; *TSM,* transparent semipermeable membrane; *VAD,* venous access device.

Modified from Infusion Nurses Society: Infusion therapy standards of practice, *J Intraven Nurs* 39(suppl 1):1S, 2016.

BOX 28.2

Standards for Reducing Occupational Exposure to Bloodborne Pathogens

- Gloves are necessary when there is a reasonable expectation that the employee may contact blood (e.g., during vascular access procedures or while changing intravenous [IV] administration sets).
- Immediately place contaminated needles, needleless devices, and other sharps in puncture-resistant, leak-proof containers properly labeled as a biohazard; when the containers are full, seal and dispose of them properly.
- Do not bend, shear, recap, or remove contaminated needles from the syringe after use.
- Occupational Safety and Health Administration (OSHA) requires reports of needlestick injuries, and the health care agency must provide medical evaluation and follow-up.
- Hepatitis B vaccinations should be made available to all employees who have occupational exposure.
- Training and education about exposure prevention and use of protective equipment must be offered to high-risk workers who initiate IV therapy.
- Each agency must have an infection control plan, including methods to reduce health care worker's exposure to biohazardous wastes.
- Agencies must have engineering and work practice controls to eliminate or minimize employee exposure. Controls may include sharps disposal containers and self-sheathing needles.

Modified from Occupational Safety and Health Administration (OSHA): Bloodborne pathogens standards, United States Department of Labor, April 3, 2012. https://www.osha.gov/pls/oshaweb/owadisp.show_document?p_table=STANDARDS&p_id=10051.

✦ SKILL 28.1 Insertion of a Short-Peripheral Intravenous Device

Purpose

Placement of an intravenous (IV) device is one of the most invasive procedures a nurse can perform, putting a patient at risk for complications associated with infusion therapy. The Infusion Nurses Society (INS) standards of practice recommend using the smallest-gauge peripheral catheter that will accommodate the prescribed therapy and patient needs (INS, 2016a). Several venous access devices (VADs) are available for use in peripheral veins (Table 28.1). Steel-winged infusion devices (butterfly needles) should be limited to single-dose IV administration and blood sample collection because they are easier to insert but may infiltrate easily (Gorski, 2018; INS, 2016a). Commonly used over-the-needle catheters (ONCs) consist of (1) a metal stylet used to pierce the skin and (2) a flexible plastic catheter made of silicone, polyurethane, polyvinyl chloride, or polytetrafluoroethylene (Teflon with a hard plastic hub that threads into the vein and provides access to deliver infusion therapy; Gorski, 2018). These flexible catheters do not dislodge from veins as easily as stainless steel needles.

Delegation and Collaboration

The skill of inserting a short-peripheral IV access device cannot be delegated to nursing assistive personnel (NAP). Delegation to licensed practical nurses (LPNs) varies by state Nurse Practice Act. The nurse instructs the NAP to:

- Notify the nurse if the patient complains of any IV site–related complications such as redness, pain, tenderness, swelling, bleeding, drainage, or leaking from under dressing.
- Notify the nurse if the patient's IV dressing becomes wet or loose.
- Notify the nurse if the level of fluid in the IV bag is low or the electronic infusion device (EID) is sounding an alarm.

Equipment

- Short-peripheral IV start kit supplies (available in some agencies): single-use tourniquet, tape, transparent semipermeable membrane (TSM) dressing or sterile gauze and sterile tape, antiseptic solution (alcoholic chlorhexidine solution preferred, 70% alcohol, povidone-iodine, or tincture of iodine), 2 × 2–inch gauze pads, and label
- Appropriate short-peripheral IV catheter with safety mechanism for venipuncture; for adults, 20- to 24-gauge catheter; for neonates, children, and older adults, 22- to 24-gauge catheter; for rapid fluid replacement, 16- to 20-gauge catheter; based on vein size for blood transfusion, 20- to 24-gauge catheter; and for short-term therapy or a single dose, steel-winged device (INS, 2016a).
- Clean gloves (latex-free for patients with latex allergy); sterile gloves if palpating the site after skin antisepsis (INS, 2016a)
- Single-use hair clippers or scissors for hair removal if indicated
- Short extension tubing with fused needleless connector or separate needleless connector (also called *injection cap, saline lock, heparin lock, IV plug, buff cap, buffalo cap,* or *PRN adapter*)
- 10-mL syringe prefilled with preservative-free 0.9% sodium chloride (normal saline [NS]; INS, 2016a)
- Antiseptic swabs
- Manufactured catheter stabilization device (if available) and polymer-based skin protectant swab
- Prescribed intravenous solution or medication
- IV administration set (IV tubing), either macrodrip or microdrip, depending on prescribed rate; if using EID, appropriate administration set
- 0.2-micron filter for nonlipid (fat emulsion) solutions (may be incorporated into the infusion set)
- Personal protective equipment: Goggles and mask *(optional based on agency policy)*
- EID and IV pole
- Vein visualization device *(optional based on agency policy)*
- Stethoscope
- Watch with second hand to calculate drip rate
- Special patient gown with snaps at shoulder seams if available
- Needle disposal container (*sharps container* or *biohazard container*)

TABLE 28.1

Intravenous Access Device Options

Type	Use	Types of Infusions
Winged infusion butterfly needle	One-time infusion, IV push administration	Solutions or medications with an osmolarity <900 mOsm/L (INS, 2016a)
Short, over-the-needle catheter (7.5 cm [<3 inches]) may be winged or nonwinged	Most common, continuous infusion, intermittent infusion, short-term duration (INS, 2016a)	Solutions or medications with an osmolarity <900 mOsm/L (INS, 2016a)
Midline peripheral catheters (7.5–20 cm [3–8 inches])	Continuous and intermittent infusions (1–4 weeks; INS, 2016a)	Solutions or medications with an osmolarity <900 mOsm/L (INS, 2016a)

IV, Intravenous.

ASSESSMENT

1. Review accuracy of health care provider's order: date and time, IV solution, route of administration, volume, rate, duration, and signature of ordering health care provider (Gorski, 2018). Follow the seven rights of medication administration (see Chapter 22). *Rationale: Before IV therapy, an order from a health care provider is needed (INS, 2016a). Verification that order is complete prevents medication errors.*
   a. Check approved online database, drug reference book, or pharmacist about IV solution composition, purpose, potential incompatibilities, adverse reactions, and side effects. *Rationale: Ensures safe and correct administration of IV therapy and appropriate selection of VAD.*
2. Obtain data from patient's electronic health record of clinical factors/conditions that will respond to or be affected by administration of IV solutions. *Rationale: Provides baseline to determine effectiveness of prescribed therapy. A systems approach*

is recommended to assess for fluid and electrolyte imbalances (Gorski, 2018).

a. Body weight. *Rationale: Changes in body weight can be an indication of fluid loss or gain (Gorski, 2018).*

b. Clinical markers of vascular volume:

(1) Urine output (decreased, dark yellow). *Rationale: Kidneys respond to extracellular volume (ECV) deficit by reducing urine production and concentrating urine. Kidney disease can also cause oliguria.*

(2) Vital signs: blood pressure, respirations, pulse, temperature. *Rationale: Changes in blood pressure may be associated with fluid-volume status (fluid-volume deficit [FVD]) seen in postural hypotension. Respirations can be altered in presence of acid–base imbalances. Temperature elevations increase need for fluid requirements (temperature of 38.3° C [101° F] to 39.4° C [103° F] require at least 500 mL of fluid replacement within a 24-hour period; Weinstein and Hagle, 2014).*

(3) Distended neck veins. (Normally veins are full when person is supine and flat when person is upright.) *Rationale: Indicator of fluid-volume status: flat or collapsing with inhalation when supine with ECV deficit; full when upright or semi-upright with ECV excess.*

(4) Auscultation of lungs. *Rationale: Crackles or rhonchi in dependent parts of lung may signal fluid buildup caused by ECV excess.*

(5) Capillary refill. *Rationale: Indirect measure of tissue perfusion (sluggish with ECV deficit).*

c. Clinical markers of interstitial volume:

(1) Skin turgor. (Pinch skin over sternum or inside of forearm.) *Rationale: Failure of skin to return to normal position after several seconds indicates FVD (Gorski, 2018).*

(2) Dependent edema (pitting or nonpitting; see Chapter 8). *Rationale: Edema is not usually apparent until 4.4 to 8.8 pounds (2 to 4 kg) of fluid is retained. A weight gain of 2.2 pounds (1 kg) is equivalent to the retention of 1 L of body water (Gorski, 2018).*

(3) Oral mucous membrane between cheek and gum (see Chapter 8). *Rationale: More reliable indicator than dry lips or skin. Dry between cheek and gums indicates ECV deficit.*

d. Thirst. *Rationale: Occurs with hypernatremia and severe ECV deficit. Not a reliable indicator for older adults (Gorski, 2018).*

e. Behavior and level of consciousness:

(1) Restlessness and mild confusion. *Rationale: Occurs with FVD or acid-base imbalance*

(2) Decreased level of consciousness (lethargy, confusion, coma). *Rationale: Occurs with severe ECV deficit. May occur with osmolality, fluid and electrolyte, and acid–base imbalances.*

3. Determine whether patient is to undergo any planned surgeries or procedures. *Rationale: Allows anticipation and placement of appropriate VAD for infusion and avoids placement in an area that will interfere with medical procedures (INS, 2016a).*

4. Assess available laboratory data (e.g., hematocrit, serum electrolytes, arterial blood gases, and kidney functions [blood urea nitrogen, urine specific gravity, and urine osmolality]). *Rationale: Helps determine priority assessments and establishes baseline for determining if therapy is effective. Laboratory values are an assessment of hydration status (Gorski, 2018).*

5. Assess patient's history of allergies, especially to iodine, adhesive, or latex. *Rationale: Equipment used during VAD insertion may contain substances to which patient is allergic. Will require use of latex-free gloves.*

6. Assess patient's arm preference for placement of IV. *Rationale: Provides patient-centered care by determining level of emotional support and instruction needed.*

7. Assess patient's or family caregiver's knowledge, experience, and health literacy regarding IV therapy. *Rationale: Ensures patient or family caregiver has the capacity to obtain, communicate, process, and understand basic health information (Centers for Disease Control and Prevention [CDC], 2016).*

STEP	RATIONALE
PLANNING	
1. Expected outcomes following completion of procedure:	
• Patient's VAD remains patent, and site is free from signs and symptoms of IV-related complications.	Ensures that patient receives prescribed infusion therapy and VAD is without complications (INS, 2016a).
• Vital signs are stable and within normal limits for patient.	Demonstrates response of body systems to fluid and electrolyte replacement (Gorski, 2018).
• Fluid and electrolyte balance returns to normal.	Proper solution is infused at proper rate and monitored, resolving fluid and electrolyte imbalance (Gorski, 2018).
• Patient is able to explain purpose and risks of IV therapy.	Demonstrates learning (INS, 2016a).
2. Provide privacy and prepare environment.	Providing privacy and preparing the environment early help the student/nurse think about the need to remove clutter from the over-bed or bedside table.
3. Perform hand hygiene. Collect and organize equipment on clean, clutter-free bedside stand or over-bed table. Be sure you have the correct infusion set for the EID that is to be used.	Reduces risk of microbial contamination and cross-contamination of equipment (INS, 2016b). Easy access to equipment improves efficiency. Ensures patient safety.
4. Select appropriate-sized catheter; open and prepare sterile packages using sterile aseptic technique (see Chapter 5).	Use smallest-gauge peripheral catheter that will accommodate prescribed therapy and patient needs (INS, 2016a).

STEP	RATIONALE
5. Help patient to comfortable sitting or supine position. Change patient's gown to one more easily removed with snaps at shoulder if available. Provide adequate lighting.	Promotes comfort and relaxation of patient. Use of this gown decreases risk of inadvertently dislodging VAD or administration set when changing gown. Aids in successful vein location.
6. Explain/instruct patient about rationale for infusion, including solution and medications ordered, procedure for initiating an IV line, and signs and symptoms of complications (e.g., redness, pain, tenderness, swelling, bleeding, drainage, or leaking from under dressing).	Provides patient with information about procedure and promotes compliance (INS, 2016a). Informing patient may minimize anxiety.

IMPLEMENTATION

STEP	RATIONALE
1. Identify patient using at least two identifiers (e.g., name and birthday or name and medical record number) according to agency policy. Compare identifiers with information on patient's medication administration record (MAR) or medical record.	Ensures correct patient. Complies with The Joint Commission standards and improves patient safety (TJC, 2019).
2. Perform hand hygiene. Prepare short extension tubing with fused needleless connector or separate needleless connector (injection cap) to attach to catheter hub.	Needleless connectors protect health care workers by eliminating needles and potential for needlestick injuries when accessing VAD (INS, 2016a).
a. Remove protective cap from needleless connector and attach syringe with 1 to 3 mL 0.9% sodium chloride (normal saline), maintaining sterility. Slowly inject enough saline to prime (fill) short extension tubing and connector, removing all air. Leave syringe attached to tubing.	Replaces air with normal saline, preventing air from entering patient's vein later during VAD insertion.
b. Maintain sterility of end of connector by reapplying end caps; set aside for attaching to catheter hub after successful venipuncture. Do not overtighten end caps.	Prevents touch contamination, which allows microorganisms to enter infusion equipment and bloodstream. Overtightening end caps will make it difficult to remove them.

Safe Patient Care *Short extension sets may be used on short-peripheral catheters. Reduces catheter manipulation. For patient safety, all connections should be of Luer-Lok type (INS, 2016a). Luer-Lok connections should be used to prevent accidental disconnection (INS, 2016a). Many agencies use short extension tubing for continuous infusions and stand-alone saline locks (capped catheters).*

STEP	RATIONALE
3. Prepare IV tubing and solution for continuous infusion.	
a. Check IV solution using seven rights of medication administration (see Chapter 22) and review label for name and concentration of solution, type and concentration of any additives, volume, beyond-use and expiration dates, and sterility state. If using bar code, scan code on patient's wristband and then on IV fluid container. Be sure that prescribed additives such as potassium and vitamins have been added. Check solution for color and clarity. Check bag for leaks.	Reviewing label for accuracy reduces risk for medication errors (INS, 2016a). Risk for medication errors can be reduced with safe medication practices, including (INS, 2016a): • Do not add medications to infusing containers of IV solutions (INS, 2016a). • Do not use IV solutions that are discolored, contain precipitates, or are expired. • Risk for transmission of infection can be reduced by not using leaking bags because integrity has been compromised.
b. Open IV infusion set, maintaining sterility. **NOTE:** EIDs sometimes have a dedicated administration set; follow manufacturer's instructions.	Prevents touch contamination, which allows microorganisms to enter infusion equipment and bloodstream.
c. Place roller clamp (see illustration A) about 2 to 5 cm (1 to 2 inches) below drip chamber and move roller clamp to "off" position (see illustration B).	Close proximity of roller clamp to drip chamber allows more accurate regulation of flow rate. Moving clamp to "off" prevents accidental spillage of IV solution during priming.
d. Remove protective sheath over IV tubing port on plastic IV solution bag (see illustration) or top of IV solution bottle while maintaining sterility.	Provides access for insertion of IV tubing spike into solution using sterile technique.
e. Remove protective cover from IV tubing spike while maintaining sterility of spike. Insert spike into port of IV bag using a twisting motion (see illustration). If solution container is glass bottle, clean rubber stopper on glass-bottled solution with antiseptic swab and insert spike into rubber stopper of IV bottle. Bottles require vented tubing.	Flat surface on top of bottled solution may contain contaminants, whereas opening to plastic bag is recessed. Prevents contamination of bottled solution during insertion of spike. If sterility of spike is compromised, discard IV tubing and obtain new one.

STEP	RATIONALE
f. Compress drip chamber and release, allowing it to fill one-third to one-half full (see illustration).	Creates suction effect; fluid enters drip chamber to prevent air from entering tubing.
g. Prime air out of IV tubing by filling with IV solution: Remove protective cover on end of IV tubing (some tubing can be primed without removing protective cover) and slowly open roller clamp to allow fluid to flow from drip chamber to distal end of IV tubing. If tubing has a Y connector, invert Y connector when fluid reaches it to displace air. Return roller clamp to "off" position after priming tubing (filled with IV fluid). Replace protective cover on distal end of tubing. Label IV tubing with date according to agency policy and procedure.	Priming ensures that IV tubing is clear of air and filled with IV solution before connecting to VAD. Slowly filling tubing decreases turbulence and chance of bubble formation. Closing clamp prevents accidental loss of fluid. Maintains sterility. Labeling IV tubing allows for recognition of length of time that tubing has in use and when to change it.

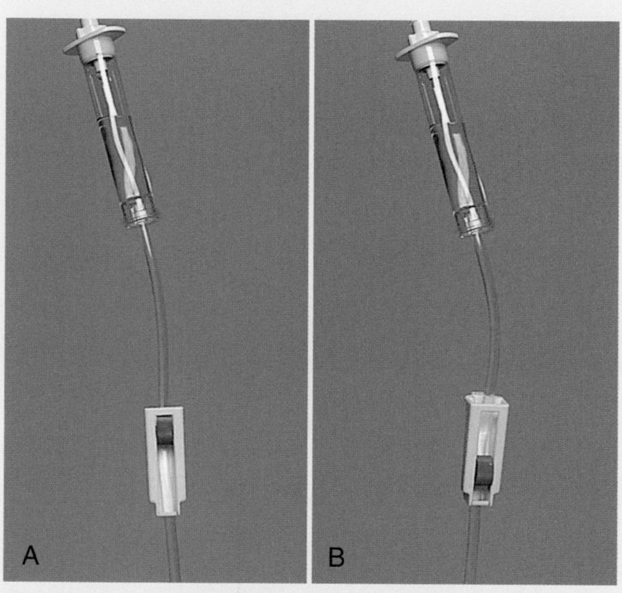

STEP 3c (A) Roller clamp in open position. (B) Roller clamp in closed position.

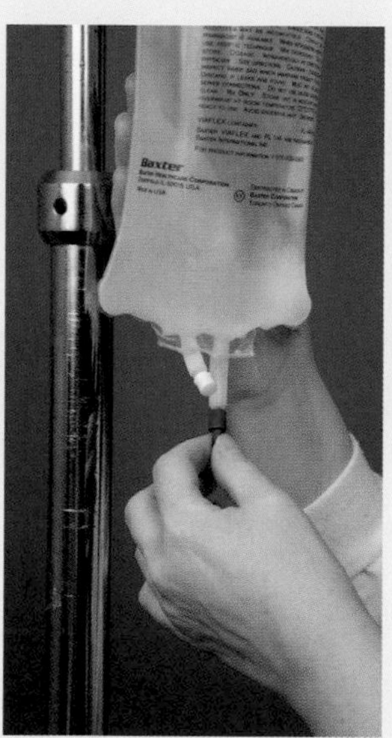

STEP 3d Removing protective sheath from intravenous (IV) tubing port.

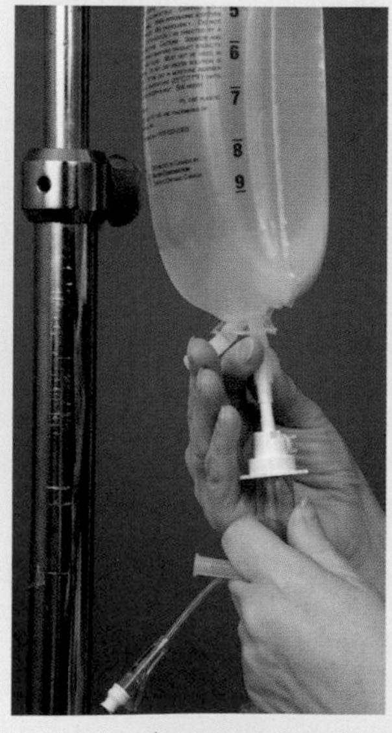

STEP 3e Inserting spike into intravenous (IV) bag.

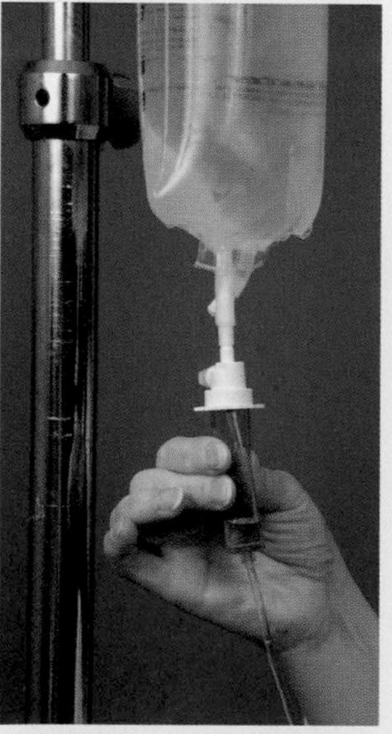

STEP 3f Squeezing drip chamber to fill with fluid one-third to one-half full.

STEP	RATIONALE
h. Be certain that IV tubing is clear of air and air bubbles. To remove small air bubbles, firmly tap tubing where they are located. Check entire length of tubing to ensure that all air bubbles are removed (see illustration).	Large air bubbles act as emboli and should be avoided (Mattox, 2017).
i. If using optional long extension tubing (not short tubing in Step 2), remove protective cover and attach it to distal end of IV tubing, maintaining sterility. Then prime long extension tubing. Insert tubing into EID with power off.	Priming removes air from long extension tubing so it does not enter patient's vascular system. Facilitates starting infusion as soon as IV site is ready.
4. Perform hand hygiene.	Decreases potential risk of microbial contamination and cross-contamination (INS, 2016a).

Safe Patient Care *Gloves are not necessary to locate vein but must be applied for VAD insertion using a no-touch technique where the site is not palpated after skin antisepsis (INS, 2016a, 2016b).*

STEP	RATIONALE
5. Apply tourniquet around upper arm about 10 to 15 cm (4 to 6 inches) above proposed insertion site (see illustration). Do not apply tourniquet too tightly. Check for presence of pulse distal to tourniquet.	Tourniquet should be tight enough to impede venous flow while maintaining arterial circulation (INS, 2016a, 2016b). If patient has fragile veins or bruises easily, tourniquet should be applied loosely or not at all to prevent damage to veins and bruising (INS, 2016a).
Option A: Apply tourniquet on top of thin layer of clothing such as gown sleeve to protect fragile or hairy skin.	Reduces trauma to skin.
Option B: Blood pressure cuff may be used in place of tourniquet: activate cuff and hold at approximately 50 mm Hg)	
6. Select vein for VAD insertion (see illustration). Veins on dorsal and ventral surfaces of arms (e.g., metacarpal, cephalic, basilic, or median) are preferred in adults.	Ensures adequate vein that is easy to puncture and less likely to rupture.
a. Use most distal site in nondominant arm if possible.	Patients with VAD placement in their dominant hand have decreased ability to perform self-care.
b. With your fingertip, palpate vein at intended insertion site by pressing downward. Note resilient, soft, bouncy feeling while releasing pressure (see illustration).	Fingertip is more sensitive and better for assessing vein location and condition.
c. Select well-dilated vein. Methods to improve vascular distention:	Increased volume of blood in vein at venipuncture site makes vein more visible.
(1) Position extremity lower than heart, have patient open and close fist slowly, and lightly stroke vein downward.	Use of gravity promotes vascular distention (INS, 2016a).

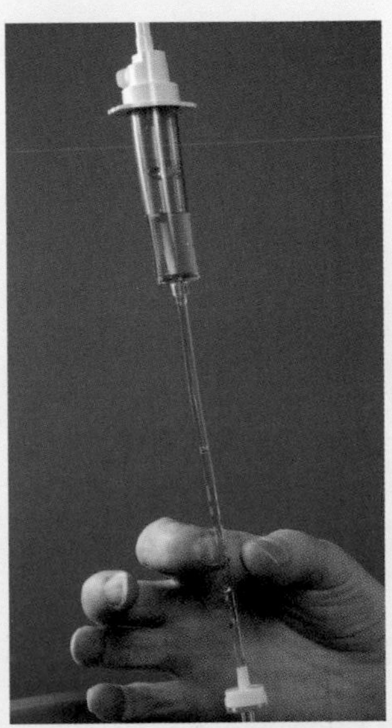

STEP 3h Removing air bubbles from tubing.

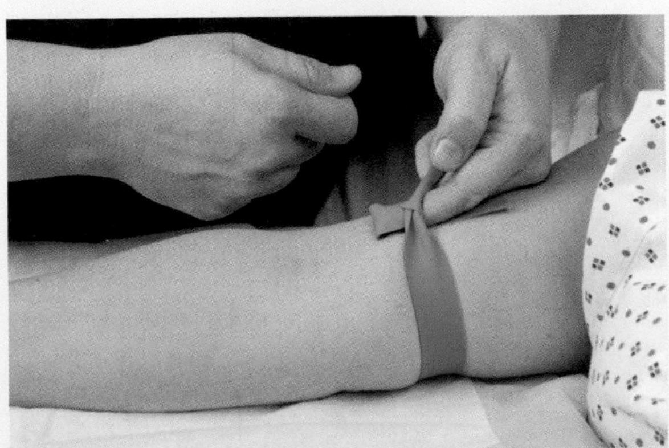

STEP 5 Tourniquet placed on arm for initial vein selection.

STEP	RATIONALE
(2) Apply dry heat to extremity for several minutes.	Dry heat has been found to increase successful peripheral catheter insertion (INS, 2016a).

Safe Patient Care *Vigorous friction, slapping, or hard tapping of a vein, especially in older adults, can cause venous constriction and/or bruising and hematoma (Weinstein and Hagle, 2014).*

STEP	RATIONALE
7. When selecting a vein:	
a. Avoid vein selection in:	
(1) Areas with pain on palpation, compromised areas, sites distal to compromised areas (e.g., open wounds, bruising, infection, infiltration, or extravasation; INS, 2016a).	It would be difficult to assess for any signs or symptoms of complications if an IV device were inserted in an area already compromised.
(2) Upper extremity on side of breast surgery with axillary node dissection or lymphedema or after radiation, arteriovenous (AV) fistulas/grafts; or affected extremity from cerebrovascular accident (CVA; INS, 2016a).	Increases risk for complications such as infection, lymphedema, or vessel damage.
(3) Site distal to previous venipuncture site, sclerosed or hardened veins, previous infiltrations or extravasations, areas of venous valves, or phlebitic vessels.	Such sites cause infiltration around newly placed VAD site and vessel damage.
(4) Fragile dorsal hand veins in older adults. Veins of lower extremities should not be used for routine IV therapy in adults because of risk of tissue damage and thrombophlebitis (INS, 2016a).	Veins have increased risk for infiltration.
(5) Areas of flexion such as wrist or antecubital area (INS, 2016a).	Veins have increased risk for occlusion, infiltration, phlebitis, or dislodgement.
(6) Ventral surface of wrist (10–12.5 cm [4–5 inches])	Venipuncture in ventral surface of wrist is painful and has potential for nerve damage (INS, 2016a).
b. Choose site that will not interfere with patient's activities of daily living (ADLs), use of assistive devices, or planned procedures.	Keeps patient as mobile as possible.
8. Release tourniquet temporarily.	Restores blood flow and prevents venospasm when preparing for venipuncture.

Safe Patient Care *If hair removal is needed, do not shave area with a razor. Shaving may increase risk of infection (INS, 2016a). Clip hair with scissors or hair clippers to prepare area for application of transparent semipermeable membrane (TSM) dressing if necessary (explain to patient).*

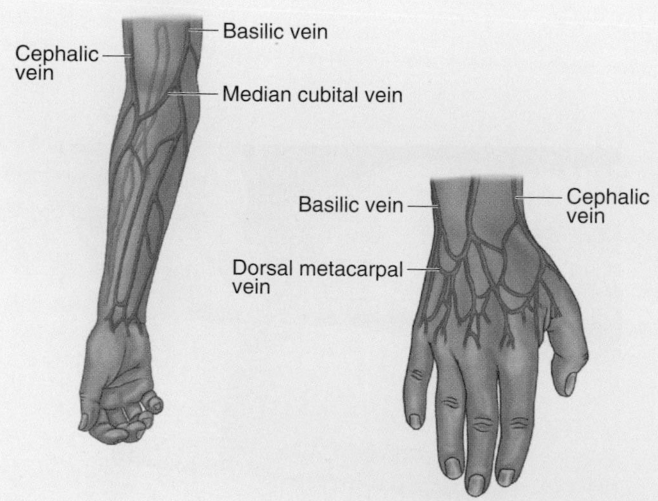

STEP 6 Cephalic, basilic, and median cubital veins are best for intravenous (IV) line placement in adults.

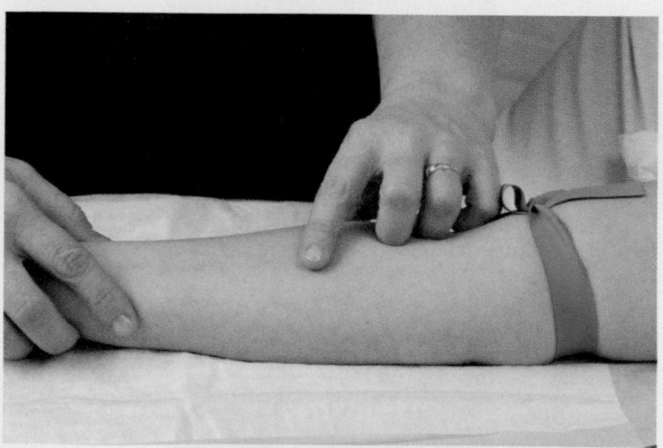

STEP 6b Palpate vein.

STEP	RATIONALE

Safe Patient Care *Local anesthetic reduces discomfort associated with placement of a VAD. Both topical and injectable drugs can be used to reduce pain and require a health care provider's order. You may apply topical local anesthetic to intended IV site 30 minutes before procedure. Follow manufacturer recommendations and monitor for allergic reaction (Gorski, 2018; INS, 2016a).*

STEP	RATIONALE
9. Perform hand hygiene and apply clean gloves. Wear eye protection and mask (see agency policy) if splash or spray of blood is possible.	Decreases potential risk of microbial contamination and cross-contamination (INS, 2016a).
10. Place adapter end of short extension set (prepared in Step 2) or needless connector (injection cap) for saline lock nearby in sterile package.	Permits smooth, quick connection of infusion to short-peripheral catheter once vein is accessed.
11. If area of insertion is visibly soiled, clean site with antiseptic soap and water first and dry. Perform skin antisepsis with alcoholic chlorhexidine solution using friction in back-and-forth motion (see illustration) for 30 seconds and allow to dry completely. If using alcohol or povidone-iodine, clean in concentric circle, moving from insertion site outward with swab. Allow drying time between agents if agents are used in combination (alcohol and povidone-iodine).	Mechanical friction in this pattern allows penetration of antiseptic solution to epidermal layer of skin. Reduces incidence of catheter-related infections (Gorski, 2018). Allow any skin antiseptic agent to fully dry for complete antisepsis; alcoholic chlorhexidine solutions for at least 30 seconds; iodophors for at least 1.5 to 2 minutes (INS, 2016a).

Safe Patient Care *If vein palpation is necessary after performing skin antisepsis, use sterile gloves for palpation or perform skin antisepsis again because touching cleaned area introduces microorganisms from your finger to site (INS, 2016a, 2016b).*

STEP	RATIONALE
12. Reapply tourniquet 10 to 15 cm (4 to 6 inches) above anticipated insertion site. Check for presence of pulse distal to tourniquet.	Pressure of tourniquet promotes vein distention. Diminished arterial flow prevents venous filling.
13. Perform venipuncture. Anchor vein below anticipated insertion site by placing thumb over vein 4 to 5 cm (1½ to 2 inches) distal to site (see illustration) and gently stretching skin against direction of insertion. Instruct patient to relax hand.	Stabilizes vein for needle insertion; prevents vein from rolling; and stretches skin taut, decreasing drag during insertion. Some devices require loosening needle (stylet) from catheter before venipuncture. Follow manufacturer directions for use.
a. Warn patient of a sharp stick. Hold VAD with needle bevel up. Align catheter on top of vein at 10- to 30-degree angle. Puncture skin and anterior vein wall (see illustration).	Accessing vein at an angle reduces risk of puncturing posterior vein wall. Superficial veins require smaller angle. Deeper veins require greater angle.

Safe Patient Care *Use each catheter only once for each insertion attempt.*

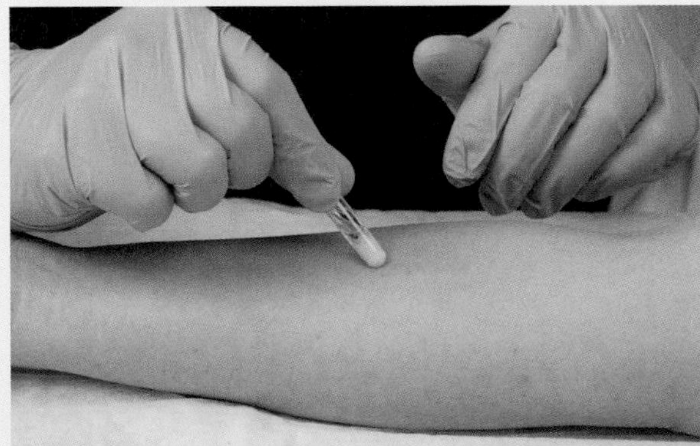

STEP 11 Clean site with antiseptic swab (alcoholic chlorhexidine solution preferred, 70% alcohol, or povidone-iodine).

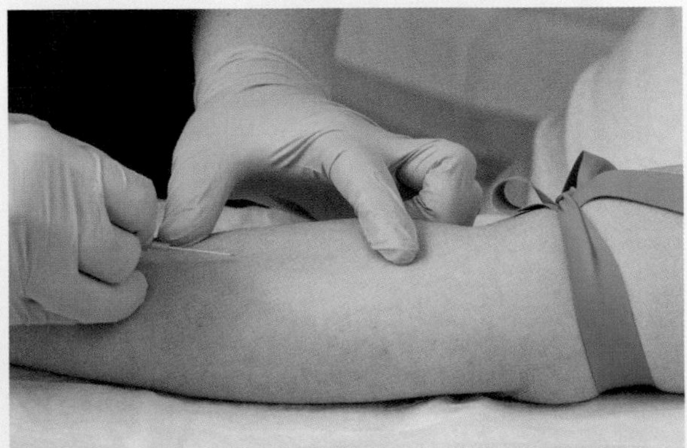

STEP 13 Stabilize vein below insertion site.

STEP	RATIONALE
14. Observe for blood return in catheter or flashback chamber of catheter, indicating that bevel of needle has entered vein (see illustration A). Advance VAD approximately ¼ inch (0.6 cm) into vein and loosen stylet (needle) of ONC. Continue to hold skin taut while stabilizing VAD and, with index finger on push-off tab of VAD, advance catheter off needle into vein until hub rests at venipuncture site (see illustration B). *Do not reinsert stylet into catheter once catheter has been advanced into vein.* Advance catheter while safety device automatically retracts stylet (techniques for retracting stylet vary with different VADs). Place stylet directly into sharps container.	Increased venous pressure from tourniquet causes backflow of blood into catheter and/or flashback chamber. Some VADs have a notch in the stylet, allowing flash of blood into catheter. Stabilizing VAD allows for placement of catheter into vein and advancement of catheter off stylet. Advancing entire stylet into vein may penetrate wall of vein, resulting in hematoma. Advancing catheter with finger on open hub causes contamination (INS, 2016a). Reinsertion of stylet can cause catheter to shear off and embolize into vein. Devices with safety mechanisms and proper sharps disposal prevent needlestick injuries (OSHA, 2012).

Safe Patient Care *A single clinician should not make more than two attempts at initiating IV access and limit total attempts to no more than four (Gorski, 2018; INS, 2016a).*

STEP	RATIONALE
15. Stabilize VAD with nondominant hand and release tourniquet or blood pressure cuff with other. Apply gentle but firm pressure with middle finger of nondominant hand 3 cm (1¼ inches) above insertion site. Keep catheter stable with index finger.	Permits venous flow and reduces backflow of blood. Digital pressure minimizes blood loss and allows attachment of extension set or needleless connector (INS, 2016b).
16. Quickly connect Luer-Lok end of short extension tubing with needleless connector to end of catheter hub. Secure connection. Avoid touching sterile connection ends. *Option:* IV tubing can be attached directly to catheter hub in place of short extension tubing or needleless connector.	Prompt connection maintains patency of vein, minimizes blood loss, and prevents risk of exposure to blood. Maintains sterility.

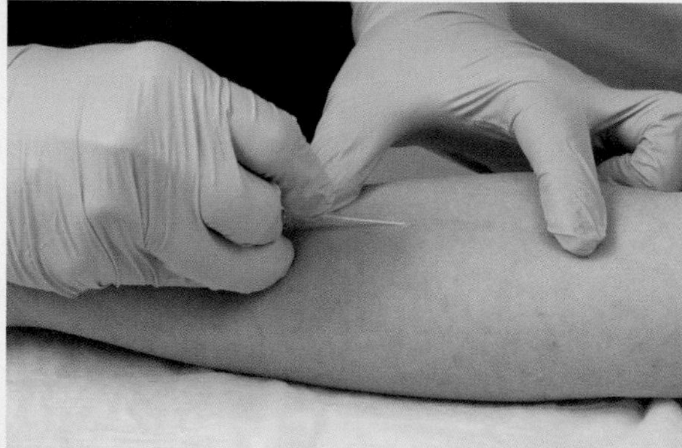

STEP 13a Puncture skin with catheter at 10- to 30-degree angle.

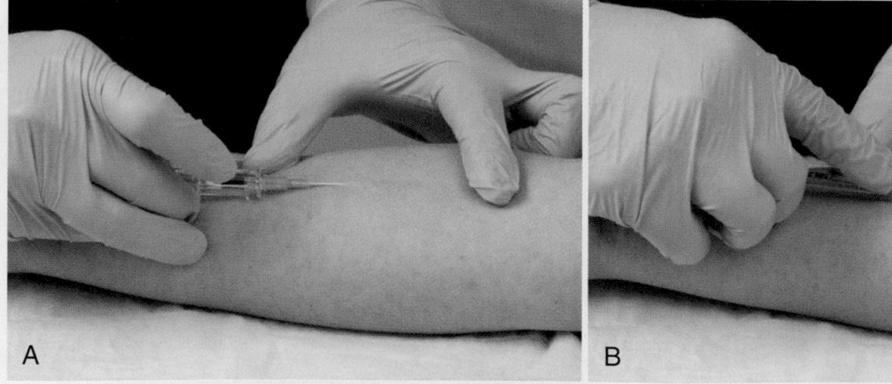

STEP 14 (A) Observe for blood return in catheter and/or flashback chamber. (B) Advance catheter into vein until hub rests at venipuncture site.

STEP	RATIONALE
17. Attach 10-mL syringe prefilled with preservative-free 0.9% sodium chloride (normal saline [NS]) to short extension set and aspirate to remove air and assess blood return. Slowly inject NS from prefilled syringe into VAD (see illustration A). Remove syringe and discard.	Aspirating air prevents air embolism. Blood return that is color and consistency of whole blood confirms placement of catheter in vein (INS, 2016a). Flushing prevents reflux of blood into catheter and occlusion (INS, 2016b).
Option: To begin primary infusion, swab needleless connector with antiseptic swab and attach Luer-Lok end of IV tubing to needleless connector (see illustration B). Open roller clamp of IV tubing, turn on EID, and program it. Begin infusion at correct rate. If using gravity flow instead of EID, begin infusion by slowly opening roller clamp to regulate rate.	Initiates flow of fluid through IV catheter, preventing clotting of device. Swelling indicates infiltration, and catheter would need to be removed. Initiates flow of fluid through IV catheter, preventing clotting of VAD.

Safe Patient Care *Needleless connectors protect health care workers and decrease risk for needlestick injuries. They have different internal mechanisms for fluid displacement and vary in the flush/clamp/disconnect sequence to prevent reflux of blood into catheter on disconnection (INS, 2016a).*

The sequence depends on the type of internal mechanism (Gorski, 2018):

- *Neutral displacement devices do not have a specified flush/clamp/disconnect sequence.*
- *For negative-pressure displacement devices, flush, clamp catheter, then disconnect syringe.*
- *For positive-pressure displacement, flush, disconnect syringe, then clamp catheter.*

STEP	RATIONALE
18. Observe insertion site for swelling.	Swelling indicates infiltration, which requires immediate catheter removal.
19. Apply sterile dressing over site.	
a. Transparent semipermeable membrane (TSM) dressing:	
(1) Continue to secure catheter with nondominant hand. Remove adherent backing. Apply one edge of dressing and gently smooth remaining dressing over IV insertion site, leaving Luer-Lok connection between tubing and catheter hub uncovered. Gently press dressing to adhere to skin. Remove outer covering and smooth dressing gently over site (see illustration).	Protects catheter insertion site and minimizes risk for infection (Gorski, 2018). Allows visualization of insertion site and surrounding area for complications (INS, 2016a). Access to Luer-Lok connection between tubing and catheter hub facilitates changing tubing if necessary.
(2) Place 2.5 cm (2-inch) piece of tape over Luer-Lok connection (see illustration). Do not apply tape on top of TSM dressing.	Removal of tape from TSM dressing can tear dressing and cause catheter dislodgement. Tape on top of TSM dressing prevents moisture from being carried away from skin.

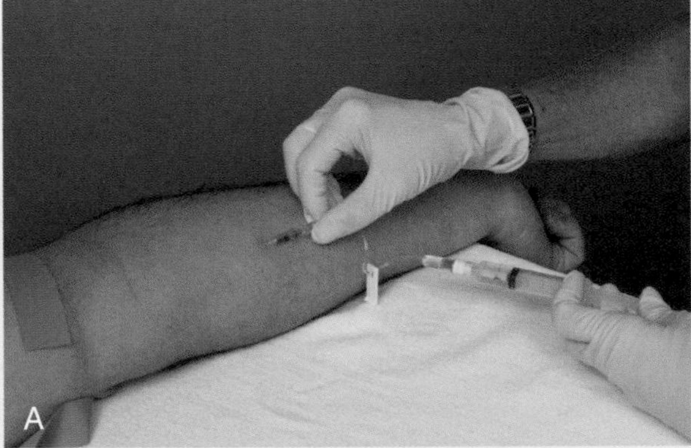

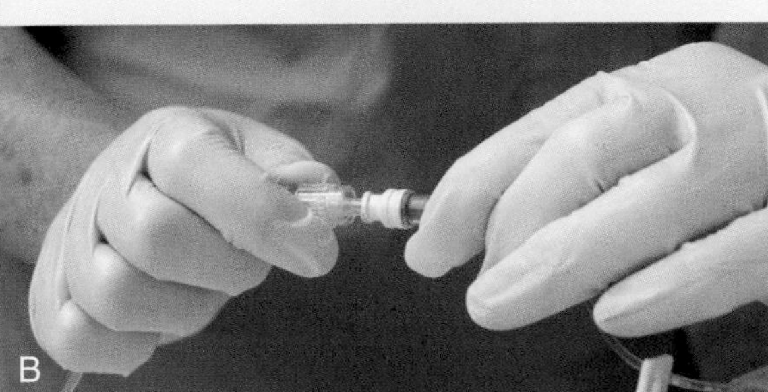

STEP 17 (A) Flush short extension set after aspirating air and assessing blood return. (B) Connect IV tubing to the short extension set that is attached to the catheter.

STEP	RATIONALE
b. Sterile gauze dressing:	
(1) Place 5-cm (2-inch) piece of sterile tape over catheter hub (see illustration).	Stabilizes catheter under gauze dressing.
(2) Place 2 × 2–inch gauze pad over insertion site and edge of catheter hub. Secure all edges with tape. Do not place tape over insertion site. Do not cover connection between IV tubing and catheter hub (see illustration).	Use gauze dressings for site drainage, excessive perspiration, or sensitivity/allergic reactions to TSM dressings (Gorski, 2018; INS, 2016a).
(3) Fold 2 × 2–inch gauze in half and cover with 10-cm (4-inch) or 1 inch–wide tape so about an inch extends on each side. Place under Luer-Lok connection (see illustration). Secure Luer-Lok connection and tubing to tape on folded gauze with 2.5-cm (1-inch) piece of tape. Avoid applying tape or gauze around arm. Do not use rolled bandages with or without elastic to secure VAD. Taping Luer-Lok connection can be eliminated if engineered stabilization device is to be used.	Tape on top of gauze makes it easier to access hub/tubing junction. Gauze pad elevates hub off skin to prevent pressure area. Prevents back-and-forth motion of catheter. Rolled bandages do not secure VAD adequately, can impair circulation or flow of infusion, and obscure visualization for complications (INS, 2016a).
20. *Option:* Secure IV catheter using engineered stabilization device (follow manufacturer directions and agency policy).	Use of engineered stabilization devices that allow visual inspection of insertion site can reduce risk of VAD complications (i.e., phlebitis, infection, migration) and unintentional loss of access (INS, 2016a).
a. Apply polymer-based skin protectant to area of skin around IV site and allow to dry completely.	Risk for medical adhesive–related skin injury (MARSI) is increased as result of age, joint movement, and edema; use of skin protectant can decrease risk (INS, 2016a).

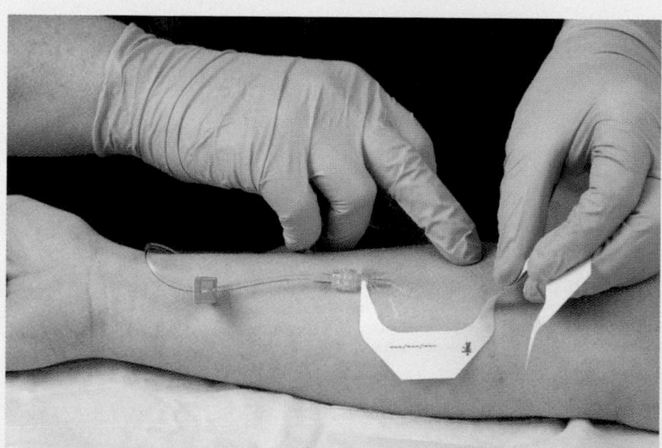

STEP 19a(1) Apply transparent semipermeable membrane (TSM) dressing.

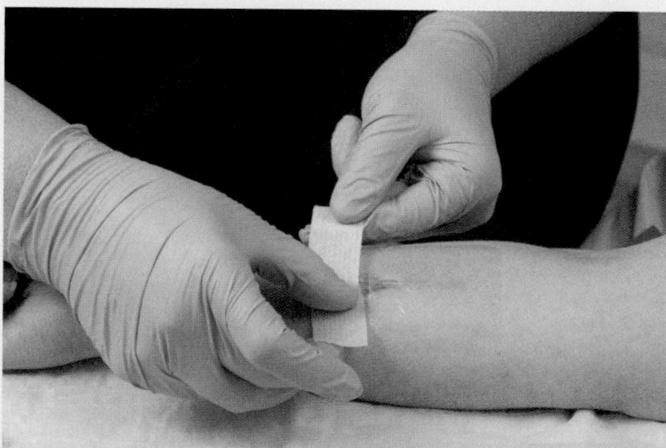

STEP 19a(2) Place tape over administration set tubing.

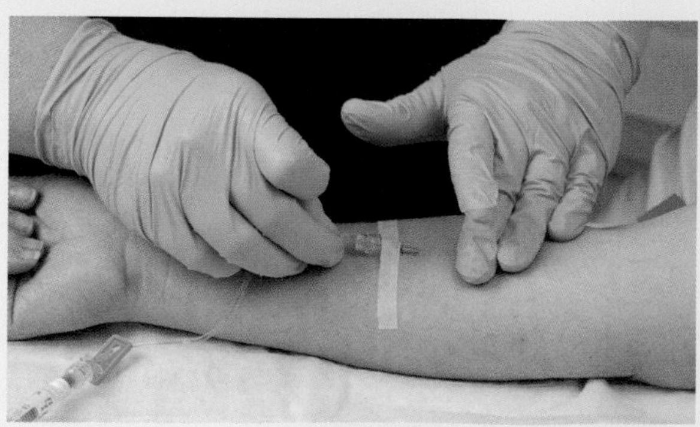

STEP 19b(1) Place sterile tape over catheter hub.

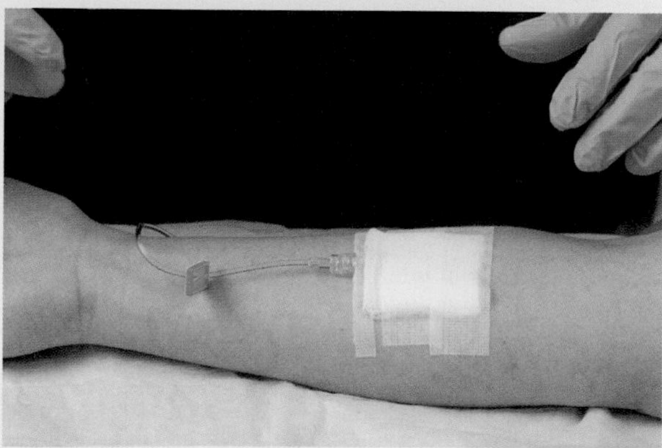

STEP 19b(2) Place 2 × 2–inch gauze over insertion site and catheter hub.

STEP	RATIONALE
(1) Align anchoring pads with directional arrow pointing to insertion site. Press device retainer over top of Luer-Lok connection while supporting underneath connection.	
(2) Stabilize catheter and peel off one side of liner and press to adhere to skin. Repeat on other side (see illustration).	
(3) Monitor for MARSI.	
21. *Option:* Apply site protection device (e.g., I.V. House Ultra Protective Dressing®).	Reduces risk of VAD dislodgement (INS, 2016a).
22. Loop extension or IV tubing alongside dressing on arm and secure with second piece of tape directly over tubing (see illustration).	Securing tubing reduces risk for dislodging catheter if IV tubing is pulled (i.e., loop comes apart before catheter dislodges).
23. Label dressing per agency policy. Include date and time of IV insertion, VAD gauge size and length, and your initials (see illustration).	Allows for recognition of type of device and length of time that device has been in place.
24. Dispose of any remaining sharps in appropriate sharps container. Discard supplies.	Prevents accidental needlestick injuries (OSHA, 2012).
25. Remove gloves and perform hand hygiene.	Reduces risk of contamination (INS, 2016b).

Safe Patient Care *Check agency policy for appropriate process for cleaning beneath nails. Do not use an orange stick or end of cotton swab; these splinters and can cause injury.*

STEP	RATIONALE
26. Assist patient to a comfortable position and instruct how to move and turn without dislodging VAD.	Prevents accidental dislodgement of catheter and minimizes risk for falls.
27. Raise bed rails (as appropriate) and lower bed to lowest position.	Minimizes risk for falls and injury.
28. Be sure nurse call system is in an accessible location within patient's reach. Instruct patient in its use.	Ensures patient can call for assistance if needed.

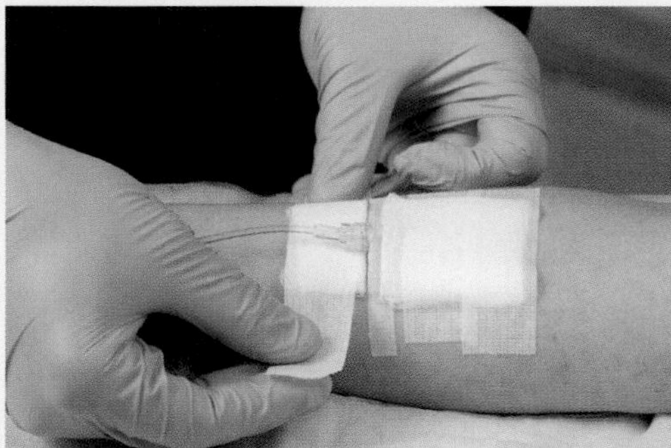

STEP 19b(3) Apply 2 × 2–inch gauze dressing under tubing junction.

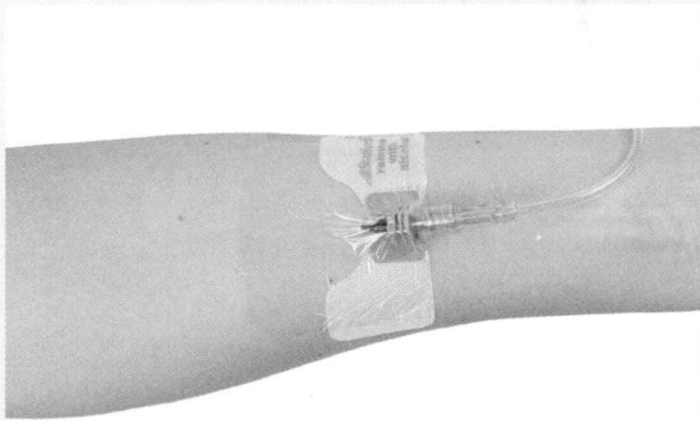

STEP 20a(2) Catheter stabilization device in place. *(Image Courtesy C.R. Bard, Inc., All rights reserved.)*

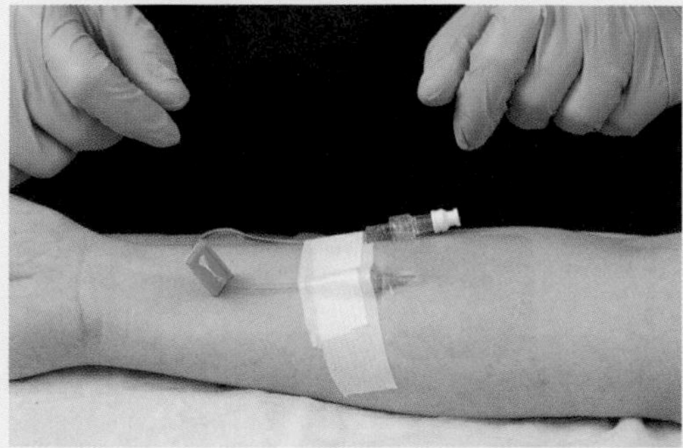

STEP 22 Loop and secure tubing.

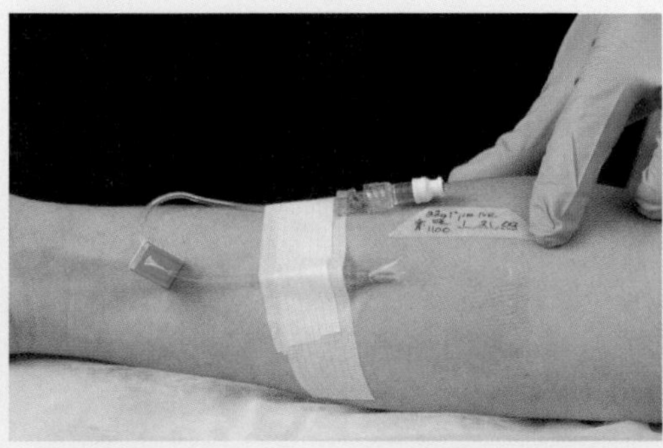

STEP 23 Label intravenous (IV) dressing.

STEP	RATIONALE

EVALUATION

STEP	RATIONALE
1. Observe patient every 1 to 2 hours, or at established intervals per agency policy and procedure, for function, intactness, and patency of IV system and for correct infusion rate and accurate type/amount of IV solution infused by observing level in IV container.	Ensures delivery of prescribed volume over prescribed time and decreases risk for fluid and electrolyte imbalance.
2. Evaluate patient to determine response to therapy (e.g., laboratory values, input and output [I&O]), weights, vital signs, postprocedure assessments).	Early recognition of complications leads to prompt treatment.
3. Evaluate patient with a short-peripheral IV at least every 4 hours, or every 1 to 2 hours for patients that are critically ill, sedated, or have cognitive deficits (INS, 2016a), or at established intervals per agency policy and procedure, for signs and symptoms of catheter-related complications. Assess the VAD catheter–skin junction site and surrounding area by visually inspecting and palpating through the intact dressing for redness, tenderness, swelling, and drainage.	Identifies complications that compromise integrity of VAD or cause inaccurate IV solution flow rate.

Safe Patient Care *If IV is positional, fluid will run slowly or stop, depending on position of patient's arm; if this continues, you may have to restart IV line.*

STEP	RATIONALE
4. **Use Teach-Back:** "I want to make sure that I explained the problems that can happen with your IV line. Tell me the signs or symptoms that you should tell me or the other nurses about." Revise your instruction now or develop a plan for revised patient/family caregiver teaching if patient/family caregiver is not able to teach back correctly.	Determines patient's/family caregiver's level of understanding of instructional topic.

Unexpected Outcomes	Related Interventions
1. Fluid and electrolyte imbalances: a. Fluid-volume deficit (FVD): decreased urine output, dry mucous membranes, decreased capillary refill, disparity in central and peripheral pulses, tachycardia, hypotension, shock b. Fluid-volume excess (FVE): dyspnea, crackles in lung, edema, and/or increased urine output c. Electrolyte imbalances: abnormal serum electrolyte levels, changes in mental status, alterations in neuromuscular function, cardiac arrhythmias, and changes in vital signs	• Notify health care provider. • Requires readjusting infusion rate. • Requires adjusting additives in IV line or type of IV fluid ordered.
2. IV-related complications a. Infiltration: pain, swelling, coolness to touch, or presence of blanching (white, shiny appearance at or above IV site) or redness (INS, 2016b)	• Stop infusion and remove IV catheter at first sign of infiltration (see Procedural Guideline 28.1). • Elevate affected extremity. • Avoid applying pressure, which can force solution into contact with more tissue, causing tissue damage. • Use standard scale for assessing and documenting infiltration (INS, 2016a).
b. Catheter occlusion can occur from bent catheter, positional catheter (catheter resting against catheter wall), kink or knot in infusion tubing, clot formation, or precipitate formation from administration of incompatible medications or solutions (Gorski, 2018).	• Determine cause and consider catheter removal. • Positional catheters can be repositioned to improve IV flow. • Remove occluded IV catheter. Occluded catheters should not be flushed because an embolus can result from dislodging a clot (Gorski, 2018).
c. Phlebitis (i.e., vein inflammation): pain, redness, warmth, swelling, induration, or presence of palpable cord along course of vein (INS, 2016a). Rate of infusion may be altered.	• Notify health care provider. • Determine cause (i.e., chemical, mechanical, bacterial) and consider removal or replacement of VAD. • *Chemical phlebitis:* Apply heat, elevate limb, consider slowing infusion rate, and determine whether catheter removal is necessary (INS, 2016a).

Unexpected Outcomes	Related Interventions
	• *Mechanical phlebitis:* Apply heat, elevate limb, monitor for 24 to 48 hours, and consider catheter removal if signs and symptoms persist (INS, 2016a). • *Bacterial phlebitis:* Remove IV catheter (INS, 2016a). • Document phlebitis using a standardized scale, including nursing interventions per agency policy and procedure (Tables 28.2 and 28.3).
d. Catheter-related infection can present as redness, swelling around or above IV site, pain, purulent drainage at insertion site, and body-temperature elevations (INS, 2016a).	• Notify health care provider. Obtain order to culture drainage (INS, 2016a). • Remove IV catheter and culture purulent drainage from around IV site (see Chapter 9; INS, 2016a).
e. Hematoma is bleeding under skin caused by trauma to vessel wall. It can occur during short-peripheral IV insertion if needle punctures either adjacent vessels or posterior vein wall or can be seen with multiple venipuncture attempts (Gorski, 2018).	• Remove IV catheter immediately and apply pressure and dry, sterile dressing. • Monitor for additional bleeding. • Elevate extremity and monitor for circulatory, neurological, or motor dysfunction (Gorski, 2018).
f. Nerve injuries during short-peripheral IV insertion can occur. Be alert for patient complaints of paresthesias, including shocklike pain, tingling or pins and needles, burning, or numbness on insertion.	• Notify health care provider of any signs and symptoms of nerve injury (INS, 2016b). • Immediately stop VAD insertion and remove device if patient complains of symptoms of paresthesias (INS, 2016a). • Continue to monitor neurovascular status (INS, 2016b)

Recording

- Record number of attempts at insertion; type of solution and additives infusing; rate and method of infusion (e.g., gravity or name of EID); purpose of infusion; insertion site by location and vessel; brand, length, and gauge of IV device; patient's response to insertion (e.g., what he or she reports); and when infusion was started.
- Document your evaluation of patient learning.

Hand-Off Reporting

- Placement of VAD with reason for insertion
- Signs or symptoms of observed or patient-reported IV-related complications (e.g., redness, tenderness, swelling, drainage, leaking from under dressing, change in flow rate, infection)
- Report to health care provider any adverse events occurring upon VAD placement (e.g., persistent pain or suspected nerve damage, hematoma formation, or arterial puncture).

TABLE 28.2

Phlebitis Scale

Score	Clinical Signs
0	No symptoms
1	Erythema at access site with or without pain
2	Pain at access site with erythema and/or edema
3	Pain at access site with erythema and/or edema Streak formation Palpable venous cord
4	Pain at access site with erythema and/or edema Streak formation Palpable venous cord >2.5 cm (1 inch) in length Purulent drainage

Data from Infusion Nurses Society (INS): 2016 infusion nursing standards of practice, *J Infus Nurs* 39(suppl 1):1S, 2016.

TABLE 28.3

Visual Infusion Phlebitis Scale

Score	Observation
0	IV site appears healthy
1	One of the following signs is evident: Slight pain near IV site *or* slight redness near IV site
2	Two of the following signs are evident: • Pain at IV site • Erythema • Swelling
3	All of the following signs are evident: • Pain along the path of cannula • Induration
4	All of the following signs are evident and extensive: • Pain along the path of cannula • Erythema • Induration • Palpable venous cord
5	All of the following signs are evident and extensive: • Pain along the path of cannula • Erythema • Induration • Palpable venous cord • Pyrexia

IV, Intravenous.

Modified from Infusion Nurses Society (INS): 2016 infusion nursing standards of practice, *J Infus Nurs* 39(suppl 1):1S, 2016.

✦ SKILL 28.2 Regulating Intravenous Infusion Flow Rates

Purpose

Accurate infusion rates in intravenous (IV) therapy are essential in the safe delivery of solutions and medications (see Chapter 22). Various factors can interfere with accuracy of infusion rates (Table 28.4). Appropriate regulation and monitoring can reduce complications (e.g., infiltration, phlebitis, occlusion of venous access device [VAD], or circulatory overload) associated with IV therapy and allow patients to achieve therapeutic outcomes (Gorski, 2018; INS, 2016b). A health care provider's order for IV therapy should specify the volume of fluid a patient is to receive within a specific time frame (INS, 2016a), such as "1 L of D_5NS over 8 hours." You must be able to calculate hourly flow rates to ensure that the prescribed amount of fluid infuses correctly over the prescribed time frame. There are a variety of flow-control devices for regulating infusion rates (i.e., manual, mechanical, and electronic infusion devices [EIDs]), and the type used should be guided by factors such as age, acuity, mobility of patient, severity of illness, type of therapy, dosing considerations, and care setting (INS, 2016a).

Delegation and Collaboration

The skill of regulating IV flow rates cannot be delegated to nursing assistive personnel (NAP). Delegation to licensed practical nurses (LPNs) varies by state Nurse Practice Act. The nurse instructs the NAP to:

- Inform the nurse when the EID alarm signals.
- Inform the nurse when the fluid container near completion.
- Report any patient complaints of discomfort related to infusion such as pain, burning, bleeding, or swelling.

TABLE 28.4

Factors That Alter Intravenous Flow Rates

Patient Factors	Mechanical Factors
Change in patient position	Height of parenteral container (should be >90 cm [36 inches] above heart)
Flexion of involved extremity	Positional access device; IV tubing size; gauge of IV device
Partial or complete occlusion of IV device	Viscosity or temperature of IV solution; occluded air vent
Venous spasm	Occluded in-line filter
Vein trauma (phlebitis)	Improperly placed IV devices
Manipulated by patient or visitor	Crimped administration set tubing; tubing dangling below bed; low battery of an electronic device

IV, Intravenous.

From Alexander M et al: *Core curriculum for infusion nursing*, ed 4, Philadelphia, 2014, Lippincott Williams & Wilkins; and Gorski L: *Phillip's manual of IV therapeutics: evidence-based practice for infusion therapy,* ed 7, Philadelphia, 2018, FA Davis.

Equipment

- Watch with a second hand
- Calculator, paper, and pencil/pen
- Label
- IV solution bag and appropriate administration set
- IV regulating device: EID *(optional)*
- Clean gloves

ASSESSMENT

1. Review accuracy and completeness of health care provider order in patient's medical record for patient name and correct solution: type, volume, additives, infusion rate, and duration of IV therapy. Follow the seven rights of drug administration (see Chapter 22). *Rationale: Ensures delivery of correct IV solution and prescribed volume over prescribed time.*
2. Identify patient risk for fluid and electrolyte imbalance given type of IV solution (e.g., neonate, history of cardiac or renal disease). *Rationale: Helps prioritize assessments. Volume control needs to be strict. Guides choice of infusion device.*
3. Perform hand hygiene and apply clean gloves. *Rationale: Reduces risk of contamination (INS, 2016b).*
4. Check infusion system from solution container down to venous access device (VAD) insertion site for integrity. *Rationale: Identifies complications that can compromise integrity of VAD and patient safety.*
   a. Assess IV container for discoloration, cloudiness, leakage, and expiration date. *Rationale: Incompatibility of solutions or medications compromises integrity of VAD and patient safety (Gorski, 2018).*
   b. Assess IV tubing for puncture, contamination, or occlusion. *Rationale: Compromised tubing results in fluid leakage and bacterial contamination.*
5. Assess the integrity, patency, and functioning of the existing VAD. Assess the VAD catheter-skin junction site and surrounding area for catheter-related complications by visually inspecting and palpating through the intact dressing for redness, tenderness, swelling, and drainage. Assess the patency of the VAD by aspiration of a blood return, absence of resistance when flushing, and complaints of patient pain or discomfort when flushing. *Rationale: Identifies complications that compromise integrity of VAD and necessitate replacement of VAD.*
6. Remove gloves and perform hand hygiene. *Rationale: Reduces risk of contamination (INS, 2016b).*
7. Assess patient's and family caregiver's knowledge, experience, and health literacy regarding how positioning of IV site affects flow rate. *Rationale: Ensures patient or family caregiver has the capacity to obtain, communicate, process, and understand basic health information (CDC, 2016).*

STEP	RATIONALE

PLANNING

1. Expected outcomes following completion of procedure:
   - Fluid and electrolyte levels remain within normal limits. — IV solution helps to maintain fluid and electrolyte levels.
   - Patient receives prescribed volume of solution over prescribed time interval. — Patient achieves therapeutic outcomes.
   - Patient's VAD remains patent, and site is free from signs and symptoms of IV-related complications. — Ensures that patient receives prescribed infusion therapy and that VAD is without complications (INS, 2016a).
   - Patient is able to explain how positioning of IV site affects rate and describe complications related to inaccurate flow rate. — Demonstrates learning (INS, 2016a).
2. Prepare and organize equipment.
   a. Have paper and pencil or calculator to calculate flow rate. — Calculating hourly flow rates ensures that the prescribed amount of fluid to be infused over the prescribed time frame is correct.
   b. Check order to see how long each liter of fluid should infuse. If hourly rate (mL/hr) is not provided in order, calculate it by dividing volume by hours. For example: — Basis of calculation to ensure infusion of solution over prescribed hourly rate.

$$\text{mL/hr} = \frac{\text{Total infusion (mL)}}{\text{Hours of infusion}}$$

$$1000 \text{ mL}/8 \text{ hr} = 125 \text{ mL/hr}$$

or if 3 L is ordered for 24 hours:

$$3000 \text{ mL}/24 \text{ hr} = 125 \text{ mL/hr}$$

Safe Patient Care *It is common for health care providers to write an abbreviated IV order such as "D_5W with 20 mEq KCl 125 mL/hr continuous." This order implies that the IV should be maintained at this rate until an order has been written for the IV to be discontinued or changed to another order.*

   c. If keep-vein-open (KVO) rate is ordered, check agency policy regarding flow rate of KVO. — Prevents catheter clotting, thus preserving venous access while infusing a minimal amount of fluid. An order for KVO rate must specify an infusion rate as required by the seven rights of medication administration (see Chapter 22). Rates may vary from 0.5 mL/hr to 30 mL/hr based on type of VAD, patient-specific therapy, and method of infusion (gravity or EID).
   d. Use hourly rate to program EID or, if gravity-flow infusion, use to calculate minute flow rate (gtt/mL), — EID automatically delivers correct minute flow rate. Gravity infusion requires calculation of gtt/mL.
   e. Know calibration (drop factor), in drops per milliliter (gtt/mL), of infusion set used by agency:
      (1) Microdrip: 60 gtt/mL: Used to deliver rates less than 100 mL/hr. — Microdrip tubing universally delivers 60 gtt/mL. Used when small or very precise volumes are to be infused.
      (2) Macrodrip: 10 to 15 gtt/mL (depending on manufacturer). Used to deliver rates greater than 100 mL/hr. — There are different commercial parenteral administration sets for macrodrip tubing. Used when large volumes or fast rates are necessary. Know drip factor for tubing being used.
   f. Select one of the following formulas to calculate minute flow rate (drops per minute) based on drop factor of infusion set: — Once you determine hourly rate, these formulas compute the correct flow rate.
      (1) $\text{mL/hr}/60 \text{ min} = \text{mL/min}$
      $\text{Drop factor} \times \text{mL/min} = \text{Drops/min}$
      Or
      (2) $\text{mL/hr} \times \text{Drop factor}/60 \text{ min} = \text{Drops/min}$
   g. Calculate minute flow rate for a bag 1000 mL with 20 mEq KCl at 100 mL/hr.
      Microdrip: — When using microdrip, milliliters per hour (mL/hr) always equals drops per minute (gtt/min).

$$100 \text{ mL/hr} \times 60 \text{ gtt/mL} = 6000$$
$$6000 \text{ gtt} \div 60 \text{ min} = 100 \text{ gtt/min}$$

      Macrodrip: — Multiply volume by drop factor and divide product by time (in minutes).

$$125 \text{ mL/hr} \times 15 \text{ gtt/mL} = 1875 \text{ gtt/hr}$$
$$1875 \text{ gtt} \div 60 \text{ min} = 31\text{–}32 \text{ gtt/min}$$

STEP	RATIONALE
3. Explain/instruct patient and family caregiver on reasons for ongoing IV therapy.	Provides patient with information about procedure and promotes compliance (INS, 2016a). Informing patient may minimize anxiety.

IMPLEMENTATION

STEP	RATIONALE
1. Identify patient using at least two identifiers (e.g., name and birthday or name and medical record number) according to agency policy. Compare identifiers with information on patient's medication administration record (MAR) or medical record.	Ensures correct patient. Complies with The Joint Commission standards and improves patient safety (TJC, 2019).

Safe Patient Care *Manual and mechanical flow-control devices may be used for infusions that do not require strict rate control (INS, 2016b). Fluids run by gravity are adjusted through use of a flow control/regulator. Manual flow regulators (e.g., roller clamp, dial, or barrel-shaped) are not recommended for use in infants and children because accuracy cannot be guaranteed (Alexander et al., 2014; Gorski, 2018) and can be affected by mechanical and patient factors. A calibrated chamber is a volume-controlled flow regulator that uses gravity to deliver only a limited amount of solution. It is placed between the IV container and the insertion spike and drip chamber of an administration set (see Chapter 24). Mechanical infusion devices (e.g., elastomeric devices, piston-driven pumps) regulate infusion rates with no outside power source (Gorski, 2018).*

STEP	RATIONALE
2. Regulate gravity infusion.	
a. Ensure that IV container is at least 76.2 cm (30 inches) above IV site for adults, and increase height for more viscous fluids (Alexander et al., 2014).	Pressure caused by gravity is necessary to overcome venous pressure and resistance from tubing and catheter.
b. Slowly open roller clamp on tubing until you can see drops in drip chamber. Hold a watch with second hand at same level as drip chamber and count drip rate for 1 minute (see illustration). Adjust roller clamp to increase or decrease rate of infusion.	Regulates flow to prescribed rate.
c. Monitor drip rate at least hourly.	Many factors influence drip rate; frequent monitoring ensures IV fluid administration as prescribed.

Safe Patient Care *An EID uses positive pressure to maintain correct flow rates and catheter patency to deliver a measured amount of fluid over a prescribed period of time (e.g., 100 mL/hr). Infusion pumps are needed for patients requiring low hourly rates, at risk for volume overload, with impaired renal function, or receiving solutions or medications that require a specific hourly volume.*

EIDs use an electronic sensor and an alarm that signals if pressure in the system changes and the desired flow rate changes. Many EIDs have operating and programming capabilities that allow for infusions of single or multiple solutions at different rates. Various detectors and alarms respond to air in IV lines, completion of infusion, high and low pressure, low battery power, occlusion, and the inability to deliver at a preset rate. The use of an EID does not absolve you from checking to ensure that the pump is functioning and infusing at the prescribed rate.

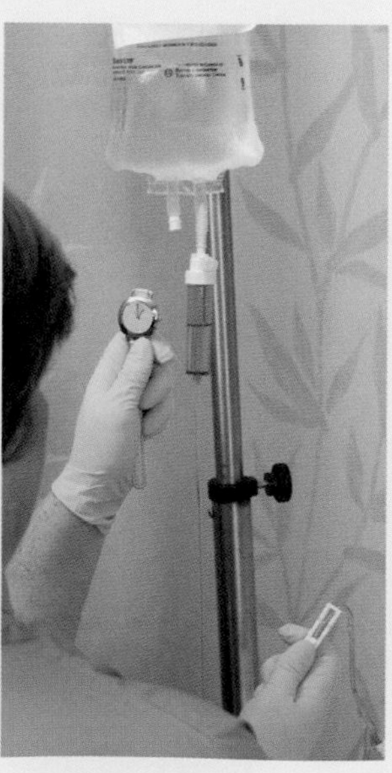

STEP 2b Nurse counting drip rate on gravity infusion.

STEP	RATIONALE
3. **Regulate EID (infusion pump or smart pump):** Follow manufacturer guidelines for set up of EID. Be sure you are using infusion tubing compatible with EID.	Smart pumps with medication safety software are designed for administration of IV fluids that contain medications.
a. Close roller clamp on primed IV infusion tubing.	Prevents fluid leakage.
b. Insert infusion tubing into chamber of control mechanism (see manufacturer directions; see illustration). Roller clamp on IV tubing goes between EID and patient.	Most EIDs use positive pressure to infuse. Infusion pumps propel fluid through tubing by compressing and milking IV tubing.
c. Secure part of IV tubing through "air in line" alarm system. Close door (see illustration A) and turn on power button, select required drops per minute or volume per hour, close door to control chamber, and press start button (see illustration B). If infusing medication, access the smart pump drug library of medications and set appropriate rate and dose limits. If smart pump alarms immediately and shuts down, your settings were outside unit parameters.	Ensures safe administration of ordered flow rate or medication dose. Smart pumps require additional information such as patient unit and medication. Computer matches pump setting against a drug database, and dose error reduction systems (DERSs) provide a means for decreasing IV medication administration errors (Giuliano, 2015).

Safe Patient Care *An anti–free flow safeguard (preventing bolus infusion in the event of machine malfunction or when tubing is removed from machine) is an important element of an EID and is required. Always check and follow manufacturer recommendations for specific device features* (Alexander et al., 2014; Gorski, 2018).

STEP	RATIONALE
d. Open infusion tubing drip regulator completely while EID is in use.	Ensures that pump freely regulates infusion rate.
e. Monitor infusion rate and IV site for complications according to agency policy. Use watch to verify rate of infusion, even when using EID.	Flow controllers and pumps do not replace frequent, accurate nursing evaluation. EIDs can continue to infuse IV solutions after a complication has developed (INS, 2016a).
f. Assess IV system from container to VAD insertion site when alarm signals.	Alarm indicates situation that requires attention. Empty solution container, tubing kinks, closed clamp, infiltration, clotted catheter, air in tubing, and/or low battery can trigger EID alarm.
4. Attach label to IV solution container with date and time container changed (check agency policy).	Provides reference to determine next time for container change, especially with keep-vein-open (KVO) rate that contains a specific infusion rate as ordered by health care provider.
5. Teach patient purpose of EID if infusion therapy is delivered by EID, purpose of alarms, to avoid raising hand or arm that affects flow rate, and to avoid touching control clamp.	Information allows patient to protect IV site and informs him or her about rationale for not altering control rate.

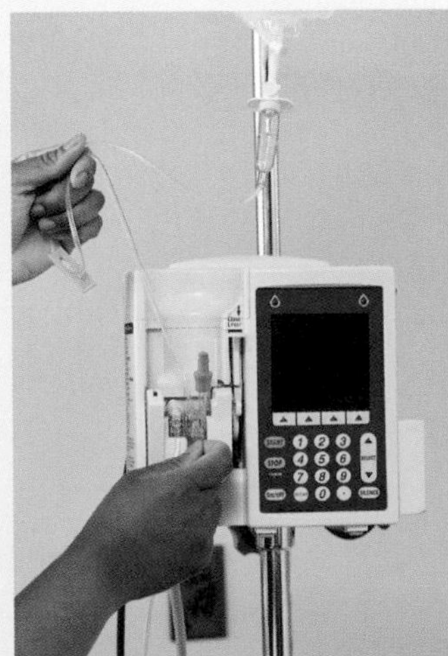

STEP 3b Insert IV tubing into chamber of control mechanism.

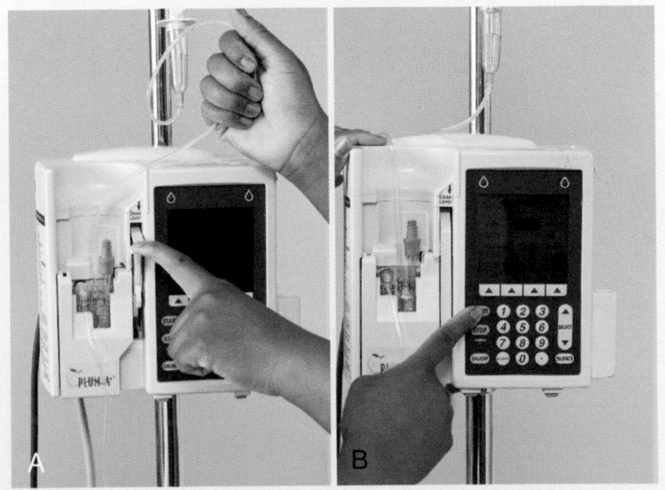

STEP 3c (A) Close door of control mechanism. (B) Select rate and volume to be infused and press start button.

STEP	RATIONALE
6. Dispose of any used supplies. Remove gloves and perform hand hygiene.	Reduces risk of contamination (INS, 2016b).
7. Assist patient to a comfortable position and instruct how to move and turn without dislodging VAD.	Prevents accidental dislodgement of catheter and minimizes risk for falls.
8. Raise bed rails (as appropriate) and lower bed to lowest position.	Minimizes risk for falls and injury.
9. Be sure nurse call system is in an accessible location within patient's reach. Instruct patient in its use.	Ensures patient can call for assistance if needed.

EVALUATION

STEP	RATIONALE
1. Observe patient every 1 to 2 hours (see agency policy), noting volume of IV fluid infused and rate of infusion.	Ensures delivery of prescribed volume over prescribed time and decreases risk for fluid and electrolyte imbalance.
2. Evaluate patient's response to therapy (e.g., laboratory values, input and output [I&O], weights, vital signs, postprocedure assessments).	Provides ongoing evaluation of patient's fluid status, including monitoring for FVE or FVD. Early recognition of complications leads to prompt treatment.
3. Evaluate patient with a short-peripheral IV at least every 4 hours, or every 1 to 2 hours for patients who are critically ill, sedated, or have cognitive deficits (INS, 2016a), or at established intervals per agency policy and procedure, for signs and symptoms of IV-related complications.	Prevents complications that compromise integrity of VAD or cause inaccurate IV solution flow rate.
4. **Use Teach-Back:** "I want to be sure that I explained the importance of your IV fluids running on time at the rate ordered. Tell me what you think may cause the pump to alarm and what you would do." Revise your instruction now or develop a plan for revised patient/family caregiver teaching if patient/family caregiver is not able to teach back correctly.	Determines patient's/family caregiver's level of understanding of instructional topic.

Unexpected Outcomes	Related Interventions
1. Solution does not infuse at prescribed rate.	
a. Sudden infusion of large volume of solution occurs; patient develops dyspnea, crackles in lung, dependent edema (edema in legs), and increased urine output, indicating fluid-volume excess (FVE).	• Slow infusion rate: KVO rates must have specific rate ordered by health care provider. • Notify health care provider immediately. • Place patient in high-Fowler's position. • Anticipate new IV orders. • Anticipate administration of oxygen per order. • Administer diuretics if ordered.
b. IV solution runs slower than ordered.	• Check for positional change that affects rate, height of IV container, kinking of tubing, or obstruction. • Check VAD site for complications. • Consult health care provider for new order to provide necessary fluid volume.
2. IV patency is lost subsequent to IV solution container running empty.	• Discontinue present IV infusion and restart new short-peripheral catheter in new site.

Recording

- Record type and rate of infusion in milliliters per hour (drops per minute in gravity flow) in patient's medical record and any ordered change in fluid rates. Document use of EID.
- Document your evaluation of patient learning.

Hand-Off Reporting

- Rate of infusion and volume left in infusion.
- Report to provider any signs or symptoms of IV rate–related complication (e.g., fluid and electrolyte imbalances).

✦ SKILL 28.3 Maintenance of an Intravenous Site

Purpose

An important component of patient care is maintaining the integrity of the intravenous (IV) system to ensure positive patient outcomes. Short-peripheral IV catheters and infusion therapy are often associated with systemic and local complications (Gorski, 2018). Appropriate ongoing management of IV sites and associated equipment can prevent or minimize these complications. Strict adherence to infection-prevention measures is required when changing infusion tubing, solution and medication containers, and short-peripheral IV dressings to prevent entry of bacteria into the bloodstream. Developing good organizational skills can help in managing equipment to coordinate tasks in an efficient manner, such as coordinating the short-peripheral IV dressing change with the administration set change and performing the administration set change when it is time to hang a new IV container.

Delegation and Collaboration

The skill of changing an IV solution, tubing, or short-peripheral IV dressing cannot be delegated to nursing assistive personnel (NAP). Delegation to licensed practical nurses (LPNs) varies by state Nurse Practice Act. The nurse instructs the NAP to:

- Inform the nurse when an IV container is near completion.
- Report any cloudiness or precipitate in the IV solution.
- Report alarm sounding on electronic infusion device (EID).
- Report any patient complaints of discomfort related to infusion, such as pain, burning, bleeding, or swelling.
- Report to the nurse any leakage from or around the IV tubing.
- Report if tubing has become contaminated (lying on the floor).
- Report to the nurse if a patient complains of moistness or loosening of an IV dressing.
- Protect the IV dressing during hygiene and activities of daily living (ADLs).

Equipment

Changing Intravenous Container

- Correct volume and type of solution (with additives if indicated) as ordered by health care provider
- Time tape
- Pen

Changing Infusion Tubing

- Clean gloves
- Antiseptic swabs (alcoholic chlorhexidine solution preferred, 70% alcohol, or povidone-iodine)
- Tubing label
- Sterile 2 × 2–inch gauze pads *(optional)*

Continuous IV Infusion

- Microdrip or macrodrip administration set as appropriate
- Add-on device as necessary (e.g., filters, extension set, needleless connector)

Intermittent Extension Set

- 10-mL syringe prefilled with preservative-free 0.9% sodium chloride (normal saline [NS]; INS, 2016a)
- Short extension tubing (if necessary), injection cap

Changing a Short-Peripheral IV Dressing

- Antiseptic swabs (alcoholic chlorhexidine solution preferred, 70% alcohol, or povidone-iodine)
- Adhesive remover *(optional)*
- Polymer-based skin protectant swab *(optional)*
- Clean gloves
- Engineered catheter stabilization device if available or precut strips of sterile nonallergic tape
- Commercially available IV site protector device *(optional)* (Fig. 28.1)
- Sterile transparent semipermeable membrane (TSM) dressing, *or*
- Sterile 2 × 2–inch gauze pads and tape

ASSESSMENT

1. Review accuracy and completeness of health care provider's order in patient's medical record for patient name and correct solution: type, volume, additives, rate, and duration of IV therapy. Follow the seven rights of drug administration (see Chapter 22). *Rationale: Ensures delivery of correct IV solution and prescribed volume over prescribed time (INS, 2016a).*
2. Check pertinent laboratory data such as potassium level. *Rationale: Compare data with baseline to determine ongoing response to IV solution administration.*
3. Determine compatibility of all IV solutions and additives by consulting approved online database, drug reference, or pharmacist. *Rationale: Incompatibilities cause physical, chemical, and therapeutic changes with adverse patient outcomes (Gorksi, 2018).*
4. Perform hand hygiene and apply clean gloves. *Rationale: Reduces risk of contamination and cross-contamination (INS, 2016b).*
5. Note date and time when IV tubing and solution were last changed. (See Table 28.5 for recommendations on administration set changes.) *Rationale: Ensures correct timing of tubing changes. Decreases risk for infection.*

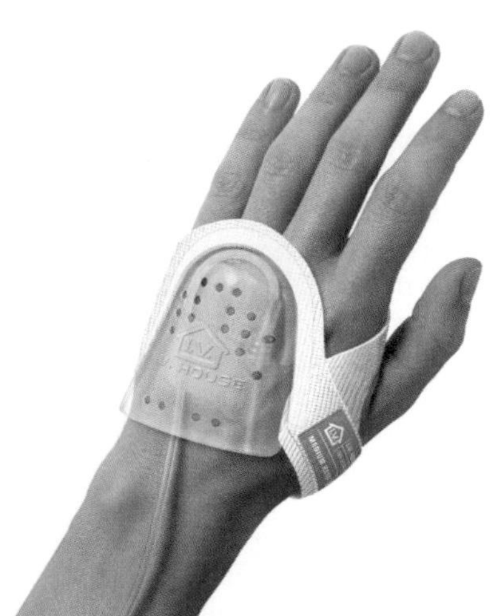

FIG 28.1 Commercially available IV site protector. *(Courtesy I.V. House.)*

6. Check infusion system from solution container down to venous access device (VAD) insertion site for integrity. *Rationale: Identifies complications that can compromise integrity of VAD and patient safety.*
   a. Assess IV container for discoloration, cloudiness, leakage, and expiration date. *Rationale: Incompatibility of solutions or medications compromises integrity of VAD and patient safety (Gorski, 2018).*
   b. Assess IV tubing for puncture, contamination, or occlusion. *Rationale: Compromised tubing results in fluid leakage and bacterial contamination.*

Safe Patient Care *If the tubing and/or IV bag becomes damaged, is leaking, or becomes contaminated, it must be changed, regardless of the tubing change schedule. If there has been a break in integrity of solution container, a new container is needed (Gorksi, 2018).*

7. Determine when dressing on VAD was last changed. Dressing should be labeled to include date and time applied, size and type of VAD, and insertion date. *Rationale: Provides information regarding length of time dressing has been in place and allows planning for dressing change.*
8. Assess the integrity, patency, and functioning of the existing VAD. Assess the VAD catheter–skin junction site and surrounding area for catheter-related complications by visually inspecting and palpating through the intact dressing for redness, tenderness, swelling, and drainage. Assess the patency of the VAD by aspiration of a blood return, absence of resistance when flushing, and complaints of patient pain or discomfort when flushing. *Rationale: Identifies complications that compromise integrity of VAD and necessitate replacement of VAD.*
9. Remove gloves and perform hand hygiene. *Rationale: Reduces risk of contamination (INS, 2016b).*
10. Assess patient's and family caregiver's knowledge, experience, and health literacy regarding protection of IV site. *Rationale: Ensures patient or family caregiver has the capacity to obtain, communicate, process, and understand basic health information (CDC, 2016).*

STEP	RATIONALE
PLANNING	
1. Expected outcomes following completion of procedure:	
• IV solution is correct, and patient receives prescribed IV therapy as ordered.	Patient receives solution ordered for treatment of diagnosis.
• Fluid and electrolyte balance returns to normal.	Patient achieves therapeutic outcomes.
• Patient's IV tubing is patent, and patient experiences no leakage of solution from or around IV tubing.	Intact system decreases risk for microbial contamination. Brief interruption of IV infusion does not result in occlusion of VAD.
• Patient's VAD remains patent, and site is free from signs and symptoms of IV-related complications.	Ensures IV access for delivery of prescribed IV therapy (INS, 2016a).
• Patient and family caregiver can explain purpose of changing IV solution, administration set, and VAD dressing.	Demonstrates learning (INS, 2016a).
2. Provide privacy and prepare environment.	Providing privacy and preparing the environment early help the student/nurse think about the need to remove clutter from the over-bed or bedside table.
3. Perform hand hygiene. Collect and organize equipment on clean, clutter-free bedside stand or over-bed table.	Reduces risk of microbial contamination and cross-contamination of equipment (INS, 2016b). Easy access to equipment improves efficiency.
a. Have next solution prepared at least 1 hour before needed. If solution is prepared in pharmacy, ensure that it has been delivered to patient care unit. Allow solution to warm to room temperature if it has been refrigerated. Check that solution is correct and properly labeled. Check solution expiration date. Ensure that any light-sensitivity restrictions are followed.	Reduces transmission of infection and contamination of equipment (INS, 2016a). Proper handling of solutions prevents IV-related complications such as occlusion. Checking that solution is correct prevents medication error and promotes patient safety.
b. Be sure you have the correct administration set for the type of infusion to be administered and electronic infusion device (EID) that is to be used. Coordinate IV tubing changes with solution changes when possible.	Ensures patient safety. Decreases number of times system is open.
c. Open and prepare sterile packages using sterile aseptic technique (see Chapter 5).	Reduces risk of microbial contamination and cross-contamination of equipment (INS, 2016b).
4. Help patient to comfortable position.	Promotes comfort and relaxation of patient. May reduce anxiety and promote cooperation.

STEP	RATIONALE
5. Explain/instruct patient and family caregiver on reasons for ongoing IV therapy. Explain patient will need to hold affected extremity still and how long procedure will take.	Provides patient with information about procedure and promotes compliance (INS, 2016a). Informing patient may minimize anxiety. Gives patient time frame around which to plan personal activities.

IMPLEMENTATION

STEP	RATIONALE
1. Identify patient using at least two identifiers (e.g., name and birthday or name and medical record number) according to agency policy. Compare identifiers with information on patient's medication administration record (MAR) or medical record.	Ensures correct patient. Complies with The Joint Commission standards and improves patient safety (TJC, 2019).
2. Changing intravenous container:	Patients receiving intravenous therapy periodically require changes of IV solutions or containers depending on the rate of infusion, volume in the container, and stability of the solution or medication (INS, 2016b). It becomes clinically appropriate to change the type of solution depending on a patient's fluid and electrolyte balance, response to therapy (e.g., therapeutic drug monitoring), and goals of therapy.
a. Change solution when fluid remains only in neck of container (about 50 mL) or when new type of solution has been ordered.	A container is changed when there is an order for a new solution or when it becomes time to add a sequential container to avoid exceeding hang time (Alexander et al., 2014). Prevents waste of solution.

Safe Patient Care *The maximum hang time for routine replacement of IV containers is established by agency policy and procedure. Maximum hang time would be based on factors such as the use of strict aseptic technique, whether the system remains closed without injection ports or add-on tubing, stability of the solution or medication being infused, and how long the solution in the IV container will last (Alexander et al., 2014). It is recommended that each container be changed within 24 hours after the administration set is added (Alexander et al., 2014; INS, 2016b). Solution and medication containers on ambulatory infusion devices may remain longer than 24 hours if aseptic technique is used, the system remains closed without injection ports or add-on tubing, and the medication is stable for the anticipated infusion time (Alexander et al., 2014).*

STEP	RATIONALE
b. Perform hand hygiene.	Reduces transmission of microorganisms.
c. Prepare new solution for changing. If using plastic bag, hang on IV pole and remove protective cover from IV tubing port. If using glass bottle, remove metal cap and metal and rubber disks.	Solution and medication containers include plastic bags, plastic bottles, and glass bottles. Permits quick, smooth, organized change from old to new container.
d. Close roller clamp on existing solution to stop flow rate. Remove IV tubing from EID (if used). Then remove old IV solution container from IV pole. Hold container with tubing port pointing upward.	Prevents solution remaining in drip chamber from emptying while changing solutions. Prevents solution in bag from spilling.
e. Quickly remove spike from old solution container and, without touching tip, insert spike into new container (see illustrations).	Reduces risk for solution in drip chamber becoming empty and maintains sterility.

Safe Patient Care *If spike becomes contaminated by touching an unsterile object, you will need a new IV tubing set.*

STEP	RATIONALE
f. Hang new container of solution on IV pole.	Gravity helps with delivery of fluid into drip chamber.
g. Check for air in IV tubing. If air bubbles have formed, remove them by closing roller clamp, stretching tubing downward, and tapping tubing with finger (bubbles rise in fluid to drip chamber; see illustration).	Reduces risk of air entering tubing. Use of an air-eliminating filter also reduces risk.
h. Make sure that drip chamber is one-third to one-half full. If drip chamber is too full, level can be decreased by removing bag from IV pole, pinching off IV tubing below drip chamber, inverting container, squeezing drip chamber (see illustration), releasing and turning solution container upright, and releasing pinch on tubing.	Reduces risk for air entering IV tubing. If chamber is filled, you cannot observe or regulate drip rate.
i. Regulate flow to ordered rate by opening and adjusting roller clamp on IV tubing or by opening roller clamp and programming and turning on EID.	Maintains measures to restore fluid balance and deliver IV solution as ordered.

STEP	RATIONALE
j. Place time label on side of container and label with time hung, time of completion, and appropriate intervals. If using plastic bags, mark only on label and not container.	Provides visual comparison of volume infused compared with prescribed rate of infusion.
k. Instruct patient on purpose of new IV solution, additives, flow rate, potential side effects, how to avoid occluding tubing, and what to report.	Information informs patient about purpose for continued IV therapy and what to report and protects VAD patency.
3. Changing infusion tubing:	

Safe Patient Care *Administration sets are the primary method to carry a solution or medication to a patient. These administration sets are considered the primary set. In addition, patients may have add-on devices (e.g., filters, extension sets), which you connect to the primary set as indicated by the prescribed therapy. Secondary sets may be used as a method to administer additional medications in conjunction with the primary infusion (e.g., antibiotics). Follow agency policy and procedures for specific requirements (Table 28.5).*

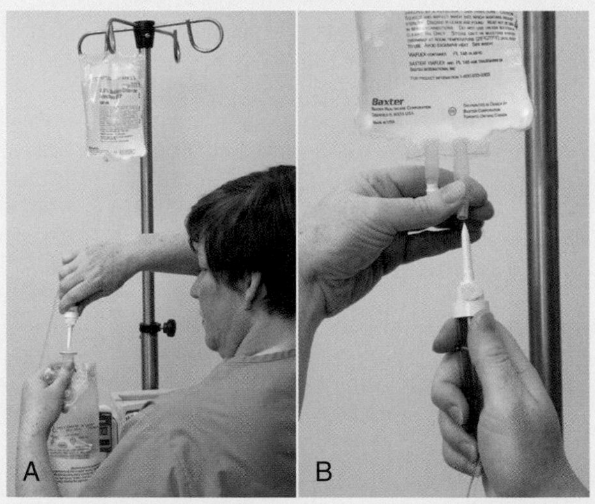

STEP 2e (A) Quickly remove spike from old solution container. (B) Without touching tip, insert spike into new container.

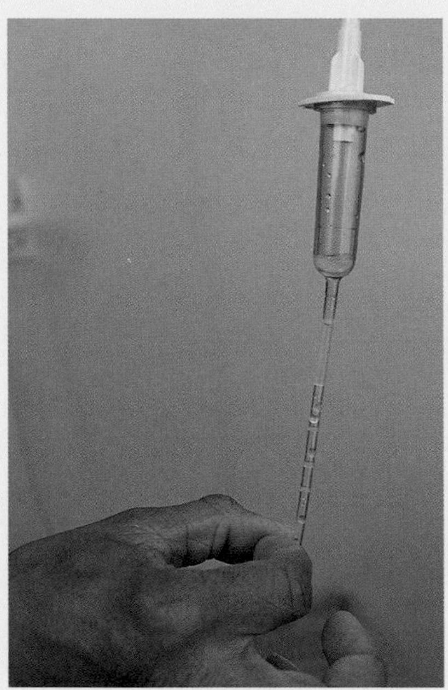

STEP 2g Tap tubing to cause air bubbles to rise up to drip chamber.

TABLE 28.5

Administration Set Changes

Primary and Secondary Continuous Infusions	Primary Intermittent Infusions	Use of Add-on Devices
• Change no more frequently than every 96 hours for solutions *other* than lipid, blood, or blood products. • In addition to routine changes, change the administration set whenever the short-peripheral IV site is changed or a new CVAD is placed. • If the secondary set is removed from the primary set, the secondary set is now an intermittent set and should be changed every 24 hours.	• Should be changed every 24 hours because of increased risk of infection with repeatedly disconnecting and reconnecting administration set. • Aseptically attach a new, sterile covering device to the Luer end of the administration set after each intermittent use. *Avoid* attaching the exposed end of the administration set to port on the same set (e.g., looping).	• Should be minimized because each is a potential source of contamination and disconnection. • Use of administration sets with devices as part of the set is preferred. • Aseptically change with insertion of new VAD or with each administration set replacement. • Change if the integrity of the product is compromised or suspected of being compromised.

CVAD, Central vascular access device; *IV,* intravenous.

Modified from Infusion Nurses Society (INS): *Policy and procedures for infusion therapy*, ed 5, Norwood, MA, 2016, The Society.

STEP	RATIONALE

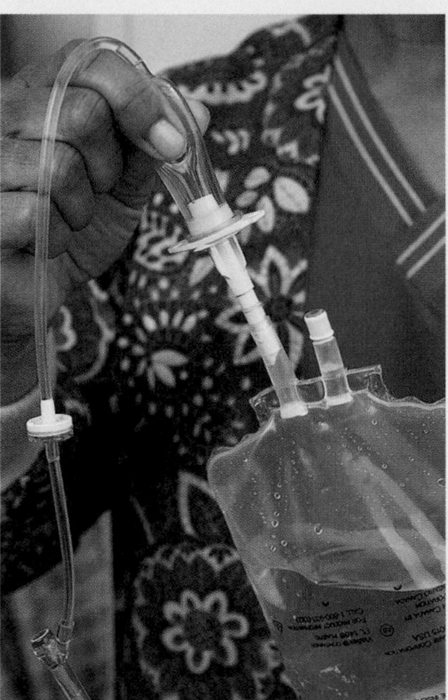

STEP 2h Squeeze drip chamber to fill with fluid. Be sure to leave chamber one-third to one-half full.

STEP	RATIONALE
a. Perform hand hygiene. Open new infusion set and connect add-on pieces (e.g., filters, extension tubing) using aseptic technique. Keep protective coverings over infusion spike and distal adapter. Place roller clamp about 2 to 2.5 cm (1 to 2 inches) below drip chamber and move roller clamp to "off" position. Secure all connections.	Close proximity of roller clamp to drip chamber allows more accurate regulation of flow rate. Securing connections reduces risk later of air emboli and infection. Protective covers reduce entrance of microorganisms. All connections should be of Luer-Lok type (INS, 2016a).
b. Apply clean gloves. If patient's IV cannula hub is not visible, remove IV dressing as described in Step 4a. Do not remove tape securing cannula to skin.	Cannula hub must be visible to provide smooth transition when removing old and inserting new tubing.
c. Prepare IV tubing with new IV container. (See Skill 28.1, Step 3.)	
d. Prepare IV tubing with existing continuous IV infusion bag.	
(1) Move roller clamp on new IV tubing to "off" position.	Prevents fluid spillage.
(2) Slow rate of infusion through old tubing to keep-vein-open (KVO) rate using EID or roller clamp.	Prevents occlusion of VAD.
(3) Compress and fill drip chamber of old tubing.	Ensures that drip chamber remains full until new tubing is changed.
(4) Invert container and remove old tubing. Keep spike sterile and upright.	Solution in drip chamber will continue to run and maintain catheter patency.
(5) Insert spike of new infusion tubing into solution container. Hang solution bag on IV pole, compress drip chamber on new tubing, and release, allowing it to fill one-third to one-half full.	Permits drip chamber to fill and promotes rapid, smooth flow of solution through tubing.
(6) Prime air out of IV tubing by filling with IV solution: Remove protective cover on end of tubing and slowly open roller clamp to allow solution to flow from drip chamber to distal end of IV tubing. If tubing has Y connector, invert Y connector when solution reaches it to displace air. Return roller clamp to "off" position after priming tubing (filled with IV solution). Replace protective cover on end of IV tubing. Place end of adapter near patient's IV site.	Priming ensures that IV tubing is clear of air before connection with VAD and filled with IV solution. Slow fill of tubing decreases turbulence and chance of bubble formation. Closing clamp prevents accidental loss of fluid. Maintains sterility. Equipment is positioned for quick connection of new tubing.

STEP	RATIONALE
(7) Stop EID or turn roller clamp on old tubing to "off" position.	Prevents fluid spillage.
e. Prepare tubing with extension set or saline lock.	Placement of a short extension tubing or loop between a catheter hub and injection cap allows manipulation of the injection cap without moving the catheter.

Safe Patient Care *The extension tubing remains attached to the short-peripheral catheter and is changed when the catheter is changed.*

STEP	RATIONALE
(1) If short extension tubing is needed, use sterile technique to connect new injection cap to new extension set or IV tubing.	Prepares extension set for connecting with IV.
(2) Scrub injection cap with antiseptic swab for at least 15 seconds and allow to dry completely. Attach syringe with 3 to 5 mL of normal saline [NS] flush solution and inject through injection cap into extension set.	Ensures effective disinfection (Gorski, 2018). Maintains patency of catheter.
f. Reestablish infusion.	
(1) Gently disconnect old tubing from extension tubing (or from IV catheter hub) and quickly insert Luer-Lok end of new tubing or saline lock into extension tubing connection (or IV catheter hub; see illustrations for example of connecting tubing to short extension set).	Allows smooth transition from old to new tubing, minimizing time system is open.
(2) For continuous infusion, open roller clamp on new tubing and regulate drip rate using roller clamp, or insert tubing into EID, program to desired rate, and push on.	Ensures catheter patency and prevents occlusion.
(3) Attach piece of tape or preprinted label with date and time of IV tubing change onto tubing below drip chamber.	Provides reference to determine next time for tubing change.
(4) Form loop of tubing and secure it to patient's arm with strip of tape.	Avoids accidental pulling against site and stabilizes catheter.
(5) If necessary, apply new dressing.	Maintains integrity of VAD site.

Safe Patient Care *You may need to assist patients with many aspects of hygiene (e.g., gown changes, bathing) while patients are receiving IV therapy. Never disconnect infusion tubing to change a gown or any article of clothing. Coordinate care so that bathing or hygiene activities are done after discontinuing an IV site and before another venipuncture is performed. If infusion cannot be discontinued, use special "IV gowns" if available.*

STEP	RATIONALE
4. Changing short-peripheral IV dressing:	The skin insertion site is the most common source of colonization for IV catheters and catheter-related infections (Alexander et al., 2014).

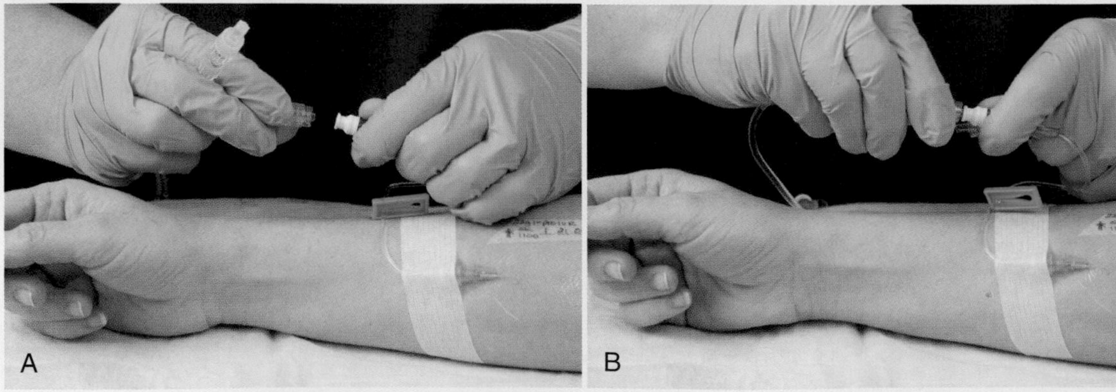

STEP 3f(1) (A) Disconnect old tubing. (B) Insert adapter of new tubing.

STEP	RATIONALE

Safe Patient Care *Short-peripheral catheter dressing changes should be performed every 5 to 7 days and gauze dressings every 2 days (INS, 2016a). Therefore, you need to securely apply catheter dressings and change dressings when wet, soiled, or loosened or if the integrity is compromised (INS, 2016b).*

STEP	RATIONALE
a. Remove existing dressing:	Technique minimizes discomfort during removal. Use alcohol swab on TSM dressing next to patient's skin to loosen dressing.
(1) For TSM dressing: Stabilize catheter with nondominant hand (see illustration). Remove dressing by pulling up one corner and gently pulling straight out and parallel to skin. Repeat on all sides until dressing has been removed.	
(2) For gauze dressing: Stabilize catheter hub while loosening tape and removing old dressing one layer at a time by pulling toward insertion site. Be cautious if tubing becomes tangled between two layers of dressing.	
b. Assess VAD insertion site for signs and symptoms of IV-related complications. If complication exists, determine if VAD requires removal. Remove catheter if ordered by health care provider (see Procedural Guideline 28.1).	Presence of complication may necessitate VAD removal.
c. If catheter is to remain in place, assess integrity of engineered stabilization device. Continue to stabilize catheter and remove as recommended by manufacturer directions for use. Inspect for signs of adhesive-related skin injury from adhesive-based engineered stabilization devices. **NOTE:** Some stabilization devices are designed to remain in place for length of time VAD is in as long as adequate stabilization is evident.	Removing stabilization device allows for appropriate skin antisepsis before applying dressing and new stabilization device (INS, 2016a). Stabilization prevents accidental dislodgement of VAD.

Safe Patient Care *Keep one finger over catheter at all times until dressing secures catheter hub. If patient is restless or uncooperative, it is helpful to have another staff member help with procedure.*

STEP	RATIONALE
d. While stabilizing IV line, perform skin antisepsis to insertion site with antiseptic wipe using friction in back-and-forth motion for 30 seconds and allow to dry completely. If using alcohol or povidone-iodine, clean in concentric circle, moving from insertion site outward with the swab. Allow antiseptic solution to dry completely.	Reduces incidence of catheter-related infections (Gorski, 2018). Allow any skin antiseptic agent to fully dry for complete antisepsis (INS, 2016a).

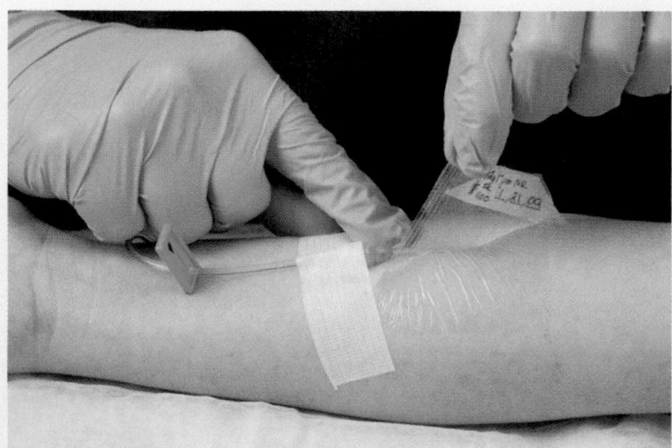

STEP 4a(1) Remove transparent semipermeable membrane (TSM) dressing by pulling side laterally.

STEP	RATIONALE
e. *Option:* Apply skin protectant to area where you will apply tape, dressing, or engineered stabilization device. Allow to dry.	Coats skin with protective solution to maintain skin integrity, prevents irritation from adhesive, and promotes adhesion of dressing.
f. While stabilizing catheter, apply sterile dressing over site (procedures differ; follow agency policy).	

Safe Patient Care *Because adhesive bandages are not occlusive and nonsterile tape increases the risk for insertion site infection, do not use either over catheter insertion points.*

STEP	RATIONALE
(1) *TSM dressing:* Apply TSM dressing as directed in Skill 28.1, Step 19a.	Protects catheter insertion site and minimizes risk for infection (Gorski, 2018). TSM dressing allows visualization of insertion site and surrounding area for complications (INS, 2016a).
(2) *Sterile gauze dressing:* Apply sterile gauze dressing as directed in Skill 28.1, Step 19b.	Only use sterile tape under sterile dressing to prevent site contamination. Gauze dressing obscures observation of insertion site and is changed every 2 days (INS, 2016a).
g. *Option: Secure with new engineered catheter stabilization device:* Apply device as directed in Skill 28.1, Step 20.	Use of engineered stabilization devices can reduce risk for VAD complications (i.e., phlebitis, infection, migration) and unintentional loss of access (INS, 2016a).

Safe Patient Care *Stabilization of short-peripheral catheters decreases risk of catheter-related complications and premature loss of access. Preferred options for stabilization include an adhesive engineered stabilization device used with a standard short-peripheral IV catheter, or an integrated feature on the IV catheter with use of a bordered polyurethane dressing (INS, 2016a). Although sterile tape or surgical strips can be used, they are not as effective as an engineered stabilization device (Gorski, 2018; INS, 2016a).*

STEP	RATIONALE
h. *Option:* Apply polymer-based site protection device (e.g., I.V. House Ultra Protective Dressing®).	Reduces risk of VAD dislodgement (INS, 2016a).
i. Anchor extension tubing or IV tubing alongside dressing on arm and secure with tape directly over tubing. When using TSM dressing, avoid placing tape over dressing.	Prevents accidental dislodgement of VAD tubing.
j. Label dressing per agency policy. Information on label includes date and time of IV insertion, VAD gauge size and length, and your initials.	Communicates type of device and time interval for dressing change and site rotation.
5. Dispose of any used supplies. Remove gloves and perform hand hygiene.	Reduces transmission of microorganisms (INS, 2016a).
6. Assist patient to a comfortable position and instruct how to move and turn properly with VAD.	Prevents accidental dislodgement of IV catheter.
7. Raise bed rails (as appropriate) and lower bed to lowest position.	Minimizes risk for falls and injury.
8. Be sure nurse call system is in an accessible location within patient's reach. Instruct patient in its use.	Ensures patient can call for assistance if needed.

EVALUATION

STEP	RATIONALE
1. Observe patient with a short-peripheral IV at least every 4 hours, or every 1 to 2 hours for patients who are critically ill, sedated, or have cognitive deficits (INS, 2016a), or at established intervals per agency policy and procedure, for the following:	Ensures delivery of infusion therapy as ordered.
a. Correct type and amount of solution infused	Ensures delivery of prescribed volume over prescribed time and decreases risk for fluid and electrolyte imbalance.
b. Leaking at connection sites	Minimizes risk of infection caused by breach in system integrity.
c. Function, intactness, and patency of IV system	Validates that IV line is patent and functioning correctly. Manipulation of catheter and tubing may affect rate of infusion.
d. IV-related complications by visually inspecting and gently palpating skin around and above IV site through the intact dressing.	Identifies complications that compromise integrity of VAD or cause inaccurate IV solution flow rate.

STEP	RATIONALE
2. Evaluate patient to determine response to therapy (e.g., laboratory values, input and output [I&O], weights, vital signs, postprocedure assessments).	Provides ongoing evaluation of patient's fluid status.
3. Monitor patient for signs of fluid-volume excess (FVE) or fluid-volume deficit (FVD) or signs and symptoms of electrolyte imbalances.	Early recognition of complications leads to prompt treatment.
4. **Use Teach-Back:** "We talked about the importance of your IV solutions running as prescribed. I want to be sure I explained this clearly. Tell me in your own words what you should do if you notice that the IV is not dripping or you notice leaking." Revise your instruction now or develop a plan for revised patient/family caregiver teaching if patient/family caregiver is not able to teach back correctly.	Determines patient's/family caregiver's level of understanding of instructional topic.

Unexpected Outcomes	Related Interventions
1. Flow rate is incorrect; patient receives too little or too much solution.	• Notify health care provider if patient's anticipated infusion is 100 to 200 mL less than or greater than anticipated (per agency policy and procedure). • Evaluate patient for signs and symptoms of adverse effects of infusion (e.g., FVD or FVE). • Consult health care provider for new order to provide necessary fluid volume. • Use EID when accurate flow rate is critical. • Determine and correct cause of incorrect flow rate (e.g., height of IV container, tubing bent or kinked, roller clamp closed). • Check for positional IV site and reposition catheter or apply new dressing if necessary. • Check IV catheter for loss of patency or dislodgement; catheter may require replacement. • Check VAD site for complications.
2. Leaking occurs at IV connection.	• Determine site of leaking and secure connection. • Apply new dressing if necessary.
3. IV catheter is removed or dislodged accidentally.	• Restart new short-peripheral IV line in other extremity or above previous insertion site if continued therapy is necessary.

Recording

- Record solution and tubing changes; type of infusion solution, including any additives; volume of container; and rate of infusion.
- Record time of discontinuing solution or IV medication and tubing or catheter flushes to include solution, volume, and concentration.
- Record time short-peripheral dressing was changed, reason for dressing change, antiseptic used, type of dressing applied, patency of system, and observation of venipuncture site.
- Document your evaluation of patient learning.

Hand-Off Reporting

- Any significant information about IV site or system; time medication or IV solution was discontinued

PROCEDURAL GUIDELINE 28.1 *Discontinuing a Short-Peripheral Intravenous Device*

Purpose

A short-peripheral intravenous (IV) catheter is discontinued when the prescribed length of therapy is completed or when a complication occurs (e.g., phlebitis, infiltration, or catheter occlusion). The technique for discontinuing a short-peripheral IV catheter follows infection-prevention guidelines to minimize the chances of the patient acquiring an infection. Care must also be taken because the risk of catheter emboli may occur if the catheter breaks off during removal.

Delegation and Collaboration

The skill of discontinuing a short-peripheral IV line cannot be delegated to nursing assistive personnel (NAP). Delegation to licensed practical nurses (LPNs) varies

Continued

PROCEDURAL GUIDELINE 28.1 *Discontinuing a Short-Peripheral Intravenous Device—cont'd*

by state Nurse Practice Act. The nurse instructs the NAP to:

- Report to the nurse any bleeding at the site after catheter has been removed.
- Report any complaints of pain or observation of redness at the site by the patient.

Equipment

Clean gloves; sterile 2 × 2–inch or 4 × 4–inch gauze sponge; antiseptic swabs (alcoholic chlorhexidine solution preferred, 70% alcohol, or povidone-iodine); tape

Procedural Steps

1. Review accuracy and completeness of health care provider's order for discontinuation of venous access device (VAD).
2. Perform hand hygiene and collect equipment.
3. Identify patient using at least two identifiers (e.g., name and birthday or name and medical record number) according to agency policy. Compare identifiers with information on patient's medication administration record (MAR) or medical record (TJC, 2019).
4. Apply clean gloves. Observe existing IV site for signs and symptoms of IV-related complications by visual inspection and palpating around and above site through the intact dressing for redness, tenderness, swelling, and drainage. Ask patient how IV site feels.
5. Assess if patient is receiving an anticoagulant or has a history of a coagulopathy.
6. Assess patient's or family caregiver's knowledge, experience, and health literacy related to IV catheter to be discontinued.
7. Explain procedure to patient before you remove catheter. Explain that patient needs to hold affected extremity still.
8. Turn IV tubing roller clamp to "off" position or turn electronic infusion device (EID) off and roller clamp to "off" position.
9. Carefully remove VAD dressing and engineered stabilization device.
10. Stabilize IV catheter hub with middle finger of nondominant hand.

Safe Patient Care *Never use scissors to remove the tape or dressing because you may accidentally cut the catheter.*

11. Place clean sterile gauze above insertion site and, using dominant hand, withdraw catheter using a slow, steady motion and keeping the hub parallel to skin (see illustration).

Safe Patient Care *Do not raise or lift catheter before it is completely out of the vein to avoid trauma or hematoma formation.*

12. Apply pressure to site for a minimum of 30 seconds until bleeding has stopped. **NOTE:** Apply pressure for at least 5 to 10 minutes if patient is on anticoagulants.
13. Inspect catheter for intactness after removal; note tip integrity and length.
14. Observe IV site for evidence of any complications, such as redness, pain, tenderness, swelling, bleeding, or drainage. Monitor for 24 to 48 hours after removal for postinfusion phlebitis.
15. Apply clean, folded gauze dressing over insertion site and secure with tape.
16. Discard used supplies, remove gloves, and perform hand hygiene.
17. Document procedure in patient's medical record in electronic health record or chart.
18. Assist patient to comfortable position.
19. Be sure nurse call system is in an accessible location within patient's reach.
20. Raise side rails (as appropriate) and lower bed to lowest position.
21. Document time short-peripheral catheter was removed, reason for removal, antiseptic used, type of dressing applied, observation of venipuncture site.
22. Notify health care provider of problems during procedure or signs of infection.

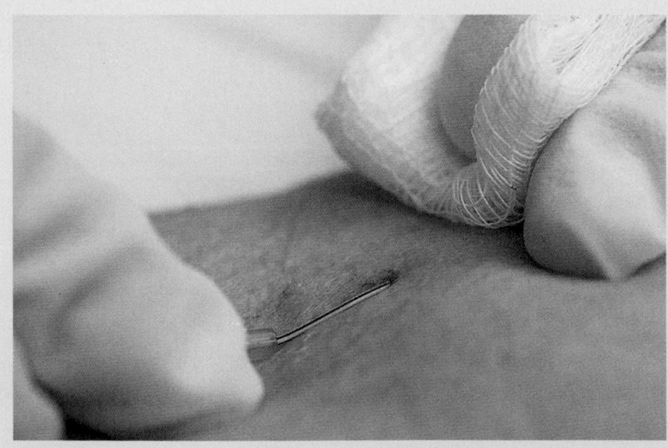

STEP 11 Intravenous (IV) catheter is removed slowly, keeping catheter parallel to vein.

✦ SKILL 28.4 Managing Central Vascular Access Devices

Purpose

The need for safe and convenient intravenous (IV) therapy has led to the development of venous access devices (VADs) designed for long-term access to the venous or arterial systems. Physicians or competently trained nurses place these devices into the central vascular system. Factors considered when determining placement of a central vascular access device (CVAD) include type and duration of infusion therapy (greater than 7 days), vascular characteristics, patient's age, co-morbidities, history of infusion therapy, and preference for VAD location (INS, 2016a). CVADs can have single or multiple lumens. The tip of a CVAD is placed in the lower third of the superior vena cava near the junction of the right atrium (Fig. 28.2) (INS, 2016a). The choice of the number of lumens

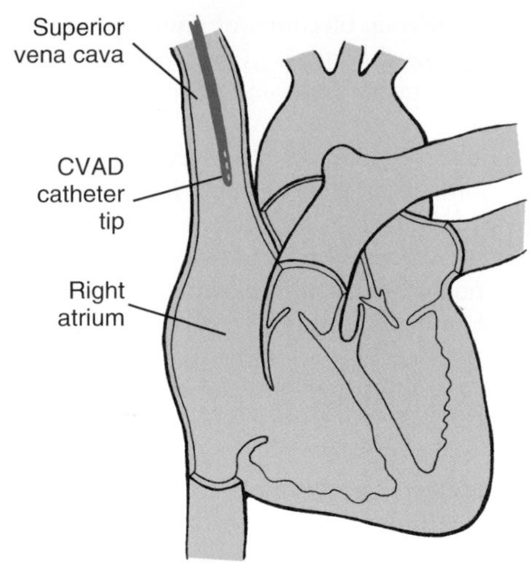

FIG 28.2 CVAD tip placement in superior vena cava.

depends on a patient's condition, prescribed therapy, and the need for numerous infusions and blood samplings. A device with more than one lumen allows for simultaneous administration of solutions and medications and for administration of incompatible solutions or medications at the same time. Your role is to anticipate the need for a CVAD, assist the health care provider in placing a CVAD, care for and maintain the device, administer solutions or medications, and assess for signs and symptoms of IV-related complications (Gorksi, 2018).

Delegation and Collaboration

The skill of managing a CVAD cannot be delegated to nursing assistive personnel (NAP). The nurse instructs the NAP to:

- Report the following to the nurse immediately: bleeding or leaking around CVAD insertion site; shortness of breath; loosened or soiled dressing; or if the patient has a fever or complains of pain at the site or catheter becomes dislodged.
- Inform nurse if the electronic infusion device (EID) alarm signals or if the fluid level in container is low or empty.
- Help with positioning patient during insertion and care.

Equipment

Insertion and Dressing Care

- Hair clippers
- Central vascular access insertion tray to include appropriate-length catheter and introducer needle, sterile gauze, sterile drapes, disposable tape measure
- Maximum barrier supplies to include head covering, sterile gowns, masks, sterile gloves (powder free), antiseptic solution (alcoholic chlorhexidine solution preferred, 70% alcohol, povidone-iodine for chlorhexidine sensitivities), large full-body sterile drape with fenestration
- Protective eyewear
- Nonsterile gloves
- Gauze pads
- Surgical towels
- 1% lidocaine (Xylocaine) for use as local anesthetic as ordered by health care provider
- 3-mL syringe and small-gauge needle for anesthetic administration
- 10-mL syringe
- Transparent semipermeable membrane (TSM) or gauze 4 × 4 dressing for catheter insertion site
- Engineered stabilization device
- Needleless connector for each lumen
- Polymer-based skin protectant swab *(optional)*
- Sterile tape
- Electronic infusion device
- Ultrasound (if available) with sterile wand cover and sterile transducer gel

Site Care and Dressing Change

- CVAD dressing change kit, which includes sterile gloves, mask, antiseptic swabs or sponge for skin disinfection (alcoholic chlorhexidine solution preferred, 70% alcohol, or povidone-iodine), TSM dressing, 4 × 4 gauze pads, tape measure, sterile tape, label
- Engineered stabilization device (if not sutured) for peripherally inserted central catheter (PICC) or nontunneled catheters (see Fig. 28.3 and Table 28.6).
- Polymer-based skin protectant swab
- Clean gloves
- Needleless injection cap(s) for each lumen(s)

Blood Sampling

- Clean gloves
- Antiseptic swabs (alcoholic chlorhexidine solution preferred, 70% alcohol, or povidone-iodine)
- 5-mL Luer-Lok syringes
- 10-mL Luer-Lok syringes
- Vacuum system or blood transfer device (see agency policy)
- Blood tubes, including waste tubes, labels
- Needleless injection cap
- Syringe (5 mL or 10 mL; see agency policy) for discarded blood
- 10-mL syringe with 5 to 10 mL preservative-free 0.9% sodium chloride (normal saline [NS])
- 10-mL syringe with heparin flush solution
- Sterile cap to maintain sterility of distal end of IV tubing

Changing the Injection Cap

- Clean gloves
- Antiseptic swabs (alcoholic chlorhexidine solution preferred, or 70% alcohol)
- Needleless injection cap(s)
- 10-mL syringe with 10 mL preservative-free 0.9% sodium chloride (NS)
- 10-mL syringe with heparin flush solution

Discontinuation of a Nontunneled Catheter

- Personal protective equipment as indicated (goggles, gown, mask, and clean gloves)
- CVAD dressing change kit, which includes sterile gloves, mask, antiseptic swabs for skin disinfection, TSM dressing, 4 × 4 gauze pads, tape measure, sterile tape, label
- Petroleum-based ointment or petroleum-based gauze, sterile
- Suture removal kit (if sutures are in place)
- Stethoscope

ASSESSMENT

1. Review accuracy and completeness of health care provider's order for insertion of CVAD for size and type. Assess treatment schedule: times for administration of IV solutions, medications, and blood sampling. Follow the seven rights of medication administration (see Chapter 22). Confirm that

informed consent has been obtained and witnessed by health care provider who will perform procedure. *Rationale: Identifies patient's need for vascular access, evaluates response to therapy, and determines education needs. Insertion of central catheter requires informed consent (INS, 2016a).*

2. Obtain data from the patient's electronic health record, including coagulopathy disorders, current anticoagulant use, respiratory diseases, and intracranial bleeding. *Rationale: Direct pressure can be applied to control bleeding in patients with coagulopathy or on anticoagulant therapy. Trendelenburg position may be contraindicated in certain patients with respiratory diseases or intracranial bleeding (INS, 2016b).*
3. Assess type of CVAD intended for placement. Review manufacturer directions concerning catheter and maintenance. *Rationale: Care and management depend on type and size of catheter or port, number of lumens, and purpose of therapy. Knowledge of how to care for CVADs can decrease the incidence of central line–associated bloodstream infection (CLABSI; Humphrey, 2015).*
4. Perform hand hygiene. Assess patient's hydration status: skin turgor, dryness of mouth, skin texture, and fluid intake and output. *Rationale: Reduces transmission of infection. Provides baseline. In addition, dehydration makes insertion of CVAD more difficult.*
5. Assess patient for any surgical procedures of upper chest or anatomical irregularities of proposed insertion site. *Rationale: Previous surgical procedures or central vascular catheterizations indicate that you should not use a particular site. Spinal deformities and contractions make positioning difficult.*
6. Assess CVAD placement site for skin integrity (open lesions) and signs of infection (i.e., redness, pain, tenderness, swelling, bleeding, or drainage). Apply gloves if drainage is present. *Rationale: Compromised skin integrity contraindicates catheter insertion and can lead to secondary complications.*
7. Assess patient for allergy to chlorhexidine gluconate (CHG), iodine, lidocaine, or latex. *Rationale: Medications, solutions used during catheter insertion, and use of gloves and tape can cause serious allergic reactions.*
8. Assess for proper function of existing CVAD before therapy: integrity of catheter, ability to flush or infuse solution without resistance, absence of patient complaint of pain or discomfort when flushing, and ability to aspirate blood. Remove and discard gloves (if worn). Perform hand hygiene. Assess the VAD catheter–skin junction site and surrounding area for catheter-related complications by visually inspecting and palpating through the intact dressing for redness, tenderness, swelling, and drainage. *Rationale: Blood return should be obtained, and patency confirmed before infusion of solutions or medications (INS, 2016a).*
9. Assess if any catheter lumens require flushing or if CVAD site needs dressing change by referring to medical record, nurses' notes, agency policies, and manufacturer-recommended guidelines for use. *Rationale: Provides guidelines for maintaining catheter patency and preventing infection.*
10. Assess patient's and family caregiver's knowledge, experience, and health literacy regarding CVAD and knowledge of purpose, care, and maintenance. *Rationale: Ensures patient or family caregiver has the capacity to obtain, communicate, process, and understand basic health information (CDC, 2016).*

STEP	RATIONALE
PLANNING	
1. Expected outcomes following completion of procedure:	
• Insertion occurs without complication.	Placement of nontunneled CVAD carries risks such as pneumothorax, hematoma, air embolism, thrombosis, and infection.
• Catheter tip placement is appropriate at or near the cavoatrial junction as confirmed by x-ray (see Fig. 28.2).	Appropriate tip placement decreases risk of thrombotic complications or arrhythmias. Confirmation of tip location is required before use of CVAD (INS, 2016a).
• CVAD site is intact, with no evidence of signs or symptoms of postinsertion complications (e.g., catheter migration, redness, swelling, aching, or pain).	Catheter is patent, properly placed, and without evidence of complications.
• Prescribed solutions and medications infuse without difficulty.	Catheter remains patent.
• Patient's CVAD is maintained routinely and remains patent; site is free from signs and symptoms of IV-related complications.	Care and maintenance of CVAD includes assessment, site care, dressing changes, injection cap changes, and flushing with aseptic technique (Alexander et al., 2014).

Safe Patient Care *Complications associated with CVADs can include local or systemic infection. A local infection can develop around the catheter insertion site. A more serious infection of the bloodstream may be caused by contamination of the catheter from the skin of the patient or poor infection-prevention practices during insertion, care, or maintenance (Gorksi, 2018). The implementation of the Institute for Healthcare Improvement (IHI) central line bundle prevents infection. The key components of the IHI central line bundle are as follows (IHI, 2012):*

- *Hand hygiene prior to catheter insertion*
- *Maximal sterile barrier precautions with insertion (Inserter wears a cap, mask, and sterile gloves and gown, and a large sterile drape is placed over patient during insertion.)*
- *CHG skin antisepsis*
- *Optimal catheter site selection, with avoidance of the femoral vein for central venous access in adult patients*
- *Necessity of daily review of condition of the line and insertion site, with prompt removal of unnecessary lines*

STEP	RATIONALE
• Blood specimens are obtained, and CVAD patency is maintained.	Catheter remains patent after blood draws.
• Patient and family caregiver are able to explain purpose of CVAD and IV-line therapy, care, and maintenance.	Demonstrates that patient and family caregiver have understanding and competency in caring for CVAD.
2. Provide privacy and prepare environment.	Providing privacy and preparing the environment early help the student/nurse think about the need to remove clutter from the over-bed or bedside table.
3. Perform hand hygiene. Collect equipment and organize on clean, clutter-free bedside stand or over-bed table.	Reduces transmission of infection and contamination of equipment (INS, 2016a).
4. Explain procedure and purpose to patient and family caregiver. Explain to patient that he or she must not move during procedure. Offer opportunity at this time to toilet, and offer pain medication (if needed).	Decreases anxiety, promotes cooperation, and prevents sudden movement during sterile procedure.

IMPLEMENTATION

STEP	RATIONALE
1. Identify patient using at least two identifiers (e.g., name and birthday or name and medical record number) according to agency policy. Compare identifiers with information on patient's medication administration record (MAR) or medical record.	Ensures correct patient. Complies with The Joint Commission standards and improves patient safety (TJC, 2019).

Safe Patient Care *Remain aware of the similarities and differences of CVADs (Table 28.6). Characteristics of the devices and the type of patient education affect care and maintenance of each. These devices are composed of silicone or polyurethane and can be coated with antibiotics, silver, minocycline/rifampin, or chlorhexidine (Gorski, 2018).*

STEP	RATIONALE
2. Catheter insertion: nontunneled device	Ultrasound-guided venous access is recommended when internal jugular vein is going to be used and equipment and clinical expertise are available. Ultrasound is also used to place PICCs using brachial or basilic vein in children and adults (Heffner et al., 2017; Sabado et al., 2018).
a. Physician, with help from nurse, positions patient in Trendelenburg's or supine position for placement in vessels above heart, unless contraindicated.	Opens angle between clavicle and first rib; dilates veins to facilitate eventual catheter insertion.

TABLE 28.6
Types of Central Vascular Access Devices

Short-Term Devices	Long-Term Devices
Nontunneled Percutaneous • Length of dwell: Days to several weeks • Insertion sites: Subclavian, external/internal jugular and femoral vein • Insertion technique: Not surgically placed, done at bedside using sterile technique, direct puncture into intended vein without passing through subcutaneous tissue • Held in place: With sutures or manufactured securement device	**External Tunneled (Hickman, Broviac)** • Length of dwell: Considered permanent • Insertion sites: Chest region through the subclavian or jugular vein • Insertion technique: Surgery required, tunneling of the proximal end subcutaneously from the insertion site and bringing it out through the skin at an exit site (Fig. 28.4) • Held in place: By Dacron cuff coated in antimicrobial solution. Scar tissue forms around cuff in about 2–3 weeks, fixing the catheter in place
PICCs (Fig. 28.3) • Length of dwell: Months or up to 1 year as long as there is no evidence of IV-related complications (see manufacturer's recommendations) • Insertion sites: Antecubital fossa or upper arm (basilic or cephalic vein) and advanced until catheter tip reaches SVC • Insertion technique: Not surgically placed, done at bedside using sterile technique, in home setting or in radiology setting • Held in place: With sutures or manufactured securement device	**Implanted Venous Ports** • Length of dwell: Considered permanent • Insertion sites: Chest, abdomen, or inner aspect of forearm • Insertion techniques: Requires surgery, catheter is placed via subclavian or jugular vein and attached to a reservoir located within a subcutaneous pocket (Fig. 28.5) • Held in place: Within reservoir pocket and accessed using a 90-degree angle noncoring needle (Fig. 28.6)

IV, Intravenous; *PICCs,* peripherally inserted central catheters; *SVC,* superior vena cava.

STEP	RATIONALE
Safe Patient Care *Trendelenburg's position is contraindicated in patients with head injuries, increased intracranial pressure, certain respiratory conditions, and spinal cord injuries.*	
(1) Nurse places rolled towel or bath blanket between patient's shoulder blades, rotating them slightly to 10-degree angle. Turn patient's head away from intended insertion site.	Head down, below heart, promotes maximum filling and distention with increase in diameter of subclavicular vein (Gorski, 2018); 10-degree tilt effectively achieves increase in diameter of vein.
b. Perform hand hygiene using antiseptic soap for 60 seconds.	Handwashing technique removes transient and resident bacteria from skin.
c. If necessary, use scissors or electric clippers to remove any hair around insertion site. Explain rationale to patient.	Transient microorganisms reside in body hair. Shaving can cause increased risk for infection (INS, 2016a).
d. Physician and nurse apply cap, mask, eyewear, surgical gown, and powder-free sterile gloves.	Maximum barrier precautions needed when inserting central vascular catheter (INS, 2016a).

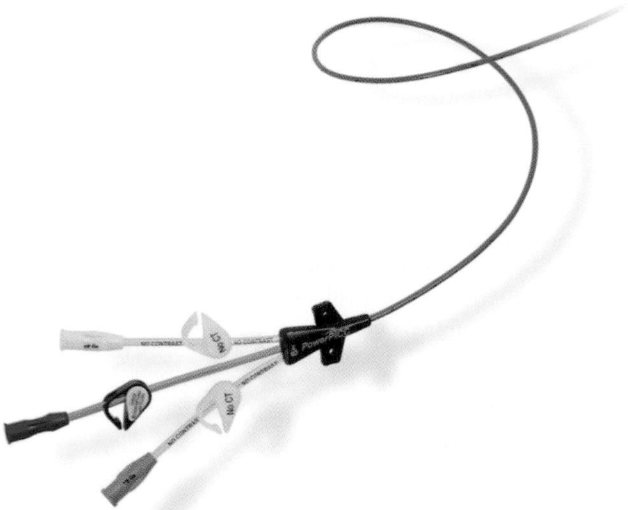

FIG 28.3 Peripherally inserted central catheter (PICC) line.

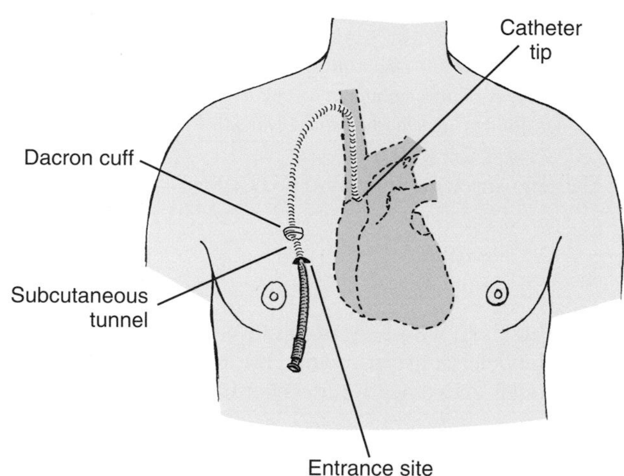

FIG 28.4 Tunneled catheter in place threaded to superior vena cava (SVC).

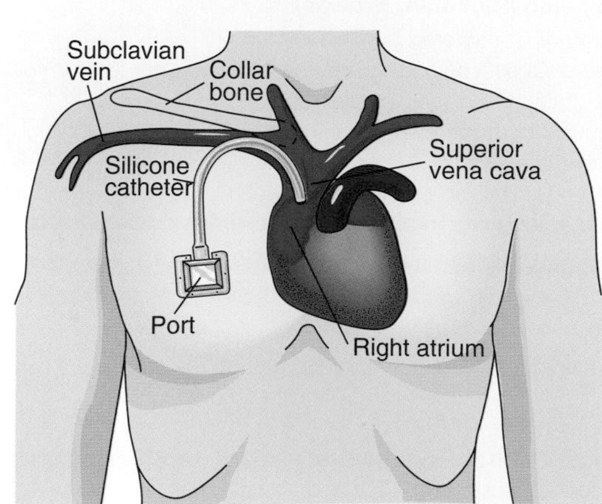

FIG 28.5 Implanted port and catheter.

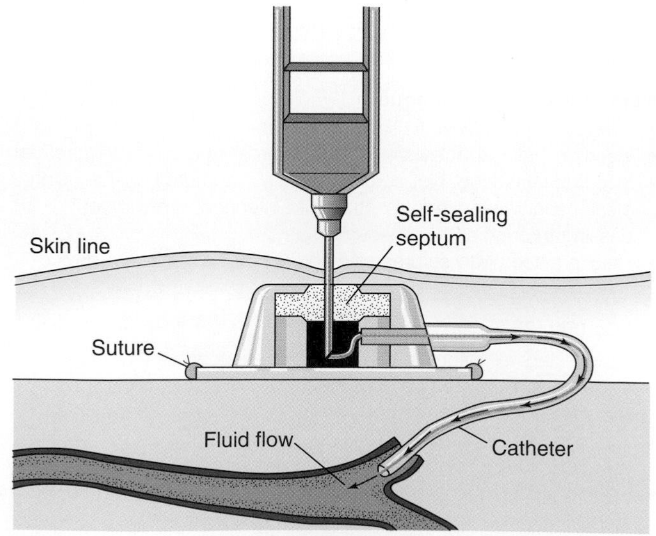

FIG 28.6 Cross section of implanted port accessed with noncoring needle.

STEP	RATIONALE
e. Physician opens central vascular access kit. May have nurse add needed sterile equipment to kit for use during insertion (see Chapter 5).	Maintains sterile field.
f. Prepare site.	Reduces incidence of catheter-related infections (Alexander et al., 2014; CDC, 2011).
(1) Perform skin antisepsis with antiseptic swab using friction in back-and-forth motion for 30 seconds and allow to dry completely.	Allow any skin antiseptic agent to fully dry for complete antisepsis (INS, 2016a).
g. After cleaning site, physician and nurse remove gloves. Physician changes into second pair of sterile gloves, and nurse performs hand hygiene. (Check agency policy because some agencies require strict precautions.)	Gloves become contaminated from surface bacteria picked up in solution. Nurse functions as nonsterile circulator whose primary role is to ensure sterility of insertion field.
h. Physician uses large sterile drape and sterile towels to create sterile field. Physician finds anatomical landmarks and places sterile fenestrated drape appropriately over proposed insertion site.	Provides sterile work space for catheter insertion (INS, 2016a).
i. Physician arranges equipment in kit in preparation for catheter insertion.	Ensures smooth, orderly procedure.
j. Nurse sets up IV bag, primes and fills tubing, and covers end of tubing with sterile cap (see Skill 28.1).	IV tubing is ready to be connected to IV catheter.
k. Nurse scrubs top of 1% lidocaine bottle with antiseptic swab, allowing to dry completely, and holds bottle upside down if not in insertion kit. *Option:* Topical local anesthetic agents can be applied before insertion with health care provider's order.	Removes surface bacteria; allows physician to withdraw lidocaine while maintaining asepsis. Lidocaine has potential for creating allergic reaction and tissue damage.
l. Physician injects needle into bottle and withdraws approximately 3 to 4 mL lidocaine. He or she injects needle into site for internal jugular puncture and anesthetizes venipuncture site, waiting 1 to 2 minutes for effect to take place.	Minimizes discomfort patient feels during venipuncture. Site has been documented to be safer for bedside insertion and ability to use ultrasound-guided insertion (Heffner et al., 2017; Sabado et al., 2018).

Safe Patient Care *Just before time of catheter insertion, ask patient to hold breath and strain. This is a Valsalva maneuver, which increases central venous pressure to prevent entry of air into the catheter. The Valsalva maneuver is the preferred method, although breath holding or humming may be a necessary option in uncooperative patients. In addition, if patient is unable to perform maneuvers, compress patient's abdomen gently.*

STEP	RATIONALE
m. Physician inserts IV catheter into internal jugular vein via ultrasound-guided access or using knowledge of vein anatomy. Usually this is done by locating vein with large-bore cannula, removing needle from cannula, threading wire into cannula and vein, removing cannula over wire, and threading central vein catheter over wire to appropriate location (Seldinger technique; Alexander et al., 2014; Heffner et al., 2017).	Large vein is selected because it will be less irritated by hypertonic solutions or medications.
n. Physician determines patency of line by withdrawing blood with 5-mL syringe, flushing with 0.9% sodium chloride, and placing needleless connectors on hub of each lumen. *Option:* VAD may be flushed with heparin based on type of catheter and agency policy and procedure.	Determines patency of device. Use of heparin, flush volume, and concentration vary by agency and type of catheter.

Safe Patient Care *Catheter tip configuration can be either open-ended or valve-ended. Open-ended devices (e.g., Hickman, Broviac) have a catheter tip that is open like a "straw." Valve-ended catheters (e.g., Groshong) have a rounded catheter tip with a three-way pressure-activated valve that prevents reflux of blood into the catheter to reduce the risk of hemorrhage, air embolism, and occlusion. This technology can also be located in the catheter hub (e.g., PASV, SOLO2). Manufacturers of valved catheters state that heparin is not needed to maintain patency and recommend flushing with only 0.9% sodium chloride (normal saline [NS]; Gorski, 2018).*

STEP	RATIONALE
o. Physician applies catheter securement device (e.g., engineered stabilization device, sutures, sterile tape, or surgical Steri-Strips) to secure central vascular catheter in place. Cover with TSM dressing.	Suturing catheter to skin at insertion site increases risk for infection. Catheter securement devices are noninvasive and preferred for preventing catheter dislodgement (INS, 2016a).
p. Physician removes sterile drapes and completes procedure. External catheter length is measured.	Measurement allows for comparison if dislodgement of CVAD is suspected (INS, 2016a).

Safe Patient Care *A central vascular access device (CVAD) differs from short-peripheral or midline catheters in that the farthest tip of the catheter ends in a larger blood vessel. The tip of a CVAD placed in the upper body should be in the lower segment of the superior or inferior vena cava at or near the cavoatrial junction (see Fig. 28.2). Those placed in the lower body should end in the inferior vena cava above the level of the diaphragm (INS, 2016a). CVADs placed in the femoral region are not recommended in adults (Ciocson et al., 2014).*

STEP	RATIONALE
q. Nurse initiates and regulates IV infusion to prescribed rate and connects to electronic infusion device after receiving a chest x-ray confirmation of appropriate tip placement. Although chest x-ray is still the gold standard for determining tip placement, it is required if other technology such as fluoroscopy or transesophageal echocardiography is not used during the procedure (INS, 2016a).	Maintains patency of VAD. Confirmation of tip placement prevents complications.
3. Insertion site care and dressing change:	
a. Position patient in comfortable position with head slightly elevated. Have arm extended for PICC or midline device.	Provides access to patient.
b. Prepare dressing materials. *TSM dressing:* change at least every 5 to 7 days *Gauze dressing:* change at least every 2 days *Gauze under TSM:* change at least every 2 days	TSM dressings have advantage of allowing visualization of IV site. Gauze dressings and TSM dressings are associated with a lower rate of catheter tip infection (Band and Gaynes, 2017; INS, 2016a).
c. Perform hand hygiene and apply mask. Instruct patient to turn head away from site during dressing change or provide mask for patient.	Reduces transfer of microorganisms; prevents spread of airborne microorganisms over CVAD insertion site.
d. Apply clean gloves. Remove old TSM dressing by stabilizing catheter with nondominant hand. Remove dressing by pulling up one corner and gently pulling straight out and parallel to skin. Repeat on all sides until dressing has been removed.	Prevents unintentional catheter removal.
e. Remove catheter stabilization device if used and requires changing. Must use alcohol to remove adhesive stabilization devices.	Allows visualization of insertion site and allows for appropriate skin antisepsis (INS, 2016a). Use of alcohol minimizes risk for medical adhesive–related skin injury (MARSI; INS, 2016a).

Safe Patient Care *If sutures are used for initial catheter stabilization and become loosened or are no longer intact, alternative stabilization measures should be used. Use of an engineered stabilization device is recommended because sutures are associated with increased risk of infection (Alexander et al., 2014; INS, 2016a).*

STEP	RATIONALE
f. Inspect catheter, insertion site, and surrounding skin. Measure external CVAD length and compare with measurement from insertion if dislodgement is suspected. For PICC and midlines, measure upper-arm circumference 10 cm above antecubital fossa if clinically indicated and compare with baseline.	Insertion sites require regular inspection for early detection of signs and symptoms of IV-related complications (INS, 2016a). Measurement of external catheter length provides comparison to determine dislodgement; arm measurement with a 3-cm increase can indicate thrombosis (INS, 2016a).
g. Remove and discard clean gloves; perform hand hygiene. Open CVAD dressing kit using sterile technique and *apply sterile gloves* (see Chapter 5). Area to be cleaned should be same size as dressing.	Sterile technique is required to apply new dressing.
h. Clean site:	Reduces incidence of catheter-related infections (Alexander, et al., 2014; Gorksi, 2018).
(1) Perform skin antisepsis with antiseptic swab using friction in back-and-forth motion for 30 seconds and allow to dry completely.	Allow any skin antiseptic agent to dry fully for complete antisepsis (INS, 2016a).

STEP	RATIONALE
(2) Povidone-iodine and alcohol may be used in some settings or if patient is sensitive to CHG (see agency policy). If using alcohol or povidone-iodine, clean in concentric circle, moving from insertion site outward with swab. Allow to dry completely.	
i. Apply polymer-based skin protectant to area and allow to dry completely so that skin is not tacky. Skin protectant must be used if adhesive stabilization device will be used.	Protects irritated or fragile skin from dressing and stabilization device, if used, and minimizes risk for MARSI.
j. *Option:* Use CHG-impregnated dressing for short-term CVADs.	CHG-impregnated dressings reduce risk of infection (INS, 2016a; Mimoz, 2015). Use with caution in premature neonates and patients with fragile skin and/or complicated skin pathologies (INS, 2016a).
k. Apply sterile TSM dressing or gauze dressing over insertion site (see Skill 28.1, Step 19a).	Protects catheter insertion site and minimizes risk for infection (Gorski, 2018). Allows for clear visualization of catheter site between dressing changes (INS, 2016b).
l. Apply new catheter stabilization device according to manufacturer directions for use if catheter is not sutured in place (see Skill 28.1, Step 20).	Use of engineered stabilization devices that allow visual inspection of insertion site can reduce risk for VAD complications (e.g., phlebitis, infection, migration) and unintentional loss of access (INS, 2016a).
m. Apply label to dressing with date, time, and your initials.	Provides information about next dressing change.
n. Dispose of soiled supplies and used equipment. Remove gloves and perform hand hygiene.	Reduces transmission of microorganisms.
4. Blood sampling:	
a. Apply clean gloves.	Reduces transmission of microorganisms. Prevents transfer of body fluids.
b. Turn off all infusions for at least 1 to 5 minutes before drawing blood and clamp the catheter if there is a clamp. **NOTE:** If you cannot stop infusion, draw blood from peripheral vein.	Prevents dilution of sample. Prevents interruption of critical IV therapy.
c. When drawing through staggered multilumen catheters, draw from distal lumen (or one recommended by manufacturer).	Distal lumen typically is largest-gauge lumen (Gorski, 2018).
d. Syringe method: **NOTE:** Check agency policy for use of vacuum tube method with CVADs.	
(1) Remove distal end of IV tubing from needleless connector or catheter hub. Cover end of IV tubing with sterile cap to keep end of tubing sterile.	Maintains sterility of end of IV tubing. Drawing from needleless connector minimizes risk of blood exposure.
(2) Scrub needleless connector or catheter hub with antiseptic swab for at least 15 seconds and allow to dry completely.	Reduces risk of infection.
(3) Attach empty 5-mL syringe, unclamp catheter (if necessary), and withdraw 4 to 5 mL of blood for discard sample.	Discard sample reduces risk of drug concentrations or diluted specimen (Gorksi, 2018). Drawing specimens for international normalized ratio (INR) studies from heparinized lines is not recommended (INS, 2016b).
(4) Clamp catheter (if necessary); remove syringe with blood and discard in appropriate biohazard container.	Valved catheters do not require clamping because clamp opens valve and allows reflux of blood into catheter.
(5) Scrub needleless connector or catheter hub with a new antiseptic swab for 15 seconds and allow to dry completely.	
(6) Attach empty 10-mL syringe(s) to obtain required volume of blood needed for specimen ordered.	Multiple syringes may be required, depending on specimens required and number of blood tubes needed.
(7) Unclamp catheter (if necessary) and gently aspirate to withdraw blood.	
(8) Once specimens are obtained, clamp catheter (if necessary) and remove syringe.	

STEP	RATIONALE
(9) Scrub catheter hub with antiseptic swab for 15 seconds and allow to dry completely.	
(10) Attach 10-mL syringe prefilled with preservative-free 0.9% sodium chloride (NS) and flush catheter using the appropriate flush/clamp/disconnect sequence based on the type of needleless connector (e.g., neutral, negative or positive pressure displacement). Ensure that clamp is engaged (if available).	Flush with minimum volume of twice the internal volume of catheter with 0.9% sodium chloride (NS; INS, 2016a). Refer to agency policy and procedure for flush volume requirements.
(11) Remove syringe and discard into appropriate biohazard container. Ensure that clamp is engaged (if available).	Reduces transmission of microorganisms. Reduces risk for catheter clotting after procedure.
e. Transfer blood using transfer vacuum device (see illustration).	Reduces risk of blood exposure.

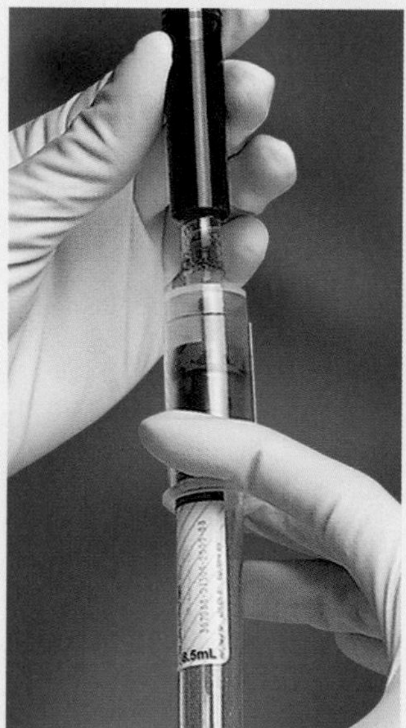

STEP 4e Blood specimen transfer device. *(Courtesy ©Becton Dickinson & Co.)*

STEP	RATIONALE
f. Flush catheter with heparin flush based on type of catheter and agency policy and procedure using appropriate flush/clamp/disconnect sequence. Ensure that clamp is engaged (if available).	Prevents clot formation. Heparin flush volume and concentration vary by agency and type of catheter. Valved catheters are flushed with 0.9% sodium chloride (NS) only and do not require heparin.

Safe Patient Care *Always use a 10-mL syringe or syringe designed to generate lower injection pressure (i.e., 10 mL–diameter syringe barrel) on central lines in adults to minimize pressure during injection (INS, 2016a).*

STEP	RATIONALE
g. Remove syringe. Scrub exposed hub with antiseptic swab for 15 seconds and allow to dry. Attach new needleless connector or IV tubing to hub of catheter. Resume infusion as ordered or clamp catheter (if necessary).	Decreases risk of contamination.
h. Dispose of soiled equipment and used supplies. Remove gloves and perform hand hygiene.	Reduces transmission of microorganisms.
5. Changing injection cap:	
a. Determine if injection caps should be changed.	Injection caps should be changed no more frequently than 9-hour intervals, with primary administration set changed for continuous infusions if it is removed for any reason, if there is residual blood or debris in it, if it becomes contaminated, or according to agency policies and procedures (INS, 2016a).

STEP	RATIONALE
b. Prepare new injection cap(s):	Understanding of types of injection caps ensures appropriate flush/clamp/disconnect sequence based on type of device (e.g., positive, negative, or neutral displacement valves; INS, 2016a).
(1) Perform hand hygiene. Apply clean gloves. Remove cap from package. Do not contaminate sterile injection port.	Reduces transfer of microorganisms. Maintains sterility.
(2) Keep protective cover on tip of injection cap.	Maintains sterility.
(3) Prime injection cap by 10-mL syringe prefilled with preservative-free 0.9% sodium chloride (NS) through cap until fluid is seen in protective cover. Keep syringe attached.	Removes air from system, preventing it from being introduced into vein (Alexander et al., 2014).
c. Based on catheter type, clamp catheter lumens one at a time by using slide or squeeze clamp, if necessary. If catheter is not clamped, ask patient to perform Valsalva maneuver as new cap is applied.	Prevents air from entering system when opened. Valsalva maneuver prevents air embolus (Gorski, 2018).
d. Scrub catheter hub and injection cap with antiseptic swab for 15 seconds and allow to dry completely. Remove and dispose of old injection cap using aseptic technique.	Reduces transmission of microorganisms.
e. Scrub exposed catheter hub with antiseptic swab for 15 seconds and allow to dry completely. Connect new injection cap(s) on catheter hub.	Drying allows time for maximum antimicrobial activity of agents.
f. Flush catheter with 10-mL 0.9% sodium chloride (NS), followed by heparin flush based on type of catheter and agency policy and procedure using appropriate sequence to clamp/flush/disconnect based on type of needleless connector (e.g., neutral, negative, or positive pressure displacement). Ensure that clamp is engaged (if available).	Prevents clot formation. Heparin flush volume and concentration vary by agency and type of catheter. Valved catheters are flushed with 0.9% sodium chloride (NS) only and do not require heparin. Engaging clamp minimizes risk if injection cap loosens or comes off, which can cause infection, air embolism, and bleeding.
g. Dispose of all soiled supplies and used equipment. Remove gloves and perform hand hygiene.	Reduces transmission of microorganisms.

Safe Patient Care *An implanted venous port (see Fig. 28.5) is a CVAD that has a reservoir placed in a pocket under the skin with the catheter inserted into a major vessel (e.g., subclavian). The CVAD has no external lumen or hub. Instead, you access an implanted venous port by inserting a special 90-degree-angle noncoring needle through the skin into the self-sealing injection port in the septum of the reservoir (see Fig. 28.6 and Table 28.7). A port may not be used for extended periods (i.e., weeks) between infusions, and it is not necessary that the port remain accessed during those periods. To maintain patency of a port, it is necessary to flush monthly with heparin solution or 0.9% sodium chloride in accordance with agency policies and procedures and manufacturer's directions for use (INS, 2016a).*

STEP	RATIONALE
6. Discontinuing nontunneled catheters:	
a. Verify health care provider's order to discontinue line. Check agency policy because most require health care providers to discontinue CVAD. In some settings advanced practice nurses or specially credentialed nurses can remove devices.	Verifies appropriateness of procedure. Only specially trained health care professional can remove CVAD.
b. If IV solutions or medications are to continue, arrange placement of a short-peripheral or midline catheter before CVAD discontinuation. **NOTE:** Be aware of pH and osmolarity of solution or medication for appropriateness of conversion to short-peripheral or midline catheter.	Prevents interruption of IV therapy.
c. Position patient in supine flat or 10-degree Trendelenburg's position unless contraindicated.	Position promotes venous filling and prevents air embolus during catheter removal.
d. Perform hand hygiene.	Prevents transmission of microorganisms.
e. Turn off IV solutions infusing through central line and convert to alternate VAD.	Prevents fluid loss during CVAD removal.
f. Place moisture-proof pad under site.	Minimizes soiling of bed linen. Provides clean environment.
g. Apply gown, clean gloves, mask, and goggles.	Prevents transmission of microorganisms and exposure to bloodborne pathogens.

STEP	RATIONALE
h. Gently remove CVAD dressing by stabilizing catheter with nondominant hand, pulling up one corner and gently pulling straight out and parallel to skin. Repeat on all sides until dressing has been removed.	Prevents skin tears. Allows inspection of CVAD insertion site before removal.
i. If catheter securement device is present, carefully remove catheter from device and remove device with alcohol.	Alcohol aids in removal of securement device without causing skin tear.
j. Remove gloves and perform hand hygiene; open CVAD dressing change kit and suture removal kit (if CVAD is sutured in place). Add items to sterile field. Apply sterile gloves.	Prevents transfer of organisms on soiled dressing to catheter insertion site.
k. Perform skin antisepsis of insertion site with antiseptic swab or sponge using friction in back-and-forth motion for 30 seconds and allow to dry completely. *Option:* If CVAD is sutured in place, remove sutures.	Reduces risk of migration of microbes into catheter tract. Allows CVAD removal.

Safe Patient Care *All CVADs require measurements of total length and external catheter on insertion. PICC lines also require measurement of upper-arm circumference.*

STEP	RATIONALE
l. Using nondominant hand, apply sterile 4 × 4–inch gauze to site. Instruct patient to take deep breath and perform Valsalva maneuver as catheter is withdrawn.	Valsalva maneuver reduces risk for air embolus by decreasing negative pressure in respiratory system.
m. With dominant hand, slowly remove catheter in smooth, continuous motion an inch at a time. Keeping fingers near insertion site, immediately apply pressure to site and continue until bleeding stops. Stop removal procedure if resistance is met while removing catheter (INS, 2016b).	Gentle removal of catheter prevents stretching and breaking it. Damaged catheter may break off and leave piece in patient's arm. Direct pressure reduces risk for bleeding and hematoma formation.

Safe Patient Care *It is often necessary to apply pressure longer if patient is receiving anticoagulation therapy or has prolonged clotting times.*

STEP	RATIONALE
n. Apply petroleum-based ointment or gauze to exit site. Apply sterile occlusive dressing such as TSM dressing or sterile gauze to site. Change dressing every 24 hours until healed.	Reduces chance of air embolism and seals skin-to-vein tract (Alexander et al., 2014). Allows for inspection of site for bleeding and infection until it is healed.
o. Label dressing with date, time, and your initials.	Identifies date of catheter removal and need for dressing change.
p. Inspect catheter integrity for intactness, especially along tip, and that length is appropriate for device. Discard in appropriate biohazard container. **NOTE:** Catheter cultures should be performed when catheter is removed for suspected catheter-related bloodstream infection (CRBSI). Catheter cultures should not be obtained routinely (INS, 2016a).	If catheter tip is broken or compromised, place in container and label for possible follow-up and notify health care provider.
q. Position patient in a supine position for 30 minutes after nontunneled CVAD removal (INS, 2016a). Be sure that short-peripheral IV line or midline is infusing at correct rate.	Reduces chance of air embolism. Maintains prescribed IV solution therapy.
7. Dispose of any used supplies and personal protective equipment. Discard sharps in sharps container. Remove gloves and perform hand hygiene.	Reduces transmission of microorganisms (INS, 2016a).
8. Assist patient to a comfortable position and instruct how to move and turn properly with VAD.	Prevents accidental dislodgement of CVAD.
9. Raise bed rails (as appropriate) and lower bed to lowest position.	Minimizes risk for falls and injury.
10. Be sure nurse call system is in an accessible location within patient's reach. Instruct patient in its use.	Ensures patient can call for assistance if needed.

STEP	RATIONALE

EVALUATION

STEP	RATIONALE
1. Consult x-ray film (or echocardiography, fluoroscopy) examination reports for catheter placement.	A routine chest x-ray film examination is still the gold standard to confirm position of catheter tip and presence of pneumothorax. However, other technologies are proving reliable.
2. Determine daily, in consultation with health care provider, the continued need for the CVAD.	Daily review of line necessity with prompt removal of unnecessary lines is practice recommended in the IHI central line–associated bloodstream infection (CLABSI) bundle (Band and Gaynes, 2017; IHI, 2012).
3. Evaluate for postinsertion complications to include:	Complications after insertion can include pneumothorax, cardiac arrhythmias, and nerve injury (Gorski, 2018). Prompt identification can allow for treatment, repositioning of catheter, or removal if necessary.
a. Auscultate breath sounds and evaluate for shortness of breath, chest pain, absent breath sounds.	Signs and symptoms of pneumothorax develop if CVAD pierces intrathoracic space.
b. Monitor vital signs, including heart rate and rhythm.	Evaluates for signs of cardiac arrhythmias.
c. Monitor patient complaints of pain, numbness, tingling, or weakness.	Signs of nerve injury from catheter insertion.
4. Evaluate patient to determine response to infusion therapy (e.g., laboratory values, input and output [I&O], weights, vital signs, postprocedure assessments).	IV solutions and additives maintain or restore fluid and electrolyte balance. Early recognition of complications leads to prompt treatment.
5. Evaluate patient at established intervals for signs and symptoms of CVAD-related complications (Table 28.7) according to agency policy and procedure.	Prevents complications that compromise integrity of CVAD or cause inaccurate IV solution flow rate and allows for prompt intervention.
6. Observe all connection points, being sure that they are secure as directed by agency policy and procedure.	An intact system prevents accidental blood loss or entrance of air or microbes into the vasculature.
7. **Use Teach-Back:** "I want to be sure that I explained the purpose and care of your intravenous catheter. This catheter is placed in a large vein in your body, and the problems we talked about can occur. Tell me in your own words the problems that might develop with your catheter and the signs and symptoms you would report to me or another nurse." Revise your instruction now or develop a plan for revised patient/family caregiver teaching if patient/family caregiver is not able to teach back correctly.	Determines patient's/family caregiver's level of understanding of instructional topic.

Unexpected Outcomes	Related Interventions
1. For catheter complications, see Table 28.7.	• See Table 28.7.
2. Patient or family caregiver is unable to explain or perform CVAD care.	• Indicates need for home care referral or additional instruction.

Recording

- Record type of CVAD, number of lumens, location and appearance of site, condition and type of dressing, procedure performed, and any signs and symptoms of complications.
- Document your evaluation of patient learning.

Hand-Off Reporting

- Report unexpected outcomes (e.g., signs and symptoms of complications), interventions, and patient's response to treatment to health care provider.

TABLE 28.7

Complications of Venous Access Devices

Complication	Assessment	Prevention	Intervention
Catheter damage, breakage, fracture	Every shift observes for pinholes, leaks, tears. Assess for drainage from site after flushing.	Follow proper clamping procedure. Avoid sharp objects near catheter. Use needleless system device. A 10-mL syringe is preferred for flushing CVADs to avoid excessive pressure and potential catheter damage. Never flush against resistance.	Clamp catheter near insertion site and place sterile gauze over break or hole until repaired. Use only repair kit that is recommended by manufacturer. Remove catheter with order.
Occlusion: thrombus, fibrin sheath, fibrin tail, precipitation, malposition	Assess insertion site and sutures. Assess for blood return. Assess for ability to infuse fluid. Assess equipment. If port is in place, reassess and verify noncoring needle placement. Assess with syringe directly on catheter. Assess for discomfort or pain in shoulder, neck, ear, or arm at insertion site. Assess for neck or shoulder edema.	Follow routine flushing with positive pressure and/or use positive-pressure valve injection cap. Secure with catheter stabilization device to prevent tension on CVAD. A 10-mL syringe is preferred for flushing CVADs to avoid excessive pressure and potential catheter damage. Do not flush against resistance. Flush between medications. Flush vigorously after viscous solutions. Avoid mixing incompatible drugs. Avoid kinking catheter.	Reposition patient. Have patient cough and deep breathe. Raise patient's arm overhead. Obtain venogram if ordered. Administer thrombolytics if ordered. Remove catheter (CVAD requires order). Obtain x-ray film as ordered. Do not use a 1-mL syringe to instill saline because pressure exceeds 200 psi.
Infection and sepsis: catheter skin junction, tunnel, thrombus, port pocket, CLABSI	Assess catheter skin junction for redness, drainage, edema, or tenderness. Assess for signs of systemic infection. Monitor laboratory findings.	Use aseptic technique. Prevent contamination of catheter hub. Adhere to dressing change technique. Apply TSM dressing over catheter skin junction.	Obtain blood cultures from peripheral and CVAD if ordered. Remove catheter (CVAD requires order). Replace catheter.
Dislodgement	Assess length of catheter daily. Inform patient of possible catheter dislodgement. Identify edema at catheter skin junction or drainage. Palpate catheter skin junction and tunnel for coiling (catheter can feel cordlike underneath the skin). Assess for distended neck veins.	Loop and tape catheter securely. Use catheter stabilization device and TSM dressing. Avoid pulling on CVAD. Avoid manipulating catheter by hand.	Insert new catheter. Secure with catheter stabilization device. Teach patient not to manipulate catheter.
Catheter migration (e.g., length of catheter moved from original position), pinch-off syndrome (e.g., compression of catheter between clavicle and first rib), port separation or catheter fracture (e.g., internal fracture or separation of catheter)	Assess for patient complaints of gurgling sounds. Assess for change in patency of catheter by evaluating change in flow rate, local irritation, swelling, occlusion, tenderness, pain, inability to aspirate fluid and/or blood. Pain at site when flushed or symptoms of embolus. Obtain x-ray film examination. Assess edema of arm and hand on side of insertion. Assess for distended neck veins. Assess for inability to infuse solutions. Assess length of catheter daily.	Avoid trauma. Avoid placement near site of local infection, scarring, or skin disorder.	Reposition under fluoroscopy as ordered. Remove catheter as ordered. Stop all fluid administration.

TABLE 28.7

Complications of Venous Access Devices—cont'd

Complication	Assessment	Prevention	Intervention
Skin erosion (e.g., mechanical loss of skin tissue), hematomas (e.g., local collection of blood), cuff extrusion (e.g., tissue at edges of insertion site separate), scar tissue formation over port	Assess for loss of viable tissue over septum site. Assess for separation of exit site edges. Assess for drainage at catheter skin junction. Assess for redness. Assess for edema, contusions. Note if tunneled catheter is exposed (Dacron cuff is visible).	Maintain nutritional status. Avoid pressure or trauma. Rotate with each port access. Do not reinsert a noncoring needle in the same "hole" of a previous insertion. This creates a permanent hole in the septum. Do not use standard needle to access port.	Remove CVAD as ordered. Improve nutrition. Provide appropriate skin care.
Infiltration, extravasation	Assess for erythema. Assess for edema. Assess for spongy feeling. Assess for swelling around IV site and at termination of catheter tip. Assess for labored breathing. Assess for aspiration of fluid and/or blood. Assess for complaints of pain with infusion of solutions or medications (e.g., burning). Assess for no free-flow IV drip.	Immediately stop vesicant administration. Administer antidote or therapeutic medications to maintain tissue integrity according to protocol.	Apply cold/warm compresses according to specific vesicant protocol. Provide emotional support. Obtain x-ray film if ordered. Use antidotes per protocol. Discontinue IV solutions.
Pneumothorax, hemothorax, air emboli, hydrothorax	Assess for subcutaneous emphysema by inspecting and palpating skin around insertion site and along arm. Inspection may reveal edema where air is located, and air may travel if skin is loose. Palpation reveals a crackling sensation such as popping plastic bubble wrap. Assess for chest pain. Assess for dyspnea, apnea, hypoxia, tachycardia, hypotension, nausea, confusion.	Use injection cap on distal end when not in use. Do not leave catheter hub open to air. If appropriate for device, be sure that clamps are engaged.	Administer oxygen as ordered. Elevate feet. Aspirate air, fluid. If air emboli suspected, place patient on left side with head down. Remove catheter as ordered. Help with insertion of chest tubes as ordered.
Incorrect placement	Assess for cardiac dysrhythmias. Assess for hypotension. Assess for neck distention. Assess for narrow pulse pressure. Assess for inadequate blood withdrawal. Assess for retrograde flow of blood (flow of blood back into tubing usually caused by decreased pressure gradient between venous system and access device unit [e.g., IV infusion, heparin lock]).	Obtain x-ray film examination after placement. Reposition catheter as warranted.	Stop all fluid administration until placement is confirmed. Discontinue catheter (requires order). Obtain x-ray film and electrocardiogram (for PICC and CVAD). Administer support medications as ordered.

CLABSI, Central line–associated bloodstream infection; *CVAD*, central vascular access device; *CVC*, central venous catheter; *IV*, intravenous; *PICC*, peripherally inserted central catheter.

✦ SKILL 28.5 Transfusion of Blood Products

Purpose

Transfusion therapy or blood replacement is the intravenous (IV) administration of whole blood, its components (e.g., packed red blood cells, cryoprecipitate, platelets), or a plasma-derived product for therapeutic purposes (Gorksi, 2018). Transfusion therapy restores intravascular volume with whole blood or albumin; restores the oxygen-carrying capacity of blood with red blood cells; and provides clotting factors and/or platelets for patients with hematological disorders, cancer, or injury or patients undergoing surgical intervention, and provides treatment for diseases related to coagulation deficiencies (AABB, 2017). The blood product can be allogeneic, blood donated from someone else, or autologous, in which a patient's own blood is collected and reinfused for intravascular volume replacement (AABB, 2017). There are three primary blood-typing systems: ABO, Rh, and human leukocyte antigen (HLA; Tables 28.8 and 28.9). These systems are used during the cross-matching procedures. A competent nurse must know not only the complexities of the ABO and Rh systems but also the numerous components of blood that can be transfused and the serious negative outcomes that can occur. The nurse should never view the transfusion of blood products as routine; overlooking a minor detail is dangerous and can be life threatening to a patient (AABB, 2017; Gorski, 2018).

Delegation and Collaboration

The skill of initiating transfusion therapy cannot be delegated to nursing assistive personnel (NAP). The skill of initiating

TABLE 28.8
Blood Typing Systems

Blood Typing System	Description	Administration Considerations
ABO	The ABO system uses the presence or absence of specific antigens on the surface of red blood cells to identify blood groups. When the type A antigen is present, the blood group is type A. When the type B antigen is present, the blood group is type B. When both A and B antigens are present, the blood group is type AB, and when neither A nor B antigens are present, the blood group is type O (AABB, 2017; Gorksi, 2018; see Table 28.9).	Antibodies that react against the A and B antigens are naturally present in the plasma of people whose red blood cells do not carry the antigen. These antibodies (agglutinins) react against the foreign antigens (agglutinogens). Incompatible red blood cells agglutinate (clump together) and result in a life-threatening hemolytic transfusion reaction. People with type A blood have anti-B antibodies; people with type B blood have anti-A antibodies. People with type AB blood have neither antibody and can receive all blood types. People with type O blood have both A and B antibodies and can receive only type O blood (AABB, 2017; Gorksi, 2018).
Rh factor	Although nearly 50 types of Rh antigen may be present on the surface of red blood cells, the type D antigen is widely prevalent and is most likely to elicit an immune response. It is the presence or absence of the D antigen that determines a person's Rh factor. A person with the D antigen is Rh positive, and a person without the D antigen is Rh negative (AABB, 2017; Gorksi, 2018).	Unlike the ABO antigens, there are not naturally occurring antibodies to the Rh(D) antigen. A person with Rh-negative blood must first be exposed to Rh-positive blood before any Rh antibodies are formed. A person with Rh-negative blood who is exposed to a large volume (200 mL or more) of Rh-positive blood will develop enough antibodies to cause a severe transfusion reaction with repeat exposure. These antibodies take up to 2 weeks to form (AABB, 2017).
Human leukocyte antigen	The human leukocyte antigen system (HLA) system is a complex set of genes that plays a role in the self-recognition of the immune system and the response to antigenic stimuli (AABB, 2017; Gorksi, 2018). The identification of HLA antibodies in donor blood can be used to perform a virtual crossmatch and minimize transfusion reactions for the recipient (AABB, 2017).	HLAs are highly immunogenic antigens that can cause serious transfusion complications. HLA antibodies are located on the cell surface of leukocytes but can be found on all cells of the body (AABB, 2017; Gorski, 2018). HLA complications most commonly seen are: • Febrile nonhemolytic reaction (FNH) • Immune-mediated platelet refractoriness • Transfusion-related acute lung injury (TRALI) • Transfusion-associated graft-versus-host disease (TA-GVHD)

TABLE 28.9
ABO System

Patient's Blood Type	Red Blood Cells Antigen	Transfusion With Type A	Transfusion With Type B	Transfusion With Type AB	Transfusion With Type O	Transfusion Options
A (+)	A	Yes	No	No	Yes	A+, A–, O+, O–
A (–)	A	Yes	No	No	Yes	A–, O–
B (+)	B	No	Yes	No	Yes	B+, B–, O+, O–
B (–)	B	No	Yes	No	Yes	B–, O–
AB (+)	AB	Yes	Yes	Yes	Yes	A+, A–, B+, B–, O+, O–, universal recipient
AB (–)	AB	Yes	Yes	Yes	Yes	A–, B–, O–
O (+)	None	No	No	No	Yes	O+, O–
O (–)	None	No	No	No	Yes	O–, universal donor

From Alexander M et al: *Core curriculum for infusion nursing*, ed 4, Philadelphia, 2014, Lippincott Williams & Wilkins; and Gorski L: *Phillip's manual of IV therapeutics: evidence-based practice for infusion therapy,* ed 7, Philadelphia, 2018, FA Davis.

transfusion therapy by a licensed practical nurse (LPN) varies by state Nurse Practice Act. After the transfusion has been started and the patient is stable, monitoring a patient by NAP does not relieve a registered nurse (RN) of the responsibility to continue to assess the patient during the transfusion. The nurse instructs the NAP about:

- Frequency of vital sign monitoring needed.
- What to observe, such as complaints of shortness of breath, hives, and/or chills and reporting this information to the nurse.
- Obtaining blood components from the blood bank (check agency policy).

Equipment

- Y-type blood administration set with standard filter and macrodrip drop factor (**NOTE:** Depending on blood product, special tubing and filters may be necessary.)
- Prescribed blood product
- IV 250-mL bag 0.9% NaCl (normal saline [NS]) IV solution
- 5- to 10-mL syringe containing NS

- Clean gloves
- Tape
- Antiseptic wipes or swabs (alcoholic chlorhexidine solution preferred, 70% alcohol, or povidone-iodine)
- Vital sign equipment: thermometer, blood pressure cuff, stethoscope, and pulse oximeter
- Signed transfusion consent

Optional Equipment

- Rapid infusion pump
- Electronic infusion device (EID; verify that infusion pump can be used to deliver blood or blood products)
- *Option:* Leukocyte-depleting filter (**NOTE:** Agency may irradiate blood products within its blood bank facility.)
- Blood warmer (used mainly when large-volume or rapid transfusion is needed)
- Pressure bag (used for rapid infusion in acute blood loss)

ASSESSMENT

1. Verify health care provider's order for:
   a. Specific blood or blood product and number of units
   b. Date and time to begin transfusion
   c. Special instructions (i.e., irradiated, leukocyte depleted)
   d. Duration
   e. Pretransfusion medications to administer
   f. Posttransfusion medications to administer
   Rationale: Verifying order helps ensure that appropriate blood component will be administered (AABB, 2017; Alexander et al., 2014; INS, 2016a). Pretransfusion medications prevent and alleviate certain transfusion-related symptoms.

Safe Patient Care *A health care provider's order must be present before transfusing a blood product. If more than one blood product is to be given, the sequence or order of transfusion should be specified. Any additional medications, such as an antihistamine (given when the history shows previous allergic response), antipyretics (given when the history shows previous febrile nonhemolytic response), or diuretics (given when the history shows potential for heart failure), or other special treatment of the components should also be included in a written transfusion order.*

2. Obtain patient's transfusion history and note known allergies and previous transfusion reactions. Verify that type and cross-match have been completed within 72 hours of transfusion. *Rationale: Identifies patient's prior response(s) to transfusion of blood components. If patient has experienced reaction in the past, anticipate similar reaction and be prepared to rapidly intervene.*
3. Assess laboratory values such as hematocrit, coagulation values, platelet count, and potassium. *Rationale: Provides baseline for later evaluation of patient response to transfusion (INS, 2016a). When blood is stored, there is continual destruction of red blood cells, which releases potassium (K) from the cells into the plasma. Often a laboratory test of a patient's K level is ordered before administering a unit of blood.*
4. Check that patient has completed and signed transfusion consent properly before retrieving blood. *Rationale: Informed consent is required before transfusion. The consent form should include risks, benefits, and treatment alternatives; right to accept or refuse transfusion; and opportunity to ask questions (AABB, 2017; INS, 2016a). Administration of albumin does not require informed consent.*

Safe Patient Care *Transfusion of blood and blood products is closely regulated and monitored. Standards of operation for all blood bank centers are set by the AABB, the Occupational Safety and Health Administration (OSHA, 2012), the U.S. Food and Drug Administration (FDA, 2015), and the American Red Cross. These standards include the collection of donor blood, distribution of the product, and standards for transfusion.*

5. Know indications or reasons for transfusion (e.g., packed red blood cells [PRBCs] for patient with low hematocrit level from gastrointestinal bleeding or surgery blood loss). *Rationale: Allows you to anticipate patient's response to therapy.*
6. Obtain and record pretransfusion baseline vital signs (temperature, pulse, respirations, and blood pressure). If patient is febrile (temperature greater than 37.8° C [100° F]), notify health care provider before initiating transfusion. *Rationale: Change from baseline vital signs during infusion alerts nurse to potential transfusion reaction or adverse effect of therapy (Gorski, 2018; INS, 2016b).*
7. Verify that IV cannula is patent and without complications such as infiltration or phlebitis. Assess the venous access device (VAD) catheter–skin junction site and surrounding area for catheter-related complications by visually inspecting and palpating through the intact dressing for redness, tenderness, swelling, and drainage. Assess the patency of the VAD by aspiration of a blood return, absence of resistance when flushing, and complaints of patient pain or discomfort when flushing. If necessary, place a VAD for transfusion purposes (see Skill 28.1). *Rationale: Patent IV ensures that transfusion will be infused within established time guidelines.*
   a. Administer blood or blood components to an adult through a 14- to 24-gauge short-peripheral catheter, with an 18- to 20-gauge catheter appropriate for the general population and a 14- to 18-gauge catheter when rapid infusion is required (Gorski, 2018; INS, 2016a). *Rationale: The gauge of the IV cannula should be appropriate for accommodating the infusion of blood and/or blood components (INS, 2016a). Large-gauge cannulas promote rapid flow of blood components.*
   b. Transfuse a neonate, pediatric, and older adult patient with a 22- to 24-gauge device (INS, 2016a). *Rationale: Use of smaller cannula gauges such as 24 gauge often requires blood bank to divide the unit so that each half can be infused within allotted time or with pressure-assisted devices.*
   c. Appropriate-gauge central vascular access device (CVAD) may also be used. *Rationale: Use of CVAD for administration of blood depends on catheter gauge and manufacturer recommendations for use (Gorski, 2018).*
8. Assess patient's need for IV fluids or medications while transfusion is infusing. *Rationale: If IV medications need to be administered during transfusion, a second IV access is necessary. No other infusions are to be administered through the same IV site as blood transfusion.*
9. Assess patient's and family caregiver's knowledge, experience, and health literacy regarding blood transfusion therapy. *Rationale: Ensures patient or family caregiver has the capacity to obtain, communicate, process, and understand basic health information (CDC, 2016).*

Safe Patient Care *Be prepared to inform your patients thoroughly about the options, benefits, and risks of transfusion and reassure them that every effort is taken to ensure a safe blood supply and transfusion. The risk of a blood recipient developing an infectious disease is lower than ever before because of improved testing of donor blood. However rare, viral, bacterial, and parasitic diseases can still be transmitted through blood. Screening of blood donors is an important first step to identify people with a medical history, behavior, or events that put them at risk of transmissible disease (Alexander et al., 2014; Simon et al., 2016) and ensure the safety, purity, and potency of blood and blood components (U.S. Food and Drug Administration [FDA], 2015). Patients should know that there is never a completely risk-free transfusion.*

STEP	RATIONALE
PLANNING	
1. Expected outcomes following completion of the procedure:	
• Patient verbalizes understanding of rationale for therapy.	Indicates patient's understanding and ability to make informed decision for consent.
• Patient experiences improved activity tolerance.	Oxygenation is improved.
• Mucous membranes are pink, and patient has brisk capillary refill.	Tissue perfusion is improved.
• Patient's cardiac output returns to baseline.	Intravascular volume is restored.
• Patient's systolic blood pressure improves, and urine output is 0.5 to 1 mL/kg/hr.	Parameters reflect optimal fluid status and adequate renal blood flow.
• Patient's laboratory values improve in targeted areas (e.g., hematocrit, coagulation values, platelet count).	Indicates that patient responds appropriately to blood or blood component infusion.
2. Provide privacy and prepare environment.	Providing privacy and preparing the environment early help the student/nurse think about the need to remove clutter from the over-bed or bedside table.
3. Perform hand hygiene. Collect equipment and organize on clean, clutter-free bedside stand or over-bed table. Apply clean gloves.	Reduces transmission of infection and contamination of equipment (INS, 2016a).
4. Explain procedure and purpose to patient and family caregiver regarding the need for blood therapy.	Decreases anxiety, promotes cooperation, and gives patient time frame around which to plan personal activities.
IMPLEMENTATION	
1. Preadministration protocol:	
a. Obtain blood component from blood bank following agency protocol (see illustration).	Timely acquisition ensures that product is safe to administer. Agency protocol usually encompasses safeguards to ensure quality control throughout transfusion process.

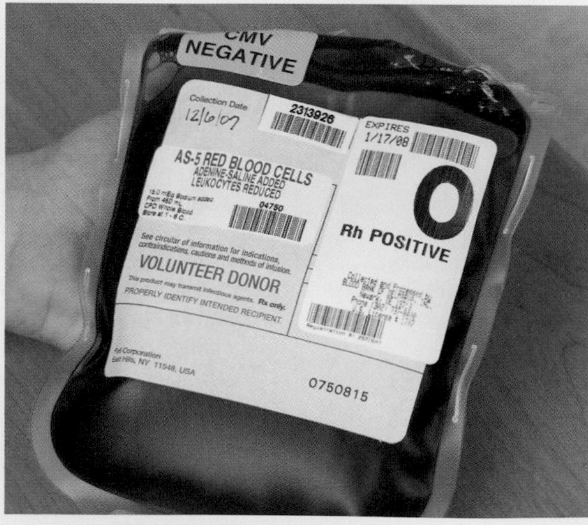

STEP 1a Unit of blood with label.

STEP	RATIONALE
b. Check blood bag for any signs of contamination (i.e., clumping/clots, gas bubbles, purplish color) and presence of leaks.	Blood should not be infused if integrity is compromised. Air bubbles, clumping, clots, and discoloration can be an indication of bacterial contamination or inadequate anticoagulation of stored component and are contraindications for transfusion of that product (Gorski, 2018). Blood serves as medium for bacterial growth.
c. Verbally compare and correctly verify patient, blood product, and type with another person considered qualified by your agency (e.g., registered nurse [RN] or licensed practical nurse [LPN]) before initiating transfusion. Check the following:	Strict adherence to verification procedures before administration of blood or blood components reduces risk for administering wrong blood to patient. Misidentification of patient is one of most important factors in transfusion errors (Gorski, 2018).
(1) Identify patient using at least two identifiers (e.g., name and birthday or name and medical record number) according to agency policy. Compare identifiers with information on patient's medication administration record (MAR) or medical record.	Ensures correct patient. Complies with The Joint Commission standards and improves patient safety (TJC, 2019).
(2) Transfusion record number and patient's identification number match.	Prevents accidental administration of wrong component.

Safe Patient Care *If you notice a discrepancy during verification procedure, do not administer the product. Notify blood bank and appropriate personnel as indicated by agency policy. The product should be returned to the blood bank until the discrepancy is resolved (Gorski, 2018; INS, 2016a).*

STEP	RATIONALE
(3) Patient's name is correct on all documents. Check patient identification number and date of birth on identification band and patient record.	
(4) Check unit number on blood bag with blood bank form to ensure that they are the same. Check expiration date and time.	
(5) Blood type matches on transfusion record and blood bag. Verify that component received from blood bank is same component that health care provider ordered (e.g., packed red cells, platelets; see illustration).	Ensures that patient receives correct therapy. Misidentification and improper labeling result in transfusing wrong ABO group (Gorski, 2018). The ABO system and Rh factor are the primary blood typing systems that ensure a close match between transfused products and a recipient's blood.
(6) Check that patient's blood type and Rh type are compatible with donor blood type and Rh type (e.g., Patient A+: Donor A+ or O+).	Verifies accurate donor blood type and compatibility.
(7) Check expiration date and time on unit of blood.	Never use expired blood because cell components deteriorate and may contain excess citrate ions. There is also a higher rate of infection with expired blood (AABB, 2017; Weinstein and Hagle, 2014).

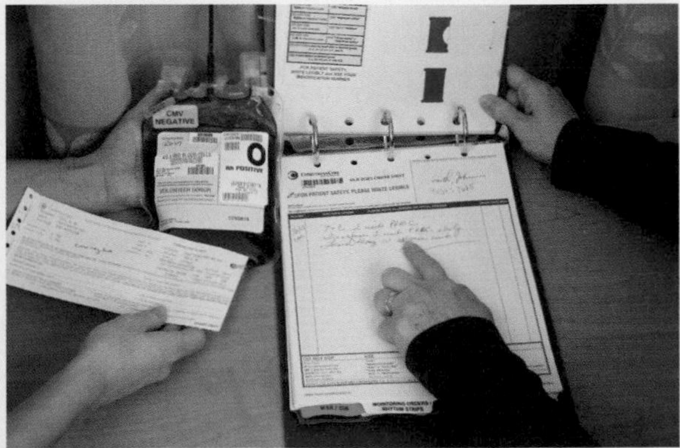

STEP 1c(5) Two clinicians verifying blood type with health care provider order.

STEP	RATIONALE
(8) Just before initiating transfusion, check patient identification information with blood unit label information (see illustration). Do not administer blood to patient without identification bracelet or blood identification bracelet (see agency policy).	Serves as last point of patient and blood confirmation (Gorski, 2018).
(9) Both individuals verify patient and unit identification record process as directed by agency policy.	Documentation is legal medical record.
d. Review purpose of transfusion and ask patient to report any changes that he or she may feel during the transfusion.	Signs and symptoms of transfusion reactions include chills, low back pain, shortness of breath, rash, hives, or itching (Gorksi, 2018; Table 28.10). Prompt notification aids in early intervention.
e. Have patient void or apply clean gloves and empty urine drainage collection container.	If transfusion reaction occurs, urine specimen containing urine produced after initiation of transfusion will be sent to laboratory (Weinstein and Hagle, 2014; see Table 28.10).

Safe Patient Care *Blood transfusion should be initiated within 30 minutes from time of release from blood bank. If this cannot be completed because of factors such as an elevated temperature, immediately return the blood to the blood bank and retrieve it when you can administer it (Weinstein and Hagle, 2014). It is important that the blood bag not be spiked until you ensure that no factors exist preventing transfusion.*

STEP	RATIONALE
2. Administration:	
a. Perform hand hygiene. Apply clean gloves. Reinspect blood product for signs of leakage or unusual appearance.	Using standard precautions reduces risk for transmission of microorganisms. Provides ongoing verification of blood product.
b. Open Y-tubing blood administration set for single unit. Use multiset if multiple units are to be transfused.	Y-tubing facilitates maintenance of IV-line access with NS in case patient will need more than 1 unit of blood.
c. Set all clamp(s) to "off" position.	Setting clamps to "off" position prevents accidentally spilling and wasting product.
d. Use aseptic technique and spike bag of 0.9% sodium chloride (NS) IV bag with one of Y-tubing spikes. Hang bag on IV pole and prime tubing. Open upper clamp on normal saline side of tubing and squeeze drip chamber until fluid covers filter and one-third to one-half of drip chamber (see illustration).	Primes tubing with fluid to eliminate air in Y-tubing. Closing clamp prevents spillage and waste of fluid.

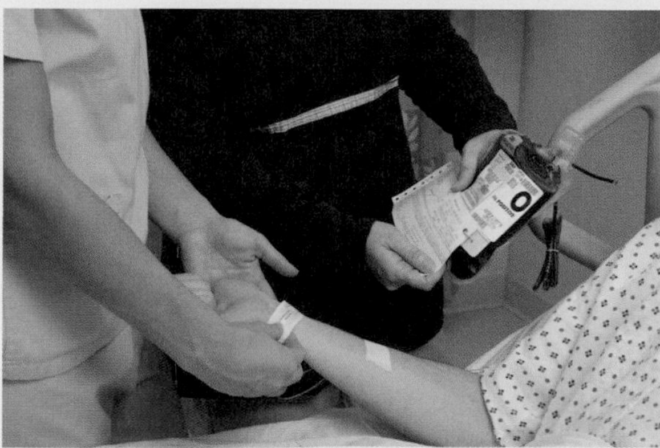

STEP 1c(8) Two clinicians verifying identification of patient and blood product.

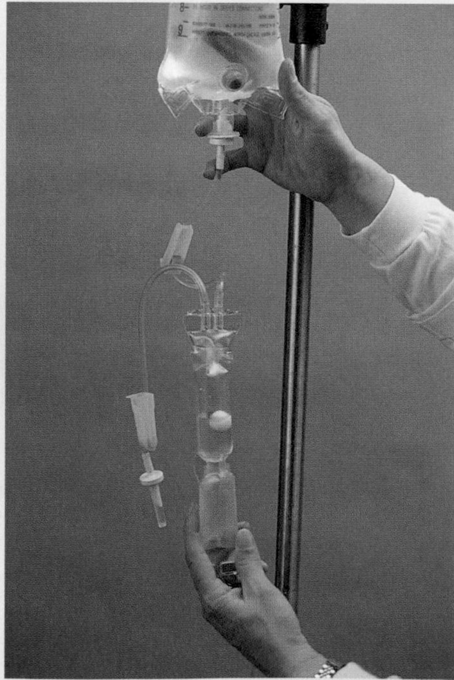

STEP 2d Blood administration set primed with normal saline.

TABLE 28.10

Transfusion Reactions

Reaction	Mechanism	Onset	Signs and Symptoms	Prevention	Nursing Intervention
Febrile, nonhemolytic	Most common type of transfusion reaction. Caused by WBC antigen-antibody reaction	May begin early in transfusion or as long as several hours after completion	Temperature increase of 1° C (2° F) or more above baseline, chills, rigors, general malaise	Premedicate as ordered with antipyretics if prior history of reaction; use leukocyte-reduced blood products	**Stop transfusion.** Change administration set and administer 0.9% sodium chloride at rate to maintain patent IV access. Institute transfusion reaction protocol. Administer antipyretics as ordered to treat fever. Document clinical symptoms, when transfusion was stopped, notification of health care provider and blood bank, nursing interventions and response to interventions, and patient teaching.
Acute hemolytic transfusion reaction	Caused by ABO, Rh incompatibility; donor red cells incompatible with recipient's plasma that can be potentially fatal with as little as 10–15 mL of incompatible blood; usually due to administration of blood with wrong ABO blood group due to misidentification or improper labeling	Within minutes of transfusion initiation	Fever with or without chills, tachycardia, hypotension, lumbar/flank pain, hemoglobinemia, hemoglobinuria, dyspnea, shock, oliguria or anuria, abnormal bleeding	Proper patient identification; proper labeling of blood sample; verification of ABO/Rh compatibility between donor and recipient before administration	**Stop transfusion.** Change administration set and administer 0.9% sodium chloride at rate to maintain patent IV access. Notify health care provider and blood bank. Monitor vital signs at least every 15 min. Administer ordered therapy to correct arterial blood pressure and coagulopathy. Insert Foley catheter. Monitor intake and output hourly. Assess for shock. Dialysis may be required. Obtain blood and urine samples and send to laboratory with unused portion of unit of blood. Document reaction according to agency policy.
Delayed hemolytic transfusion reaction (extravascular)	ABO, Rh incompatibility. Caused by donor plasma incompatible with recipient's red cells usually due to improperly identified blood sample, blood unit, or patient	Several hours after transfusion	Unexplained fever, unexplained decrease in Hgb/Hct, increased bilirubin levels, jaundice	Proper patient identification; proper labeling of blood sample	**Stop transfusion if in progress.** Change administration set and administer 0.9% sodium chloride at rate to maintain patent IV access. Notify health care provider and blood bank immediately. Monitor laboratory values for anemia. (Recognition is important because subsequent transfusions may cause an acute hemolytic reaction.) Most delayed hemolytic reactions require no treatment.
Allergic reaction (mild to moderate)	Thought to be caused by sensitivity reaction to foreign plasma protein in transfused product	Within minutes of transfusion initiation	Local erythema, hives, and urticaria, itching or pruritus	May administer antihistamines before transfusion if prescribed	**Stop transfusion.** Change administration set and administer 0.9% sodium chloride at rate to maintain patent IV access. Notify health care provider and blood bank. Administer antihistamines as ordered. Monitor and document vital signs every 15 min. Transfusion may be restarted if fever, dyspnea, and wheezing are not present.
Allergic reaction (severe)	Usually idiopathic and idiosyncratic. Rarely caused by recipient allergy to a donor antigen (usually IgA) Agglutination of RBCs obstructing capillaries and blocking blood flow, causing symptoms to all major organ systems	Within minutes of transfusion initiation	Coughing, nausea, vomiting, respiratory distress, wheezing, hypotension, loss of consciousness, possible cardiac arrest	Transfusion of saline-washed or leukocyte-depleted RBCs	**Stop transfusion.** This is a life-threatening reaction. Change administration set and administer 0.9% sodium chloride at rate to maintain patent IV access. Notify health care provider and blood bank. Administer antihistamines, corticosteroids, epinephrine, and antipyretics as ordered. Monitor and document vital signs until stable. Initiate cardiopulmonary resuscitation if necessary.

Continued

TABLE 28.10

Transfusion Reactions—cont'd

Reaction	Mechanism	Onset	Signs and Symptoms	Prevention	Nursing Intervention
Graft-versus-host disease	Donor lymphocytes are destroyed by recipient's immune system. In immunocompromised patients the donor lymphocytes are identified as foreign; however, patient's immune system is not capable of destroying, and in turn patient's lymphocytes are destroyed.	8 to 10 days after transfusion	Skin rash, diarrhea, fever, jaundice caused by liver dysfunction, bone marrow suppression	Administration of irradiated blood and leukocyte-depleted RBC products as prescribed	Administer methotrexate and corticosteroids as ordered for treatment of symptoms.
Circulatory overload	Occurs with transfusion of excessive volume or excessively rapid rate; can lead to pulmonary edema.	Anytime during or within 1–2 hours after transfusion	Dyspnea, cough, crackles at lung bases, tachypnea, headache, hypertension, tachycardia, increased central venous pressure, distended neck veins	Administer blood or component at prescribed rate, usually no greater than 2–4 mL/kg/hr; particular attention paid to rate and volume in older adults, young children, and patients with cardiac and renal disorders. Administer PRBCs instead of whole blood. Minimize amount of saline infused with transfusion.	Slow or stop transfusion as ordered. Elevate patient's head. Notify health care provider. Administer oxygen and diuretics as ordered. Monitor and document vital signs including a cardiac and respiratory assessment
Infectious disease transmission	Microorganism contamination of infused product	During transfusion to 2 hours after transfusion Complete transfusion within 4 hours	High fever, chills, abdominal cramping, vomiting, diarrhea, profound hypotension, flushed skin, back pain	Proper care of blood or blood product from time of procurement through end of administration	**Stop transfusion.** Change administration set and maintain patent IV access. Notify health care provider and blood bank. Monitor and document vital signs. Obtain samples for blood culture and Gram stain from recipient. Administer IV fluids, broad-spectrum antimicrobials, vasopressors, and steroids as ordered.
Iron overload	Iron from donated blood binds to protein and is not eliminated	May occur with multiple transfusions or chronic transfusion therapy	Cardiac dysfunction, SOB, arrhythmias, heart failure, increased serum transferrin, increased liver enzymes, jaundice	Chelation, phlebotomy, monitor serum iron levels	Monitor patient for heart failure, cardiac disorder, liver disorder, serum transferrin.

HF, Heart failure; *Hct*, hematocrit; *Hgb*, hemoglobin; *Ig*, immunoglobulin; *IV*, intravenous; *PRBCs*, packed red blood cells; *RBC*, red blood cell; *SOB*, shortness of breath.

Data modified from Alexander M et al: *Core curriculum for infusion nursing*, ed 4, St. Louis, 2014; American Association of Blood Banks (AABB): *Technical manual of the American Association of Blood Banks,* ed 19, Bethesda, MD, 2017; and Gorski L: *Phillip's manual of IV therapeutics: evidence-based practice for infusion therapy,* ed 7, Philadelphia, 2018, FA Davis.

STEP	RATIONALE
e. Maintain clamp on blood product side of Y-tubing in "off" position. Open common tubing clamp to finish priming tubing to distal end of tubing connector. Close tubing clamp when tubing is filled with saline. All three tubing clamps should be closed. Maintain protective sterile cap on tubing connector.	This will completely prime tubing with saline, and IV line is ready to be connected to patient's VAD.
f. Prepare blood component for administration. Gently invert bag two or three times, turning back and forth. Remove protective covering from access port. Spike blood component unit with other Y-connection. Close normal saline clamp above filter, open clamp above filter to blood unit, and prime tubing with blood. Blood will flow into drip chamber (see illustration). Tap filter chamber to ensure that residual air is removed.	Gentle agitation suspends red blood cells in anticoagulant. Protective barrier drape may be used to catch any potential blood spillage. Tubing is primed with blood unit and ready for transfusion into patient.

Safe Patient Care *Sodium chloride (NS) is compatible with blood products, unlike solutions that contain dextrose, which cause coagulation of blood. Only use 0.9% NS to administer blood. No other solutions are to be administered with blood (piggybacked; AABB, 2017; INS, 2016a).*

STEP	RATIONALE
g. Maintaining asepsis, attach primed tubing to patient's VAD by first cleansing the catheter hub with an antiseptic swab. Then quickly connect NS-primed blood administration tubing directly to patient's VAD.	Reduces transmission of microorganisms from catheter hub. This initiates infusion of blood product into patient's vein. Avoid use of needleless connectors for rapid flow rates for red blood cell infusion, which can greatly reduce blood flow (INS, 2016a).
h. Open common tubing clamp and regulate blood infusion to allow only 2 mL/min to infuse in initial 15 minutes. Remain with patient during first 15 minutes of transfusion. Initial flow rate during this time should be 1 to 2 mL/min or 10 to 20 gtt/min (using macrodrip of 10 gtt/mL).	Many transfusion reactions occur within first 15 minutes of transfusion (Gorski, 2018). Infusing small amount of blood component initially minimizes volume of blood to which patient is exposed, thereby minimizing severity of reaction (Gorski, 2018).

Safe Patient Care *If signs of a transfusion reaction occur,* ***stop the transfusion,*** *start 0.9% sodium chloride (NS) with a new primed tubing attached directly to the VAD hub, and notify the health care provider immediately (see Table 28.10). Do not discard the blood product or tubing because they need to be returned to the blood bank. Do not infuse saline through existing tubing because it will cause blood in tubing to enter patient.*

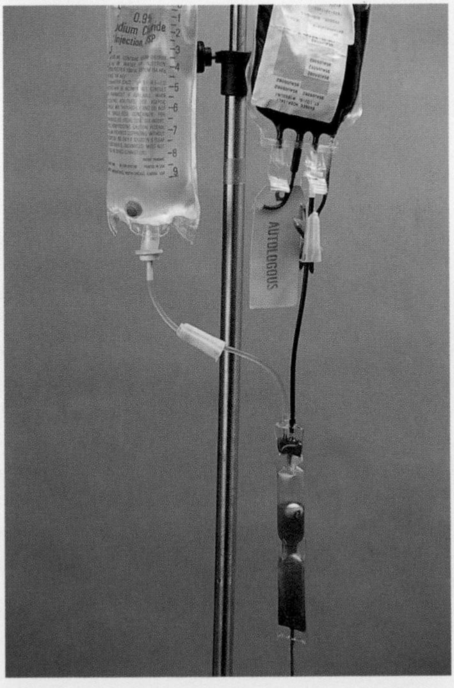

STEP 2f Unit of blood connected to Y-tubing setup.

STEP	RATIONALE
i. Monitor patient's vital signs within 5 to 15 minutes of initiating transfusion and at completion of transfusion (AABB, 2017; Gorski, 2018) or according to agency policy.	Frequently monitoring patient helps to quickly alert you to transfusion reaction (Weinstein and Hagle, 2014). The three most common causes of transfusion-related mortality are transfusion-related acute lung injury (TRALI), hemolytic transfusion reaction (HTR), and transfusion-associated circulatory overload (TACO; AABB, 2017).
j. If there is no transfusion reaction, regulate rate of transfusion according to health care provider's orders based on drop factor for blood administration tubing.	Maintaining prescribed rate of flow decreases risk for fluid-volume excess while restoring vascular volume. Drop factor for most blood tubing is 10 gtt/mL.

Safe Patient Care *A single unit of whole blood or blood components should be infused within a 4-hour period (AABB, 2017). When a longer transfusion time is indicated clinically, the unit may be divided by the blood bank, and the part not being transfused can be properly refrigerated (Gorski, 2018). Administration sets should be changed at the completion of each unit or every 4 hours to reduce bacterial contamination (INS, 2016a). Blood should only be stored in a refrigerator specific for blood or blood products to maintain appropriate temperature controls.*

Safe Patient Care *Medications and solutions should not be infused into the same IV line with a blood component because of the possibility of incompatibility unless the drug or solution has been approved by the FDA for use with blood administration. Maintain a separate IV access if patient requires IV solutions or medications (Gorski, 2018).*

STEP	RATIONALE
k. After blood has infused, clear IV line with 0.9% sodium chloride (NS) and discard blood bag according to agency policy. When consecutive units are ordered, line patency with 0.9% NS at keep-vein-open (KVO) rate as ordered by health care provider and retrieve subsequent unit for administration.	Infusing IV NS allows remainder of blood in IV tubing to infuse and maintains IV line patency for supportive measures in case of transfusion reaction (Gorski, 2018). KVO rate must specify infusion rate as required by the seven rights of medication administration (see Chapter 22).
3. Dispose of any used supplies and personal protective equipment. Discard sharps in sharps container. Remove gloves and perform hand hygiene.	Reduces transmission of microorganisms (INS, 2016a).
4. Assist patient to a comfortable position and instruct on signs or symptoms to report regarding transfusion-related reactions.	Ensures early reporting of signs or symptoms of transfusion-related reactions.
5. Raise bed rails (as appropriate) and lower bed to lowest position.	Minimizes risk for falls and injury.
6. Be sure nurse call system is in an accessible location within patient's reach. Instruct patient in its use.	Ensures patient can call for assistance if needed.

EVALUATION

STEP	RATIONALE
1. Observe IV site and status of infusion each time vital signs are taken.	Detects presence of IV-related complications and verifies continuous and safe infusion of blood product.
2. Observe for any signs of transfusion reactions such as chills, flushing, itching, dyspnea, or rash.	Compare presenting signs and symptoms to baseline assessment of patient before transfusion. These are early signs of transfusion reaction (see Table 28.10).
3. Observe patient and assess laboratory values to determine response to administration of blood component.	Aids in determining whether goals of therapy have been reached or if further blood component therapy will be required. Laboratory results may not reflect transfusion reaction for several hours.
4. Use Teach-Back: "I want to be sure that I explained the reason for your blood transfusion, including the risks and benefits. How can this transfusion help you?" Revise your instruction now or develop a plan for revised patient/family caregiver teaching if patient/family caregiver is not able to teach back correctly.	Determines patient's/family caregiver's level of understanding of instructional topic.

Unexpected Outcomes	Related Interventions
1. Patient displays signs and symptoms of transfusion reaction such as chills, flushing, itching, dyspnea, or rash.	• Stop transfusion immediately. • Disconnect blood tubing at VAD hub and cap distal end with sterile connector to maintain sterile system. • Connect new normal saline solution and primed tubing directly to VAD hub to prevent any subsequent blood from infusing into patient from tubing. • Keep vein open with slow infusion of normal saline at 1 to 2 mL/min to ensure venous patency and maintain venous access for medication or to resume transfusion. • Notify health care provider. • See Table 28.10 for interventions.
2. Patient develops infiltration or phlebitis at venipuncture site.	• Transfusion should be stopped at first sign of infiltration, and IV line removed (see Procedural Guideline 28.1). • Insert new VAD in area above previous location or opposite arm. • Restart product if remainder can be infused within 4 hours of initiation of transfusion. • Institute nursing measures to reduce discomfort at infiltrated or phlebitic area.
3. Fluid-volume overload occurs, and/or patient exhibits difficulty breathing or has crackles on auscultation of lungs.	• Slow or stop transfusion, elevate head of bed, and inform health care provider of physical findings. • Administer diuretics, morphine, and/or oxygen as ordered by health care provider. • Continue frequent assessments and closely monitor vital signs and intake and output.

Recording

- Pretransfusion medications, vital signs, location and condition of IV site, and patient education
- Type and volume of blood component, ABO group and Rh, blood unit/donor/recipient identification, compatibility, and expiration date according to agency policy, along with patient's response to therapy
- Volume of normal saline and blood component infused with start time, stop time, and duration of infusions
- Amount of blood received by autotransfusion and patient's response to therapy
- Vital signs before, within 15 minutes after initiation, and after transfusion
- Transfusion-related adverse events and any intervention
- Document your evaluation of patient learning.

Hand-Off Reporting

- Report signs and symptoms of a transfusion reaction immediately to the health care provider.
- Report to health care provider any intratransfusion/posttransfusion deterioration in cardiac, pulmonary, and/or renal status.

SPECIAL CONSIDERATIONS

Patient-Centered Care

- The ability to recognize diversity in patients, whether age, gender, race, ethnicity or culture, sexual orientation, linguistic, religious, or caused by past experiences, will prepare you to be confident in providing intravenous therapy to patients.
- Communication is essential when delivering infusion therapy; if the patient does not speak English, have a professional interpreter present or available.
- Patients should participate in creating the plan of care, and patient preferences as to the degree of active involvement in the care process should be respected. Although the skills in this chapter are performed by the nurse, engaging the patient in the decision-making process can give the patient a sense of control.
- Reduce anxiety and fear during insertion of a VAD by preparing patients before insertion of a short-peripheral IV catheter. Place patients in a comfortable position, speak directly to them, and answer questions as honestly as possible. Ask patients if they have had IV therapy in the past. Know what their concerns and expectations are. Have a patient use diversional techniques, such as deep breathing, avoiding looking at a catheter during insertion, and focusing on pleasant images or past experiences (Gorski, 2018).
- When preparing for insertion, use techniques that minimize discomfort. Consider using anesthetic agents (see agency policy) based on patient condition, needs, risks, benefits, and the anticipated discomfort of the procedure (INS, 2016a).
- Some of the skills in this chapter include hands-on patient care, which may pose a problem in certain cultures where touching is not acceptable. Before implementing any of these skills, explain what touching is involved and what the patient may experience.
- Allow the patient to have a family caregiver present and provide privacy during the procedure; if possible, assign same-sex caregivers to avoid opposite-sex touching.
- Pain is also expressed differently in different cultures, and you may see some cultures that encourage expressiveness and others that encourage stoicism; this is important to keep in mind when performing skills that may elicit a response to the pain of insertion of or the removal of the tape and dressing from a VAD (Galanti, 2015).
- Consider patients' religious beliefs, especially when locking VADs with heparin. Heparin is derived from animal products (e.g.,

porcine, bovine) and may be a conflict with some religious beliefs (INS, 2016a).
- When administering blood products, you need to consider a patient's values and cultural and religious beliefs about blood therapy. A person's perception of his or her disease or health condition affects how receptive he or she is to receiving blood. Blood transfusion is often equated to severity of illness.
- Allay patient anxieties when possible and acknowledge their beliefs. Certain religions do not allow blood transfusions or organ donation if it involves blood exchange or the blood has not been removed from the organ (Galanti, 2015). Be familiar with agency policies and procedures to follow when patients refuse blood transfusions, and inform the health care provider of a patient's decision.
- By law, parents have the primary obligation to care for and make decisions about their minor children. However, the legal principle of parens patriae says that the state has an overriding interest in the health and welfare of its citizens. The parents' refusal can be interpreted as neglect. The nurse's role is to advocate for the patient and family, and the nurse may need to identify new, alternative methods of transfusion. If necessary, the nurse coordinates with officials to petition juvenile or family court for temporary guardianship of the child.
- Another aspect of patient-centered care is safety, specifically the prevention of transfusion-related complications. Transfusion-related reactions occur most commonly from human error. To ensure safe patient outcomes, the NQF endorses a list of serious reportable events (SREs), which outlines 28 events that are preventable. Regarding transfusion therapy, any "patient death or serious disability associated with a hemolytic reaction due to the administration of ABO/HLA–incompatible blood or blood products" is considered a Care Management Event and must be reported (NQF, 2011).

Patient Education

- Patient education includes clear and concise terms for all aspects of IV therapy and individualized training that include self-care practices (Gorski, 2018).
- Patient teaching should also include care of the VAD, infection prevention, and potential VAD complications and signs and symptoms to report (INS, 2016a).
- Explain the necessity for infusion, how long the device will remain in place, and what signs and symptoms need to be reported (Weinstein and Hagle, 2014).
- Patients with CVADs require health education and teaching about infection-prevention practices and skin care.
- Instruct patient regarding rationale for transfusion and anticipated amount of time for completion of transfusion.
- Discuss with patient and family caregiver the rationale for patient monitoring throughout transfusion.
- Inform patient and family caregiver to notify nurse if patient experiences itching, swelling, dizziness, dyspnea, low back pain, and/or chest pain because these may indicate a transfusion reaction.
- Instruct patient to inform nurse if redness, pain, tenderness, swelling, bleeding, drainage, or leaking from under dressing occurs at IV site.

Age-Specific

Pediatric

- In addition to the usual venipuncture sites, the four scalp veins are used in infants and toddlers and, if not walking, the dorsum of the foot.
- Needle selection is based on age: 26- to 24-gauge needle for neonates; 24- to 22-gauge needle for children (Hockenberry and Wilson, 2017).
- Perform venipuncture in a neutral space to allow the child's room to be a safe place.
- Apply latex-free tourniquet or rubber band or use a blood pressure cuff inflated to just below the patient's diastolic blood pressure (BP).
- Allow older children to select IV site to increase cooperation so that they believe that they have some control over their treatment.
- Use local anesthetics and distraction strategies to minimize the distress associated with venipuncture (Alexander et al., 2014).
- To maintain safety in positioning, have extra help when starting an IV on a child. Use therapeutic hugging, usually in a sitting position, to provide close contact (Hockenberry and Wilson, 2017). NAP can help with positioning.
- Choose age-appropriate activities compatible with the maintenance of the IV infusion to maintain normal growth and development.
- Maintain skin integrity, especially in neonates. Use adhesives such as tape sparingly and remove tape gently.
- Stabilization is essential, especially in young children who cannot comprehend the importance of not "playing" with the IV device.
- Do not use containers exceeding 150 mL in children younger than 2 years old, exceeding 250 mL in children younger than 5 years, or exceeding 500 mL in children younger than 10 years. Always use tamper-resistant, volume-controlled EIDs to ensure accurate fluid delivery (Alexander et al., 2014; Hockenberry and Wilson, 2017).
- Use commercially available IV site protectors to cover and protect the IV site in young active children. Ensure that identification band is visible and nonrestricting (INS, 2016b).
- Use chlorhexidine gluconate with care in premature infants and those under 2 months of age due to the risk of skin irritation and chemical burns (INS, 2016a).
- CVADs are available in smaller diameters and shorter lengths for children and infants (Gorski, 2018). Amount and dosage of flush solution (heparin/saline) varies with age and size of catheter.
- Take care to secure infant catheters in a manner that does not allow them to twist. Small-diameter catheters are fragile, and twisting them will cause them to tear.
- Dried povidone-iodine should be removed with sodium chloride or sterile water for neonates with compromised skin integrity (INS, 2016b).
- Record volume of blood draws on intake and output record.
- Pediatric blood units are prepared in special units (aliquots) and usually equal half the volume of a conventional adult unit (AABB, 2017).
- Usual dose of PRBCs is 10 to 15 mL/kg (Alexander et al., 2014).
- Administer 5% to 10% of total transfusion volume the first 15 minutes of transfusion; then, if no adverse effects, increase administration rate to 2 to 5 mL/kg/hr (Alexander et al., 2014).
- Umbilical catheters or catheters placed in the small saphenous veins may be used in infants and/or pediatric patients (Alexander et al., 2014).

Gerontological

- Older adults have less subcutaneous tissue, making veins more prominent. To prevent bruising, skin tears, and vein damage, the length of time and tension of tourniquet should be limited when applying the tourniquet. Place tourniquet over clothing to prevent bruising or skin tears. Attempt to insert catheter without the use of a tourniquet if veins are visible (INS, 2016c).

- As older adults lose subcutaneous tissue, the veins lose stability and roll away from the needle. To stabilize the vein, pull the skin taut and toward you with your nondominant hand and anchor the vein with your thumb. Minimize the use of tape directly on the skin, and apply skin protectant before applying tape.
- Use of smaller-gauge devices is recommended; ideal size is 22 or 24 gauge (Alexander et al., 2014; INS, 2016a, 2016c). Smaller-gauge catheters are less traumatizing to the vein but still allow blood flow to provide increased hemodilution of the IV solutions or medications (Alexander et al., 2014).
- If possible, avoid the back of the older adult's hand or the dominant arm for venipuncture because the use of these sites interferes with the older adult's independence.
- Vigilance in monitoring an access site during transfusion is vital in an older adult who may be less sensitive to the symptoms of infiltration and the generalized symptoms of a transfusion reaction (INS, 2016c). Infiltration may go unnoticed because of the decreased elasticity of the skin and loose skin folds. Because of decreased tactile sensation, a large amount of fluid may infiltrate before the patient experiences pain (INS, 2016c). Phlebitis may develop without pain but with significant inflammation resulting from the decreased sensitivity of the nerve endings of the skin.
- Use an EID with an appropriate infusion tubing to administer IV solutions. Carefully monitor patient's clinical status, vital signs, electrolyte levels, blood urea nitrogen (BUN), creatinine, weight gain or loss, and I&O (Alexander et al., 2014; INS, 2016a, 2016c).
- Infusing dextrose too rapidly may cause cerebral edema more readily in older patients. NS given to an older patient with impaired renal function can cause hypernatremia (Alexander et al., 2014).
- Some older adults have difficulty with lying flat in bed, and a modification of the totally supine position during CVAD insertion or removal is often necessary.
- PICC insertion may provide an alternative route of administration and reduce the risk of complications associated with subclavian or jugular insertion.
- Some older adults have decreased cardiac function, thus requiring a slower length of time for blood transfusions. Half units may be obtained if a patient is unable to tolerate the volume in a whole unit of blood or blood component. Regulate flow rate to 1 mL/kg/hr to reduce the risk of circulatory overload.

Home Care

- Initiate early referral for discharge planning to social services, counselor, or home care coordinator for assessment of resources.
- Ensure the ability and willingness of the patient or family caregiver to administer and monitor IV therapy in the home, including an ambulatory infusion pump. Determine whether patient or family caregiver has the manual dexterity and cognitive ability to manage the infusion or seek assistance in an emergency for equipment malfunction (Gorski, 2018).
- Assess home environment and determine suitable area for storage of medications and equipment, performing IV therapy, and performing dressing changes and areas to avoid where contaminants are potential hazards.
- Ensure availability of 24-hour assistance with provider of home infusion therapy pharmaceuticals and equipment, including written instructions regarding infusion procedure and pump use. Provide telephone numbers for 24-hour service and emergencies.
- A nurse should be in the home during initiation of IV therapy to ensure correct pump settings for solution, rate, time, and alarms.
- Instruct patient and family caregiver on performing hand hygiene, flushing the VAD, and aseptic technique for changing IV site dressing.
- Patients often have ambulatory infusion pumps. Most pumps weigh less than 2.7 kg (6 pounds) and range from palm to backpack size. They function on battery power, allowing patients the freedom to perform normal daily activities. Programming options include automatic rate adjustments, remote site adjustments via a telephone modem, and therapy-specific settings such as patient-controlled analgesia (see manufacturer directions; Fig. 28.7).
- Provide appropriate information about home disposal of sharps and equipment contaminated by blood, which are disposed of in leak-proof, puncture-resistant containers with lids (see Chapter 32; OSHA, 2012).
- Teach patient to keep site dry during bath (preferred) or shower by wrapping in plastic bag and occlusive taping. Ensure EID or ambulatory infusion pump safety during hygiene activity.
- Provide education to the patient and family caregiver on how to recognize signs and symptoms of IV-related complications, actions to take, how to report, and methods for preservation of CVADs (Gorski, 2018; see Table 28.7). If the catheter comes out, instruct caregiver to apply gauze pressure dressing and notify home care nurse. Provide patient with Kelly clamp without teeth (bulldog clamp) that can be used in the event of catheter rupture to prevent air embolism, and instruct patient on use.
- Patients who have had prior transfusion reactions, acute angina, or heart failure are not considered good candidates for home blood transfusions.
- When blood sample is obtained for blood typing and cross-matching, attach identification band to patient with full name

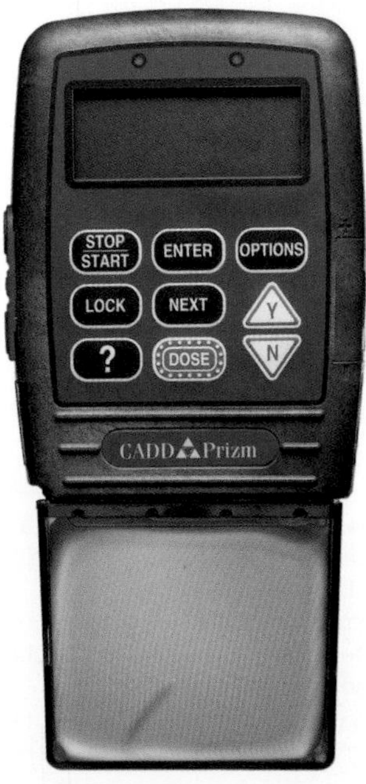

FIG 28.7 Patient-controlled ambulatory infusion pump. *(Courtesy Smiths Medical ASD, Inc., St. Paul, MN.)*

and identification number used by laboratory. This provides clear identification of patient when blood component transfusion is initiated.
- Blood and blood products must be transported in a container with appropriate coolant. Verify and record the temperature at the time of delivery.
- Initiate the transfusion as soon as possible after component is obtained from blood bank.
- Nursing personnel must be present for the entire blood transfusion process and for 30 to 60 minutes after transfusion.
- Posttransfusion instructions must be given in writing, and the patient or family caregiver must be provided with names and phone numbers of individuals available to be called in the event of a delayed problem (e.g., unexplained fever, malaise, jaundice). Complications may occur days to weeks after transfusion.
- Instruct patient and family caregiver regarding signs and symptoms of adverse outcomes (infectious disease transmission) or transfusion reactions (delayed hemolytic) that can occur hours to weeks after patient has received transfusion and may become evident in the home setting and steps to be taken should they occur.
- Return the container, empty bags, and tubing to the home care agency after completion of the transfusion.

✦ PRACTICE REFLECTIONS

A patient with diabetes mellitus is admitted to the health care agency for treatment of osteomyelitis of the right foot that resulted in a transmetatarsal amputation. After surgery, a PICC line is placed in the left upper arm for several weeks of IV antibiotic therapy. After 1 week of IV antibiotics and wound care, arrangements are being made for the patient to be discharged and continue IV antibiotics and wound care at home.

1. What are some techniques you used when caring for your patient's central vascular access device (CVAD)?
2. What advice would you give someone who has never cared for a PICC line before?
3. What did you do to help meet your patient's needs?

✦ CLINICAL REVIEW QUESTIONS

1. An elderly patient is showing signs of dehydration due to fever from a urinary tract infection and poor oral intake. Intravenous fluids are ordered for D_5 0.45% NS to infuse continuously at 60 mL/hr. If the drop factor on the patient's infusion tubing is 10 gtt/mL, what would the rate of infusion be in drops per minute (gtt/min)?
2. Place the steps for changing a central line dressing over a PICC line in the correct order.
   1. Perform hand hygiene, apply sterile gloves, and cleanse insertion site and surrounding area with antiseptic swab.
   2. Inspect catheter insertion site for IV-related complications and remove the transparent dressing.
   3. Apply new transparent semipermeable membrane (TSM) dressing.
   4. Measure external PICC length and upper arm circumference.
   5. Label dressing with date, time, catheter gauge size, and initials.
   6. Perform hand hygiene, collect supplies, and apply mask and clean gloves.
3. Which of the following steps are necessary when initiating a transfusion of packed red blood cells (PRBCs)? (Select all that apply.)
   1. Verify the health care providers order for PRBCs, number of units, date and time to give, duration, and pretransfusion medications.
   2. Ensure the patient has a patent, working VAD, and then obtain PRBCs from blood bank.
   3. Verify the correct product was obtained, patient's ABO and Rh types are compatible, and match product obtained with another qualified person (i.e., nurse).
   4. Prior to initiating transfusion, check product expiration date, patient identification number matches transfusion number, and PRBC unit number matches blood bank form with another qualified person (i.e., nurse).
   5. Aseptically spike a bag of D_5W with one of the Y-tubing spikes on the blood administration set, prime the tubing with D_5W, and spike the PRBC bag with the other spike on the administration set.
   6. Administer PRBCs over 4 hours, taking vital signs before, 15 minutes after beginning transfusion, and at completion of transfusion.

Answers and Rationales for Clinical Review Questions can be found on the Evolve website.

REFERENCES

Alexander M, et al: *Core curriculum for infusion nursing*, ed 4, Philadelphia, 2014, Lippincott Williams & Wilkins.

American Association of Blood Banks (AABB): *Technical manual*, ed 19, Bethesda, MD, 2017, Author.

Band J, Gaynes R: Prevention of intravascular catheter-related infections, 2017. http://www.uptodate.com/contents/prevention-of-intravascular-catheter-related-infections.

Centers for Disease Control and Infection (CDC): Guidelines for the prevention of intravascular catheter-related infections, 2011. https://www.cdc.gov/infectioncontrol/guidelines/pdf/bsi/bsi-guidelines-H.pdf.

Centers for Disease Control and Prevention (CDC): What is health literacy? 2016. https://www.cdc.gov/healthliteracy/learn/index.htmlde.

Ciocson M, et al: Central vascular access device: an adapted evidence-based clinical practice guideline, *J Assoc Vasc Access* 19(4):221–237, 2014.

Galanti GA: *Caring for patients from different cultures*, ed 5, Philadelphia, 2015, University of Pennsylvania Press.

Giuliano KK: IV smart pumps: the impact of a simplified user interface on clinical use, *Biomed Instrum Technol* 49(S4):13, 2015.

Gorski L: *Phillip's manual of IV therapeutics: evidence-based practice for infusion therapy*, ed 7, Philadelphia, 2018, FA Davis.

Heffner A, et al: Overview of central line care, October 24, 2017. http://www.uptodate.com/contents/overview-of-central-venous-access?source=search_result&search=central+line&selectedTitle=1%7E150.

Helton J, et al: Peripheral IV site rotation based on clinical assessment vs. length of time since insertion, *Medsurg Nurs* 25(1):44, 2016.

Hockenberry M, Wilson D: *Wong's essentials of pediatric nursing*, ed 10, St. Louis, 2017, Elsevier.

Humphrey JS: Improving registered nurses' knowledge of evidence-based practice guidelines to decrease the incidence of central line-associated bloodstream infections: an educational intervention, *J Assoc Vasc Access* 20(3):143, 2015.

Infusion Nurses Society (INS): Infusion therapy standards of practice, *J Infus Nurs* 39(IS):S11, 2016a.

Infusion Nurses Society (INS): *Policy and procedures for infusion therapy*, ed 5, Norwood, MA, 2016b, Author.

Infusion Nurses Society (INS): *Policy and procedures for infusion therapy of the older adult*, ed 3, Norwood, MA, 2016c, Author.

Institute for Healthcare Improvement (IHI): *How-to guide: prevent central line-associated bloodstream infections*, Cambridge, MA, 2012, Author. http://www.ihi.org/resources/Pages/Tools/HowtoGuidePreventCentralLineAssociatedBloodstreamInfection.aspx.

Kamboj M, et al: Use of disinfection cap to reduce central-line–associated bloodstream infection and blood culture contamination among hematology–oncology patients, *Infect Control Hosp Epidemiol* 36(12):1401, 2015.

Mattox EA: Complications of peripheral venous access devices: prevention, detection, and recovery strategies, *Crit Care Nurse* 37(2):e1, 2017.

Mimoz O, et al: Skin antisepsis with chlorhexidine-alcohol versus povidone iodine-alcohol, with and without skin scrubbing, for prevention of intravascular-catheter-related infection (CLEAN): an open-label, multicenter, randomized, controlled, two-by-two factorial trial, *Lancet* 386(10008):2069, 2015.

National Quality Forum (NQF): *Serious reportable events in healthcare—2011 update: a consensus report*, Washington, DC, 2011, Author. http://www.qualityforum.org/Publications/2011/12/Serious_Reportable_Events_in_Healthcare_2011.aspx.

Occupational Safety and Health Administration (OSHA): Bloodborne pathogens standards, United States Department of Labor, April 3, 2012. https://www.osha.gov/pls/oshaweb/owadisp.show_document?p_table=STANDARDS&p_id=10051.

Oncology Nurses Society (ONS): *Access device standards of practice for oncology nursing*, Pittsburgh, PA, 2017, Author.

Sabado J, et al: Principles of ultrasound-guided venous access, 2018. http://www.uptodate.com/contents/principles-of-ultrasound-guided-venous-access. Last amended January 8, 2018.

Simon T, et al: *Rossi's principles of transfusion medicine*, ed 5, West Sussex, UK, 2016, Wiley-Blackwell.

The Joint Commission (TJC): Sentinel event alert: managing risk during transition to new ISO tubing connector standards, Oakbrook Terrace, IL, 2014. https://www.jointcommission.org/assets/1/6/SEA_53_Connectors_8_19_14_final.pdf.

The Joint Commission (TJC): *2019 National Patient Safety Goals*, Oakbrook Terrace, IL, 2019, The Commission, p 2018. http://www.jointcommission.org/standards_information/npsgs.aspx.

U.S. Food and Drug Administration (FDA): Requirements for blood and blood components intended for transfusion or for further manufacturing use, final rule, *Fed Register* 80(99):12228, 2015. https://www.gpo.gov/fdsys/pkg/FR-2015-05-22/html/2015-12228.htm.

Weinstein S, Hagle M: *Plumer's principles and practice of infusion therapy*, Philadelphia, 2014, Lippincott William & Wilkins.

29 Preoperative and Postoperative Care

SKILLS AND PROCEDURES

EVOLVE WEBSITE/RESOURCES LIST

http://evolve.elsevier.com/Perry/nursinginterventions

Audio Glossary • Case Study • Checklists • Clinical Review Questions • Answers and Rationales for Clinical Review Questions

INTRODUCTION

Surgical care of patients is currently in a state of advancement in technology, which results in less invasive surgery and shortened length of stays. Surgery takes place in a variety of settings, including hospitals, ambulatory surgery centers, health care providers' offices, and even mobile units. The principles of caring for perioperative patients are basically the same, regardless of the setting, except for the timing and extent of therapy.

During preoperative preparation, a nurse focuses on physical, psychological, sociocultural, and spiritual preparation; assessment and validation of existing information; reinforcement of teaching that applies to the perioperative period; and provision of nursing care to complete preparation for the surgical experience (American Society of PeriAnesthesia Nurses [ASPAN], 2017). Postoperative care involves stabilizing a patient's physical condition, educating a patient and family, and preparing them for effective management of the condition during recovery. The care of postoperative patients returning from the operating room (OR) requires the nurse to complete a thorough assessment, provide ongoing monitoring and, finally, education of both the patient and the family caregiver.

PRACTICE STANDARDS

- American Society of PeriAnesthesia Nurses (ASPAN), 2017: 2017–2018 perianesthesia nursing standards, practice recommendations and interpretive statements—Periaensthesia nursing standards of practice during recovery
- Berrios-Torres et al., 2017: Centers for Disease Control and Prevention guideline for the prevention of surgical site infection—Steps to prevent SSI
- The Joint Commission, n.d.: The universal protocol for preventing wrong site, wrong procedure, and wrong person surgery™: guidance for health care providers—Prevention of surgical errors
- The Joint Commission, 2017: Surgical site infections (SSIs)—Prevention of surgical site infections
- The Joint Commission, 2019: National Patient Safety Goals—Patient identification

EVIDENCE-BASED PRACTICE

Surgical Site Infections

A surgical site infection (SSI) is a post-surgical infection that develops at the surgical location (Centers for Disease Control and Prevention [CDC], 2017). SSIs develop in 2% to 5% of the more than 30 million patients who have inpatient surgery annually (Anderson and Sexton, 2017) and contribute to longer lengths of stay, cost, and associated interventions. The rate of SSIs varies depending on several factors, such as procedure type, surgeon experience, type of hospital and length of stay, the patient's presentation (e.g., smokers and those with diabetes, malnutrition, or obesity are at higher risk for SSI), and surveillance methods (Anderson and Sexton, 2017). Most SSIs are largely preventable. The following evidence-based strategies are available to guide providers of care in reducing their occurrence (Berrios-Torres et al., 2017):

- Prior to surgery, patients should shower or take a full-body bath with soap (antimicrobial or nonantimicrobial) on at least the night before the operative day.
- Follow antibiotic prophylaxis procedures based on published clinical practice guidelines so that bactericidal concentration of agents is in the blood and tissues when the surgeon incises the tissue. (Antimicrobial prophylaxis should be administered before skin incision in cesarean section procedures.)
- Use alcohol-based antiseptics for skin cleansing in the operating room unless contraindicated.
- Additional prophylactic antimicrobial agent doses should *not* be administered after the surgical incision is closed in the operating room, even in the presence of a drain, for clean and clean-contaminated procedures.

- Antimicrobial sealant (topical) agents applied to areas of surgical incision are not necessary to prevent SSI.
- Glycemic control should be implemented during surgical procedures using blood glucose target levels less than 200 mg/dL.
- Perioperative normothermia (normal temperature) should be maintained in all patients.
- Increased fraction of inspired oxygen should be given during surgery and after extubation in the immediate postoperative period for individuals with normal pulmonary function who have general anesthesia with endotracheal intubation.
- Transfusion of blood products should not be withheld from surgical patients in order to prevent SSI.

SAFETY GUIDELINES

Preparing patients to undergo surgery and anesthesia involves important skills and a thorough preoperative assessment. Regardless of the setting, the preoperative assessment forms the basis for a plan of care that will follow a patient during and after surgery. Safety guidelines include the following:

- Follow safety measures such as verifying correct patient, correct procedure, and correct surgical site; obtaining signed consent and recording thorough documentation (e.g., history and physical examination, nursing assessment, and preanesthesia assessment); and ensuring the availability of required blood products, implants, devices, or special equipment for the procedure.
- Timing and duration of antibiotic administration and proper surgical site preparation are essential to prevent SSIs.
- The surgical site must be marked before surgery by the licensed independent practitioner who is ultimately accountable for the procedure (and who will be present during surgery) to allow staff to identify clearly the intended site for the procedure. It is optimum to have the patient—if able—mark the site, also (TJC, 2017, 2019).
- A time-out must be performed immediately before beginning the procedure to ensure right patient and right site (TJC, n.d., 2019).
- Patient assessment in the immediate postoperative recovery phase emphasizes the ABCs—*A*, airway; *B*, breathing; and *C*, circulation. Postoperative patients are still under sedation and can become hypoxic. Nurses routinely monitor oxygen saturation levels and provide supplemental oxygen (when ordered) for as long as needed.
- During the postoperative period, assess the wound size, location, and depth, all of which influence the type and amount of drainage. It is important to know which type of drainage to anticipate from the dressing, tubes, and catheters to differentiate what is expected from what is abnormal.
- Implement prophylactic venous thromboembolism measures as ordered.
- Remove wound drains as clinically indicated and ordered to prevent SSI.
- Patients who are overweight or obese have increased risk of postoperative complications such as obstructive sleep apnea (OSA), which predisposes them to airway management problems in the postanesthesia care unit (PACU) and possible postoperative pulmonary complications. Longer lengths of stay and unanticipated postoperative intensive care admission may be required for these patients.
- A patient having surgery performed in an ambulatory surgery center must be accompanied by a family member or friend to allow for discharge after the procedure.

✦ SKILL 29.1 Preoperative Assessment

Purpose

Nurses must perform thorough preoperative assessments to provide a baseline for intraoperative and postoperative care. Many health care agencies have a designated department devoted to completing thorough preoperative screening and testing before a patient is admitted for surgery. Laboratory tests, electrocardiograms (ECGs), chest x-ray films, and other tests are often obtained in these facilities 1 to 2 weeks in advance of the scheduled procedure so that abnormalities can be addressed before surgery. During this screening, provide privacy and a location free of interruption to encourage open communication. It is not unusual for a patient to remember and report facts that may not have previously been reported to the surgeon. A nurse will again assess patients 1 to 2 hours before the actual surgical procedure to ensure that there are no medical changes. A preprocedure verification process should be followed (TJC, 2017).

Delegation and Collaboration

The surgeon and anesthetist will complete their own assessments, and a consent form is signed. The skill of preoperative assessment cannot be delegated to nursing assistive personnel (NAP). If a patient is stable, the nurse instructs the NAP to:

- Obtain vital signs and height and weight measurements.

Equipment

- Stethoscope
- Blood pressure monitoring equipment
- Pulse oximetry
- Thermometer
- Watch or clock with a second hand
- Scale to measure height and weight
- Access to laboratory, ECG, x-ray films, and other diagnostic equipment
- Preprocedure checklist
- Preoperative assessment form

ASSESSMENT

1. Identify patient using at least two identifiers (e.g., name and birthday or name and medical record number) according to agency policy. *Rationale: Ensures correct patient. Complies with The Joint Commission standards and improves patient safety (TJC, 2019).*
2. Perform hand hygiene. Prepare equipment and room for assessment. *Rationale: Reduces transmission of microorganisms. Makes assessment more efficient.*
3. Determine if patient has any communication impairment (e.g., blindness, hearing loss), can read and understand English, and is competent to make autonomous decisions. For example, give patient an informational brochure and have him or her explain part of the contents. Obtain a professional interpreter if needed. *Rationale: Patient may not fully comprehend a diagnosis, understand proposed treatment, or effectively consider alternatives that are presented without*

effective communication. Family members should never be used as interpreters.

4. Assess patient's understanding of the intended surgery and anesthesia. Ask patient to offer a description rather than asking a simple yes-or-no question (e.g., "Tell me what your surgery will involve"). Ask about patient's and family caregiver's expectations of surgery and care. Include questions concerning fears, cultural practices, and religious or spiritual beliefs. *Rationale: Patients may have misconceptions and incomplete knowledge. Asking about fears, cultural practices, and religious or spiritual beliefs allows you to anticipate priorities of care and adapt teaching and support accordingly.*
5. Ask about advance directives (see Chapter 31) and be sure these are accessible via the electronic health record (EHR). *Rationale: Advance directives protect patient's rights by communicating patient's treatment preferences if he or she is unable to communicate. This should be readily available in case decisions need to be made during the surgical procedure that involve the patient's wishes.*
6. Collect nursing history and identify surgical risk factors. *Rationale: Allows for anticipation of possible complications and planning for interventions to reduce risks.*

Safe Patient Care *If patient is having emergency surgery, focus on assessment of primary body systems affected.*

a. Patient's condition requiring surgery. *Rationale: Allows you to anticipate postoperative needs and possible complications.*

b. Chronic illnesses and associated risk (e.g., diabetes may hinder wound healing; asthma may impair ventilation; history of methicillin-resistant *Staphylococcus aureus* may impair wound healing and increase risk for sepsis). *Rationale: Chronic conditions increase risk for complications associated with surgery and anesthesia.*

c. Screen for obstructive sleep apnea (OSA). Many heath care agencies use the STOP-BANG assessment tool **(any question answered Yes is a risk factor)**:

STOP
- Do you SNORE loudly (louder than talking or loud enough to be heard through closed doors)?
- Do you often feel TIRED, fatigued, or sleepy during the daytime?
- Has anyone OBSERVED you stop breathing during your sleep?
- Do you have or are you being treated for high blood PRESSURE?

BANG
- Body mass index (BMI) more than 35 kg/m^2
- Age over 50 years old
- Neck circumference >40 cm (16 inches)
- Gender: Male

Rationale: In the surgical population, a STOP-BANG score of 5 to 8 identifies patients with high probability of moderate/severe OSA. The STOP-BANG score helps the health care team to stratify patients for unrecognized OSA, practice perioperative precautions, or triage patients for diagnosis and treatment (Chung et al., 2016). Patients with OSA require special anesthesia precautions. Patients with OSA are often sensitive to sedative medications, especially if the OSA is untreated. Even minimal sedation can cause airway obstruction and ventilatory arrest, thus requiring close monitoring postoperatively (Ogan and Plevak, n.d.).

Safe Patient Care *If patient has a score of high probability for OSA, alert the health care team so that anesthesia precautions and close monitoring can be undertaken.*

d. Last menstrual period (for female patients in childbearing years). *Rationale: Anesthetic agents and other medications could injure fetus.*

e. Previous hospitalizations. *Rationale: Provides information about existing medical conditions and previous surgeries that pose surgical risks.*

f. Full medication history, including prescription, over-the-counter (OTC), and vitamin and herbal remedies, and date and time of last doses. *Rationale: Patient may not report OTC medications and vitamin and herbal remedies unless specifically asked. These may interact with anesthetic agents or other medications given during surgery. The surgeon will instruct the patient about whether or not to take routine blood pressure, cardiac, or seizure medications on the day of surgery. Changes in dosages of oral diabetic agents or insulin may be ordered.*

g. Previous experience with surgery and anesthesia; have patient clarify if any undesirable outcomes occurred. *Rationale: Information helps to prevent recurrent problems, particularly if the patient had problems with anesthesia or delayed wound healing.*

h. Family history of complications from surgery or anesthesia. *Rationale: Family history of reactions to anesthetic agents may indicate a familial condition such as malignant hyperthermia, which is life threatening.*

i. Patient history of chronic pain disorders and treatments used at home. *Rationale: Preoperative assessment is essential to identify signs and symptoms of opioid abuse and later, postoperatively, opioid withdrawal, which can complicate patient pain management postoperatively (Coluzzi et al., 2017).*

j. Allergies to medications, food, or tape, including specific questions about natural rubber latex (using both words so that patient understands that rubber and latex are the same thing). Ask patients if they have had any problem with medication or anything placed on their skin (e.g., adhesive). *Rationale: Allergies to medications or latex can be life threatening. Prevention of latex allergy in sensitized patients requires specific precautions. Sensitivity to adhesive should be noted so that tissue integrity is considered when caring for a wound.*

k. Physical limitation or impairment (e.g., paralysis, reduced range of motion). *Rationale: Limited mobility can lead to problems with positioning and risk for pressure injury formation. Communicate this information to the operating room (OR) nurse because these patients may need special positioning or OR bed surfaces.*

l. Presence of prostheses and implants (e.g., implantable medication-delivery pump, dentures, hearing aid, pacemaker, internal defibrillator, hip prosthesis). *Rationale: These items could become damaged or malfunction for various reasons during surgery. Report this information to the OR nurse.*

m. History of smoking, alcohol, and drug use. *Rationale: Preoperative alcohol consumption is associated with an increased risk of general postoperative morbidity, general infections, wound complications, pulmonary complications, prolonged stay at the hospital, and admission to an intensive care unit (Rotevatn et al., 2017). Preoperative use of illicit drugs can lead to pulmonary complications, poor pain control, and withdrawal symptoms. Smoking can lead to cardiopulmonary complications.*

n. Patient's occupation. *Rationale: Anticipates how postoperative restrictions may affect patient's ability to return to work.*

7. Obtain weight, height, and vital signs (see Chapters 7 and 8). *Rationale: Height and weight are used to calculate drug dosages. Vital signs provide a baseline for postoperative comparison in determining change in patient condition.*

Safe Patient Care *Some patients with OSA are morbidly obese, placing them at increased risk for aspiration of acidic gastric fluid at the time of anesthesia induction. These patients may be prescribed medications by their health care provider to suppress gastric acid production, neutralize the acid, or stimulate emptying of the stomach preoperatively.*

8. Assess respiratory status. Auscultate lungs and note adventitious sounds; assess character and rate of respirations, oxygen saturation, ability to breathe lying flat, use of oxygen or continuous positive airway pressure (CPAP) at home, and chest x-ray film report. *Rationale: Compromised respiratory status can affect patient's response to general anesthesia. Use of CPAP may indicate that patient has OSA, which increases patient's postoperative risk factors.*
9. Auscultate heart sounds and evaluate circulatory status, including apical pulse, ECG report, and peripheral pulses (see Chapter 8). *Rationale: Certain cardiac problems that may contraindicate surgery. Circulation may be a factor in positioning patient on OR table.*
10. Assess for risk factors for preoperative venous thromboembolism (e.g., older adults, immobilized patients, patients with personal or family history of blood clots, use of birth control pills or hormones). Ask about leg pain; observe calves for symmetry, swelling, warmth, and redness; palpate pedal pulses. *Rationale: Circulation slows after general anesthesia, increasing tendency for blood clot formation. Immobilization during surgical procedure increases risk for venous stasis. Manipulation and positioning can cause accidental trauma to leg veins.*

Safe Patient Care ***Do not routinely assess for Homans' sign; stop patient's calf movement immediately if any pain is noted.*** *If you suspect a deep vein thrombosis (DVT), notify the surgeon and refrain from manipulating the extremity any further. Surgery will usually need to be postponed. Antiembolism stockings or venous flexus foot pump (Fig. 29.1) may be ordered for patients at risk for thrombus formation (see Chapter 18).*

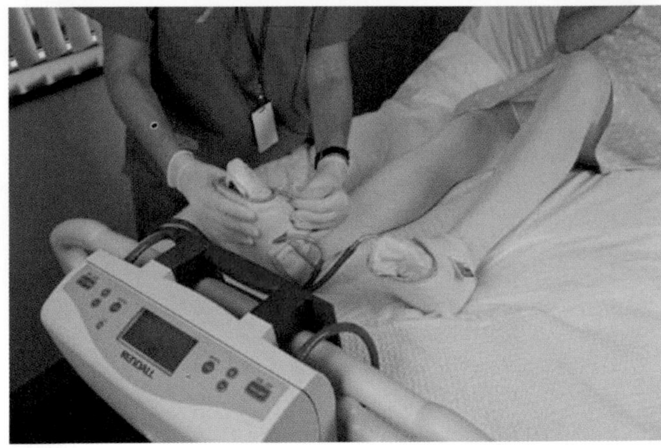

FIG 29.1 Venous plexus foot pump with bedside controls. *(Courtesy Tyco Healthcare Group LP.)*

11. Complete a gastrointestinal assessment; if surgery is scheduled for that day, identify time of patient's last intake of food or drink (see Chapter 8). See agency policy for nothing-by-mouth (NPO) restrictions. *Rationale: The esophageal sphincter relaxes in the presence of general anesthesia, so if stomach contents are present, they can be aspirated. The American Society of Anesthesiologists (ASA) guidelines note that unnecessarily prolonged fasting can be avoided by allowing patients to have clear liquids with the minimal fasting time of only 2 hours (ASA Committee, 2017).*
12. Complete a full neurological assessment; determine patient's level of consciousness (LOC), cognitive function, and sensation and note neurological deficits (see Chapter 8). *Rationale: Patient's neurological status may indicate conditions such as a stroke. This assessment also reflects attentiveness to instruction and offers important baseline information for postoperative evaluation.*
13. Assess patient's musculoskeletal system, including range of motion (ROM) of joints (see Chapter 8). *Rationale: If ROM is limited, extra care is needed to prevent injury during surgical positioning.*
14. Carefully inspect all areas of the skin; identify breaks in skin integrity and determine level of hydration (see Chapter 8). *Rationale: If skin is thin, broken, or bruised, extra padding is needed in surgery. It is also important to document all skin observations that were present before surgery and hospitalization. Hydration may affect skin integrity.*
15. Assess patient's emotional status, including anxiety, coping mechanisms, and family caregiver support. Consider using Hospital Anxiety and Depression Scale (HADS). Assess for presence of, or potential for, abuse or neglect from partner or family caregiver. *Rationale: If patient has high level of anxiety or fear, consultation with social worker, pastoral care, or advanced practice nurse might be useful.*
16. Review results of laboratory tests, including complete blood count, electrolytes, urinalysis, and other diagnostic tests. *Rationale: Laboratory work provides information about important body systems and can indicate presence of abnormalities that may affect the surgical process or outcome.*
17. Assess patient's or family caregiver's knowledge, experience, and health literacy. *Rationale: Ensures patient or family caregiver has the capacity to obtain, communicate, process, and understand basic health information (CDC, 2016).*

STEP	RATIONALE

PLANNING

Step	Rationale
1. Expected outcomes following completion of procedure:	
• Patient understands the surgical rationale, preparation, and procedure.	Identifies patient's knowledge of preoperative plan of care.
• Patient remains alert and appropriately responsive to assessment questions.	Identifies patient readiness to learn.
• Patient's risks for postoperative complications are identified.	Thorough assessment reveals surgical risks.
• Patient does not incur positional or skin injury during preoperative preparation in OR.	Precautions taken as a result of assessment findings prevent positional and skin injury.
2. Provide privacy; set up any equipment or learning materials needed.	Protects patient's privacy; reduces anxiety. Ensures more efficiency when completing patient teaching.
3. Explain to patient and family caregiver how the preoperative assessment will be used in patient's care.	Empowers the patient and family caregiver by knowing value of information shared; reduces anxiety.

IMPLEMENTATION

Step	Rationale
1. Communicate to the preoperative team risk factors that have the potential for making the patient vulnerable to intraoperative complications.	Limitations in mobility and sensation should affect how patient is positioned for surgery. Presence of OSA and any cardiopulmonary abnormalities can influence anesthesia approach.

Safe Patient Care *Even though the surgeon and anesthesia provider will conduct separate assessments, your findings may reveal surgical risk factors not identified previously.*

Step	Rationale
2. Based on the patient's cognitive status, level of health literacy, and nature of planned surgery, present preoperative instruction to patient and family caregiver (see Skill 29.2).	Assessment findings influence approach to personalize the plan of care.
3. After completion of assessment, appropriately dispose of supplies and equipment.	Reduces transmission of microorganisms.
4. Be sure nurse call system is in an accessible location within patient's reach.	Ensures patient can call for assistance if needed.
5. Raise side rails (as appropriate) and lower bed to lowest position.	Ensures patient safety.

EVALUATION

Step	Rationale
1. Determine if patient information is complete so that plan of care can be established. Validate unclear information with family caregiver.	Validates preoperative baseline assessment data.
2. Evaluate patient's ability to cooperatively interact (e.g., makes eye contact, answers appropriately) and level of health literacy.	Establishes patient's ability to participate in assessment and understand teaching.
3. **Use Teach-Back:** "I want to be sure I explained what you need to know about your intended surgery and anesthesia. Tell me when your surgery is scheduled and the reason you are having surgery." Revise your instruction now or develop a plan for revised patient/family caregiver teaching if patient/family caregiver is not able to teach back correctly.	Determines patient's/family caregiver's level of understanding of instructional topic.

Unexpected Outcomes	Related Interventions
1. Patient does not understand what surgery will be performed.	• Notify surgeon. Clarification will need to be provided by the surgeon, and informed consent may need to be obtained again.
2. Patient reports allergy to latex.	• Remove all supplies containing latex from patient's room. • Post latex precautions sign on door and stretcher and in other places as needed per agency protocol. • Notify surgeon, anesthesia provider, OR nurse, and other members of the interprofessional intra- and postoperative team.

Recording

- Document assessment findings in the designated area of the patient's record.
- Document evaluation and evidence of patient learning.

Hand-Off Reporting

- Report abnormal laboratory values or other operative risks to the surgeon, anesthesiologist, and OR nurse. If patient has known history of opioid use for pain control, communicate to health care provider.

✦ SKILL 29.2 Preoperative Teaching

Purpose

Comprehensive preoperative patient education has traditionally been provided to patients with the intent of improving patients' knowledge, health behaviors, and health outcomes. The content of preoperative education varies across settings but frequently includes discussion of presurgical procedures, the actual steps in a surgical procedure, postoperative care (e.g., monitoring, positioning, exercises), potential stressful scenarios associated with surgery, potential surgical and nonsurgical complications, postoperative pain management and physical movements to avoid post-surgery, and how to eliminate high-risk behaviors (Association of periOperative Registered Nurses [AORN], 2015; McDonald et al., 2014).

Provide privacy, and tailor teaching based on the preoperative assessment. Select the best learning method for a patient, which may include videotape or streaming videos and written materials. Involve the family caregivers whenever possible. Plan to have the patient demonstrate expected postoperative skills to allow for practice and facilitate understanding. To decrease anxiety, teach about expected perioperative sensations, and set postoperative expectations about pain management and average length of surgery so that the patient knows what to expect during the postoperative recovery phase.

Delegation and Collaboration

The skills of preoperative teaching cannot be delegated to nursing assistive personnel (NAP). NAP can reinforce and help patients perform postoperative exercises. The nurse instructs the NAP about:

- Any precautions or safety issues unique to the patient (e.g., falls, mobility limitations, bleeding precautions).
- Informing the nurse of any identified concerns (e.g., inability to perform exercise).

Equipment

- Pillow
- Incentive spirometer
- Preoperative education flow sheet
- Positive expiratory pressure (PEP) device
- Stethoscope

ASSESSMENT

1. Identify patient using at least two identifiers (e.g., name and birthday or name and medical record number) according to agency policy. *Rationale: Ensures correct patient. Complies with The Joint Commission standards and improves patient safety (TJC, 2019).*
2. Perform hand hygiene. Ask about previous experience with surgery and anesthesia; have patient clarify if any undesirable outcomes occurred. *Rationale: Reduces transmission of microorganisms. Information helps to prevent recurrent problems, particularly if the patient had problems with anesthesia or delayed wound healing.*
3. Assess patient's understanding of the intended surgery and anesthesia. Ask patient to offer a description rather than asking a simple yes-or-no question (e.g., "Tell me what your surgery will involve"). Ask about patient's and family caregiver's expectations of surgery and care. Include questions concerning time frame for surgery and recovery, fears, cultural practices, and religious or spiritual beliefs. *Rationale: Patients may have misconceptions and incomplete knowledge. Asking about fears, cultural practices, and religious or spiritual beliefs allows you to anticipate priorities of care and adapt teaching and support accordingly.*
4. Identify patient's cognitive level, language, and culture. If patient does not speak English, have a professional interpreter available to assist you. *Rationale: These factors may alter patient's ability to understand meaning of surgery and can affect postoperative healing if full understanding is not present.*
5. Assess patient's risk factors for postoperative respiratory complications (see Skill 29.1). Check nursing history for patient's height and age. *Rationale: General anesthesia predisposes patient to respiratory problems (see Chapter 16). Presence of underlying respiratory conditions or patient's inability to perform postoperative respiratory exercises increases the risk for pulmonary complications. Height and age are used to set incentive spirometer parameters.*
6. Assess patient's anxiety related to surgery. *Rationale: Directs you to provide additional emotional support, which may be needed to facilitate the patient's readiness to learn.*
7. Assess family caregiver's ability and willingness to learn and support patient following surgery. *Rationale: Family caregiver's presence after surgery is an important factor in patient recovery. Caregiver can coach patient through postoperative exercise, help with medication administration, and observe for postoperative complications.*
8. Assess patient's medical record for type of surgery and approach. *Rationale: The surgical procedure itself may require patients to limit activities postoperatively. Anticipating any limitations that might affect how patient can perform postoperative exercises allows you to adapt your instruction preoperatively.*
9. Assess patient's or family caregiver's knowledge, experience, and health literacy. *Rationale: Ensures patient or family caregiver has the capacity to obtain, communicate, process, and understand basic health information (CDC, 2016).*

STEP	RATIONALE
PLANNING	
1. Expected outcomes following completion of procedure:	
• Patient demonstrates eye contact and asks and answers questions appropriately.	Identifies patient's readiness to learn and investment in postoperative self-care.
• Patient correctly performs splinting, turning and sitting, breathing exercises, and leg exercises.	Patient will be prepared to perform postoperative exercises following surgery.
• Family caregiver identifies location of waiting room and time frame when they can expect status updates on their family member.	Family caregiver anxiety may be reduced with operative expectations clearly provided.
• Family caregivers verbalize understanding of and ability to help prepare patient at home before surgery.	Family caregivers are able and adequately prepared to assist patient with necessary preparations before surgery at home.
2. Provide privacy. Organize and set up any equipment/materials needed to perform preoperative teaching.	Protects patient's privacy; reduces anxiety. Ensures efficiency when completing preoperative teaching.
3. Perform hand hygiene. Assist patient to a comfortable position in bed or chair.	Reduces transmission of microorganisms. Comfort improves ability to attend.
4. Instruct patient and family caregiver about preoperative processes.	Empowers the patient and family caregiver with information; reduces anxiety.
IMPLEMENTATION	
1. Inform patient and family caregiver of date, time, and location of surgery; anticipated length of surgery; additional time in postanesthesia recovery area; and where to wait.	Reduces transmission of infection. Accurate information helps reduce stress of uncertainty associated with surgery.
2. Encourage and answer questions patient and family caregiver ask.	Responding to patient and family caregiver questions helps to decrease anxiety and demonstrates your concern for them.
3. Instruct patient about preoperative bowel or skin preparations as needed. Check medical orders and agency policy regarding number of preoperative showers and agent to be used for each shower (2% chlorhexidine gluconate is used most often). Following each preoperative shower, instruct patient to rinse the skin thoroughly and dry with a fresh, clean, dry towel. Patient should don clean clothing.	Proper skin preparation is a critical element in preventing surgical site infections (SSIs). Rinsing skin removes residual antiseptic preparation that may cause skin irritation. After use, towels contain microorganisms that can grow in presence of moisture. Using fresh towel after each shower and donning clean clothing minimizes risk of reintroducing microorganisms to clean skin (AORN, 2015; Berrios-Torres et al., 2017).
4. Instruct patient about extent and purpose of food and fluid restrictions for period specified before surgery (e.g., no clear liquids at least 2 hours before surgery, no light meal [e.g., toast and a clear liquid] 6 hours or more before surgery, no meat or fried foods 8 hours before surgery, unless otherwise specified by surgeon or anesthesiologist; ASA, 2017).	During general anesthesia, muscles relax; gastric contents can reflux into esophagus, leading to aspiration. Anesthetic eliminates patient's ability to gag.
5. Describe perioperative routines (e.g., time-out procedure, operative site marking, intravenous [IV] therapy, urinary catheterization, hair clipping or removal, laboratory tests, transport to operating room [OR]).	Allows patient to anticipate and recognize routine procedures, reducing anxiety. Empowers patient with information about what staff does to keep patient safe for operative process.
6. Describe planned effect of preoperative medications.	Provides information about what to expect, decreasing anxiety.
7. Review which routine medications patient needs to discontinue before surgery.	Some medications are discontinued before surgery to minimize effects that can cause surgical risks. For example, anticoagulants may increase bleeding and are usually discontinued several days before surgery. Insulin dosages are usually adjusted because of reduced intake of food before surgery.
8. Describe perioperative sensations and sounds (e.g., blood pressure cuff tightening, electrocardiogram [ECG] leads, cool room, and beep of monitor).	Misconceptions and concerns about perioperative sensations and sounds have been ranked high among preoperative patients. Knowing what to expect lessens anxiety.
9. Describe pain-control methods to be used after surgery. Many patients have a patient-controlled analgesia (PCA) pump (see Chapter 15).	Patients are fearful of postoperative pain. Explaining pain-management techniques reduces this fear. This helps the nurse understand what degree of pain the patient feels is acceptable and educates the patient that although he or she will not be pain-free, his or her pain will be managed.

STEP	RATIONALE
10. Describe what patient will experience after surgery (e.g., where patient will be upon awakening; that frequent vital signs will be taken; presence of dressing, catheters, drains, tubes; alternating pressure from sequential compression device; postoperative exercises that will need to be done).	Provides objective description of what patient can expect after surgery so that patient is prepared.
11. Teach turning:	
a. Instruct patient on turning and sitting up (especially suited for abdominal and thoracic surgery):	Promotes circulation and ventilation.
(1) Have patient turn onto right side, assume supine position, and move to side of bed (in this case left side) if permitted by surgery. Instruct patient to move by bending knees and pressing heels against mattress to raise and move buttocks (see illustration). Top side rails on both sides of bed should be in upright position.	Positioning begins on side of bed so that turning to other side does not cause patient to roll toward edge of bed. Buttocks lift prevents shearing force against sheets. If patient's bed has a turn-assist feature, use it to help position him or her.
(2) Have patient splint incision with right hand or with right hand with pillow over incisional area; keep right leg straight and flex left knee up (see illustration); grab right side rail with left hand, pull toward right, and roll onto right side. Reverse process to turn to left side.	Supports incision and decreases discomfort while turning.
(3) Instruct patient to turn every 2 hours from side to side while awake. Often patient requires assistance with turning after surgery.	Reduces risk of vascular, pulmonary, and pressure injury complications.

Safe Patient Care *Some patients, such as those who have had back surgery or vascular repair, are restricted from flexing their legs after surgery. Some patients are restricted from turning or may need help for positioning (see Chapter 18).*

STEP	RATIONALE
(4) Sit up on right side of bed. Elevate head of bed and have patient turn onto right side. While lying on right side, patient pushes on mattress with left arm and swings feet over edge of bed with nurse's help. To sit up on left side of bed, reverse this process.	Sitting position lowers diaphragm to permit fuller lung expansion.

Safe Patient Care *Caution patient to always use the nurse call system to ask for assistance to reduce risk of a fall.*

STEP	RATIONALE
12. Teach coughing and deep breathing:	Patient may hesitate to take deep breaths because of weakness or pain. Collection of secretions in the base of the lungs increases risk of pulmonary atelectasis and pneumonia. This is especially important for patients with a history of smoking, pneumonia, or chronic obstructive pulmonary disease (COPD) or patients who are confined to bed rest.
a. Assist patient to high-Fowler's position in bed with knees flexed, or have patient sit on side of bed or chair in upright position.	Sitting position facilitates diaphragmatic expansion.
b. Instruct patient to place palms of hands across from one another lightly along lower border of rib cage or upper abdomen (see illustration).	Allows patient to feel rise and fall of abdomen during deep breathing.

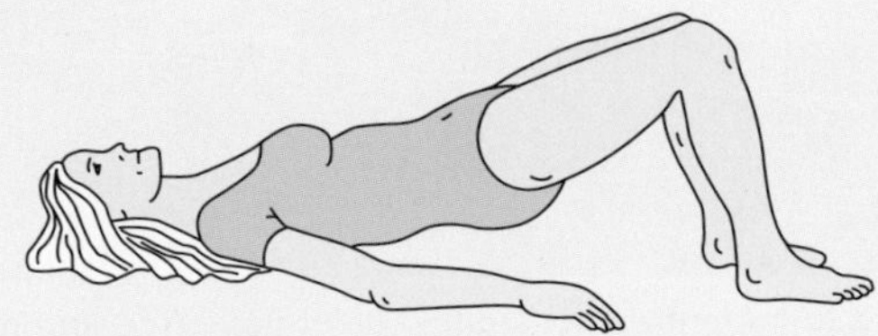

STEP 11a(1) Buttocks lift for moving to side of bed.

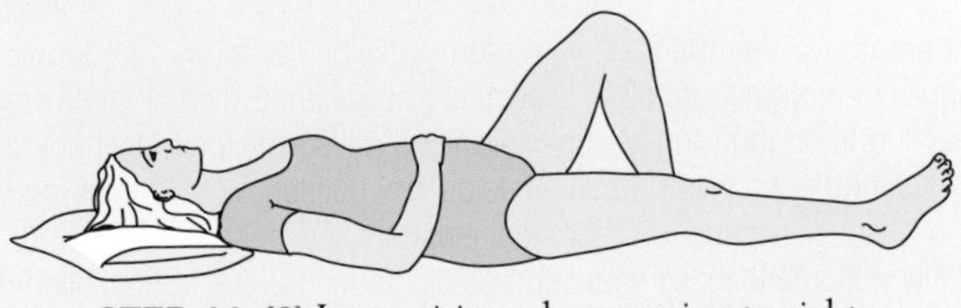

STEP 11a(2) Leg position when turning to right.

STEP	RATIONALE
c. Have patient take slow, deep breaths, inhaling through nose. Explain that patient will feel normal downward movement of diaphragm during inspiration. Demonstrate as needed.	Helps to prevent hyperventilation or panting. Slow deep breath allows for more complete lung expansion.
d. Have patient avoid using chest and shoulder muscles while inhaling.	Increases unnecessary energy expenditure and does not promote full lung expansion.
e. After patient takes slow, deep breath through the nose; hold for count of 3 seconds; and slowly exhale through mouth as if blowing out candle (pursed lips).	Resistance during exhalation helps to prevent alveolar collapse.
f. Have patient repeat breathing exercise 3 to 5 times.	Repetition reinforces learning.
g. Have patient take two slow, deep breaths, inhaling through nose and exhaling through pursed lips.	Deep breaths expand lungs fully to aid gas exchange and remove anesthetic agent so that patient regains consciousness (Lewis et al., 2017). Deep breaths also move air behind mucus to facilitate coughing.
h. Have patient inhale deeply a third time and hold breath to count of 3. Cough fully for two to three consecutive coughs without inhaling between coughs.	Deep breathing and coughing prevent alveolar collapse and move respiratory secretions to larger airways for expectoration (Lewis et al., 2017).
i. Caution patient against just clearing throat without deep breathing.	Clearing throat does not remove mucus from deeper airways.
j. Have patient practice several times. Instruct patient to perform turning, coughing, and deep breathing every 1 to 2 hours (Lewis et al., 2017). Have family caregiver coach patient to exercise.	Allows for full chest expansion and increased perfusion of both lungs (Lewis et al., 2017). Decrease risk of postoperative pneumonia developing.
13. Teach use of an incentive spirometer:	Provides visual aid of respiratory effort. Encourages deep breathing to loosen secretions in lung bases.
a. Position patient in sitting position in chair or in reclining position with head of bed elevated at least 45 degrees.	Facilitates diaphragm lowering and lung expansion.
b. Set targeted tidal volume on the incentive spirometer according to manufacturer directions. Explain that this is the volume level to be reached with each breath.	Establishes goal of volume level necessary for adequate lung expansion. Manufacturers determine target on basis of patient height and age.
c. Explain how to place mouthpiece of incentive spirometer so that lips completely cover mouthpiece (see illustration). Have patient demonstrate until position is correct.	Validates patient's understanding of instructions and evaluates psychomotor skills.
d. Instruct patient to exhale completely, then position mouthpiece so that lips completely cover it, and inhale slowly, maintaining constant flow through unit until reaching targeted tidal volume (see illustration).	Promotes complete inflation of lungs and minimizes atelectasis. Aiming toward target volume offers visual feedback of respiratory effort.

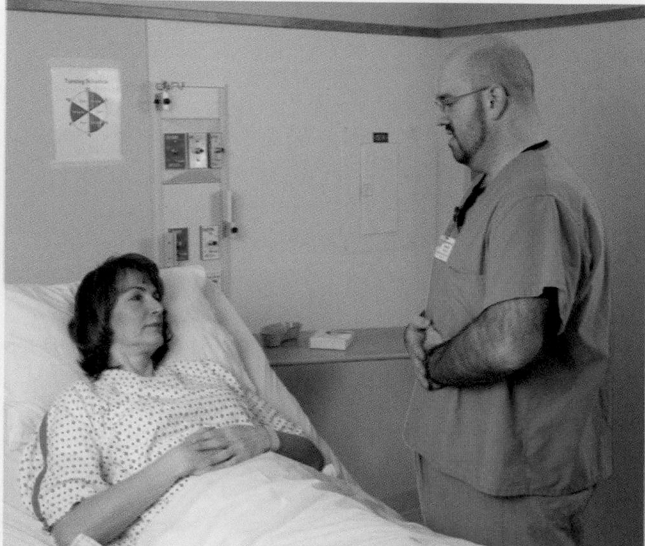

STEP 12b Deep-breathing exercise—placement of hands on upper abdomen during inhalation.

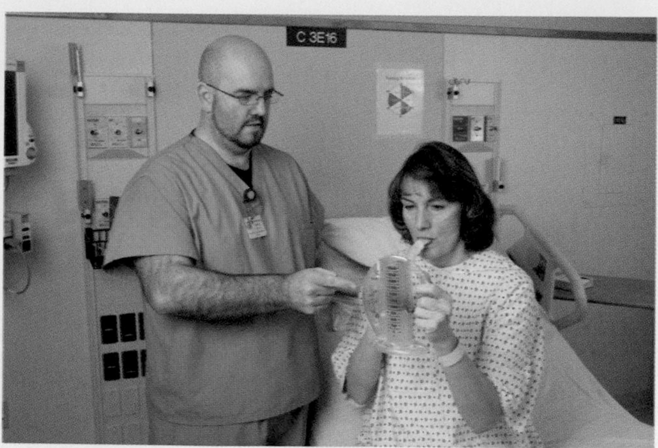

STEP 13c Patient demonstrates use of incentive spirometry.

STEP	RATIONALE
e. Once maximum inspiration is reached, have patient hold breath for 2 to 3 seconds and exhale slowly.	Promotes alveolar inflation.
f. Instruct patient to breathe normally for short period between each of the 10 breaths taken on incentive spirometer. Repeat every hour while awake.	Prevents hyperventilation and fatigue.
14. Teach positive expiratory pressure (PEP) therapy:	
a. Set PEP device for setting ordered.	Higher settings require more effort.
b. Instruct patient to assume semi-Fowler's or high-Fowler's position in bed or to sit in a chair and place nose clip on patient's nose (see illustration).	Promotes optimum lung expansion and expectoration of mucus.
c. Have patient place lips around mouthpiece. Instruct patient to take full breath and exhale 2 or 3 times longer than inhalation. Repeat pattern for 10 to 20 breaths.	Ensures that patient does all breathing through mouth. Ensures that patient uses device properly.
d. Remove device from mouth and have patient take slow, deep breath and hold for 3 seconds.	Promotes lung expansion before coughing.
e. Instruct patient to exhale with a deep cough. Repeat exercise every 2 hours while awake.	Coughing promotes bronchial hygiene by increasing expectoration of secretions.
15. Teach controlled coughing:	Deep breaths expand lungs fully so that air moves behind mucus and facilitates effective coughing.
a. Explain importance of maintaining upright position in bed or chair; have patient lean slightly forward.	Position facilitates diaphragm excursion and enhances thorax and abdominal expansion.
b. Demonstrate coughing. Fold arms across abdomen and breathe in slowly through the nose.	Expands lungs.
c. To exhale: lean forward, pressing your arms against your abdomen. Cough 2 to 3 times without inhaling between coughs. Cough through a slightly open mouth. Coughs should be short and sharp (Cleveland Clinic, 2017; see illustration).	Clearing throat does not remove mucus from deeper airways. Full, forceful cough is most effective in removing mucus.
d. Breathe in again by "sniffing" slowly and gently through the nose.	Prevents mucus from moving back down airways.
e. Caution patient against just clearing throat instead of coughing deeply. Have patient rest a few minutes and repeat exercise.	Clearing throat does not remove mucus from deeper airways.
f. If surgical incision is thoracic or abdominal, teach patient to place either hands or pillow over incisional area and place hands over pillow to splint incision (see illustration). During breathing and coughing exercises, press gently against incisional area for splinting and support.	Surgical incision cuts through muscles, tissues, and nerve endings. Deep-breathing and coughing exercises place additional stress on suture line and cause discomfort. Splinting incision with hands or pillow provides firm support and reduces incisional pulling and pain.
g. Instruct patient to cough 2 to 3 times every 2 hours while awake and to continue to practice coughing exercises, splinting imaginary incision (see illustration).	Deep coughing with splinting effectively expectorates mucus with minimal discomfort.

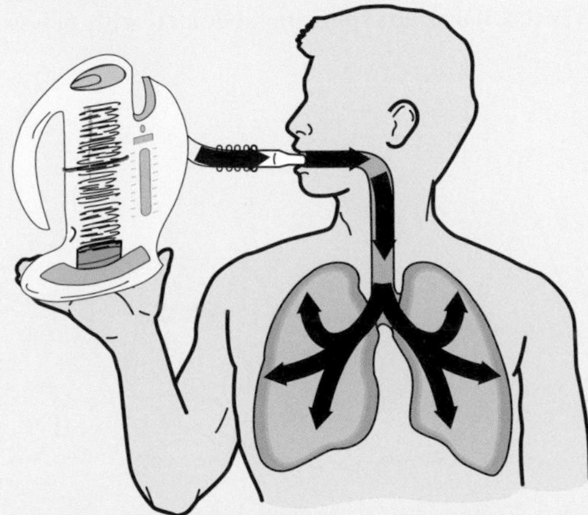

STEP 13d Diagram of use of incentive spirometer.

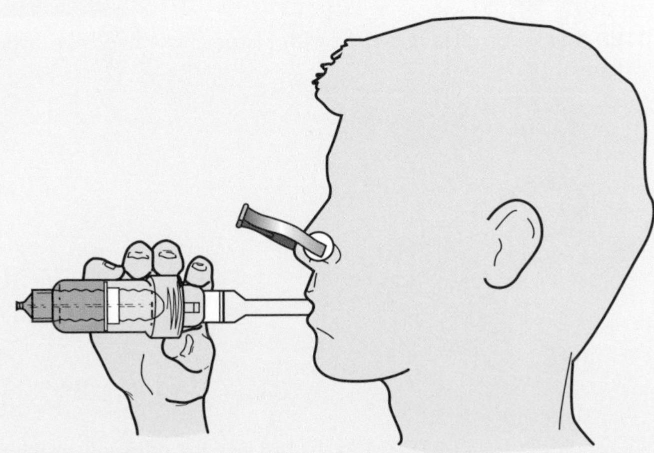

STEP 14b Diagram of use of positive expiratory pressure device.

STEP	RATIONALE
h. Instruct patient to examine sputum for consistency, odor, amount, and color changes and notify a nurse if any changes are noted.	Sputum consistency, odor, amount, and color changes may indicate presence of pulmonary complication such as pneumonia.
16. Teach leg exercises:	

Safe Patient Care *Leg exercises are recommended for patients restricted to bed or during times when patients are ambulatory but resting in bed or in a chair. The ideal exercise to promote venous return and improve lung vital capacity is early mobility (see Chapter 18).*

STEP	RATIONALE
a. Instruct patient to perform leg exercises every 1 to 2 hours while awake: ankle rotation, dorsiflexion and plantar flexion, leg extension and flexion, and straight leg raises.	Leg exercises facilitate venous return from lower extremities and reduce risk of circulatory complications such as venous thromboembolism.
b. Position patient supine.	
c. Instruct patient to rotate each ankle in complete circle and draw imaginary circles with big toe 5 times (see illustration).	Promotes joint mobility.
d. Alternate dorsiflexion and plantar flexion while instructing patient to feel calf muscles tighten and relax. Repeat 5 times (see illustration).	Helps maintain joint mobility and promote venous return to prevent thrombus formation.
e. Perform quadriceps setting by tightening thigh and bringing knee down toward mattress and relaxing. Repeat 5 times (see illustration).	Quadriceps-setting exercises contract muscles of upper legs, maintain knee mobility, and improve venous return to heart.
f. Instruct patient to alternate raising legs straight up from bed surface. Leg should be kept straight. Repeat 5 times (see illustration).	Causes quadriceps muscle contraction and relaxation, which help promote venous return.

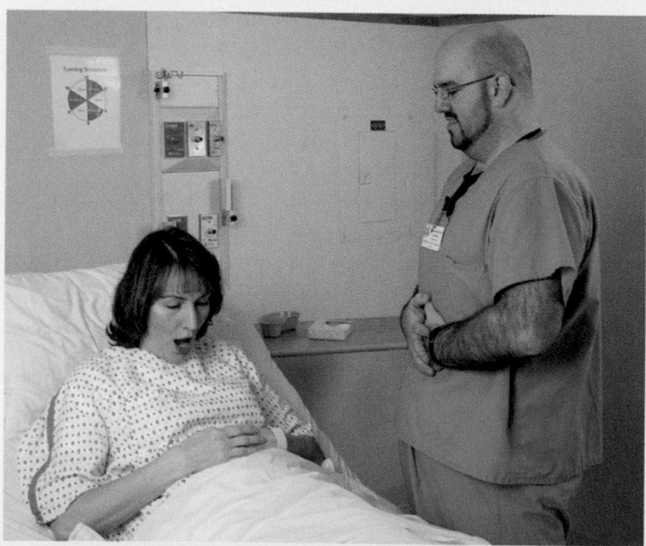

STEP 15c Controlled coughing with placement of hands on upper abdomen.

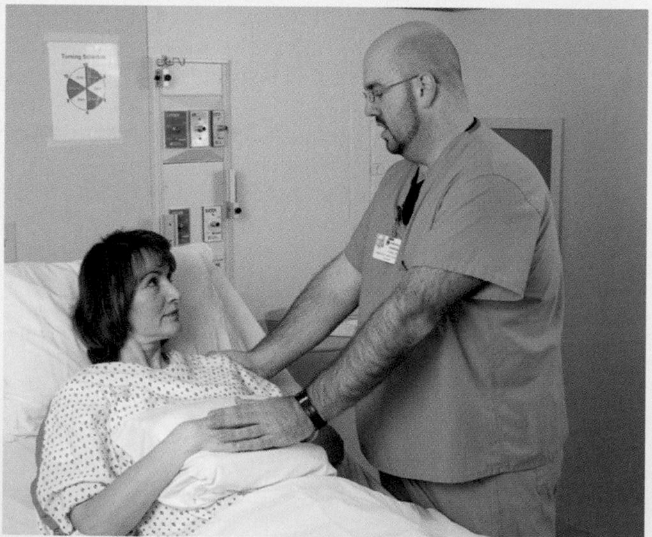

STEP 15f Patient splinting abdomen with pillow.

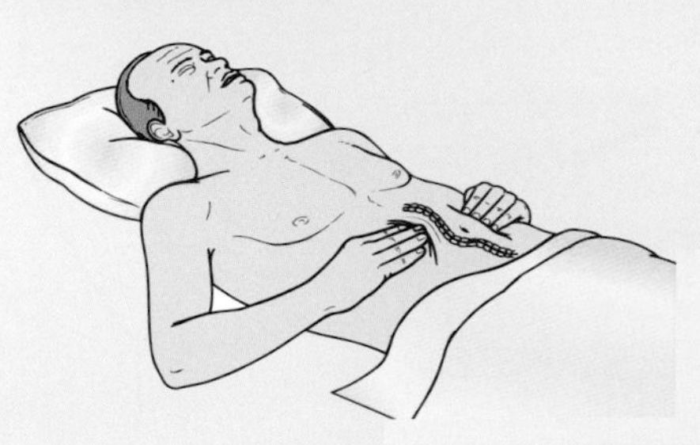

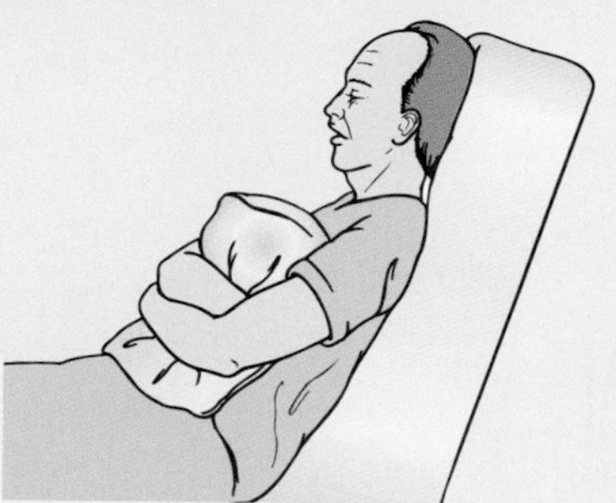

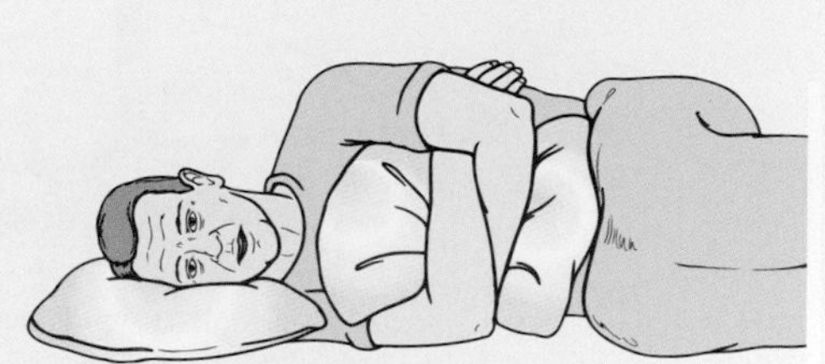

STEP 15g Techniques for splinting incisions. *(From Lewis SL, et al: Medical-surgical nursing: assessment and management of clinical problems, ed 8, St Louis, 2011, Mosby.)*

STEP	RATIONALE

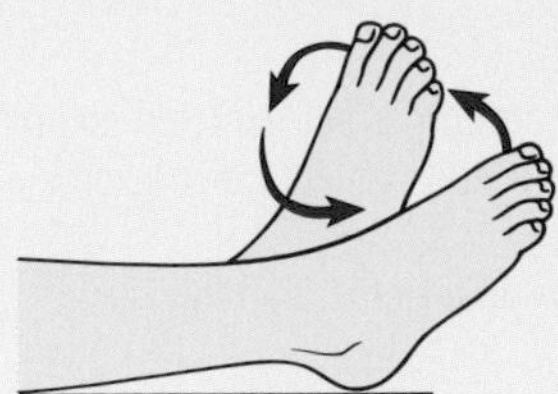

STEP 16c Foot circles. *(From Lewis S et al: Medical-surgical nursing: assessment and management of clinical problems, ed 9, St. Louis, 2014, Mosby.)*

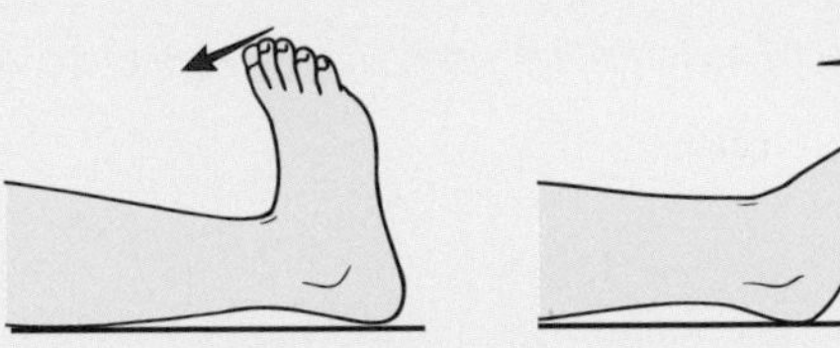

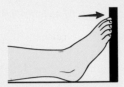

STEP 16d Alternate dorsiflexion and plantar flexion. *(From Lewis S et al: Medical-surgical nursing: assessment and management of clinical problems, ed 9, St. Louis, 2014, Mosby.)*

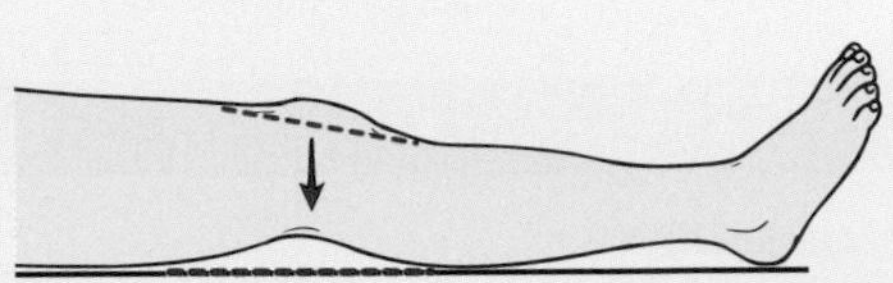

STEP 16e Quadriceps (thigh) setting. *(From Lewis S et al: Medical-surgical nursing: assessment and management of clinical problems, ed 9, St. Louis, 2014, Mosby.)*

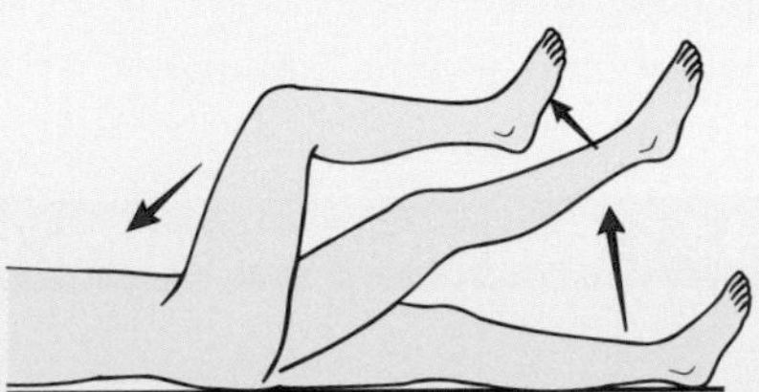

STEP 16f Hip and knee movements. *(From Lewis S et al: Medical-surgical nursing: assessment and management of clinical problems, ed 9, St. Louis, 2014, Mosby.)*

STEP	RATIONALE
17. Have patient continue to practice exercises before surgery at least every 2 hours while awake. Teach patient to coordinate turning and leg exercises with diaphragmatic breathing and use of incentive spirometer.	Leg exercises stimulate circulation, which prevents venous stasis to help prevent formation of deep vein thrombosis (DVT). Coordinating exercises help patient continuously work toward best outcomes for recovery.
18. Answer questions and verify patient's expectations of surgery. Coach expectations as needed.	Can reduce postoperative anxiety or anger.
19. Reinforce therapeutic coping strategies (e.g., meditation, calming conversation [Aust et al., 2016], listening to music).	Therapeutic coping strategies that self-distract patients from thinking about surgery reduce preoperative anxiety.
20. Help patient to a comfortable position.	Gives patient a sense of well-being.
21. Be sure nurse call system is in an accessible location within patient's reach.	Ensures patient can call for assistance if needed.
22. Raise side rails (as appropriate) and lower bed to lowest position.	Ensures patient safety.
23. After completion of preoperative teaching, appropriately dispose of supplies and equipment and perform hand hygiene.	Reduces transmission of microorganisms.

EVALUATION

STEP	RATIONALE
1. If possible, observe patient demonstrating splinting, turning and sitting, deep breathing, use of incentive spirometer, PEP therapy, and leg exercises.	Validates patient's ability to correctly perform postoperative exercises and use devices.
2. Ask family member(s) to identify location of surgical waiting room and time frame when they can expect status updates on their family member.	Demonstrates learning.
3. Ask family caregiver to describe how he or she can coach patient with exercises at home prior to surgery.	Demonstrates understanding of role family member can play to support patient.
4. **Use Teach-Back:** "I want to be sure I explained what you need to know about the exercises we want you to perform after surgery. Tell me which exercises you will do and how to do them." Revise your instruction now or develop a plan for revised patient/family caregiver teaching if patient/family caregiver is not able to teach back correctly.	Determines patient's/family caregiver's level of understanding of instructional topic.

Unexpected Outcomes	Related Interventions
1. Patient identifies incorrect surgical procedure, site, date, or time of surgery.	• Provide correct information verbally and in writing for patient and family caregiver.
2. Patient incorrectly performs/describes postoperative exercise(s).	• Explain and demonstrate correct exercise technique. • Explain importance of the postoperative exercise as it pertains to patient recovery. • Instruct patient to repeat demonstration.

Recording

- Document preoperative teaching on the appropriate place within the patient's record. There is often a preoperative education flow sheet or designated agency form where this information should be documented.
- Document evaluation of patient learning.

Hand-Off Reporting

- Report patient's inability to identify procedure and site of surgery, as well as understanding of postoperative exercise(s) and teaching. to health care provider.

✦ SKILL 29.3 Patient Preparation Before Surgery

Purpose

Preparation of a patient for surgery involves confirming key assessment factors, providing ordered preoperative procedures, verifying patient understanding, verifying that required procedures and tests have been performed, and documenting care in the patient's record. Preparation begins when the patient is admitted to the surgical center and continues to transfer to the operating room. The physical care procedures depend on the type of surgery being performed and the risks involved. For example, compression stockings, intermittent compression devices (ICDs), and the venous foot pump are frequently used for adult patients undergoing surgery that will last several hours and require a long period of immobilization afterward. Bowel preparation such as an enema, laxative, or cathartic (which is done at home by patients admitted the morning of surgery) may be required for abdominal surgery involving the intestine. Regardless of the type of surgery, the goal of physical preparation is to place the patient in the best condition possible to minimize the risks of the planned surgery and achieve subsequent best outcomes.

The World Health Organization (WHO, n.d.) offers a Surgical Safety Checklist (Fig. 29.2) that ensures effective communication and safe practices during three perioperative periods: prior to administration of anesthesia, prior to skin incision, and prior to the patient leaving the operative area. Hospitals and surgical outpatient centers can modify or add to the checklist based on their practice guidelines.

Delegation and Collaboration

The skill of coordinating a patient's preparation for surgery cannot be delegated to nursing assistive personnel (NAP). However, the NAP may administer an enema or douche, obtain vital signs in stable patients, apply antiembolic stockings, and help patients remove clothing, jewelry, or prostheses (see agency policy). The nurse instructs the NAP about:

- Using basic infection control practices and proper precautions when preparing a patient for surgery.
- Observing and using precautions if the patient has an intravenous (IV) catheter or other invasive device in place.

Equipment

NOTE: Equipment varies by procedure.

- Vital sign equipment: Stethoscope, blood pressure (BP) cuff, thermometer, pulse oximeter
- Oxygen equipment
- Suction equipment as ordered
- Hospital gown and disposable head cover
- IV solution and equipment (see Chapter 28)
- Skin cleansing solution
- Compression (antiembolism) stockings (see Chapter 18)
- Intermittent compression devices (ICD)
- Venous foot pump
- Urinary catheterization kit (see Chapter 19)
- Preoperative checklist
- Medications (e.g., sedative)
- Clean gloves

ASSESSMENT

1. Identify patient using at least two identifiers (e.g., name and birthday or name and medical record number) according to agency policy. *Rationale: Ensures correct patient. Complies with The Joint Commission standards and improves patient safety (TJC, 2019).*
2. Perform hand hygiene. Complete preoperative assessment (see Skill 29.1); confirm patient procedure, presence of allergies, any airway or bleeding risks (WHO, n.d.). *Rationale: Provides baseline assessment data for surgical team.* **NOTE:** *Assessment conducted at time of admission to surgery center may differ from that performed preoperatively. Confirms patient risks.*
3. Assess and record patient's heart rate, blood pressure, respiratory rate, oxygen saturation, and temperature. *Option:* Keep oximeter attached to patient (WHO, n.d.). *Rationale: Provides baseline for patient's preoperative status. Continuous oximetry monitoring will occur during surgery.*
4. If patient is same-day admit or ambulatory patient, validate that admission preparations (e.g., enema, shower with antiseptic, withholding medications) were completed at home as ordered. Ensure that patient has followed appropriate fluid and food restrictions per surgeon or anesthesiologist order (see Skill 29.2). *Rationale: Failure to complete preparation could lead to perioperative or postoperative complications and may necessitate postponement or cancellation of surgery.*
5. Ask if patient has advance directive. If so, be certain a copy is available in the patient's health record. *Rationale:*

World Health Organization

SURGICAL SAFETY CHECKLIST (FIRST EDITION)

Before induction of anaesthesia ▸▸▸▸▸▸▸▸▸	Before skin incision ▸▸▸▸▸▸▸▸▸▸▸▸▸▸	Before patient leaves operating room
SIGN IN	**TIME OUT**	**SIGN OUT**
☐ **PATIENT HAS CONFIRMED** • IDENTITY • SITE • PROCEDURE • CONSENT ☐ **SITE MARKED/NOT APPLICABLE** ☐ **ANAESTHESIA SAFETY CHECK COMPLETED** ☐ **PULSE OXIMETER ON PATIENT AND FUNCTIONING** **DOES PATIENT HAVE A: KNOWN ALLERGY?** ☐ NO ☐ YES **DIFFICULT AIRWAY/ASPIRATION RISK?** ☐ NO ☐ YES, AND EQUIPMENT/ASSISTANCE AVAILABLE **RISK OF >500ML BLOOD LOSS (7ML/KG IN CHILDREN)?** ☐ NO ☐ YES, AND ADEQUATE INTRAVENOUS ACCESS AND FLUIDS PLANNED	☐ **CONFIRM ALL TEAM MEMBERS HAVE INTRODUCED THEMSELVES BY NAME AND ROLE** ☐ **SURGEON, ANAESTHESIA PROFESSIONAL AND NURSE VERBALLY CONFIRM** • PATIENT • SITE • PROCEDURE **ANTICIPATED CRITICAL EVENTS** ☐ **SURGEON REVIEWS:** WHAT ARE THE CRITICAL OR UNEXPECTED STEPS, OPERATIVE DURATION, ANTICIPATED BLOOD LOSS? ☐ **ANAESTHESIA TEAM REVIEWS:** ARE THERE ANY PATIENT-SPECIFIC CONCERNS? ☐ **NURSING TEAM REVIEWS:** HAS STERILITY (INCLUDING INDICATOR RESULTS) BEEN CONFIRMED? ARE THERE EQUIPMENT ISSUES OR ANY CONCERNS? **HAS ANTIBIOTIC PROPHYLAXIS BEEN GIVEN WITHIN THE LAST 60 MINUTES?** ☐ YES ☐ NOT APPLICABLE **IS ESSENTIAL IMAGING DISPLAYED?** ☐ YES ☐ NOT APPLICABLE	**NURSE VERBALLY CONFIRMS WITH THE TEAM:** ☐ **THE NAME OF THE PROCEDURE RECORDED** ☐ **THAT INSTRUMENT, SPONGE AND NEEDLE COUNTS ARE CORRECT (OR NOT APPLICABLE)** ☐ **HOW THE SPECIMEN IS LABELLED (INCLUDING PATIENT NAME)** ☐ **WHETHER THERE ARE ANY EQUIPMENT PROBLEMS TO BE ADDRESSED** ☐ **SURGEON, ANAESTHESIA PROFESSIONAL AND NURSE REVIEW THE KEY CONCERNS FOR RECOVERY AND MANAGEMENT OF THIS PATIENT**

THIS CHECKLIST IS NOT INTENDED TO BE COMPREHENSIVE. ADDITIONS AND MODIFICATIONS TO FIT LOCAL PRACTICE ARE ENCOURAGED.

FIG 29.2 World Health Organization's Surgical Safety Checklist. (*Courtesy World Health Organization: Surgical safety checklist, n.d. http://www.who.int/patientsafety/safesurgery/tools_resources/SSSL_Checklist_finalJun08.pdf.*)

Document conveys patient's wishes if life-support measures are necessary.

6. Ask if patient has any final questions about procedure. *Rationale: Provides opportunity to clarify any misunderstanding.*

7. Assess patient's or family caregiver's knowledge, experience, and health literacy. *Rationale: Ensures patient or family caregiver has the capacity to obtain, communicate, process, and understand basic health information (CDC, 2016).*

STEP	RATIONALE
PLANNING	
1. Expected outcomes following completion of procedure:	
• Patient can state which surgical procedure is being performed and risks and benefits of surgery.	Identifies understanding and readiness to sign informed consent.
• Patient states that anxiety is managed.	Managed anxiety increases patient confidence and participation in own care.

STEP	RATIONALE
2. Perform hand hygiene. Provide privacy. Organize and set up any equipment needed.	Reduces transmission of microorganisms. Protects patient's privacy; reduces anxiety. Ensures more efficiency when completing preoperative procedures.
3. Instruct patient and family caregiver about purpose of physical preparation for surgery.	Empowers the patient and family caregiver with information; reduces anxiety.

IMPLEMENTATION

STEP	RATIONALE
1. Perform hand hygiene. Help patient put on hospital gown and remove personal items. Before any procedure, decrease anxiety by explaining how equipment or preparation will feel (e.g., cold, tight) before touching patient.	Reduces transmission of microorganisms. Decreases anxiety by allowing patient to orient to surroundings and understand pre-surgical procedures.
2. Instruct patient to remove makeup, nail polish, hairpins, and jewelry. **NOTE:** This is usually recommended earlier when patient receives initial preoperative instruction.	Hair appliances and jewelry anywhere on body may become dislodged and cause injury during positioning and intubation. Rings decrease circulation in fingers. Makeup, nail polish, and artificial nails impede assessment of skin and oxygenation. Artificial nails harbor pathogenic organisms (Rothrock, 2015).
3. Ensure that money and valuables have been locked up or given to a family caregiver.	Patient may not return to same location after surgery. Prevents valuables from being misplaced or lost.
4. Verify again the presence of allergies and ensure that allergy/sensitivity band or other safety armbands are present.	Alerts surgeons and health care team to potential allergies.
5. Verify that patient has followed instructions about omission or ingestion of medications as instructed.	Misuse or inaccurate medication dosage could precipitate complications.
6. Assess patient's fall risks; apply fall risk armband if appropriate.	Alerts all health care providers to patient's risk for falling.
7. Verify that bowel preparation (e.g., laxative, cathartic, enema) has been completed by patient or family caregiver at home if ordered.	Proper bowel evacuation is needed for surgery to be performed to decrease the chance for postoperative ileus.

Safe Patient Care *In some situations, additional enemas and/or cathartics are ordered. Emptying the bowel is necessary for bowel surgery and to decrease the risk of postoperative ileus. Enemas are used when surgery is near the lower intestine.*

STEP	RATIONALE
8. Ensure that medical history and physical examination results are in patient's record.	Ensures that pertinent data are available and that all preoperative preparations are completed.
9. Verify that surgical consent, anesthesia consent, and consent for blood transfusion are complete. The name of procedure; name of surgeon; date; name of person authorized to obtain surgical consent; signature of surgeon (or authorized person) obtaining consent, anesthesia provider delivering anesthesia, and witness (often the nurse); and patient's signature all should be present.	Ensures patient's agreement to undergo intended procedure. In most settings, the surgeon obtains consent, and the nurse verifies that it is complete and consistent with patient's understanding (refer to agency policy).
10. Ensure that necessary laboratory work, electrocardiogram (ECG), and chest x-ray film studies are completed and results are available in the chart.	Diagnostic test results provide information necessary during surgical procedure and provide data to monitor for postoperative comparison (Nagelhout and Elisha, 2017).
11. Verify that blood type and cross-match are completed as ordered or per agency protocol, and that blood transfusions are available as needed.	In many cases surgery cannot begin without availability of blood units.
12. Instruct patient to void.	Prevents risk of bladder distention or rupture during surgery.
13. Perform hand hygiene. Apply clean gloves. Start IV line; refer to unit standards or surgeon's orders (see Chapter 28). Connect to ordered IV fluid and maintain at keep-open rate. Remove and dispose of gloves.	IV line provides access for fluids and medications to be administered when in operating room (OR).
14. Administer preoperative medications as ordered (e.g., preoperative antibiotics, prophylactic agents).	Preoperative medications are used for various reasons and should be administered as ordered for maximum effectiveness.

STEP	RATIONALE
15. Apply compression stockings (see Chapter 18).	Compression stockings promote circulation during periods of immobilization, reducing risk of embolism.
16. Apply intermittent compression devices (ICDs) if ordered. **NOTE:** ICDs may or may not be used in combination with compression stockings. Verify order.	ICDs push blood from superficial veins into deep veins, decreasing venous stasis.

Safe Patient Care *ICDs do not provide effective venous thromboembolism prophylaxis if the device is not applied correctly or if the patient does not wear the device continuously except during bathing, skin assessment, and ambulation. ICDs are not to be worn when a patient has a deep vein thrombosis (DVT) because of the risk for pulmonary embolism.*

STEP	RATIONALE
17. Perform hand hygiene. Apply clean gloves. Clean and prepare surgical site as ordered. Remove and dispose of gloves.	This step is more likely to be performed in the operating suite. Cleaning with antimicrobial soap decreases bacterial flora on skin. Reduces transmission of microorganisms.
18. Perform hand hygiene. Apply sterile gloves. Insert urinary catheter as ordered (see Chapter 19). **NOTE:** There are times when urinary catheter is placed in OR. Remove and dispose of gloves.	Maintains bladder decompression and provides for monitoring output during surgery.
19. Allow patient to wear eyeglasses or hearing aid as long as possible before surgery so that patient is able to sign consents and read materials. Remove contact lenses, eyeglasses, hairpieces, and dentures just before surgery (see checklist completed before surgery noting that all items are removed before proceeding to OR).	These aids facilitate patient cooperation by ensuring that patient has clear vision and maximal auditory perception throughout preoperative phase.
20. Place head cover over patient's head and hair.	The cap contains hair and minimizes contamination during surgery. Plastic or reflective caps reduce heat loss during surgery.
21. Place patient on bed rest with nurse call system within reach and inform him or her not to get out of bed without help. Allow family members to remain at bedside until patient is transferred to surgical area. Maintain quiet and relaxing environment. If patient is sedated, do not leave patient.	Increases safety and allows patient to have the comfort of loved ones present as long as possible. There is increased chance of injury by trying to ambulate to void when patient is sedated and unattended, so never leave patient unattended once sedating medication has been administered.
22. Transfer patient via stretcher bed to OR. Raise side rails appropriately.	Facilitates transportation to OR suite. Provides patient safety.
23. Dispose of supplies and equipment in preoperative bay. Perform hand hygiene.	Reduces transmission of microorganisms.

EVALUATION

1. Have patient describe surgical procedure and its benefits and risks.	Confirms level of knowledge needed to sign informed consent.
2. Have patient repeat preoperative instructions.	Provides evidence that patient understands instructions.
3. Monitor patient for signs and symptoms of anxiety and ask how patient and family caregivers are feeling.	Increased heart rate and blood pressure, dilated pupils, dry mouth, increased sweating, and muscle rigidity or shaking may indicate stress and anxiety. Asking patient and family caregivers about feelings gives permission to express concerns, which can be further explored.
4. Confirm IV is infusing at a keep-open or ordered rate.	Patent and functional IV is needed when patient enters operating room suite.
5. **Use Teach-Back:** "I want to be sure you are ready for surgery. Tell me what you expect to happen once you get to the recovery room." Revise your instruction now or develop a plan for revised patient/family caregiver teaching if patient/family caregiver is not able to teach back correctly.	Determines patient's/family caregiver's level of understanding of instructional topic.

Unexpected Outcomes	Related Interventions
1. Patient is unable to give consent, and family member is unavailable.	• In emergency situations, strictly follow agency policy. This may involve obtaining consent from power of attorney. • If agency policy allows for oral consent to be obtained from power of attorney, document explanation of situation and fact that oral consent was obtained and witnessed by two people (or per agency policy). • At earliest opportunity, follow agency policy to obtain written consent from the person who gave oral consent. Signed telegram or signed fax may also be considered oral consent.
2. Patient did not maintain nothing-by-mouth (NPO) status, which may place him or her at risk for aspiration and may indicate that he or she did not understand instructions or forgot.	• Notify surgeon and anesthesiologist. Surgery may be postponed or canceled.
3. Informed consent has not been signed and witnessed. Surgeon and anesthesiologist did not provide information and/or ensure that consent forms were signed.	• Patient is not ready for surgery. Patient must sign consent before administration of preoperative medications or any medication that alters central nervous system. Notify surgeon and anesthesiologist.

Recording

- Document preoperative physical preparation.
- Document that informed consent has been completed.

Hand-Off Reporting

- Report to nursing staff receiving patient in OR that preoperative physical preparation has been successfully completed, any deviations from appropriate preparation, and that completed informed consent is available in the patient's record.

✦ SKILL 29.4 Providing Immediate Anesthesia Recovery in the Postanesthesia Care Unit (PACU)

Purpose

There are three phases of anesthesia recovery. Phase I recovery begins when a patient leaves the operating room (OR). It extends from the time a patient leaves the OR to the time he or she is stabilized in the PACU, meets discharge criteria, and is transferred to a nursing unit or other location. During Phase I, close monitoring is required; for the first 1 to 2 hours the focus is on assessing for the aftereffects of anesthesia, including airway clearance, cardiovascular complications, fluid management, temperature control, and neurological function. A patient's condition can change rapidly; assessments must be timely, knowledgeable, and accurate. Table 29.1 provides an overview of common postoperative complications and interventions, including expected monitoring following anesthesia. When a patient has progressed beyond these elements of care, the patient can progress to the Phase II level of care, in which plans and care are provided to progress the patient to home (ASPAN, 2018). This care may be provided in the same physical location as Phase I care. Many PACUs provide blended levels of care, in which both levels of care are provided in the same location (ASPAN, 2018). For example, if a patient is ready to ambulate to the bathroom and is awake and stable enough, the patient is not necessarily a Phase I patient anymore; the patient has progressed to the Phase II level of care even if he or she is in the same location (ASPAN, 2018).

During anesthesia recovery, quick judgment regarding the most appropriate interventions is essential. You need to be aware of the common complications and problems associated with specific types of anesthesia (Table 29.2). A patient is usually ready for discharge to a general patient care unit in a hospital when specific standardized criteria are met. The Aldrete score (Table 29.3) and the Postanesthetic Discharge Scoring System (PADSS) are types of scoring systems for assessment. The Aldrete score uses parameters of activity, respiration, circulation, consciousness, and oxygen saturation. A score of 8 or less indicates additional monitoring is required. A score of 10 indicates the full recovery of a patient.

Recovery from ambulatory surgery requires the same assessments. However, the depth of general anesthesia may be less because the surgery is less involved and of shorter duration. Some patients have only IV moderate (conscious) sedation, and intensive monitoring is required for a shorter time period. As soon as the patient is stable and alert, give instructions for home care to the patient and family caregiver, including demonstrations and written instructions.

Delegation and Collaboration

The skill of initiating immediate anesthesia recovery of a patient cannot be delegated to nursing assistive personnel (NAP). The NAP may provide basic comfort and hygiene measures. The nurse instructs the NAP by:

- Explaining any restrictions for how to provide comfort measures
- Offering instruction in providing needed supplies to nurse

Note: NAP may be allowed to do more in ambulatory surgery recovery (see agency guidelines),

Equipment

- Blood pressure monitoring equipment
- Oxygen equipment such as mask, oxygen regulator and tubing, and positive-pressure delivery system

TABLE 29.1

Postanesthesia Complications and Intervention

Condition	Interventions
Airway	
Mechanical obstruction: Decreased LOC and/or use of muscle relaxants result in flaccid muscles and tongue blocking airway	Hyperextend neck; pull mandible forward; use nasal or oral airway; encourage deep breathing.
Retained thick secretions: Irritation from anesthetic; anticholinergic medications; history of smoking	Suction; encourage coughing.
Laryngospasm: Stridor from excessive secretions or airway irritation	Encourage to relax and breathe through the mouth. If extreme, may require positive-pressure ventilation with oxygen, small dose of muscle relaxant (ordered by anesthesiologist), and intubation.
Laryngeal edema: Allergic reaction, irritation from ET tube, fluid overload	Administer humidified oxygen, antihistamines, steroids, sedatives; in some cases, perform reintubation.
Bronchospasm: Preexisting asthma, anesthetic irritation (expiratory wheeze)	Administer bronchodilators as ordered.
Aspiration: Vomiting from hypotension, accumulated gastric secretions and delayed gastric emptying, pain, fear, position changes	Position on side; suction airway; administer antiemetic as ordered.
Breathing: Hypoventilation/Hypoxemia	
CNS depression: Anesthesia, analgesics, muscle relaxants (respiratory rate shallow)	Encourage to cough and deep breathe; use mechanical ventilator; administer narcotic antagonist and muscle relaxant reversal agent.
Mechanical chest restriction: Obesity, pain, tight cast or dressings, abdominal distention	Reposition; administer analgesic; loosen cast or dressings; implement measures to reduce gastric distention (e.g., NG intubation, NG suction).
Circulation	
Hypovolemia: Blood loss, dehydration	Administer IV fluids or blood replacement.
Hypotension: Anesthesia/drug effects, vasodilation (possibly from spinal anesthesia); opioids	Elevate legs; give oxygen, IV fluids, or blood replacement; administer vasopressors; monitor I&O, stimulation, hemoglobin, and hematocrit.
Cardiac failure: Preexisting cardiac disease; circulatory overload; excessive/too-rapid fluid replacement	Provide digitalization and diuretics; monitor ECG.
Cardiac arrhythmias: Hypoxemia; MI; hypothermia; imbalance of potassium, calcium, magnesium	Administer IV fluid replacement; monitor ECG and urine output; identify and treat cause.
Hypertension: Pain; distended bladder; preexisting hypertension; vasopressor drugs	Compare with preoperative baseline; identify and determine cause.
Compartment syndrome: Pressure from edema causing enough compression to obstruct arterial and venous circulation resulting in ischemia, permanent numbness, loss of function; forearm and lower leg most often affected	Obtain compartment pressures to diagnose, and elevate extremity no higher than heart level; remove or loosen bandage or cast to relieve compression; if left untreated, amputation may be required. Do not apply ice.

CNS, Central nervous system; *ECG,* electrocardiogram; *ET,* endotracheal; *I&O,* intake and output; *IV,* intravenous; *LOC,* level of consciousness; *MI,* myocardial infarction; *NG,* nasogastric.

TABLE 29.2

Focused Assessment of Patient Problems Related to Anesthesia Type

Anesthesia Type	Focused Problem Assessment
General	Hypotension; changes in heart rate or rhythm; lowered body temperature; respiratory depression; emergence delirium in the form of shivering, trembling, confusion, or hallucinations; malignant hyperthermia
Spinal	Headache, hypotension, decreased cardiac output, cyanosis, difficulty breathing
Neuromuscular blocking drugs (NMBDs)	Intraocular pressure, intracranial pressure
Local	Skin rash; allergic reaction with edema of the face, lips, mouth, or throat; restlessness; bradycardia; hypotension; ischemic necrosis at injection site; hypertension if given with a vasoconstrictor
Moderate (conscious) sedation	Assess for liver or kidney impairment since this is commonly used across the life span, and older patients may respond differently; Respiratory depression, bradycardia, hypotension, nausea and vomiting
Spinal or epidural	Cyanosis, breathing difficulties, decreased heart rate, irregular heart rate, pale skin color, nausea and vomiting

Data from Lilley LL, Rainforth Collins S, Snyder J: *Pharmacology and the nursing process,* ed 8, St. Louis, 2017, Elsevier.

TABLE 29.3

Aldrete Score for Postanesthesia Monitoring

		Score
Activity (able to move voluntarily or on command)	4 extremities	2
	2 extremities	1
	0 extremities	0
Respiration	Able to deep breathe and cough freely	2
	Dyspnea or limited breathing	1
	Apneic	0
Circulation	BP + 20 mm Hg of preanesthetic level	2
	BP + 20–50 mm Hg of preanesthetic level	1
	BP + 50 mm Hg of preanesthetic level	0
Consciousness	Fully awake	2
	Arousable on having name called	1
	Not responding	0
Oxygen saturation	Able to maintain oxygen saturation >92% on room air	2
	Needs oxygen to maintain oxygen saturation above 90%	1
	Oxygen saturation <90% even with oxygen	0

BP, Blood pressure.

From American Society of PeriAnesthesia Nurses (ASPAN): *2017-2018 perianesthesia nursing standards, practice recommendations and interpretive statements,* Cherry Hill, NJ, 2017, Author.

- Various types and sizes of artificial airways
- Constant and intermittent suction
- Pulse oximeter
- End-tidal carbon dioxide (CO_2) monitor
- Electrocardiogram (ECG) monitor
- Portable ultrasound to assess pulses
- Thermoregulation equipment, including thermometers, blanket warmers, and cooling devices
- Bladder scanner
- IV supplies (if ordered) (see Chapter 28)
- Adult and pediatric emergency cart with defibrillator
- Stock supplies (e.g., facial tissues, dressings, bedpans, urinals, emesis basin)
- Adjustable lighting
- Personal protective equipment
- Latex-free supplies and equipment

ASSESSMENT

1. Identify patient using at least two identifiers (e.g., name and birthday or name and medical record number) according to agency policy. *Rationale: Ensures correct patient. Complies with The Joint Commission standards and improves patient safety (TJC, 2019).*
2. Receive hand-off report from circulating nurse and anesthesia provider, including procedure performed, range of vital signs, any complications, estimated blood loss (EBL), other fluid loss, fluid replacement during surgery, type of anesthesia, medications given, type of airway and size, extent of surgical wound, restrictions to movement of position during surgery, and any preoperative medical and/or nursing diagnoses. *Rationale: Determines patient's general status and allows you to anticipate ongoing assessment needs, the need for special equipment, potential treatment measures, and nursing care interventions in PACU.*
3. On patient's arrival in PACU, review surgeon's orders. *Rationale: Places focus on priority interventions; assists you in organizing your care.*
4. Consider type of surgical procedure, restrictions to movement, and type of anesthesia used. *Rationale: Influences type of assessments necessary, complications for which to observe, and specific nursing interventions needed.*
5. Perform hand hygiene. Perform thorough patient assessment, including vital signs, pulse oximetry, and pain and assessment of body systems, including respiratory, cardiac, neurological, gastrointestinal (GI), genitourinary (GU), metabolic, and fluid status. Assess patient's surgical site and drains, skin integrity, safety, and anxiety level. *Rationale: Reduces transmission of infection. Provides baseline for ongoing postoperative evaluations. Identifies priority nursing interventions.*
6. Take vital signs and monitor pulse oximetry during initial stabilization (ASPAN, 2017). *Rationale: Monitors patient stability.*
7. Discharge from Phase I level of care is based on specific criteria, not a time limit. Criteria should address assessment of airway patency, oxygenation, hemodynamic stability, thermoregulation, neurological stability, intake and output, tube patency, dressings, pain and comfort management, and postanesthesia scoring system if used. Each agency defines frequency of assessment. *Rationale: Discharge instructions are developed in consultation with anesthesia department.*

Safe Patient Care *Be sure to turn patient on side (when possible) to observe underlying skin and accumulation of blood or serous drainage not visible otherwise.*

STEP	RATIONALE

PLANNING

STEP	RATIONALE
1. Expected outcomes following completion of procedure: • Patient's airway remains clear; respirations are deep, regular, and within normal limits by time of transfer. Oxygen saturation remains greater than 95% (see agency policy).	No occurrence of pulmonary changes except those expected from effects of anesthetic or analgesic. Agency standards may vary; 90% or greater oxygen saturation may be considered a safe normal range. Range may be based on patient's normal baseline.
• Patient's blood pressure (BP), pulse, and temperature remain within previous baseline or normal expected range by time of transfer.	No occurrence of cardiovascular, pulmonary, or thermoregulatory changes except those expected from effects of anesthetic or analgesic.

STEP	RATIONALE
• Dressings are clean, dry, and intact by discharge from recovery.	Indicates wound stabilization without signs of bleeding or infection.
• Intake and output (I&O) are within expected parameters by discharge from PACU.	Adequate urinary elimination maintained. Fluid intake (IV and/or by mouth [PO]) adequately maintained.
• Patient reports relief of discomfort after analgesia or other pain-relief measures by time of transfer from immediate recovery area (usually 1 to 2 hours).	Pain-relief measures effectively alter patient's reported pain.
• Postoperative assessments are within expected normal postoperative parameters.	Indicates stability and readiness for Phase III postoperative recovery (see Skill 29.5).
2. Provide privacy. Perform hand hygiene; organize and set up equipment for continued monitoring and care activities.	Protects patient's privacy. Reduces transmission of infection and promotes readiness for next priorities of care.
3. Explain PACU activities to the patient (as able) and family caregiver (when allowed into recovery).	Empowers the patient (as able) and family caregiver with information; reduces anxiety.

IMPLEMENTATION

STEP	RATIONALE
1. Perform hand hygiene. While receiving hand-off report as patient enters PACU on stretcher/bed, immediately attach oxygen tubing to regulator, hang IV fluids, and check IV flow rates. Connect any drainage tubes to gravity drainage or continuous or intermittent suction as ordered. Attach cardiac monitor. Ensure that indwelling catheter and bag are in drainage position and patent.	Reduces transmission of microorganisms. Maintaining oxygenation and circulation are priorities according to airway, breathing, and circulation. Inhaled oxygen improves percentage of oxygen delivered to alveoli. IV fluids maintain circulatory volume and provide route for emergency drugs. Drainage tubes must remain patent and in proper position to allow fluid to drain.
2. Apply clean gloves. Perform thorough patient assessment; collect vital signs, pulse oximetry, and/or end-tidal CO_2; assess pain perception and management. Assess surgical site and drains, skin integrity, safety, and anxiety level.	Reduces transmission of microorganisms. Provides baseline for ongoing postoperative evaluations. Indicates areas for priority nursing interventions.
3. Continue ongoing assessment of all vital signs every 5 to 15 minutes until patient stabilizes or more frequently if clinically indicated (ASPAN, 2017b; see agency protocol). Compare findings with patient's baseline. Provide warm blankets or use active rewarming device as needed for patient comfort.	Vital signs reveal stability or onset of postoperative complications from surgery or anesthesia (see Table 29.1). Acute blood loss may lead to hypovolemic shock with signs of reduced BP, elevated heart and respiratory rates, pale skin, and restlessness. General anesthetic may affect temperature-regulating center and lower metabolic rate, causing hypothermia. Malignant hyperthermia is a rare inherited condition that develops after receiving an anesthetic and is a medical emergency (Rothrock 2015; Schick and Windle, 2016).

Safe Patient Care *If patient underwent a short procedure under procedural sedation, check agency policy for sedation recovery guidelines. The perianesthesia registered nurse (RN) monitoring a patient who receives procedural sedation/analgesia should have no other responsibilities that compromise continuous patient monitoring (ASPAN, 2017). Monitor oxygenation until patients are no longer at risk for hypoxemia. Monitor ventilation and circulation at regular intervals until patients are suitable for discharge (ASPAN, 2017).*

STEP	RATIONALE
4. Maintain patent airway:	Ensures appropriate oxygenation.
a. Keep patient positioned on side with head facing down and neck slightly extended (see illustration). Never position patient with hands over chest because this reduces chest expansion.	Extension prevents occlusion of airway at pharynx. Downward position of head moves tongue forward, and mucus or vomitus can drain out of mouth, preventing aspiration.

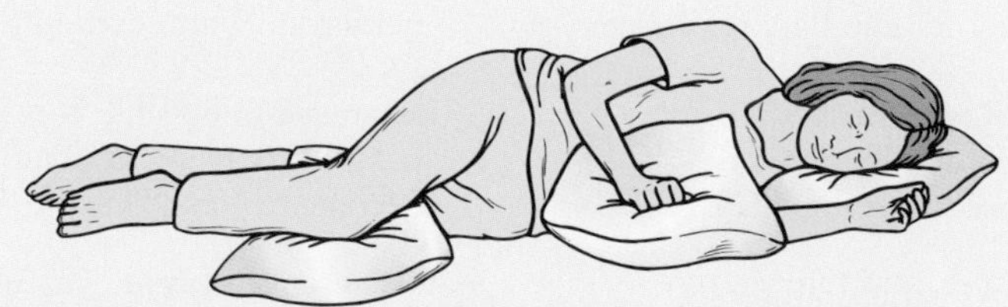

STEP 4a Position of patient during recovery from general anesthesia.

STEP	RATIONALE

Safe Patient Care *Always stay with a patient who has been sedated until respirations are well established. Patients with an artificial airway may gag and vomit, become restless, or stop breathing. Closely monitor patients with a history of obstructive sleep apnea.*

STEP	RATIONALE
b. Place small folded towel or small pillow under patient's head. If patient is restricted to supine position, elevate head of bed approximately 10 to 15 degrees, extend neck, and turn head to side. Have emesis basin available if patient becomes nauseated.	Supports head in extended position. Prevents aspiration if patient should vomit.

Safe Patient Care *If patient is not able to extend neck, turn head to side if possible; suction oropharynx (see Chapter 16) frequently.*

STEP	RATIONALE
c. Encourage patient to cough and deep breathe as instructed on awakening and every 15 minutes.	Promotes lung expansion and expectoration of mucus secretions.
d. Suction artificial airway and oral cavity as secretions accumulate.	Clears airway of secretions.
e. Once gag reflex returns, have patient spit out oral airway (see illustration). Do not tape oral airway.	Indicates that patient can clear airway independently. If airway is taped, patient will gag, which can lead to airway obstruction.

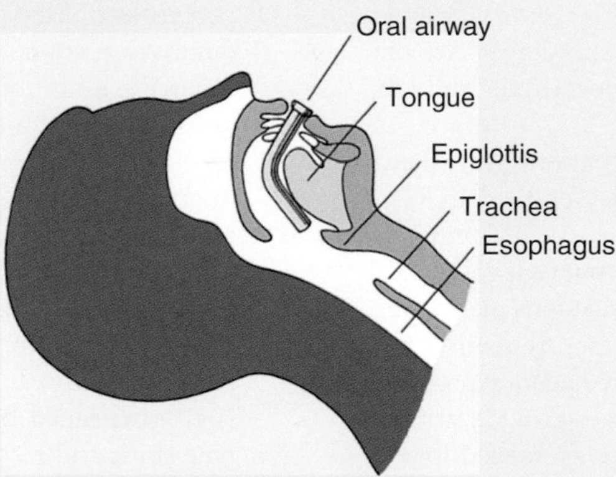

STEP 4e Oral airway position before removal.

STEP	RATIONALE
f. Avoid rapid position changes in patients who had spinal anesthesia, which can cause changes in patient's BP. Good body alignment is needed. Maintain IV fluid infusion. Encourage fluid intake (only if patient can take fluids, such as with ambulatory surgery).	Rapid movements are avoided to avoid spinal headache from loss of cerebrospinal fluid. Increased fluids help body replace cerebrospinal fluid.

Safe Patient Care *Because of shorter half-life of drugs, patients often have oral airway removed before leaving the OR. However, the PACU nurse must assess that respiratory effort is adequate; otherwise, the airway may need to be replaced, and the patient may need a ventilator if respiratory status declines.*

STEP	RATIONALE
5. Call patient by name in normal tone of voice. If there is no response, attempt to arouse patient by touching or gently moving a body part. Introduce yourself, explain that surgery is over, and orient to surroundings in the recovery area.	Determines patient's level of responsiveness. Provides early orientation to surroundings.
6. Assess circulatory perfusion by inspecting color of nail beds and capillary refill, mucous membranes, and skin. Palpate for skin temperature. Test for capillary refill (see Chapter 8).	Pink or normal color of skin, nail beds, and mucous membranes and brisk (3 seconds or less) capillary refill indicate adequate perfusion. Warm extremities reveal adequate circulation.
7. Assess closely for any behavioral or clinical changes reflecting potential cardiovascular and pulmonary complications of general anesthesia (see Table 29.1). Monitor laboratory findings.	Alerts nurse to possible postoperative emergencies or complications. Postoperative patients who are sedated may become hypoxic.
8. *If patient had general anesthesia:* As patient arouses, introduce yourself and orient him or her to surroundings.	

STEP	RATIONALE
9. *If patient had spinal or epidural anesthesia:* monitor sensory, circulatory, pulmonary, and neurological responses:	Reflects return of spinal function.
a. Monitor for hypotension, bradycardia, and nausea and vomiting.	Blockage of sympathetic nervous system results in vasodilation of major vessels and systemic hypotension.
b. Maintain adequate IV infusion.	Maintains BP by increasing fluid volume and fills temporarily expanded vascular space.
c. Keep patient supine or with head slightly elevated and maintain position.	Minimizes risk of postspinal anesthesia headache from leakage of spinal fluid at injection site, with increased pressures caused by elevation of upper body. Headache is more common with spinal than epidural anesthesia (Lewis et al., 2017).
d. Observe patients in PACU until they regain movement in extremities.	Alerts nurse to possible complications; can alleviate anxiety because patients often fear permanent loss of function.
e. Assess respiratory status, level of spinal sensation, and mobility in lower extremities. Drowsiness will be apparent after IV sedation. Level of anesthesia depends on location of sensation change. Have patient close eyes and use alcohol wipe to test sensation along sensory dermatomes. Have patient identify if warm or cold. *If patient had spinal anesthesia:* Remind that loss of extremity sensation and movement is normal and will return in several hours.	Spinal block is set within 20 minutes of onset. However, if level of anesthesia moves above sixth thoracic vertebra (T6), respiratory muscles are affected. Patients often feel short of breath and may require mechanical ventilation if respiratory muscles are severely affected.
10. Monitor sources of intake and output:	
a. Observe dressing and drains for any evidence of bright red blood. Inspect surgical incision for swelling or discoloration. Note condition of surgical dressing, including amount, color, odor, and consistency of drainage. Mark dressing with circle around drainage using black pen. Place time of marking and check area every 10 to 15 minutes, marking changes and noting vital signs.	Determines extent of fluid loss and condition of underlying wound. Size, location, and depth of wound influence amount of drainage. Marking dressing provides baseline reference.
b. Reinforce a pressure dressing or change simple dressing if ordered (see Chapter 27). Continue to monitor condition of incision, surrounding tissue, and amount and color of any drainage if incision is exposed or covered with transparent dressing.	Pressure dressing should not be removed because it helps to maintain hemostasis (termination of bleeding) and absorb drainage. Changing dressings immediately after surgery can disrupt wound edges and aggravate drainage. First dressing changes most often occur 24 hours after surgery and are usually done by surgeon. Minor surgical wounds may not have dressings but simply skin closure, or wounds may be covered with transparent dressing, which allows for observation of incision and surrounding tissue (Rothrock, 2015).
c. Inform surgeon of unexpected bloody drainage and reinforce dressing as indicated. Apply direct pressure. Assess underneath patient for pooling of bloody drainage. Monitor for decreased BP and increased pulse.	Progressive increase or changes in characteristics of drainage could indicate hemorrhage (Lewis et al., 2017; Schick and Windle, 2016). Hemorrhage from surgical wound is most likely within first few hours, indicating inadequate hemostasis during surgery. As dressing becomes saturated, blood often oozes down patient's side and collects underneath.
d. Inspect condition and contents of drainage tubes and collecting devices. Note character and volume of drainage.	Determines patency of drainage tube and extent of wound drainage.
e. Observe amount, color, and appearance of urine from indwelling Foley catheter (if present).	Urine output of less than 30 mL/hr is sign of decreased renal perfusion or altered renal function.
f. If nasogastric (NG) tube is present, assess drainage. If not draining, check placement and irrigate if necessary with normal saline (see Chapter 20).	Maintains patency of tube to ensure gastric decompression. Expected drainage is dark or pale, yellow, or green and 100 to 200 mL/hr. Bloody drainage occurs after some surgeries.
g. Monitor and maintain IV fluid rates. Observe IV site for signs of infiltration (see Chapter 28).	Provides adequate hydration and circulatory function.

STEP	RATIONALE
11. Promote comfort:	
a. Provide mouth care by placing moistened washcloth to lips, swabbing oral mucosa with dampened swab or soft toothbrush, or applying petrolatum to lips.	Mouth may be dry from NPO status and preoperative anticholinergics.
b. Provide warm blanket or active rewarming therapy to promote warmth and minimize shivering (ASPAN, 2017).	General anesthesia impairs thermoregulation, OR environment is cold, and exposure of body cavity results in internal heat loss. Shivering increases oxygen consumption, predisposes patient to arrhythmias and hypertension, impairs platelet function, alters drug metabolism, impairs wound healing, and increases hospitalization costs because of cumulative adverse outcomes (ASPAN, 2017).
c. Assist with position changes and provide supportive pillows.	Improves chest expansion for better ventilation and promotes circulation.
12. Continue assessing for pain as patient awakens and until transfer to surgical unit or discharge, including quality, severity, and location (see Chapter 15). Do not assume that all postoperative pain is incisional pain.	Pain may not be directly related to surgical procedure (e.g., chest pain [myocardial infarction or pulmonary embolism] or muscle pain [trauma from positioning]). Referred pain in shoulder often occurs after laparoscopy. Continuous assessment of pain helps patients achieve functional status.
a. Administer pain medication as ordered when vital signs have stabilized.	Promotes patient comfort.
13. Explain patient's condition to patient and inform of plans for transfer to nursing unit or discharge. In ambulatory surgery, family will be permitted to be with patient at this time.	Decreases anxiety that can interfere with recovery process.
14. When patient's condition stabilizes, contact surgeon to approve transfer to nursing unit or release to home.	Surgeon is responsible for authorizing transfer or discharge.
15. Before discharge to home from ambulatory surgery unit, provide verbal and written instructions (Box 29.1).	Patients and family care providers must be aware of potential complications and follow-up care.
16. For patients transferring to the next point of care by stretcher, raise side rails and request transport team. Appropriately dispose of supplies and equipment used in PACU setting. Perform hand hygiene.	Ensures patient safety. Reduces transmission of microorganisms.

Safe Patient Care *If patient is to be discharged to home, ensure that patient has someone to drive him or her home. A cab driver is usually not allowed. Observe for signs and symptoms of complications prior to discharge. Review with patient and driver reportable signs and symptoms and emergency care needed.*

EVALUATION

1. Compare all vital sign assessment measurements with patient's baseline and expected normal levels.	Evaluates patient's respiratory, cardiovascular, and thermoregulatory status throughout recovery.
2. Inspect surgical wound and dressings for drainage. Assess for wound drainage under patient.	Measures progress of wound healing. Checking underneath patient gives visualization if drainage has pooled.
3. Measure I&O. Urine output should be at least 30 to 50 mL/hr.	Low urine output indicates onset of fluid imbalances.

BOX 29.1

Postanesthesia and Ambulatory Surgery Discharge Criteria

Postanesthesia Discharge Criteria

- Patient awake (or returns to baseline)
- Vital signs stable
- No excess bleeding or drainage
- No respiratory depression
- SaO_2 greater than 90%
- Pain controlled
- Hand-off report given

Ambulatory Surgery Discharge Criteria

- All postanesthesia care unit (PACU) discharge criteria met
- No intravenous (IV) opioids for past 30 minutes
- Minimal nausea and vomiting
- Pain controlled
- Voided (if appropriate to surgical procedure/orders)
- Able to ambulate if age appropriate and not contraindicated
- Responsible adult present to accompany patient
- Discharge instructions given and understood

STEP	RATIONALE
4. Auscultate bowel sounds and ask if patient has passed flatus.	Evaluates return of peristalsis and diet tolerance.
5. Measure patient's perception of pain after implementing pain-relief measures such as positioning and use of analgesics.	Determines level of comfort achieved and effectiveness of pain-relief measures.
6. Complete system-specific assessments according to patient's unique type of surgery (e.g., craniotomy—neurological assessment; neck surgery—airway status; vascular surgery—circulation and bleeding; orthopedic surgery—neurovascular status and immobility or positioning).	Evaluates course of recovery.
7. **Use Teach-Back:** "I want to be sure you know what to expect when you go home. Tell me the signs and symptoms to expect if you were to get an infection." Revise your instruction now or develop a plan for revised patient/family caregiver teaching if patient/family caregiver is not able to teach back correctly.	Determines patient's/family caregiver's level of understanding of instructional topic.

Unexpected Outcomes	Related Interventions
1. Patient exhibits respiratory depression (pulse oximetry < 95%, respiratory rate < 10 breaths/min or shallow; see agency standards for range). Serious hypoxemic episode: oxygen saturation < 90% for ≥ 1 hour (Khanna et al., 2017). **NOTE:** A combination of "too much anesthesia" from excessive opioid use, inadequate reversal of neuromuscular blockade agents, or prolonged persistence of these agents in the system as a result of liver or renal disease is common for respiratory depression in the PACU (Khanna et al., 2017).	• Promptly report assessment findings to surgeon. • Administer oxygen as ordered by nasal cannula. Give patients with chronic obstructive pulmonary disease (COPD) 2 L/min or less of oxygen to prevent hypercapnia. • Encourage deep breathing every 5 to 15 minutes. • Position to promote chest expansion (on side or semi-Fowler's). • Administer prescribed medications (e.g., epinephrine, narcotic reversal agent).

2. Patient exhibits signs of hypovolemia related to internal or incisional hemorrhage.	• Elevate patient's legs enough to maintain downward slope toward trunk of body. Do not lower head past flat position because this position increases respiratory effort and may decrease cerebral perfusion.
	• Promptly report patient's status to surgeon.
	• Administer oxygen at 6 to 10 L/min by mask per order.
	• Increase rate of IV fluid or administer blood products as ordered.
	• Monitor BP and pulse every 5 to 15 minutes.
	• Apply pressure dressings as follows per order:
	  • *Abdominal dressing:* Cover bleeding area with several thicknesses of gauze compresses and place tape 7 to 10 cm (3 to 4 inches) beyond width of dressing with firm, even pressure on both sides close to bleeding source. Maintain pressure as you tape entire dressing to maximize pressure at source of bleeding.
	  • *Dressing on extremity:* Apply rolled gauze, pressing gauze compress over bleeding site. Refrain from taping around entire extremity.
	  • *Dressing in neck region:* Cover with several thicknesses of gauze and place tape 7 to 10 cm (3 to 4 inches) beyond width of dressing. Apply with pressure, but do not occlude carotid artery or airway. Assess every 5 to 15 minutes for carotid pulse and evidence of airway obstruction.
	• Maintain NPO status because it is often necessary to return to surgery for control of bleeding.

3. Patient reports severe incisional pain.	• Administer analgesics as ordered before pain becomes severe. • For patients with patient-controlled analgesia (PCA), assess for correct use of device. Teach family caregiver not to manipulate PCA. • *Orthopedic surgery:* Earliest symptom of compartment syndrome in extremity is pain unrelieved by analgesics. Other symptoms include numbness, tingling, pallor, coolness, and absent peripheral pulses. Surgeon *must* be notified immediately. Do not elevate extremity above level of heart because this increases venous pressure. Application of ice is contraindicated because vasoconstriction will occur (Lewis et al., 2017).

Recording

- Document patient's arrival time at PACU; include vital signs and assessment findings, level of consciousness (LOC), and pain severity. Record presence of dressings and tubes, character of drainage, and all nursing interventions initiated with patient response as appropriate.
- Document vital signs and I&O on appropriate flow sheets.

Hand-Off Reporting

- Report any abnormal assessment findings and signs of complications to surgeon.

✦ SKILL 29.5 Providing Early Postoperative (Phase II) and Convalescent Phase (Phase III) Recovery

Purpose

Early postoperative (Phase II) anesthesia recovery focuses on preparing a patient for self-care, care by family members, or care in an extended care environment (ASPAN, 2018). A patient is discharged to Phase II recovery when intensive monitoring is no longer needed, and patients are transported to a step-down or discharge area and the patient becomes more alert and functional (AORN, 2005). Convalescent (Phase III) anesthesia recovery focuses on providing ongoing care for patients who require extended observation or intervention after transfer from Phase I or Phase II. Interventions are directed toward preparing the patient for self-care or care by family members. Phases of recovery are not locations but levels of care (ASPAN, 2018).

Teaching is also important to promote patient independence, inform the patient and family caregiver about limitations and restrictions, and provide resources needed to achieve an optimal state of wellness. This level of care occurs during the early postoperative recovery period, which extends from the time a patient is discharged from the PACU to the time he or she is discharged or moved to the next point of care. Patients who have outpatient surgery undergo convalescence at home. Individualize your nursing care depending on the type of surgery, preexisting medical conditions, the risk for or development of complications, and the rate of recovery. Many health care agencies have developed enhanced recovery after surgery (ERAS) protocols. The protocols are interprofessional and based on published scientific evidence. Elements of an ERAS protocol might include minimally invasive surgical approaches instead of large incisions, management of fluids to seek balance rather than large volumes of intravenous fluids, avoidance of or early removal of drains and tubes, early mobilization, and serving of drinks and food the day of an operation (Ljungqvist et al., 2017).

Delegation and Collaboration

The skill of patient assessment and coordination of anesthesia recovery during the Early postoperative (Phase II) and Convalescent (Phase III) cannot be delegated to nursing assistive personnel (NAP). NAP may obtain vital signs when a patient has stabilized, apply nasal cannula or oxygen mask (but not adjust oxygen flow), provide hygiene and repositioning, and assist with early ambulation. The nurse instructs the NAP by:

- Explaining the frequency needed for vital signs.
- Reviewing specific safety concerns and what to observe and report back to the nurse.
- Explaining any precautions that affect how to provide basic hygiene and comfort measures.

Equipment

- Postoperative bed (recliner for day surgery recovery)
- Stethoscope, sphygmomanometer, thermometer, pulse oximeter
- Bladder scanner
- Intravenous (IV) fluid poles and infusion pumps as needed
- Emesis basin
- Washcloth and towel
- Waterproof pads
- Equipment for oral hygiene
- Pillows
- Facial tissue
- Oxygen equipment and bag-valve masks
- Emergency cart with defibrillator available for adults and children
- Suction equipment (to suction airway)
- Dressing supplies
- Intermittent suction (to connect to nasogastric [NG] or wound drainage tubes)
- Orthopedic appliances (if needed)
- Clean gloves
- Personal protective equipment as indicated
- Malignant hyperthermia cart (Rothrock, 2015; Schick and Windle, 2016)
- Latex-free supplies and equipment
- Transport equipment, including wheelchairs and carts

ASSESSMENT

1. Obtain phone report from postanesthesia care unit (PACU) nurse summarizing patient's current status. *Rationale: Allows you to prepare hospital room, supplies, and equipment for patient's specific needs.*
2. Perform hand hygiene and arrange equipment at bedside. *Rationale: Reduces transmission of microorganisms. Improves efficiency of care activity.*
3. If patient has been transported by stretcher, prepare for transfer with bed in high position (level with stretcher), with sheet folded to side and room for stretcher to be placed beside bed easily (see Chapter 17). Transfer patient to bed. *Rationale: Arrangement of equipment facilitates safety and smooth transfer process.*
4. Identify patient using at least two identifiers (e.g., name and birthday or name and medical record number) according to agency policy. *Rationale: Ensures correct patient. Complies with The Joint Commission standards and improves patient safety (TJC, 2019).*

5. Collect detailed hand-off report from nurse accompanying patient. *Rationale: Helps you plan appropriate assessment and nursing care measures. Data provide baseline from which to detect any change in patient's condition.*
6. Collect an initial set of vital signs. *Rationale: Allows for comparison with patient's status in operating room (OR) and PACU.*
7. Review electronic health record for information pertaining to type of surgery; complications; medications administered; preoperative medical risks; baseline vital signs, PACU vital signs; and patient's usual medications given/not given before surgery. Compare and validate with information from hand-off report. *Rationale: Surgical review identifies intraoperative complications and presence of medical risks that dictate complications for which to observe. Vital signs provide way to detect postoperative changes. List of patient's usual medications may necessitate call to surgeon or hospitalist for orders concerning timing and dose of drugs not given before surgery.*
8. Review postoperative medical orders. *Rationale: Offers additional information regarding type of care to provide.*
9. Assess patient's and family's knowledge and expectations of surgical recovery. *Rationale: Patient will be better prepared to participate in care.*
10. Assess patient's or family caregiver's knowledge, experience, and health literacy. *Rationale: Ensures patient or family caregiver has the capacity to obtain, communicate, process, and understand basic health information (CDC, 2016).*

STEP	RATIONALE
PLANNING	
1. Expected outcomes following completion of procedure:	
• Patient's breath sounds remain clear bilaterally.	No occurrence of pulmonary changes except those expected from effects of anesthetic or analgesic.
• Patient's vital signs remain within normal limits consistent with preoperative baseline.	No occurrence of cardiovascular, pulmonary, or thermoregulation changes except those expected from effects of anesthetic or analgesic.
• Incision wound edges are well approximated; no drainage is noted.	Indicates wound healing without signs of bleeding or infection.
• Fluid balance is evident by intake and output (I&O) records.	Adequate urinary elimination maintained. Fluid intake (IV and/or by mouth [PO]) adequately maintained.
• Patient describes pain as less than 4 on scale of 0 to 10 while engaged in moderate activity by discharge.	Pain-relief measures effectively alter patient's reception or perception of pain.
• Normal bowel sounds are present after bowel surgery or general anesthesia within 48 to 72 hours after surgery.	Indicates return of peristalsis.
• Patient or family caregiver describes signs that need to be reported, dietary modifications, and activity restrictions. Identifies plans for follow-up visit and demonstrates incision care.	Involves patient and family caregiver in plan of care and minimizes anxiety. As recovery progresses, patient is able to make more choices regarding how procedures should be performed. Family caregiver can serve as coach or provide direct assistance and help patient remember explanations given.
2. Provide privacy. Attach any existing oxygen tubing, position IV fluids, verify IV flow-rate settings on infusion pump, and check drainage tubes (e.g., Foley catheter or wound drainage).	Protects patient's privacy. Provides continuity of therapies.
3. Plan for appropriate postoperative teaching for the patient and family caregiver. Gather any needed teaching materials.	Empowers the patient and family caregiver with information; reduces anxiety.
IMPLEMENTATION	
1. Perform hand hygiene. Apply clean gloves for any necessary procedures.	Reduces transmission of microorganisms.
2. **Early Recovery Initial Postoperative Care (Phase II recovery):**	
a. Maintain airway. If patient remains sleepy or lethargic, keep head extended and support in side-lying position.	Minimizes chances of aspiration and obstruction of airway with tongue.
b. Conduct initial assessment of level of consciousness (LOC) and continue measuring vital signs per frequency of agency policy or health care provider order. Compare findings with vital signs taken in recovery area and patient's baseline.	Patient's status may change during transfer. Movement of patient and pain level influence stability of vital signs. Change in vital signs may reveal onset of postoperative complications.
c. Encourage coughing, deep breathing, and use of incentive spirometry and positive expiratory pressure (PEP) device (see Skill 29.2).	Anesthesia, medications, and intubation irritate airways, resulting in secretions and atelectasis. Coughing and use of devices expand chest, aerate lungs, and mobilize secretions.

STEP	RATIONALE
d. Assess gastrointestinal system (GI) for return of bowel sounds and note if patient begins to pass flatus.	Indicates return of peristalsis.
e. If NG tube is present, check placement and irrigate (see Chapter 20). Connect to proper drainage device. Connect all other drainage tubes to appropriate suction or collection device. Secure to prevent tension on tubing.	Transfer and movement may dislodge tubes, which interferes with drainage.
f. Assess patient's surgical dressing for appearance, presence, and character of drainage. Unless contraindicated by surgeon, outline drainage along edges with pen and reassess in 1 hour for change. Check under patient for pooling. If no dressing is present, inspect condition of wound (see Chapter 25).	Wound can hemorrhage quickly during early postoperative period. Assessment of wound and dressings provides data to measure progress of wound healing. Checking under patient is important to note whether drainage has pooled.

Safe Patient Care *If unable to change dressing, mark area of drainage and label with time, date, and initials. Record frequency of reinforcement. Never use felt-tip marker to mark dressing because ink can bleed into gauze, contaminating the incision site.*

STEP	RATIONALE
g. If patient has not voided for 4 hours, use a bladder scanner to detect for bladder distention. If Foley catheter is present, check placement. Ensure that it is draining freely and properly secured. Patient may have continuous bladder irrigations or suprapubic catheter (see Chapter 19).	Anesthesia often contributes to urinary retention. Urinary stasis increases risk for urinary tract infection.

Safe Patient Care *For surgical patients who have an indication for an indwelling catheter, remove the catheter as soon as possible postoperatively, preferably within 24 hours, unless there are appropriate indications for continued use (Gould et al., 2010; Lo et al., 2014). This action is a practice standard for preventing catheter-associated urinary tract infection.*

STEP	RATIONALE
h. If no urinary drainage system is present, explain that voiding within 8 hours after surgery is expected. Male patients may void more successfully if allowed to stand. Try interventions that promote normal micturition (see Chapter 19).	Anesthetics and analgesics depress sensation of bladder fullness. Patient may still have no sensation below level of spinal or epidural anesthetic.
(1) If the patient has not voided within 4 hours and there is more than 600 mL of urine on bladder scan, a one-time catheterization is recommended.	Many factors contribute to postoperative urinary retention (POUR) (e.g., older age, male gender). Catheterization prevents overdistention of the bladder (Glick et al., 2018).
i. Measure all sources of fluid I&O (including estimated blood loss during surgery).	Altered fluid and electrolyte balance is a potential complication of major surgery.
j. Describe purpose of equipment and frequent assessments to patient and family caregivers.	Unfamiliar sights (e.g., equipment, patient's appearance) can provoke anxiety. Providing information decreases anxiety.
k. Position patient for comfort, maintaining correct body alignment. Avoid tension on surgical wound site.	Reduces stress on suture line. Helps patient relax and promotes comfort.
l. Place nurse call system within reach and raise side rails (as appropriate). Instruct patient to call for help to get out of bed.	Promotes patient's safety as effects of anesthesia continue to diminish. Patient is a fall risk. Raising all side rails may be considered physical restraint.
m. Assess patient's level of pain on age-appropriate pain scale. Assess last time analgesic was given. Patient-controlled analgesia (PCA) may be used for pain control (see Chapter 15). Medicate patient as ordered either around the clock or prn as ordered during first 24 to 48 hours. Explain pain-management measures to patient. Know the symptoms of opioid use and withdrawal (Table 29.4).	Determines level of discomfort. Adequate pain control is needed to permit patient to participate fully with recovery activities. Consider time of the last opioid dose; withdrawal symptoms will occur upon abrupt discontinuation of opioids or when opioid antagonists are administered (Coluzzi et al., 2017).
3. Continued Postoperative Care (Phase III recovery):	
a. Continue to assess vital signs at least every 4 hours or as ordered.	Temperature greater than 38° C (100.4° F) in first 48 hours may indicate atelectasis, the normal inflammatory response, or dehydration. Temperature greater than 37.8° C (100° F) after first 48 hours (postop day 3) often indicates wound infection, pneumonia, or phlebitis (Lewis et al., 2017). Altered blood pressure or pulse is associated with cardiovascular complications (see Table 29.1).

TABLE 29.4

Signs and Symptoms of Opioid Abuse and Opioid Withdrawal

Opioid Abuse	Opioid Withdrawal
Vomiting	Dysphoric mood
Pruritus	Nausea or vomiting
Sweating	Lacrimation
Twitching	Rhinorrhea
Miosis (contracted pupils)	Muscle aches
Loss of appetite	Pupillary dilation
Drowsiness	Piloerection
Respiratory depression	Sweating
Coma	Diarrhea
Needle marks	Yawning
	Fever
	Insomnia

STEP	RATIONALE

Safe Patient Care *Malignant hyperthermia (MH) causes a rapid rise in core body temperature to 40.5° C or higher and severe muscle contractions (Lewis et al., 2017). Know your patient's risks and have an MH emergency cart available.*

STEP	RATIONALE
b. Closely monitor progress of wound healing and change dressings as ordered.	Wound infection occurs most often within 3 to 6 days after surgery. Wound dehiscence occurs most often 3 to 11 days after surgery (see Chapter 25).
c. Continue to monitor drainage (see illustration A) and maintain wound drainage devices such as Jackson-Pratt, Hemovac, or Penrose drains. Jackson-Pratt and Hemovac drainage systems must be emptied when they are half full of drainage or air and recharged (compressed to discharge air; see illustration B).	Wound drainage devices promote healing from inside to outside and relieve pressure on suture line. Compressing flexible closed container and then plugging drainage hole creates negative suction pressure.

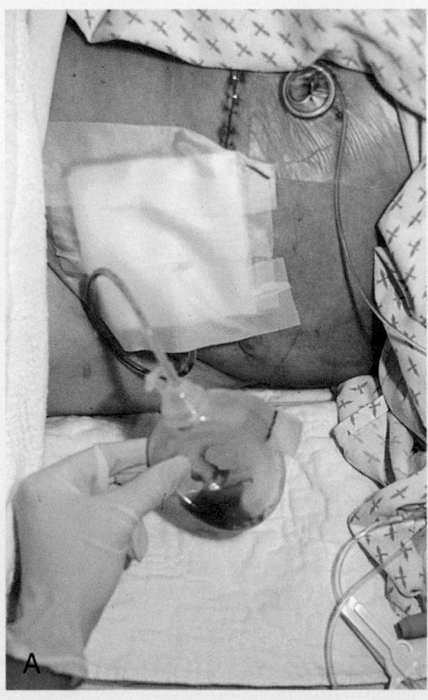

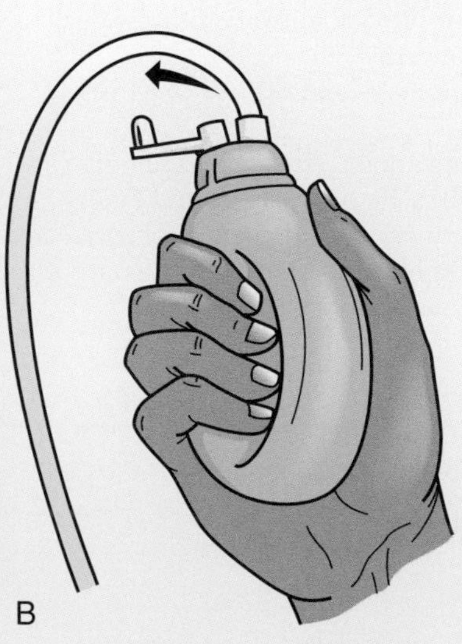

STEP 3c (A) Note color of drainage from device. (B) Charging Jackson-Pratt drainage system.

STEP	RATIONALE
d. Provide oral care at least every 2 hours as needed. If permitted, offer ice chips or advance to clear liquids if ordered.	Medication given before surgery can make mouth dry. Oral care and ice chips promote comfort. Adequate oral care is associated with lesser chance of respiratory infection.
e. Encourage patient to turn, cough, deep breathe, and use incentive spirometer and PEP device at least every 2 hours (see Skill 29.2).	Promotes adequate ventilation and minimizes hypoventilation and atelectasis.
f. Monitor function of sequential compression devices. If ordered, apply elastic stockings to lower extremities (see Chapter 18). Explain to patient that compression device will inflate and deflate intermittently.	Elastic stockings increase venous return (Elisha et al., 2015). Explanation decreases anxiety and fosters cooperation.
g. Promote early ambulation per agency protocol (see Chapter 18). Assess vital signs before and after activity to assess tolerance. Patients are often ambulating within first 12 hours of arrival to patient care unit. Set goals for patient to increase ambulation progressively.	Early ambulation is critical to prevent deconditioning and resultant postoperative complications (Grass et al., 2018; Whitcomb and Psaila, 2015). Mobility promotes circulation, lung expansion, and peristalsis. Postural hypotension is caused by sudden position changes.
h. Progress from clear liquids to regular diet as ordered and tolerated if nausea and vomiting do not occur.	Appropriate nutrition aids in postoperative healing process. Nausea and vomiting are associated with anesthesia and surgery, so clear liquids must be introduced first after surgery. IV fluids are usually discontinued when oral intake is tolerated.
i. Include patient and family caregiver in postoperative instruction and decision making; answer questions as they arise.	Promotes patient's sense of control and independence and improves self-esteem.
j. Provide opportunity for patients who must adjust to change in body appearance or function to verbalize feelings.	Radical surgery, amputation, or inoperable cancer often results in anxiety and depression. Grief response to loss of body organ is common and should be expected.
4. **Convalescent Phase (Phase III):**	
a. Assess patient's home environment for safety, cleanliness, and availability of community resources and patient assistance. (**NOTE:** This may be done by a case manager and not a staff nurse.) Use the information to revise teaching as needed.	Provides information about patient's environment after discharge and the possible need for home care. Verifies patient's and family caregiver's level of knowledge and any additional teaching needs for discharge. Helps to facilitate transition management and patient's independence and participation in care.
b. Provide instruction on care activities that patient or family caregiver will perform at home (e.g., dressing change, medication administration, exercises, IV therapy).	Enables patient to participate in self-care at home.
c. Keep patient and family caregiver informed of progress made toward recovery. Explain time expected for discharge from hospital. Provide answers to individual patient questions or concerns.	Decreases anxiety and helps patient know what to anticipate in preparation for discharge planning.
5. Following any procedure, remove and dispose of gloves; perform hand hygiene.	Reduces transmission of microorganisms.
6. Prepare patient for discharge home (this may occur after Phase II or during Phase III). Be sure patient and family caregiver have all necessary printed instructions. Provide a hand-off report if patient is being discharged to an agency such as extended care or nursing home.	Ensures continuity of care.

EVALUATION

1. Auscultate breath sounds bilaterally.	Determines status of airways.
2. Monitor trends in vital signs.	Provides data to evaluate postoperative status.
3. Evaluate I&O records. Note time of patient's first postoperative urination.	Indicates onset of postoperative urination.
4. Auscultate bowel sounds.	Establishes time of return of peristalsis.
5. Ask patient to evaluate pain on a scale of 0 to 10 after moderate activity.	Determines level of comfort achieved and effectiveness of pain-relief measures.

STEP	RATIONALE
6. Inspect incision (wound edges well approximated; no drainage noted).	Provides data to measure progress of wound healing.
7. Have patient or family caregiver describe incision care, dietary modifications or restrictions, activity restrictions, medication schedule, and plans for follow-up visit.	Identifies need for further teaching.
8. **Use Teach-Back:** "I want to be sure I explained what you need to know about your postoperative activity level. Explain for me how you will increase your activity level during the first week at home." Revise your instruction now or develop a plan for revised patient/family caregiver teaching if patient/family caregiver is not able to teach back correctly.	Determines patient's/family caregiver's level of understanding of instructional topic.

Unexpected Outcomes	Related Interventions
1. Vital signs are above or below patient's baseline or expected range. Initially this could be related to anesthesia effects, pain, hypovolemic shock, airway obstruction, fluid and electrolyte imbalance, or hypothermia.	• Identify contributing factors. • Notify surgeon.
2. Patient reports severe incisional pain.	• Report to surgeon; discuss alternative analgesic option. • Try nonpharmacological pain control measures (see Chapter 15).

Recording

- Document patient's arrival at nursing unit; record vital signs, assessment findings, and all nursing interventions initiated. Document every 4 hours or more frequently as patient's condition warrants.
- During ongoing recovery, document all assessment findings, vital signs, and I&O on appropriate record.
- Document any abnormal assessment findings and/or signs of complications.
- Document evaluation of patient learning.

Hand-Off Reporting

- Report onset of any postoperative complications to surgeon or other health care provider immediately.
- During hand-off report, communicate patient's assessment findings pertinent to surgery, patient response, and progress with postoperative instruction.
- If transitioned to any other environment than home, report preoperative course and postoperative summary, as well as current status, to receiving nurse.

SPECIAL CONSIDERATIONS

Patient-Centered Care

- Spiritual/religious training or support specific to a patient's faith and beliefs can be effective in reducing preoperative anxiety.
- Patients may follow spiritual practices such as receiving sacraments immediately before surgery and wearing religious medals or undergarments until just before surgery.
- Communicating all information pertaining to specific patient preferences, practices, and beliefs to all members of the interprofessional health care team is important and improves the likelihood that each patient receives personalized, comprehensive, holistic care to help reduce health disparities (Diaz et al., 2015).
- A recent study shows that nurse leaders need to continually assess nursing staff cultural awareness (McElroy et al., 2016) so that ongoing educational opportunities can be appropriately constructed and delivered to enhance understanding.
- For information collected preoperatively, collaborate with the patient and family to have cultural and spiritual needs available immediately prior to and following surgery (e.g., planning for dietary needs; arranging for presence of spiritual leader of the patient's choice).

Patient Education

- Whenever you provide printed educational materials about a patient's surgery or recovery process, be sure the materials are age appropriate and at the patient's literacy level.
- It is important that any preoperative educational strategy focuses on improving a patient's sense of empowerment.
- Patient teaching for ambulatory surgical patients should include:
  - Surgeon's office and surgery center 24-hour telephone number
  - Follow-up appointment date and time
  - Review of prescribed medications and dosage schedules
  - Activity or diet restrictions related to specific surgery
  - Dressing and wound care
  - Pain control
  - Warning signs of possible anesthesia effects
  - Signs and symptoms of complications
- Teach patients and their family caregivers the signs and symptoms and appropriate actions to take for infection and respiratory, circulatory, or gastrointestinal difficulties.

Age-Specific

Pediatric

- Preoperative education involving use of videos, multifaceted programs, and interactive games to reduce preoperative anxiety in children undergoing elective surgery have been found most effective, whereas music therapy and Internet programs are less effective (Chow et al., 2016; Hockenberry and Wilson, 2017).
- When preparing a child for surgery, keep parent–child separation to the minimum.

- Consider a child's developmental level when performing preoperative assessment and preparation.
- Maintenance of body temperature in infants and children after surgery is a priority because of their immature temperature-control mechanisms.
- Infants and children normally have higher metabolic rates and differences in physiological makeup compared with adults, resulting in greater oxygen, fluid, and calorie needs. Vomiting is a concern because of increased risk for fluid and electrolyte imbalances and risk for aspiration.

Gerontological

- If age-related changes have resulted in diminished short-term memory, perform additional assessment and provide additional teaching time as appropriate.
- An older patient with limitations in ROM may require adaptations in how to perform postoperative exercises. Also communicate information to OR nurse so that surgical position can be modified.
- Reinforce teaching with older adults. Offer audiovisual (AV) or other media resources, demonstrations, and more verbal explanation. Consider vision and hearing deficits when providing written and verbal instructions.

Home Care

- Be sure family caregivers have access to resources at home that are needed to support recovering patient in the home (e.g., bandage supplies, assist devices, bedside toilet).
- Assess early in hospitalization if patient is eligible for home care.
- If patient is discharged with dressing changes, the bedroom or bath is usually ideal for the procedure. Have patient and family caregiver perform a return demonstration of dressing change before discharge from hospital (if possible).
- Explain to patients and family caregivers the options for pain management, but encourage patients to take analgesics as ordered. Pain control is critical, and if patients cannot achieve pain relief, a return visit to a health care provider is essential. Patients should not try to self-medicate.

✦ PRACTICE REFLECTIONS

Consider caring for a 72-year-old patient who is coming to the health care agency for a right-knee replacement. The patient has not had surgery in the past. You are talking with the patient and his wife in the preoperative screening department 2 weeks before the procedure.

1. What should you consider when providing preoperative instruction for this patient compared with one who is 15 years younger?
2. In what ways can the patient's wife assist the patient's recovery postoperatively?
3. If you were the nurse caring for the patient in Phase I recovery, what would be your priorities?

✦ CLINICAL REVIEW QUESTIONS

1. A nurse is responsible for properly instructing patients on breathing exercises before surgery. Place the following steps for deep breathing and coughing in the correct order.
   a. Have patient place palms of hands across from each other lightly along lower border of rib cage or upper abdomen.
   b. Have patient take slow, deep breath; hold for count of 3 seconds; and exhale.
   c. Have patient sit in high-Fowler's position with knees flexed.
   d. Have patient take slow, deep breaths, inhaling through nose.
   e. Have patient repeat breathing exercise three to five times.
   1. a, c, b, d, e
   2. c, a, d, b, e
   3. b, c, a, d, e
   4. c, b, a, d, e
2. Which assessment findings in a patient in the PACU need to be reported to the surgeon? (Select all that apply.)
   1. Respiratory rate less than 10 per minute with shallow breathing
   2. Bright red wound drainage saturating dressing
   3. Pain rating of 3 on a scale of 0 to 10
   4. Scattered crackles in posterior lung bases
   5. Intravenous infusion rate at time patient enters the PACU
3. The nurse has provided preoperative teaching when the patient states, "I don't understand this surgery, and I don't think I want it done." Which responses are appropriate for the nurse to make? (Select all that apply.)
   1. "That was a lot of information to take in at one time. You're having a knee replacement."
   2. "Let me start over and teach you again."
   3. "I'll contact the surgeon to go over the procedure with you."
   4. "Don't worry about it; I will make sure your family caretaker knows about your surgery."
   5. "It sounds like you are concerned about having surgery."

Answers and Rationales for Clinical Review Questions can be found on the Evolve website.

REFERENCES

American Society of Anesthesiologists (ASA) Committee: Practice guidelines for preoperative fasting and the use of pharmacologic agents to reduce the risk of pulmonary aspiration: application to healthy patients undergoing elective procedures, an updated report by the American Society of Anesthesiologists task force on preoperative fasting and the use of pharmacologic agents to reduce the risk of pulmonary aspiration, *Anesthesiology* 126(3):376, 2017.

American Society of PeriAnesthesia Nurses (ASPAN): *2017-2018 perianesthesia nursing standards, practice recommendations and interpretive statements*, Cherry Hill, NJ, 2017, Author.

American Society of PeriAnesthesia Nurses (ASPAN): Frequently asked questions, 2018. http://www.aspan.org/Clinical-Practice/FAQs.

Anderson D, Sexton DJ: Overview of control measures for prevention of surgical site infection in adults, 2017. https://www.uptodate.com/contents/overview-of-control-measures-for-prevention-of-surgical-site-infection-in-adults.

Association of periOperative Registered Nurses (AORN): AORN guidance statement postoperative patient care in the ambulatory surgery setting, *AORN J* 81(4):881, 2005.

Association of periOperative Registered Nurses (AORN): *Perioperative standards and recommended practices*, Denver, CO, 2015, Author.

Aust H, et al: Coping strategies in anxious surgical patients, *BMC Health Serv Res* 16:250, 2016.

Berrios-Torres S, et al: Centers for Disease Control and Prevention guideline for the prevention of surgical site infection, *JAMA Surg* 152(8):784, 2017.

Centers for Disease Control and Prevention (CDC): What is health literacy? 2016. https://www.cdc.gov/healthliteracy/learn/index.html.

Centers for Disease Control and Prevention (CDC): FAQs about "surgical site infections," 2017. https://www.cdc.gov/hai/pdfs/ssi/ssi_tagged.pdf.

Chow CHT, et al: Systematic review: audiovisual interventions for reducing preoperative anxiety in children undergoing elective surgery, *J Pediatr Psychol* 41(2):182, 2016.

Chung F, et al: STOP-BANG questionnaire: a practical approach to screen for obstructive sleep apnea, *Chest* 149:631, 2016.

Cleveland Clinic: Coughing: controlled coughing: management and treatment, 2017. https://my.clevelandclinic.org/health/diseases/8697-coughing-controlled-coughing/management-and-treatment.

Coluzzi F, et al: The challenge of perioperative pain management in opioid-tolerant patients, *Ther Clin Risk Manag* 13:1163, 2017.

Diaz C, et al: Cultural competence in rural nursing education: are we there yet?, *Nurs Educ Perspect* 36(1):22, 2015.

Elisha S, et al: Venous thromboembolism: new concepts in perioperative management, *AANA J* 83(3):211, 2015.

Glick D, et al: Overview of post-anesthetic care for adult patients, *UpToDate* 2018. https://www.uptodate.com/contents/overview-of-post-anesthetic-care-for-adult-patients.

Gould CV, et al: Guideline for prevention of catheter-associated urinary tract infections 2009, *Infect Control Hosp Epidemiol* 31(4):319, 2010.

Grass G, et al: Feasibility of early postoperative mobilisation after colorectal surgery: a retrospective cohort study, *Int J Surg* 56:161, 2018.

Hockenberry MJ, Wilson D: *Wong's essentials of pediatric nursing*, ed 10, St. Louis, 2017, Mosby.

Khanna A, et al: Respiratory depression: beyond the PACU, before ICU, *Soc Crit Care Anesthesiol* 28(1):4, 2017.

Lewis S, et al: *Medical-surgical nursing: assessment and management of clinical problems*, ed 10, St. Louis, 2017, Elsevier.

Ljungqvist O, et al: Enhanced recovery after surgery: a review, *JAMA Surg* 152(3):292, 2017.

Lo E, et al: Strategies to prevent catheter-associated urinary tract infections in acute care hospitals: 2014 update, *Infect Control Hosp Epidemiol* 35(5):464, 2014.

McDonald S, et al: Preoperative education for hip or knee replacement, 2014. http://www.cochrane.org/CD003526/MUSKEL_preoperative-education-hip-or-knee-replacement.

McElroy J, et al: Cultural awareness among nursing staff at an academic medical center, *J Nurs Adm* 46(3):146, 2016.

Nagelhout JJ, Elisha S: *Nurse anesthesia*, ed 6, St. Louis, 2017, Saunders.

Ogan OU, Plevak DJ: Anesthesia safety always an issue with obstructive sleep apnea, American Sleep Apnea Association, n.d. http://www.apsf.org/newsletters/html/1997/summer/sleepapnea.html.

Rotevatn TA, et al: Alcohol consumption and the risk of postoperative mortality and morbidity after primary hip or knee arthroplasty: a register-based cohort study, *PLoS ONE* 12(3):e0173083, 2017.

Rothrock JC: *Alexander's care of the patient in surgery*, ed 15, St. Louis, 2015, Mosby.

Schick L, Windle P: *PeriAnesthesia nursing core curriculum: preoperative, phase I and phase II PACU nursing*, ed 3, St. Louis, 2016, Saunders.

The Joint Commission (TJC): The universal protocol for preventing wrong site, wrong procedure, and wrong person surgery™: guidance for health care professionals, n.d. https://www.jointcommission.org/assets/1/18/UP_Poster1.PDF.

The Joint Commission (TJC): Surgical site infections (SSIs), 2017. https://www.jointcommission.org/topics/hai_ssi.aspx.

The Joint Commission (TJC): *2019 National Patient Safety Goals*, 2019. Oakbrook Terrace, IL, The Commission. http://www.jointcommission.org/standards_information/npsgs.aspx.

Whitcomb W, Psaila J: Early mobility program, *Hospitalist* 2015. https://www.the-hospitalist.org/hospitalist/article/122012/early-mobility-program.

World Health Organization: Surgical safety checklist, n.d. http://www.who.int/patientsafety/safesurgery/tools_resources/SSSL_Checklist_finalJun08.pdf.

30 Emergency Measures for Life Support in the Hospital Setting

SKILLS AND PROCEDURES

EVOLVE WEBSITE/RESOURCES LIST

http://evolve.elsevier.com/Perry/nursinginterventions

Audio Glossary • Animations • Case Studies • Checklists • Nursing Skills Online • Clinical Review Questions • Answers and Rationales for Clinical Review Questions • Video Clips

INTRODUCTION

Emergency measures for life support are those interventions designed to maintain or improve cardiopulmonary function. Cardiac arrest is the cessation of circulating blood flow. To survive a cardiac arrest, a patient must receive cardiopulmonary resuscitation (CPR), which includes airway, breathing, and circulation. Timely emergency measures are critical for improving patient outcomes.

PRACTICE STANDARDS

- American Heart Association, 2017: Get with the guidelines: resuscitation recognition criteria—Resuscitation guidelines
- Neumar et al., 2015: American Heart Association guidelines update for cardiopulmonary resuscitation and emergency cardiovascular care—Resuscitation guidelines

EVIDENCE-BASED PRACTICE

Maintaining High-Quality CPR

Every 5 years, the American Heart Association (AHA) reviews all the resuscitation science to provide the latest recommendations for basic, adult, pediatric, and neonatal life support (Neumar et al., 2015). Research demonstrates that early, high-quality CPR and early defibrillation are the primary components influencing survival. Measurements such as end-tidal carbon dioxide (CO_2) and arterial pressures (when available) provide valuable information as to the quality of chest compressions and ventilations during CPR. Guidelines for maintaining high-quality CPR include the following:

- Immediate recognition of cardiac arrest and activation of emergency medical response are critical.
- Early CPR and recommended health care team–level coordination that switches the provider who performs chest compressions every 2 minutes improves the performance of high-quality CPR (AHA, 2017).
- Ensure proper hand position.
- Provide compressions at adequate rate and depth.
- Minimize interruptions in chest compressions.
- The AHA (2017) Get With the Guidelines—Resuscitation Recognition Criteria (2017) expect hospitals and first responders to deliver the first electrical shock to patients in ventricular fibrillation or pulseless ventricular tachycardia in less than 2 minutes and 59 seconds (AHA, 2017).
- Maintain end-tidal CO_2 greater than 20 (normal is 35 to 45 mm).
- Avoid excessive ventilation. Focus on chest compressions.
- Consider post–cardiac arrest hypothermia, to preserve neurological functioning (Callaway et al., 2015; Rittenberger and Callaway, 2018) (Box 30.1).

SAFETY GUIDELINES

- Know patient's current and baseline vital signs and fluid and electrolyte status.
- Know patient's advanced directives pertaining to life-saving measures.
- Be aware of patient's history of and type of cardiac rhythm irregularities and specific treatments (e.g., medications, past defibrillation).
- The treatment for lethal arrhythmias, such as ventricular fibrillation (V Fib; VF) or ventricular tachycardia (V Tach; VT) requires an externally applied electrical shock called defibrillation to a patient's chest (see Skills 30.2 and 30.3). When electrical energy is used during an emergency, certain safety steps must be taken to avoid the release of live electricity into the environment and possibly causing others in the room to be shocked.

BOX 30.1

Targeted Temperature Management

- Hypothermia or targeted temperature management is effective in reducing neurological deficits in selected patients following cardiac arrest (Callaway, 2017). Neurological deficits are the most common cause of mortality and morbidity following cardiac arrest.
  - Targeted temperature 32° to 36° C for 24 hours
  - Targeted temperature 32° to 34° C for 21 to 24 hours
  - Followed by gradual rewarming (0.25° C/hr; Rittenberg and Callaway, 2018)
- Monitor patient's acid–base balance, complete blood count, serum lactate, and other laboratory markers as indicated by patient status
- Maintain oxygen saturation (SpO_2) > 94%.
- Positive outcomes are associated with patients who had out-of-hospital cardiac arrest with an initial shockable rhythm (Donnino et al., 2016).

- Steps to provide safe defibrillation include the following:
  - Good skin contact between the defibrillation pad and the patient's chest.
  - Pressing the shock buttons only when the pads are in contact with the patient's chest.
  - Clear communication to everyone in the room not to touch the patient or the patient's bed during defibrillation.
- Other safety steps involved with basic life-support measures include the following:
  - Proper hand position when performing chest compressions ensures effective perfusion while minimizing internal injury to a patient.
  - A mask with a one-way valve provides a safety barrier between the patient and the rescuer, protecting both from direct contact during mask-to-mouth ventilation.

✦ SKILL 30.1 Inserting an Oropharyngeal Airway

Purpose

Insertion of an oropharyngeal airway keeps a patient's oral airway open by displacing the tongue or soft palate from the pharyngeal air passages. An oropharyngeal airway or oral airway is a semicircular-shaped, minimally flexible, curved piece of rigid plastic (Fig. 30.1). *These airways should only be placed in an unconscious patient without a gag reflex.*

The oral airway is available for adults and children in various sizes (Table 30.1). It is important to select the correct size for each patient. When inserted, it extends from just outside the lips, over the tongue, and into the pharynx (Fig. 30.2). If it is too small, it may push the base of the tongue into the airway. If it is too large, the device itself may obstruct the airway. The proper length of the airway can be estimated by placing it on the face with one end at the angle of the jaw and the other end parallel to the front teeth (Fig. 30.3). If the airway fits within this length, it should fit in the patient's actual oropharyngeal space.

Equipment

- Appropriate-sized oral airway (see Table 30.1)
- Clean gloves
- Gown if needed
- Tissues or washcloths
- Suction equipment if indicated
- Nonallergic tape
- Face shield if indicated
- Tongue blade
- Stethoscope

TABLE 30.1

Oral Airway Guidelines for Size[a] by Age

Size	Age
30 mm or size 000	Premature neonates
45 mm or size 00	Newborn
55 mm or size 0	Newborn to 1 year
60 mm or size 1	1–2 years
70 mm or size 2	2–6 years
80 mm or size 3	6–18 years
90 mm or size 4	Adult medium
100 mm or size 5	Adult large
110 mm or size 6	Adult extra large

[a]Measure from the corner of the mouth to the angle of the jaw just below the ear for size estimation (see Fig. 30.3).

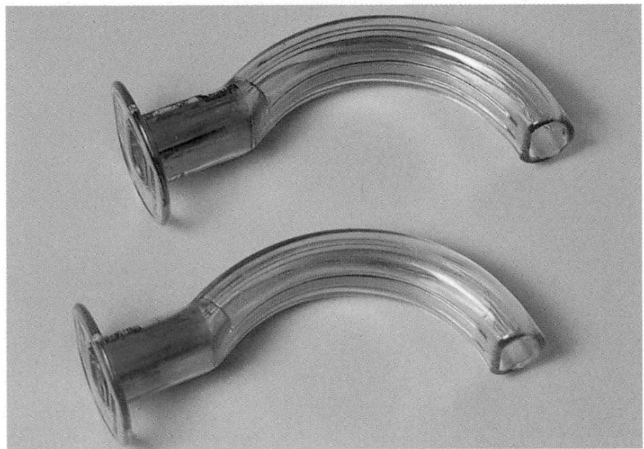

FIG 30.1 Oral airways.

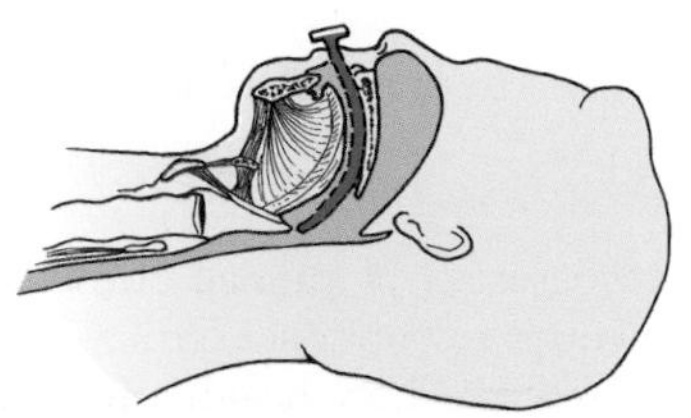

FIG 30.2 Placement of oral airway.

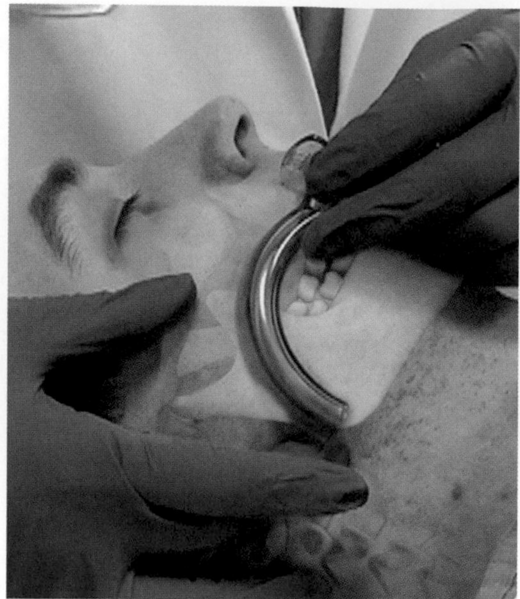

FIG 30.3 Measuring for an oral airway. *(From Roberts JR, et al:* Roberts and Hedges' clinical procedures in emergency medicine and acute care, *ed 7, Philadelphia, 2019, Elsevier.)*

ASSESSMENT

1. Identify need to insert an oropharyngeal airway. Signs and symptoms include upper airway gurgling with breathing, absent cough or gag reflex, increased oral secretions, excessive drooling, grinding teeth, clenched teeth, biting endotracheal or gastric tubes, and labored respirations. *Rationale: These conditions place patient at risk for obstruction of the upper airway.* **NOTE**: *Use oropharyngeal airways only in unconscious patients. They may stimulate vomiting or laryngospasm if inserted in a semiconscious or conscious patient.*
2. Determine factors that may contribute to upper airway obstruction, such as age (children have a proportionally larger tongue) or presence of a nasal or oropharyngeal airway and drainage tubes (swallowing is more difficult with tubes in place). *Rationale: Allows you to accurately assess potential need for oropharyngeal airway placement. Patients at greater risk for upper airway obstruction are infants; children; and adults with upper airway congestion, loss of consciousness, seizure disorders, neuromuscular diseases, or increased oral secretions.*
3. Perform hand hygiene. Ensure that patient does not have dentures in place before attempting an oropharyngeal airway insertion. *Rationale: Reduces transmission of microorganisms. Oropharyngeal airway insertion can dislodge dentures and cause worsening airway obstruction.*

Safe Patient Care *Never insert an oropharyngeal airway in a conscious patient or a patient with recent oral/facial trauma, oral surgery, or loose teeth. Never force an airway into place.*

4. Assess family caregiver's knowledge, experience, and health literacy. *Rationale: Ensures family caregiver has the capacity to obtain, communicate, process, and understand basic health information (Centers for Disease Control and Prevention [CDC], 2016).*
5. Assess family caregiver's knowledge of procedure. *Rationale: Identify learning needs of family. Patient will be unconscious.*

STEP	RATIONALE
PLANNING	
1. Expected outcomes following completion of procedure:	
• Patient's respiratory status improves, as evidenced by respirations with normal rate, easier removal of secretions, and lack of gurgling noise in throat with respirations.	Airway is clear of secretions.
• Patient is not able to grind teeth or bite tubes.	Oropharyngeal airways can also act as a bite block to provide airway tube patency.
• Patient's tongue does not obstruct airway.	Oropharyngeal airway keeps tongue in correct position to maintain patent airway.
• Family caregiver can verbalize understanding of need for oropharyngeal airway.	Teaching was successful.
2. Position unconscious patient in semi-Fowler's position if possible.	Provides easy access to oral cavity.
IMPLEMENTATION	
1. Perform hand hygiene and apply clean gloves and face shield (when possible).	Reduces transmission of microorganisms.
2. Whenever possible, use padded tongue blade to open patient's mouth; if necessary, use thumb and forefinger of nondominant hand to open jaws and teeth.	Provides access to oral cavity.

Safe Patient Care *To avoid a bite, do not insert your fingers into patient's mouth. Use extreme caution if manually opening patient's jaw and teeth.*

STEP	RATIONALE
3. Insert oropharyngeal airway.	When inserting airway, take care not to push patient's tongue into pharynx.

STEP	RATIONALE
a. Hold oropharyngeal airway with curved end up and insert distal end until airway reaches back of throat; then turn airway over 180 degrees and follow natural curve of tongue. *Option:* Hold airway sideways, insert halfway, and rotate 90 degrees while gliding it over natural curvature of tongue. Make sure that outer flange is just outside patient's lips.	Proper insertion of airway prevents displacement of patient's tongue into posterior oropharynx. Secure oropharyngeal airway with tape on upper and lower flange.

Safe Patient Care *In a* ***pediatric patient, DO NOT rotate*** *the oropharyngeal airway on insertion because the airway tip will damage the soft palate.*

STEP	RATIONALE
4. Suction secretions as needed.	Removes secretions; maintains patent airway.
5. Reassess patient's respiratory status; auscultate lungs.	Verifies respiratory status and patent airway.
6. Clean patient's face with soft tissue or washcloth.	Promotes hygiene.
7. Discard tissue into appropriate receptacle, place washcloth in dirty or soiled linen bag, remove gloves and face shield and discard in appropriate receptacle, and perform hand hygiene.	Reduces transmission of microorganisms.
8. Be sure nurse call system is accessible within patient's reach. When patient regains consciousness, instruct patient in its use.	Provides patient safety and allows patient/family to call nurse for assistance.
9. Administer mouth care frequently.	Increases patient comfort and removes debris. It also provides moisture to oral mucosal tissues.

Safe Patient Care *Oropharyngeal airway will need to be removed, discarded, and replaced in patients with excessive oral secretions. Frequent suctioning of the oral cavity may be required. Oropharyngeal airways are not a long-term solution. They can create pressure on underlying tissue and cause significant lip and tongue erosion, which can result in a medical device–related pressure injury (MDPI; Pittman et al., 2015).*

EVALUATION

STEP	RATIONALE
1. Observe patient's respiratory status and compare respiratory assessments before and after insertion of oral airway.	Identifies patient's response to insertion of airway.
2. Evaluate that airway is patent and that patient's tongue does not obstruct it.	Ensures route for oxygen delivery to patient.
3. Observe adjacent and underlying tissue for signs of tissue injury, such as redness, abrasion, or bruising.	Identifies early signs of MDPI.
4. Observe for patient pushing airway out with tongue or coughing.	Patient's ability to clear his or her own airway may have returned. Indicates reassessment of need for oropharyngeal airway.
5. **Use Teach-Back:** "I want to be sure I explained why your loved one needs this oral airway. Tell me why it is important." Revise your instruction now or develop a plan for revised family caregiver teaching if family caregiver is not able to teach back correctly.	Determines family caregiver's level of understanding of instructional topic.

Unexpected Outcomes	Related Interventions
1. Patient continually coughs and gags when airway is inserted.	• Do not continue inserting airway. Stimulation of gag reflex can cause vomiting and aspiration. • Remove oral airway and position patient on side. • Reassess need for artificial airway prn.
2. Airway obstruction not relieved.	• Obtain immediate assistance from rapid response team or available health care provider. • Determine from health care provider if another form of airway is needed. • Assess for other causes of obstruction.
3. Patient pushes airway out of place or out of mouth.	• Reassess patient's need for oral airway.
4. Unable to insert oral airway, patient is combative, or you are unable to open his or her mouth.	• Get help. • Reassess patient's need for oral airway. • Provide sedation as ordered.

Recording

- Record assessment findings while inserting oral airway; size of oral airway; placement; any other procedures performed at same time, especially positioning; secretions obtained; and patient's tolerance of procedure.
- Document evaluation of family caregiver learning.

Hand-Off Reporting

- Report any airway obstruction or changes in secretions or patient's tolerance of airway (e.g., pushing airway out).

✦ SKILL 30.2 Using an Automated External Defibrillator

Purpose

An automated external defibrillator (AED) provides early defibrillation. It advises the user to provide a shock or no shock to an unconscious, pulseless patient. It analyzes the patient's heart rhythm using a computerized algorithm. This eliminates the need for the user to have to interpret an electrocardiogram (ECG) and thereby makes it possible for a CPR-trained user to defibrillate a patient promptly. An AED can be a stand-alone box (Fig. 30.4) with a very simple three-step function, or it can be incorporated into a manual defibrillator. If a shock is advised, the device automatically charges and gives the user audible and visible prompts to press the shock button.

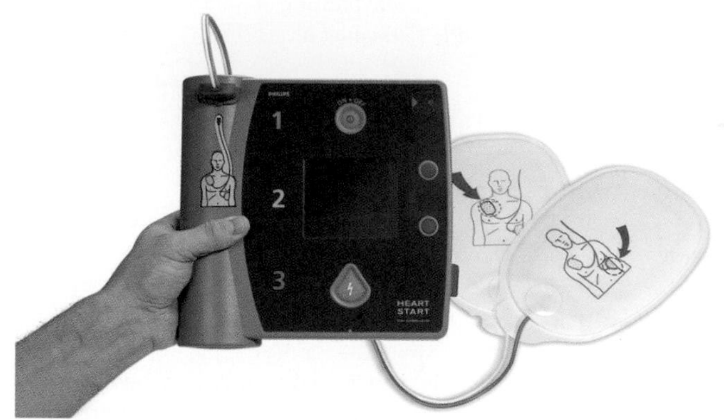

FIG 30.4 Automated external defibrillator (AED) device. *(Courtesy Philips Medical Systems.)*

Equipment

- AED
- Pair of AED adhesive pads

ASSESSMENT

1. Establish patient's unresponsiveness, if patient is unconscious, by shaking him or her and shouting, "Are you OK?" Call for help. (In community settings, have someone call 911. In the hospital setting, activate the resuscitation or code team.) *Rationale: Confirms that patient is unresponsive rather than intoxicated, sleeping, or hearing impaired. Substance abuse, hypoglycemia, toxicities, seizures, trauma, ketoacidosis, and shock also can cause unconsciousness.*
2. Palpate for carotid pulse on adult or child; use brachial or femoral pulse in infant. Palpate for no more than 10 seconds (Kleinman et al., 2015). *Rationale: Carotid pulse is the easiest to locate in adults and children. Femoral pulse may also be palpated in child or infant.*

Safe Patient Care *An AED should be applied only to a patient who is unconscious, not breathing, and pulseless. For children younger than 8 years old, AED pads designed for children should be used. When child pads are not available, use adult AED pads (Atkins et al., 2015).*

3. Establish absence of respirations and lack of circulation within 10 seconds: no pulse, no respirations, no movement. *Rationale: Indicates need for emergency measures, including AED.*

STEP	RATIONALE
PLANNING	
1. Expected outcomes following completion of procedure:	
• Patient's cardiac rhythm is converted back to stable rhythm.	Defibrillation provides electrical shock to convert lethal arrhythmias.
• Patient regains pulse and respirations.	CPR and defibrillation were successful.
2. Position patient on back.	Facilitates correct placement of AED pads.
IMPLEMENTATION	
1. Reassess patient for unresponsiveness. If no pulse, start chest compressions and continue until AED is attached to patient and verbal prompt of device advises you, "Do not touch the patient."	Chest compressions should be provided while AED pads are applied and until the AED is ready to analyze the heart rhythm.

STEP	RATIONALE
Safe Patient Care *Be sure that the code or Rapid Response Team is notified according to agency policy.*	
2. Place AED next to patient near chest or head.	Ensures easy access to device.
Safe Patient Care *If the AED is immediately available, attach it to patient as soon as possible. The faster defibrillation is delivered, the better the survival rate (Kleinman et al., 2015).*	
3. Turn on power (see illustration).	Turning on power begins verbal prompts to guide you through the next steps.
4. Attach device. The device is attached to a patient's chest via two adhesive pads with conductive gel. Place first AED pad on upper right sternal border directly below clavicle. Place second AED pad lateral to left nipple with top of pad a few inches below axilla (see illustration). Ensure that cables are connected to AED.	Conductive gel facilitates transmission of electric shock. Alternative placement of AED pads is not recommended. AEDs analyze most heart rhythms using lead II.
Safe Patient Care *Do not attach pads to wet skin, over a medication patch, or over a pacemaker or implanted defibrillator. Improper application reduces the likelihood of a successful defibrillation attempt and may result in complications.*	
5. Do *NOT* touch patient when AED prompts you. Direct all rescuers and bystanders to avoid touching patient by announcing "Clear!" Allow AED to analyze the rhythm. Some devices require that an analysis button be pressed. The AED takes approximately 5 to 15 seconds to analyze the rhythm.	Each brand of AED is different; thus, familiarity with the specific model that you are using is important. Avoid contact with the patient to prevent rhythm analysis errors and prevent accidental shocking of bystanders (Kleinman et al., 2015).

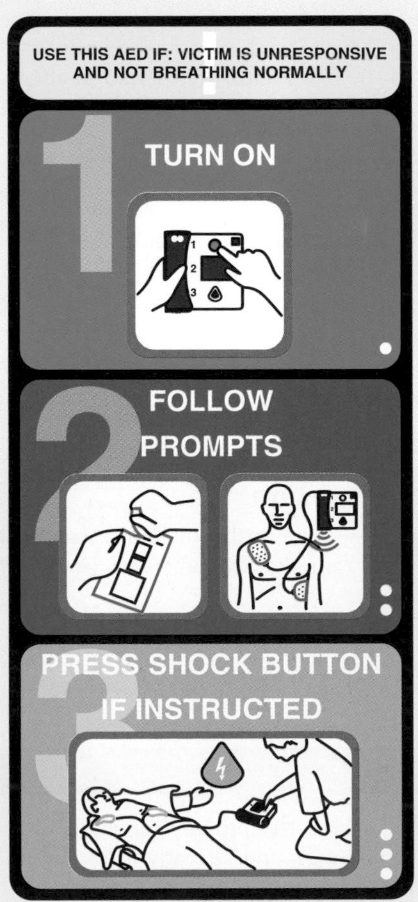

STEP 3 Power panel with automated external defibrillator (AED) prompts. *(Courtesy Philips Medical Systems.)*

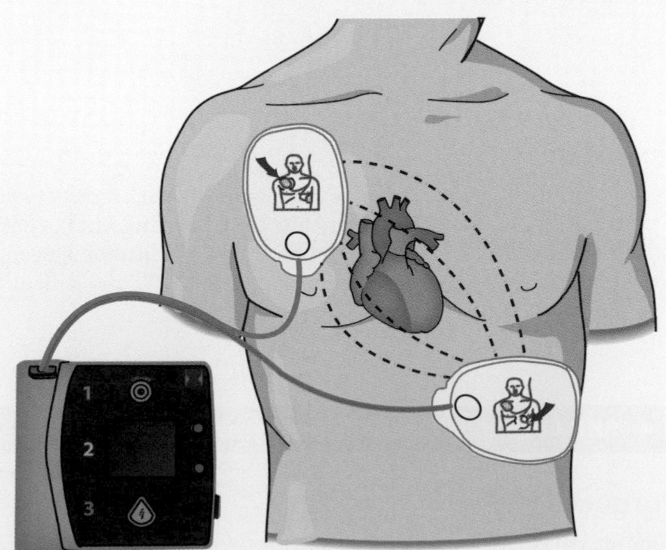

STEP 4 Placement of automated external defibrillator (AED) pads with device next to patient.

STEP	RATIONALE
6. Before pressing the shock button, announce loudly to "Clear" the victim and perform a visual check to ensure that no one is in contact with him or her. Then press the shock button.	Clearing patient ensures extra safety check for those involved in rescue efforts. Shock delivers electrical current.
7. Immediately begin chest compression after the shock and continue for 2 minutes with a ratio of 30:2 (30 compressions and 2 breaths). Do *NOT* remove pads.	Creates blood flow by increasing intrathoracic pressure and directly compressing the heart, which results in critical blood flow and oxygen delivery to the heart and brain.
8. Deliver 2 breaths after every 30 chest compressions using mouth-to-mouth with barrier device or bag-valve-mask device. Watch for chest rise and fall.	In a hospital setting where protected methods of artificial ventilation are available, mouth-to-mouth without a barrier device is not recommended because of risk for microbial contamination.
9. After 2 minutes of CPR, AED will prompt you not to touch patient and will resume analysis of patient's rhythm. This cycle will continue until patient regains a pulse or a health care provider determines death.	The AED will continue to provide analysis of the patient's heart rhythm during these 2-minute cycles. Remember to maintain chest compressions until the AED advises NOT to touch the patient. This will minimize CPR interruption time.

EVALUATION

1. Inspect pad adhesion to the chest wall. If pads are not in good contact with chest wall, remove them and apply a new set. Attach new pads to the AED.	Poor pad–skin contact reduces effectiveness of the shock, causes skin burns, or increases chance of shocking those involved in the rescue efforts. Always apply a new set of pads. Do *NOT* reuse.
2. Check for palpable pulse or patient movement. Continue resuscitative efforts until patient regains pulse or health care provider determines death.	Evaluates circulatory status.
3. Provide updates to family on patient's status.	Use resources to keep family informed, including providers, chaplain, and social workers. Screen family for possible family presence in the room during resuscitation efforts.

Unexpected Outcomes	Related Interventions
1. Patient's heart rhythm does not convert into stable rhythm with pulse after defibrillation.	• Assess pad contact on patient's chest wall. • Do not touch patient during AED rhythm analysis. • Avoid placing AED pads over medication patches, pacemaker, or implantable defibrillator generators.
2. Patient's skin has burns under AED pads.	• Assess AED pad contact on chest. • Ensure that chest is dry before applying pads to chest. • Apply skin care as indicated if patient is resuscitated successfully.

Recording

- Record onset of arrest, time and number of AED shocks (you will not know the exact energy level used by the AED), time and energy level of manual defibrillations, medications given, procedures performed, cardiac rhythm, use of CPR, and patient's response.

Hand-Off Reporting

- Provide an up-to-date cardiopulmonary assessment and patient response to all resuscitation interventions.

✦ SKILL 30.3 Code Management

Purpose

Code management includes a team of providers trained in both basic and advanced life support. However, it is the first responder (usually a nurse inside a hospital) who makes the biggest difference using basic life-support (BLS) skills. These BLS skills include the first responder making the primary survey of C (circulation), *A* (airway), *B* (breathing), and *D* (early defibrillation). This survey continues and repeats until the code team arrives.

The code team immediately determines the patient's cardiac rhythm, and the advanced life-support team or code team leader will determine the next interventions according to AHA (2015)

TABLE 30.2

Adult, Child, and Infant Cardiopulmonary Resuscitation Techniques (Health Care Providers [HCPs])

Technique	Adult	Child (1 Year to Puberty)	Infant (Under 1 Year—Does Not Include Newborns)
Compression initiation	Begin compressions if unresponsive, no breathing or only gasping breaths, and no pulse palpated within 10 seconds. Child and infant: Begin compressions, if HR <60 bpm and signs of poor perfusion.		
Chest compression hand placement	2 hands on the lower half of sternum	2 hands or 1 hand (for very small child) on the lower half of sternum	One rescuer: 2 fingers in center of chest just below the nipple line Two rescuers: 2 thumb-encircling hands in the center of the chest, just below the nipple line
Chest compression depth, rate, and ratio	Compress 2–2.4 inches deep at a rate of 100–120/min One to two rescuers: 100–120/min, 30 compressions to 2 breaths (30:2)	Compress at least $\frac{1}{3}$ depth of chest (2 inches) at a rate of 100–120/min One rescuer: 30 compressions, 2 breaths (30:2) Two rescuers: 15 compressions, 2 breaths (15:2)	Compress 1 inch at a rate of 100–120/min One rescuer: 30 compressions, 2 breaths (30:2) Two rescuers: 15 compressions, 2 breaths (15:2)
Defibrillation	Use adult pads. AED should be applied as soon as available, and shock as soon as advised.	Use child pads whenever possible. If none, use adult pads, but do not overlap them. Apply AED as soon as available, and shock as soon as advised.	If there is a shockable rhythm, use manual defibrillation.
Ventilation rate with compressions and advanced airway	Give 1 breath every 6 seconds (10 breaths/min) via resuscitation bag. Do not interrupt chest compressions to deliver breaths.		

AED, Automated external defibrillator; *HR,* heart rate.

Data from Kleinman ME, et al: American Heart Association Guidelines for cardiopulmonary resuscitation and emergency cardiovascular care. Part 5: Adult basic life support, *Circulation* 132(suppl 2):S414, 2015; and Atkins DL, et al: American Heart Association Guidelines for cardiopulmonary resuscitation and emergency cardiovascular care. Part 11: Pediatric basic life support and cardiopulmonary resuscitation quality, *Circulation* 132(suppl 2):S519, 2015.

guidelines (Table 30.2). Code team members are trained in the performance of the secondary survey: C (continued quality chest compressions and rhythm analysis of cardiac rhythm), A (advanced airway placement), B (confirmation of airway and ventilation), and D (defibrillation and differential diagnosis of the cause for the arrest). Both primary and secondary surveys must be reassessed continually and managed throughout the code situation until the patient responds or a determination of death is made.

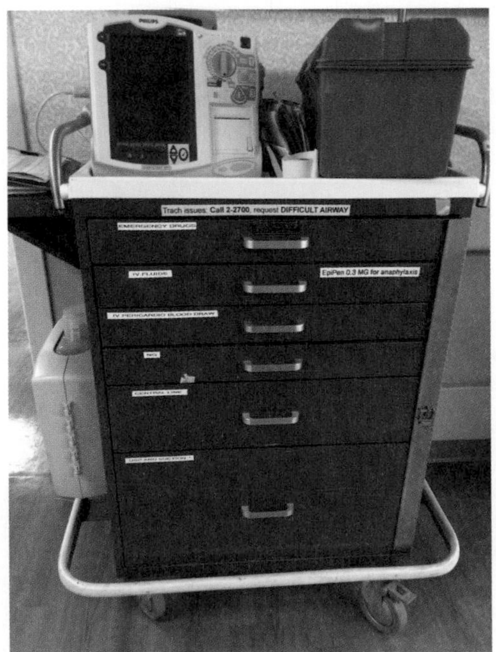

FIG 30.5 Emergency code cart.

Equipment

- Code cart (Fig. 30.5)—most adult code (crash) carts have the following equipment:
  - Clean and sterile gloves, gown, protective eyewear
  - Oxygen source
  - Bag-valve-mask device or resuscitation bag
  - Oral airways
  - Laryngoscope, handle, and straight and curved laryngoscope blades
  - Endotracheal (ET) tube, various sizes (6 to 9 mm for adults; 0 to 4 mm for pediatrics)
  - End-tidal CO_2 detector or monitor
  - Tape or commercial ET tube holder
  - Backboard
  - Automated external defibrillator (AED) and/or manual defibrillator with AED/defibrillator pads.
  - Intravascular needles (14 to 22 gauge) and possibly intraosseous needles
  - Central vascular access kit
  - Intravenous (IV) tubing, fluids (9% normal saline, D_5W)
  - Syringes
  - Laboratory specimen tubes
  - Arterial blood gas kit
  - Emergency medications
  - Advanced cardiac life support (ACLS) guidelines or algorithms
  - Suction equipment, wall or portable suction

ASSESSMENT

1. Determine whether patient is unconscious by shaking him or her and shouting, "Are you OK?" Assess patient unresponsiveness. *Rationale: Confirms that patient is unresponsive rather than intoxicated, sleeping, or hearing impaired. Substance abuse, hypoglycemia, toxicities, seizures, trauma, ketoacidosis, and shock also can cause unconsciousness.*

Safe Patient Care *If an unresponsive person has adequate respirations and pulse, remain until further help is present. Place victim in a modified lateral recovery position (see illustration). Continue to assess for the presence of respirations and pulse because a recurrent arrest may develop.*

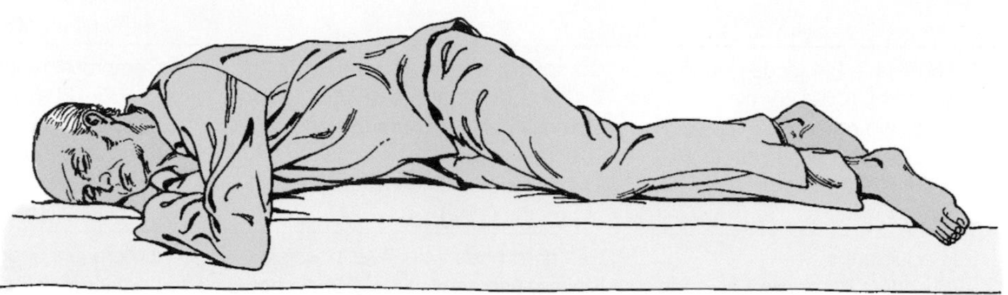

STEP 1 Recovery position.

STEP	RATIONALE

PLANNING

STEP	RATIONALE
1. Expected outcomes following completion of procedure:	
• Patient regains pulse and respirations.	Cardiopulmonary resuscitation (CPR) was successful.
• Patient maintains a stable cardiac rhythm and blood pressure.	Stabilizing treatment is successful.
• Patient transported to intensive care unit (ICU) for post-resuscitation care.	Ongoing treatment and support needed.
2. Immediately activate the hospital's code team or emergency medical services (EMS). Tell co-workers or bystanders to bring AED (if available) and crash cart to bedside.	Ensures timely delivery of defibrillation, chest compressions, and ACLS to arrest victim.
3. As soon as possible, apply clean gloves and face shield.	Reduces transmission of microorganisms.

IMPLEMENTATION

Primary Survey: *C* (Circulation); *D* (Defibrillation [as Soon as Device Is Available])

STEP	RATIONALE
1. Check carotid pulse on adult or child; use brachial or femoral pulse in infant. Palpate for no more than 10 seconds (Kleinman et al., 2015; Pozner et al., 2018).	Carotid pulse is the easiest to locate in adults and children. Femoral pulse may also be palpated in child or infant.
2. Position patient supine on hard surface, such as backboard over mattress, floor, or ground. Victim must be flat. Logroll victim to flat, supine position using spine precautions if trauma is suspected.	Facilitates external compression of the heart. Heart is compressed between sternum and spinal vertebrae, which must be on hard and firm surface. Do NOT delay the start of CPR. Positioning patient on hard surface may take more than one or two rescuers. You may need to wait to safely move him or her. Place backboard or position patient as soon as appropriate assistance is present.

Primary Survey: *A* (Airway)

STEP	RATIONALE
3. Open airway:	
a. Head tilt–chin lift (no history of cervical trauma; see illustration) *or*	Tongue is most common cause of blocked airway in unresponsive patient.

STEP	RATIONALE
b. Jaw thrust (cervical trauma is suspected; see illustration)	Suspect spinal cord injury in patients with trauma. Jaw-thrust maneuver prevents head extension and neck movement which may cause further injury. Apply rigid cervical collar and immobilize patient as soon as possible to reduce cervical spine motion.
4. Assess for spontaneous respirations.	Determines level of resuscitation required.

Primary Survey: *B* (Breathing)

STEP	RATIONALE
5. Attempt to ventilate patient with 2 breaths using one of these methods.	Slow breaths deliver air at low pressure to reduce risk of gastric distention.
a. Mouth-to-mouth using barrier device.	Forms airtight seal to prevent air from escaping through nose.
b. Mouth-to-mask using pocket mask (see illustration).	Provides secure seal and permits use of supplemental oxygen.
c. Resuscitation bag and mask (see illustrations).	Gives breaths with enough force to make chest rise.
6. If the tongue to obstructing the airway, consider inserting oropharyngeal airway (see Skill 30.1).	Maintains tongue on anterior floor of mouth and prevents obstruction of posterior airway by tongue.
7. Suction secretions if necessary or turn victim's head to one side unless trauma is suspected.	Suctioning prevents airway obstruction. Turning patient's head to one side allows gravity to drain any secretions, decreasing risk of aspiration.

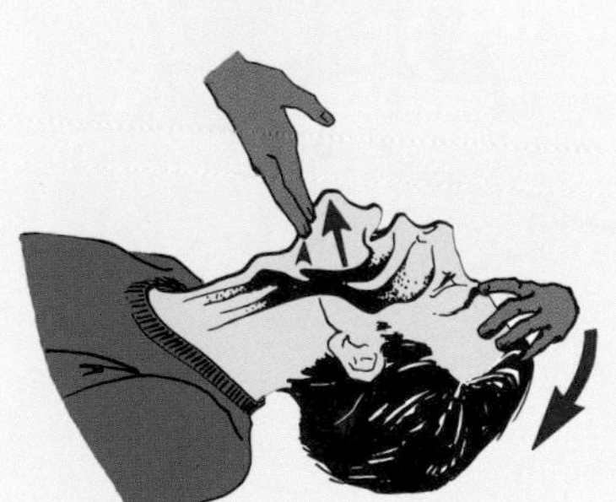

STEP 3a Head tilt–chin lift. *(From Sorrentino S: Mosby's textbook for nursing assistants, ed 7, St. Louis, 2008, Mosby.)*

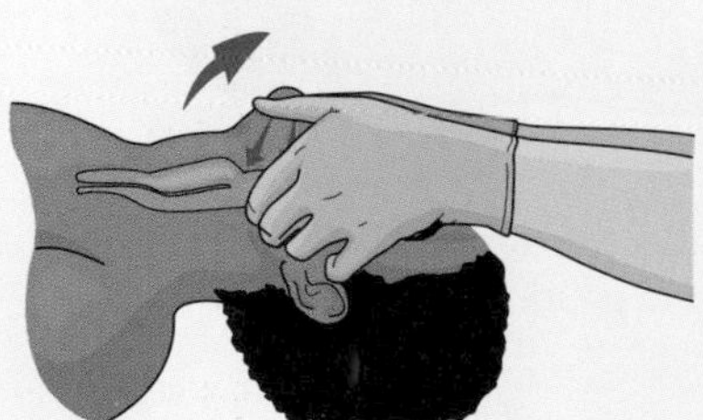

STEP 3b Jaw thrust without head tilt.

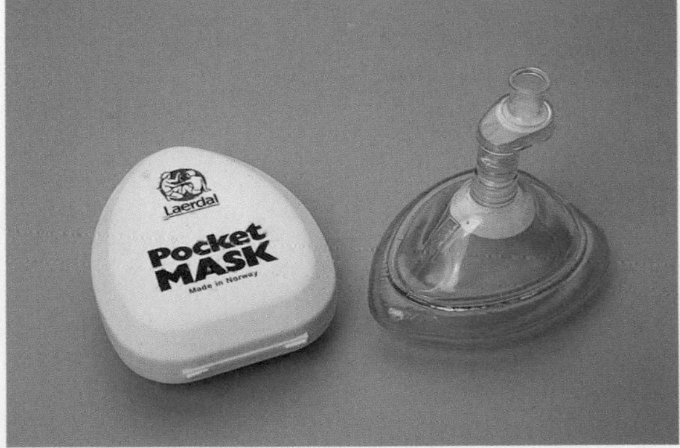

STEP 5b Pocket mask.

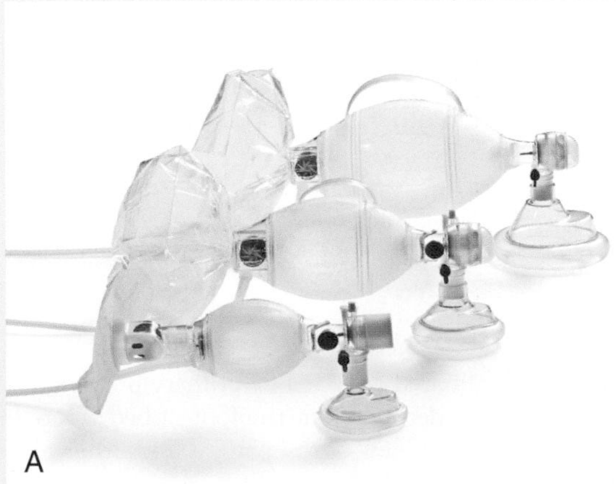

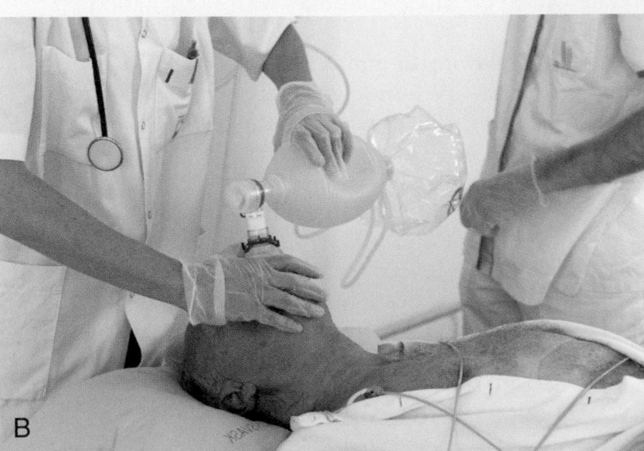

STEP 5c (A) Bag-valve-mask device. (B) Two-rescuer breathing with bag-valve-mask device. *(Courtesy Ambu A/S.)*

STEP	RATIONALE

Primary Survey: *D* (Defibrillation)

8. If pulse is absent and AED is available, apply AED immediately as appropriate (see Skill 30.2).
   a. After first shock, immediately resume CPR for 5 cycles or approximately 2 minutes. One cycle is considered 30 compressions: 2 breaths for adults. Every 2 minutes, perform rhythm analysis and possible shock if appropriate (see Table 30.2).

A shock followed by chest compression provides sufficient blood flow and perfusion before another is delivered (Kleinman et al., 2015; Pozner et al., 2018). Energy is delivered in prescribed doses for different age groups and devices. Manual biphasic devices deliver shocks at a lower level (200 joules); monophasic waveforms use 360 joules.

9. If pulse is absent and an AED is unavailable, immediately initiate chest compressions.
   a. Assume correct hand position and compression ratio (30:2 adult) for patient (see illustrations).

Specific hand position, compression depth, and ratio are different for adults, children, and infants to avoid injury to heart, lung, or liver (see Table 30.2).

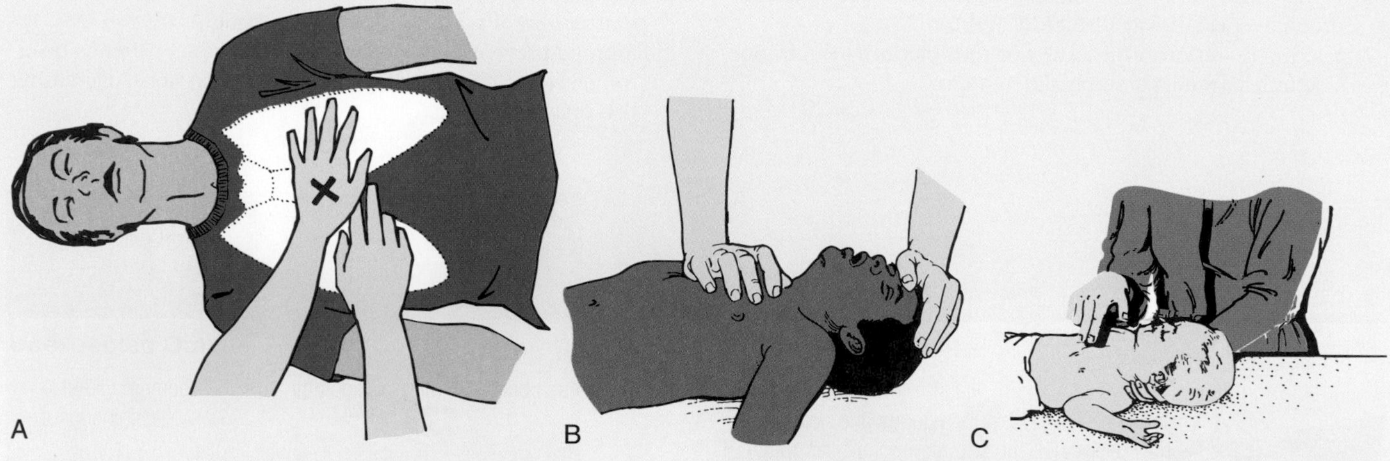

STEP 9a (A) Proper hand position—adult. (B) Proper hand position—child. (C) Proper hand position—infant.

Secondary Survey: Implementation

10. Give code leader brief verbal report of events just prior to the patient's discovery and any interventions performed before code team's arrival (e.g., age, admit diagnosis, how patient was found, interventions).

This information is critical to give the code team a brief overview of the patient and what steps to take next.

11. On arrival of sufficient personnel, delegate tasks as appropriate while core group continues with resuscitation efforts.

Delegation of duties is essential to meet the emergent needs of patient and his or her family in timely matter.

   a. Delegate the following to nurses in the room:
      - Bedside nurse—performs tasks such as medication administration, vital signs, and helping with procedures
      - Crash cart nurse—prepares medications and gets supplies from crash cart to hand off to code team members
      - Recorder—ensures accurate documentation of events of code, medications, and treatments administered

These three roles are essential to cover most of the actions needed during an arrest. Each nurse needs to communicate clearly to each other and the code team leader.

   b. Other code team members will assume the following roles:
      - Code team leader: physician or advanced practice nurse
      - Anesthesiology staff
      - Respiratory therapy (RT)

Ensures a coordinated code led by primary physician.

Code team leader is best at the foot of bed where he or she can have a clear view of the patient and other team members.

Anesthesiology staff is best at the head of the bed to place advanced airway. Respiratory therapy will be assisting anesthesia.

STEP	RATIONALE
c. Other nurses or ancillary help can assist with the following: • Safely move the roommate and unneeded staff away from the code scene. • Assign pastoral care or other nurses to communicate with patient's family. • Consider allowing family to witness resuscitation (see agency policy). • Access the patient's chart at the bedside. • Removal of excess furniture or equipment from the room.	Family members who were allowed to witness resuscitation efforts have been found to have a significant reduction in posttraumatic stress and also self-report a greater sense of resolution and fulfillment (American Association of Critical-Care Nurses [AACCN], 2016). Chart will provide more information on the patient's medical condition, code status, and presence of any allergies

Secondary Survey: *C* (Continued Compressions and Analysis of Cardiac Rhythm)

STEP	RATIONALE
12. Attach manual defibrillator/monitor to patient using electrocardiogram (ECG) electrodes or "hands-off" defibrillator pads to visualize cardiac rhythm (see illustration).	Cardiac rhythm monitoring devices provide immediate rhythm display for analysis without disruption of rescue breathing and chest compression.

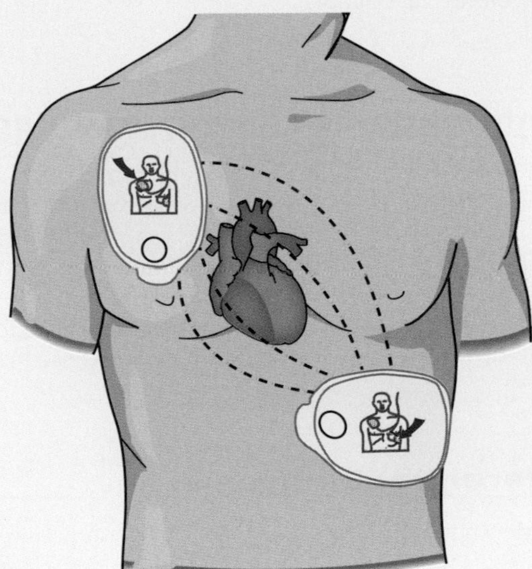

STEP 12 Secondary Survey C, Step 3: Paddle placement for defibrillation.

STEP	RATIONALE
13. If cardiac rhythm is "shockable," continue CPR and help code team with manual defibrillation.	
a. Turn on defibrillator and select proper energy level following agency policy and equipment directions.	Energy is delivered in prescribed doses. Manual biphasic devices deliver shocks at a lower level (200 joules); monophasic waveforms use 360 joules.
b. Apply conductive gel or gel pads to patient's chest where defibrillator paddles will be placed. Most defibrillators use "hands-off pads" that are applied to patient's chest and directly connect to manual defibrillator.	Good skin-to-paddle/pad contact ensures appropriate discharge of current and decreases chance of skin burns (Link et al., 2015).
c. Verify that no one is in physical contact with patient, bed, or any item contacting patient during defibrillation. A warning must be called out before initiating charge.	Prevents accidental delivery of shock or injury to personnel.
14. Establish IV access with large-bore IV needle (14 to 20 gauge) and begin infusion of 0.9% normal saline (NS; see Chapter 28).	Provides a route for rapid drug administration and access for blood samples and fluid administration. Physiological saline is isotonic. Rapid fluid infusion facilitates dispersal of medication throughout cardiovascular system.

STEP	RATIONALE
a. If you cannot obtain peripheral intravenous (IV) access, health care provider may pursue central venous or intraosseous (IO) access.	Administration of emergency medications is dependent on vascular or IO access.
15. Help with procedures as needed.	Most equipment needed for special procedures during code is on the crash cart. Knowledge of crash cart contents is very helpful in the code to provide personnel with appropriate equipment.
16. Switch chest compressors every 2 minutes to maintain quality CPR.	Chest compressor switch-outs usually occur at the 2-minute pulse check/rhythm check and should not exceed 10 seconds (Kleinman et al., 2015; Pozner et al., 2018).

Secondary Survey: *A* (Advanced Airway Placement)

STEP	RATIONALE
17. Assist anesthesia or RT personnel in performing endotracheal (ET) intubation or other advanced airway placement.	Intubation provides a patent airway and facilitates pulmonary ventilation. Laryngeal mask airway or esophageal-tracheal Combitube can also be used to provide advanced airway support.
a. Have available laryngoscope handle, laryngoscope blades, curved and straight blades, ET tubes, stylet, suction, and tape or ET tube holder. Ensure that light source on laryngoscope is functional.	Light is necessary on laryngoscope to visualize vocal cords and intubate trachea. Batteries may need to be changed.

Secondary Survey: *B* (Confirmation of Airway and Ventilation)

STEP	RATIONALE
18. Assist in confirming that the advanced airway has been placed in the trachea by auscultating lungs for bilateral breath sounds and monitoring the carbon dioxide (CO_2) detector (Link et al., 2015; Pozner et al., 2018).	Auscultation of lungs and monitoring of exhaled CO_2 provides two methods of immediate placement verification. Chest x-ray film is obtained after patient has been stabilized to confirm placement of advanced airway and central venous catheters.
19. Ventilate using resuscitation bag upon advanced airway placement. Avoid hyperventilation. Give 1 breath every 6 seconds.	Increased intrathoracic pressure caused by hyperventilation results in reduced cardiac output (Link et al., 2015).

Secondary Survey: *D* (Differential Diagnosis)

STEP	RATIONALE
20. Obtain ordered laboratory and diagnostic studies.	Aids in determination of cause of arrest.

EVALUATION

STEP	RATIONALE
1. Reassess primary and secondary surveys throughout code event.	Keeps process organized and addresses immediate needs of patient.
2. Palpate carotid pulse at 5 cycles or 2 minutes of CPR.	Documents adequacy of external cardiac compressions. Use of a feedback device is encouraged.
3. Observe for spontaneous return of respirations or heart rate every 2 minutes.	Assessment of heart rate, pulse, respirations, and cardiac rhythm occurs every 2 minutes during a brief interruption of chest compressions and ventilation.
4. Ensure that interruptions in CPR are minimized.	Interruptions are associated with reduced coronary artery perfusion pressure and lower mean coronary perfusion pressure (Link et al., 2015; Pozner et al., 2018).
5. **Use Teach-Back:** "I want to be sure I clearly explained what has happened to your loved one and why we performed CPR. In your own words, tell me why we had to perform CPR." Revise your instruction now or develop a plan for revised family caregiver teaching if family caregiver is not able to teach back correctly.	Determines family caregiver's level of understanding of instructional topic. Understanding the situation fully may be difficult for family due to emotional stress. Keep instructions very simple and straightforward.

Unexpected Outcomes	Related Interventions
1. Patient develops skeletal injury such as fractured ribs or sternum or internal organ injury such as lacerated lung or liver as result of chest compressions.	• Obtain appropriate diagnostic tests to document injuries. • Assess patient's post-arrest breathing for symmetry and pain. • Assess for intrathoracic or intraabdominal bleeding (hematomas, increasing abdominal girth).
2. Patient's CPR is unsuccessful.	• Contact chaplain services. • Contact social worker. • Complete postmortem care on patient (see Chapter 31). • Notify coroner and organ procurement agency in accordance with local hospital or state law. • Provide privacy for patient's family to grieve and mourn loss of loved one.

Recording

- Record the timeline of events, in this order: time of patient discovery, time of first chest compression, time of first shock (if delivered), time of first assisted ventilations. Other documentation should include number of AED shocks (you need to know the device-specific energy level delivered by the AED), time and energy level of manual defibrillations, medications given, procedures performed, cardiac rhythm strips, use of CPR, and patient's response. Most hospitals use a form designed specifically for arrests that prompts the recorder to enter appropriate information.

Hand-Off Reporting

- Report relevant cardiac arrest history and patient response.
- Report cardiac arrhythmias and response to interventions.

SPECIAL CONSIDERATIONS

Patient-Centered Care

- Advance directives are unique for each patient, and these directives offer valuable information about a patient's decisions regarding resuscitation efforts. Nurses may be involved in coordinating meetings between providers and family or assist in completion of the patient's advance directive document or provider's order to not resuscitate. Advance directive documents can help minimize confusion as to what resuscitation efforts should be avoided.

Patient Education

- For select patients, teach family members how to use an AED; use a practice model, and verify competency via return demonstration.
- Educate patients and family members about the importance of keeping emergency numbers taped to phone programming them into the speed-dial function on both home and mobile phones.
- Stress the use of 911 versus driving family member to the hospital.

Age-Specific

Pediatric

- Infants and children experience respiratory arrest more frequently than full cardiopulmonary arrest.
- Oropharyngeal airways are seldom used in the treatment of airway obstruction in children and infants. A child's airway is narrow; thus, oropharyngeal airways are often more occlusive than beneficial (Atkins et al., 2015). A nasopharyngeal airway may be tolerated by children better than an oropharyngeal one (Ralston et al., 2018).
- For infants and small children, sliding the oropharyngeal airway along the side of the mouth rather than with the tip up is recommended because the soft palate is easily injured.
- Many AEDs are equipped to deliver energy suitable for infants and children younger than 8 years old using specific pads for children. Adult pads can be used if child pads are unavailable, but be sure not to overlap or cut the pads. If using a manual defibrillator, an energy setting of 2 to 4 J/kg is recommended for infants (Atkins et al., 2015; Scarfone et al., 2018).

Gerontological

- Older adults, especially older adults with osteoporosis, are at greater risk for rib fractures.
- Remove loose-fitting dentures to avoid airway obstruction during CPR and airway insertions. Leave properly fitting dentures in place because they assist in ensuring a tight seal during artificial ventilation.

Home Care

- AEDs are available for use in the community and home setting.
- A family member living in the home must know how to use the AED and be willing to use this device as needed.

✦ PRACTICE REFLECTIONS

A patient with a history of heart failure is admitted to the cardiology unit and is on telemetry. As the heart failure worsened, pulmonary edema resulted.

1. You find the patient lying on the floor of the bathroom. What is your priority action? Why?
2. The patient goes into cardiac arrest. You activate the emergency response code team. After the code team arrives, you are responsible for code management. What tasks will you delegate to ancillary staff?
3. You become the crash cart nurse. What are your responsibilities and tasks?

✦ CLINICAL REVIEW QUESTIONS

1. Place the steps for inserting an oral airway in the correct order.
   1. Perform hand hygiene and don appropriate PPE.
   2. Hold airway curved end up and insert until airway reaches back of the throat.
   3. Rotate airway 180 degrees.
   4. Position patient.
   5. Allow airway to follow natural curve of tongue.
   6. Reassess patient's respiratory status.
   7. Suction secretions as needed.
2. Automated external defibrillators (AEDs) are used to halt lethal cardiac arrhythmias. Which of the following features apply to AEDs? (Select all that apply.)
   1. Does not require user to make rhythm analysis
   2. Used in unconscious patients
   3. Guide the user with verbal prompts
   4. One pad placed on upper right sternal border
   5. Quicker defibrillation correlated with better survival
   6. Second pad placed on left sternal border
3. Which of the following techniques ensures the highest quality chest compressions? (Select all that apply.)
   1. Minimizing interruption in chest compressions
   2. Avoiding full chest recoil
   3. Providing excessive ventilations
   4. Ensuring adequate depth and rate of compression
   5. Ensuring AED in place

Answers and Rationales for Clinical Review Questions can be found on the Evolve website.

REFERENCES

American Association of Critical-Care Nurses (AACCN): Practice alert: family presence during resuscitation and invasive procedures, *Crit Care Nurse* 36(1):e11, 2016.

American Heart Association (AHA): Get with the guidelines—resuscitation recognition criteria, 2017. http://www.heart.org/HEARTORG/HealthcareResearch/GetWithTheGuidelines/GetWithTheGuidelines-Resuscitation/Get-With-The-Guidelines-Resuscitation-Recognition-Criteria_UCM_433238_Article.jsp.

Atkins DL, et al: American Heart Association guidelines for cardiopulmonary resuscitation and emergency cardiovascular care. Part 11: pediatric basic life support and cardiopulmonary resuscitation quality, *Circulation* 132(suppl 2):S519b, 2015.

Callaway CW: Targeted temperature management after cardiac arrest finding the right dose for critical care interventions, *JAMA* 318(4):334, 2017.

Callaway CW, et al: Part 8: post-cardiac arrest care: American Heart Association guidelines update for cardiopulmonary resuscitation and emergency cardiovascular care, *Circulation* 132(suppl 1):S465, 2015.

Centers for Disease Control and Prevention: What is health literacy? 2016. https://www.cdc.gov/healthliteracy/learn/index.html.

Donnino MW, et al: Temperature management after cardiac arrest: an advisory statement by the advanced life support task force of the international liaison committee on resuscitation and the American Heart Association Emergency Cardiovascular Care Committee and the Council on Cardiopulmonary, Critical Care, Perioperative and Resuscitation, *Resuscitation* 98:97, 2016.

Kleinman ME, et al: American Heart Association guidelines for cardiopulmonary resuscitation and emergency cardiovascular care. Part 5: adult basic life support and cardiopulmonary resuscitation quality, *Circulation* 132(suppl 2):S414a, 2015.

Link MS, et al: Part 7: adult advanced cardiovascular life support: American Heart Association guidelines for cardiopulmonary resuscitation and emergency cardiovascular care, *Circulation* 132(suppl 2):S444, 2015.

Neumar RW, et al: Part 1: executive summary: 2015 American Heart Association guidelines update for cardiopulmonary resuscitation and emergency cardiovascular care, *Circulation* 132(18 suppl 2):2015.

Pittman J, et al: Medical device related hospital-acquired pressure ulcers, *J Wound Ostomy Continence Nurs* 42(2):151, 2015.

Pozner C, et al: Basic life support (BLS) in adults, *UpToDate* 2018. https://www.uptodate.com/contents/basic-life-support-bls-in-adults#!

Ralston M, et al: Basic airway management in children, *UpToDate* 2018. https://www.uptodate.com/contents/basic-airway-management-in-children#!

Rittenberger JC, Callaway CW: Post-cardiac arrest management in adults, *UpToDate* 2018. https://www.uptodate.com/contents/post-cardiac-arrest-management-in-adults.

Scarfone R, et al: Defibrillation and cardioversion in children (including automated external defibrillation), *UpToDate* 2018. https://www.uptodate.com/contents/defibrillation-and-cardioversion-in-children-including-automated-external-defibrillation#!

31 | End-of-Life Care

SKILLS AND PROCEDURES

EVOLVE WEBSITE/RESOURCES LIST

http://evolve.elsevier.com/Perry/nursinginterventions

Audio Glossary • Checklists • Clinical Review Questions • Answers and Rationales for Clinical Review Questions

INTRODUCTION

Nurses play a vital role in helping patients with chronic, life-limiting illnesses maintain the best possible quality of life (QOL) by providing expert palliative care. Palliative care is defined by the World Health Organization (WHO, 2018) as approaches that improve the quality of life of patients and their families facing the problem associated with life-threatening illness. This is accomplished through the prevention and relief of suffering by means of early identification and thorough assessment and treatment of pain and other physical, psychosocial, and spiritual problems. Members of the palliative care team manage symptoms, facilitate person-centered communication, promote decision making, and coordinate care across settings throughout the disease trajectory (National Consensus Project for Quality Palliative Care [NCP], 2018). Ideally, patients who receive palliative care would move seamlessly into hospice care when they no longer benefit from curative treatments (Fig. 31.1). End-of-life care encompasses the care and support provided to patients during the time surrounding death, not only in the moments before breathing stops, to help patients reach peaceful deaths at the end of life (National Institute on Aging [NIA], 2017).

PRACTICE STANDARDS

- National Consensus Project for Quality Palliative Care (NCP), 2018: Clinical practice guidelines for quality palliative care—Care guidelines
- National Institute on Aging (NIA), 2017: What is end-of-life care?—Palliative and end-of-life support for patients and families
- The Joint Commission (TJC), 2019: National Patient Safety Goals—Patient identification

EVIDENCE-BASED PRACTICE

Self-Care and Compassion Satisfaction

There is an abundance of research on compassion fatigue in palliative care and end-of-life care in relation to health care providers. Health care providers are invaluable to the patients and families they care for but are at risk for burnout and other psychological effects due to constantly dealing with death and dying. Recent research examined ways to support health care providers so that they can experience compassion satisfaction rather than compassion fatigue and develop tools to deal with these high-stress work environments (Salmond et al., 2017; Sansó et al., 2015). Evidence-based guidelines for self-care and compassion satisfaction include the following:

- To nurture your capacity to remain empathically engaged with patients and family members, you must also care for yourself physically, spiritually, and emotionally.
- Self-care helps health care providers cope with frequent exposure to death and dying. Self-care was found to be a necessity for providers within these high-stress and emotionally charged environments, where spiritual and existential issues are often encountered (Salmond et al., 2017; Sansó et al., 2015).
- Participants who scored greater levels of self-awareness also had greater scores in competence in coping with death (Sansó et al., 2015).
- Providers' ability to cope with death was positively related to compassion satisfaction and negatively related to burnout and compassion fatigue. There was also a strong relationship between the ability to cope with death and the providers' own quality of life (Salmond et al., 2017; Sansó et al., 2015).

SAFETY GUIDELINES

- Patients who are seriously ill experience decreased muscle strength and limited endurance. However, they may prefer to get out of bed for meals or to walk to the bathroom as long as possible. Have them sit on the side of the bed for a minute before getting up. Guard against falls by having patients use appropriate assistive devices for walking (see Chapter 18). Remain with patients until they are safely seated or lying down (American Cancer Society [ACS], 2017).

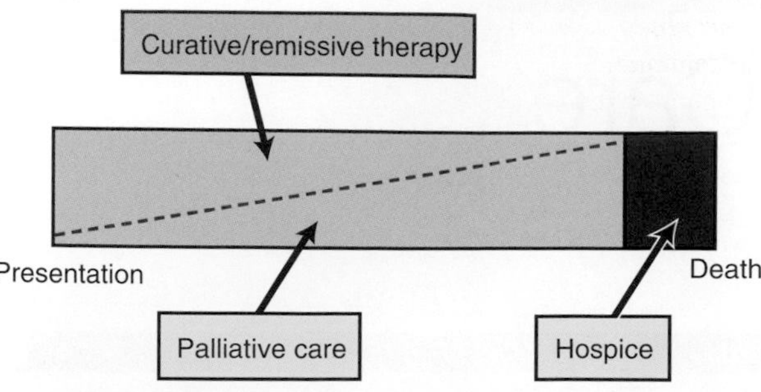

FIG 31.1 Palliative care and hospice. *(From Emanuel L et al.: The education in palliative and end of life care [EPEC] curriculum: The EPEC Project, 2003, Northwestern University Feinberg School of Medicine.)*

- Place a patient who wants to eat or drink in an upright position and offer small bites of food or sips of water slowly to avoid aspiration (see Chapter 13).
- Be sure that the nurse call system is in an accessible location within the patient's reach at all times, and consider calls as a high priority.
- In some agencies, patients who have a do-not-resuscitate (DNR) order wear a wrist bracelet that alerts care providers that they should not start cardiopulmonary resuscitation (CPR) when the patient's heart or breathing stops. Identify a patient with DNR status by using two identifiers (i.e., name and birthday or name and account number, according to agency policy) (TJC, 2019). Compare identifiers with information on the patient's identification bracelet. Placing a DNR bracelet on the wrong patient may lead to unintentional death or the resuscitation of a patient against his or her wishes.
- In the case of a patient's death, identify patient using at least two identifiers (e.g., name and birthday or name and medical record number) according to agency policy. Compare identifiers with information on the patient's identification bracelet before sending a body to the morgue. Improper identification of a body may lead to a serious miscommunication with family members.
- After a death, communicate to others who will care for the patient's body (e.g., transporters, morgue attendants, and funeral home employees) any potential infection risks. The bodies of patients that pose a high infectious risk should be carefully marked, and the body should be prepared after death to avoid leakage of infectious body fluids.

PROMOTING NURSES' SELF-CARE

Nurses who are routinely involved in the care of seriously ill and dying patients will experience a wide range of emotional experiences (Ingebretsen and Sagbakken, 2016). Although they value the strong bond they develop with patients and family caregivers, nurses have identified that they also need to be cautious and not get overwhelmed by the experiences and that they must balance their emotions with those of their patients. Compassion fatigue is often reported, which may leave you feeling isolated, confused, and spiritually exhausted, leading to an inability to relate well to the people in your care (Salmond et al., 2017).

Self-care for nurses in these experiences can be enhanced by talking about your feelings and experiences with a trusted friend or peer. Identify ways in which you can work with others to address workplace barriers to effective self-care. Sometimes a debriefing after a particularly long or difficult death helps you feel support and gain perspective. Regularly practice stress management techniques such as relaxation techniques when feeling stressed, physical exercise, nutritious eating patterns, humor, hobbies, and adequate sleep. Strengthen yourself spiritually with meditation, prayer, or consultation with a spiritual care provider. It may help to attend the funeral of a patient with whom you shared special bonds. You might also gain insight by reflecting on your own personal beliefs and feelings about death and loss.

✦ SKILL 31.1 Supporting Patients and Families in Grief

Purpose

For cases in which patients require palliative care or in end-of-life situations, patients and family members experience intense feelings such as anxiety, sadness, regret, or relief. They ask questions of spiritual significance about the meaning of life, pain, suffering, and loss of personal power and control. In short, they experience grief, an intense emotional and behavioral response to perceived and actual losses. Grief experiences often begin during chronic illness and before a patient dies. Survivors grieve as they anticipate a loss and continue to feel grief after the patient dies.

Delegation and Collaboration

The skills of assessing patients' or family members' grief reactions and designing appropriate interventions cannot be delegated to nursing assistive personnel (NAP). The nurse directs the NAP to:

- Inform the nurse when a patient or family member exhibits behavior commonly associated with grief (e.g., crying, anger, withdrawal).
- Form supportive relationships with patients and families and inform the nurse when patients or family members have questions or concerns.
- Alert the nurse to the arrival of family members so that the nurse can discuss the plan of care and offer support.

ASSESSMENT

1. Identify patient using at least two identifiers (e.g., name and birthday or name and medical record number) according to agency policy. *Rationale: Ensures patient safety. Complies with The Joint Commission standards and improves patient safety (TJC, 2019).*
2. Sit near patient in a quiet, private location. Center yourself and establish a quiet presence. Establish eye contact. Be aware that use of eye contact in some cultures conveys disrespect or discomfort. *Rationale: Presence expresses caring and creates healing moments (Arbour and Wiegand, 2014). Privacy protects confidentiality and promotes a sense of safety for patient when expressing thoughts and emotions.*
3. Consider the influence of patient's cultural background on communication. Apply principles of plain language and health literacy during assessment (NCP, 2018). *Rationale: Individual differences influence patient's grief response and communication style (Selman et al., 2014).*
4. Assess patient's or family caregiver's knowledge, experience, and health literacy level. *Rationale: Ensures patient has the capacity to obtain, communicate, process, and understand basic health information (Centers for Disease Control and Prevention [CDC], 2016).*

5. Listen carefully to patient's story about illness/sense of loss. Observe patient responses. Use open communication. *Rationale: Develops trust in a caring relationship. Actively listening to patient's concerns and verbalizing patient's needs conveys empathy and compassion (Doherty and Thompson, 2014).*
6. Determine meaning of the loss to patient: its type, suddenness, and when it occurred. Use open-ended questions such as:
   - "Tell me how your loss affects your family."
   - "You said your illness was unexpected. Describe how that made you feel."

   Rationale: The type, meaning, suddenness, and time elapsed since the loss influence the grief experience and coping methods.
7. Combine knowledge of grief theory with observation of patient behaviors. Validate observations by sharing them with patient; paraphrase, clarify, or summarize, as in the following examples:
   - "You've mentioned several times that you feel hopeless."
   - "It seems that this is hard for you to talk about."
   - "You look sad. Is there something in particular that brought on your tears?"

   Rationale: Use information about type and stage of grief to guide discussion, not to judge patient's responses. Confirms accuracy of your observations and validates patient's feelings. Prompts patient to continue.
8. Encourage patient to describe impact of loss on daily life (e.g., "You said your diagnosis changed your life forever. Tell me more"). *Rationale: Listening to patient's description helps to minimize assumptions.*
9. Ask patient to describe the coping strategies that he or she uses most often in difficult times (e.g., "What or who helps you in times of crisis?"). *Rationale: Familiar, effective coping strategies are often helpful in the current crisis, loss, or grief experience.*
10. Assess family caregivers' unique needs and resources. Note if patient receives care at home and who gives the care. *Rationale: Illness significantly affects family relationships. Family caregivers need support and guidance to aid in processing emotions and any fears they may have related to end-of-life care (Given and Reinhard, 2017).*
11. Assess patient's spiritual needs, beliefs, and resources. Focus on aspects likely to be involved (e.g., trust, life purpose, faith/belief, and hope). *Rationale: Identifies patient's spiritual beliefs and values. Enables patient autonomy by identifying beliefs and preferences for care or rituals related to faith and/or spirituality. Offers a greater understanding of patient's culture and values, leading to patient-centered care (Hodge, 2015).*

STEP	RATIONALE
PLANNING	
1. Expected outcomes following completion of procedures:	
• Patient maintains relationships with patient-identified significant people.	Patient in grief or loss retains connections with social network.
• Patient expresses grief in keeping with his or her cultural and religious practices.	Patient receives support necessary to retain cherished values and ways of being.
• Patient uses effective coping strategies.	Patient identifies sense of relief.
• Patient maintains normal life routines.	Patient adjusts to life-changing circumstances and maintains sense of control.
IMPLEMENTATION	
1. Show an empathic understanding of patient's strengths and needs.	Promotes nurse–patient trust, caring, compassion, and empathy (Doherty and Thompson, 2014).
2. Offer information about patient's illness and treatment. Clarify misunderstandings or misinformation. Use culturally appropriate language and simple terms.	Misunderstanding adds to patient's uncertainty, anxiety, and suffering.
3. Encourage patient to sustain relationships with others to help maintain independence and receive necessary help. Include patient-identified support people in discussions.	Affiliation with others offers support and helps patient stay engaged in life.
4. Help patient achieve short-term goals (e.g., symptom relief, task completion, resolution of relational problems).	Helping patients identify and meet their personal goals contributes to their quality of life.
5. Provide frequent opportunities for patient and family members to express their fears and concerns. Be attentive to expressions of intense emotions.	Emotions change quickly and frequently during stress and complicate communication for nurses and patients.
6. Educate and support patient and family about plan of care and anticipated changes. Use interprofessional team to support patient's needs and preferences.	Provides emotional support and comfort, decreases anxiety, and allows patient to rest. Advocating for patient encourages patient autonomy and incorporates patient preferences into plan of care (Arbour and Wiegand, 2014).
7. Instruct patient in relaxation strategies: mindfulness-based stress reduction, guided imagery, meditation, hand massage, healing touch (see Chapter 15).	Complementary nonpharmacologic therapies aim to reduce suffering and enhance patient comfort, promoting dimensions of healing in the face of serious or life-threatening illness (Hospice and Palliative Care Nurses Association [HPNA], 2015)

STEP	RATIONALE
8. Encourage visits with loved ones, life review with stories or photographs, or projects such as organizing photo albums or journal writing.	Reviewing positive and negative events in one's life allows a person to find meaning in his or her experiences, resolve conflicts, and come to a place of acceptance (Keall et al., 2015).
9. Facilitate patient's religious/spiritual practices and connections with higher power or religious community (e.g., prayer or music) and provide a listening presence. Make a referral to a spiritual care provider if appropriate.	Spiritual interventions help patients maintain hope and connect with the core of their identity. Spiritual interventions can decrease anxiety, promote a sense of peace, and help patient find meaning in his or her life (Kisvetrova et al., 2013; Wynne, 2013).

EVALUATION

1. Note patient descriptions of relationships and activities with others.	Provides information on extent to which patient retains relational ties.
2. Observe patient's behaviors during ongoing interactions.	Demonstrates patient's ability to express grief and coping.
3. Elicit patient perceptions of benefit gained from use of coping interventions.	Evaluates efficacy of interventions.
4. Discuss progress toward performing routine activities at home.	Evaluates patient's achievement of desired goals or need for goal revision.

Unexpected Outcomes	Related Interventions
1. Patient does not acknowledge loss and shows signs of extreme sorrow, anger, withdrawal, or denial.	• Consider referral to grief specialist professional (e.g., nurse practitioner, psychologist, spiritual care provider).
2. Family and patient relationships do not give patient needed support.	• Share and validate observations of family strain or patient concern over family interactions. • Consider family–patient discussion with health care team.

Recording

- Record in nurses' notes interventions for psychological and spiritual grief responses, including patient response, patient and family preferences, family presence and involvement, and evidence of unresolved issues and concerns.

Hand-Off Reporting

- Report to other health care providers patient's current emotional status and when a patient or family member requests therapeutic intervention from social worker, counselor, or spiritual care provider.

✦ SKILL 31.2 Symptom Management at End of Life

Purpose

Symptom management at the end of life involves caring for the whole person—body, mind, and spirit. Relief of symptoms is balanced with the possible side effects of medications (Pirschel, 2016). Patients and family caregivers often identify relief from pain and other troublesome physical symptoms as a high priority in end-of-life care. Lessen the fear and uncertainty often associated with the dying process by helping patients and family members understand and anticipate the common physical changes associated with impending death (Table 31.1).

Delegation and Collaboration

Supportive care for symptom management can be delegated to nursing assistive personnel (NAP). However, the nurse must conduct the initial assessments of symptoms and determination of therapies. The nurse directs the NAP to:

- Notify the nurse if patient reports new symptoms or if existing symptoms worsen or change.
- Provide basic comfort care, such as positioning, room temperature control, hygiene measures.
- Report possible adverse effects of drug therapy as instructed by the nurse.
- Speak to unconscious or dying patients because hearing is the last sense to diminish.

Equipment

- Personal care items most preferred by patient
- Comfort and hygiene products
- Clean gloves

ASSESSMENT

1. Identify patient using at least two identifiers (e.g., name and birthday or name and medical record number) according to agency policy. *Rationale: Ensures correct patient. Complies with The Joint Commission standards and improves patient safety (TJC, 2019).*

TABLE 31.1

Physical Changes Commonly Associated With Impending Death

Signs and Symptoms	Interventions
Coolness and color changes in extremities	Use slippers or socks; cover person with light blankets, tucked loosely over toes.
Increased periods of sleeping and unresponsiveness	Sit with patient, perhaps holding a hand and talking quietly; speak to patient even though there may be a lack of response.
Bowel or bladder incontinence	Change bedding as appropriate, use bed pads, and provide frequent skin care. Use external urinary catheters. An indwelling urinary catheter may be indicated because of patient fatigue or skin breakdown.
Decreased urine output	Consider advocating for the removal of indwelling urinary catheters. Change bed pads as needed.
Pulmonary congestion and increased secretions	Explain, especially to family members, that noisy breathing is not uncomfortable for patient. Elevate head of bed; turn the head to drain secretions. Avoid suctioning.
Altered breathing patterns (i.e., apnea, labored, and irregular breathing)	Elevate the head, hold a hand, and use quiet voice tones. Administer prescribed anxiolytics and opioids for pain and apprehension. Explain to family members common changes in breathing patterns at end of life to decrease concerns.
Restlessness or disorientation	Speak calmly. Gently massage hands or feet. Play soothing music and lower lights.
Decreased intake of food or fluids	Do not force patient to eat or drink. Offer ice chips, ice pops, or sips of fluid. Apply lip balm and provide oral care.

2. Ask patients to describe symptoms in their own words. Use open-ended prompts such as "Describe your leg pain to me," or "Tell me about how you are sleeping since you started taking this medicine." *Rationale: Symptoms are personal perceptions and only experienced by the patient (Nunn, 2014).*
3. Allow sufficient time for patients to describe their symptoms and encourage them to say more. *Rationale: Ethical dilemmas can arise when communication breaks down, patient autonomy is compromised, and ineffective symptom management occurs. Ensure enough time to allow patients to speak and be listened to (Pirschel, 2016).*
   - "Is there anything else bothering you?"
   - "You've told me about your ____ pain. Do you have pain anywhere else?"
4. Assess patient's psychological, social, and spiritual needs (American Association of Colleges of Nursing [AACN], 2016). *Rationale: Emotional conditions have potential to worsen fatigue in patients with cancer (American Cancer Society [ACS], 2016). A holistic assessment can help to improve quality of life for patients with serious illness and their families (AACN, 2016).*
5. Perform hand hygiene and apply clean gloves. Inspect and palpate areas where patient reports pain. Assess patient's pain severity on a pain scale of 0 to 10 (see Chapter 15). If patient cannot self-report pain, observe for these symptoms (ACS, 2016):
   - Noisy breathing—labored, harsh, or rapid breaths
   - Making pained sounds—including groaning, moaning, or expressing discomfort
   - Facial expressions—looking sad, tense, or frightened; frowning or crying
   - Body language—tension, clenched fists, knees pulled up, inflexibility, restlessness, or looking like he or she is trying to get away from area of discomfort
   - Body movement—changing positions to get comfortable but cannot

   Rationale: Reduces transmission of microorganisms. Clarifies area of discomfort. Consistent use of a standard pain scale helps assess changes in patient pain levels and evaluate effectiveness of pain interventions (Paice, 2015). The use of a pain scale is recommended by the ACS (2016) as a helpful way to describe patients' responses to pain-relief measures. Patients unable to report or verbalize pain show nonverbal signs of pain.
6. Assess for feeling of breathlessness (whether patient feels that he or she is getting enough air), respiratory rate, breathing patterns, and lung sounds. Assess for presence of airway secretions. *Rationale: Dyspnea, air hunger, or shortness of breath results from metabolic or respiratory changes. Near the end of life, Cheyne-Stokes respirations are common and are characterized by alternating periods of apnea and hyperpnea.*
7. Observe condition of skin, especially back, heels, and buttocks (see Chapter 8). *Rationale: Decreased peripheral circulation and activity level contribute to skin breakdown.*
8. Inspect patient's oral cavity, including mucosa, tongue, and teeth (see Chapter 8). *Rationale: Dehydration, difficulty swallowing, and inflammation of mouth are common at end of life.*
9. Assess bowel function (see Chapter 20). *Rationale: Patients experience constipation because of decreased oral intake, immobility, and medications such as opioids (Clark and Currow, 2014). Patients who have diarrhea are at risk for dehydration.*
   a. Determine usual bowel elimination pattern (frequency, character, usual time of day) and effectiveness of usual bowel-management routines.
   b. If patient is passing liquid stool, assess for presence of fecal impaction (see agency policy). *Rationale: Watery stool leaking around blockage indicates fecal impaction.*
   c. Review medication regimens, prescriptions, and over-the-counter drugs known to cause constipation (e.g., opioids, antacids). *Rationale: Medications can alter bowel elimination patterns. Diarrhea results from infections, diseases, or medications (e.g., antibiotics or chemotherapy). Change in therapy might be necessary.*
   d. Identify typical food and fluid intake over 1 week and patient's activity levels. *Rationale: Oral intake and activity levels influence bowel elimination patterns.*
10. Assess urinary elimination (see Chapter 19) and ability to control urination. If incontinent, assess for skin breakdown

or patient discomfort. *Rationale: Urinary incontinence results from patient's disease process, altered level of consciousness, or medications (e.g., diuretics, anticholinergics, opioids).*

11. Assess patient's appetite, gag reflex, and ability to swallow, and assess for presence of nausea or vomiting. Use standardized tool for assessment if available. Consider presence of nausea in patients receiving enteral feedings. *Rationale: Medications, pain, depression, disease progression, or decreased blood flow to digestive organs near death often contribute to nausea, vomiting, and decreased appetite. Patients who have decreased consciousness are unable to report nausea. Patients who have difficulty swallowing are at risk for aspiration.*
12. Assess daily food and fluid intake in relation to patient's condition and preferences. Consult with registered dietician as indicated. *Rationale: Nutrition screening helps to identify deficits and allows for interventions to be carried out to improve nutritional status (Shaw and Eldridge, 2015).*
13. Use descriptive scale to assess fatigue (e.g., scale with descriptors *none, moderate, severe*). Ask if fatigue limits patient's ability to perform desired activities. *Rationale: Metabolic demands of a disease, anemia as a result of chemotherapy, treatments, and cumulative effects of other symptoms cause weakness and fatigue (ACS, 2016).*
14. Remove and dispose of gloves. Perform hand hygiene. *Rationale: Reduces transmission of microorganisms.*
15. Assess for terminal delirium in patient near death (e.g., confusion, restlessness, and/or agitation, with or without day–night reversal). Attempt to define cause in effort to reduce medication use (Bailey and Harmon, 2017). *Rationale: May be the first sign to signal that patient may have a difficult road to death. There is a need to educate and support family caregivers to understand its causes, the finality and irreversibility of the situation, and approaches to its management (Emanuel et al., 2015).*
    a. Consider if patient has pain, nausea, dyspnea, full bladder or bowel, poor sleep patterns, anxiety, or joint pain from immobility. *Rationale: Risk factors for presence of delirium are common physical problems that need to be treated or ruled out as causative factors.*
    b. Review medical record for hypercalcemia, hypoglycemia, hyponatremia, or dehydration. *Rationale: Metabolic imbalances cause restlessness or delirium.*
    c. Review patient's medications. *Rationale: Unintended responses to medications result in changed activity states.*
    d. Determine whether patient has unresolved psychosocial or spiritual issues. *Rationale: Spiritual distress contributes to restlessness or increased pain.*
    e. Assess family caregiver's knowledge of end-of-life-related symptoms.

STEP	RATIONALE
PLANNING	
1. Expected outcomes following completion of procedure:	
• Patient reports acceptable level of pain.	Indicates pain control.
• Patient reports feeling warm and comfortable.	Warming interventions help reverse effects of reduced peripheral circulation.
• Patient reports comfort with eating and drinking patterns.	Optimal food and fluid intake is based on patient preferences and comfort.
• Patient has soft, formed bowel movements.	Indicates adequate bowel function and peristaltic activity.
• Skin remains free of irritation or breakdown.	Interventions to protect skin from bowel or urinary incontinence are effective.
• Patient is not restless.	Therapies have calming effect.
• Patient reports less distress from fatigue.	Energy conservation methods are effective; patient adjusts to changes in activity level.
• Patient experiences less respiratory distress.	Patient is less apprehensive and breathes easily.
IMPLEMENTATION	
1. Perform hand hygiene.	Reduces transmission of microorganisms.
2. Provide pain relief. Use multimodal interventions (combining pharmacologic and nonpharmacologic measures):	Management of symptoms should be multimodal (NCP, 2018).
a. Administer ordered analgesics and adjuvants. Confer with health care provider and recommend an around-the-clock (ATC) dosing schedule, especially if pain is anticipated for majority of day. A variety of extended- or controlled-release oral opioid formulations (dosing intervals of 8, 10, 12 or 24 hours) and transdermal patches (72 hours) are effective.	Opioids should be given on a fixed dosage schedule ATC rather than prn, with doses given before pain returns (Burchum and Rosenthal, 2016). An ATC medication lessens the severity of end-of-dose pain, allowing a patient to sleep through the night and reduce "clock watching" for the next dose. Extended-release medications maintain constant serum opioid concentration, minimizing toxic and subtherapeutic concentrations (Burchum and Rosenthal, 2016).
b. Provide nonpharmacological interventions such as mindfulness-based stress reduction, relaxation exercises, and guided imagery (see Chapter 15).	Nonpharmacological measures supplement pain medication and can increase patient comfort (Hall, 2014; Nunn, 2014).

STEP	RATIONALE
c. Provide patient and family caregiver education on causes and patterns of pain and safety of opioid use and explain interventions.	Encourages patient autonomy and reduces emotional distress, clarifying misinformation about opioid therapies.
3. Provide general comfort measures.	
a. Provide bath and skin care based on patient's preferences and hygiene needs (see Chapter 11). **NOTE:** Daily baths are not always desired or necessary at end of life if they cause discomfort, fatigue, or increased pain.	Clean skin promotes comfort.
b. Provide eye care and use artificial tears in patients with decreased consciousness (see Chapter 12).	Eye irritation causes pain. Blink reflex diminishes near death, causing drying of cornea.
c. Reposition frequently; do not position on tubes or other objects.	Prolonged pressure, even slight, from weight of patient's body or objects causes skin injury.
4. Provide oral hygiene after meals and at bedtime while awake and more frequently in mouth-breathing or unconscious patients (see Chapter 11).	Oral mucosa integrity is needed for normal swallowing and to minimize anorexia and malnutrition. Mouth rinses remove oral debris and clean the mouth. Dehydration develops as patient experiences metabolic changes and fluid intake declines.
a. Use antifungal oral rinses as prescribed, sodium bicarbonate, or normal saline rinses.	Patients near death breathe through the mouth, drying oral mucosa.
b. Moisten lips with nonpetroleum balm.	Prevents skin breakdown.
5. Initiate bowel-management regimen to reduce risk for constipation or diarrhea:	Interventions improve peristalsis in constipation, soften fecal mass, and decrease abdominal discomfort (Bruera et al., 2018; Clark and Currow, 2014; Santucci and Battista, 2015).
a. Give patient whatever fluids he or she enjoys if medically tolerated. Near end of life, patient may refuse fluids. Do not force fluid intake.	Decreased blood flow to intestines at end of life causes anorexia.
b. Encourage regular physical activity (e.g., walking) if tolerated.	Exercise promotes peristalsis.
c. Administer daily stool softener or laxative, especially in patients using opioids for pain management.	Opioids cause constipation.
d. In case of diarrhea, provide low-residue diet; administer antibiotics to treat infections or discontinue medications if possible. Administer antidiarrheal medications.	Treatments reduce incidence and severity of diarrhea, which can lead to dehydration. Patients with chronic diarrhea require rigorous skin care to promote comfort.
6. Manage urinary incontinence with intervention appropriate for patient's conditions (e.g., condom catheter, adult incontinence pads [see Chapter 19]).	Urinary output declines near death, making it possible to manage incontinence without an indwelling catheter.

Safe Patient Care *Consider an indwelling catheter only if skin integrity, patient preference, or fatigue from bed changes becomes an issue.*

STEP	RATIONALE
7. Offer patient favorite foods in amount and at time he or she desires. Do not overly encourage patient to eat.	Patients may be experiencing gastrointestinal (GI) distress, dry mouth, or other symptoms related to the disease process, which may contribute to decreased oral intake. In addition, patients nearing final hours of life decrease their oral intake as a result of slowing of bodily functions and/or altered level of consciousness (Bruera et al., 2018; Gillespie and Raftery, 2014).
a. Treat nausea by administering antiemetics intravenously or rectally as prescribed. As nausea subsides, offer clear liquids and ice chips. Avoid caffeinated liquids, milk, and fruit juices.	GI mucosa tolerates clear liquids more readily. Certain liquids increase stomach acidity.
8. Manage fatigue.	Taking rest breaks during activity will help conserve energy (Bruera et al., 2018; Koornstra et al., 2014). Tired patients need help and monitoring to ensure patient safety.
a. Help patient identify valued or desired tasks, how to perform tasks, and preferred time of day to perform tasks. Help with activities of daily living. Eliminate extra steps in activities.	Approaches conserve energy.
b. Explain care activities before performing them and include patient in setting daily schedule.	Minimizes anxiety and maintains patient's autonomy and involvement.

STEP	RATIONALE
c. Discuss with patient easy ways to incorporate exercise (e.g., yoga, walking, biking, and swimming) into daily activities.	Research has shown that, even for people with advanced-stage cancer, exercise can lessen pain and decrease anxiety, stress, depression, shortness of breath, and fatigue (Bruera et al., 2018).
9. Support patient's breathing efforts.	
a. Position for comfort in semi-Fowler's or Fowler's position.	Promotes maximal ventilation, lung expansion, and drainage of secretions.
b. Elevate head to facilitate postural drainage. Turn from side to side to mobilize and drain secretions. Suction only if necessary.	Deep airway suctioning causes discomfort and is not effective in reducing airway noise or secretion clearance (Bailey and Harmon, 2017).
c. Provide ordered antimuscarinic medications.	Anticholinergic medications reduce saliva and excessive secretions (Bruera et al., 2018; Nunn, 2014), thus decreasing noisy respirations.
d. Stay with patients experiencing dyspnea or air hunger. Use interventions that patients perceive as relieving their shortness of breath (choice of oxygen-delivery modes, fan near face, body position). Administer opioids or anxiolytics as prescribed. Benzodiazepines may also be administered for anxiety related to dyspnea. Keep room cool with low humidity.	Sharing control with patients reduces anxiety that contributes to feelings of air hunger. Anticholinergic medications are the drug of choice for dyspnea, decreasing respiratory rate and decreasing anxiety. Use of oxygen has little benefit unless patient feels better using it (Bruera et al., 2018).

Safe Patient Care ***Caution:*** *The use of benzodiazepines in very elderly patients can result in a paradoxical agitation.*

STEP	RATIONALE
10. Manage restlessness.	
a. Keep patient's room quiet with soft lighting and at comfortable temperature. Offer family members opportunities to maintain close contact. Encourage use of soft music, prayer, or reading from patient's favorite book.	Reduces unnecessary external stimulation and provides comforting space. Privacy allows family members chance to provide verbal assurances and touch. Presence of a family member to hold a hand provides a calming effect.
b. Use least-sedating pharmacological options to control restlessness. Consult with interprofessional team about titrating a medication (e.g., lorazepam). Discontinue all nonessential medication. Use subcutaneous, transdermal, sublingual, or rectal medication delivery routes.	Reduce delirium without making patient unconscious. Control of restlessness relieves family members' concern that patient is in pain or distress.
11. Manage anxiety.	
a. Provide counseling and supportive therapy. Consult with prescribing health care provider for benzodiazepines, the drugs of choice. Offer available counseling services (e.g., pastoral care, psychologist, social worker).	Counseling improves patient/family understanding of the disease and its expected course and identifies strengths and coping strategies. Chaplains, psychologists, child life specialists, and social workers can assist nurses to support patients and family caregivers (Pirschel, 2016).
12. Educate family caregivers on symptom management interventions and why they are necessary to increase patient comfort.	Family caregivers usually do not have time to prepare for this role or receive training before they take on this role. Education is therefore essential as soon as possible to prepare and support family caregivers (Given and Reinhard, 2017).

EVALUATION

1. Ask patient to rate pain on scale of 0 to 10 (see Chapter 15) and evaluate pain characteristics 1 hour after administering analgesics or other pain therapies. Assess behavior in nonverbal patients.	Determines extent of pain relief.
2. Ask patient to describe mouth comfort and inspect oral cavity.	Evaluates condition of oral cavity and ability to chew or swallow.
3. Evaluate frequency of defecation; after patient defecates, inspect feces.	Determines status of bowel function and character of stool.
4. Observe skin condition.	Determines whether skin tears or areas of pressure or maceration are present.
5. Ask patient to rate fatigue (scale from none to moderate to severe) and compare with baseline. Observe for fatigue or shortness of breath when patient performs activities.	Determines whether patient is less distressed with activity.

STEP	RATIONALE
6. Observe patient's respiratory patterns and ask if breathing is easy and comfortable.	Determines whether respiratory distress is relieved.
7. Observe patient's behavior or ask family to report on it. Note level of restlessness.	Determines level of comfort and extent of restlessness.
8. **Use Teach-Back:** "I want to be sure I explained how we want to control your pain, and this requires you to describe it. Tell me what the numbers on the pain scale mean. Tell me when it is a good time to let me know about your pain before it gets too severe." Revise your instruction now or develop a plan for revised patient/family caregiver teaching if patient/family caregiver is not able to teach back correctly.	Determines patient's/family caregiver's level of understanding of instructional topic.

Unexpected Outcomes	Related Interventions
1. One or more symptoms remain unresolved, with patient reporting little or no relief.	• Increase frequency of or change an intervention. • Try combination therapies.
2. Patient becomes anxious, fearful, or exhausted because of continued symptoms.	• Give patients therapy choices and try different interventions. • Explain goals of therapies and possible reasons for symptoms. • Answer nurse call system quickly and explain plan of care throughout the day.

Recording

- Record interventions for pain and symptom management, including patient response; changes in physical, mental, emotional, or spiritual status; patient and family preferences; family presence and involvement; and evidence of unresolved issues and concerns with physical care or patient symptoms.

Hand-Off Reporting

- Report when a previously alert patient becomes unresponsive.

✦ SKILL 31.3 Care of the Body After Death

Purpose

After a patient dies, the designated health care provider, often a physician or nurse practitioner, certifies the death and records the time and actions taken at the time of death in the medical record. The health care provider may request permission from the family for an autopsy or postmortem examination, although this is less likely with an anticipated death or when the cause of death is known. An autopsy consent form must be signed by the appropriate family member and the health care provider. Autopsies normally do not delay burial. You are responsible for providing respectful, thorough care of the body after death.

Delegation and Collaboration

The skill of care of a body after death can be delegated to nursing assistive personnel (NAP). However, it is often easier for the nurse and NAP to work together in providing postmortem care. The nurse directs the NAP to:

- Follow agency policy in cases of autopsy or organ and tissue donation.
- Honor family cultural or religious rituals when performing postmortem care (see Box 31.2).
- Handle the body with dignity and respect for privacy.

Equipment

- Clean gloves, gown, and other personal protective equipment
- Clean gown or disposable gown for body (consult agency policy)
- Washbasin, washcloth, warm water, and bath towel
- Absorbent pads
- Plastic bag for hazardous waste disposal
- Body bag or shroud kit (consult agency policy)
- Paper tape and gauze dressing
- Bag or receptacle for patient's clothing and other items to be returned to family members
- Envelope for valuables
- Identification tags as specified by agency policy

ASSESSMENT

1. Identify patient using at least two identifiers (e.g., name and birthday or name and medical record number) according to agency policy. Tag the body and leave tag on the body as directed by agency policy. *Rationale: Ensures correct patient. Complies with The Joint Commission standards and improves patient safety (TJC, 2019).*
2. Ask health care provider to establish time of death and determine whether he or she has requested an autopsy. If an autopsy is planned or a possible crime is involved, use special precautions to preserve evidence (see agency policy). *Rationale: Certifies patient's death. Autopsy can determine cause of death and reveal more about a disease. Patient's legal representative and the health care provider or designated requester must sign an autopsy consent form.*

3. Determine whether family members or significant others are present and whether they have been informed of the death. Identify patient's surrogate (next of kin or durable power of attorney [DPOA]). *Rationale: Verifies that family has been notified of patient's death to avoid inappropriate communication of this sensitive information.*
4. Determine whether patient's surrogate has been asked about organ and tissue donation and validate that donation request form has been signed. Notify organ request team per policy. *Rationale: Federal guidelines require documentation that request has been made.*
5. Provide family members and friends a private place to gather. Allow them time to ask questions (including those about medical care) or discuss grief. *Rationale: Creates safe environment for grieving family. Questions provide information about how they are coping with loss and their needs.*
6. Ask family members whether they have requests for preparation or viewing of the body (e.g., washing the body, position of body, special clothing, shaving). Determine whether they wish to be present or help with care of the body. *Rationale: Respects individuality of patient and family and supports their right to having cultural or religious values and beliefs upheld. Provides closure for those who wish to help with body preparation (Hadders et al., 2014).*
7. Contact support person (e.g., pastoral care, social work) to stay with family members not helping to prepare the body. Implement in timely manner a bereavement care plan after patient's death when family remains the focus of care (NCP, 2018). *Rationale: Provides family support during an emotional time.*
8. Consult health care providers' orders for special care directives or specimens that are to be collected. *Rationale: Specimens may be used in determining cause of death.*
9. Perform hand hygiene; apply clean gloves, gown, or protective barriers. *Rationale: Reduces transmission of microorganisms.*
10. Assess general condition of the body and note presence of dressings, tubes, and medical equipment. *Rationale: Validates whether tissue damage was present before postmortem care.*

STEP	RATIONALE
PLANNING	
1. Expected outcomes following completion of procedure:	
• Body is free of new skin damage.	Careful handling of body prevents lacerations, bruises, or abrasions during postmortem care.
• Significant others able to express grief.	Significant others feel supported through their loss.

Safe Patient Care *Immediately after death and before proceeding with other activities, place body in supine position and elevate head of bed 30 degrees to decrease livor mortis.*

STEP	RATIONALE
2. Position patient supine in bed, arms at side, in a private room if possible. If patient has a roommate, explain and move him or her to another location temporarily. If leaving room, remove personal protective equipment and perform hand hygiene.	Provides staff with larger area for postmortem care and for family members to gather in a private setting.
3. As soon as possible, a patient's death must be "pronounced" by someone in authority (e.g., physician in hospital or hospice nurse). This person completes forms certifying the cause, time, and place of death. The legal form is necessary for life insurance and financial and property issues. If hospice is helping, a plan for what happens after death is already in place (NIA, 2017).	These steps make it possible for an official death certificate to be prepared.
4. Direct NAP to gather needed equipment and arrange at bedside.	Because this is often an emotional time for family members, organized and efficient care is important.
IMPLEMENTATION	
1. Help family members notify others of the death. Promptly notify the mortuary, as chosen by the family, and discuss plans for postmortem care.	Following a death, grieving persons have difficulty focusing on details and often need guidance. Being informed increases a sense of control.
2. If patient has made tissue donation, consult agency policy for guidelines for care of the body.	Retrieval of tissues (e.g., eyes, bone, skin) may require special procedures.
3. Perform hand hygiene; apply clean gloves, gown, or protective barriers.	Reduces transmission of microorganisms.

Safe Patient Care *Have family caregivers helping in postmortem care wear a gown and gloves to protect them from body fluids.*

STEP	RATIONALE
4. Remove indwelling devices (e.g., urinary catheter, endotracheal tube). Disconnect and cap off (no need to remove) intravenous lines. *Do not remove indwelling devices in cases of autopsy* (follow agency policy). Be mindful about removing tubes from patients with increased bleeding times.	Creates normal appearance for family viewing of body. Removing intravenous catheters allows fluids to leak. Removal of tubes and lines is contraindicated if an autopsy is planned. Increased bleeding times may increase bleeding at removal site.
5. Clean the mouth and clean and replace dentures as soon as possible. If dentures cannot be replaced, send them with body in clearly labeled denture cup and transport with body to mortuary (Greenway and Johnson, 2016). If culturally appropriate, close mouth with rolled-up towel under chin.	Gives face more natural appearance. If dentures are not replaced, it can be very difficult later for workers at funeral home to place dentures.
6. Place small pillow under head or position according to cultural preferences. Do not tie hands together on top of body. Check agency policy regarding need to secure hands and feet. Use only circular gauze bandaging on body.	Patient appears natural. Weight of limp arms causes skin damage and discoloration if hands are tied. Some agencies require securing appendages to prevent tissue damage when body is being moved.
7. Close eyes by applying light pressure for 30 seconds. Use saline-moistened gauze if corneal or eye donation is to take place (Greenway and Johnson, 2016). Some cultures prefer that eyes remain open.	Closed eyes convey to some people a more peaceful and natural appearance. Gauze prevents corneal drying.
8. Groom and arrange hair into preferred style, if known. Remove any clips, hairpins, or rubber bands. Do not shave patient. Some cultures or faith groups prohibit shaving.	Hard objects damage or discolor face and scalp. Shaving too soon after death can cause bruising, so this is done by the funeral director. Explain this to the family if they request shaving (Greenway and Johnson, 2016).
9. Wash soiled body parts. Some cultural practices require that family members clean the body.	Prepares body for viewing and reduces odors. Mortuary personnel provide complete bath.
10. Remove soiled dressings and replace with clean dressings, using paper tape or circular gauze bandaging.	Changing dressings controls odors and creates more acceptable appearance. Paper tape minimizes skin damage when tape is removed.

Safe Patient Care *Turning a recently dead body to the side sometimes causes the flow of exhaled air. This is a normal event and not a sign of life.*

STEP	RATIONALE
11. Place absorbent pad under buttocks.	Relaxation of sphincter muscles at time of death causes release of urine or feces.
12. Place clean gown on body. Some agencies require gown removal before placing body in shroud (see agency policy).	Provides privacy and prepares body for viewing.
13. Identify personal belongings that stay with body and those to be given to family.	Prevents loss of valuable or meaningful property.
14. If family requests viewing, respect individual cultural practices. Otherwise, place clean sheet over body up to chin with arms outside covers. Remove medical equipment from room. Provide soft lighting and chairs.	Maintains respect for patient and those viewing body. Prevents exposure of body parts. Removing medical equipment provides more peaceful, natural setting.
15. Allow family time alone with body and encourage them to say goodbye with religious rituals and in a culturally appropriate manner. Some families want time to sit quietly with the body, console each other, and share memories (NIA, 2017). Some cultural practices include maintaining silence at the time of death, whereas others express grief with intense emotional displays. Do not rush any grieving process.	Compassionate care provides family members with meaningful experience during early phase of grief. Ensure privacy and a safe environment. Provide chair at bedside for family member who might collapse.
16. After viewing, remove linens and gown per agency policy. Place body in shroud provided by the agency (see illustration).	Shroud prevents injury to skin, avoids exposure of body, and provides barrier against potentially contaminated body fluids.
17. Place identification label on outside of shroud if required by agency policy. Follow agency policy for marking a body that poses an infectious risk to others. Remove and dispose of personal protective equipment and perform hygiene.	Ensures proper identification of body. Reduces exposure of morgue and mortuary staff to contamination. Reduces transmission of microorganisms.

STEP	RATIONALE

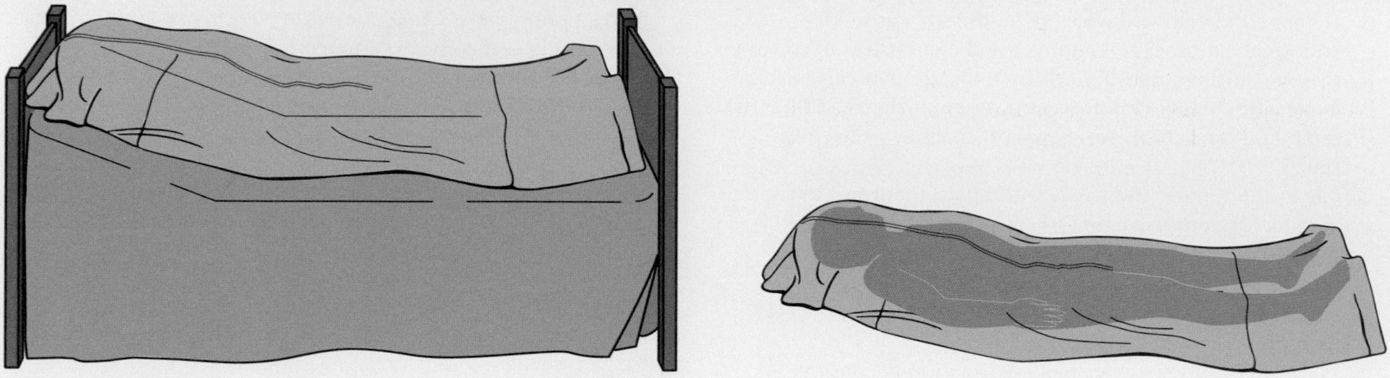

STEP 16 Body in shroud.

STEP	RATIONALE
18. Arrange prompt transportation of body to the mortuary. If you anticipate a delay, transport body to the morgue.	Mortuary personnel get best results if embalming occurs before full rigor mortis (i.e., stiffening of body after death) occurs.

EVALUATION

1. Observe family members', friends', and significant others' response to the loss.	The need for referral or help is based on evaluation of person's unique response to loss.
2. Note appearance and condition of patient's skin during preparation of the body.	Provides information for postmortem care documentation.

Unexpected Outcomes	Related Interventions
1. A family member becomes immobilized with grief and has difficulty functioning.	• Enlist the help of a family member or trusted friend to provide direction and support. • Offer assistance from a counselor, social worker, or pastoral care.
2. A family member becomes agitated and threatens or strikes out against others.	• Call for assistance from a psychiatric nurse practitioner, spiritual care provider, or social worker who has a relationship with the family. • Enlist help from security staff or crisis intervention professional if safety is a concern.

Recording

- Record the date and time of death as determined by designated health care professional. Include the time professional notified, name of professional pronouncing death, completion of postmortem care, identification and disposition of body, information provided to significant others, whether autopsy consent (if needed) was signed, and how valuables and personal belongings were handled and who received them. Secure signatures as required by agency policy.

Hand-Off Reporting

- Report any new marks, bruises, or wounds on body before death or observed during care of body.

SPECIAL CONSIDERATIONS

Patient-Centered Care

- End of life is a sacred time; nurses are fortunate to be present with patients and family caregivers (Pirschel, 2016).
- Patients of all ages with any diagnosis can receive symptom management with palliative care throughout the duration of their illness, even as they seek treatment and curative interventions.
- Each person will die in his or her own way, influenced by religion, ethnicity, availability of financial resources, belief systems, and key relationships.
- As the plan of care shifts toward patient comfort and QOL, think creatively about how to help patients live as well as possible as they approach the end of life. For example, listen carefully to patients' and family members' descriptions of their needs and wishes, and set nursing care priorities accordingly; consider extending visiting hours in a hospital setting to meet the needs of a family to be together as a loved one dies.
- Develop an ability to understand, acknowledge, and be present with people experiencing intense and changing emotional reactions to their situation. Compassion and attentiveness are conveyed in many ways, including the therapeutic use of touch (Fig. 31.2), active listening, or silently sitting with a patient.
- Spiritual concerns arise in situations of serious illness and impending death. All patients, including individuals who do not practice a particular religion, have spiritual strengths, needs, and practices. Explore a patient's spirituality by organizing a patient-centered nursing assessment focused on four conceptual

areas: meaning, hope, community, and a sense of the Holy Other (Box 31.1).

- Cultural sensitivity is crucial in providing patient-centered care at the end of life. A patient's culturally influenced health care beliefs and practices, communication patterns, and family structures affect the dying process (AACN, 2016).
- Be especially aware of religious diversity in end-of-life care (Box 31.2). People with the same religion have varying beliefs or practices and may adhere more or less strictly to their beliefs.
- A patient-centered care approach allows patients to communicate their preferences clearly for end-of-life care. An advance directive provides a patient with a mechanism to make personal values and wishes known and guide others in making care decisions when the patient can no longer participate (e.g., overwhelming illness, unconsciousness, or sedating drugs).
- Advance directives are written documents such as living wills or durable powers of attorney for health care, which designate a patient-appointed representative. In a living will, patients express their wishes concerning the use of extraordinary medical procedures, artificial nutrition and fluids, comfort measures, life-support interventions, or other care preferences.
- Patients should give copies of completed advance directives to their health care providers and responsible family members and request that their advance directives be placed in their medical record. If a patient expresses his or her wish to forgo CPR in an advance directive, a health care provider must also write a DNR order in the medical chart.

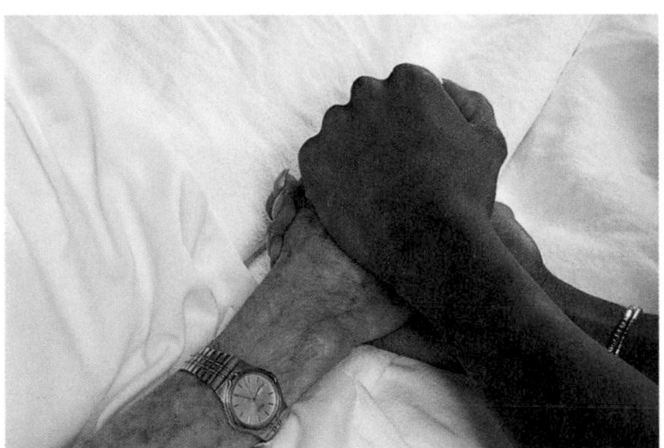

FIG 31.2 Touch can communicate caring and compassion.

BOX 31.1

Assessing the Spiritual Dimension

Meaning

- What gives your life meaning and purpose in your current situation?
- What are your goals? What do you still want to achieve?
- What do you live for now?

Hope

- What do you hope for right now?
- How have your hopes changed?
- What gives you hope during difficult times?

Community

- Who are the people most important to you?
- Who gives you comfort in difficult times?
- Are you able to participate in community activities (i.e., church, family, friends)?

Sense of Holy Other or God

- What is God like for you? What is your concept of that which is larger than yourself?
- Is religion or God significant to you? If yes, describe how.
- What religious practices or spiritual rituals are meaningful to you?

BOX 31.2

Some Religious Practices Related to Death and Dying

Judaism

Persons dying may want to hear prayers and scripture at the time of death. After death, there should be minimal handling of the body by non-Jews. A family member may stay with the body until burial. Close the eyes after death. It is customary for burial to occur within 24 hours except on the Sabbath. Families participate in a mourning period during which grief is expressed openly and in keeping with ritual. Because life is valued as a gift of God, all efforts to continue life are supported, even when it appears that there is no hope, especially in Orthodox Judaism. In some, but not all, types of Judaism, cremation, autopsy, and embalming are avoided.

Christianity

Christians believe in life after death and eternal life. Some may request rituals of confession, laying on of hands, anointing the sick, baptism, or Holy Communion. Prayer and reading from the Bible may be appropriate. There may be a period of viewing the body or a wake before burial, and funerals or memorial services are common. Cremation, autopsy, and embalming are usually permitted.

Islam

Muslims believe in eternal life and the will of God (Allah). Patients may wish to face Mecca (the East) as they are dying. Cleanliness and modesty are very important. Help patient continue regular prayer five times a day as long as possible. Loved ones usually remain with the dying person 24 hours a day. Non-Muslims should wear gloves when touching the body. Cover the body with a plain sheet until a person of Muslim faith can give the ritual bath and wrap the body in a white cloth. Burial is usually in a Muslim cemetery within 24 hours. Autopsy is usually forbidden, but organ donation is becoming more acceptable.

Hinduism

Hindus believe in one supreme deity and in lesser gods with powers and interests in specific areas of life. Core beliefs include community connectedness, reincarnation, and karma (how one has lived in this world affects how one might return in the next one). Patients may want the presence of a Brahmin priest who may chant prayers. Only the family should touch the body after death, and they are responsible for washing and preparing it. Cremation is traditional, but autopsy and organ donation are not commonly practiced.

Buddhism

In Buddhism, the state of the mind at the time of death is relevant in the person's rebirth into a new life. The goal of life and death is to reach the eternal state of nirvana, or inner peace and happiness. A patient may want to remain conscious to be able to meditate or contemplate the dying process. Allow for a peaceful environment at the time of death, and notify a Buddhist priest. Time from death to burial varies from 3 to 7 days. Mourners wear white to the funeral. Cremation and autopsy are usually allowed.

Adapted from Sherman D, Free D: Culture and spirituality as domains of quality palliative care. In Matzo M, Sherman D, editors: *Palliative care nursing: quality care to the end of life*, ed 4, New York, 2014, Springer.

BOX 31.3

Similarities and Differences Between Palliative Care and Hospice Care

Similarities

- Prioritize for quality of life and relief from pain and other distressing symptoms
- Integrate physical, psychological, social, and spiritual dimensions into plan of care
- Affirm life and regard dying as a normal process
- Involve the patient and family members as active participants in all decisions and care
- Rely on the expertise of an interdisciplinary team for planning and implementing care
- Appropriate for all patients, regardless of diagnosis, age, or setting

Differences

- Palliative care is used in varying extent at any time during an illness. Hospice care is designed exclusively for patients near the end of life.
- Palliative care is often used in conjunction with curative interventions, whereas patients who receive hospice care can no longer pursue curative care.
- Palliative care helps people living with chronic illness over an extended period of time rather than the shorter time frame (approximately 6 to 12 months) designated for hospice.

- Because discussions about care decisions are very sensitive and emotional for patients and families, provide a quiet setting for conversation and participate when your involvement is appropriate. Recognize that cultural, ethnic, and religious values influence the likelihood that a patient will complete an advance directive (NIA, 2017).
- End-of-life care poses many challenging ethical questions, including a patient's right to have assisted dying, use of artificial food and hydration, pain management, and the appropriate use of technology. To ensure that you are providing patient-centered care in ethical deliberations, listen carefully and nonjudgmentally to concerns of patients and family caregivers.
- Patients, family caregivers, and members of the interprofessional team determine the best course of action by having meaningful conversations together.

Patient Education

- Patients, family members, and health care providers sometimes resist palliative care because of a lack of understanding about its benefits or the mistaken belief that palliative care is used only at the end of life (NIA, 2017). Offer care alternatives and meaningful education to help patients and family caregivers understand the similarities and differences between palliative and hospice care (Box 31.3).

Age-Specific

Pediatric

- Encourage parents to share information about their child's coping style and the degree of openness with which death is addressed in the family.
- Decisions to end treatment can be very difficult when children are involved.
- Many children know they are dying and can have age-appropriate conversations about their feelings and fears. Consider child's age and developmental level in care planning, symptom management, and sibling support (Hockenberry et al., 2017).
- Treat family and child as one unit. Encourage parents to stay with child and participate in care as much as desired or possible.
- Parents need the opportunity to hold their deceased child and help with body preparation.
- If parents agree, assess siblings' developmental level and readiness to view their brother's or sister's body.
- In cases of neonatal deaths or stillbirths, many parents appreciate having a picture or lock of hair from their child as a remembrance.

Gerontological

- Older adults have experienced multiple losses in their lives, which may affect their reactions to subsequent losses and their grief response.
- Do not assume that older adults accept or have addressed their feelings about death.
- Older adults may have fewer relatives and friends available to offer support. The nurse may be the person who stays with the patient in the final stages of life.
- Older patients may have more than one disease process and multiple physical symptoms and medications.
- Drug metabolism changes with increased age, requiring careful monitoring to determine proper dose.
- Older adults may experience pain, respiratory distress, and confusion at the end of life but may receive less-than-optimal symptom management.
- For older adults who live in an extended care facility, the residents and staff are often regarded as family members and should be notified of the patient's death.

Home Care

- Family caregivers need ongoing education on hospice care, end-of-life comfort measures, signs of impending death, whom to call for help with symptom control, what to do and whom to call at the time of death, and how to arrange for transportation of the body.
- Family members may have ambivalent feelings about having a loved one die at home. Encourage them to express their concerns.
- Family members need respite care to meet caregiving demands and to attend to their own grief and responses to loss.

✦ PRACTICE REFLECTIONS

A 78-year-old female patient with metastatic bone cancer was recently admitted to your unit. The patient had recently undergone aggressive chemotherapy treatments at the urging of her young adult daughter and was admitted for dehydration and pain control. The patient cried as she explained to you that she could no longer tolerate these treatments and wanted to be kept comfortable, but her daughter could not cope with the thought of her dying and kept pushing her to agree to more treatments.

1. What can you do to help this patient communicate her wishes to her daughter?
2. Do you have any ethical concerns about this family situation?
3. How will you provide supportive care to this patient?

✦ CLINICAL REVIEW QUESTIONS

1. Unless there are cultural practices that prohibit certain care practices, a nurse will expect to do which of the following when performing postmortem care? (Select all that apply.)
   1. Tie hands together at the top of the body.
   2. Shave facial hair and trim eyebrows.
   3. Replace dentures if able to insert.
   4. Close the eyes by applying light pressure.
   5. Wash soiled body parts.
2. When providing support to family caregivers who are grieving, what is the nurse's first priority?
   1. Encourage other family members to visit.
   2. Begin education on ways to cope with grief.
   3. Demonstrate empathy and understanding.
   4. Refer family caregivers to spiritual counseling.
3. Which physical symptoms are associated with impending death? (Select all that apply.)
   1. Warmth of the skin
   2. Bladder incontinence
   3. Increased food intake
   4. Labored breathing
   5. Restlessness

Answers and Rationales for Clinical Review Questions can be found on the Evolve website.

REFERENCES

American Association of Colleges of Nursing (AACN): CARES: competencies and recommendations for educating undergraduate nursing students, 2016. http://www.aacnnursing.org/Portals/42/ELNEC/PDF/New-Palliative-Care-Competencies.pdf.

American Cancer Society (ACS): Physical symptoms in the last 2 to 3 months of life, 2016. https://www.cancer.org/treatment/end-of-life-care/nearing-the-end-of-life/physical-symptoms.html.

American Cancer Society (ACS): Avoiding and dealing with falls during cancer treatment, 2017. https://www.cancer.org/treatment/treatments-and-side-effects/physical-side-effects/falls.html.

Arbour R, Wiegand D: Self-described nursing roles experienced during care of dying patients and their families: a phenomenological study, *Intensive Crit Care Nurs* 30:211, 2014.

Bailey F, Harmon S: Palliative care: the last hours of day and life, *UpToDate* 2017. http://www.uptodate.com/contents/palliative-care-the-last-hours-and-days-of-life.

Bruera E, et al: Overview of managing common non-pain symptoms in palliative care, *UpToDate* 2018. https://www.uptodate.com/contents/overview-of-managing-common-non-pain-symptoms-in-palliative-care.

Burchum JR, Rosenthal LD: *Lehne's pharmacology for nursing care*, ed 9, St. Louis, 2016, Elsevier.

Centers for Disease Control and Prevention (CDC): What is health literacy, 2016. https://www.cdc.gov/healthliteracy/learn/index.html.

Clark K, Currow D: Advancing research into symptoms of constipation at the end of life, *Int J Palliat Nurs* 20(8):370, 2014.

Doherty M, Thompson H: Enhancing person-centered care through the development of a therapeutic relationship, *Br J Community Nurs* 19(10):502, 2014.

Emanuel L, et al: The last hours of living: practical advice for clinicians, 2015. http://www.medscape.com/viewarticle/716463_4.

Gillespie L, Raftery A: Nutrition in palliative and end-of-life care, *Br J Community Nurs* S15(suppl):2014.

Given BA, Reinhard SC: Caregiving at the end of life: the challenges for family caregivers, *Generations* 41(1):50, 2017.

Greenway J, Johnson P: How to care for a patient after death in the community, *Nurs Stand* 30(37):34, 2016.

Hadders H, et al: Relatives' participation at the time of death: standardisation in pre- and post-mortem care in a palliative medical unit, *Eur J Oncol Nurs* 18:159, 2014.

Hall A: An overview of end-of-life care in the community setting, *J Clin Nurs* 28(6):36, 2014.

Hockenberry MJ, et al: *Wong's essentials of pediatric nursing*, ed 10, St. Louis, 2017, Mosby.

Hodge D: Administering a two-stage spiritual assessment in healthcare settings: a necessary component of ethical and effective care, *J Nurs Manag* 23(1):27, 2015.

Hospice and Palliative Care Nurses Association (HPNA): HPNA position statement complementary therapies in palliative nursing practice, 2015. http://hpna.advancingexpertcare.org/wp-content/uploads/2015/08/Complementary-Therapies-in-Palliative-Nursing-Practice.pdf.

Ingebretsen LP, Sagbakken M: hospice nurses' emotional challenges in their encounters with the dying, *Int J Qual Stud Health Well-being* 11:2016.

Keall R, et al: Therapeutic life review in palliative care: a systematic review of quantitative evaluations, *J Pain Symptom Manage* 49(4):747, 2015.

Kisvetrova H, et al: Spiritual support interventions in nursing care for patients suffering death anxiety in the final phase of life, *Int J Palliat Nurs* 19(12):599, 2013.

Koornstra R, et al: Management of fatigue in patients with cancer—a practical overview, *Cancer Treat Rev* 40:791, 2014.

National Consensus Project for Quality Palliative Care (NCP): Clinical practice guidelines for quality palliative care, ed 4, 2018. https://www.nationalcoalitionhpc.org/wp-content/uploads/2018/10/NCHPC-NCPGuidelines_4thED_web_FINAL.pdf.

National Institute on Aging (NIA): What is end-of-life care? 2017. https://www.nia.nih.gov/health/what-end-life-care.

Nunn C: It's not just about pain: symptom management in palliative care, *Nurse Prescrib* 12(7):338, 2014.

Paice J: Pain at the end of life. In Ferrell B, et al, editors: *Textbook of palliative nursing*, ed 4, New York, 2015, Oxford University Press.

Pirschel C: Ethical dilemmas at the end of life, *ONS Connect* 31(9):10, 2016.

Salmond E, et al: Experiences of compassion fatigue in direct care nurses: A qualitative systematic review protocol, *JBI Database System Rev Implement Rep* 15(7):1805, 2017.

Sansó N, et al: Palliative care professionals' inner life: exploring the relationships among awareness, self-care, and compassion satisfaction and fatigue, burnout, and coping with death, *J Pain Symptom Manage* 50(2):200, 2015.

Santucci G, Battista V: Methylnaltrexone for opioid-induced constipation in patients at the end of life, *Int J Palliat Nurs* 21(4):162, 2015.

Selman L, et al: Holistic models for end-of-life care: establishing place of culture, *Prog Palliat Care* 22(2):80, 2014.

Shaw C, Eldridge L: Nutritional considerations for the palliative care patient, *Int J Palliat Nurs* 21(1):7, 2015.

The Joint Commission (TJC): *2019 National Patient Safety Goals*, Oakbrook Terrace, IL, 2019, The Commission. http://www.jointcommission.org/standards_information/npsgs.aspx.

World Health Organization (WHO): WHO definition of palliative care, 2018. http://www.who.int/cancer/palliative/definition/en/.

Wynne L: Spiritual care at the end of life, *Nurs Stand* 28(2):41, 2013.

32 Home Care Safety

SKILLS AND PROCEDURES

EVOLVE WEBSITE/RESOURCES LIST

http://evolve.elsevier.com/Perry/nursinginterventions
Audio Glossary • Checklists • Clinical Review Questions • Answers and Rationales for Clinical Review Questions

INTRODUCTION

In the home setting, the recipient of care is commonly referred to as the *client* rather than *patient* because of the collaborative nature of the relationship. Clients and family caregivers need instruction so that they are prepared to assume self-care in the home and can function safely in their environment, adjust to health-related restrictions, and access available education programs and resources in the community. Home care instruction begins at the time of admission to a health care agency and continues in the home setting. In both settings, instruction includes multiple topics, such as health care promotion (e.g., exercise or diet), coping with impaired function (e.g., making adaptive changes in the home), and restoration of health (e.g., learning how to take medicines or perform exercises; recognizing risks to recovery).

PRACTICE STANDARDS

- Centers for Disease Control and Prevention (CDC), 2017: Medication safety program—Medication safety guidelines
- The Joint Commission (TJC), 2019: National Patient Safety Goals—Patient identification

EVIDENCE-BASED PRACTICE

Medication Management

There are unique challenges with medication management in the home setting for clients and caregivers. Seniors in particular face unique challenges because they manage multiple medications for more than one chronic illness. Recent research explored factors that affect this complex issue in home care and discovered ways to support clients and caregivers. Strategies to promote medication adherence and safety include:

- Six patterns of medication management safety have been identified: vulnerabilities that impact safe management and storage, sustaining adequate support, degrees of shared accountability, systems of variable effectiveness, poly-literacy requirements, and maintaining medication safety (Lang et al., 2015).
- Clients and family caregivers may have cognitive impairment, dexterity issues, illnesses, or risky storage practices (Lang et al., 2015).
- Medication errors include dosage errors, omitted administration, wrong medication, and wrong time or route of administration (Parand et al., 2016).
- The age, education level, and time/other responsibilities of the caregiver can be individual contributing factors to medication errors (Parand et al., 2016).
- Psychosocial factors also contribute to medication errors, such as panic/cognitive failure, fear of spillage of medication, and communication issues between the caregiver and client (Parand et al., 2016).
- Caregivers may refuse help or have difficulty sharing accountability (Lang et al., 2015).
- Caregivers often develop their own workarounds for labeling medications. Varying systems were also found for documentation and tracking (Lang et al., 2015).
- Solutions focused on the following areas: adapting medication administration to the home setting, developing tools to support safe medication administration, and strengthening health systems integration (Lang et al., 2015).
- There is an ongoing need to train caregivers, support communication with the health care team, and ensure appropriate supplies and equipment are used along with the correct medications (Parand et al., 2016).

SAFETY GUIDELINES

Home safety modifications affect all people living in a home. You must include the client and family caregiver in all discussions. The Joint Commission (TJC, 2019) identified five goals related to client safety in home care, focusing on problems in safety and how to solve them:

- Identify clients correctly—follow procedure to ensure clients receive the correct medications.
- Use medicines safely—ensure a client has one up-to-date medication list and understands his or her medications.
- Prevent infection—apply hand hygiene principles when providing care in the home.
- Prevent falls—recognize fall risks and implement preventive strategies.
- Identify client safety risks—identify specifically risks associated with the use of oxygen therapy.

✦ SKILL 32.1 Home Environment Assessment and Safety

Purpose

The home environment includes external (e.g., community) and internal (e.g., indoor living) physical spaces and should be a place in which individuals feel comfortable and safe. Older adults are at risk for threats to safety because of physiological changes associated with aging and may benefit from the use of assistive devices. For example, a hearing loss prevents a client from hearing a smoke alarm, whereas a cognitive deficit affects a person's ability to organize or store medications properly. Clients of all ages can be at risk for safety due to external forces, such as violence in their communities; this violence can also affect the home care nurse in the community. *Healthy People 2020* (U.S. Department of Health and Human Service [HHS], 2017) has a goal for the prevention of injury and violence, highlighting the impact and effects of injuries and violence (Box 32.1).

Delegation and Collaboration

The skill of conducting an initial home safety assessment cannot be delegated to nursing assistive personnel (NAP). The nurse instructs the NAP to:

- Inform the nurse of suggestions for ways to make the home safer.

Equipment

- Home safety checklist (Table 32.1)

ASSESSMENT

1. Perform hand hygiene. Assess client for risk factors that predispose clients to accidents within the home and community:
   a. Known visual impairment (e.g., glaucoma, cataracts, diabetic retinopathy, diabetic macular edema, macular degeneration). *Rationale: Reduced visual function alters client's balance, depth perception, or adaptation to dark or glaring light (Touhy and Jett, 2018).*
   b. Hearing impairment (e.g., hearing loss, tinnitus). *Rationale: Diminishes quality of life. Associated with decreased function, increased likelihood of hospitalizations, miscommunication, depression, falls, loss of self-esteem, safety risks, and cognitive decline (Touhy and Jett, 2018).*
   c. Neuromuscular alterations (e.g., lower-extremity weakness, unsteady gait, impaired balance, poor ankle dorsiflexion). *Rationale: Factors predispose clients to falls. Recurrent falls are associated with difficulty standing up from chair (Touhy and Jett, 2018).*
   d. Reduced energy or fatigue. *Rationale: Predisposes clients to falls.*
   e. Incontinence or nocturia. *Rationale: Frequent trips to bathroom often cause client with other deficits to accidentally trip or fall over barriers. Dementia affects client's ability to find bathroom and recognize need to void (Touhy and Jett, 2018).*
   f. History of stroke, parkinsonism, delirium, seizures, dementia, syncope. *Rationale: Gait disorders make clients vulnerable to tripping and falling (Touhy and Jett, 2018). Age-related changes of neurological system include slowing of reaction time (Meiner and Yeager, 2019). Present multiple reasons for falls, including impaired gait and coordination, visual changes, diminished cognition, pain, muscle weakness, and polypharmacy (Touhy and Jett, 2018).*
   g. Cardiopulmonary conditions (e.g., postural hypotension, arrhythmias, palpitations, difficulty breathing, or shortness of breath). *Rationale: Dizziness, fatigue, and light-headedness predispose to falls (Touhy and Jett, 2018) and cause client to be unsteady and compensate for difficulties.*
   h. Medication usage and history, including polypharmacy and use of sedatives, antihypertensives, antidepressants, and diuretics. *Rationale: Medications that alter sensorium affect balance and judgment (Touhy and Jett, 2018).*
   i. History of previous fall—obtain detailed description of previous fall (see Chapter 4). *Rationale: Increases risk for future fall, even if previous fall did not result in injury. Falls contribute to a loss of confidence and increased fear of falling (Touhy and Jett, 2018).*
   j. Susceptibility to violence and crime. *Rationale: Older adults may feel more vulnerable because of frailness, disability, and living alone. Assessing client's perception and risk will assist in exploring ways to help older adults protect themselves (Touhy and Jett, 2018).*
   k. Assess client's or family caregiver's knowledge, experience, and health literacy level. *Rationale: Ensures client or family*

BOX 32.1

Prevention of Injury and Violence

- Unintentional injuries and those caused by acts of violence rank in the top 15 killers for Americans of all ages.
- Injuries are the leading cause of death for ages 1 to 44 years; they are a leading cause of disability for all ages, regardless of sex, race/ethnicity, or socioeconomic status.
- Injuries and violence contribute to premature death, poor mental health, high medical costs, and loss of productivity.
- The effects of injuries and violence affect the victim of violence and family members, friends, co-workers, employers, and communities.

Adapted from U.S. Department of Health and Human Services (HHS): *Healthy People 2020:* injury and violence prevention, 2017. https://www.healthypeople.gov/2020/topics-objectives/topic/injury-and-violence-prevention.

TABLE 32.1
Home Safety Checklist

Safety Criteria	Yes	No
Front and Back Entrances		
1. Walkways and steps are smooth and well lighted. Sturdy handrail is on both sides of stairs to entrance.	___	___
2. If client lives in an apartment or assisted-living facility, elevators are in working order.	___	___
3. Nonskid strips/safety treads or bright paint is used on outdoor steps. All steps have the same rise and depth (standard: 7-inch rise and 11-inch depth).	___	___
4. A shelf or bench is kept by front and back doors to place grocery bags or packages if needed.	___	___
5. Doormats are in good condition.	___	___
Kitchen		
1. Client wears clothes with short or close-fitting sleeves when cooking.	___	___
2. Stove control dials are easy to see and use, and stovetop and oven are clean and grease-free.	___	___
3. A working refrigerator is present.	___	___
4. Items in kitchen cabinets and shelves are easy to reach; expiration dates on food items are appropriate.	___	___
5. Lighting over sink, stove, and work areas is bright.	___	___
6. Client stays in kitchen while cooking.	___	___
7. Fire extinguisher is functional, available, and easy to handle and use.	___	___
Floors		
1. All carpeting and mats are secure. Skid backing is present under area rugs, or throw rugs are removed.	___	___
2. Walkways are free of clutter.	___	___
Bathrooms		
1. Door lock can be unlocked from both sides.	___	___
2. Tub or shower has nonskid mats or abrasive strips. Floor mats have nonskid backing.	___	___
3. Tub or shower has at least one grab bar kept free of towels or other items.	___	___
4. Shower has a stable stool or chair and handheld sprayer.	___	___
5. Cold and hot water faucets are clearly marked and functional, and temperature on water heater is 120°F (49°C) or lower.	___	___
6. An automatic nightlight is present and functional.	___	___
Bedroom		
1. Client can turn on light without having to get out of bed in the dark. Lighting is adequate for clear vision.	___	___
2. Furniture is arranged to provide clear path from bed to bathroom.	___	___
3. Phone with large-print emergency numbers is within easy reach of bed.	___	___
4. Alarm systems are available. There are listening devices for invalid clients.	___	___
Living Room/Family Room		
1. Light can be turned on without having to walk into dark room.	___	___
2. Lamp, extension, or phone cords are kept out of traffic ways.	___	___
3. Furniture is arranged so that it can be walked around easily, and walking paths are free of clutter.	___	___
Fire Safety		
1. Sufficient numbers of working smoke detectors are in appropriate locations.	___	___
2. Emergency exit plans are in place in case of fire.	___	___
3. Family has determined a meeting place outside the house.	___	___
4. Portable space heaters have a UL certification mark and are placed on flat, level surfaces 3 feet away from flammable items.	___	___
5. Furnace area is free of things that can catch on fire.	___	___
6. Furnace and chimney are checked annually by a qualified professional. Wood fireplaces are cleaned regularly of ash and soot.	___	___
7. Emergency numbers for police, fire, and poison control are posted near phone.	___	___
8. Fire extinguisher is functional, available, and easy to handle and use.	___	___

TABLE 32.1

Home Safety Checklist—cont'd

Electrical Safety		
1. Electrical cords are in good condition and not frayed, spliced, or cracked.	___	___
2. Electrical cords are kept away from water.	___	___
3. Extension cord/outlet extenders have built-in circuit breaker or fuse; outlets are not overloaded.	___	___
4. Wall outlets and switches have cover plates.	___	___
5. Light bulbs are of correct wattage for each fixture.	___	___
6. Fuse box is easily accessible and clearly labeled.	___	___
7. Lamp switches are easy to turn on to avoid burns from hot light bulbs.	___	___
Carbon Monoxide Prevention		
1. Furnace flues are checked regularly for patency.	___	___
2. Battery-operated carbon monoxide detector is in home. Battery is checked regularly each spring and fall.	___	___

Modified from Meiner S, Yeager J: *Gerontologic nursing*, ed 6, St. Louis, 2019, Elsevier.

BOX 32.2

Fall/Near-Fall Diary

- Keep a notebook and create across the longest edge of the paper these headings: "Date," "Time of Fall," "Activity at Time of Fall," "Symptoms," and "Injury."
- As soon as possible after a fall, have client or family caregiver complete information under each heading.
- List emergency contact numbers at the bottom of the fall diary for client to call in case a fall results in serious injury.
- Instruct client to bring the diary to the health care provider's office at the next scheduled visit or share information with home care nurse on next home visit.

Modified from Meiner S, Yeager J: *Gerontologic nursing*, ed 6, St. Louis, 2019, Elsevier.

caregiver has the capacity to obtain, communicate, process, and understand basic health information (CDC, 2016a).

2. If client has fallen in home or had other injuries within home, use the mnemonic SPLATT for a complete assessment (Meiner and Yeager, 2019). *Rationale: Key symptoms are helpful in identifying cause of fall and how to prevent future falls. SPLATT test allows client to explain symptoms in own words; it is important to understand circumstances around fall (Meiner and Yeager, 2019).*
   - Symptoms at time of fall
   - Previous fall
   - Location of fall
   - Activity at time of fall
   - Time of fall
   - Trauma after fall
3. Have client who has had a near fall or actual fall maintain a fall diary (Box 32.2). *Rationale: Information is very helpful in determining what happened prior to the fall and consequences of falling (Meiner and Yeager, 2019).*
4. Conduct the timed "get up and go" (TUG) test for basic mobility (see Skill 4.1 in Chapter 4). *Rationale: Simple screening examination may be used as a guide for initial falls screening to categorize high and low physiological fall risks (Singh et al., 2015).*
5. Determine whether client has fear of falling. Possible indicators include apprehension during ambulation (observed in facial expressions); sweating or trembling while ambulating; clutching people or objects while ambulating; reluctance to change position or ambulate; and new onset of wobbly, reduced mobility after fall. *Rationale: Fear of falling occurs variably in older adults. Some clients may restrict mobility and participation in activities of daily living (ADLs) or instrumental activities of daily living (IADLs) because of fear of falling (Hill and Fauerbach, 2014).*

Safe Patient Care *In addition to the client, include family caregivers as a resource in assessments because they may witness accident trends or patterns.*

6. Partner with client and family caregivers to conduct home safety assessment. *Rationale: Provides comprehensive review of all areas within home that pose hazardous situations.*
   a. Front and back entrances:
      (1) Are walkways to front/back door even and free from holes or cracks? *Rationale: Entrances pose barriers in surfaces over which client must walk. Uneven pavement and holes may not be seen by client, causing tripping and falls.*
      (2) Are home entrances, including walkways, well lit? *Rationale: Poorly lit areas prevent individuals from seeing variations in walking surface.*
      (3) Does client have nonskid strips/safety treads or bright-colored paint on outdoor steps? Which colors are most easily seen by client? Are these colors used? *Rationale: Nonskid surfaces cause fewer slips on stairs. Color on steps permits individual to see edges, accommodating for any reduced depth perception.*
      (4) Are doormats in good repair, with nonskid backing and tapered edge? *Rationale: Raised edges pose risk for tripping. Doormats without nonskid backing slide when stepped on, causing client to lose balance.*
      (5) Are doors in good repair, and do they open and close easily? Can client open and close all doors easily? *Rationale: Act of opening and closing door is difficult if grasp is weak. Tripping may occur during opening and cause a fall.*
      (6) Is there a sturdy handrail on both sides of stairs leading to entrance? *Rationale: Handrails provide greater support while ascending and descending stairs.*

(7) Are steps in good condition with even, flat surfaces? *Rationale: Uneven surfaces predispose to tripping.*
(8) Are doorways and stairs free of clutter? *Rationale: Reduces risk for tripping and/or falling.*

b. Kitchen. *Rationale: Cooking equipment was one of the major causes of home fire fatalities from 2010 through 2014 (National Fire Protection Association [NFPA], 2016).*
(1) Does client wear clothing with short or close-fitting sleeves when cooking? *Rationale: Short or close-fitting sleeves are less likely to accidentally catch on fire when person works at stove.*
(2) Does client always stay in kitchen when cooking? *Rationale: Lack of attention when cooking with fire is a risk.*
(3) Does client have loud timer to signal when food is cooked? *Rationale: Prevents burning food and risk for fire.*
(4) Does client keep stovetop and oven clean and grease-free? *Rationale: Grease is highly flammable.*
(5) Are stove control dials easy to see and use? *Rationale: Client may accidentally use higher flame than is necessary for cooking safely.*
(6) Is charged, easy-to-use fire extinguisher close at hand? *Rationale: Extinguisher should be ready for use at all times.*

Safe Patient Care *Have client demonstrate steps of how to use fire extinguisher.*

(7) Are emergency numbers for police, fire, and poison control posted on or near telephone or in an easily accessible place? If client uses cell phone, ask if client keeps phone on or near him or her. *Rationale: Emergency phone numbers and extinguisher ensure quick response if fire occurs. If client only uses cell phone, ensure that phone is charged and kept on or near him or her so that it can be accessed at any time.*
(8) Can items in kitchen cabinets and shelves be reached without climbing on stool or chair? *Rationale: Climbing on step stools or chairs creates risks for falls.*
(9) Is there adequate lighting over sink, stove, and work areas? *Rationale: Poor lighting makes it difficult to see control knobs or dials and provides inadequate illumination when using sharp knives or utensils (Touhy and Jett, 2018).*
(10) Are kitchen throw rugs and mats slip resistant? *Rationale: Rugs or mats that are not slip resistant can easily slide on tile or wood floors.*
(11) Assess food safety: Are perishable foods in refrigerator and nonperishable foods safe to eat? Is food stored appropriately? Are expiration dates past? Is there evidence that food has spoiled? Does client know how to prepare and store food safely? *Rationale: Proper food storage and preparation can prevent foodborne illnesses. Foods are properly cooked when they are heated for long enough time and at high enough temperature to kill harmful bacteria that cause foodborne illness (Foodsafety.gov, 2017). Eating foods that have spoiled or with expiration dates that have passed puts client at risk for foodborne illness (e.g., food poisoning).*

c. Bathroom:
(1) Can client unlock bathroom door from both sides of door? *Rationale: Functional locks prevent person from being trapped in bathroom.*
(2) Is tub or shower equipped with nonskid mats, abrasive strips, or surfaces that are not slippery? *Rationale: Bathrooms are hazardous. Wet floors and tub or shower bottoms can be very slippery, creating risk for falls.*
(3) Does bathroom floor have nonslip surface or rug with nonskid backing? *Rationale: Slippery tile predisposes to falls (Touhy and Jett, 2018).*
(4) Does client avoid using slippery bath oils when bathing? *Rationale: Use of bath oils makes tub surface slippery and increases risk for falls.*
(5) Do bathtub and shower have at least one grab bar or handrail placed where client can reach it? *Rationale: Grab bars provide extra support while maneuvering into and out of tubs or showers. Grab bars placed correctly where client can safely reach them help to steady gait and lessen chance of falls (Meiner and Yeager, 2019).*
(6) Is client careful not to place towels on grab bars? *Rationale: Some clients accidentally grab towel instead of bar when needing support. Towel can slip off bar.*
(7) Does shower have stable stool or chair and handheld sprayer? Is shower easy to access (walk-in versus step-in tub area)? *Rationale: Shower stool allows client to sit while showering.*
(8) Are cold and hot water faucets clearly marked, and is temperature on water heater 48.8°C (120°F) or lower? *Rationale: Accidental burns can occur from exposure to hot water.*

d. Bedroom:
(1) Is night-light placed in bedroom and/or bath? *Rationale: Older adults have altered night vision.*
(2) Is working smoke detector just outside bedroom door? *Rationale: Alarm situated just outside bedroom can awaken person early enough to escape fire.*
(3) Can client turn on light without having to get out of bed in dark? Is flashlight available at bedside? Flashlight can be attached to walker or cane. *Rationale: Getting out of bed without proper lighting or ability to adjust to light changes and reaching for necessary objects puts client at risk for falls (Touhy and Jett, 2018).*
(4) Is furniture arranged to provide clear path from bed to bathroom? *Rationale: Obstructed path creates barrier that causes tripping and falls.*
(5) Is phone with emergency numbers within easy reach of bed? *Rationale: If clients develop physical symptoms while in bed, they need to be able to reach phone without having to get out of bed.*
(6) Are other alarm systems available? Push buttons that call for help? Nursery listening devices for cognitively impaired or nonambulatory clients? *Rationale: Can alert family caregivers when person requires immediate help. Bedside phone, cordless phone, intercom buzzer, or lifeline can be placed in readily accessible location (Touhy and Jett, 2018).*

e. Living room/family room:
(1) Are electrical or extension cords removed from under furniture and carpeting? Kept out of way of traffic? *Rationale: Clients can easily trip or fall over electrical cords. Hidden cords are trip and fire hazards.*
(2) Can client turn on light without having to walk into dark room? *Rationale: Darkened room can disorient and prevent client from seeing uneven surfaces.*
(3) Are hallways and walkways free from objects and clutter? *Rationale: Objects and clutter in common walkway can cause client to trip, resulting in falls.*

(4) Are loose area rugs securely attached to floor and not placed over carpeting? (For best safety, consider removing throw rugs.) *Rationale: Loose edges of rugs are easy for persons to trip over (Touhy and Jett, 2018).*
(5) Is furniture arranged in each room so that client can walk around easily? *Rationale: Furniture creates obstacles to walking in room.*
(6) Is all furniture steady and without sharp edges? *Rationale: Clients often use edge of furniture for support when standing.*

f. Around the house:
(1) Are all living areas and stairways well lit? *Rationale: Helps people see any barriers or uneven walking surfaces.*
(2) Is flooring or carpeting throughout house in good repair? *Rationale: Frayed carpet or irregular surfaces can cause tripping and result in fall.*
(3) Are all thresholds level with floor or no more than 1.27 cm (0.5 inch) in height? *Rationale: Uneven thresholds can cause tripping.*
(4) Is light switch at both top and bottom of stairs? *Rationale: Prevents individual from having to walk part of stairs in dark.*
(5) Does lighting produce glare or shadows on stairs or floor surfaces? *Rationale: Older adults are sensitive to glare because their visual pathway becomes distorted.*
(6) Do handrails run continuously from top to bottom of flights of stairs? *Rationale: Handrails provide source of physical support when ascending and descending stairs.*
(7) Are handrails securely attached to wall? *Rationale: Handrails should be installed at least on one side of hallway or stairwell (Touhy and Jett, 2018).*
(8) Are step coverings in good condition? *Rationale: Loosened covering can cause tripping.*
(9) Are guns kept in house? Are trigger locks installed on all guns? Are guns stored unloaded? Is ammunition in locked secure location? Is ammunition stored in a different place than the guns? *Rationale: Questions are important to assess understanding of and compliance with gun safety. Following gun safety standards decreases risk for injury and death related to gun use (National Rifle Association [NRA], 2017).*

g. General fire safety:
(1) Does client have properly working smoke detectors with fresh batteries? *Rationale: Smoke alarms properly located, functioning well, and with batteries replaced twice a year can provide timely alert for fire.*

Safe Patient Care *There are many different smoke-alarm products. Assess the type your client has to determine if it is battery operated, hard-wired, multifunctional (e.g., can also detect carbon monoxide), or a smart detector (which can communicate through apps; Safewise, 2017). Batteries will need to be changed according to type; some batteries last for 6 months, whereas newer detectors can last 10 years. Check to see when smoke-alarm battery was last changed and instruct clients to change battery according to the type of smoke detector.*

(2) Does client have several emergency exit plans in case of fire? *Rationale: Exit plan helps people anticipate route of escape when fire does occur. Exit should not have locks that are difficult to open or any physical barriers.*
(3) Has family determined meeting place in event of emergency, such as at mailbox in front of home? *Rationale: Use of common emergency meeting location is efficient method for determining that all family members are safely out of house.*
(4) Does client use portable space heaters? Are they kept at least 1 meter (3 feet) away from flammable items? *Rationale: Heaters, furnaces, and chimneys pose risks for fire.*
(5) Is a three-foot area around furnace kept clear of items that can catch on fire (U.S. Fire Administration, n.d.)? *Rationale: Heating equipment was second-most common cause of home fire fatalities from 2010 through 2014 (NFPA, 2016). This can be a particular problem for people who are hoarders.*
(6) Does a qualified professional check furnace and chimney annually? Is there a CO_2 detector? *Rationale: Buildup of creosote within chimney can catch on fire. Overheated motor in furnace can burn out and possibly cause fire.*
(7) Does client who smokes report smoking in bed? *Rationale: Smoking materials were the leading cause of home fires in 2010 through 2014 (NFPA, 2016). Smoking in bed has added risk of client falling asleep while cigarette is lit.*

h. General electrical safety:
(1) Are electrical cords in good condition (i.e., not frayed, spliced, or cracked)? *Rationale: Damaged cords can short circuit and lead to fire.*
(2) Are electrical cords kept away from water? *Rationale: Use of any appliance or device that is exposed to water creates risk for electrical shock.*
(3) Does client use extension cord/outlet extenders with built-in circuit breaker or fuse? *Rationale: Prevents overloading of circuit that can lead to fire.*
(4) Do all wall outlets and switches have cover plates? *Rationale: Prevents physical contact with wiring.*
(5) Does client use light bulbs of correct wattage for each fixture? *Rationale: Use of excessive wattage can lead to fire.*
(6) Is main electrical fuse box for home easily accessible and clearly labeled? *Rationale: In event of emergency, fuse box should be easy to access so that proper circuit can be cut off.*

i. Carbon monoxide prevention:
(1) Are furnace flues checked regularly for patency? *Rationale: Obstructed flues are common cause of carbon monoxide toxicity.*
(2) Is there a working carbon monoxide detector in home? *Rationale: The warning signs for carbon monoxide poisoning can be subtle. People who are sleeping in particular may not be aware of a problem (Mayo Clinic, n.d.).*

7. Assess client's financial resources; determine monthly income used for ongoing expenses. *Rationale: Determines potential for making repairs to home. Reveals need for low-cost community service support.*
8. Assess client for need of additional supportive services (e.g., physical therapy, speech, therapy, occupational therapy, social services). *Rationale: Promotes an interprofessional collaborative approach to client care; helps ensure all needs are met.*
9. Assess client's and family caregiver's willingness to make changes. Has client accepted limitations that pose risk for injury? *Rationale: Some clients perceive attempts to improve safety within home as intrusive. If you show that necessary revisions to home environment will preserve independence, client will participate more willingly.*

STEP	RATIONALE
PLANNING	
1. Expected outcomes following completion of procedure:	
• Client and/or family caregiver describes potential environmental risks within and outside home that predispose to accidents or injuries.	Demonstrates client's and family caregiver's recognition of safety risks that are of greatest concern.
• Client and/or family caregiver initiate actions to correct environmental risks, making home safer.	Client sees value in altering living environment.
• Client remains free of injury.	Environmental barriers are reduced or removed to minimize injuries.
2. Prioritize with client and family caregiver environmental barriers that pose greatest risk.	Client's own physical and/or cognitive deficits make certain environmental risks more hazardous. Prioritization helps client make best choices.
3. Recommend calling in reliable contractor if major home repairs are necessary and acceptable to client and family.	Ensures that repairs are made safely and correctly.
IMPLEMENTATION	
1. **General home safety:**	
a. Provide direct light source in areas where client reads, cooks, uses tools, or conducts hobby work. High-intensity light on object or surface that is involved works best.	Visual impairment in older adults usually is a result of cataracts, macular degeneration, glaucoma, or diabetic retinopathy (Touhy and Jett, 2018).
Safe Patient Care *Avoid fluorescent lighting because it creates excessive glare.*	
b. Consider satin and nonglossy finishes for walls, cabinets, and countertops in kitchen. Have sheer curtains or adjustable shades in other living areas.	Reduces glare for older adults.
c. Apply colored tape or paint to color code controls of stove, oven, dryer, toaster, and other appliances.	Clients with reduced visual acuity may adjust appliance to wrong setting, creating potential risk for fire or burning.
d. Consider installing Lazy Susan or pull-out drawers with glide mechanisms in kitchen cabinets. Install C-ring handles in lower cabinets.	Makes access to food and kitchen supplies easier.
e. Install automatic door openers, level doorknob handles, and hook-and-chain locks.	Devices may be easier to grasp and use. Remote-controlled door locks can also provide additional security (Touhy and Jett, 2018).
f. Consider external home environment safety measures (such as an alarm system, video camera monitoring, community watch group, motion detection lighting, floodlights).	Provides sense of security for clients. Helps monitor conditions outside the home and recognize potential threats.
2. **Fall prevention steps:**	
a. Paint edges of concrete stairs bright yellow, orange, or white.	Client can see edge of stairs more clearly.
b. Install treads with uniform depth of 22.5 cm (9 inches) and 22.5-cm (9-inch) risers (vertical face of steps).	If stairs are of uniform size, client does not have to continually adjust vision or stride.
c. Rearrange furniture to open up space through hallways and major rooms.	Creates unobstructed pathway for ambulation.
d. Reduce clutter within living areas (e.g., footstools, flower pots, extension cords, children's toys, stacked newspapers or magazines).	Mobility hazards resulting from clutter are especially risky at night.
e. Secure all carpeting, mats, and tile; place nonskid backing under small rugs and doormats. Remove throw rugs/mats in nonessential (dry) areas.	Reduces chance of client slipping when stepping on rug surface (Touhy and Jett, 2018).
f. Pad floor and use specialized tile that absorbs impact of falls.	Cushions person's fall.
g. Use low-rise beds, futon beds, or mattress on floor if not contraindicated.	Lowers distance to floor surface.
h. Have enough electrical outlets installed to be able to plug light or electronic device (e.g., television, video) into nearby outlet. Secure electrical cords against baseboards.	Prevents need to run extension cords across walkways.

STEP	RATIONALE
i. Install nonskid strips on surface of bathtub and/or shower stall. Be sure that floor is clean and dry.	Reduces chances of slipping on tub/shower stall surface.
j. Have grab bar installed in studs at tub, toilet, and/or shower (see illustration). Have client select vertical or horizontal placement if choice available. Be sure that bar is different color than wall and easy to see.	Bar provides stability for maneuvering in bathroom (Touhy and Jett, 2016). Grab bars placed in correct place where client can safely reach them help to steady stance and gait and lessen chance of falls (Meiner and Yeager, 2019).
k. Have handrails installed along side of any stairway (see illustration). Be sure that stairways are well lit, with switches at top and bottom of steps.	Ideally, handrails on both sides of stairwell provide greatest stability for client. If entrance space does not allow this, install at least on one side to prevent fall from imbalance (Touhy and Jett, 2016). Older adults have difficulty seeing edges of stairs.
l. Install appropriate broad-beam lighting for outside walkways.	Provides full illumination.
m. Keep lighted phone easily accessible, next to client's bed. If client only uses a cell phone, make sure it is charged and kept next to bed; ensure that charging cord is not an obstacle.	Prevents client from having to get up out of bed, often in dark.
n. Install motion-sensor exterior lighting for walkways/driveway.	Reduces risk for client falls caused by dark surroundings.
o. Have client use padding or types of clothing that will cushion bony prominences, especially high-risk bony prominences (e.g., hips). Specially designed hip protectors are available.	For clients with a history of hip fracture, who are frail, or who have degenerative disease, hip protectors are recommended (Hester, 2015).
3. Prevent spread of infection:	
a. Teach client and family caregiver cleaning practices to prevent spread of infection (e.g., cleaning kitchen countertops before and after food preparation; use correct cleaning solutions and keep solution in original container).	Ensures more consistent infection control practices in the home. Solutions in original containers avoid confusion of products and risk of combining chemicals.
b. Instruct client not to share eating and drinking utensils.	Some infections are spread by saliva.
c. Instruct client to clean appliances and cooking surfaces daily.	Regular cleaning prevents risk for contamination and spread of infection.

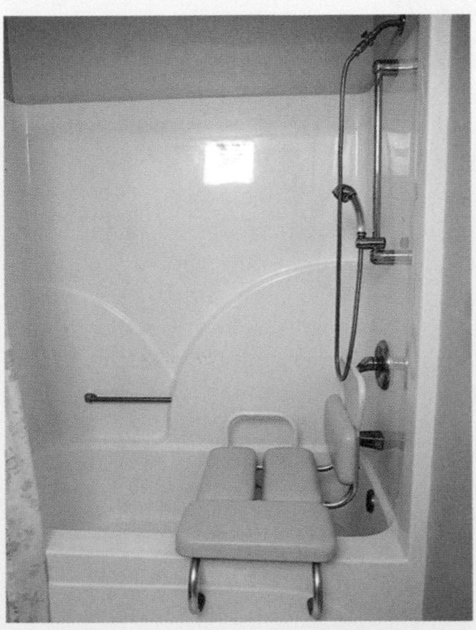

STEP 2j Grab bars and safety seat installed in shower.

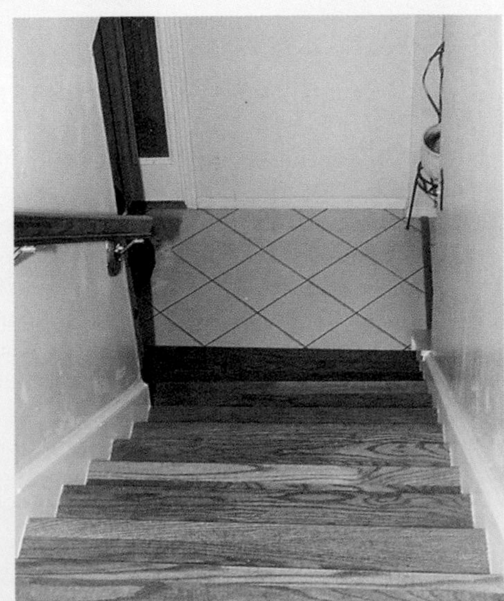

STEP 2k Handrails installed along stairways provide security for clients with visual, balance, and coordination problems.

STEP	RATIONALE
d. Instruct client in safe food preparation and storage. Refer to guidelines at Foodsafety.gov for a complete list of tips and techniques to keep food safe.	Ensures safe thawing and cooking of foods (Foodsafety.gov, 2017).
For example: • 4- to 12-lb turkey can safely be thawed in refrigerator for 1 to 3 days or in cold water for 2 to 6 hours; cook poultry to 165°F.	
• Bacon can be stored in refrigerator for 7 days and freezer for 1 month; hamburger and other ground meats can be stored in refrigerator for 1 to 2 days and in freezer for 3 to 4 months.	Safe storage times for food in refrigerator and freezer help prevent foodborne illnesses (Foodsafety.gov, 2017).
4. Fire safety:	
a. Have smoke detectors installed near each bedroom, in kitchen, and in basement. Be sure that detector is on each floor of home. Alarm should be close to alert client and family when sleeping.	Fires most frequently start in basement near furnace, dryer, or electrical wiring; kitchen; or living areas where there is extensive wiring.
b. Have client select fire extinguisher that is easy to handle and manipulate (see illustration). Ask him or her to read instructions and demonstrate its proper use.	Some older adults or clients with disabilities have difficulty gripping mechanisms on certain extinguishers.

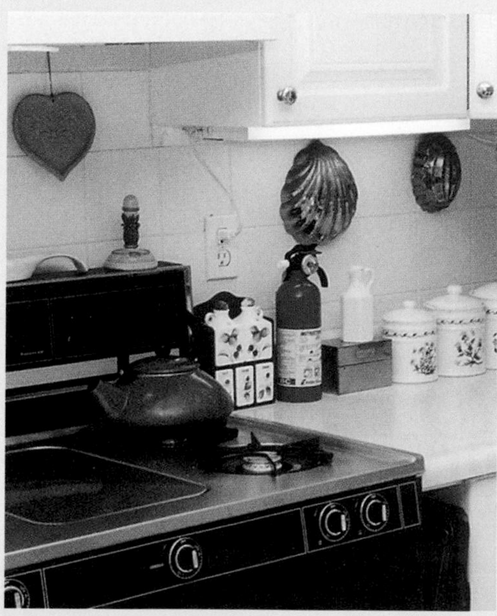

STEP 4b Fire extinguisher accessible in kitchen.

STEP	RATIONALE
c. Have area around furnace cleared 3 feet of any flammable items (e.g., boxes, papers).	Reduces risk for fire.
d. Instruct client to be sure that portable space heater has emergency shut off and that the equipment housing and electrical cords are intact (Meiner and Yeager, 2019).	Space heaters can be overturned by accident, which can cause fire; safety mechanism on newer models will turn unit off immediately (Meiner and Yeager, 2019).
e. Have client make appointments for maintenance of furnace and chimney cleaning in appropriate season.	Furnace maintenance prevents short circuits and fires. Accumulation of creosote on chimney walls can lead to fire.
f. Have client check light-bulb wattage in all fixtures.	Ensures proper wattage being used; wattage that exceeds recommendation can cause fire.
g. Have client establish routine during cooking that keeps him or her in kitchen. Be sure that cooking range is clean and items such as potholders and towels are away from burners.	Food cooking on stove can easily boil over or begin to burn when unattended.
h. If client is a smoker, review need to keep ashtrays clean and emptied. Placing small amount of water or sand in bottom of ashtray is useful if client is visually impaired.	Clients with reduced vision may be unable to tell if cigarette, cigar, or match has extinguished.

STEP	RATIONALE
i. Strongly discourage smoking in bed, smoking in chair when there is possibility of falling asleep, and smoking after taking medication that diminishes alertness. Instruct client/family caregiver to put cigarette or cigar out at first sign of feeling drowsy (Meiner and Yeager, 2019).	Risks factors for burns and fire. Client's reaction time may be slower when tired.
j. Recommend that client install power strips or surge protectors for plugging in multiple appliances/devices.	Prevents risk for electrical short, which can cause fire.
5. **Burn safety:**	
a. Have setting on hot water heater adjusted to 49° C (120° F) or lower.	Prevents scalding burns (Meiner and Yeager, 2019).
b. Instruct client to always turn cold water on first.	Prevents direct exposure to hot water.
c. Install touch pads on lamps.	Light is easy to turn on without risk of touching hot light bulb.
d. Use color codes of red for hot and blue for cold on water faucets. (If client has difficulty distinguishing these colors, choose two that are easily distinguished.)	Prevents accidental burning from turning on wrong faucet.
6. **Carbon monoxide safety:**	
a. Have condition of furnace venting checked annually just before turning on furnace.	Improper venting prevents escape of carbon monoxide, a poisonous gas that alters hemoglobin to prevent formation of oxyhemoglobin and reduces oxygen supply to tissues.
b. Caution clients against using gas stove or barbecue grill for heating inside home.	Both are sources of carbon monoxide (Meiner and Yeager, 2019).
c. Have battery-operated carbon monoxide detector installed in home; check or replace battery when you change your clocks in fall and spring (see illustration).	Detector alarms when carbon monoxide reaches unsafe levels. Battery operation is not affected by power outages (Meiner and Yeager, 2019).

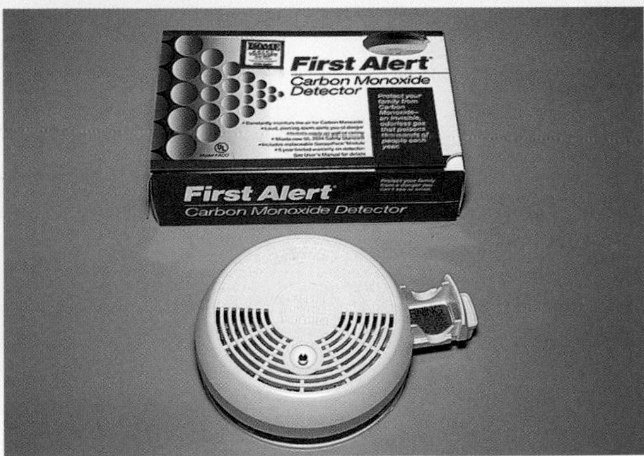

STEP 6c Carbon monoxide detector.

STEP	RATIONALE
7. **Firearm safety:**	
a. Teach client about dangers associated with keeping guns in home.	Risk of suicide increases in homes with firearms (Edelman et al., 2014). Increased risk for accidental shootings.
b. If guns are in home, teach client to install trigger locks and store them unloaded in locked cabinet. Teach client to store ammunition in secured area separate from guns. Store keys in place inaccessible to children.	Following gun safety standards decreases risk of injury and death related to gun use (Hockenberry et al., 2017).

EVALUATION

1. Have client and family caregiver(s) identify safety risks revealed in home safety assessment.	Demonstrates what client recognizes as risk and its relative importance for changing.
2. During follow-up visit or call to home ask client to discuss plans for making any modifications and observe changes client has implemented.	Evaluates extent to which client sees risks as potentially harmful and complies with suggested changes.
3. During follow-up visits or calls, ask if client has experienced any falls or other injuries within or outside of the home.	Reveals new risks and/or if risks have been eliminated, depending on client's previous history of injury.

STEP	RATIONALE
4. During subsequent home visits, reassess for progression of dementia.	Evaluates for potential new risks to client and caregiver.
5. Use Teach-Back: "I want to be sure I explained why you need to make modifications in your home. Tell me why this is important." Revise your instruction now or develop a plan for revised client/family caregiver teaching if client/family caregiver is not able to teach back correctly.	Determines client's/family caregiver's level of understanding of instructional topic.

Unexpected Outcomes	Related Interventions
1. Client and family caregiver do not acknowledge risks identified from home safety assessment.	• Determine reason client is reluctant to make changes. Consider limited resources, disbelief concerning need to make changes, fear of loss of autonomy, or other reasons. • Review implications of risks to client's safety and welfare.
2. Client fails to make changes agreed on in previous plan.	• Determine reason for failure to make changes. • Help prioritize greatest risks. • Suggest making a single change and gauge client's response.
3. Client suffers fall or burn within home.	• Conduct assessment of contributing factors and conditions in environment at time of injury. • Make revisions based on assessment findings.

Recording

- Record assessment of physical and cognitive status, home barriers or risks, recommended interventions, instruction provided, response of client or family caregiver, and changes client makes to home environment.
- Document your evaluation of client learning.

Hand-Off Reporting

- Report any physical or cognitive changes not previously identified and remaining barriers in the home environment.

✦ SKILL 32.2 Adapting the Home Setting for Clients With Cognitive Deficits

Purpose

It is a myth that all older adults experience cognitive dysfunctions; however, older adults are more likely to develop them. Clients with cognitive impairments and their family caregivers need assistance in making adaptations to preserve the client's ability to function safely within the home and understand changes in cognition. To be safe, a person needs to be able to perform routine activities of daily living (ADLs) and instrumental activities of daily living (IADLs; e.g., check writing, buying groceries) and make sound decisions. When there are cognitive limitations, a person's independence is threatened.

Delegation and Collaboration

The skill of adapting the home environment for clients with cognitive deficits cannot be delegated to nursing assistive personnel (NAP). The nurse is responsible for the assessment of cognitive function. The nurse directs the NAP to:

- Inform the nurse when there is a change in client's mood, memory, and ability to maintain the home or perform self-care.

Equipment

- Mini-Mental State Examination (MMSE)
- Calendar
- Paper for making lists
- Bulletin board or poster board *(optional)*
- Motion detector *(optional)*

ASSESSMENT

1. Identify client using at least two identifiers (e.g., name and birthday or name and medical record number) according to agency policy. *Rationale: Ensures client safety. Complies with The Joint Commission standards and improves client safety (TJC, 2019).*
2. Assess client over several short periods of time and be ready to adapt assessment if client has sensory disabilities. *Rationale: Respects human dignity of client. Improves likelihood of gathering relevant data.*
3. Assess client's or family caregiver's knowledge, experience, and health literacy level. *Rationale: Ensures client has the capacity to obtain, communicate, process, and understand basic health information (CDC, 2016a).*
4. Be sure that room in which you meet with client and family is well lit, with minimal outside noises or interruptions. Listen carefully and speak clearly and in normal tone of voice. *Rationale: Optimal environment for assessment of client's cognitive and mental status provides more valid assessment.*
5. Ask client to describe own level of health and have him or her describe how it affects ability to perform ADLs and IADLs. Ask family caregiver (if available) to confirm description. Screen for risky behaviors (e.g., medication nonadherence, unsupervised use of stove). *Rationale: Question requires client to focus on one topic. Allows you to assess attention and concentration. Also determines whether client is fully perceptive of physical and cognitive capabilities.*

Safe Patient Care *Be aware of your communication with the client and family caregivers. Do not make the client think that you are not listening to his or her views. The additional person supplements answers with client's consent, but the client remains the focus of the interview.*

6. Ask how client is handling home-management responsibilities: "Tell me which bills you pay each month. Can you tell me what each one is for?" Ability to perform ADLs: "Can you tell me about your normal day? When do you get up, eat meals, dress? Tell me what you do to dress or bath each morning." *Rationale: Provides good comparison of client and family perceptions. Interaction helps measure short-term memory, judgment, and problem solving.*
7. Assess client's adherence to taking medications. *Rationale: Medication administration in the home presents unique challenges.*
   a. Review number and type of medications being taken, client's understanding of purpose as prescribed (or as chosen for over-the-counter [OTC] medications), time of day taken, and dosages. *Rationale: Keeping list of medications allows health care provider easy access to medication history and assists the nurse in education of client and family caregiver.*
   b. Conduct pill count over course of a week (family caregiver may need to help). *Rationale: A pill count helps to validate medication adherence and identify when a medication is omitted.*
   c. Assess where client stores medications. *Rationale: Ensures medications are kept in secure and appropriate place.*
   d. Give special attention to pain medications, anticonvulsants, antihypertensives (especially beta-adrenergic blockers), diuretics, digoxin, aspirin, and anticoagulants. Have client or family caregiver keep updated list of medications that can be brought to emergency department if needed. Ask to see medications and/or list used. *Rationale: Keeping a list of medications gives health care providers easy access to medication history.*
8. Determine whether client has family caregiver who helps with self-care or home-management responsibilities. Consider asking the following questions: What level of support does caregiver provide? How frequently is caregiver available? Does client perceive satisfaction in caregiver's support? What level of satisfaction does caregiver perceive? Does caregiver have access to and/or take advantage of respite care? *Rationale: Relationship between family caregiver and client helps define how difficult it is to provide caregiving support. Role of family caregiver is often stressful, particularly if individual has other responsibilities, such as parenting, work, or school. Determines availability of resource to client and quality of that support.*
9. During discussion, observe client's dress, nonverbal expressions, appearance, and cleanliness. *Rationale: Conditions such as depression and dementia can result in client's inability to attend to personal appearance.*

Safe Patient Care *Do not confuse behavioral changes with lack of available resources to maintain hygiene. Also, be aware of signs and symptoms of abuse or neglect (see Chapter 8). Report suspected abuse to appropriate social service agency.*

10. Observe immediate home environment. *Rationale: Behavioral changes associated with cognitive dysfunction are evident in disorderly home and inappropriate placement of objects (e.g., carton of orange juice placed inside kitchen cabinet instead of in refrigerator).*
11. If you suspect cognitive or mental status change:
    a. Complete Dementia Severity Rating Scale (DSRS) for dementia. *Rationale: Test screens orientation, memory, judgment, home activities, personal care, speech and language recognition, and incontinence. If client scores higher than 4, it generally indicates cognitive impairment that requires further evaluation (Meiner and Yeager, 2019).*
    b. Complete Short Geriatric Depression Scale (SGDS) for depression. (**NOTE:** Other depression scales, such as the Beck Depression Inventory [BDI], are available.) *Rationale: SGDS is recommended because it takes 5 minutes to administer and has been tested, validated, and used extensively for depression in older adults (Touhy and Jett, 2018).*
12. If you suspect that client is at risk for wandering or is wandering, observe for the following behaviors (family caregivers might provide information as well):
    - Repeated shadowing or seeking whereabouts of caregiver
    - Revisiting one destination many times
    - Inability to locate landmarks or getting lost in familiar setting
    - Going into unauthorized or private places
    - Searching for "missing" people or places
    - Walking with no apparent destination or purpose
    - Haphazard or continuous moving, walking, or pacing
    - Walking that cannot easily be redirected

    Rationale: Alerts family and caregivers to potential safety risks. When wandering extends outside safe environment, client is at increased risk for injury or death.
13. Assess which current environmental strategies family caregivers are using to deal with wandering (e.g., latches and alarms on doors, visual cues such as STOP signs, constant supervision, and wearing identification band). *Rationale: Helps determine level of intervention necessary. Allows for assessment of how family is dealing with issues of wandering and need for additional outside support.*
14. Assess family caregiver for signs and symptoms of stress. *Rationale: Helps determine whether family caregiver is feeling burdened or overwhelmed and needs help.*

STEP	RATIONALE

PLANNING

1. Expected outcomes following completion of procedure:
   - Client is able to complete home-management responsibilities within existing limitations. — Modifications are made that help client apply remaining cognitive functions.
   - Client receives appropriate combination of medications for diagnosed conditions. — Assistive devices enable client to adhere to prescribed medication regimen.

STEP	RATIONALE
• Client is able to perform self-care activities or receives appropriate help.	Interventions preserve client's autonomy and maximize his or her functionality.
• Family caregivers describe steps to take to minimize wandering.	Instruction prepares family caregivers with wandering-management strategies.
• Client experiences fewer episodes of wandering.	Wandering-management strategies are effective.
• Family caregiver identifies community resources for support.	Services available can include respite care, adult day care programs, and support groups.
2. If client has difficulty with self-care or fine-motor skills, refer family to occupational therapy, homemaker services, or respite care as appropriate.	Occupational therapists provide assistive devices and recommend self-care adaptations. Homemaker services provide added resource for meal preparation and home cleaning. Respite care provides family caregiver temporary rest away from continuous responsibilities.
3. Consider client's level of cognitive impairment when making changes in his or her living environment. Some clients may require only minor adaptations, and others will depend more on help of family caregivers.	Retention of client's independence and autonomy is ultimate goal.
4. Determine best time of day for approaches that result in desired response.	Some clients are more alert and responsive in morning versus afternoon or vice versa.

IMPLEMENTATION

STEP	RATIONALE
1. If client has difficulty remembering when to perform tasks (e.g., paying bills, making appointments), help to create list or post reminder notes or calendar in conspicuous location (e.g., bulletin board, front of refrigerator).	Lists and organizers help client cope with memory loss and still safely perform activities.
2. If client has difficulty remembering when to take medicines, help to create list or reminder note, provide medication container organized by days of week, or recommend wristwatch with alarm or schedule of text messages to signal medication administration times.	There is no gold standard for improving medication adherence. Reminder systems have benefit if client or family caregiver is motivated and/or desires to adhere to them.
3. When client has difficulty completing tasks such as writing checks for bills or bringing groceries into home from store, reduce steps it takes to complete task. Consolidate steps or simplify task (e.g., consider a grocery delivery service, or engage family caregiver to assist with bill paying).	Prevents frustration in completing task and/or forgetting step that leads to task being unfinished.
4. If client has difficulty bathing, dressing, writing, and feeding, offer assistive devices (see illustrations).	Assistive eating devices have larger handles, cup handles, or plate edges to help with meals. Assistive dressing devices use Velcro, large zippers, and elastic to facilitate independence when dressing.

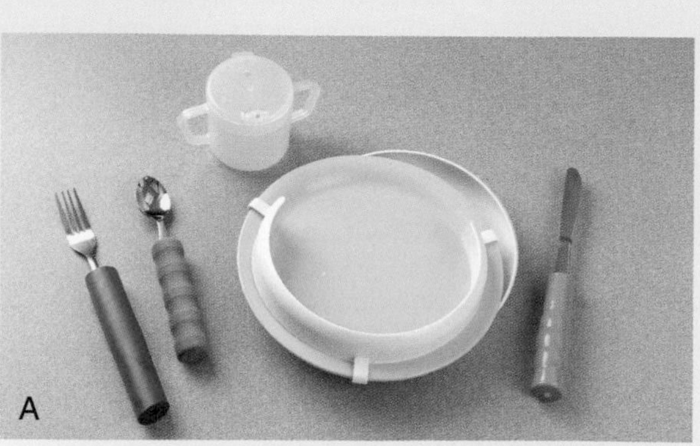

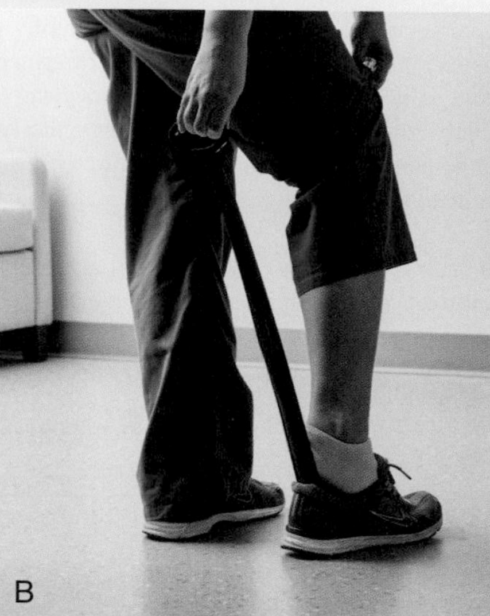

STEP 4 (A) Assistive feeding devices. (B) Assistive device to help put on shoes. *(Image A used with permission ArcMate Manufacturing Corporation. All rights reserved.)*

STEP	RATIONALE
5. Help client and family caregiver determine routine schedule for ADLs such as eating, bathing, daily exercise, home cleaning, and napping. Have large calendar posted in conspicuous area to write in appointments or special planned events.	Consistency creates sense of security and keeps client oriented to daily activities. Routines are important in providing security, but client also needs to have option of making changes as necessary (Touhy and Jett, 2016).
6. Instruct family caregiver to focus on client's abilities rather than disabilities. Use abilities in modifying approaches to perform daily activities (e.g., if client has limited use of right hand, try approaches that maximize use of left hand).	Retains client's autonomy and sense of self-worth.
7. Have family caregiver help set up activities so that client can complete tasks (e.g., chopping vegetables before cooking, placing wash basin on table in bedroom for sponge bath, placing clothes to wear for day on bed, unpacking groceries on countertop for eventual storage, arranging food on plate with items in clockwise orientation [vegetables at 9, salad at 3, meat at 6]).	Helps client master task even though unable either physically or cognitively to perform all steps.
8. Discuss with client, family caregiver, pharmacist, and health care provider options for scheduling multiple medications:	Drugs sometimes cause physiological changes that create risk for injury.
a. Have medications that are likely to cause confusion prescribed to be given at bedtime.	Reduces risk for confusion during waking hours that contribute to disorientation and risk for falling.

Safe Patient Care *Do not recommend this if client has nocturia because client will be at greater risk for falling when getting out of bed.*

STEP	RATIONALE
b. Space antihypertensives and antiarrhythmics at different times to minimize side effects.	These drugs cause blood pressure changes and dizziness, thus increasing risk for falls.
c. When possible reduce number of pain medications used.	Drugs create sedative effects, increasing risk for falls.
d. Have diuretics taken early in day and not at night.	Ensures diuretic effect will occur during day while client is awake.
e. Discuss with health care provider possibility of taking medications at same time.	If safe and appropriate, taking medications at same time will alleviate problem of client remembering multiple administration times.
f. Discuss use of medication organizer and dispenser (see illustration).	Organizing medication in daily dispenser helps client and caregiver avoid medication errors of duplicating or missing medications.

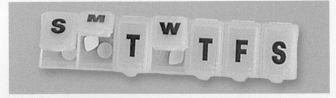

STEP 8f Weekly medication organizer.

STEP	RATIONALE
9. Teach family caregiver how to use simple and direct communication:	Relays care and support through therapeutic communication techniques.
a. Sit or stand in front of client in full view.	Promotes reception of verbal and nonverbal messages.
b. Face client with hearing impairment while speaking; do not cover mouth, and do not speak in a loud tone.	Client can see speaker's lips. Prevents voice distortion.
c. Use calm and relaxed approach.	
d. Use eye contact and touch.	Helps reinforce messages.
e. Speak slowly, in simple words and short sentences.	Enhances understanding of messages.
f. Use nonverbal gestures that complement verbal messages.	Provides clear messages.
10. Place clocks, calendars, and personal mementos (e.g., pictures, scrapbooks) throughout rooms within home. Enhance environment with addition of tactile boards or three-dimensional art.	Maintaining familiar surroundings maximizes cognitive function.

STEP	RATIONALE
11. Have family caregiver routinely orient client to who family caregiver is and which activities he or she is going to complete.	This strategy is useful in clients with progressive dementia. Behavioral symptoms in later stages include delusions, agitation, and hallucinations (Alzheimer's Association, 2017).
12. Be sure that client has regular naps or rest periods during day.	Fatigue adds to any mental status changes. Provides client energy to perform planned activities.
13. Have family caregiver encourage and support frequent visits by family and friends. Teach family caregiver how to use humor and reminiscing about favorite stories to promote social interaction.	Participation in social activities prevents boredom and restlessness.
14. Provide safe place for person to wander (e.g., large family room or fenced yard).	Reduces risk for injury and leaving residence (Touhy and Jett, 2016).
15. Recommend that family of wandering client install door locks or electronic guards.	Reduces chance of client exiting home unsupervised.
16. Create calm, safe setting that is appropriate for client's abilities (Alzheimer's Association, 2017).	Prevents falls and minimizes behavioral symptoms.
17. Monitor client for personal comfort (e.g., hunger, thirst, constipation, full bladder, and comfortable temperature; Alzheimer's Association, 2017).	Reduces stimuli that prompt wandering.
18. Keep list of places to which client may wander (e.g., former homes or workplaces).	Client may seek a familiar place.
19. Consider having client wear global positioning system (GPS) device to help manage location. Install motion detector near exit site, with portable alarm that can accompany family caregiver.	Alerts family caregiver to client's attempt to exit residence (Alzheimer's Association, 2017).
20. Consider need for full-time care.	Caregiving contributes significant mental and physical stress on family caregivers.

EVALUATION

Step	Rationale
1. During follow-up visits, ask client to review home-management activities completed the morning of that day and previous day.	Determines client's ability to recall events and evaluates if client completed planned activities.
2. Review with client and family caregiver revised schedule for medication administration.	Evaluates understanding of regimen.
3. Check pill count you asked client/family caregiver to maintain for a week.	Tracking doses confirms if client is adherent to regimen.
4. Ask family caregiver to describe ways that will increase client's success in completing home-management and self-care activities.	Measures learning.
5. Have family caregiver show schedules of daily routines and review specific approaches used. Observe environment for presence of reality-orientation cues.	Determines family caregiver's success in applying information and making environmental changes.
6. Have family caregivers describe options for minimizing wandering.	Measures learning.
7. Have family caregivers report number of occurrences of wandering.	Determines whether reduction in wandering has occurred.
8. **Use Teach-Back:** "I want to be sure I explained how you can help minimize your husband's wandering. Tell me some ways you can do this." Revise your instruction now or develop a plan for revised family caregiver teaching if family caregiver is not able to teach back correctly.	Determines family caregiver's level of understanding of instructional topic.

Unexpected Outcomes	Related Interventions
1. Client is unable to complete ADLs/IADLs as planned.	• Further modifications are sometimes necessary. • Reassess what occurred when task was not completed. • Have family caregiver offer suggestions.

Unexpected Outcomes	Related Interventions
2. Family caregiver is unable to describe/implement techniques that will improve client's orientation and ability to complete activities.	• Reinstruction and discussion are necessary. • Support for family caregiver is sometimes necessary before caregiver can learn how to support someone else.
3. Client's wandering increases.	• Consider that family caregiver is not able to provide necessary support; need to analyze other options. • Family caregiver may not have resources available to adapt environment. • Discussion is necessary to reconsider strategies used. • Reassess factors prompting wandering.

Recording

- Record cognitive abilities and mental status, recommended interventions, and responses of client and family caregiver.
- Document your evaluation of family caregiver learning.

Hand-Off Reporting

- Report change in cognitive or mental status to health care provider.

✦ SKILL 32.3 Medication and Medical Device Safety

Purpose

Medication safety in the home requires clients and family caregivers to understand how to store and prepare medications correctly, follow a medication schedule, administer medications correctly (Fig. 32.1), and dispose of unused or expired medications properly. Clients also need to know how to store and handle medical devices properly and dispose of medical waste properly to prevent infection and avoid injury (U.S. Environmental Protection Agency [EPA], 2017). Be mindful that clients with special needs, because of acute sensory or neurological impairment, chronic illnesses, and physical limitations, may have difficulty manipulating medical devices and handling medications.

Delegation and Collaboration

The skill of assessing for and monitoring medication and medical device safety cannot be delegated to nursing assistive personnel (NAP). The nurse directs the NAP to:

- Make suggestions that further ensure client safety regarding the use of basic infection control practices.
- Make suggestions as to how to properly dispose of sharps, needles, and contaminated supplies in the home.

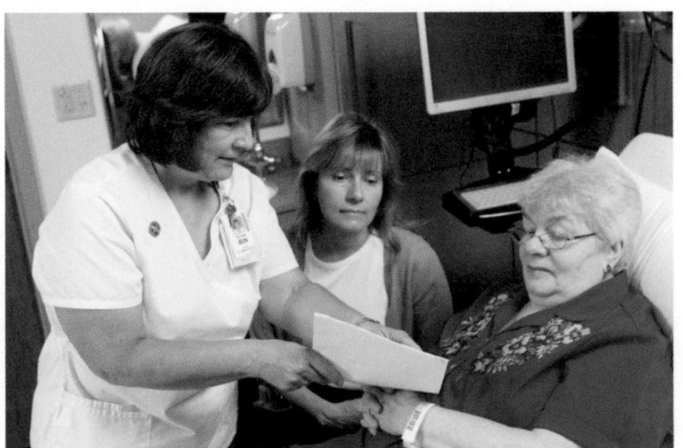

FIG 32.1 A family caregiver or other caregiver often needs to learn about prescribed medications.

Equipment

- Written instructions or charts
- Medications
- Pill organizer for daily or weekly medication preparation
- Measuring devices (e.g., medicine cup, teaspoon, syringe) if needed
- Colored marking pens
- Labels
- Assistive device (e.g., syringe magnifier) or medical device (e.g., blood glucose monitor)
- Puncture-resistant sharps container or hard plastic bottle (e.g., laundry detergent or fabric softener bottle) with cap

ASSESSMENT

1. Identify client using at least two identifiers (e.g., name and birthday or name and medical record number) according to agency policy. *Rationale: Ensures client safety. Complies with The Joint Commission standards and improves client safety (TJC, 2019).*
2. Assess client's sensory, musculoskeletal, and neurological function (see Chapter 8), specifically hand strength, ability to read labels on containers, ability to read doses on syringe, and ability to prepare medicine in a syringe. *Rationale: Reveals any deficits that will affect preparation and use of medications or medical devices.*
3. If family caregiver provides routine help, ask caregiver if there are any concerns about his or her ability or willingness to care for client. *Rationale: Assesses family caregivers' health and willingness to care for client. Information can help you educate family caregivers as to need for help and provide information to avoid injury to client (Clark, 2015).*
4. Assess client's medication regimen and length of time that client has been receiving each drug. Ask client to describe doses taken daily for each medication. Query family caregiver if necessary. *Rationale: Determines complexity of medication regimen and how familiar client or family caregiver is with regimen.*
5. Assess client's or family caregiver's knowledge, experience, and health literacy level. *Rationale: Ensures client and family*

caregiver has the capacity to obtain, communicate, process, and understand basic health information (CDC, 2016a).

Safe Patient Care *Be sure that medication labels are not confusing for a client. For example, the Spanish word for "eleven" is written as "once." A Spanish-speaking client could confuse a medication direction that requires them to take a medication 1 time a day as 11 times a day.*

6. Ask client to show you where medications are stored in home. Look at each container. *Rationale: Determines condition and labeling of containers.*
7. Assess temperature of storage area. *Rationale: Medication should not be stored in extreme heat. Insulin should not be stored near extreme heat or cold (ISMP, 2018).*
8. Assess client's daily schedule for drug administration. Ask client to describe schedule and whether there are any problems in following that schedule. *Rationale: Helps reveal client's adherence to or misunderstanding of instructions.*
9. If client self-administers injections, ask to see a demonstration of the injection, where he or she stores supplies, and what he or she uses to dispose of used syringes and needles. Plan a visit at the time an injection is needed. *Rationale: Determines correct injection method, sterility of equipment, and whether method of disposal creates risk to client or family for needlestick injuries.*
10. If client uses glucose-monitoring device, ask client to demonstrate use, and ask to see where monitor, lancets, and glucose strips are stored. Also ask about how client disposes of lancets. *Rationale: Allows you to examine client's technique, cleanliness of equipment, sterility of lancets, and condition of glucose strips. Sharps should be disposed of in puncture-proof container.*

STEP	RATIONALE
PLANNING	
1. Expected outcomes following completion of procedure:	
• Client and family caregiver identify principles of medication safety.	Client education includes information and techniques for safe medication administration.
• Client and family caregiver prepare medications independently.	Adaptations successfully accommodate client's and/or family caregiver's deficits in handling and manipulating equipment.
• Client and family caregiver identify correct conditions for storing medications, medical devices, and supplies.	Instruction focuses on ensuring infection control measures.
• Client and family caregiver dispose of used medical equipment and supplies correctly.	Appropriate receptacles and methods for disposal are made available and used.
IMPLEMENTATION	
1. Teach client and family caregiver the following principles to ensure that medications are used and stored safely:	
a. Instruct client and family caregiver how to perform hand hygiene before and after medication administration.	Helps prevent spread of infection and/or contamination of medication or medical devices.
b. Never take medicine prescribed for another member of household (CDC, 2017).	Medications must be of full strength and used for appropriate pharmacological reason to have therapeutic benefit.
c. Do not take any medicine that is more than 1 year old or past expiration date on container.	Expired medication is sometimes toxic or no longer effective.
d. Do not place different medicines in same container.	Prevents accidental "mix-up" of medications and medication error.
e. Do not place medications in pill containers different from their original ones.	Prevents accidental "mix-up" of medications and confusion as to expiration dates.
f. Always finish prescribed medication; do not save for future illness.	Prevents underdosing or inappropriate dosing.
2. Recommend approaches for preparation of medications:	
a. For clients with weakened grasp or pain in hands and fingers, have local pharmacist place medications in screw-top container.	Tops of childproof containers are difficult to remove, especially if hand and finger grasp is weakened.

Safe Patient Care *If client has children or grandchildren, be sure that medications are put up and away, out of reach and out of sight of children, and put away every time* (CDC, 2016b).

STEP	RATIONALE
b. For clients with visual alterations, have pharmacy type larger labels for all medication containers.	Ensures that client is able to read drug name and dosage schedule clearly.
c. For clients who are legally blind, have Braille labels placed on medication containers.	Labels embossed with drug name, strength, and prescription numbers are easy to read for client trained in use of Braille.

STEP	RATIONALE
d. For clients taking multiple medications, ask if they wish to try to introduce color-coding system. Use same color for drugs that client needs to take at same time. Mark tops of bottle caps with colored marking pen.	Technique helps client take correct drugs and doses at correct times of day. Best used when client is reliable in self-administration.
e. Provide specially designed syringes with large numerals or syringe magnifier for clients with visual alterations (see illustration).	Ensures that accurate dose of drug is prepared in syringe.

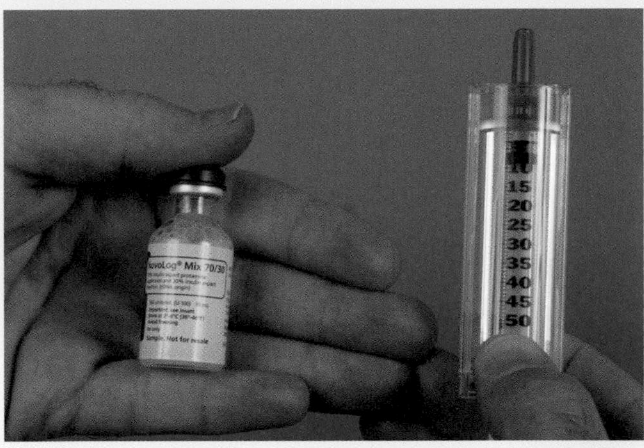

STEP 2e Syringe with magnifier.

STEP	RATIONALE
f. For clients who have difficulty manipulating syringes, offer spring-loaded needle insertion aid.	Delivers injection safely without manipulation of plunger.

Safe Patient Care *Teach family caregivers what to do following a needlestick injury. Wash the affected area thoroughly with soap and water and dry. If client has acquired immunodeficiency syndrome (AIDS), hepatitis, or other communicable disease, caregivers should seek medical attention immediately.*

STEP	RATIONALE
g. Teach family caregivers how to properly draw up prescribed volume of medication into syringe. When necessary, have family caregiver prepare extra prefilled syringes for client's use when caregiver is absent.	Ensures that family caregiver knows proper preparation techniques and that client has access to injections. Watch client and/or family caregiver draw up and dispense medications to determine whether more teaching is needed.
3. Recommend approaches for medication and supply storage:	
a. Store medications in safe, dry place, preferably in kitchen.	Moisture in bathroom may cause medications to decompose.
b. Keep liquid medications and parenteral drugs, especially insulin, in cool place.	Prevents decomposition of drug.

Safe Patient Care *Although manufacturers recommend storing insulin in the refrigerator, injecting cold insulin can sometimes make the injection more painful. To avoid this, store the bottle of insulin being used at room temperature. Insulin kept at room temperature will last approximately 1 month. However, remember to store extra bottles in the refrigerator if a client buys more than one bottle at a time to save money (ISMP, 2018). If insulin is stored in refrigerator, be sure that drug is in a bin or container, away from food.*

STEP	RATIONALE
c. Keep medical supplies such as syringes, dressing supplies, and glucose meter in airtight container (e.g., plastic storage bin) and store in cool place such as bedroom closet.	Ensures that supplies are not exposed to moisture or other contaminants.
d. Instruct client and family caregiver to use new needle with each medication administration.	Multiple use of same needle puts client at risk for infection.
4. Review for client and family caregiver proper techniques for disposal of medications, "sharps," and disposable medical supplies:	Proper practices necessary to prevent client injury.
a. Discard unused parts of drugs or outdated drugs properly, using these guidelines from the U.S. Food and Drug Administration (FDA, 2018).	

STEP	RATIONALE
(1) DO NOT FLUSH unused medications. However, although rule of thumb is not to flush, the U.S. Food and Drug Administration (FDA, 2018) has determined that certain medications should be flushed because of their abuse potential. Read the instructions on your medication and talk to your pharmacist.	Recent environmental impact studies report that flushing medications down toilet could be having an adverse impact on environment (FDA, 2018).
(2) When tossing unused medications, protect children and pets by crushing solid medications or dissolving them in water (this applies for liquid medications as well) and mix with kitty litter, coffee grounds, or sawdust (e.g., any material that absorbs dissolved medication and makes it less appealing for pets or children to eat); place in sealed plastic bag BEFORE tossing in trash.	Ensures that no one in household uses drug not prescribed for their use or drugs that will be ineffective pharmacologically.
(3) Remove and destroy ALL identifying personal information (prescription label) from medication container.	Ensures safe disposal to prevent outsider from acquiring medications.
(4) Check for approved state and local collection programs or with area hazardous waste facilities regarding proper way to dispose of waste, including some medications.	In certain states, you may be able to take your unused medications to your community pharmacy (FDA, 2018). Most communities have strict guidelines for waste and medication disposal.
b. Obtain sharps container from medical supply store or IV equipment supplier. (If finances are limited, have client use small-neck plastic bottle such as soda bottle.) Dispose of all needles and lancets in container.	Puncture-proof container prevents exposure to contaminated needlestick. Small-neck container makes it difficult for anyone to easily retrieve used needle or sharp.
c. Caution against filling sharps container to point where needles protrude out opening. Discard when three-fourths full, securing top with duct tape or adhesive tape.	Prevents needlesticks.
d. Store sharps container in area inaccessible to children.	Prevents injury to child.
e. Dispose of soiled dressings, used glucose testing reagent strips, and intravenous (IV) tubing in separate, sealed, plastic garbage bag. Place in second plastic bag (double bagged) and discard appropriately as trash.	Prevents contamination of other items in home. Minimizes chances of caregiver being exposed to infectious waste.

EVALUATION

1. Have client and/or family caregiver describe steps to take to ensure that medications are safe to use.	Demonstrates learning.
2. Observe client and/or caregiver prepare and administer medication dose.	Evaluates ability to physically manipulate medications and necessary equipment.
3. Observe home setting for location of medications and supplies.	Evaluates client's and/or family caregiver's adherence to recommendations.
4. Have client describe how sharps or medical equipment is discarded.	Demonstrates learning.
5. Do pill counts (pills remaining in containers) at successive intervals, such as twice a week for 2 weeks.	Helps verify that client takes correct number of medications over period of time.
6. **Use Teach-Back:** "I want to be sure I explained the importance of disposing of your fingerstick lancet appropriately. Tell me how to dispose of your lancets correctly and why this is important." Revise your instruction now or develop a plan or revised client/family caregiver teaching if client/family caregiver is not able to teach back correctly.	Determines client's/family caregiver's level of understanding of instructional topic.

Unexpected Outcomes	Related Interventions
1. Client and/or family caregiver is unable to recall principles for safe use of drugs.	• Reinstruction is necessary, or client and caregiver need chance to ask more questions regarding benefit of precautions. • Offer simple, plain-language and/or written instructions.

Unexpected Outcomes	Related Interventions
2. Client and/or family caregiver has difficulty or is unable to prepare and self-administer medication.	• Offer further help to set up equipment. • Offer assistive aids. • Reinstruct in steps used to prepare and/or administer medication. • Review with client and family caregiver daily drug prescribed. • Reevaluate use of dosage reminders. • Notify health care provider.
3. Medications and medical devices are not stored in secure or appropriate location or are not disposed of properly.	• Assess whether client chooses to store items conveniently rather than safely or has limited resources. • Reinstruction and discussion are necessary. • Arrange to provide appropriate containers.

Recording

- Record all instructions given, including details of medication administration and use of medical devices.
- Document your evaluation of client or family caregiver learning.

Hand-Off Reporting

- Report client's inability to adhere to medication safety plan to health care provider.

SPECIAL CONSIDERATIONS

Client-Centered Care

- If client speaks a different language than you do, have a professional interpreter present or available by phone.
- Nurses must step outside of their biases and accept that clients may have different values, choices, and priorities. Practice in a culturally competent manner with respect for all persons (Touhy and Jett, 2018).
- Home care is part of the continuum of care. Nurses are instrumental in helping clients to achieve their maximum functional ability and adjust to changes when back in their home.
- Accident prevention begins with making timely and adequate home repairs; however, it may also be necessary to modify the home to make it more accessible for the client.
- Be prepared to discuss concerns about the number of modifications required, costs of modifications, and change in home decor. The goal is to provide an environment in which the client or the family caregiver can provide care safely and effectively.
- Let the client be the final decision maker in the types of changes to be made whenever possible. Consider the client's physical strengths and remaining functional abilities, not just the disabilities.

Client Education

- The capacity for learning new information remains as an adult ages (in the absence of dementia). Additional time is needed to accomplish learning; allow adequate time and number of teaching sessions to support successful learning. Consider learning style as well as barriers to learning.
- Frail older clients should not ride in the passenger side of the car if the car has airbags. Teach the client and family caregivers that client should sit in the back seat or at least 10 inches away from the airbag.
- Refer family caregivers to resources for safety, caregiver support, and communication tips and to organizations such as the Alzheimer's Association.
- Educate family caregivers about the importance of preserving client autonomy.

Age-Specific

Pediatric

- Keep all medications, medical supplies, and equipment safely out of reach of children. Children are curious and put things in their mouths; risk is high for accidental poisoning (CDC, 2017).
- Tell family caregivers not to refer to medications as treats; this could add to risk of child overdosing by mistaking medicine for candy (CDC, 2017).
- Ensuring the safety of children in the home is based on child's developmental level. Instruct families to use safety devices as applicable (Hockenberry et al., 2017).
- Suggest that parents get down on the floor to look at the environment from child's view to identify dangers present in the home (Hockenberry et al., 2017).
- Children with cognitive impairments often are unaware of dangers normally present during play and daily activities. Adult supervision is critical.
- Children imitate and copy what they see and hear. Instruct parents that practicing safety teaches safety (Hockenberry et al., 2017).

Gerontological

- Instruct caregivers to keep medications locked in a secure place for clients with cognitive impairment.
- Many clients experience progressive loss of function, requiring continuous adaptations and adjustments. If client becomes unable to complete any ADLs or experiences major behavioral changes (e.g., excessive wandering), you may need to help family caregiver determine need for alternative living arrangements.
- Older adults can be at greater risk for environmental hazards and mistreatment/abuse as they age.

✦ PRACTICE REFLECTIONS

A few years ago, as a home health care nurse arrived for a client home visit at a home she had been to several times in the past few months, she was met by a group of strangers in front of the home. As the nurse began to park her car, some members of this group began to approach the car, speaking in loud and threatening tones. The nurse hesitated for a moment to leave without seeing the client because she knew he was waiting for her, but she felt uncomfortable getting out of the car and decided it was best to return to the home care agency rather than attempt to go into the client's home.

1. What about this experience was concerning?
2. Was the nurse right to return to the agency without visiting this client?
3. What strategies can a home care nurse use to ensure safety while visiting clients in their homes?

✦ CLINICAL REVIEW QUESTIONS

1. During an initial home care visit to an elderly client, the nurse discovers several safety concerns in the client's kitchen. Which of the following findings are of concern? (Select all that apply.)
   1. Thick layer of grease on the stovetop
   2. Loud food timer on the kitchen counter
   3. Stove control dials behind the burners
   4. Fire extinguisher uncharged, hanging near the stove
   5. Bright lighting over the cooking area
2. The home care nurse is visiting a client who was recently diagnosed with diabetes and began taking insulin. Which of the following observations would be the first priority to address during the home visit?
   1. The client's wife and grown children insist on being present during the entire home visit.
   2. The client removes a prefilled syringe from the refrigerator, preparing to immediately inject it.
   3. The children express concern that they do not have enough supplies for their father, such as an extra sharps container.
   4. The client tells you he is feeling sad about his recent diagnosis and is concerned about the effect on his wife.
3. When assessing a client with cognitive deficits, the nurse should do which of the following? (Select all that apply.)
   1. Plan for a one-time, longer visit.
   2. Speak loudly and quickly.
   3. Limit outside noises and distractions.
   4. Ask family caregiver to be present.
   5. Pose questions only to the caregiver.

Answers and Rationales for Clinical Review Questions can be found on the Evolve website.

REFERENCES

Alzheimer's Association: Alzheimer's and dementia basics, 2017. http://www.alz.org/alzheimers_disease_what_is_alzheimers.asp.

American Diabetes Association (ADA): Living with diabetes: insulin storage and syringe safety, 2014. http://www.diabetes.org/living-with-diabetes/treatment-and-care/medication/insulin/insulin-storage-and-syringe-safety.html.

Centers for Disease Control and Prevention (CDC): What is health literacy, 2016a. https://www.cdc.gov/healthliteracy/learn/index.html.

Centers for Disease Control and Prevention (CDC): Put your medicines up and away and out of sight, 2016b. http://www.cdc.gov/features/medicationstorage/.

Centers for Disease Control and Prevention (CDC): Medication safety program, 2017. http://www.cdc.gov/medicationsafety/.

Clark MJ: *Population and community health nursing*, ed 6, Hoboken, NJ, 2015, Pearson.

Edelman CL, et al: *Health promotion throughout the lifespan*, ed 8, St. Louis, 2014, Mosby.

Foodsafety.gov: Keep food safe, 2017. https://www.foodsafety.gov/keep/index.html.

Hester AL: Preventing injuries from patient falls, *Am Nurse Today* 10(7):36, 2015.

Hill E, Fauerbach LA: Falls and fall prevention in older adults, *J Legal Nurs Consult* 25(2):24, 2014.

Hockenberry MJ, et al: *Wong's essentials of pediatric nursing*, ed 10, St. Louis, 2017, Mosby.

Institute for Safe Medication Practices (ISMP): Insulin storage, 2018. http://www.consumermedsafety.org/insulin-safety-center/item/420.

Lang A, et al: Seniors managing multiple medications: using mixed methods to view the home care safety lens, *BMC Health Serv Res* 15:548, 2015.

Mayo Clinic: Carbon monoxide poisoning, n.d. http://www.mayoclinic.org/diseases-conditions/carbon-monoxide/basics/symptoms/con-20025444.

Meiner S, Yeager J: *Gerontologic nursing*, ed 6, St. Louis, 2019, Elsevier.

National Fire Protection Association (NFPA): Home structure fires, 2016. http://www.nfpa.org/news-and-research/fire-statistics-and-reports/fire-statistics/fires-by-property-type/residential/home-structure-fires.

National Rifle Association (NRA): NRA gun safety rules, 2017. https://gunsafetyrules.nra.org/. (Accessed 17 July 2017).

Parand A, et al: Carer's medication administration errors in the domicillary settings: a systematic review, *PLoS One* 11(12):1, 2016.

Safewise: Top smoke alarms, 2017. https://www.safewise.com/resources/smoke-alarm-buyers-guide.

Singh DK, et al: Association between physiological falls risk and physical performance tests among community-dwelling older adults, *Clin Interv Aging* 10:1319, 2015.

The Joint Commission (TJC): *2019 National Patient Safety Goals*, 2019, Oakbrook Terrace, IL, The Commission. http://www.jointcommission.org/standards_information/npsgs.aspx.

Touhy TA, Jett K: *Ebersole and Hess' gerontological nursing & healthy aging*, ed 5, St. Louis, 2018, Elsevier.

Touhy TA, Jett K: *Ebersole and Hess' toward healthy aging: human needs and nursing response*, ed 9, St. Louis, 2016, Elsevier.

U.S. Department of Health and Human Services (HHS): *Healthy People 2020*: injury and violence prevention, 2017. https://www.healthypeople.gov/2020/topics-objectives/topic/injury-and-violence-prevention.

U.S. Environmental Protection Agency (EPA): Medical waste, 2017. http://epa.gov/wastes/nonhaz/industrial/medical/.

U.S. Fire Administration: Basement fire safety, n.d. https://www.usfa.fema.gov/downloads/pdf/publications/basement_fire_safety_flyer.pdf.

U.S. Food and Drug Administration (FDA): Where and how to dispose of unused medication, 2018. https://www.fda.gov/forconsumers/consumerupdates/ucm101653.htm.

Appendix A Integrative Practice Reflections

Apply your knowledge from what you have learned about all the nursing skills to reflect on the following integrative practice reflections.

GERONTOLOGICAL FOCUS

An 80-year-old patient recently underwent hip replacement surgery and is currently recovering in the post anesthesia care unit (PACU). The patient has an intravenous (IV) running in the left hand of D5½NS at 75 mL/hr and has a left hip soft silicone dressing in place. Current vital signs include temperature of 37°C (98.6°F), heart rate 88 beats/min, respiratory rate 18 breaths/min. Pain assessment is currently 4 on a 0-to-10 scale after having received 8 mg IV morphine sulfate 30 minutes ago. The patient will be transferred to the rehabilitation unit within the health care agency within 36 hours. Consider the complexity of care for the gerontologic patient and reflect on the following questions.

1. What safety concerns do you have for this patient?
2. What assistive devices would you expect this patient to need?
3. What risks for infection does this patient have, and what infection control practices might be put in place?
4. What factors influence this patient's pain perception, and what would be your pain management plan for this patient?
5. What would be the essential components of the hand-off report for this patient from the PACU to the rehabilitation unit?

Related Chapters: 2, 4, 5, 15, 18, 29

HOME CARE FOCUS

A 62-year-old patient was recently discharged to home and has a 5-year history of type 1 diabetes mellitus and a new colostomy. Prior to discharge, the patient teaching focused on a review of current medication regimen and colostomy site care (e.g., normal output, skin care, stoma care, colostomy supplies). It was noted that the patient's wife was concerned about her husband's nutrition/diet needs. This is the first home care visit since discharge, and you are meeting with the patient and his wife.

1. Prior to your first visit, where would you search for best practice guidelines for management of the stoma?
2. What are the home care safety needs for this patient?
3. What safe medication practices would you review with this patient and his wife?
4. What type of nutrition/diet teaching might you consider for this patient?
5. What health-related complications might you be concerned about for this patient?

Related Chapters: 1, 13, 21, 22, 24, 25, 32

Appendix B Abbreviations and Equivalents

ABBREVIATIONS FOR CONVERSION USING HOUSEHOLD MEASURES

1 drop (gtt) = 1 minim
1 teaspoon (1 tsp) = 5 mL
3 tsp = 1 tablespoon (tbsp)
1 cup = 8 oz
16 oz = 1 pound (lb)

STANDARD EQUIVALENTS, ABBREVIATIONS, AND CONVERSIONS

1000 mg = 1 g
1000 mL = 1 liter (L)
2.2 lb = 1 kilogram (kg) = 1000 g
1 tsp = 5 mL
1 dr = 4 mL
mEq: milliequivalent
mcg: microgram

SYMBOLS

/ Per
≤ Equal to or less than
≥ Equal to or more than
≅ Approximately equal to
+/−, ± Plus or minus
♂ Male
♀ Female
1° Primary; first degree
2° Secondary; second degree
3° Tertiary; third degree
↑ Up; increase
↓ Down; decrease

ABBREVIATIONS

ā: before
abd: abdomen
ABGs: arterial blood gases
ac: before meals
ad lib: as desired
ADH: antidiuretic hormone
ADLs: activities of daily living
AFB: acid-fast bacillus (related to tuberculosis)
AIDS: acquired immunodeficiency syndrome
ALL: acute lymphoblastic leukemia
AMB: ambulatory
AP (and lateral chest): anterior and posterior
ASA: aspirin
ASHD: arteriosclerotic heart disease
ax: axillary
BE: barium enema
bid: twice a day
BM: bowel movement
BP: blood pressure
BPH: benign prostatic hypertrophy
BR: bed rest
BRP: bathroom privileges
BSE: breast self-examination
BSI: body substance isolation
BUN: blood urea nitrogen
bx: biopsy
c̄: with
C&S: culture and sensitivity
CA: cancer
CABG: coronary artery bypass graft
CAD: coronary artery disease
cap: capsule
CBC: complete blood count
CBI: continuous bladder irrigation
CBR: complete bed rest
CC: chief complaint
CDC: Centers for Disease Control and Prevention
CHF: congestive heart failure
Cl: chloride
CN: cranial nerve
CNS: central nervous system
c/o: complains of
CO_2: carbon dioxide
COPD: chronic obstructive pulmonary disease
CPM: continuous passive motion
CPR: cardiopulmonary resuscitation
CSF: cerebrospinal fluid
CT: computed tomography
CVA: cerebrovascular accident (stroke)
CVP: central venous pressure
D5NS, D_5NS: 5% dextrose in 0.9% (normal) saline
DAT: diet as tolerated
DM: diabetes mellitus
DNR: do not resuscitate
DSD: dry sterile dressing
DTR: deep tendon reflex
DVT: deep venous thrombosis
dx: diagnosis
EC: enteric coated
ECG, EKG: electrocardiogram
elix: elixir
ER: extended release
ESR: erythrocyte sedimentation rate

ESRD: end-stage renal disease
ET: enterostomal therapist
FUO: fever of unknown origin
fx: fracture
g: gram
GI: gastrointestinal
gtt: drops
GU: genitourinary
Hb, Hgb: hemoglobin
HBV: hepatitis B virus
HCO_3^-: bicarbonate
Hct: hematocrit
HCV: hepatitis C virus
HEPA: high-efficiency particulate air
HIV: human immunodeficiency virus
h/o: history of
HOB: head of bed
HR: heart rate
hs: at bedtime
HTN: hypertension
I&O: intake and output
ICP: intracranial pressure
ICU: intensive care unit
IDDM: insulin-dependent diabetes mellitus
IM: intramuscular
IPPB: intermittent positive-pressure breathing
IV: intravenous
JVD: jugular vein distention
K: potassium
KUB: kidney, ureter, bladder
KVO: keep vein open (run IV very slowly)
LLQ: left lower quadrant
LMP: last menstrual period
LOC: level of consciousness
LR: lactated Ringer's solution lytes: electrolytes
MAP: mean arterial pressure
MCHC: mean corpuscular hemoglobin concentration
MCV: mean corpuscular volume
MI: myocardial infarction
N: nitrogen
Na: sodium
NaCl: sodium chloride
neg: negative
NG: nasogastric
NPO: nothing by mouth
NS: normal saline
NSAIDs: nonsteroidal antiinflammatory drugs
O_2: oxygen
OOB: out of bed
OR: operating room
OT: occupational therapy
OTC: over-the-counter (medicine available without prescription)
P: pulse
PACU: postanesthesia care unit
pc: after meals
PCA: patient-controlled analgesia
PE: pulmonary embolism
PID: pelvic inflammatory disease
PMH: past medical history
PMI: point of maximal impulse
PO: by mouth
postop: after surgery
preop: before surgery
prn: as needed
pt: patient
PT: physical therapy
PT: prothrombin time
PTT: partial thromboplastin time
PVD: peripheral vascular disease
q: each
q_h (fill in the number of hours), e.g., q3h: every 3 hours
qs: sufficient quantity
R: respirations
RA: rheumatoid arthritis
RBC: red blood cells
R/O: rule out (eliminate possibility of a condition)
ROM: range of motion
ROS: review of systems
r/t: related to
RUQ: right upper quadrant
Rx: treatment
$\bar{s}$: without
sl (SL): sublingual
SOB: shortness of breath
sp gr: specific gravity
SR: sustained release
STAT: immediately
STD: sexually transmitted disease
supp: suppository
susp: suspension
sx: symptoms, signs
T: temperature
T&C: type and crossmatch
Tab: tablet
TB: tuberculosis
TCDB: turn, cough, deep breathe
tid: three times a day
TPN: total parenteral nutrition
TPR: temperature, pulse, respirations
TURP: transurethral resection of prostate
UA: urinalysis
up ad: up as desired
URI: upper respiratory infection
US: ultrasound
UTI: urinary tract infection
VS: vital signs
VTBI: volume to be infused
WBC: white blood cell
WC: wheelchair
WNL: within normal limits
wt: weight

Official "Do Not Use" List[a]

Do Not Use	Potential Problem	Use Instead
U (unit)	Mistaken for "0" (zero), the number "4" (four), or "cc"	Write "unit"
IU (International Unit)	Mistaken for IV (intravenous) or the number 10 (ten)	Write "International Unit"
Q.D., QD, q.d., qd (daily) Q.O.D., QOD, q.o.d., qod (every other day)	Mistaken for each other Period after the Q mistaken for "I" and the "O" mistaken for "I"	Write "daily" Write "every other day"
Trailing zero (X.0 mg)[b] Lack of leading zero (.X mg)	Decimal point is missing	Write X mg Write 0.X mg
MS MSO_4 and $MgSO_4$	Can mean morphine sulphate or magnesium sulphate Confused for one another	Write "morphine sulphate" Write "magnesium sulphate"

Official "Do Not Use" List, Joint Commission on Accreditation of Healthcare Organizations, February 2012; www.jointcommission.org.

[a]Applies to all orders and all medication-related documentation that is handwritten (including free-text computer entry) or on preprinted forms.

[b]**Exception**: A "trailing zero" may be used only where required to demonstrate the level of precision of the value being reported such as for laboratory results, imaging studies that report size of lesions, or catheter/tube sizes. It may not be used in medication orders or other medical-related documentation.

Additional Abbreviations, Acronyms, and Symbols (for possible future inclusion in the Official "Do Not Use" List)

Do Not Use	Potential Problem	Use Instead
> (greater than) < (less than)	Misinterpreted as the number "7" (seven) or the letter "L" Confused for one another	Write "greater than" Write "less than"
Abbreviations for drug names	Misinterpreted due to similar abbreviations for multiple drugs	Write drugs names in full
Apothecary units	Unfamiliar to many practitioners Confused with metric units	Write drugs names in full
@	Mistaken for the number "2" (two)	Write "at"
cc	Mistaken for U (units) when written poorly	Write "mL" or "milliliters"
µg	Mistaken for mg (milligrams), resulting in one thousand-fold overdose	Write "mcg" or "micrograms"

Official "Do Not Use" List, Joint Commission on Accreditation of Healthcare Organizations, February 2012; www.jointcommission.org, accessed December 15, 2014.

Index

b indicates boxes, *f* indicates illustrations, and *t* indicates tables.

Index of Skills